Basic
Medical-Surgical
Nursing

Basic Medical-Surgical Nursing

5th Edition

Mildred A. Mason, R.N., Ed.D.

*Late Associate Professor
and
Program Area Leader,
Health Occupations Education,
Old Dominion University,
Norfolk, Virginia*

Grace Fleet Bates, R.N., M.S.

*Acting Assistant Dean of Instruction
and
Lecturer in Practical Nursing
Department of Practical Nursing
Kapiolani Community College
Honolulu, Hawaii*

Macmillan Publishing Company
NEW YORK

Collier Macmillan Canada, Inc.
TORONTO

Collier Macmillan Publishers
LONDON

Macmillan Publishing Company
866 Third Avenue, New York, New York 10022

Collier Macmillan Canada, Inc.
Collier Macmillan Publishers • London

Library of Congress Cataloging in Publication Data

Mason, Mildred A.
  Basic medical-surgical nursing.

  Includes bibliographies and index.
  1. Practical nursing. I. Bates, Grace Fleet.
II. Title. [DNLM: 1. Nursing, Practical. WY 195 M411b]
RT62.M3 1984   610.73   83–11284
ISBN 0–02–376980–7
Printing: 2 3 4 5 6 7 8   Year: 5 6 7 8 9 0 1 2

Preface to the Fifth Edition

A change in the format of the fifth edition reflects the authors' belief in the importance of nursing observations as a basis for establishing a nursing diagnosis and selecting appropriate nursing interventions. A head-to-toe sequence of observing is emphasized since this method is used frequently by nurses in clinical practice. Each chapter contains a description of observations that can be seen by the nurse when the patient has a disease affecting that body system. Also integrated into this framework are the patient's symptoms, experiences, and reports. These are followed by a description of common nursing interventions related to hygiene, food and fluids, exercise, drug therapy, and similar activities. Integrated into this framework are medical treatment plans as they affect the patient and the nurse. These two components form the basis of the nursing care plan.

A new chapter on cultural components of illness has been added to assist the licensed practical/vocational nursing student or LPN/LVN to give culturally sensitive care. This chapter reflects the growing body of knowledge and interest in transcultural nursing. Nursing interventions for pain relief have been incorporated into a new chapter to help the student develop the knowledge and skill necessary to help the patient in pain.

As in the fourth edition, each chapter begins with an outline, followed by expected behavioral outcomes designed for the practical/vocational nursing student to use as educational guides. Vocabulary development, which includes prefixes, suffixes, and combining forms, appears next and is followed by a review of structure and function in those chapters pertaining to body systems. Each chapter is concluded by one or more case studies, review questions, suggestions for further study, and additional readings of up-to-date clinical articles and books. The case studies include questions designed primarily to facilitate the nursing student's ability to use nursing knowledge as a basis for nursing action. A glossary is included in the back matter of the book.

Supplementary materials to reinforce the text include a teacher's manual, a newly revised workbook for students (Mason, Bates, and Smola's *Workbook in Basic Medical-Surgical Nursing*, 3rd ed., 1984), and an answer key to the workbook.

MILDRED A. MASON

GRACE FLEET BATES

Several months after the completion of the fifth edition, Dr. Mildred A. Mason, the senior author, died in Norfolk, Virginia. Readers may be interested to learn that Dr. Mason was a pioneer in practical/vocational nurse education. Her interest and commitment to practical/vocational nursing students, graduates, and educators began in the 1940s and continued throughout her life. The first edition, published in 1959, was the first textbook of medical-surgical nursing for practical/vocational nursing students. In addition, Dr. Mason cofounded the first periodical for practical nurses, *Practical Nurse Digest*. These and other accomplishments were made possible by Dr. Mason's unique combination of superior ability, genuine caring, sense of humor, and very hard work. Thus, she was both respected and loved. This edition is lovingly dedicated to her.

GRACE FLEET BATES

Acknowledgments

This volume has been made possible by interactions with innumerable practical/vocational nursing students, licensed practical nurses/licensed vocational nurses (LPN/LVNs), and practical nursing educators throughout the United States of America. The strong desire of practical nursing students and LPN/LVNs to give the best care possible to medical and surgical patients served as a motivating factor for the first edition. Continuing contacts with practical nursing students, practical nursing educators, and LPN/LVNs to determine their needs and interests have served as the basis for the addition and/or deletion of content in this edition. These interactions have been invaluable to the authors, who want to express appreciation to past and future generations of LPN/LVNs.

Nine chapters in this fifth edition had at least one contributing author, who was selected for her clinical expertise as well as nursing and teaching experience. The names and affiliations of these contributing authors are listed on the opening pages of chapters, and their invaluable assistance is gratefully acknowledged.

Appreciation is also expressed to the following colleagues, who reviewed portions of the manuscript and offered helpful comments and criticisms:

Mrs. Vivian Barnum Cabaniss, R.N.
Wethersfield, Connecticut

Barbara Molina Kooker, R.N., M.S., M.P.H.
Maternal-Child Health
Department of Obstetrics and Gynecology
Mercy Hospital
San Diego, California

Joan Takao Matsukawa, R.N., M.S., M.P.H.
Chairperson, Department of Practical Nursing
Kapiolani Community College
Honolulu, Hawaii

Judith A. Mullen, R.N.C., M.S.
Clinical Nurse Specialist
Medical-Surgical, Psychiatric–Mental Health Nursing
Kaiser Foundation Clinics
Waipahu, Hawaii

Gail Zukosky, R.N., M.S.
Clinical Instructor
Fairfax County School of Practical Nursing
Falls Church, Virginia

Preparation of the manuscript was greatly facilitated by Gloria Rudibaugh, R.N., M.S., who, in addition to serving as coauthor of two chapters, provided assistance with selection of suggested references. The authors also wish to express appreciation to Karen Dyer Allen for her expert secretarial assistance in typing the manuscript. Photographic expertise provided by Mr. Frank Matthews of Norfolk, Virginia, is gratefully acknowledged.

The cooperation and encouragement of the faculty in the Department of Practical Nursing, Kapiolani Community College, Honolulu, Hawaii, facilitated completion of the manuscript.

The authors also wish to express appreciation to their families and friends, who helped in numerous ways throughout the revision.

It is difficult to put into a few words the contributions made by Charles Kirk Bates. His continued encouragement and loving support were vital ingredients in the preparation of the fifth edition.

Special recognition is extended to Sara N. Boggs for her continued encouragement, support, and innumerable kindnesses.

Revision of this edition was made possible by Joan C. Zulch, Vice President, Macmillan Publishing Company. Miss Zulch arranged for a smooth transition to Mrs. Carol Wolfe, Senior Editor–Nursing, whose understanding, insight, and expert guidance provided the technical support system necessary for final completion of the manuscript.

Contents

Basic Medical-Surgical Nursing

Chapter 1

The Impact of Illness
on an Individual

Expected Behavioral Outcomes

Minimum objectives referred to as expected behavioral outcomes have been designed for the practical/vocational nursing student to use as guides in studying this chapter. The student should read these expected outcomes before studying the chapter. The objectives can be used as guides for study.

Using the content of this chapter, the student should return to the objectives and evaluate the ability to:

1. *Describe how one's own life would change if hospitalized tomorrow.*
2. *Describe the action that one would take if a terminally ill patient threw a lunch tray on the floor.*
3. *Demonstrate ability to use the observation guide by simulating a practical situation.*
4. *Describe six nursing actions that communicate a caring attitude to the patient.*
5. *Compare personal feelings of anxiety associated with a recent examination with those that might be experienced by a newly admitted patient.*

Vocabulary Development

The following prefixes, suffixes and combining forms pertain to this chapter. By learning and/or reviewing their meanings, the practical/vocational nursing student will have the keys needed to unlock many exciting new medical terms.

Discover the meaning of these keys in a medical dictionary or in the content of this chapter. How does each key pertain to this chapter? In your notebook write the correct meaning of each prefix, suffix, or combining form listed below. Illustrate each key with an example.

con—with together. Ex. *Conversion*—emotional conflicts expressed with physical symptoms.

act-	ec-	psych-	therap-
con-	im-	re-	vers-
dis-	pro-	somat-	

Introduction

A patient is an individual who needs assistance from members of the health team or health care delivery system in order to adapt to a changed health status. All human beings have certain basic needs. For purposes of understanding and study, basic human needs have been further separated into physical needs and psychological needs. Physical needs include such elements as oxygen, food, and water which the body needs for survival. *Somat* refers to the body. Psychological needs include love and affection, respect and approval, safety and security, and self-development. *Psyche* refers to the mind. Although separate categories may help us in our study and understanding, it is important to remember that the human individual is not separated but whole. Throughout life, there is constant and continuous interaction of the mind and the body in all persons.

Recently, scientific interest in the continuous mind-body interaction has increased. Research shows that certain forms of mental relaxation result in changes in heart and respiratory rates and oxygen consumption. *Biofeedback* is a new technique that enables the individual to control certain physiologic processes that were previously considered automatic. The person receives information about a specific physiologic process such as blood pressure via electronic equipment. Although the exact mechanism is not yet understood, with practice some persons can learn to alter blood pressure. Psychosomatic medicine is a special branch of medicine that develops from the realization that illness must be considered and treated in relation to the whole person. The term "psychosomatic" implies that the mind cannot be sick without affecting the physical body or the physical body be sick without affecting the mind.

A person's mind and body influence health. It is very important that assistance given to a patient by the nurse and all members of the health team contain both a physical and psychological component. For example, Mr. Land, a student LPN/LVN, is assisting Ms. Raymond with breakfast. While buttering the toast and stirring the coffee, Mr. Land initiates conversation with the patient. Such assistance contains a physical component, buttering the toast and stirring the coffee, as well as a psychological component, and so he recognizes Ms. Raymond as a whole person. In the hospital, most activities directly concern only physical aspects of the patient. Knowledge, skill, and a real commitment to the patient are required to carry out those activities in a way that recognizes and cares for the whole person.

Experiences Common to Illness

Illness interrupts usual ways of living and brings new and often unpleasant change. One of the first changes an individual who is ill experiences is a change in behavior.

Behavior consists of actions taken to meet the requirements of living. The specific actions a person takes depend upon many factors, including age, sex, education, income, and the group, family, or society. For example, all persons require water to live. Mr. Jones drinks coffee. Mrs. Jones, who grew up in England, prefers tea, and their daughter, Suzanne, aged 10, drinks milk. Similarly, all persons have the need to develop according to their talents and abilities. Mr. Jones builds model cars; Mrs. Jones restores antique furniture; Suzanne plays baseball.

In selecting specific actions, each person decides which needs are the most important and takes actions to meet those needs first. The selection process may be conscious or unconscious. In other words, the person may be aware or not aware of choosing. For example, Mrs. Black burns her arm while reaching over the stove to rescue her daughter. Mrs. Black's action is automatic, taken without much awareness of the possible consequences to herself. Later the same week, Mrs. Black cancels a doctor's appointment because there is no one to care for her daughter. Mrs. Black is aware that postponing this appointment may be risky, but the care of her daughter is more important than the risk. Mrs. Black's acts are based on what she considers important and not necessarily what the nurse, doctor, or other hospital representatives think is important. The nurse shows respect for the individual by acting in a way that recognizes each person's right to choose the way in which basic human needs are met. This does not mean necessarily that the nurse agrees with the patient's choices.

Each person is unique and thus responds to illness in a special way. A variety of behaviors can be expected of the individual who faces the threat of pain, disability, loss of income, separation from family and/or friends, loss of limb or other body part, or loss of life. Changes in behavior may be a direct result of the disease or be associated with the frustration of illness. The changes in behavior also may be a combination of both.

The case of Mr. Thompson is an example of a behavior change that was a direct result of disease. This patient was recuperating from a stroke (cerebral accident). On one occasion, after the nurse and the orderly had assisted him in walking to a chair, he cried. This middle-aged man had not wept since he was a boy. In a few minutes he was laughing and talking. The nurse had learned that sudden emotional outbursts, such as crying and laughing, are associated with a stroke. Since the nurse understood the relationship of emotional reactions to the physical condition of a patient with a stroke, seeing the emotional reaction of Mr. Thompson was not surprising. The nurse can easily understand that the entire individual is affected, not just the diseased area of the brain.

Another example of disease affecting the entire individual is the case of Mr. Adams, who was in a body cast because of three fractured vertebrae. He appeared depressed to the practical nursing student during his daily bath. Mr. Adams responded to the kindly attitude of the nurse by talking about his family and his job as a truck driver. The patient seemed most concerned about the welfare of his wife and four children while he was unable to earn a livelihood. It is evident that Mr. Adams' depressed mood was associated with his illness. He was suffering from depression as well as from fractured vertebrae.

A pattern of behaviors developed over a lifetime is called *life-style*: a person's usual way of living. The nurse studies an individual's life-style for many reasons. First, a person's life-style may have contributed to or caused illness or disease. For example, a person who smokes is more likely to develop emphysema than one who does not. Second, knowledge of a person's life-style enables the nurse to assess the meaning of a person's illness. For example, some persons believe that illness is punishment for wrongdoing. The personal meaning attached to illness can have a profound effect on the way the patient behaves and can influence the course and outcome of that illness. Third, care that is planned with a person's life-style in mind is likely to reduce the anxiety and stress associated with illness. Last, extensive or prolonged illness may necessitate a permanent change in goals, plans and activities. Knowledge of the person's life-style enables the nurse to suggest alternate ways of doing things which the patient can accept and use.

Personal autonomy is the power we all have to take care of ourselves and control aspects of our lives. (Figure 1.1). Illness often results in considerable changes in the patient's personal autonomy. Consider Mr. Jones who recently has been hospitalized because of chest pain. His activity is restricted to bedrest, the diet is changed to low salt, and visiting is restricted to immediate family only. These are three of many activities Mr. Jones no longer can control while hospitalized. Simply coming to the hospital requires Mr. Jones to relinquish considerable personal autonomy. The nurse who understands the changes in personal autonomy that illness brings, creates every opportunity for Mr. Jones to control his own life. He can choose which low-salt foods to eat, when to bathe, and when to sleep. Through these and other similar opportunities, Mr. Jones learns that he retains considerable influence and control, even though ill.

In our minds, we carry a mental picture of what we look like. This picture is called *body image*. Close your eyes and let the picture of yourself come into focus: the color of your hair, the shape of your body, the way you walk and talk. Some experts believe that body image exerts a very powerful influence over the choices we make and the way we live.

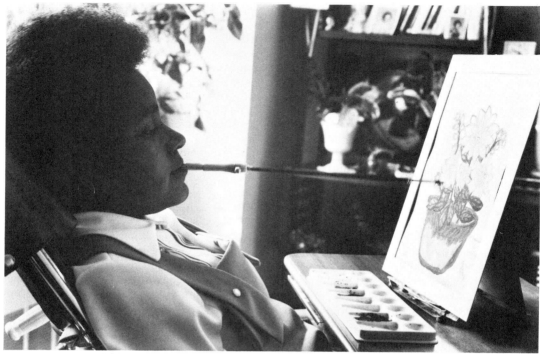

FIGURE 1.1   This person has made an exceptional adjustment in personal autonomy and life-style. (Courtesy of Bergen Pines County Hospital School of Practical Nursing, Paramus, New Jersey.)

Illness and disease disturb a person's usual body image temporarily or, at times, permanently. Surgery, illness, and drugs are components of illness and disease that can force a person to change a mental picture. Also, some parts of a person's body may be more important than others. For example, to many men and women the female breast represents femininity, sexuality, and attractiveness. A woman who has a breast removal (mastectomy) may feel that she is no longer as feminine, sexual, or attractive as she was prior to the surgery.

When a person loses a body part because of disease or accident, there is grieving over that important loss just as if a friend or family member had died. The grieving process is described later in this chapter.

The nurse has many ways to help a person adjust to a changed body image. Touching the body during care shows acceptance of the changed body appearance. Encouraging participation in care helps the patient to become familiar with and accepting of the new body appearance. In helping the patient adjust to a changed body image, the nurse can remember that each individual changes in a unique way and pace.

In some cases, the patient may benefit by associating with others who have experienced a similar loss. Patients who have undergone removal of the voice box (laryngectomy) may find help in belonging to the Lost Cord Club. The person with a colostomy or ileostomy may find support in an organization called the United Ostomy Association. The patient who has had a recent removal of the breast (mastectomy) may be helped by a visit from a woman who has recovered from such an operation. Reach to Recovery is a program in which volunteers visit recent mastectomy patients. The nurse should know what programs are available in the community and the referral procedures to be used.

Another common experience of the individual who is ill is *fatigue* and *sleep disruption*. Sleep consists of regularly occurring cycles which last from 70 to 90 minutes. Each cycle has several distinct parts that can be demonstrated by recording the brain waves (by an electroencephalogram or EEG). One part of the cycle, lasting about 60 minutes, is known as NREM sleep (nonrapid eye movement). There seems to be general agreement among experts that the function of NREM sleep is physical rest. The other part of the cycle, lasting from 10 to 30 minutes, is known as REM sleep (rapid eye movement). Although still controversial, REM sleep has been associated with dreaming and dream recall, but the exact relationship is unknown. Some experts have suggested that REM sleep plays a role in integrating current experiences with those of the past.

Sleep deprivation is a very common experience of the individual under nursing care. When deprived of sleep, an individual can be expected to demonstrate one or more of the following characteristics:

- Increased sensitivity to pain
- Feelings of irritability and disorientation
- Impaired learning and performance

Many of the factors that disturb sleep are known and some can be controlled by the nurse: noise in the environment, many interruptions for medication, treatments, and vital signs, worry over events of the day, and pain. Some specific interventions by the nurse that can reduce disturbances in the patient's sleep considerably include:

- Preparation for sleep including hygiene, ventilation, temperature, and lighting
- Organization of care so that the number of disruptions is minimized; example, give medication and take vital signs at the same time
- Appropriate administration of pain medication
- Reduction of noise in the environment

Pain and suffering are common experiences of the individual who is ill. More complete information about the individual in pain is in Chapter 7. Although still the subject of considerable research, it is known that pain involves the entire person and, thus, includes a physical component and a psychological component. Because each person's pain experience is different, the nurse is challenged to choose interventions based on the unique qualities of that individual. In addition, it is known that the nurse's relationship with the patient can enhance or diminish the effectiveness of pain remedies. For example, Mrs. Chin is a 75-year-old woman experiencing pain in the right knee from osteoarthritis. Mrs. Chin, who follows many Chinese healing practices, has been applying an herbal pack obtained from a neighborhood healer. After consulting with the physician and the registered nurse, the student LPN/LVN selects the following interventions:

- Assist Mrs. Chin to reapply the herbal pack.
- Change Mrs. Chin's position in bed.
- Administer oral pain medication.
- Spend 10 minutes talking with Mrs. Chin about other methods which she finds useful in pain relief.

It is important to note that the student LPN/LVN has used knowledge from several equally important sources: what is known about pain, what is known about Mrs. Chin's medical condition (osteoarthritis), and what is known about Mrs. Chin as a person. Thus, the interventions selected seem likely to relieve pain.

The healthy individual has many channels in which to direct efforts and interest. Many of these channels are closed when a person becomes ill. The physical confinement of the patient to a small unit of living, the loss of energy associated with disease, and the patient's concern over his or her welfare are important factors in the narrowing of personal interests. The person who focuses mainly on the self is said to be *self-centered* or *egocentric*.

This may be illustrated by the illness of Mrs. East. She and her husband lived in a newly acquired brick home. Mrs. East had joined several of the local community clubs and was especially interested in the garden club. She spent many happy hours digging, planting, and caring for her flower garden. The night after she had planted several rose bushes she started having chills and fever. The next day she was admitted to the hospital for observation. During this period of observation, Mrs. East spent many long hours looking at the four walls of the hospital room. Her thoughts were centered on herself. She wondered what was causing her illness, when she would be feeling better, and whether she was going to get well. Before this, Mrs. East had had many interests other than herself. Being sick caused her to focus her thoughts primarily on herself. She was temporarily egocentric, or self-centered. As Mrs. East improved, she became less self-centered, and her interest in outside activities returned.

Patients frequently lose interest in things that previously have been important. This loss may be slight in the case of one person and markedly greater in another. Factors that may seem unimportant to the well person frequently become extremely important to a patient. An example of this is seen in the patient's diet, which often assumes greater importance during illness. Mealtime becomes one of the anticipated highlights of the day. The patient usually can depend on the diversion of having a tray served three times a day. The nurse needs to realize that the patients look forward to mealtime as a break in an otherwise monotonous day but often do not feel hungry. For this reason, some patients can be expected to be overly critical of the food. This should be a challenge to the nurse to do whatever possible to make the meal more appetizing.

Patients who are ill may focus a great deal of attention on bodily needs. The healthy person does not think much about bodily needs. Breathing, eating, urination, and resting are automatic. Illness often means a sudden awareness that help is needed even for these simple activities.

Mr. Smith has been told to drink a glass of water every hour. However, the water pitcher is empty and he cannot get the water himself. He is on bedrest. Now he is worried because he cannot drink the water he is supposed to drink. Mrs. Jones has had a heart attack. As she lies in bed, she can feel her heart beat. She wonders if the beat is normal, too fast, or too slow. The nurse can do much to relieve the patients' worries by meeting physical needs safely, promptly, and comfortably. In addition, the psychological component is communicated by the nurse's calm, accepting attitude which invites the patient to talk over concerns.

Frequently, illness represents a crisis or turning point in the life of a person and family. For example, what happens to the family when the father has a heart attack? What is the impact of a life-threatening disease on the family of a young mother with five children?

The individual who is ill can be expected to experience a variety of *emotions* during the crisis of illness. Emotions are feelings that arise from living one's life and can be viewed as barometers of the weather in our lives from stormy to sunny. When a person experiences a feeling, there are body changes associated with that feeling. Pulse and respiratory rates, blood pressure, and blood supply to vital organs are examples of physical characteristics strongly influenced by a person's emotions. This is another example of the continuous mind-body interaction described earlier in this chapter.

All patients can be expected to show signs of anxiety. *Anxiety* is a state of mental uneasiness or worry that can result from a person's inability to meet his needs. Anxiety also is associated with illness. The patient may have a feeling of danger and lack of control. The body responds to anxiety by increasing the output of epinephrine. This, in turn, causes the pulse and respiratory rates to increase, the blood pressure to rise, and the blood supply to the central nervous system, heart, and muscles to increase. The blood supply to the gastrointestinal tract is decreased. The person may experience a loss of appetite, abdominal cramps, nausea, vomiting, insomnia, and diarrhea. The patient's face may become pale or flushed, the skin may feel moist. Frequent voiding generally is associated with anxiety. In other words, the body is prepared to escape the danger or to fight the danger.

Everyone has experienced anxiety at one time or another. The nursing student may feel a mild amount of anxiety before taking an examination, meeting a new patient, or starting a new clinical rotation. Severe anxiety or panic may cause a person to behave irrationally or to be unable to move. The nurse who observes severe anxiety or panic in the patient should report it to the appropriate member of the health team. Panic can aggravate an individual's illness. For example, Dr. Jones decided to cancel Mrs. Smith's surgery after the nurse reported that Mrs. Smith was in a state of panic. Anxiety is also known as a group phenomenon. In other words, anxiety can be transmitted from one person to another. For example, the patient can communicate the feeling of anxiety to the family or the nurse, or the nurse to the family.

Prolonged anxiety and the body changes associated with it are believed to be important factors in the development and/or outcome of many illnesses. The nurse can reduce many of the anxieties that accompany illness by a calm manner, simple explanations, and treating the patient as a unique individual. As a person becomes less anxious, more mental and physical energy is available for other activities.

Fear is an emotion that accompanies illness. A person who is ill is likely to have many fears. Some of the difficulties a patient may fear are death, loss of a body part, loss of job, paying the hospital bill, paying a loan, being a burden on the family, pain, surgery, and being in a strange place. The physiologic changes associated with fear are similar to those of anxiety. The nurse can help the patient who is afraid by explaining that it is normal for a person who is ill to be afraid and that talking about it sometimes helps. The nurse can offer to listen.

Depression is a state of feeling sad. The depressed individual feels lonely and empty and lacks self-esteem. The nurse, in listening to the patient, may hear such words as sad, blue, despondent, "down-in-the-dumps," lonely, gloomy, discouraged, unhappy, low, disgusted, or downhearted. Depression may be associated with the loss of a loved one, a part of the body, an ability, or the function of a part of the body. It may be associated also with some other personal disaster, or it may be a symptom of a psychiatric condition. Many factors can lead to depression.

The depressed person may lose interest in usual activities, lose weight, become constipated, experience fatigue and loss of appetite, and cry easily. Personal appearance may be neglected, sleep habits may be disturbed often by early morning wakening, and memory may be affected. The person also may be shy and oversensitive. Suicide may be considered. Anytime a person expresses the desire to "end it all" or to "do away with myself," the threat should be taken seriously. The physician should be notified. The patient may need protection from self-injury and/or suicide.

When ill, a person frequently feels a greater need for *spiritual help*. During illness, a person may derive reassurance, support, comfort, and courage from religious faith. This seems to be especially true when medical science is failing. The patient's rabbi, minister, or priest is an important member of the health team. Many large hospitals have chaplains of various faiths who minister to the patient's spiritual needs. The nurse acknowledges and respects the patient's beliefs by providing privacy when the chaplain or patient's spiritual advisor visits, by developing a knowledge of the resources available for spiritual support, and by meeting the patient's request for spiritual support as promptly as if it were a request for pain medication.

Defense Mechanisms

The person confronted with illness uses methods of adjustment used previously to adjust to other stressful situations. Defense mechanisms or mental mechanisms are mental processes that help a person adapt to the changes in life. They can be used consciously or unconsciously. The nursing student can learn to recognize these mechanisms in self and others. No attempt should be made to change these mechanisms in others. A patient uses a defense mechanism as a protection from things considered injurious or harmful. Understanding the patient's feelings enables the nurse to deal more effectively with behavior that provokes the nurse's own feelings of discomfort or anger. Such behavior often is not directed toward the nurse personally but simply reflects the patient's struggle to adapt to changes that illness brings.

A defense mechanism can be considered a sign of illness if it is used too frequently and if its use does not result in an adaptation that is consistent with reality.

DENIAL

The mental mechanism of denial is one in which the person refuses to face some part of reality. The individual using denial is usually unaware of the existence of wishes, needs, ideas, or actual incidents that are unacceptable. For example, the patient may deny illness or the presence of certain symptoms.

However, denial also may be on a conscious level. For example, the nursing student may deny being afraid of doing tracheostomy care for the first time. In this case, admitting fear may have been damaging to self-esteem.

The patient who refuses to admit to feeling ill and will not discuss it is said to be adjusting by denial. Another patient may say that illness or symptom is due to a harmless cause. For example, Mr. Carson has marked anemia accompanied by extreme fatigue. Mr. Carson says that he is just lazy. Some patients ignore the disability and pay little attention to it. For example, Mr. Danders, a cardiac patient, refuses to follow the doctor's orders for prescribed bed rest. He gets out of bed when no one is around and goes to the bathroom. The man with a marked facial scar who refuses to shave and thus avoids looking in the mirror is another example.

By recognizing that denial is a method of adjustment or a defense mechanism, the nurse is in a better position to accept fully this patient and this behavior. At times, denial saves the patient from more serious actions such as suicide or a serious personality disorder. The patient frequently needs time to work through the shock of knowing about a serious condition. When denial is harmful to the patient, the health team attempts to find out why the patient is responding in this manner.

REPRESSION

An individual using repression unconsciously excludes from consciousness unbearable ideas, thoughts, and feelings. Repression is an unconscious process of forgetting. In other words, the person walls off certain thoughts and feelings from the conscious. This frequently used method of adjustment serves to protect the person from painful thoughts. Repression is often used when feelings of shame, guilt, and anger are involved.

Mr. and Mrs. Freeman have decided not to have a baby until Mr. Freeman finishes college next year. However, Mrs. Freeman forgets to take her birth control pills for three days.

IDENTIFICATION

A person who unconsciously adopts the characteristics or traits of another is using the mechanism of identification. For example, the student nurse unconsciously adopts the professional and warm attitude of an admired instructor.

COMPENSATION

The defense mechanism of compensation is one in which anxiety is relieved by making up for a real or imagined personal lack or feeling of inadequacy. When using compensation, the individual emphasizes some personal, social, or physical attribute so that it overshadows the inadequacy. Compensation can take place on either a conscious or unconscious level. In other words, the person may or may not be aware of this mechanism.

Mr. Golack always has been an avid skier. Now he is paralyzed from the waist down. He works hard to develop the muscles of his arms and chest and eventually joins a basketball team in which all of the team members are confined to a wheelchair.

Mr. Golack has compensated for the inability to use his legs by developing unusual strengths and skill in the use of his arms.

REGRESSION

Regression refers to a return to previous methods of coping with stress. Regression occurs in varying degrees with almost every illness. The patient retreats from the present to a more satisfying form of behavior from the past. This behavior causes less conflict and anxiety.

Perhaps the most common expression of regression is seen in the patient's dependence on others for various activities necessary to life. As the patient improves, there may be a reluctance to resume responsibility for these activities. Although regression is common, it is serious when extreme.

PROJECTION

When using projection, the individual unconsciously rejects an unacceptable idea or feeling and identifies it as coming from another person. The person's own faults or shortcomings are attributed to others.

Mr. Acton has been told by his physician that he will need an operation. He is feeling anxious and afraid when his wife arrives. He tells her there is no reason to be afraid and to stop wringing her hands, and to go home if she cannot control her nerves.

RATIONALIZATION

Rationalization is a frequent, unconscious mental mechanism in which the person finds a good reason for doing or not doing something. An acceptable reason is substituted for the behavior in place of the real reason.

The student nurse fails a test in anatomy and physiology. Although she did not study for the test, she tells classmates that she "never was any good at remembering a lot of terms that had no meaning."

CONVERSION

Conversion occurs when a person expresses strong emotional conflicts through physical symptoms. Such a person unconsciously converts anxiety into a physical symptom which has no physical basis. Blindness and paralysis without physical cause are two examples.

The Impact of Death

In order to help the patient and/or family cope with disturbing thoughts and feelings of death, the nurse must first examine personal feelings and attitudes. Perhaps one of the best ways to deal with one's attitudes about death is to discuss the first death you can recall with a classmate or instructor. One of the senior author's first recollections of death occurred as a child when her uncle who lived in the same household died. He had been ill with cancer for a long time, and when he died the small child was told that her uncle had gone to heaven to live with God.

The grieving process is a series of steps during which a person and loved ones respond to the threat of impending death. The five stages described by Kübler-Ross are (1) denial, (2) anger, (3) bargaining, (4) depression, and (5) acceptance.

Similar stages have been observed in patients who face the loss of a body part. Just as each person responds to illness in his or her own way at his own pace, each person grieves in his or her own way and at his or her own pace.

When caring for the grieving patient and/or family, members of the health team do not attempt to change the ways or time of grieving. Rather, they provide time for, a place for, and acceptance of thoughts and feelings that the dying patient and his loved ones are experiencing. The nurse can expect to grieve along with other members of the health team when facing the loss of a patient. Children also grieve. Although they may not be able to talk about their fears and feelings, children often draw pictures that symbolize their fear of dying.

When faced with the prospect of losing a part of one's body, life, or a loved one, an individual can be expected to respond initially with a type of *denial*. For example, when the patient and/or family is told of a diagnosis that leads to death, the frequent response is "No, it can't be!" The family may refuse to believe the disastrous news and insist that everything is all right. The patient may maintain that everything is fine and that the doctor has made a mistake. By denying or refusing to believe disastrous news, the person allows time to make an adjustment. Denial helps one to keep from "falling to pieces." When dealing with a patient or family who is denying an actual situation, the nurse should accept this response. Lengthy discussions about the facts at this time will go unheard. Denial frequently is associated with feelings of numbness.

When caring for the patient who is grieving over the loss of a body part or impending death, the nurse and other members of the health team should allow time to experience each phase of the process. The time needed varies with the person. There needs to be time to think, be alone, cry, be angry, and still be accepted fully by the nurse. Usually, this stage draws to a close when the person feels ready to cope with the reality of the loss.

The second stage of *anger* and hostility is exemplified by such questions as "Why does it have to happen to me?" "What have I done to deserve this?" During this stage, the patient and/or family may express dissatisfaction with the nursing care, food, doctor, or financial burden. The nurse should listen to complaints without being defensive. Of course, complaints that can be corrected should be taken care of immediately. The nurse needs to remember that during this stage the bitterness and anger are not directed at anyone personally.

The third stage of *bargaining* follows anger and usually is short. The patient and/or family may make deals to obtain more time or permission to accomplish a certain goal. For example, Mrs. Ganson who had an incurable illness wanted to go home one more time and celebrate Christmas with her husband and children.

Depression is the stage in which the person experiences a great feeling of sadness. The patient and/or family already may have experienced many losses and realize that more will come or that the total loss is imminent. During this stage, the nursing student can communicate the feeling of caring by being quietly present or by a gentle touch with the hand. The patient and family may need to be protected from the well-meaning visitor who wants to spread cheer.

When nursing the patient whose depression is due to impending loss or loss of a body part, the student should not expect a rapid response. The patient should not be hurried or pushed. Superficial conversation and overcheerfulness should be avoided. The student may need to learn to work with the patient without unnecessary conversation.

The final stage is *acceptance*. The dying person seems to have a decreased intensity of emotion and may appear to have little feeling. This, however, is no time for the patient to be left alone. It is important that family members and the health team maintain contact. Sometimes words are needed;

sometimes not. Hearing appears to be the last sense to leave the body. Knowledge of this enables the nurse to continue speaking in low tones to the patient. The family also is encouraged to continue to communicate with the dying loved one. Other activities that grieving families sometimes find helpful include participating in certain aspects of physical care such as washing the face or massaging the back. These activities have the advantage of encouraging the family to touch their loved ones. As the importance of language diminishes, touch often is a more effective way of communicating. Some families find comfort in reading the Bible or praying together.

As death approaches, both the patient and the family need a trusting relationship with the physician and nursing staff. The family needs the reassurance that everything possible is being done for their loved one. This is not time for false reassurance. The patient and family respond to the emotional atmosphere created by those caring for the patient. Every person has the right to a dignified death. When death occurs, the family needs a supportive, understanding nurse. The family can be expected to need time to express feelings. The silent, accepting, and supporting presence of the nurse will be an important source of assistance to the family. In general, the grieving family is helped most by honesty accompanied by warmth and caring. For example, sometimes a patient dies and family members are not at the bedside. If it is necessary to call them at home, the family should be told of the death of their loved one. To say instead that the loved one has "taken a turn for the worse" may result in unpleasant consequences. The family rushing to the bedside could have an auto accident. Family members may later be haunted by persistent feelings of guilt for failing to get to the bedside in time for a last goodbye. Often, the nurse is asked by the family if they should view the body. Generally, the family who expresses an interest in viewing the body should be encouraged to do so. This helps family members acknowledge the loved one's death and begin their own grieving.

Each member of the family deals personally with the loss. Feelings of shock, disbelief, and numbness are frequently followed by discussions of the loved one. Positive feelings about the deceased are highlighted. This phase may continue for many weeks, months, or longer. The loss is said to be resolved when the grieving person can remember both pleasant and unpleasant aspects of the relationship with the deceased.

Nurses also grieve when a patient dies. Because nurses view themselves as helpers, they may not be aware that they, too, sometimes need help when grieving. Self-understanding and self-awareness are qualities that enable the nurse to reach out for help if overwhelmed by grief. As a result, the nurse approaches the grieving patient and family instead of avoiding them.

Recent developments in the care of the dying have resulted in new resources and options for patients, families, and nurses. There are nurses with additional education in the care of the dying patient and the grieving process. Such nurses are available to assist the patient, the family, and the nursing staff with grieving. In some cases, the nurse may work directly with the patient and/or family. In other cases, the nurse helps the nursing staff to develop and implement nursing care plans for a patient where the goal is a peaceful death. In still other cases, the nurse assists the nursing staff with its own grieving process.

A second important development is known as *hospice care*. Hospice care generally provides direct and indirect support services for the dying patient and family. A variety of hospice care is available. A patient wishing to die at home may be provided with support services in the home. Some general hospitals have set aside special units for hospice care. In addition, there are some individual hospitals that provide only hospice care. Finally, there are hospice programs in which dying patients are enrolled and that offer support to the patient in every location— home, hospitals, nursing home. A final feature is that hospice care is usually given by a *multidisciplinary* health team that has special interest and additional education in the care of the dying patient. Multidisciplinary refers to professionals from many different fields who use their special knowledge and skill to care for the dying patient. This team usually includes the nurse, physician, pharmacist, dietitian, clergyperson, social worker, physical therapist, and others as needed.

An additional resource is support groups composed of grieving persons who meet regularly for the purpose of sharing their experiences, developing healthy coping skills, and deriving comfort. The grieving patient, family, or nurse may benefit from using one or more of these resources.

The Role of the Nurse

The nurse has a vital part to play in the patient's illness. Many services received by the hospitalized patient come directly or indirectly from the nurse. Thus, the nurse has considerable impact.

One valuable part the nurse plays is that of the patient's assistant, helping with those activities a person with sufficient knowledge and skill and physical ability normally does alone. For example, all persons must excrete urine in order to rid the body of waste products. Normally, a person takes care of this function alone. During certain illnesses, a catheter is inserted into the urinary bladder to drain urine. This requires special knowledge and skill the patient does not have. The nurse's assistance is needed. Similarly, all persons need to exercise and move about. Normally, a person walks and exercises in the process of living every day. Following surgery, the patient feels weakened and tired but still needs to walk. Because the patient cannot do this alone, the nurse's assistance is needed.

Another part the nurse has to play involves the medical treatment plan devised by the physician. The nurse is the key person who carries out many aspects of diagnosis and treatment. For example, the nurse collects specimens vital to the diagnosis of the patient's illness. The nurse administers medication to treat the disease. Another vital part in the medical treatment plan played by the nurse is as an on-the-spot continuous observer and recorder of the patient's response to illness and treatment. Changes brought by illness can occur very rapidly and can threaten life. The nurse's role as an observer, reporter, and recorder is crucial both to the patient and other members of the health team.

Nursing observations are made by looking, listening, touching, and smelling. A systematic method of observing usually yields more complete, accurate, and discriminating information. One guide that the beginning nursing student may find helpful is a systematic observation from head to toe of the individual (see Table 1.1).

In addition to the head-to-toe observation described above and in Table 1.1, knowledge of an individual's life-style is needed for a complete observation. Life-style was discussed earlier in this chapter. Many persons believe that matters of life-style are private. Every individual has a right to certain privacies. No one surrenders the right to privacy simply because of illness. Members of the health team must be very careful not to intrude on an individual's privacy in collecting information related to life-style. In addition, there is variation among individuals about just which facts are considered private. Many persons, for example, are unwilling to discuss matters such as family relationships, political or church involvement, or age.

The life-style guide provided in Table 1.2 is to assist the nurse in identifying those characteristics of life-style that affect and are affected by illness.

In addition to observation of the effect of illness and treatment on the patient, it is very important to report the effect of worries, fears, anxieties, and problems. This information, when reported to the team leader or head nurse, is transmitted to the doctor and other team members. Sometimes, the problem can be solved. For example, a patient with diabetes spoke to the LPN/LVN of the fear of injecting insulin. This was reported to the head nurse. After discussing the problem with the physician, the head nurse and team leader began teaching the patient how to inject insulin. Teaching was begun early because of the LPN/LVN's report.

Another role of the nurse is coordinator of the patient's daily activities. Laboratory studies, x-rays, physical therapy, mealtimes,

TABLE 1.1
A HEAD-TO-TOE GUIDE FOR NURSING OBSERVATION

WHAT TO OBSERVE	OBSERVATIONS
1. Hair	Combed or uncombed—clean or dirty
Eyes	Closed or open—puffy or sunken—reddened or yellowed sclera—wearing glasses, contact lens, or artificial eye—makes eye contact or avoids eye contact—brows knitted
Face	Shaved or unshaved
Mouth	Smiling, frowning, grimacing, breathes through mouth—lips moist or dry—color of lips—dentures present or absent—teeth clean or unclean—teeth present or absent—odor of breath—fetid, sweet, fruity—color of mucous membranes inside mouth
Nose	Breathes through nose—nostrils flaring—color reddened, pale
Speech	Talkative or silent, accent or language spoken, slurred speech, speaks very fast or very slow, initiates questions or discussion, responds only when spoken to, responses appropriate to conversation, doesn't speak
2. Neck and chest	Respirations rapid or slow, even or uneven, coughing—for a more detailed observation, see Chapter 14
3. Abdomen	Soft, taut, flat, distended
4. Extremities	Color, warmth, pulses present or absent, strong or weak, regular or irregular, body movements quick, slow, smooth, jerky, wringing hands. Fingernails and toenails clean or dirty, wearing a prosthesis
5. Skin	Color, scars, warts, moles, wounds, freckles, birthmarks, operative scars, warm or cool to touch, moist or dry, perspiring, presence of body odor, clean or dirty
6. Posture	Erect or slumped, gait steady or unsteady, uses cane or walker
7. Dress	Comfortable, appropriate, color, clean, adequate for weather condition

TABLE 1.2
LIFE-STYLE GUIDE

1. Health habits
   - Eating and sleeping patterns
   - Bowel and bladder habits
   - Dental care
   - Medical care
   - Present medications
   - Exercise patterns
2. Family relationships, role in family
   - Family recreation patterns
   - Type of dwelling occupied by family
3. Community relationships, hobbies or other interests
   - Participation in community activities such as clubs, church, and political involvement
4. Occupational relationships, type of work
   - Work-related plans and goals

and medications are only a few examples of activities coordinated by the nurse. Successful coordination requires considerable skill as the nurse interacts not only with the patient but with many other persons. Viewing the patient as a whole person with basic human needs enables the nurse to act for the patient's benefit.

Besides the role already described, the nurse provides a new and vital channel to the world outside the sick world at a time when other channels have been closed. Thus, the patient may ask the nurse's opinion about the weather, a recent news event, or even about the nurse's social life. Often the patient's intent is not to pry but only to establish contact with the nonsick world via the nurse.

The Nursing Process

As the roles of the nurse became more numerous and complex, it became necessary to develop a systematic method of caring for the individual. That systematic method has come to be called *nursing process*. There are variations among nurses using this method, but most follow the same general plan. Nursing process is composed of several interrelated steps or phases.

The first step or phase is collecting information, also known as *nursing history*. Since history refers to events in the past, one helpful way of learning about this phase

is by asking the question: where did the person come from? Information is available from many sources including the patient, family, medical history, laboratory studies, and the nurse's own observation. The student LPN/LVN may wish to review the observation and life-style guides at this time. The information generally is recorded on a nursing history form and placed in the patient's record.

After the information has been collected, it is necessary to determine what will be achieved as a result of nursing care. This is the second phase or step, often called *nursing goals* or *objectives*. The learning question to be asked in this phase is: where is the person going? When the goal is very complex, it is usually helpful to break it down into smaller parts. For example, an appropriate goal for a patient following hip surgery could be unassisted walking. Examples of two smaller parts of unassisted walking include moving from bed to chair and walking with assistance.

It is very important that the goals reflect and be consistent with the needs and desires of the patient. Thus, the nurse makes considerable effort to learn about the patient's needs and goals. In the ideal situation, the nurse and the patient set the goals together. Goals to be meaningful should be as specific as possible. For example, a time frame should be specified. Are the goals to be achieved within two days, one week, or by discharge?

The next phase or step is often called *implementation*. The learning question to be answered by this phase is: how will the nurse help the patient reach the goal? As in the previous phase, the interventions are described as specifically as possible.

Interventions, sometimes known as *nursing orders*, are specified by how often they will be done, by whom, and for how long. An example of a complete nursing order designed to reach the goal of unassisted walking might be.

- LPN/LVN to supervise patient ambulating with walker from bed to nurse's station tid × 24 hours.

The final step in the nursing process is known as *evaluation and revision*. The learning questions to be answered in this step are: has the goal been reached, and where do we go from here? If the goal has not been reached, some revision of the goals and/or interventions is indicated.

One important requirement of the nursing process is that it must be recorded. Just as the physician must document the medical care plan on the patient's record, the nurse also must document the nursing care plan. Most agencies provide special forms on which to record the nursing care plan (Figure 1.2).

Common Nursing Practices

There are hundreds, perhaps thousands, of specific nursing interventions. In learning about the use of specific interventions, the student LPN/LVN may find it helpful to develop a perspective on common nursing practices.

All nursing care takes place in the context of an interpersonal relationship between the patient and the nurse. A very important part of nursing is developing a *therapeutic relationship*. A therapeutic relationship is one that is perceived by the patient as being helpful. As the nursing student learns more about the development of a therapeutic relationship, it may be helpful to review the earlier section describing psychological and physical needs of individuals. A very simple way to begin a therapeutic relationship is to meet patient's physical needs promptly. A patient lying in a wet bed or suffering from pain that the nurse is aware of and does not remedy promptly cannot be expected to perceive the nurse-patient relationship as caring or beneficial. The act of keeping a person waiting communicates unfriendliness in our culture. Waiting adds to the patient's frustration and very often diminishes the senses of personal autonomy and self-worth. Thus, the wise student nurse develops a practice of meeting patients' needs promptly. When this is not possible, the patient should be notified and the delay explained.

Every day in every way, we communicate our attitude or our opinion about the world and the people in it to those around us. Attitudes basic to developing a therapeu-

tic relationship are the nurse's friendliness, warmth, interest, and acceptance.

Acceptance is basic to a therapeutic relationship. *Acceptance* is a way of expressing belief in the intrinsic value of an individual. Each patient is a unique and valuable person. Perhaps the best way to identify degrees of acceptance is to select several classmates or friends who make you feel that you are unique and important. How do they convey this feeling to you? Do you have similar feelings about others? How do you feel when you fully accept another human being?

In addition to an unconditional acceptance of the patient as a worthy human being, another factor is important. Helping the patient retain individuality is beneficial to a therapeutic relationship. Speaking and referring to the patient by name at all times, pronouncing the name correctly, introducing the patient to staff members in another department such as x-ray, and handling the patient's possessions carefully are examples of strategies that recognize each person's individuality. Caring for the patient according to the nursing care plan developed to meet individual needs acknowledges that person's individuality. A practice to be avoided is the habit of referring to a patient by diagnosis or bed number.

One skill essential to developing a therapeutic relationship is *communication*, a process of exchanging ideas, beliefs, thoughts, and feelings between two or more people. Communication involves a message, a sender, and a receiver. The person who has a message is the sender and the one to whom it is sent is the receiver. The sender and receiver change roles frequently while communicating.

The types of communication of primary concern to the nursing student are the verbal and nonverbal. Verbal refers to the written and spoken word. Examples of nonverbal communication are body position, facial expression, gestures, clenched jaw, raised eyebrows, signs, symbols, crying, wheezing, coughing, moaning, screaming, groaning, humming, manner of walking, whistling, and silence.

Listening to the patient is an essential part of communication. In learning to make

[*Text continued on page 18*]

CASTLE MEDICAL CENTER
KAILUA, HAWAII

NURSING CARE PLAN

PATIENT HISTORY   DATE: CONDITION:

Family/Guardian _____   Religion _____   Pastoral Care/Date _____
                                                          (Sacraments of the Sick)
Phone No. _____   Language _____   Dialect _____

Support Person _____   Phone No. _____

PERTINENT HEALTH HISTORY

SPECIAL INFORMATION:

___ Glasses
___ Contact Lenses
___ Hearing Aid
___ Prosthesis - type
___ Dentures - upper ___ lower ___
___ Removable bridge
___ Eating patterns
___ Elimination patterns
___ Sleep patterns

SAFETY MEASURES

___ Side rails
___ Posey belt
___ Soft restraints
___ Seizure precautions
___ Trach at bedside
___ Special Equip.
___ Smoking precaution

ISOLATION

DISCHARGE PLAN	Completion Date	By Whom
Needs		

OB INFORMATION

PARA ___ GRAV ___ RH ___ RUBELLA ___
Delivery Date _____   Time _____
Baby's # _____
___ Boy ___ Girl ___ Breastfeed ___ Bottle
___ Epis. ___ Hemm. ___ Sitz Bath
___ Heatlamp ___ Other

REV 3/82 NS-15

15

LONG TERM OBJECTIVES: _____

DATE	PROBLEMS	EXPECTED OUTCOMES/GOALS	DEAD-LINES	NURSING ORDERS/ACTIONS	I.D.

SURGERY: _____ DATE: _____

ADMITTING DIAG: _____ DATE OF ADM: _____

TIME OF ADM: _____

CONSULTATIONS _____

ROOM # _____   PTS. NAME: _____   DR: _____   ALLERGIES: _____

16

VITAL SIGNS
TPR _____ B.P. _____
Breath Sounds
Weight q
CVP _____ SG _____ Art. Line
Neuro signs
Other pulses
Cardiac Monitor _____ Telemetry

ACTIVITY
_____ Bedrest
_____ Dangle _____ Chair/WC
_____ Ambulate _____ Assist
_____ BRP _____ Commode
BATH
_____ Bed _____ Assist _____ Sitz
_____ Shower _____ Tub

DIET & FLUIDS
Type _____
_____ Tea _____ Coffee _____ Sanka
_____ Feed _____ Assist _____ Self
_____ Tube _____ Gomco
_____ NPO
_____ Intake _____ Output
_____ IV's _____ cc/hr

BLADDER AND BOWEL CARE
_____ Cath prn
_____ Foley Cath _____ Date in _____
_____ G.U. irrigant
_____ Bladder training
Check for BM's or impactions:
M T W T F S SU
_____ Enemas

SKIN CARE
_____ Dressing Chg.
_____ Sheep skin
_____ Pressure matress
_____ Special skin care

REHAB MEASURES
_____ Footboard _____ Foot Cradle
_____ Bedboard _____ Overhead bar
_____ ROM to
_____ Traction
_____ Cardiac Rehab
_____ Pulmonary Rehab
_____ Other

X-RAYS, EKG'S, SPECIAL PROCEDURES

DATE	PROCEDURE	TO BE DONE	DATE	PROCEDURE	TO BE DONE

	TREATMENT		DATE	TREATMENT	

DATE	LAB WORK	TO BE DONE	DATE	LAB WORK	TO BE DONE

CULTURES

FIGURE 1.2 The nursing care plan provides written record of the nursing process. (Courtesy of Castle Medical Center, Kailua, Hawaii.)

nursing observations, the nurse must develop good listening skills. Listening can be considered a golden key to understanding. The term *listening* is not used in this text to imply an entirely one-sided conversation from the patient to the nurse. It means that the nurse speaks *with* rather than *to* the patient.

A good listener can lighten another person's burden; relief is obtained when an individual finds an interested and understanding listener. Although a person may not find a solution to worries and problems, talking about them and sharing the burden often bring feelings of serenity and lightness. Listening does not necessarily indicate agreement. It does mean that a good listener tries to understand what is being said. The person who feels criticized and judged instead of listened to and understood may either stop talking or start defending.

Genuine interest is a basic requirement for developing the art of listening and leads to understanding. All of us have had the experience of talking with someone who did not appear interested in what we were saying. That person was not listening to us because of lack of interest. Interested remarks injected appropriately into the conversation show the patient that the nurse is really listening. A nurse who chatters persistently is usually not listening and therefore, cannot understand the patient.

Words and gestures are indications of a person's thoughts and feelings. For example, Mr. Branch, a preoperative patient, asked Mrs. Lake, the nurse, several times if she knew the surgeon who was to operate on him that morning. Since Mrs. Lake was really listening, she understood that Mr. Branch's repeated question probably indicated apprehension. She reported the observation to the head nurse who asked the surgeon to stop by and see Mr. Branch before surgery. Mrs. Lake contributed to Mr. Branch's emotional and physical well-being because she was able to listen with interest and understand.

The nurse who has developed the arts of listening and communicating is often able to provide valuable *reassurance* to the patient. Reassurance enables the patient to develop or regain the confidence needed to face the future. Understanding and trust are two important requirements for reassurance. The patient needs to feel understood as an individual by members of the health team. In addition, the patient needs to trust those who are providing care.

A false idea about reassurance is to tell a person not to worry or to say that everything will be all right. Telling an individual not to worry may be compared with trying to stop the flow of a stream. The tension produced by the worry cannot be reduced by telling it to stop, just as the power of a flowing stream cannot be stopped by telling it to stop. Frequently, the tension produced by worry can be reduced or relieved by talking. The nurse should realize that this does not necessarily mean the problem has been solved. It does mean that the nurse who is a good listener helps the patient reduce tension or "let off steam" by talking. This, in turn, helps the patient feel reassured because of being understood. For example, Mr. Carter told Mr. Benite, the student LPN/LVN, about his invalid wife at home. Mr. Benite, expressing a genuine interest, asked Mr. Carter who was caring for his wife. This simple question gave Mr. Carter an opportunity to talk about his worry, which had caused several sleepless nights. Before Mr. Carter's illness, he took care of his wife. Now, a son and daughter-in-law were providing care. Although it might have seemed to Mr. Benite that there was nothing to worry about, Mr. Carter believed that there was. Some of Mr. Carter's tension was relieved just by talking about his wife. Subsequently, Mr. Carter felt reassured by the nurse's understanding of him as an individual.

There are many other ways to reassure a patient, such as telling the patient where you will be, when you will return, and how to reach you. Frequent visits by the nurse also provide reassurance.

The presence of a kindly and understanding person can be reassuring. For example, a patient transferred to the operating room may be reassured by the presence of the nurse who has been providing care.

Another important intervention used by the nurse every day is *touching*. The sensation of touch is vital to every person from birth throughout the life cycle. Insufficient tactile stimulation (touching) has been associated with a variety of abnormal conditions such as failure of infants to thrive. Touch contains both a physical and psychological component, as described earlier in this chapter. For example, the nurse uses touch to detect physical abnormalities such as full bladder, cool and clammy skin, or pulse rate. When giving a back rub, the nurse uses touch to promote circulation. The nurse also uses touch purposefully to communicate caring, concern, or encouragement. Sometimes when words fail, touch is a more effective way to communicate (Figure 1.3). One of the authors recently used touch to calm a patient who was experiencing panic. In patient teaching, the nurse's touch can be used to guide the inexperienced hand in injecting insulin. However, touch may also be harmful if used inappropriately. The rules about appropriate touching vary among cultures. For example, in native Hawaiian culture, the human head is considered the dwelling place of the person's spirit as well as the temporary home for the ancestor gods. Touching from the head to the shoulders, except when absolutely necessary, is inappropriate. Touching also communicates sexuality and inappropriate touching may send

that message. Finally, inappropriate touching can transmit disease from one person to another via the nurse's hand if scrupulous handwashing practices are not followed. The general questions below guide the nurse in the use of touch as a nursing intervention.

- When, what, and where is it all right to touch and not right to touch?
- Who may touch and who may not touch?
- What specific meaning is conveyed by touching and what meaning is conveyed by not touching?

Another very important nursing intervention is the creation of a *therapeutic environment*. A therapeutic environment generally is one that is safe, clean, and organized. Such an environment minimizes the stress of illness and contributes to the patient's sense of well-being. As mentioned earlier, when ill, a person experiences a certain sense of internal disorganization and loss of control. The orderly, well-maintained environment may act as an outside stimulus to assist the patient to reorganize.

The last major category of interventions can be called *technological skills*. Procedures such as vital signs, catheterization, dressing changes, and sterile techniques are exam-

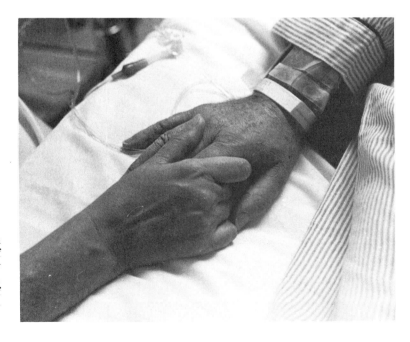

FIGURE 1.3 Touching can be an effective way of communicating. (Courtesy of Henrico County–St. Mary's Hospital School of Practical Nursing, Richmond, Virginia.)

ples of technological interventions. The student expends considerable time and energy perfecting these skills.

Just as the patient is a whole person, so is the nurse. The nurse who is overly concerned with procedures rather than the patient receiving them has lost sight of the wholeness of two very important individuals, the patient and the nurse. Similarly, the nurse who is so busy listening that a medication or treatment is late or missed has made the same error. It is important to master technological skills so well that attention can be focused on the whole person. Thus, the patient obtains maximum benefit from the nurse's assistance.

Case Study Involving Impact of Illness on an Individual

Mrs. Smith is 70 years old. Mrs. Smith was active in community activities such as volunteer work in the local hospital, housework, shopping, and traveling until two years ago. At that time, one of her primary interests was skiing. She was an active participant on frequent occasions. Two years ago Mrs. Smith suffered a cerebrovascular accident. As a result of the stroke, Mrs. Smith was paralyzed on her right side. She is predominantly right-handed.

Mrs. Smith was married when she was 18 years of age to a young student who became a physician in a cosmopolitan community. They had four children, three boys and one girl. Mrs. Smith became a widow when she was 60 years of age. Her husband was killed in an automobile accident 10 years ago.

At the present time, Mrs. Smith lives with her daughter and her son-in-law. Her daughter has three children of her own ranging in age from 8 to 15 years. Mrs. Smith has made little progress since her cerebrovascular accident two years ago.

Mrs. Smith was admitted to the hospital for a cardiac work-up. Prior to being hospitalized, Mrs. Smith was taking digoxin, 0.5 mg daily, and methyldopa (ALDOMET), 250 mg qid. When admitting Mrs. Smith to her room, the nurse noticed that she appeared disoriented to time, place, and her reason for being in the hospital. When talking with Mrs. Smith's daughter, the nurse learned that Mrs. Smith had refused most of her meals during the past few weeks. She seemed to prefer to remain in bed with her shades drawn. Mrs. Smith has remained in bed most of the time during the past year. The nurse noticed that Mrs. Smith had reddened areas on the back of her heels, her sacrum, her elbows, and both hips.

QUESTIONS

1. What losses has Mrs. Smith suffered during the past 10 to 20 years?
2. Is Mrs. Smith grieving? If so, is her grieving adaptive (leading to a conclusion in which she will accept the losses)? Is Mrs. Smith experiencing a grief that is maladaptive in that it is self-perpetuating?
3. What factors could have contributed to Mrs. Smith's general state of disorientation? (Hint: Please note Mrs. Smith's medication and nutritional status.)
4. Which factors, such as physical and mental characteristics, should be included in Mrs. Smith's nursing care plan?
5. Mrs. Smith has been placed in a private room at the request of her daughter. What are some of the advantages of a private room in this case? What are some of the disadvantages?
6. The nurse notices a gradual improvement in the orientation of Mrs. Smith and in her physical condition. Mrs. Smith is now able to use the bathroom with assistance and feed herself with the use of special utensils that have been fitted to her hand. One day the nurse goes into the room during lunch and notices Mrs. Smith's daughter feeding her.
   A. Why should Mrs. Smith be fed by her daughter when she is capable of doing it herself?
   B. What possible needs of the daughter are being met by Mrs. Smith's dependency upon her?
   C. What are the possible impacts or implications of Mrs. Smith's current illness with apparent improvement having on her daughter?

Suggestions for Further Study

1. Demonstrate an observable amount of anxiety to several of your classmates or other friends without telling them the adjustment mechanism that you are portraying. Have them identify the mechanism.
2. Can a person who has gone through one state of the grieving process and reached another one go back to the one through which he has already passed? For example, if he has gone through the anger phase can he go back to the denial stage?
3. In one expected behavioral outcome you were directed to observe an assigned patient or classmate playing the part of a patient. In your opinion, what impact did illness have on this person?
4. Have you ever thought of one of your patients as a "ruptured appendix" or a "broken leg"?

If so, compare your ideas with those presented in this chapter.

5. Mason, Mildred A.; Bates, Grace F.; and Smola, Bonnie K.: *Workbook in Basic Medical-Surgical Nursing*, 3rd ed. Macmillan Publishing Company, New York, 1984, Exercise 1.

Additional Readings

Billings, Carolyn Veronica: "Emotional First Aid." *American Journal of Nursing*, 80:2006–2009 (Nov.), 1980.

Dubree, Marily, and Vogelpohl, Ruth: "When Hope Dies—So Might the Patient." *American Journal of Nursing*, 80:2046–49 (Nov.), 1980.

Groff, Ben: "Death and I." *American Journal of Nursing*, 82:1080–84 (July), 1982.

Knowles, Ruth Dailey: "Preventing Anger." *American Journal of Nursing*, 82:118 (Jan.), 1982.

Krieger, Dolores: *Foundation for Holistic Health Nursing Practices: The Renaissance Nurse.* J. B. Lippincott Co., Philadelphia, 1981, pp. 249–72.

McCann, Elva J.: "Of Pillows and Pineapple Juice." *American Journal of Nursing*, 81:1354 (July), 1981.

Rambo, Beverly J., and Wood, Lucile A. (eds.): *Nursing Skills for Clinical Practice*, 3rd ed. W. B. Suanders Co., Philadelphia, 1982, pp. 567–75 and 777–87.

Raymond, Marsha Croy: "Time to Say Good-Bye." *American Journal of Nursing*, 82: 933–35 (June), 1982.

Self, Pamela R., and Viaw, Jeffrey: "4 Steps for Helping a Patient Alleviate Anger." *Nursing 80*, 10:66 (Dec.), 1980.

Smitherman, Colleen: "Your Patient's Angry: What Should You Do?" *Nursing 81*, 11:96–97 (Nov.), 1981.

Chapter 2

Cultural Components
of Illness*

Expected Behavioral Outcomes

Minimum objectives referred to as expected behavioral outcomes have been designed for the practical/vocational nursing student to use as guides in studying this chapter. The student should read these expected outcomes before studying the chapter.

The objectives can be used as guides for study. Using the content of this chapter, the student should return to the objectives and evaluate the ability to:

   1. Describe the four characteristics basic to all cultures.

   2. Identify possible portions of five of the major theories of disease causation found in today's society.

   3. Determine the cultural orientation of at least one classmate.

   4. Discuss the nursing implications for each cultural factor obtained from your classmate.

Vocabulary Development is not included in this chapter because of the nature of the contents.

*Written by Alice Z. Welch, R.N., M.S.N., in cooperation with the authors. Ms. Welch is Assistant Professor of Nursing, University of Utah, Salt Lake City, Utah.

Introduction

The world's population has become increasingly mobile during the past decade. This increase in mobility is in part caused by technological development, employment opportunities, refugee resettlement, and world travel as a life-style. One of the outcomes of increasing mobility of the world's people is the development of multicultural societies—societies composed of people from many lands.

The United States' population is composed of fifteen major cultural groups (Blacks, Whites, American Indians, Chinese, Filipinos, Japanese, Vietnamese, Koreans, Mexican-Americans, Samoans, Guamanians, and Asian-Indians) and is considered a multicultural society. Clientele of health care facilities located in metropolitan areas usually represents a cross-section of the overall population.

We are living in an age when culture/ethnicity is highly valued. Many cultural groups no longer believe in the "melting pot" theory. These groups prefer to be viewed and respected as each "vegetable" is viewed and valued in a "salad bowl." Clients of the nation's health care institutions expect health workers to be knowledgeable about their basic culture and to seek information from them that will aid in visualizing the world and illness as it is seen by them.

Cultural concepts will be very important to you because a large segment of the population's beliefs and health care practices are very different from your own. As a nurse, you may expect to provide care for at least four different cultural groups during an eight hour tour of duty (Figure 2.1). You may anticipate that two of the cultural groups will speak very little or no English. This knowledge will facilitate your understanding of "strange" behavior and attitude. It will also provide a basis for developing respect and valuing other cultural groups. Cultural knowledge of dominant ethnic groups in your geographic area will *restrain* your impulses to impose your health care beliefs and practices on your clients (cultural imposition) because you think your beliefs and practices are superior to others (ethnocentrism). An understanding of cultural concepts will increase your awareness of the need to elicit certain information before administering care to people when their ethnic and cultural backgrounds are different from your own.

Learning about your client's culture will impress upon you the need to assess hygiene, eating, dressing, and elimination patterns so that you may adapt your care to be consistent with another's beliefs and lifestyle. A brief introduction to the basic concepts of culture will provide a background for understanding your client's views and responses to illness.

Culture and Subculture

As stated in Chapter 1, the impact of illness on an individual is influenced by the many factors that cause that person to be unique. One of these major factors is culture. *Culture* may be thought of as a group's blueprint for living. Culture consists of patterns of behavior based upon traditional ideas, beliefs, and values. This patterned behavior is transmitted through symbols, language, art, and rituals from one generation to another. Culture provides rules or standards of behavior that members of a society consider acceptable and proper. Culture defines the child-rearing practices as well as the roles of individuals for both sexes at various ages within the family and community. Culture influences one's expressions of joy, sorrow, and pain. It teaches beliefs about environment (water, earth, and wildlife), health, illness causation, aging, and death. An individual's culture colors one's entire existence.

Within cultures, groups of individuals

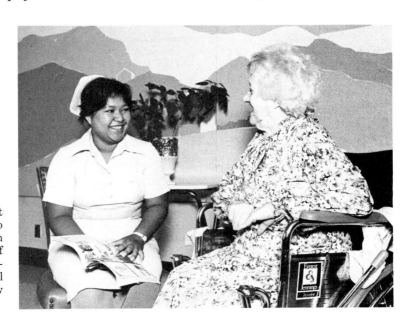

FIGURE 2.1 Mutual trust and respect are essential to creating a bridge between cultures. (Courtesy of Bergen Pines County Hospital School of Practical Nursing, Paramus, New Jersey.)

share different beliefs, values, and attitudes. Their differences occur because of
ethnic origin, religious beliefs, education,
occupation, age, and sex. Such groups functioning within a large culture are known as
subculture. Examples of subcultures in
America are Amish, Mormons, military, gay
community, Afro-American Blacks, Span-
ish-American, Native American and Ko-
rean-Americans.

Certain characteristics are basic to all
cultures: (1) culture is learned, (2) culture is
shared, (3) culture is based upon symbols,
and (4) culture is integrated.

CULTURE IS LEARNED

By growing up in it, the individual learns
culture and transmits it from one generation
to another. The process of learning one's
cultural system of thinking and acting is
known as *enculteration*. As a child grows up
in a culture, expected behaviors for specific
roles and occasions are learned. One must
not confuse behaviors and needs. Each person has need for sleep, food, safety, shelter,
and sexual fulfillment. How these needs are
satisfied are culturally learned behaviors.
Examples of culturally learned behaviors to
satisfy the need for sleep include: sleeping
on single cots in a dorsal recumbent position
with arms folded across the chest (American
Indian), sleeping on the floor with close body
contact with other family members (Vietnamese), and, sleeping in elevated beds in individual rooms (Anglo-American). The way
an individual experiences culture during for-
mative years will influence one's personality
and responses to life situations. Life situations include responses to illness, teachings
about prevention, as well as compliance with
medical regime.

CULTURE IS SHARED

Individual behavior does not constitute
culture. The group must share common beliefs and behaviors. Common behavior provides predictability of each other's actions in
given situations. It also increases the feeling
of safety and security within the group.

CULTURE IS BASED ON SYMBOLS

Examples of symbols include language,
money, and religious artifacts. Language is
considered the most important symbol in a
culture. Through language, a person communicates ideas, feelings, and emotions.
Words are substituted for objects. Symbols
are mandatory for the operation of political,
economic, religious, and organizational
structures of culture.

Culture must adapt to change to remain
relevant and viable. Members of a culture
have the *responsibility* to provide ways for
new members to join the group. They also
must be capable of maintaining a relationship with other groups. Cultural survival depends on motivation of its members to per-
petuate its cultural heritage and system.

Common Sociocultural Beliefs Concerning Disease and Illness Causation

Human beings throughout history have
attempted to understand illness and disease.
Theories have been formulated based upon
religious beliefs, social circumstances, and
level of knowledge. Many theories have been
discarded and aspects of others have been
incorporated into present-day theories of
disease causation. The purpose of this section is to highlight common theories of disease causation held by major cultural groups
within the United States. Tables 2.1 and 2.2
compare some cultural concepts between
common cultural groups in the United
States.

WITCHCRAFT

Witchcraft is one of the oldest theories of
disease causation. Witches are individuals
indentified by the community as possessing
supernatural power, capable of causing
good, evil, and illness. Witchcraft is based
upon sympathetic magic. Sympathetic
magic is believed to be the *connections* that
join all things together in the universe.
Knowledge of these connections is used to
interpret, manipulate, and control events in
the environment.

There are two types of sympathetic
magic: imitative and contagious. In *imitative magic*, the individual imitates what he/
she wishes to achieve. An example of imita-
[Text continued on page 28]

TABLE 2.1
COMPARISON OF THREE CULTURAL GROUPS, BELIEFS, VALUES, AND HEALTH PRACTICES

COMPONENTS	WHITE AMERICAN	BLACK AMERICAN	SPANISH-AMERICAN
1980 population	188,340,790	26,488,218	14,605,883
Traditional family structure	Nuclear (immediate) family	Nuclear/extended nuclear	Extended—patriarchal
Basic values and behavior	Health, rugged individualism, materialism, personal achievement, youth, social and geographic mobility, competitive and aggressive behavior	Family, community, religion, health, work, sense of discipline, shares with family and friends	Harmony in interpersonal relationships, shares with family and friends
Decision-maker	Husband	Parents with consultation with significant others	Father
Languages spoken	English	English/Black dialect	Spanish/English
Communication style	Direct	Direct/indirect	Indirect
Use of touch and gestures			
Privacy and personal space			Privacy not valued, means loneliness
Concept and use of time	Future oriented, time highly valued, planning important, all activities regulated by clock	Present oriented, spontaneous use of time, little value in planning ahead, event begins when people arrive	Present oriented, little value in planning ahead, right now means now or later
Beliefs—disease causation	Germ theory and divine punishment	Imbalance between body-mind-spirit, divine punishment, witchcraft, germ theory	Magical fright, divine punishment, hot-cold imbalance, environmental hazard
Prevention of illness	Proper diet, rest, and exercise	Good food, living right, and keeping system cleaned out	Charms, amulet, crucifix
Folk healers	Spiritualist	Root doctor, spiritualist	Folk health specialist, family
Use of health system	Professional health system	Self-care first, folk system, professional health system	Professional and folk system simultaneously
Dietary patterns	American	Soul foods: fried foods, fish, chicken, pork, greens, grits, sweet potatoes, corn, biscuits	Mexican foods—tomatoes, green peppers, onion, chili
Dietary restrictions during illness			Hot-cold foods, depending on food and disease classification
Expression of pain	Expressive—open	Vocal outcries with divine petition for assistance, varying degree stoicism	Expressive

TABLE 2.2
COMPARISON OF THREE CULTURAL GROUPS, BELIEFS, VALUES, AND HEALTH PRACTICES

COMPONENTS	FILIPINO-AMERICAN	AMERICAN INDIAN—NAVAHO	VIETNAMESE
1980 population	774,640	1,418,195 (total American Indian)	261,714
Traditional family structure	Extended—family includes friends and neighbors; egalitarianism	Extended—matriarchal	Extended
Basic values and behavior	Family, children, harmony in interpersonal relationships, respect for authority, sharing of possessions with family and friends, saving of face, group and family more important than individual, religious education	Family, individual rights, food, money, personal possession valued only when shared with others	Large families, health education, responsibility for each other
Decision-maker	Shared husband and wife	Maternal grandmother with family consultation	Husband
Languages spoken	Tagalog, dialect of province, English	Navaho/English	Vietnamese and/or ethnic dialect
Communication style	Indirect. avoid confrontation	Indirect	Indirect, avoid confrontation, gender affects which topic can be discussed
Use of touch and gestures	Touch denotes caring, very important	Gestures used to communicate, avoid direct eye contact	Avoid touching of head, and touching one shoulder—touching one shoulder disturbs genie; touching the head linked with ancestors

Privacy and personal space	Modesty required for dressing	Modesty required for dressing	
Concept and use of time	Adaptable, desire to please	Time is continuous—no beginning or end, being is important, activities not regulated by clock	Past important/present
Beliefs—disease causation	Supernatural causes, divine punishment, environmental hazards, taking baths on Friday	Out of harmony with nature	Disharmony with universe, ill winds, object intrusion, evil spirits
Prevention of illness	Wearing of crucifix, cross, charms, amulets, plenty of garlic	Sprinkling of corn	Rituals to appease evil spirits, amulets, proper diet
Folk healers	Faith healers and herbalist	Medicine man, herbalist, singer	Home remedies first, herbalist
Use of health system	Western medical system/folk remedies	Indian medicine/Anglo medical system	
Dietary patterns	Ethnic Filipino—rice, pork, chicken, vegetables, fresh fruits, garlic	Ethnic—squash, corn, goat, lamb, and fried bread	Ethnic Vietnamese—rice, soup, fish, pork, coagulated animal blood, vegetables, fruits, green tea
Dietary restrictions during illness	Hot-cold food, depending on classification of illness		Hot-cold foods depending on classification of illness
Expression of pain	Varying degrees of stoicism, strong desire to meet health worker's expectations	Stoicism	Varying degrees of stoicism

tive magic is the woman in labor with a knife under the bed to cut the labor pains.

Contagious magic advances the idea that an item, once physically connected to a living being, can never be separated. This concept implies that harm to the part affects the whole. Witches use the part-whole concept to inflict harm to individuals. They use discarded portions of finger and toenails, strands of hair, or used menstrual pads to harm individuals. Research has shown witchcraft is a prevalent belief of disease causation among Mexican-Americans, Puerto Ricans, Americans, Trinidadians, Haitians, and American Blacks.

DIVINE PUNISHMENT

Divine punishment is the belief that disease is caused by the wrath of God. This belief can be traced to Biblical times. Illness caused by sin is treated by atonement and sacrifices by the offender. Illness caused by the wrath of God is a common belief of members of Holiness, Pentecostal, and Fundamental Baptist Churches as well as Appalachian Whites, Mexican-Americans, and Blacks.

GERM THEORY

The germ theory is a commonly accepted theory in the Western world. It states a specific microorganism must enter the body, overpower natural resistance, and cause an inflammatory response in the development of each infectious disease. According to germ theory, diseases are treated by identification of the causative microorganism and administration of the appropriate drug to which the organism is sensitive.

YIN-YANG

The yin-yang theory is an ancient Chinese theory of disease causation. It has been used continuously for the past 5000 years. The theory states that all organisms and things in the universe consist of yin and yang energy forces. The seat of the energy forces are within the autonomic nervous system. *Health* is a state of perfect balance between yin and yang. When one is in balance, a feeling of inner and outer peace is experienced. *Illness* represents an imbalance of yin

and yang. Balance may be restored by herbs, acupuncture (insertion of fine needles into points along the body's meridians), or acupressure (application of pressure or massage to the same meridian points).

Yin energy forces represent the female and negative forces, such as emptiness, darkness, and cold. *Yang* forces are male and positive, emitting warmth and fullness. The autonomic nervous system is composed of the sympathetic and parasympathetic systems. The sympathetic system controls the body's defenses. It prepares the body for fight and flight. The sympathetic nervous system represents yang energy forces. Too much yang causes rapid heartbeat, tenseness, irritability, fever, dehydration, and increased blood pressure.

The parasympathetic nervous system represents yin forces. Yin forces control body function and conserve energy. An excess of yin causes gastrointestinal illness, colds, and apprehension.

The yin-yang theory is practiced throughout Asia and is gaining acceptance in the United States. It is often called Eastern or Chinese medicine. It is practiced in conjunction with Western medicine in the United States by Asian clients.

Foods are classified as hot and cold under this theory. Foods are believed to be transformed into yin and yang energy when metabolized by the body. Yin foods are cold and yang foods are hot. Cold foods are eaten with a hot illness, and hot foods are eaten with a cold illness.

Other social cultural beliefs concerning illness causation include soul loss, object intrusion, and sorcery.

ENVIRONMENTAL HAZARDS

Exposure to environmental hazards of cold, damp night air, and vapors rising from the ground following a heavy rain are believed by certain cultural groups to cause illness and disease. Other environmental hazards include impurities of the air, water, and food.

HARMONY WITH THE ENVIRONMENT

To Native Americans, religion and medicine are indistinguishable. They believe humankind lives in harmony with the environment, taking only from the environment that which is essential to sustain life. *Illness* is a sign that the individual is out of harmony with the environment.

The treatment of disease and illness involves use of the Western medicine system and tribal healing ceremonies. Tribal healing ceremonies include chants, rituals, and sandpainting by a specialist from the traditional culture. Healing ceremonies may last from 30 minutes to two hours, if performed in the hospital. Elaborate ceremonies to restore balance require from one to nine days and usually occur on the reservation.

HOT-COLD THEORY

The hot-cold theory of disease is based upon an ancient Greek theory (humoral) of disease causation, formulated during the fourth century. *Health* was defined as a balance between the four humors of the body, and *illness* resulted when an imbalance occurred.

The four humors of the body were blood, phlegm, black bile, and yellow bile. Their major purposes were to regulate the basic functions. The humors were described in terms of temperature, dryness, and moisture. *Blood* was believed to be hot and wet; *yellow bile* was hot and dry; *phlegm* was considered cold and wet; *black bile* was cold and dry. The treatment of disease consisted of addition or subtraction of cold, heat, dryness, or wetness to restore the balance of the humors.

Beverages, food, herbs, medicines, and other substances were classified as hot or cold. The classification was based upon the believed effects upon the body and not upon its physical texture, form, color, or temperature. There is little agreement among members of individual communities or between geographic areas as to which foods are hot and which are considered cold.

Illness believed to be caused by cold entering the body includes chest cramps, earache, paralysis, stomach cramps, rheumatism, and tuberculosis. Examples of illnesses believed to be caused by overheating include dysentery, abscessed teeth, sore throats, kidney ailments, and rashes. Diarrhea, toothache, and enteritis were thought to be caused by hot or cold. Recent research revealed hot-cold concepts are spread throughout the world. Individuals of Asian, Spanish, Latin, Black, Mexican, Arab, Muslim, South American, Cuban, and Puerto Rican ancestry still adhere to the basic concepts of hot-cold theory.

Hospitalization: A Form of Culture Shock

Culture shock is a feeling of confusion, frustration, and bewilderment caused by unfamiliarity and loss of environmental clues. Separation from familiar sounds, odors, language, family members, friends, and food can cause individuals to experience culture shock.

Admission to the hospital causes clients to experience many of the same feelings individuals have when traveling to a strange country and are unable to speak the language. The sights, sounds, hospital jargon, and role relationships are very frightening to clients, regardless of their ethnic or social class. The "stripping" of personal belongings and issuing of the short, split-down-back hospital gown dehumanize many individuals. The gown causes anxieties for individuals who value modesty. Hospitalization forces the individual to assume a dependent role. Patients must push buttons and ask permission to meet their most basic needs—food, water, and elimination.

Role and role relationships are altered with hospitalization. The authority figures are the hospital personnel such as doctors, nurses, nurse aides, and clerks. The doctor is at the top of the hierarchy and the patient is at the bottom, regardless of previous educational achievement. The patient is expected to be dependent, nonaggressive, and subordinate.

In large metropolitan health care settings, clients are expected to request, to question, and to evaluate therapy. This expectation can cause role conflict for Asian clients. Elderly Filipino clients believe it is disrespectful to tell the nurse or doctor how to do their jobs. Questioning health care workers about reasons for specific treatment is viewed as lack of confidence or trust in the individual's ability.

Hospital jargon impairs communication between nurse and client. The use of abbreviations such as BMs, ECG, PRN, and SOB causes confusion and further prolongs cultural shock. Until the client learns the hospital jargon, the ability to give information requested is limited.

A client shared the following hospital experience when asked what was most stressful about the hospital experience.

A loud voice came over the public address system: "DR Red! DR Red room 215 East Wing." Suddenly the sound of doors closing was heard. Then my room and bathroom door closed automatically. I could hear people scurrying around. No one came in to say anything. Suddenly, I felt real panicky, I thought, what if it's a fire! Where are my clothes? Then the voice came over the PA saying , All is clear, all clear. I pushed my button and my room door opened. I sure was relieved. Nurse, what do you think was happening?

The hospital environment is loaded with mechanical devices that the client must master in order to make personal needs known. A single device contains six to eight buttons that control the lights, door, television, intercommunication system, and the call bell.

Hospitalization causes separation from family, friends, and one's support system. Rules regarding numbers of visitors and hours of visitation cause cultural conflict between clients and health care workers.

In the American Indian, Filipino, and rural Black cultures, family members are expected to assist with physical care during illness, bathing, feeding, giving backrubs, and changing linen. Friends and members of the community are also expected to visit and take turns sitting with the relatives for support throughout illness. Family members and friends usually sit quietly at the bedside or just outside the door. Hospital rules cause feelings of abandonment by clients and feelings of guilt, anger, and shame by friends and family.

Hospitalization as a form of culture shock occurs in three phases. The *first phase* is characterized by asking what, why, and when questions regarding hospital routines and expectations of self. *Phase two* is the disenchantment phase. The patient becomes frustrated with the unfamiliarity of the hospital environment and becomes hostile, de-

pressed, and withdrawn. *Phase three* begins when the client learns the hospital jargon and routines and is able to interject humor when interacting with members of the health care team.

Nursing Implications of Cultural Concepts

Being aware of the meaning of culture, the nurse is more accepting of behavior and requests for modifying routines. Learning about another's cultural background promotes respect, even if many of the practices are nonscientific. Nursing interventions are likely to be more effective when consistent with the patient's cultural values. In addition, culturally insensitive care may place additional stress on the client and interfere with recovery.

When collecting information for the nursing history, the nurse may use Tables 2.3 and 2.4 to obtain important cultural data for a basis to plan nursing interventions.

TABLE 2.3
ASSESSMENT OF A CLIENT'S CULTURAL ORIENTATION

Since a person's ethnic identity strongly influences behavior, responses to illness, and treatment regimes, a systematic planned strategy is necessary for eliciting cultural data. The cultural tool may be a separate form or incorporated into the overall nursing history form. Information from the following areas should be included in the cultural assessment tool:
1. Name—how the client wishes to be addressed
2. Cultural/ethnic group orientation
3. Communication patterns—language spoken, use of touching and gesturing
4. Type of food—ethnic or American foods avoided during illness
5. Health care patterns—beliefs concerning disease and illness causation, folk health practices, people consulted during illness, rituals and ceremonies required to restore health
6. Caring beliefs—behaviors that indicate caring and noncaring
7. Relationship to people—individualistic or group oriented
8. Taboos—restrictions regarding body parts, exposure, and handling
9. Roles—women, men, family, and neighbors during illness and health

TABLE 2.4
SAMPLE CULTURAL ASSESSMENT TOOL

1. Name _____
2. How do you wish us to address you? (First or last name—Miss, Mrs., Mr., etc.)
3. With what ethnic/cultural group do you identify? _____
4. Which languages do you speak and/or understand? _____
5. Does it make you uncomfortable for people to maintain eye contact during conversation? _____
6. Which kinds of behaviors by health care workers indicate they care about you? _____
7. Which kinds of behaviors by health care workers indicate noncaring to you? _____
8. Do you have reservations or strong feelings about male or female health workers giving you direct care? _____
9. Are there restrictions regarding touching certain parts of your body or gesturing? _____
10. Are there cultural restrictions pertaining to bathing during illness? _____
11. Are there body parts that I should avoid exposing during treatments, daily hygiene, etc.? _____
12. Are family members or friends expected to participate in providing care for you? (Bathing, feeding, etc.) _____
13. What do you believe caused you to become sick? _____
14. Who did you consult first when you became ill? (Family members, neighbor, healer, physician, pharmacist, herbalist, friend, etc.) _____
15. What herbs, teas, overcounter drugs, or other substances did you take for treatment of symptoms prior to hospitalization? _____
16. Are you wearing special metals, charms, objects, or garments that should not be removed during hospitalization? _____
17. Which foods do you avoid during illness? _____
18. Which foods and beverages do you prefer during illness? _____
19. Are there rituals associated with your religion that you will be engaging in during this hospitalization? _____
20. Will a private room be necessary for the ritual or ceremony? _____
21. Will other family members and friends be participating in ritual? _____
22. Who makes the decisions in the family in times of emergency (permission for surgery or treatments)? _____
23. Are there days in the week or month which are considered "bad luck days"? Ones in which we should avoid scheduling tests, surgery, and other treatments? _____
24. If surgery is required, is there a special request concerning disposal of removed body parts? _____
25. Does pain have a special meaning to you? _____
26. How do you expect pain to be controlled in the hospital? _____
27. Can we expect you to request something for pain? _____

DEVELOPING A THERAPEUTIC RELATIONSHIP

As mentioned in Chapter 1, all nursing care takes place in the framework of a relationship between the nurse and the patient. Creating an environment of acceptance and respect of another's beliefs and behavior is basic to the development of a therapeutic nurse-patient relationship. Trust is kindled when individuals feel safe, respected, and accepted. Only then will they risk sharing taboos, folk health practices, and reasons for not adhering to the medical regime (Figure 2.2).

Words and phrases have cultural meanings. Used inappropriately, words can impede the development of a therapeutic relationship. Words and phrases such as "you people," "poor thing," "gal," "boy," and

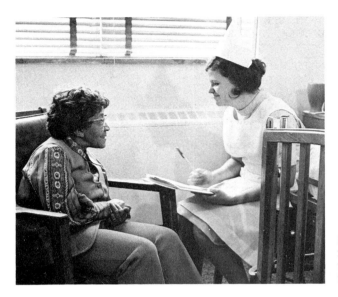

FIGURE 2.2 The nurse's warmth, friendliness, and acceptance are essential when collecting information about the patient's culture.

"Gramps" may incite anger and hostile feelings. Addressing the client inappropriately by using the first name, last name, or omitting Mr., Mrs., or Miss may be considered disrespectful and culturally insensitive. A more sensitive approach is to ask the client during the initial greeting about the name or title preferred.

A sample cultural assessment tool is shown in Table 2.4.

Establishing an effective communication system can be both a challenge and a learning experience when the client speaks little or no English. Interpreters are often unable to remain at the bedside on a 24-hour basis. Initially, the nurse can use sign language, point, mimic, and observe body language for responses. Puzzled or bland expressions, inappropriate smiles, head nods, and repeated "yes" responses my indicate lack of understanding. "Yes" responses often mean "I hear you" or "I am listening." Yes does not always mean "I agree or understand."

The nurse can develop bilingual flash cards to facilitate communication with the clients in their own language. Some of the phrases or words that can be placed on the cards are: point to the area of pain, do you want to use the bedpan?, do you want me to sit with you?, cold, hot, sit, stand, and brush your teeth.

Attempting to speak to the client in his/her own language builds mutual interest, trust, and respect. This, in turn, facilitates the establishment of a therapeutic nurse-client relationship. A balance in the nurse-patient relationship develops when the client becomes the teacher and the nurse becomes the learner. Phrase books, interpreters, family members, and the client may be consulted in the development of the phrase cards.

Using the following guidelines will improve communication with clients that understand minimal English:

• Speak slowly, using normal voice tones.
• Use simple phrases— "Are you cold?"
• Use sign language—pointing, mimicking.
• Use pictures and diagrams that illustrate procedures step by step.
• Allow adequate time for the client to comprehend your message and formulate an answer.
• Provide pencil and paper—many clients can communicate by writing or drawing.

Eye contact has different cultural meanings. To the Anglo-American, maintenance of eye contact means I am interested, paying attention, or not lying. In the Navaho culture, looking the individual in the eye is considered as taking one's soul away. Filipinos consider it disrespectful. It will be helpful for the nurse to consciously use eye contact only with clients in which it is culturally appropriate.

ASSISTING WITH HYGIENE

Cultural knowledge will be helpful when preparing to assist your client with daily hygiene. Some clients will refuse to take daily baths. Many Anglo-Americans have cultural values of cleanliness accomplished by bathing, brushing of teeth, and application of deodorant. These values may not be shared by other cultural groups. American Indians and Asian clients do not perspire often and seldom have body odor. This is due to a small number of sweat glands. Nigerian people value natural body odor and have difficulty comprehending why Americans are preoccupied with bathing and application of perfumes and deodorants. Assessment of the client's cultural beliefs will help to assist with daily hygiene without experiencing frustration caused by cultural differences.

During the bath, charms, crosses, metals, objects or small bags of ingredients which the client is wearing should not be removed. Usually, they have cultural significance. Allow family members and significant others to assist with bed making, oral hygiene, bathing, ambulation, and intake and output. This inclusion of significant others in the daily care reduces anxiety of the client and family. It also permits fulfillment of cultural expectations.

Modesty is a dominating value for many cultural groups. Disrobing in front of family and strangers is very stressful. Cultural sensitivity to these values causes the nurse to knock before entering the client's room and to ask permission before handling a body part.

ASSISTING WITH FOOD AND FLUIDS

Each ethnic group has special ways of preparing foods to obtain its characteristic flavor. The flavor is what satisfies one's taste and craving for food. Hospital menus and standard food exchange lists seldom include ethnic foods. This contributes to poor appetite, inadequate intake, and social withdrawal.

When talking with clients about eating habits, the nurse should elicit the following information: (1) the number of meals eaten per day, (2) foods the client enjoys most, (3) food preferences of others who routinely share meals with the client, (4) methods used for preparing foods, and (5) dominant seasoning used. Encouraging family members to talk with the dietitian and using ethnic cookbooks for special diets increases the likelihood of success in following a special diet.

Culture will affect the type and temperature of fluids consumed by some clients. Mormon clients will refuse tea and coffee because their religion forbids the consumption of caffeine. Korean individuals will often request a cup of warm water with meals. Individuals who believe in the hot-cold theory of disease causation will have restrictions on foods and fluid consumption depending on the classification of illness.

Some cultural groups have difficulty metabolizing milk once adulthood is reached. Their inability to digest milk is caused by a deficiency of intestinal lactose. Milk consumption causes abdominal cramps, distention, diarrhea, flatus, and colitis. Alaskan Indians, Asians, and Blacks may be lactose intolerant.

ASSISTING WITH PATIENT TEACHING

Many cultural groups do not work by the clock and schedules. Time is used spontaneously. Life is regulated by human and bodily needs (American Indians, Mexican-Americans, and Blacks). Persons from these cultural groups may not appear for an appointment or may come several hours later. Understanding that time is viewed differently by cultural groups will enable the nurse to listen to the client's reason for the broken appointment and withhold judgment. When teaching persons with a time perspective that is immediate, the nurse uses visual material and written information (in the patient's primary language, when possible). This information can be taken home so that it can be used as the need arises.

A person is considered ill in the Black culture when unable to function—eat, talk, walk, and work. Knowledge of this concept of illness helps one understand why many Blacks delay seeking medical assistance until they are far advanced in the illness cycle. Patient teaching for persons in this cultural group may be presented in terms of its effect on eating, talking, walking, and working.

Case Study Involving Cultural Components of Illness

Nye thi Linda, a 65-year-old Vietnamese grandmother is admitted to your unit with a diagnosis of bilateral lower lobe pneumonia. She has been living in the United States for six months. She resides with her daughter and family. She speaks Vietnamese and an ethnic Chinese dialect. She can say a few English words. Upon entering the room, you observe that Mrs. Nye is sitting in the middle of the bed on her "haunches," head resting on her knees, and arms supporting her flexed knees. This is Mrs. Nye's first hospital admission in the United States. She has been seen at the local health department for initial refugee screening. She refused to have her blood drawn in the Emergency Department.

The physician left the following orders:

- Bed rest with bathroom privileges
- Soft select diet
- Force fluids
- Vital signs q shift
- Chest physiotherapy qid
- Arterial blood gases this PM
- SMA-18 today
- Chest x-ray this PM
- Sputum for C & S × 3 days
- Cool mist vaporizer continuously

QUESTIONS

1. Describe how you should vary the usual admitting process for Mrs. Nye. Discuss your plans for admitting the client to the unit.
2. How can you communicate wth the client to obtain admission vital signs?
3. How should the nurse explain the cool mist vaporizer?
4. What information should the nurse obtain from the client and/or family before beginning comfort and hygiene measures?
5. What are the beliefs in the Vietnamese culture related to causes of disease and pain?
6. How can the nurse include Vietnamese food for meal selection?
7. What are the touching restrictions in the Vietnamese culture?
8. What cultural concepts may account for client's refusal for having blood drawn?
9. At what high-low level will you position the client's bed? Use a cultural concept to support your choice.
10. What biologic variation accounts for very little or absence of body odor in Asian clients?

Suggestions for Further Study

1. Answer the questions found on the cultural assessment form found in this chapter. Using the same form, interview a classmate or neighbor of a different cultural group from your own. What are the similarities and differences in your beliefs, expectations, and health practices?
2. Contact your local health department and inquire about the refugee program. What services are available, what cultural groups are serviced, and what are the prevalent illnesses?
3. What are the sources for obtaining interpreters in your community? For what languages are interpreters available?
4. Contact the local diabetes and heart associations to inquire about exchange lists and diets for ethnic groups.
5. Find out what programs are available in your community for learning English as a second language.
6. Make a list of the dominant cultural groups in your state. Develop a plan for obtaining information concerning their dominant values, beliefs, food patterns, and health care practices.
7. Enroll in a conversational language class. (Spanish is the largest non-English language spoken in the United States.)
8. Enroll in a basic cultural and/or social anthropology course. These courses are taught in most community colleges and universities.
9. Attend ethnic festivals when held in your area.
10. Read travel magazines.
11. Mason, Mildred A.; Bates, Grace F.; and Smola, Bonnie K.; *Workbook in Basic Medical-Surgical Nursing*, 3rd ed. Macmillan Publishing Company, New York, 1984, Exercise 2.

Additional Readings

Abu-Saad, Huda, and Kayser-Jones, Jeanie: "A Multicultural Approach." *Journal of Nursing Education*, 21:3 (Sept.), 1982.
Abu-Saad, Huda; Kayser-Jones, Jeanie; and Tien,

Juliet: "Asian Nursing Students in the United States." *Journal of Nursing Education,* 21:11–15. (Sept.), 1982.

Carter, Frances Monet: *Psychosocial Nursing,* 3rd ed. Macmillan Publishing Co., Inc., New York, 1981, pp. 35–41, 52–55, 74–75, and 99–104.

Kahn, Rita Ann: "Patients Are People." *Journal of Nursing Care,* 13:10–11 (May), 1980.

Kayser-Jones, Jeanie; Abu-Saad, Huda; and Akinnaso, Niyi: "Nigeria: The Land, Its People, and Health Care." *Journal of Nursing Education,* 21:32–37 (Sept.), 1982.

Krieger, Dolores: *Foundations for Holistic Health Nursing Practices: The Renaissance Nurse.* J. B. Lippincott Co., Philadelphia, 1981.

Leininger, Madeline M.: *National Transcultural Nursing Conference, 1st–4th. College of Nursing, University of Utah, 1975–1978.* Masson International Nursing Publications, New York, 1979.

_____: *Transcultural Nursing: Concepts, Theories, and Practices.* John Wiley and Sons, New York, 1978.

Robinson, Corinne H.: *Basic Nutrition and Diet Therapy,* 4th Ed. Macmillan Publishing Company, New York, 1980, pp. 155–165.

Robinson, Corinne H., and Lawler, Marilyn R.: *Normal and Therapeutic Nutrition,* 16th ed. Macmillan Publishing Company, New York, 1982, pp. 284–98 and 419.

Weiss, M. Olga: "Cultural Shock." *Nursing Outlook,* 19:40–43, 1971.

Chapter 3

The Aging Individual

Expected Behavioral Outcomes

Minimum objectives referred to as expected behavioral outcomes have been designed for the practical/vocational nursing student to use as guides in studying this chapter. The student should read these expected outcomes before studying the chapter. The objectives can be used as guides for study.

Using the content of this chapter, the student should return to the objectives and evaluate the ability to:

1. *Describe similarities and differences between feelings and the actual characteristics of the elderly individual.*
2. *Give an appropriate nursing action for each deficit when given a list of sensory deficits.*
3. *Record observations of an elderly patient when given a nursing observation guide.*
4. *Discuss the grieving process in relation to an elderly patient's admission to a nursing home.*
5. *Relate four nursing actions that provide for safety in relation to body changes in the aging process.*
6. *Describe a nursing action appropriate for an elderly person for each of the psychologic needs.*
7. *Describe the nursing responsibilities for drug therapy in relation to the aging individual.*
8. *List four nursing measures that prevent skin breakdown in the aging individual.*
9. *Describe a nursing measure for each body change associated with skin breakdown in the aging individual.*

Vocabulary Development

The following prefixes, suffixes, and combining forms pertain to this chapter. By learning and/or reviewing their meanings, the practical/vocational nursing student will have the keys needed to unlock many exciting new medical terms.

Discover the meaning of these keys in a medical dictionary or in the content of this chapter. How does each key pertain to this chapter? In your notebook write the correct meaning of each prefix, suffix, or combining form listed below. Illustrate each key with an example.

dis—apart, away from. Ex. *disability*—away from a normal function.

hom-	pro-
inter-	psych-
-mittent	re-
oss-	sta-
ost-	ur-

The Elderly Individual

The elderly individual is generally described as a person who is 65 years of age or older. The average life expectancy in the United States has increased steadily and now is about 74 years. Thus, there is an increased number of aged persons in the population and the trend is expected to continue. Most of us can expect to experience the effects of aging.

The large number of elderly persons in the population has stimulated many changes in health care. Government at the federal, state, and local levels has legislated funds for health care, research, and education that total billions of dollars. Universities and medical centers around the United States are devoting large amounts of money and personnel to the study of the physical and psychological effects of aging. The nursing student can expect to care for more hospitalized elderly patients in the future. All health team members will want to remain informed as the amount of knowledge about the aged increases.

The person who has experienced satisfying relationships with others and adapted to the ups and downs of life approaches aging with the ability to see life in its relation to a flow of history. Preparation for aging is a continuous process that begins early in life with the development of satisfying relationships and the necessary adjustments mentioned above.

Basic human needs in the elderly are the same as for other age groups. The expression of those needs in everyday life may be slightly different because of body changes associated with aging and because of the wealth of knowledge, skills, and attitudes developed through the life span. Increasing self knowledge, developing a satisfying inner life, and finding ways to contribute a lifetime of experience and wisdom to others are expressions of basic human needs in the elderly individual. The person in later years also needs to strengthen ties with relatives and friends, maintain good health, and adjust to retirement and a reduced income. Finally, the elderly person needs to face and accept declining speed, flexibility, and strength as well as death and the loss of loved ones.

In learning about elderly persons and caring for them, the student is likely to become aware of certain common *prejudices*. A *prejudice* is an opinion or belief about a person or subject that is based on incomplete knowledge.

Many prejudices surround the elderly individual. Perhaps you have always believed that all old people have some kind of damage to the brain. There are changes in the nervous system that are associated with aging; however, there is no evidence to suggest that elderly persons have brain damage unless they have a disease that results in injury to the cells.

Many people believe that intelligence and learning ability decline with age. Actually, intelligence does not appear to change much with age when factors such as interest, motivation, and education are considered. Information that interests the elderly individual and is presented in ways that consider the effects of aging is likely to be learned.

Another common prejudice about elderly persons is the notion that an aged person cannot change and has a rigid outlook on life. Actually, old age is a period of numerous changes. Consider Mr. Tompkins, aged 77. Mr. Tompkins retired at age 65 from factory work. Mrs. Tompkins died two years ago and Mr. Tompkins moved into his daughter's home. Two weeks ago, Mr. T. fell and fractured his left hip. His fracture was reduced in surgery. Mr. T. now is using a walker and will be transferred to a nursing home within six weeks. Consider the number of major changes in Mr. Tompkin's life since he reached 65.

1. Retired from work
2. Lost spouse
3. Changed residence
4. Entered hospital
5. Had surgery
6. Entered nursing home

As discussed in Chapter 4, major life-change events often precede illness. This enables the nurse to understand that the later years may be far from serene and tranquil.

Most of the changes listed above can be viewed as causes of stress.

Some people believe erroneously that all elderly persons are benevolent, kindly, and tranquil. The elderly person who has experienced persistent feelings of anger, hostility, depression, or guilt throughout life is not likely to be benevolent, kindly, and tranquil during old age without professional help. In other words, the elderly person can be expected to show personality traits and behavior patterns that were a part of earlier life.

Another common belief about the elderly is that most are sick, in nursing homes, and abandoned by families and friends. In fact, most aged persons remain in their communities and live either alone or with a family member. Less than 5 percent reside in nursing homes. Most elderly persons are in reasonably good health and a fair number have part-time jobs. Members of the health team often see only the elderly who are sick, alone, and disabled. This may explain one reason for the development of this erroneous belief.

Prejudice is very damaging to the individual and may at times be fatal. Prejudice may prevent the nurse from making accurate and complete observations. The nurse who expects the elderly person to look, feel, think, or act a certain way may overlook important information that should be reported. For example, if the nurse believes that most elderly persons are confused, this information may not be observed or reported about a specific patient. Such a patient could die unnecessarily from an undetected brain tumor, blood clot, or other fatal disease. Other serious consequences may include inaccurate or inadequate care, accidents, faulty diagnosis, increased pain, or higher cost.

Another type of damage occurs when the elderly individual believes the same prejudices and needlessly narrows opportunities for growth and development. For example, the elderly person who believes that learning declines with age is unlikely to take advantage of senior citizen discounts on college courses at a nearby school.

Fortunately, increasing numbers of elderly persons are aware and concerned about these widespread prejudices. Many elderly persons have organized to fight injustices in employment, housing, and health care which they have experienced simply because they are old. As the elderly population increases, the nurse can expect a corresponding increase in the impact made by them.

Because of the widespread and potentially damaging effects of prejudices, it is important for nurses to examine their own attitudes about the elderly. As a first step, the student may find it helpful to recall previous interactions with elderly persons in the home, neighborhood, or community. Were they positive or negative? How have they influenced the nurse's present attitudes? As a second step, the student may talk to elderly persons themselves for information on favorable and unfavorable aspects of growing old.

Looking at the elderly individual in terms of a life span enables the nurse to appreciate the rich and unique contributions the aged person offers to each of us. The authors vividly remember conversations with Mrs. S., an 80-year-old patient who accompanied her physician father on horse-and-buggy house calls in New England in the late 1880s. Mrs. S. loved to compare the remedies and treatments of the past with those of the present. Through her contribution, the authors also developed an appreciation of the treatments and remedies of yesterday and today.

The nurse cares for the elderly person at home, in the hospital, in a nursing home, or a residential care home. The elderly individual under nursing care may be healthy, ill, disabled, or handicapped. Thus, the nurse has many possible contributions to make. For example, the nurse is an important member of the health team in a community. The nurse's treatment of each person as a unique individual has a positive effect on prejudices associated with aging.

The nurse's knowledges and skills about the effects of aging on physical and psychological function are used to assist elderly persons with self-care activities such as bathing, elimination, and ambulating. The same knowledge when shared with elderly persons and their families helps to develop safer and healthier coping with changes that aging brings.

The nurse uses active listening and communication skills to develop a therapeutic relationship with the elderly person. The person then feels accepted, understood, and reassured. The nurse's caring reduces the isolation and loneliness that many elderly persons experience.

The nurse's knowledge of the relationships between aging and disease contributes to early diagnosis and treatment. Keen observation and conscientious reporting by the nurse are often the first step in diagnosing disease in the elderly.

The Aging Process

Aging is a natural process that begins at birth. *Senescence* is the period in one's life during which the greatest amount of aging occurs. *Gerontology* is the science that deals with aging. *Geriatrics* generally refers to medical treatment of disease conditions common to old age.

At the present time, research data do not support a general theory of aging although several have been proposed. Some recent theories attribute aging to the loss of irreplaceable neurons from the body, changes in the immune system, and some combination of neuroendocrine and immune system interaction. One difficulty in research is distinguishing normal aging processes from disease processes.

Whatever the cause, the aging process is generally characterized by fewer cells, loss of functional reserve, and diminished effectiveness of homeostasis. Every system in the body is affected by the aging process. However, since each person is unique, the characteristics of aging must be viewed as they apply to a particular patient receiving nursing care.

The aging process as it affects the body and mind is described under separate headings in this chapter. The reader will remember from Chapter 1, however, that there is constant and continuous mind-body interaction throughout the life cycle. The student uses information collected from and about a specific patient together with knowledge about the aging process and nursing knowledge in order to select appropriate nursing interventions.

BODY CHANGES ASSOCIATED WITH THE AGING PROCESS

NERVOUS SYSTEM. The aging process affects the nervous system in a variety of ways. There are fewer brain cells and they are smaller, especially in the frontal lobe. Changes in the circulatory system result in slower blood flow to and from the brain. The nerves exhibit less irritability and conduction is slowed. Changes occurring in important brain structures such as the hypothalamus and thymus glands affect temperature regulation and the immune response. These changes within the nervous system may result in diminished pain perception, slower reaction time, and decreased need for sleep. The elderly individual may be slower to detect temperature changes of objects in contact with the skin. Memory for recent events may be diminished. Equilibrium and motor coordination may be altered.

DIGESTION. The salivary glands secrete less saliva containing fewer enzymes in the elderly individual. The senses of smell and taste decrease. Fewer digestive enzymes and less hydrochloric acid are present in the stomach. The total capacity of the stomach decreases. Diminished peristalsis and thinning of the gastrointestinal lining occur during aging. There are fewer liver cells, more variable bile flow. The changes in the digestive tract can result in changes in bowel habits such as constipation. Indigestion, abdominal distention, and flatus appear to be more common among elderly individuals. Significant changes in drug absorption, detoxification, and elimination may occur during aging. Poor dental health in youth may result in fewer natural teeth in later years.

CIRCULATORY SYSTEM. The heart's ability to beat stronger and faster during exercise declines with aging. Cardiac output is decreased. More time is required for the heart to return to the resting stage. Blood vessels are less elastic. Fewer blood cells are produced. Blood pressure may rise as a person ages. Circulation to body parts may decline because of both diminished elasticity of blood vessels and fewer red blood cells. Fewer white cells are produced, and the body's response to inflammation and healing may be slower.

ENDOCRINE SYSTEM. Body metabolism slows down with age and can result in a poor adjustment to temperature change. Hormone production declines and the endocrine glands themselves are smaller. The metabolism of glucose changes with age as well as regulation of electrolytes such as sodium, potassium, and calcium. The ovaries in the female and the testes in the male cease functioning.

Changes in the endocrine system affect every other body system.

URINARY SYSTEM. There are fewer cells in the kidney in the aged individual. Changes in the circulatory system result in diminished blood flow to the kidney. The bladder is less elastic and the urethra has less muscle tone. Nocturia (increased voiding at night) may occur. Hypertrophy (enlargement) of the prostate gland, which surrounds the bladder neck in men, may obstruct the flow of urine. Urine may be more concentrated in the elderly individual.

RESPIRATORY SYSTEM. Changes in the larynx and pharynx may result in voice changes. The voice change is more apparent when it is accompanied by a hearing loss. Lung tissue, particularly the alveoli, becomes less elastic. Decreased blood flow within the lung results in rising carbon dioxide levels in the aged person. The diaphragm and intercostal muscles have decreased muscle tone.

MUSCULAR AND SKELETAL CHANGES. Muscle tone decreases with age. The muscles themselves are smaller, and less glycogen can be stored there. Tendons and ligaments are less elastic. Waste products such as lactic acid and carbon dioxide are retained in larger amounts. Endurance and agility diminish. Muscle spasms may occur more frequently.

As mineral salts move from bone to blood, the bones become more porous. Cartilage contracts and may harden, causing a decrease in height. Degenerative changes may occur in the joints, causing them to become less mobile.

REPRODUCTIVE SYSTEM. When the hormonal activities of the reproductive organs cease, changes occur in secondary sexual characteristics such as size of external genitalia and distribution of hair. Mucous membranes lining the vagina may become thinner and less moist. Conception is no longer possible. However, the elderly individual who is in good health does not necessarily lose the ability to function sexually.

SKIN. The elderly individual has fewer skin cells and less subcutaneous fat. The skin is less elastic. Secretions of sweat and oil from sebaceous glands diminish, causing dryness and thickening of nails and hair. The blood flow to the skin decreases. Skin pigmentation may increase. Body temperature is more difficult to maintain because of the loss of subcutaneous insulation as well as fewer sweat glands.

SPECIAL SENSES. Vision declines. Cataracts and glaucoma may occur. The eyes adjust more slowly to changes of light as the person ages. Drooping of the eyelids may develop.

Hearing may be affected gradually. The ability to perceive high notes frequently becomes impaired first. Decreased ability to hear low notes may follow.

The special senses of touch, smell, and taste become less acute. As mentioned earlier, the older person has a decreased ability to detect changes of temperature in objects touching the skin. Also, the perception of pain may decrease.

PSYCHOSOCIAL CHANGES ASSOCIATED WITH AGING

THINKING AND LEARNING. Although popular prejudices about the elderly include the belief that thinking and learning decline with age, research indicates that this is not the case. Intelligence as measured by standard tests remains relatively stable throughout life. Speed of comprehension may decline with age but retention and interpretation may actually improve. Pacing of learning, motivation to learn, and method of presentation seem to be more important influences on thinking and learning than age.

EMOTIONS. Individuals experience similar emotions throughout the life span. However, certain emotions such as anxiety, loneliness, and depression may occur more frequently with age. Anxiety may be characterized by insomnia, withdrawal, pacing, chain smoking, wringing the hands, fighting, or picking at bedclothes. Loneliness can result from such factors as death of loved ones and pets, changes in the environment, and diminished opportunities to begin new relationships. Depression is the third example of an emotion commonly associated with aging. Behaviors that may indicate depression are loss of interest in usual activities, neglect of personal appearance, withdrawal from personal relationships, and refusal to eat. In some cases, depression may become severe enough to require psychotherapy and/or drug therapy. The problem of suicide in the elderly is described later in this chapter.

SOCIAL INTERACTION. A variety of changes in social interaction may occur during the later years. Retirement, death of loved ones, ill health, and reduced income are factors that can contribute to diminished social interaction. On the other hand, the increased amount of leisure time available stimulates many elderly persons to initiate, renew or strengthen relationships with others via church or club educational or political activities. Although there are increasing numbers of programs directed specifically toward the older age group, some elderly persons have spoken out publicly against such programs, especially in areas such as housing and recreation, claiming that they isolate the elderly from others in the community. Associating with persons in a variety of age groups enables the elderly person to benefit from support, shared common experiences, and stimulating new experiences. Even more important, the variety of opinions about social interaction during later years illustrates the need for a highly individualized nursing care plan.

Retirement can be expected to result in considerable changes in social interaction between husband and wife. The amount of time spent together usually increases suddenly, requiring adjustment by both partners. For example, a wife who is used to eight or more hours per day that can be arranged according to her own desires may feel resentment when a retired husband suggests "more efficient" ways to organize the time. Similarly, a husband who is used to certain personal services after a long day's work may be surprised that such services are not provided at all times now that he is retired.

Sexuality. Perhaps because of our own prejudices, it is difficult for many of us to think of elderly persons as having sexual interest, sexual feelings, and sexual relationships. Although the aging process results in considerable changes in the reproductive and endocrine systems, research indicates that many elderly persons maintain interest and the capacity to participate and enjoy sexual activity into the ninth decade.

Factors that influence sexual behavior in later years include general health, availability of an interested and interesting partner, and previous levels of interest, enjoyment, and frequency. In general, elderly persons who are reasonably healthy, have an interested and interesting partner, and who have enjoyed sexual activity regularly throughout life continue to do so during senescence.

A factor that greatly affects sexuality in the elderly is drug therapy. Many drugs commonly prescribed for the elderly affect sexual interest and performance. Examples of these drugs include propranolol (INDERAL), furosemide (LASIX), digoxin (LANOXIN), and diazepam (VALIUM). When sexuality is adversely affected by drug therapy, another drug often can be substituted. Nursing interventions that may be helpful to the patient include the following:

- Inform the patient when drugs are known to affect sexual interest or performance.
- Encourage the patient to report changes in sexual interest and performance so that substitute drugs may be prescribed, if available.
- Teach the patient that alcohol combined with drugs known to affect sexuality may worsen symptoms.
- Record and report information obtained from the patient related to problems with sexuality.

Aging and Illness

Although aging is a normal process, senescence (aging in one's later years) is associated with an increased frequency of illness of all kinds. Illness in an elderly person is likely to be more severe and prolonged. Chronic diseases occur more frequently in the elderly. Information about specific diseases can be located in chapters of this text that discuss the main body system affected.

PHYSICAL PROBLEMS

Accidents are common among the elderly. Aging in the musculoskeletal, nervous and sensory, and circulatory systems can result in weakness, tremors, and postural hypotension. Falls and burns are frequent accidents. Failing vision and hearing also contribute to accidents. When falls do occur, changes in body structure make fractures more likely.

Changes in metabolism and the endocrine system can result in vaginitis in females. Diabetes mellitus is more likely to occur.

Changes in the digestive system can result in constipation, anorexia (poor appetite), anemia, indigestion, and weight loss.

Alterations in the blood vessels may result in intermittent claudication (pain when walking), hypertension, or cardiovascular disease (Figure 3.1).

Respiratory illnesses such as influenza, pneumonia, and pulmonary emphysema appear to affect the elderly individual more seriously than other age groups.

Changes in the urinary and muscular systems may result in urinary incontinence, stress incontinence, frequency, or nocturia.

There may be partial or complete loss of hearing and/or vision.

Changes in the immune system can result in increased susceptibility to infection, autoimmune diseases, neoplasm, and chronic low-grade tissue damage such as atherosclerosis. The elderly person who develops illness can be expected to heal slower, have more complications, and experience a longer recovery period.

PSYCHOSOCIAL PROBLEMS

As mentioned earlier, the elderly individual has the same needs as other persons for safety and security, love and affection, respect and self-esteem, and self-development. The widespread effects of aging can result in psychological problems.

Safety and security may be threatened when the elderly person has to depend on others for physical care, transportation, or financial assistance.

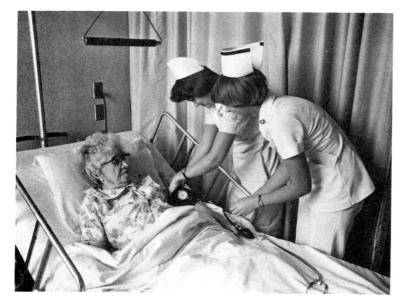

FIGURE 3.1 The blood pressure should be checked regularly during senescence. (Courtesy of Marian S. Whelen School of Practical Nursing, Geneva, New York.)

The loss of spouse or friends and other significant persons may reduce sources of love and affection that have sustained a person throughout life. Loneliness can be a real problem. The loss of a mate frequently terminates a sexual relationship that has been a vital element in the person's life. Opportunities to meet and form new friendships may decline in later life. Elderly persons may be separated from family members who live far away.

Respect and self-esteem can decline during senescence due to loss of loved ones, health, and productivity. Other factors that lower a person's self-esteem and respect include being dependent on others, income insufficient for one's needs and life-style, and being treated as a baby or as incompetent by others.

Feelings of anxiety and depression are common when a person's basic needs are not met. The elderly individual is not immune to mental illness. The suicide rate among elderly individuals is presently being studied. Unfortunately, symptoms of mental illness in the aged person are easily overlooked due to widespread prejudices described earlier in this chapter. Self-destructive behavior in the elderly is described later in this chapter.

Grieving frequently can be observed in the elderly individual who has lost a spouse or other significant person. Moving to a smaller dwelling due to finances may involve the loss of certain valued objects such as furniture, tools, or books that have been collected over a lifetime.

Disorientation can be a problem in the aged individual. Disorientation is not neces-sarily a part of the aging process. Rather, it is a symptom of illness or disease. When the elderly person is disoriented, a careful investigation of its causes is necessary. No one should assume that a person is disoriented simply because of age. Nursing interventions for the elderly individual who is disoriented are discussed later in this chapter.

Nursing Observations

When an elderly patient is under nursing care, the effect of the aging process on that person must be considered. Complete and accurate observation and recordings are essential.

Because of prejudices described earlier in this chapter, important observations may be overlooked. The aged person and family members, also victims of the same prejudices, may not recognize the significance of certain symptoms. For example, Mrs. Fulton is the 81-year-old neighbor of a nurse in California. The nurse noticed that Mrs. Fulton had developed persistent hoarseness. This observation was shared with Mrs. Fulton's son, who had also noticed the change but thought it was "just a part of getting old." The symptom in this patient was associated with polyps on the vocal cord. A polyp is an abnormal growth of tissue that resembles a mushroom. When the polyps were removed, the hoarseness disappeared.

Table 3.1 contains an observation guide related to the elderly person, and Table 3.2 contains a guide to understanding vital signs in the elderly.

TABLE 3.1
OBSERVATION GUIDE FOR THE ELDERLY INDIVIDUAL
When caring for the elderly person, develop the practice of systematic head-to-toe observations. Examples of nursing implications are included.

HEAD-TO-TOE OBSERVATION	COMMON CHANGES	EXAMPLES OF NURSING IMPLICATIONS
Hair	Thinning and graying	May need help in grooming
Eyes	Eyeglasses and/or contact lenses used	Safekeeping
	Eyelids drooping, inverted, and/or everted	Observe for interference with vision
	Normal flow of tears may be increased or decreased	Person may need help in instilling artificial tears for irritating dryness of eyes
Ears	Turning one ear toward person speaking	Look at individual when talking and speak distinctly

TABLE 3.1 (*Continued*)
OBSERVATION GUIDE FOR THE ELDERLY INDIVIDUAL

HEAD-TO-TOE OBSERVATION	COMMON CHANGES	EXAMPLES OF NURSING IMPLICATIONS
Face	Hearing aid used	May need help in caring for hearing aid
	Wrinkles; facial hair may be noticeable in women	Women may need help in removing facial hair if desired
	Overgrowth of beard in men	Men may need help in shaving or grooming beard
Mouth	Replacement of natural teeth with partial or full dentures	May need help with oral hygiene
		Provide safekeeping for removable dentures
	Mucous membrane may be dry	Report to appropriate person as this may indicate dehydration
Speech	Softer	
	Hoarseness, slurring, hesitation, or other changes	Report
Neck and chest	Atropy, wasting away of tissue of neck and breast	Use nonirritating soap for bath and dry thoroughly
	Wrinkles, especially of neck	
	Fullness of neck veins	
Abdomen	Skin growths	Describe size, shape, color, location, and other relevant factors
Extremities	Thickened nails and skin cracks	Look for signs of decreased circulation, such as change in skin color from paleness to blueness
		Observe for corns, calluses, and other lesions that can exert enough pressure to compromise circulation to underlying tissues
		Provide and/or arrange for appropriate care
Skin	Increased deposits of pigment	Report pigments that are raised, blue, black, hairy, or bleeding
		Observe such areas for change
Posture and movement	Loss of height may cause extremities to appear larger by comparison	
	Slower movement	Allow time for movement
	Use of aids, such as cane or walker	Place walking aid within reach of person

TABLE 3.2
GUIDE TO UNDERSTANDING VITAL SIGNS IN THE ELDERLY

Temperature	The body adapts more slowly and less intensely to stressors. Body temperature regulation is affected by aging in the hypothalamus, circulatory system, and by loss of subcutaneous fat. Even small changes in temperature may indicate possible disease or illness and should be reported
Pulse	Resting pulse rate should be measured before exertion such as climbing on an examination table. Following exertion, heart takes longer to return to normal. Pulse rate should be regular, but premature beats occur more often in the elderly
Respirations	Elderly person normally should not have shortness of breath except during exertion such as walking uphill or climbing stairs
Blood pressure	There should be no more than a 20 mm Hg difference between both arms. Systolic pressure generally rises until late in the 70s, then declines. Diastolic pressure usually rises until the sixth decade and then declines. The American Heart Association recommends that persons over 40 years old with a blood pressure greater than 160/95 see a physician

Life-style was discussed in Chapter 1. The reader may want to review the importance of knowing a person's life-style. In caring for an elderly person, knowledge of life-style is essential. Changes in behavior are difficult to assess in the elderly individual without knowing the usual way of living. For example, Mr. Norris was accustomed to living in the well-kept environment of a home for retired men. Mr. Norris usually was clean, well groomed, and appropriately dressed. After admission to the hospital for high blood pressure, Mr. Norris began to exhibit characteristics of poor hygiene. This change of behavior is not consistent with Mr. Norris's usual life-style and should be reported.

The life-style guide in Table 3.3 has been developed from the general guide in Chapter 1 in order to assist the student nurse to develop complete and accurate observations related to the elderly individual. Obtaining the information suggested in the guide and other relevant data over a period of time can serve several purposes. The process of talking with the elderly person aids in communication and the development of a therapeutic relationship. The process of obtaining information about life-style provides the client an opportunity to discuss facts and activities

TABLE 3.3
LIFESTYLE GUIDE FOR THE ELDERLY INDIVIDUAL

Eating patterns	Kinds of foods usually eaten daily
	Who shops and prepares food
	Usual mealtimes and where food is eaten
	Meal eaten alone or with whom
	Problems verbalized by patient
Sleeping patterns	Usual bedtime and awakening time
	Where the person sleeps
	How long it usually takes to get to sleep
	Number of times a person wakes up during night and why
	Naps per day and how long
	Bedtime routines if any
	Use of sleeping aids
	Sleeping problems verbalized by patient
Dental hygiene	Natural teeth or dentures
	How often cleaned and with what
	How often dentist consulted
	Bleeding gums, loose teeth
	Dental problems verbalized by patient
Medical care	Name of usual physician
	How often physician is consulted
	Who does person talk to about sickness (friends, neighbors, family members, nurses, healers, ministers)
Present medications	Medicine prescribed by physician
	Medicine bought from the drugstore
	Medicines borrowed from friends
	Special herbs or plants
Exercise patterns	Kind of exercise
	How often
	What exercise did person do earlier in life and why was it stopped
Urination	How often person urinates, urgency, frequency, burning, itching
	Gets up at night to urinate
	Incontinence
	Problems verbalized by patient
Bowel pattern	Frequency of bowel movement
	Foods that patient associates with constipation or diarrhea
	Laxatives and how often taken
	Problems verbalized by patient

TABLE 3.3 (*Continued*)
LIFESTYLE GUIDE FOR THE ELDERLY INDIVIDUAL

Family relationships	Members of family who reside with patient
	Friends—how many, how often seen, and/or phoned
	What family does when together, type of dwelling in which patient resides
	How many rooms, steps, and stairs
	Who cleans house
	Potential safety hazards such as unsecured scatter rugs and bath mats (home visit)
	Who the patient is most likely to talk to when troubled
Interests, hobbies, activities	Activities in typical day, week, month
	Church, club, political memberships and how often attended
	Usual pattern of in-home versus out-of-home activity
General areas	What would the person like to be doing
	What are the obstacles that prevent the above activity
	What problems does the person want help with

that are personally important. In addition, this information provides a valuable basis for discussing and planning nursing care.

Nursing Interventions

DEVELOPING A THERAPEUTIC RELATIONSHIP

As mentioned in Chapter 1, all nursing care occurs in the context of an interpersonal relationship between the nurse and the patient. The effects of aging may indicate the need for special forms of listening and communication in order to develop a therapeutic relationship (Figure 3.2).

Patients with hearing losses due to aging normally have trouble hearing sounds such as *sh, ch,* and *s.* Noise is often misinterpreted and hearing loss may be greater in some situations than others. Facing the person, using simple words spoken in distinct normal tones, and not covering one's mouth are examples of altered speaking methods that enhance communication with the elderly person who is hearing-impaired. The person with a hearing aid may need assistance to use it or have it repaired. A practice to be avoided is carrying on private conversations in low tones in the patient's presence.

The person with visual impairment should wear the glasses prescribed for its correction. Some elderly persons wear nonprescription glasses purchased at a variety

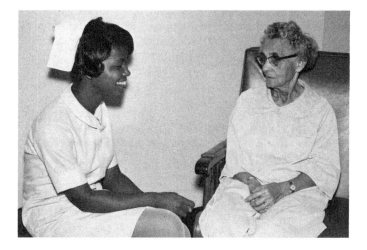

FIGURE 3.2 The nurse plays an important role in caring for the aged patient. This practical/vocational nursing student is learning the importance of talking with the patient. In some cases, the nurse may be the main link between the elderly patient and the world outside. (Courtesy of Suffolk City Schools and Louise Obici Memorial Hospital School of Practical Nursing, Suffolk, Virginia.)

store. Another common practice is to wear one's old glasses, someone else's glasses, or use a magnifying glass. When communicating with a visually impaired elderly person, the nurse should stand in good light, avoid shadows, and stand in the person's line of vision rather than at the side. At times, the patient may experience perceptual distortions that are puzzling or frightening. For example, Mrs. Marlowe was in bed with the siderails up as a safety precaution. Mrs. Marlowe, seeing the bars on the siderails, thought that she was in jail. The nurse was able to correct this distortion by showing Mrs. Marlowe that the rail could be raised and lowered. A practice to be avoided is moving familiar objects and furniture.

Other skills in communicating with the elderly include posing one thought or question at a time, providing increased time for the patient to respond, and repeating the question or information when appropriate.

Touch is another important form of communication between the elderly individual and the nurse. The nurse must use knowledge of the patient's preferences before touching the patient. In some cases, touch may irritate the patient and should be avoided. Chapter 1 contains questions to guide the nurse in selecting touch as an intervention.

Music is another way of promoting communication and group interaction. The authors recall one practical nursing student who sang a favorite hymn with an elderly patient. The student helped the patient to remember forgotten words and they both had a great time. Music also may be used to encourage patients to exercise and move about, or to encourage a person to identify and express feelings. Music therapy is the controlled use of music by a specially trained professional to treat individuals with physical, emotional, or mental illness.

Another special form of communication the nurse uses to develop a therapeutic relationship is to encourage reminiscence. *Reminiscence* or life review is a process of remembering, thinking about, and feeling emotions associated with past experiences. Elderly persons often engage in this process. Experts believe that reminiscing is a healthy activity that helps the person adapt and compensate for present inadequacies. In assisting the elderly person to reminisce, the nurse's goal is to encourage expression of feelings associated with that event. When feelings are identified and expressed, it usually is possible to gain a new perspective on the experience. Specific actions the nurse can take to encourage reminiscence include:

- Initiate reminiscence by asking the person about past events or customs.
- Participate in reminiscence by asking open-ended questions that encourage the person to expand a description.
- Choose words that encourage the person to identify and express feelings about the event or experience, even though those feelings may be painful.
- Explain the importance of this process to family members and friends who may be concerned that the patient is living in the past.

MAINTAINING SAFETY

Maintaining a safe environment is an important intervention when caring for the elderly person. For example, the flooring should be nonslip, and grab bars should be located at strategic places. The temperature of the room should be stable and comfortably warm. An adjustable hospital bed left in a conveniently low position allows the ambulatory patient more ease in getting in and out. Raised siderails for the patient in bed serve as reminders for the location of the edges of the bed.

Objects the patient may need, such as eyeglasses, water pitcher, and tissues, should be located within easy reach. The call bell should also be nearby. Some patients may want to hold the call bell or have it pinned to the gown. This may be a clue to the nurse that the person is particularly frightened of being alone. Accidents may happen when needed objects are constantly moved from place to place. The nurse and the patient can plan the location of needed items so that unnecessary reaching and searches can be avoided. If locations are recorded on the nursing care plan, other nursing personnel can cooperate in this effort.

Improper footwear can cause falls. The elderly person sometimes resorts to slippers when swelling or bony growths make other shoes painful or ill fitting. Sneakers can be a solution to this problem. The rubber soles are nonskid surfaces. Canvas tops and laces allow for swelling and foot deformities. Robes and gowns that are too long can also result in tripping and falls. Failure to use eyeglasses and/or hearing aids is another cause of accidents. If a cane or walker is needed for ambulation, one should be provided.

Remembering that the older patient generally responds slowly enables the nurse to plan increased time for daily activities such as bathing, dressing, and eating. Many accidents occur when elderly persons hurry or are rushed by others in the busy hospital environment.

A practice the student should develop is a systematic visual inspection of the patient's environment from the ceiling to the floor in order to detect and correct potential safety hazards.

ASSISTING WITH PERSONAL HYGIENE

When the elderly individual is being assisted with personal hygiene, less soap usually is needed because the skin tends to be thin and dry. All soap should be completely rinsed before the skin is dried gently and completely. Although fewer baths may be indicated, the elderly may need help to wash body areas that are hard to reach such as external genitalia, the back, and the feet. Assistance may be needed with nail care, especially toenails. Thick nails may be softened by soaking them in warm water before trimming. In some cases, professional care from a podiatrist may be needed.

A lubricating lotion may be used to reduce the dryness and itching (pruritus) that sometimes accompany old age. Men may need assistance with shaving. Women may need help to put on makeup.

The patient may require help with dental hygiene. Dentures should be brushed after meals. They should be stored in a covered container in a safe location when not in use.

ASSISTING WITH FOOD AND FLUIDS

The elderly person needs an appetizing and nourishing diet with sufficient calories, vitamins, essential amino acids, fiber, water, and essential elements (Figure 3.3). Nutritional deficiencies, particularly of calories, calcium, and vitamins, are common in elderly persons and may contribute to problems such as mental confusion and osteoporosis. Besides the aging process, factors that influence the dietary intake of the

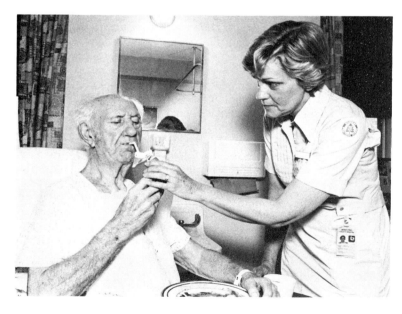

FIGURE 3.3 The nurse's company and assistance during meals encourage the patient to eat a nourishing diet. (Courtesy of Bergen Pines County Hospital School of Practical Nursing, Paramus, New Jersey.)

elderly are income, social interaction, previous food habits, transportation, living situation, and drug therapy. Aspirin, mineral oil, anticonvulsants, indomethacin (INDO-CIN), and cortisone or prednisone are examples of drugs that can contribute to nutritional deficiency even when dietary intake is adequate.

It is important to observe the tray both before and after the person eats. How much food the patient has eaten and which foods have been eaten should be observed. The tray provides important clues to the nurse whose goal is to improve the patient's nutrition. For example, the student frequently observed an unopened carton of milk on Mrs. Land's tray following the meal. In talking with the patient, the student learned that Mrs. Land had never liked the taste of milk. The student reported this information to the dietitian who was able to provide other sources of calcium for the patient. Finely chopped foods may be needed by the patient with poorly fitting dentures. Frequent small meals may be more appealing to a patient whose appetite is poor. More flavorings and spices may be added to compensate for the decline in taste and smell. Company and conversation during the meal are helpful.

ASSISTING THE PATIENT TO EXERCISE

The need for exercise does not diminish simply because a person ages. Regular exercise improves blood flow to body parts, improves peristalsis, slows the normal loss of calcium from bones, improves muscle strength and flexibility, and enhances a person's self-image. Conditions associated with aging that may be prevented or alleviated by regular exercise include joint stiffness, constipation, osteoporosis, anxiety, and sleep disturbances. The most effective exercise programs are practiced at least three times per week and are strenuous enough to get oxygen to the smallest capillary. Despite the known benefits of exercise, most elderly people lead sedentary life-styles. A number of reasons may account for this. Some elderly persons believe they are too frail or old for an exercise program. Others may accept old age as a time to take it easy. Still others

may feel awkward and embarrassed to exercise. Lack of transportation or exercise facilities also is an obstacle to such a program.

A person who wishes to begin a strenuous exercise program should first see a physician to determine if there are medical problems that might limit or alter the program. Certain cardiac arrhythmias, ventricular aneurysm, and severe emphysema are examples of medical conditions that impose strict limits on exercise. Generally, elderly persons who are beginning an exercise program should participate in supervised programs such as those offered by the YMCA or the YWCA. The nurse encourages the elderly patient to exercise by explaining the benefits of exercise, advising medical supervision, and developing a knowledge of community resources that have supervised exercise programs. Strenuous exercise should be avoided for two hours after a meal. When illness or hospitalization prevents the elderly person from participating in a program, the nurse can develop, demonstrate, and assist with alternate exercises.

A comprehensive active or assisted range-of-motion program practiced three or four times daily or more can maintain or increase flexibility. Small weights obtained from the physical therapy department assist the elderly patient to maintain or improve muscle strength in the upper extremities. Muscle-setting exercises are done by alternately tightening and relaxing certain muscle groups without moving the joint. These exercises build and strengthen muscles. Deep-breathing exercises bring air to deeper portions of the lung. Exercises should be practiced as many times as possible during the day and may be done in bed or wheelchair. Families can learn to assist the elderly member with exercises.

POSITIONING THE ELDERLY PATIENT

Changing the position of the elderly person at frequent intervals is an important nursing intervention. Prolonged immobility has special hazards for the elderly individual, such as pneumonia, decubiti (pressure sores on the skin), and decreased circulation to body parts. Studies show that sitting positions usually harmless to younger persons interfere with blood flow to the skin in elderly persons within a short time. Loss of subcutaneous fat and reduction of muscle mass causes increased pressure on the skin over bony prominences such as the sacrum. Blood flow to and from the legs is reduced, causing pain and edema (swelling). Thus, elderly persons should avoid sitting for long periods. Rocking chairs reduce potential hazards from sitting. Rocking alternates pressure areas on the buttocks, improves circulation to the lower extremities, and exercises the hip flexor muscles.

Good nutrition, adequate hydration, regular change of position, and massage to pressure areas are the four cornerstones in preventing skin breakdown in the elderly individual (see Figure 3.4).

ASSISTING WITH DRUG THERAPY

Careful observation of the elderly person's response to drug and fluid therapy is needed. The aging process affects the body's ability to absorb, metabolize, detoxify, and eliminate medications. For this reason, certain drugs such as barbiturates may accumulate in the body and cause toxic effects. The reduction in body weight and body fluids may result in overdosage with routine amounts of medication. In addition, fewer cells are available in the aged individual to act as receptor sites for drugs. For example, digitalis derivatives are frequently administered to elderly individuals to improve myocardial efficiency. Digitalis intoxication can be fatal and occurs more frequently among the aged population. The nurse should be thoroughly familiar with the signs of digitalis toxicity and should be especially alert to changes in pulse regularity, appetite, and visual disturbances in patients receiving this drug.

Drug interactions occur more frequently in elderly persons for several reasons. Because elderly persons experience more chronic illness, medication is likely to be needed over a much longer time. Elderly persons are more likely to take more than one drug. As the number of drugs taken increases, the likelihood of drug interaction also increases. Some drugs also affect laboratory values which are also influenced by aging. As mentioned earlier, vitamin deficiencies may be caused by or exacerbated by certain drugs. Changes in the heart and circulatory system can alter the body's response to fluid therapy. Intravenous fluids must be carefully regulated. The elderly per-

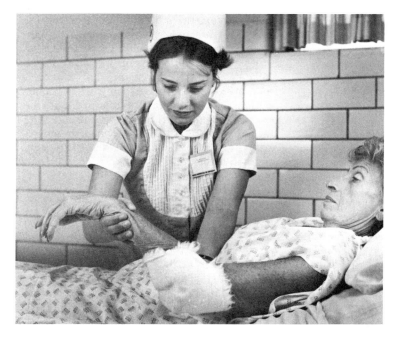

FIGURE 3.4 Regular changes of position, massage to bony prominences, and lamb's wool protection help to prevent skin breakdown in the elderly patient. (Courtesy of Shapero School of Nursing, Sinai Hospital of Detroit, Detroit, Michigan.)

son must be frequently observed for signs of circulatory overload when receiving intravenous fluids.

Reduced income, transportation problems, and life-style are three common factors that cause many elderly persons to turn to self-medication with home remedies and over-the-counter (nonprescribed) drugs. The nurse, as an important member of the health team and community, should be aware of the dangers of self-medication, especially to the elderly. A complete list of medications should be kept at home and attached to the patient's record when hospitalized. In some cases, the elderly person is discharged from the hospital, nursing home, or extended care facility with insufficient knowledge to take medication safely.

Poor vision may prevent reading instructions in small print. Decreased finger mobility may prevent the person from opening a container with a safety cap. Hand tremors or poor vision can result in wrong dosages. The elderly person may forget to take the medication or may not recognize side effects. The nurse can render lifesaving assistance in this important area. A family member may be instructed if the patient's condition prevents taking medication safely. In some cases, referrals may be needed to other community agencies such as a visiting nurse for continuing supervision. Nurses who care for the elderly in nursing homes and extended care facilities must remain especially observant of the effects of medication. Medical supervision is often less close in these facilities. The physician relies on the observations and reports of nursing personnel to keep informed of the elderly person's response to drug therapy. In addition, the elderly individual's length of stay in these facilities is likely to be longer than in a hospital. The cumulative effect and interactions of drug therapy can be more closely observed.

Drugs administered during surgery, such as anesthetic agents, can have a profound effect on the elderly individual due to the changes associated with aging. Recovery time from anesthesia may be lengthened. Dosages of postoperative medications such as opiates may be adjusted for the elderly patient's needs. Postoperative care of the elderly patient is described later in this chapter.

Nonbarbiturate sedative such as flurazepam (DALMANE), 15 mg, may be prescribed if absolutely necessary for sleep. The elderly individual may experience a change in sleep pattern as a part of the aging process.

The nurse's relationship with a patient may enhance or detract from the effectiveness of drug therapy (Figure 3.5). For example, Mrs. Soltis is a 76-year-old hospitalized patient. Mrs. Jones is the nurse who usually administers the appetite stimulant one-half hour before lunch. She then returns for a few minutes of conversation with Mrs. Soltis during her meal. Usually, Mrs. Soltis eats a hearty lunch. On the other hand, Mrs. Crocker is the nurse who administers the same drug one-half hour before supper. Mrs. Crocker never has time for a smile or conversation. Mrs. Soltis eats her supper alone and frequently leaves most of it on her plate.

ASSISTING WITH ELIMINATION

The elderly individual often experiences problems with normal elimination. Urinary and fecal incontinence and constipation are the three most common problems with elimination.

A pattern of incontinence in the elderly individual can result in damage to skin, increased likelihood of infection, and lowered self-esteem. Every effort should be made to locate the cause of incontinence and correct it.

Constipation is an insufficient number of hard stools which cause pain on defecation. Common causes of constipation are insufficient amounts of fluid, exercise, and dietary bulk. Fecal incontinence (loss of feces control) may occur if constipation is so severe that overflow of liquid stool leaks through the sphincter. Other causes of fecal incontinence include decreased sensitivity of sphincter control mechanisms and underlying disease. In addition to encouraging sufficient amounts of fluid, exercise and dietary bulk, the nurse also can help the patient to develop a regular schedule for bowel movements. When possible, the schedule should be compatible with the person's life-style.

For example, Mr. Long is an elderly patient who resides in a nursing home. For 40

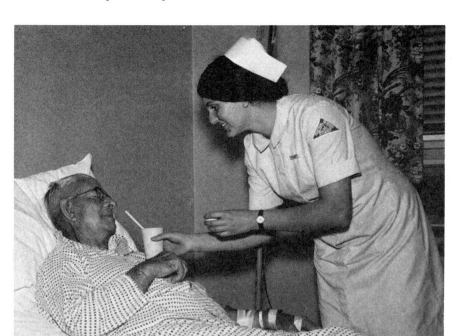

FIGURE 3.5   The nurse's warmth and friendliness enhance the effect of drug therapy. (Courtesy of Suffolk City Schools and Louise Obici Memorial Hospital School of Practical Nursing, Suffolk, Virginia.)

years he has had a daily bowel movement after breakfast. The nursing staff is not aware of this part of Mr. Long's life-style. Now, he is unable to get to the bathroom by himself. The nurses are very busy, and Mr. Long sometimes waits for 30 minutes for help to get to the bathroom. Mr. Long is frequently constipated and requires a laxative.

Loss of urine control (urinary incontinence) is not a normal part of aging. Factors that contribute to urinary incontinence include chronic illness, limitations of mobility, urinary tract infections, and prolapse of nearby organs on the bladder. In assisting the patient to correct urinary incontinence, an early intervention is to encourage an adequate fluid intake. The elderly person who has urinary incontinence needs about 2 to 3 liters of fluid per day in order to fill the bladder sufficiently to signal stretch receptors in the bladder wall. There is lack of agreement at this time about the value of restricting fluids at night to prevent incontinence. Generally, this practice is avoided when it

results in insufficient fluid intake. Another intervention is to ensure that the elderly person is not too far from toilet facilities to use them. The patient's call bell should be within easy reach.

Habit training is a process of discovering the patient's voiding pattern and developing a schedule of toileting at those times. Pelvic floor exercises, when practiced regularly over a period of months, improve voiding muscles as well as recognition of voiding sensations. One exercise is to squeeze the muscles around the urine outlet to stop urine flow for several seconds, then release the muscle, restarting the flow. A second exercise is to repeat the above process when not voiding. The amount of practice suggested varies from 20 to 60 tightenings per hour.

Catheterization as an intervention for urinary incontinence is a practice which is generally avoided because of the high incidence of bladder infection and increased susceptibility of the elderly to infection.

ASSISTING WITH SURGICAL CARE

The care of the surgical patient is described in detail in Chapter 6. Although a number of factors contribute to the increased risk of surgery to the elderly individual, age alone does not contraindicate surgery. Some of the factors known to increase surgical risk in the elderly individual include:

- Adaptive mechanisms work more slowly and are less intense.
- There is an increased susceptibility to infection.
- There is an increased sensitivity to drug therapy.
- Nutritional and fluid imbalances are more common.
- Underlying disease in vital organs (heart and lungs) occurs more frequently.
- Life changes and loss of loved ones common during later years frequently result in a less optimistic mental perspective.

In general, the nurse caring for the elderly can expect a longer recovery period and more frequent complications. The nurse's observations and interventions are keys to preventing complications.

The preoperative period may be longer for the elderly patient as the surgeon is particularly careful to identify and correct underlying conditions such as vitamin deficiency, dehydration, hypertension, urinary tract infection, and heart and lung disease which increase the surgical risk. It is especially important during the preoperative period to observe what the elderly person is eating and drinking. As mentioned previously, preoperative diagnostic tests often require the patient to refrain from eating and drinking for hours. The elderly person can become dehydrated and/or undernourished very quickly under diagnostic conditions. The nurse may consult with the dietitian to create appealing, nourishing dietary supplements.

Another area which merits the nurse's special attention at this time is medications the patient uses regularly. Drug therapy in the elderly was detailed in an earlier section. Prior to surgery, it is important to obtain and examine the complete list of prescribed and nonprescribed medications the elderly

person is using. Even one dose of aspirin doubles the person's bleeding time for about four to seven days and many elderly persons take aspirin daily. Undiscovered practices of self-medication represent a real danger to the elderly person facing surgery. When a list of medications has been obtained on admission, a safe nursing practice is to review the list with the patient or family before surgery. Self-medication with nonprescribed drugs is common among the elderly. Therefore, when nonprescribed drugs are not mentioned by the patient, the nurse asks about them. The elderly patient may not consider these "real medicine" or may not know the potential for harm.

During the preoperative period, the nurse has the opportunity for patient teaching. As mentioned in Chapter 6, studies show that patients who have received preoperative instruction have shorter recovery periods and fewer complications. Understanding the effects of aging enables the nurse to plan for instruction that includes small amounts of information at a time, repetition of information, demonstration of skills, patient practice sessions, and time for questions. The patient's family may participate by encouraging and supervising practice in activities such as turning, coughing, breathing, and leg exercises as described in Chapter 6.

Preoperative medication may be adjusted for the elderly person. Generally, barbiturates are avoided in the elderly because they often cause excitement rather than relaxation. When tranquilizers are prescribed as a preoperative medication, the nurse should be alert for possible hypotension. When opiates are prescribed, the nurse should be especially alert for signs of respiratory depression.

During the operative period, certain interventions reduce complications associated with surgery. Understanding the effect of positioning on blood flow and bony prominences enables the operating room nurse to pad bony prominences and ensure that extremities are not dangling or supporting body weight during the surgical procedure.

Although smaller dosages of anesthesia are generally used for the elderly patient in surgery, the patient may spend a longer time in the recovery room. Vital signs may take longer to stabilize and the patient may regain consciousness more slowly. Narcotics for pain during the recovery room phase of postoperative care are generally avoided when possible. These drugs may cause marked respiratory depression and hypotension, reducing blood flow to the surgical area and delaying wound repair. When other measures fail and narcotics must be administered, recovery room time is generally prolonged while vital signs are closely monitored.

Because postoperative complications occur more frequently in the elderly, nursing measures related to prevention and early detection are very important. In addition to the postoperative measures described in Chapter 6, the nurse concentrates special attention on deep breathing and coughing, fluids and nutrition, and early ambulation. The nurse is challenged to create many opportunities for the patient to breathe deeply, eat and drink, and move about. Although the patient may prefer to be left alone, prevention measures are more effective when used frequently with rest periods interspersed. Withdrawal is a normal protective response to severe stress. However, this response may be harmful to the elderly person during the postoperative period.

As part of discharge planning, the elderly patient should be told to expect a longer recovery period. Special instructions for drug therapy, wound care, and activity should be written in language and print which the patient can understand and see.

As a general rule, discharge information should include when sexual activity may be resumed. When this is not known, the discharge instructions may refer the patient to the surgeon. This approach makes discussion of the topic available to patients who might otherwise not ask.

It is especially important to caution the elderly patient about the hazards of inactivity following discharge. A helpful intervention is to ask the patient to imagine and describe a typical day following discharge. The patient has an opportunity to think ahead about specific ways to implement discharge instructions. The nurse has the opportunity to discover and correct errors of knowledge about discharge instructions.

ASSISTING THE CONFUSED ELDERLY PATIENT

The elderly person who is confused merits the nurse's careful consideration. Meticulous and complete observations demonstrate the nurse's understanding that confusion is not a normal part of aging but a symptom of possible mental and/or physical illness. The person who is confused generally has a memory loss, impaired ability to think clearly, and a short attention span. The patient may misinterpret stimuli from the environment and may experience hallucinations. Disorientation to time, place, and person is another aspect of confusion.

It is important to identify and correct the causes of confusion as early as possible. Continued confusion usually worsens, reduces the quality of the patient's life, and may be life-threatening. The progression of undetected underlying disease is an additional hazard. Besides disease, other factors known to cause confusion include undernutrition, dehydration, and drug therapy. Tranquilizers, opiates, barbiturates, and antihistamines are examples of drugs associated with confused states in the elderly patient. Drug interaction, described in earlier sections is also known to cause confusion. Diseases such as tumor, stroke, arteriosclerosis, and pneumonia can cause disorientation. Brain syndromes such as organic brain syndrome and Alzheimer's syndrome are associated with severe mental confusion. Details of Alzheimer's syndrome can be located later in Chapter 21. Unmet psychological needs, social isolation, and inadequate sensory stimulation are examples of physiological and social factors associated with confusion.

When observing the confused patient, the nurse's first step is to describe related aspects such as time of day, subject matter, memory involvement, associated activity, and persons involved. Presence or absence of eyeglasses or hearing aids if used should be noted. The specific behavior is described. These facts are recorded and reported to the physician, head nurse, or team leader. Generally, simple nursing measures are used to assist the elderly confused patient before more complex ones are considered. When inappropriately used, a nursing measure may aggravate the patient's confusion.

For example, Mr. Graves became disoriented one night. The nurse, after notifying the physician, applied restraining devices to prevent the patient from falling out of bed. The nursing action was taken without a complete investigation of causes and resulted in more disorientation. Another nurse discovered that Mr. Graves was in unfamiliar surroundings, unable to change his position, and needed to urinate. In this instance, the use of restraining devices actually prevented solving the problem since they were unfamiliar to Mr. Graves; he remained unable to change position or to void. When these needs were met, Mr. Graves became oriented and went back to sleep. Another example is Mrs. Gerson who received a sedative at bedtime and later became restless and disoriented. Although there was a physician's order for additional sedative if necessary, the nurse decided to use another intervention first. This intervention included approaching the bedside in a calm manner, speaking to Mrs. Gerson by name, and increasing the room lighting. The nurse established contact through an introduction and by touching Mrs. Gerson's hand. After Mrs. Gerson received a glass of warm milk and a back rub, the call bell was placed within easy reach. The nurse promised to return in 20 minutes. After 20 minutes elapsed, the nurse returned and observed that the patient was asleep. Knowing that sedatives often produce restlessness and confusion in the elderly patient enables the nurse to select a simpler, safer, effective nursing intervention.

Reality Orientation. The process of structuring the confused patient's daily living experience in a way that promotes remembering, mental clarity, and participation is known as reality orientation. This therapeutic intervention is more effective when practiced by every person who interacts with the elderly patient.

Two important components of reality orientation are creating a consistent environment and developing a planned approach for interaction with the patient. Clocks, calendars, and current events bulletin boards are placed in the patient's immediate environment as visual reminders. It is very important that all visual stimuli be large enough to compensate for the declining eyesight which often occurs because of aging. A regular routine is developed for each patient that avoids monotony but provides both similarities and differences. For example, a group exercise program in a nursing home takes place every afternoon at 4 o'clock. Participants wear exercise clothes and gather in the activities room which has been prepared with floor mats. The daily hour provides consistency, and changing clothes and moving to a different room provide differences. In developing a consistent environment, practices to be avoided are transfers to other areas, moving the patient's personal articles and furniture, and frequent changes of staff members who interact with the patient.

Reality-orienting interactions with the confused patient are very important. In general, the confused patient benefits from an increase in the number of interactions and by interacting with the same people regularly. A therapeutic interaction begins when the nurse calls the patient by name, introduces her- or himself, and states the purpose for the contact. This information is repeated at regular intervals during the interaction. For example, Mr. Reed, the student nurse, approaches Mr. Fish, a confused elderly gentleman, slowly from the front and says: "Good morning Mr. Fish. My name is Mr. Reed. I am a student nurse. It's 10 o'clock, time for your bath now. How can I help you get ready?" During the bath, the student nurse engages the patient in a conversation about the water temperature of the bath, the distance of the bath from the patient's room, the patient's preference for bath versus shower, and morning bath versus evening bath. At regular intervals the student calls Mr. Fish by name. The student speaks slowly, uses short sentences, and a tone of voice which indicates that a reply is expected. The student nurse and all staff members who interact with the elderly should wear large nametags with large print and contrasting lettering. Each interaction with the confused elderly patient should begin with an introduction and calling the patient by name.

It is important to help family members learn and practice reality-orienting interactions. Mental confusion of a loved one is a very distressing experience for the family. Some of that distress is diminished when family members learn and practice positive, effective ways to communicate.

LONG-TERM ASSISTANCE TO THE ELDERLY INDIVIDUAL

Illness or the changes brought about by aging may result in a need for long-term or permanent nursing assistance to an elderly person. Often such assistance means that the individual must move from a private home or apartment occupied for many years to a nursing home, retirement home, or other type of residential care facility. The nurse can anticipate the need for additional creative interventions to help the elderly person in the new environment.

Changing one's residence can be considered a major life-changing event as described in Chapter 1. The nurse may anticipate, understand, and accept that the loss of familiar objects such as books and furniture collected over a lifetime is likely to result in grieving. Separation from family, friends, and the community may be losses from which the person is unable to recover. Thus, it is very important that the number of losses be minimized whenever possible.

One way to minimize losses is to consider ways in which the environment can be adapted to the individual. For example, space can be allotted for favorite books, photographs, or a rocking chair. A portion of the grounds can be set aside for small gardens. A piano might be available for piano players and singers. Some studies suggest that pets provide important health benefits. Pets provide opportunities to touch and care for another living being. Although additional research continues, careful thought should be given to the possibility of pets in the long-term care facility.

Knowledge of community resources and a person's life-style is a tool the nurse uses to create beneficial opportunities for the elderly (Figure 3.6). Living in a community involves a balance between giving and receiving. In long-term facilities, elderly persons often have reduced opportunities for giving, and the balance is upset. A person who only receives may experience unfavorable changes in the self-concept with feelings of helplessness and worthlessness. Thus, the nurse is challenged to use this knowledge in ways that promote or restore the balance between giving and receiving.

In some communities, elderly persons act as foster grandparents to children whose natural grandparents are not available. This enables the elderly individual to remain involved and helps the child develop an appreciation of the wisdom or values of older persons. Senior citizens groups and volunteer groups are other opportunities for the elderly individual to develop satisfying relationships and help others at the same time. Even a person who is too ill or frail to participate in most group activities can benefit from helping one other person. For example, Mrs. Jones, a frail elderly woman, is teaching Mrs. Pine how to knit. Both are benefitting from this interaction which was arranged by the nurse.

The need for satisfying sexual intimacy is often overlooked in the aged person. When the nurse recognizes and provides privacy for elderly couples, these needs can be met. Most programs that discuss sexuality are well attended by elderly persons. The nurse could consider developing an afternoon or evening program with a guest speaker invited to describe the effects of aging on sexuality. A question and answer period might follow the speaker. Questions could be prepared in advance and submitted in writing if desired.

Feelings of adequacy, achievement, and mastery are conducive to self-esteem. Other factors that contribute to self-esteem are respect, attention, recognition, and appreciation from others. The nurse may need to help the patient concentrate on strengths and support areas of declining abilities. A practice to be avoided when abilities decline is automatic decision-making on the pa-

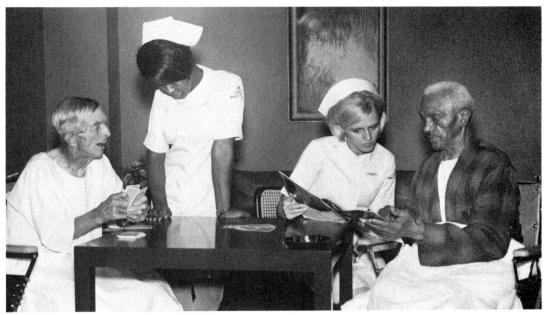

FIGURE 3.6   When possible, efforts should be made to enable the aging patient to continue activities that he has enjoyed previously. (Courtesy of Suffolk City Schools and Louise Obici Memorial Hospital School of Practical Nursing, Suffolk, Virginia.)

tient's behalf. Unless unable to do so, the patient continues to maker decisions about life goals, plans, and activities. At times, the nurse's encouragement and assistance are needed. One type of assistance is to help the patient identify the potential advantages and disadvantages of a particular decision. Another type of assistance is to explore possible alternatives in the situation under discussion.

Occasionally, a decision may have to be made for the elderly person by others. If this occurs, a complete discussion with the patient is indicated. For example, Mrs. Winston's smoking became a safety hazard to herself and others in the extended-care facility where she lives. In order to protect Mrs. Winston and others from injury, Mrs. Green, the head nurse, decided to restrict the patient's smoking to the activity and dining rooms where supervision is available. Mrs. Green discussed the need for the smoking restriction with Mrs. Winston and the family. Mrs. Winston continued to make decisions about other aspects of living such as food selection, what to wear, and bedtimes. Mrs. Green did not assume that the patient

was unable to make all decisions, only the one about safe places for smoking.

Assisting the elderly person to identify and/or develop talents can be a real challenge to the nurse. A knowledge of community resources, as well as a knowledge of the person's life-style, again may help the nurse to be creative in this area. Some community colleges and senior citizens groups offer courses designed especially for the elderly person. In some nursing homes and extended-care facilities, elderly persons make objects and sell them at church bazaars. Some elderly may be able to offer the benefit of years of experience in business or other related fields to younger persons. The nurse who perceives the elderly person as a valuable national resource that has been largely untapped can find many ways to help elderly persons continue to grow.

In nursing homes and extended-care facilities, the need for communication may increase because of fewer relationships with other persons. In some cases, the nurse may be the elderly person's only link to the world outside the institution. This is especially true if vision or hearing losses prevent watching television, listening to the radio, or reading the newspaper. A well-informed nurse can provide information about community, national, international, and sports events that enlarges the patient's world.

Taking pleasure in everyday activities, regarding life as meaningful, having a positive self-image, feeling successful in achieving major goals, and having a positive attitude about life are five positive indicators of well-being in the elderly person.

A nursing care plan is especially important for the long-term care of the aged. The plan for nursing care is widely used in hospitals but is not as common in nursing homes or extended-care facilities. A nursing care plan helps to individualize care, enables the nursing staff to establish priorities for the patient's care, facilitates communication between all members of the nursing staff, contributes to the continuity of patient care, and serves as a guide in evaluating patient care. Such a plan is even more important for the elderly person unable to recognize or communicate personal needs to the nursing staff. For example, the patient who cannot see well enough to check the menu for the desired foods may ask a busy member of the health care system to check it, and as a result the patient's choices are disregarded. In some cases, the person who is especially independent may refuse to ask for help even when it is needed. The nurse may want to review Chapter 1 for more detailed information about developing a nursing care plan.

One feature that distinguishes the plan for long-term assistance from that for shorter periods is the need for regular revisions. It is especially important to set dates for the achievement of goals in long-term assistance to the elderly. For example, if nursing interventions have been successful in achieving a goal of mental clarity or urinary continence, many new goals become possible. The individual who is mentally clear can participate in all kinds of new activities. The individual who is continent likewise can participate in different activities. Regular revisions of the nursing care plan demonstrate the nurse's continuous attention to and appreciation of the patient's capacity for growth and development.

Interested nurses may obtain additional information about long-term care of the elderly by writing to:

National Clearing House on Aging
Department of Health and Human Services
Washington, D.C. 20201

SELF-DESTRUCTIVE BEHAVIOR IN THE ELDERLY

The number of elderly persons who engage in self-destructive behavior is a cause for great concern. Statistical studies show a higher suicide rate for the ages between 65 and 84 than for all other age groups. Some elderly persons who commit suicide are suffering from mental illness which can be treated. Misconceptions about suicide among the elderly may result in missed observations and cries for help that go unrecognized. Most people who attempt suicide give warnings about their intentions. Anytime a person gives a warning, it should be taken seriously and reported at once to the head nurse, team leader, and/or physician. The fact that so many persons do give a warning demonstrates uncertainty about the choice made and a willingness to be helped. Many suicide wishes are temporary, resulting from illness, loss of hope, or an emotional upset. Recent losses, changes in health that involve pain or an alteration in body image are times when the elderly person is more likely to consider suicide.

Some experts have suggested that certain behaviors frequently observed in the elderly are actually indicators of deep depression and a death wish. Thus, the nurse's careful observations and recordings of the patient's behavior are important. Behaviors that are possible danger signals include:

- Persistent firm refusal to eat or drink sufficient food and fluids
- Refusal to take medication, forgetting medication, errors in taking medication
- Repeated accidents despite safety precautions

In addition to observing and reporting behavior that indicates possible suicide, the nurse can take many other preventive measures. A warm caring relationship between the elderly patient and another person is one of the most important preventive measures available. That other person can be the nurse. Opportunities for the elderly person to contribute, grow, and change can reduce feelings of helplessness, worthlessness, and isolation common to depressed patients. Interventions that teach the elderly person how to compensate for declining physical abilities are helpful in preventing depression. The nursing care plan that is tailored to the person's uniqueness, revised on a regular basis, and shared with the patient provides a sense of direction and achievement.

Case Study #1 Involving an Elderly Patient

Mr. Jones is 75 years old and has been admitted to the hospital for a possible operation for benign prostatic hypertrophy. Mr. Jones is an active, elderly gentleman with an apparently good sense of humor. He is frequently found in other patients' rooms joking with them and talking. From the nursing history, the nurse learns that Mr. Jones lost his wife more than 20 years ago. She died suddenly from an acute myocardial infarction. He has two children who are married and seven grandchildren. Both children and all grandchildren live more than 500 miles away. They see him only on holidays. Mr. Jones lives with a woman who is 66 years of age, Mrs. Gardner.

Mr. Jones is scheduled for a transurethral resection of the prostate gland the following day. On the morning of surgery, the nurse observes that Mr. Jones appears to be disoriented. He received diazepam (VALIUM), 10 mg, the previous night to help him sleep. Mr. Jones also received secobarbital (SECONAL), 32 mg at 7 A.M.

QUESTIONS
1. What factors could have caused Mr. Jones's disorientation?
2. Should the surgeon be notified of the change in orientation of Mr. Jones?
3. How can the nurse help Mr. Jones become re-oriented?
4. Mr. Jones asked the nurse if the operation would affect his sexual performance. Will it?
5. The nurse overheard another nurse refer to Mr. Jones as a dirty old man. In talking with

the other nurse, the nurse asked her why she felt that way. The second nurse responded that Mr. Jones was living with a woman and that they were not married. The second nurse stated further that a man 75 years of age should know better. Investigate the present Social Security laws to determine if there is a reason why an arrangement such as the one between Mr. Jones and Mrs. Gardner might be preferable to marriage.
6. According to the rules of the hospital in which Mr. Jones is having surgery, he will be permitted to have only the immediate family present during his surgery. Mr. Jones's immediate family lives a long distance from him. They will not be present at the time of surgery. Mrs. Gardner would like to visit Mr. Jones prior to visiting hours, which start at 7 P.M. Mr. Jones was returned to his room at 4 P.M. Should a visit between Mrs. Gardner and Mr. Jones be arranged?

Case Study #2 Involving an Elderly Patient

Mr. Johnson, a 73-year-old man, was admitted to an extended care facility. He stated that his wife had died two years ago and he had been living alone in their house since her death but is unable to care for himself any longer. Their only child, a son, lives many miles away and returned to help dispose of the house and other belongings as well as arrange his father's admission to the nursing home. Mr. Johnson stated that his eyesight was failing but he was otherwise in good health. He also said that he takes furosemide (LASIX), 40 mg daily, and is on a salt-free diet because of "heart trouble." Mr. Johnson smokes a cigarette after each meal and occasionally drinks a beer after working in his garden. Until he retired at age 65, Mr. Johnson was a welder in a large factory.

QUESTIONS
1. Describe the safety precautions that should be taken for Mr. Johnson.
2. Describe the possible effects of furosemide (LASIX) on this elderly individual.
3. List appropriate nursing actions related to the sensory deficit Mr. Johnson has experienced.
4. What changes of behavior can be expected as Mr. Johnson adjusts to his new situation?
5. What will Mr. Johnson do with his time while residing in the nursing home?
6. What changes will occur in Mr. Johnson's lifestyle as a result of living in a nursing home?

Suggestions for Further Study

1. Discuss the physical and emotional needs of the aging with an older member of your community.
2. When should a person start planning for old age?
3. Invite an elderly retired nurse to your class to discuss the differences between nursing of the past and present.
4. Mason, Mildred A.; Bates, Grace F.; and Smola, Bonnie K.: *Workbook in Basic Medical-Surgical Nursing*, 3rd ed. Macmillan Publishing Company, New York, 1984, Exercise 3.

Additional Readings

Allen, Marcia: "Drug Therapy in the Elderly." *American Journal of Nursing*, 80:1474–75 (Aug.), 1980.

Bozian, Marguerite W., and Clark, Helen: "Counteracting Sensory Changes in the Aging." *American Journal of Nursing*, 80:473–76 (Mar.), 1980.

Conlin, Judith B.: "A Hotel or a Hospital: Applying the Principles of Reality Orientation." *Journal of Practical Nursing*, 31:25–26 and 57 (July–Aug.), 1981.

Gasek, George: "How to Handle the Crotchety, Elderly Patient." *Nursing 80*, 10:46–48 (Mar.), 1980.

Gault, Patricia L.: "Plan for a Patchwork of Problems When Your Patient Is Elderly." *Nursing 82*, 12:50–54 (Jan.), 1982.

Gioiella, Evelynn Clark: "Give the Older Person Space." *American Journal of Nursing*, 80:898–99 (May), 1980.

Gray, Peggy L.: "Gerontological Nurse Specialist: Luxury or Necessity?" *American Journal of Nursing*, 82:82–85 (Jan.), 1982.

Hays, Antoinette: "Caring for the Hospitalized Elderly." *American Journal of Nursing*, 82:930–31 (June), 1982.

Heller, Barbara R.: "Needs of the Hospitalized Geriatric Patient." *Journal of Nursing Care*, 14:22–25 (Apr.), 1981.

Krieger, Dolores: *Foundations for Holistic Health Nursing Practices: The Renaissance Nurse*. J. B. Lippincott Co., Philadelphia, 1981, pp. 231–48.

Lee, Margaret M.: "Caring for and about the Elderly." *Journal of Nursing Care*, 14:10–13 (Feb.), 1981.

Lomy, Peter P.: "Drugs and the Elderly." *Journal of Practical Nursing*, 30:15–19 (Aug.), 1980.

Ramos, Linda Yoder: "Oral Hygiene for the Elderly." *American Journal of Nursing*, 81:1468–69 (Aug.), 1981.

_____: "Oral Hygiene for the Elderly." *Journal of Practical Nursing*, 32:29–30 (Apr.), 1982.

Robinson, Corinne H.: *Basic Nutrition and Diet Therapy*, 4th ed. Macmillan Publishing Co., Inc., New York, 1980, pp. 132–35.

Rose, Joan: "Back to Basics: Skin Care in the Elderly." *Journal of Practical Nursing*, 30:20–21 (Apr.), 1980.

Tapley, Katherine: "Psychosocial Needs and the Geriatric Patient." *Journal of Practical Nursing*, 32:22–23 and 48 (July–Aug.), 1982.

Williams, Emily: "Food for Thought: Meeting the Nutritional Needs of the Elderly." *Nursing 80*, 10:60–63 (Sept.), 1980.

Witte, Natalie Slocumb: "Why the Elderly Fall." *American Journal of Nursing*, 79:1950–52 (Nov.), 1979.

Chapter 4

Causes of Disease and Methods of Treatment

Expected Behavioral Outcomes

Minimum objectives referred to as expected behavioral outcomes have been designed for the practical/vocational nursing student to use as guides in studying this chapter. The students should read these expected outcomes before studying the chapter. The objectives can be used as guides to study.

Using the contact of this chapter, the student should return to the objectives and evaluate the ability to:

1. *Describe one other factor associated with stressors causing disease when given a list of agents that can cause disease.*
2. *Discuss the nursing action in three diagnostic procedures.*
3. *Describe the nurse's role in six treatment methods.*

Vocabulary Development

The following prefixes, suffixes, and combining forms pertain to this chapter by learning and/or reviewing their meanings, the practical/vocational nursing student will have the keys needed to unlock many exciting new medical terms.

Discover the meaning of these keys in a medical dictionary or in the content of this chapter. How does each key pertain to this chapter? In your notebook write the correct meaning of each prefix, suffix, or combining form listed below. Illustrate each key with an example.

gno—know. Ex. dia*gno*sis—knowing the nature of a disease.

hered-	path-
iatr-	pharmac-
intra-	psych-
-ject-	therap-
nutri-	zo-
or-	

Introduction

The individual with a disease has an impairment of normal physical and/or mental function. Recent theories suggest that disease results from a complex interaction of many factors.

Man lives in a constantly changing environment. *Homeostasis* refers to the ability of man to maintain an internal body environment that is relatively stable and that promotes growth, development, and function. Through the action of many adjustment mechanisms, man is protected from extremes outside and inside the body. Thus, homeostasis, a stable internal environment, is maintained.

The defense mechanisms detailed in Chapter 1 can be considered as adjustment mechanisms because they protect the person from perceived threats. An example of a physical adjustment mechanism is the role of the skin and blood vessels in maintaining a stable body temperature. Blood vessels underneath the skin dilate in response to orders from the autonomic nervous system, and heat is lost from the body. Other body organs have similar adjustment mechanisms. The heart may speed up or slow down.

Thus, the healthy person is able to adapt to a changing world. At any time, there are one or more agents inside and/or outside our bodies that are known to be capable of causing disease. Yet most of us are healthy most of the time.

A recent finding is that *life-change events* appear to be closely associated with disease in some unknown way. Marriage, divorce, and death of a spouse are examples of life-change events. Researchers observed that people who are ill have often experienced one or more major life-change events in the 12 to 18 months prior to illness. These observations have led to suggestions that persons who have major life changes are more likely to develop disease. Some health professionals are using these findings to assist clients who have experienced major life changes.

In studying disease, the student will discover many terms used to describe dimensions of a disease more completely. Some of the more common terms are defined below.

- An *acute* disease is one that has a short and relatively severe course.
- A *chronic* disease is one that persists over a long time.
- An *exacerbation* is an increase in the severity or symptoms of disease.
- *Prognosis* is a forecasting of the probably outcome of illness or disease made by the physician.
- *Recurrent* disease is one that returns after an intermission.
- *Remission* is the period in which signs and symptoms diminish or disappear.

- *Self-limited* disease is one that runs a definite limited course.
- *Signs* of disease are objective evidences of that disease or of the patient's condition.
- *Symptoms* of disease are subjective evidences of disease or of the patient's condition.
- *Syndrome* is a set of signs and symptoms that occur together.

Stress

The term *stress* has been used so often in recent years that it has different meanings for different people. Dr. Hans Selyé, a medical scientist, first described stress as the rate of wear and tear on the body caused by life. Later, Dr. Selyé modified that definition describing stress as a nonspecific response of the body to demands placed on it. The stress mechanism is an example of the adaptive mechanisms described in the previous section. Two components of stress are *stressors* and a *stress response*.

A *stressor* can be defined as any agent inside or outside the body that influences homeostasis. A stressor can be favorable when it promotes normal growth, development, and function. A stressor can be unfavorable when it stops, slows down, or excessively speeds up normal growth and development. The same stressor can be favorable to one individual and unfavorable to another. For example, a plant is given to Mrs. Jones and she derives a great deal of pleasure from it. Her roommate in the hospital, Mrs. Smith, is allergic to the plant. Her body has had a different reaction to the same stressor. Her eyes are watery and puffy; her nose is itchy and congested.

Many factors influence whether a stressor is favorable or unfavorable. These include heredity, culture, nutritional status, living habits, emotional state, fatigue, age, and sex. It is the interaction of these and other factors with an agent known to be capable of causing disease that may determine the development and/or outcome of disease. Specific stressors known to be capable of causing disease are described later in this chapter.

When exposed to a stressor, the person has two different methods of adapting. One method is known as the general adaptation syndrome (GAS). This syndrome involves the whole body response to a stressor. Shock is a general adaptation syndrome. In addition, there is a local adaptation syndrome (LAS) which occurs in a single organ or system. It is important to understand that LAS refers only to a type of response to a stressor. It does *not* mean that a part of the person is responding. The whole person is affected by and responds to illness and disease. Inflammation is a local adaptation syndrome which responds to tissue injury. A discussion of care of the patient with an inflammation is in Chapter 5.

Both syndromes are believed to develop in similar stages. The first stage is known as the *alarm reaction*. Body defenses are mobilized at this time. The second stage is called *resistance*. During this stage, body defense systems are working hard to adapt to the stressor. The third and final stage is called *exhaustion*. This stage occurs when the stressor continues, but body defenses have been exhausted. Death usually occurs in this case. Successful adaptation generally depends on the influence of factors such as heredity, diet, and past experience with stressors. Understanding the stress mechanism enables the nurse to appreciate the view of some researchers who explain disease as an inability to adapt to stressors.

Both syndromes are regulated and controlled primarily by the endocrine system and the central and autonomic nervous systems. Regulation and control are accomplished mainly by hormones—powerful chemical messengers. Two very important hormones related to the stress responses are *glucocorticoids* and *mineralocorticoids*. Glucocorticoids act to inhibit a person's inflammatory response, and therefore are also known as anti-inflammatory hormones. Mineralocorticoids act by stimulating body defenses and are also known as proinflammatory hormones. Additional information about these important hormones is provided in subsequent chapters.

Many diseases are believed to result from disturbances in the operation of the stress mechanism. Hypertension, heart disease, ulcerative colitis, and stomach ulcers are a few examples. As mentioned earlier, stress is an adaptive mechanism that enables the body to respond rapidly to changes in the internal and external environment, either by fighting or fleeing. In modern life, many daily events may trigger the stress mechanism releasing one or more of the stress hormones described earlier. Although the body is ready, it is not always possible to fight or flee. Thus, there is no release of the tension and energy made available to the body for adaptation. Over a period of years, cumulative stress is believed to play a very important role in the development of disease, both by causing changes in the person's body tissue and by weakening the immune system, a major body defense.

It is possible for an individual to influence the operation of the stress mechanism in two major areas. As mentioned earlier, stressors may be favorable or unfavorable, depending on a number of factors. A person can act to neutralize, avoid, or modify known unfavorable stressors. For example a person can avoid smoking and shorten exposure to smoke. Emotional stressors that are unfavorable also can be modified. For example, a person can learn to accept, avoid, or modify situations that consistently bring about inappropriate emotional responses.

The stress response can also be influenced by the individual. A relaxation response has been identified and can be controlled by the individual using the instructions in Table 4.1. When practiced regularly, mental and physical factors such as anxiety and blood pressure can change. Other factors that affect the stress response such as diet and exercise are also controlled by the individual.

When a person is ill, the nurse often assists in identifying avoiding, or modifying unfavorable stressors. Attention to the common nursing practices described in Chapter 1 enables the nurse to recognize and influence unfavorable stressors. Reducing noise in the patient's environment, active listening, and explaining diagnostic tests are examples of nursing activities that modify unfavorable stressors. Because of the effect on pulse rate, blood pressure, and other physical measurements, the individual who is ill

TABLE 4.1
INSTRUCTIONS FOR A RELAXATION
EXERCISE*

1. Sit quietly in a comfortable environment.
2. Close your eyes.
3. Beginning at the feet, deeply relax all your muscles by first tightening the muscle and then relaxing it. Move slowly and systematically from the feet toward the head. Include face muscles in the relaxation process.
4. When possible, breathe through the nose and count silently to yourself each time you breathe out.
5. Continue this process for about 20 minutes, but do not use an alarm to check the time. After finishing the exercise, sit quietly for several minutes before getting up from the chair.
6. Practice once or more daily but not within two hours of a meal. Do not worry about the level of relaxation. Ignore distracting thoughts, and return to counting when you become aware of them.

* Adapted from Benson, H.: *The Relaxation Response.* Avon Books, New York, 1976.

should check with the physician before beginning programs of relaxation and exercise.

STRESSORS THAT CAUSE DISEASE

An individual develops an *infection* when living microorganisms enter the body, overpower natural resistance, and cause an inflammatory process to develop. Examples of these microorganisms are bacteria and viruses. A boil or carbuncle is caused by bacteria, while the common cold is caused by viruses. The inflammatory process that results because of the invasion of bacteria and viruses is discussed in detail in Chapter 5.

A *neoplasm*, which is also known as a tumor, is a new growth or an abnormal growth of cells. As a rule these cells row faster than normal. A neoplasm may be either *benign* or *malignant*. Diseases caused by an abnormal growth of cells are known as *neoplastic diseases*, discussed in Chapter 9. Examples of neoplastic diseases are cancer, leukemia, and moles or nevi that appear on the skin.

The patient with an *allergy* has an abnormal reaction to certain substances that ordinarily have no effect on other individuals.

The hives or urticaria that appears when some persons are exposed to poison ivy is an example of an allergy. The rejection of another person's heart that is transplanted into a recipient is still another example of an allergic reaction. A discussion of these conditions is included in Chapter 10.

Injury or *trauma* from mechanical violence causes disease. For example, the bone of a person's leg may be fractured as a result of an automobile accident.

Injury can also be caused by *physical agents* such as electricity, extreme heat, and excessive cold. Excessive radiation is another physical agent that can cause injury to the body. Some *chemicals* injure the body when they come into contact with it; for example, undiluted phenol burns the body's tissues. Chemicals such as drugs can poison the body when used improperly.

A *congenital defect* can be the result of faulty transmission of genetic information from DNA to the offspring or it can be associated with the environment of the fetus in the uterus. Examples of genetic defects are Down's syndrome (mongolism), trisomy 16–18 (Edward's syndrome), phenylketonuria (PKU) and sickle cell anemia. An example of a defect associated with the environment of the fetus in the uterus is congenital syphilis. In other words, the embryo or fetus became infected with syphilis while in the uterus. Infection by the virus causing German measles can cause the embryo or fetus to be born with such defects as blindness, deafness, and congenital heart disease.

Genetics is the study of the role that heredity plays in causing disease. A defective gene can be transmitted from parent to child, or the cell can have an abnormal number of chromosomes. A *chromosome* is a rod-shaped body located in the nucleus of the cell. Chromosomes serve as vehicles to carry the basic units of heredity from parent to child. *Genes* are the biologic units of heredity that are located on definite places on the chromosome. *Deoxyribonucleic acid*, abbreviated *DNA*, is a complex protein present in chromosomes. DNA is considered a chemical carrier of genetic information.

Medical genetics is an area in which new information is being made available rapidly by research. The practical nursing student should watch with interest reports of new developments in this area.

Degeneration occurs in every person who becomes older. The normal structure of the body's cells breaks down slowly as one ages. This group of disease processes develops earlier in some than in others. Frequently these changes develop in the blood vessels and joints. Thus, arteriosclerosis (hardening of the arteries), atherosclerosis (accumulation of fat-containing material within or on the innermost surfaces of blood vessels), and arthritis are more common in older people.

Metabolism is the process by which foodstuffs are used to produce energy, changed into tissue elements, and stored in the cells of the body. It includes the changes that occur to food after it is digested and the complex chemical activities that take place within the individual cells. A disease caused by a change of metabolism is known as a metabolic disorder. An example of this is seen in a person who is unable to use glucose because of an insufficient amount of insulin or because of the body's inability to utilize insulin. This condition results in a metabolic disease known as *diabetes mellitus*. Nutritional deficiencies are closely related to this group of diseases. A person will no longer be healthy if the diet lacks the essential substances. For example, rickets will develop in an individual whose diet is deficient in vitamin D. A person who is in a poor nutritional state will recover from illness or surgery more slowly than a well-nourished person.

Emotions are defined, as one's feelings, such as love, hate, fear, anxiety, worry, anger, jealousy, disgust, depression, and joy. The nurse can readily understand how emotions can cause disease by recalling some of the body changes experienced as a result of anxiety or fear of a final examination. One student notices a pounding heart and clammy hands. A classmate reports an upset or tight stomach. It may be noticed that another student goes to the bathroom more often before an examination. These symptoms or changes develop as a result of emotion. The students became tense because of their emotion regarding the examination. Usually bodily symptoms disappear after the examination, and, if controlled, are of no lasting significance.

Realizing that bodily changes are caused by an emotional reaction enables the nurse to understand better how strong and persistent emotional conflict over a period of time can disturb the functioning of various organs. A person is said to have a *functional disease* when there is no pathologic change in either the organ or the system to account for the symptoms. the nurse needs to know that the patient with a functional disorder can suffer as much as the patient with an organic disease in which there is an actual pathologic change in the organ or body. Frequently emotional tension plays an important role in certain organic diseases, especially of the circulatory system and the digestive system. For example, emotional tension may be considered a causative factor in some patients with high blood pressure or a peptic ulcer.

Certain *pollutants* in the environment are known to cause disease. The waste products from automobiles and factories have profoundly altered our environment and, in some cases, caused disease. For example, asbestosis is a lung disease caused by the inhalation of asbestos particles.

Iatrogenic diseases are those caused by the physician in an effort to treat the patient. For example, pulmonary edema can be considered iatrogenic when it results from overload of the circulatory system with intravenous fluids. Serum hepatitis is considered iatrogenic when it results from a blood transfusion.

Prevention

One very important activity of the nurse is to assist the individual to prevent disease. To prevent disease means to avert its occurrence.

Primary prevention includes activities that promote health and a sense of well-being. Some specific factors believed to influence health promotion and well-being are exercise, diet, stress management, immunization, and accident prevention.

Secondary prevention refers to early diagnosis and treatment of disease for the purpose of stopping its spread and curing it. Screening tests are examples of secondary prevention.

Tertiary prevention refers to activities directed toward assisting the individual to regain the maximum skills possible. Rehabilitation is an example of this type of prevention.

One very effective way to assist individuals with prevention is to set a good example. The nurse who exercises regularly, maintains proper nutrition, and practices stress management is in a better position to understand and assist the patient to develop these practices.

Because of the nurse's knowledge and skill, friends, family, and neighbors often seek information and advice. In these situations the nurse has the responsibility to provide accurate information and advice. For example, the nurse may inform a friend or neighbor about the importance of monthly breast self-examination. The technique for such an examination may be demonstrated correctly. However, if a neighbor or friend reports finding a breast lump, the correct advice is to encourage that person to obtain immediate medical attention.

In carrying out everyday activities, the nurse has opportunities to explain good health practices. For example, while caring for Mr. Jones, the student remarked about the many times a day, handwashing was necessary. The nurse also related that whether at home or in the hospital frequent handwashing reduces the spread of infection. When asked what is to be served for breakfast, the nurse can describe not only the specific food but the major nutrient it contains: orange juice for vitamin C, an egg for protein. When assisting the patient to ambulate, the nurse has an opportunity to explain the benefits of exercise.

Diagnosis

The word *diagnosis* comes from a Greek word that means "to know." A diagnosis is a statement or conclusion about the nature or cause of disease. In order to diagnose, the physician collects and interprets information from a variety of sources and compares it to what is known about disease and what is known about the person. Thus, the whole person is considered. After the diagnosis has been made, the physician usually informs and explains it to the patient and/or family.

The computer is an important new diagnostic tool having many impacts on both the patient and the nurse. Currently, computers are used extensively to process a wide variety of information, screen persons for possible disease, automate patient monitoring, nurse's notes and laboratory functions, and for noninvasive testing. One potential advantage of the computer to the nurse is that more time is available to spend directly with the patient at the bedside rather than indirectly. The use of computers in all phases of patient care is expected to increase rapidly. The nurse will find it important and interesting to follow developments in this field.

Diagnostic procedures are expensive, often time consuming, uncomfortable, and sometimes painful and dangerous. In addition to experiencing the symptoms of illness, the patient usually is apprehensive about the outcome of the tests, the diagnosis, the testing procedures or all of those factors. The nurse who understands the patient's situation, provides valuable assistance by carrying out relevant nursing activities correctly, promptly, and with a warm caring attitude.

The nurse's activities are very important to correct diagnosis. Keen observations, reporting, and recording of the patient's symptoms, signs, and behavior provide information crucial to the diagnosis. The nurse uses the same methods to assess the patient's response to certain diagnostic tests. The nurse's participation may be direct or indirect. An example of direct participation in diagnostic tests is correctly collecting, labeling, and transporting laboratory specimens. The nurse assists indirectly by preparing the patient for certain diagnostic tests according to hospital or agency procedures.

Some patients feel much less anxious and fearful after the nurse explains the test. Guidelines the nurse can use when explaining a diagnostic test include:

- Name the test using terms the patient can understand. (Example: cardiogram or heart tracing rather than ECG).
- Generally explain the purpose of the test in a positive or neutral way. (Example: "The test is to look at the electrical activ-

DIAGNOSIS 67

ity in your heart," rather than "To see if you have an arrhythmia.")

- Explain where, when, and by whom the test will be done when known. (Example: "Sometime this morning in your room by Mr. Smith, the technician.")
- Describe what the patient will see, hear, feel, smell, and taste and how the test will proceed. (Example: "You'll be lying in bed and Mr. Smith will attach small metal disks with special jelly to your arms and legs. It won't hurt but you'll have to lie still for about 10 minutes.")
- Explain that the patient should ask the doctor about the test results. (Example: "You can ask Dr. Gray about the results of your cardiogram this evening.")

Generally, the physician orders tests according to a plan. Risk to the patient, usefulness of the information in establishing a diagnosis, technical difficulty in doing a particular test, and cost are some of the criteria the physician uses in developing a plan. Some patients and families feel better when

they know what the plan is and approximately how long the diagnostic testing will take.

HISTORY AND PHYSICAL EXAMINATION

One of the first studies done to diagnose disease is the history and physical examination. This is considered vital to the diagnosis and treatment of disease. A history of health and illness is obtained from the patient and/or the family by the physician. By talking with the patient and/or family members, valuable information can be obtained.

During the physical examination, additional information is gathered about body structure and function by four methods.

1. Inspection—A process of looking for abnormalities that can be seen with the eyes. Certain instruments, such as an otoscope or ophthalmoscope, are needed to visualize smaller areas inside the ear and eye (Figure 4.1).

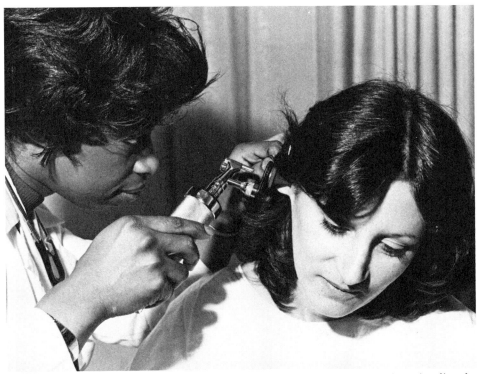

FIGURE 4.1 Examination by inspection. An ophthalmoscope is being used to visualize the ear canal and eardrum.

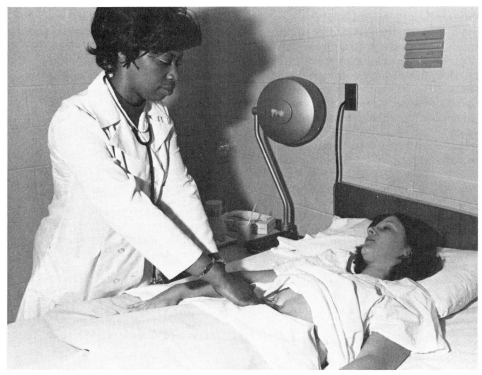

FIGURE 4.2   The physician is using the fingers to palpate the abdomen.

2. Palpation—A process of feeling with the fingers for abnormal growths and/or swelling (Figure 4.2).
3. Percussion—A process of tapping body surfaces with the fingers or an instrument. Sounds are produced by the tapping, which the examiner interprets (Figure 4.3).
4. Auscultation—A process of listening to sounds arising from within the body. The stethoscope is an instrument frequently used in auscultation (Figure 4.4).

LABORATORY ANALYSIS

Normal and abnormal body constituents are frequently examined in the laboratory. Blood, urine, sputum, feces, tissue, and other fluids are some examples of material studied in the laboratory.

Sometimes a surgical procedure is necessary to obtain specimens of tissue or fluid for laboratory examination. A biopsy is the surgical removal of tissue for laboratory examination. Needle biopsy refers to obtaining a small piece of tissue by aspirating it into a needle.

Nurses frequently assist in the collection of specimens for laboratory analysis. Specimens that are improperly collected or labeled may yield information that is inadequate or inaccurate. The collection and examination may have to be repeated, causing added expense and discomfort to the patient. The nurse should be thoroughly familiar with the procedures for the collection and labeling of specimens in the agency or institution.

ROENTGENOGRAMS (X-RAYS)

Roentgenograms or x-rays are still pictures that show structures such as bones and other body organs. Air and/or fluid within the body can be seen on x-ray.

Fluoroscopy is a special x-ray technique that allows the roentgenologist (radiologist) to see certain body parts while they are in motion.

Sometimes radiopaque substances are introduced into the body that outline the area to be examined. Barium enema, cholecystograms, and bronchograms are examples of these studies.

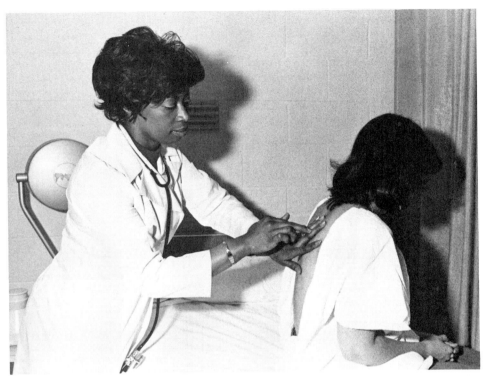

FIGURE 4.3 Examination by percussion. The physican produces sounds by tapping body surfaces with the fingers and then interprets the sounds.

Radiopaque dye can be injected into arteries and/or veins. As the dye is carried by the blood vessels within the organ being studied, x-ray films called arteriograms or angiograms are made. Blood vessels are studied.

Special preparation and patient consent are needed for these studies. Hemorrhage, dye allergy, and embolus or thrombus can be complications when large blood vessels are entered for diagnostic procedures.

Body section roentgenograms such as laminograms, tomograms, and planigrams are special x-rays taken at different levels or planes of the body until the area being studied comes clearly into focus. They are particularly helpful in studying areas that might otherwise be hidden or blurred by other body structures.

Usually, it is the responsibility of the nurse to prepare the patient for an x-ray. Knowing that metal objects are visible on an x-ray enables the nurse to remember to help the patient remove jewelry and clothing with metal fasteners. Some hospitals use

special x-ray gowns with ties rather than metal fasteners. The patient should also wear footwear and have a blanket in order to avoid accidents and chills in drafty corridors.

Fasting, cathartics, and enemas prior to or following x-ray procedures are common types of additional preparation in which the nurse usually is involved. Inadequate preparation of the patient may result in poor-quality x-rays which need to be repeated. This may be costly, uncomfortable, and tiring to the patient. Most agencies have information readily available to the nurse in order to assure adequate preparation of the patient for an x-ray procedure.

RADIOISOTOPE TRACER STUDIES

Minute amounts of radioisotope elements can be injected or swallowed by the patient. The material circulates through the body and concentrates in particular organs and tissues. Then, a sensitive device (scanner) is used to measure and record the distribution of the isotopes in the area being studied. In

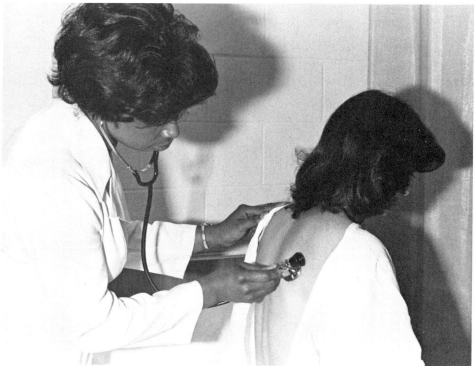

FIGURE 4.4   The physician is listening to sounds within the body by using a stethoscope. This is known as auscultation.

other words, a kind of map is made. Lung, bone, and brain are a few organs that can be studied using this method.

Since very small doses of radioisotopes are needed for these studies, the cells are not damaged. The procedure itself is painless but may be tiring since the patient must lie on a table for some time while the scanning is done.

ELECTRICAL STUDIES

Electricity released by body organs can be measured and recorded by placing small metal conductors (electrodes) on the skin. The electrocardiogram (ECG, EKG) is a record of the electrical activity in the heart. The electroencephalogram (EEG) is a record of the electrical activity within the brain.

ECHOGRAMS

Ultrasound waves can be transmitted to certain parts of the body. The waves are reflected or echoed back to a special receiver that records the pattern of the waves. The pattern is then analyzed by an expert to determine abnormalities. Pulmonary echograms and echoencephalograms are examples of these studies.

DIRECT VISUALIZATION STUDIES

Many parts of the body can be examined directly with special instruments. The nurse can generally recognize these studies by the suffix -oscopy, which appears after the name of the area to be studied. Similarly, the instrument used to examine can be recognized by the suffix -scope. The lighted hollow instrument, the endoscope, is passed into the area to be studied. The physician then looks through the endoscope at the area to be examined. Bronchoscopy, gastroscopy, and sigmoidoscopy are examples of direct visualization studies. Tissue or fluid can be withdrawn through the instrument for laboratory examination. Many direct visualization procedures require special patient preparation and/or consent prior to the examination. The nurse may be requested to observe and position the patient during and following the procedure. In some studies, a special camera is attached to the endoscope and pictures for later study are taken, as described in Chapter 15.

COMPUTERIZED AXIAL TOMOGRAPHY

Also known as a CT scan or CAT scan is a new type of scan that enables the physician to obtain detailed cross-sectional views of certain body organs and systems that previously could not be visualized. While the scanner takes views with an x-ray beam, a computer collects, analyzes, and makes a picture of the varying amounts of x-ray absorbed by the tissue. The scanner moves systematically around the person until the designated area has been scanned. The patient must lie still alone in a room with large equipment making clicking noises during the scan. A contrast dye is sometimes injected, and the scan is repeated. Normally, the procedure is not painful or dangerous. The nurse should ask the patient about iodine allergy before an iodine contrast dye is used (Figures 4.5, 4.6, 4.7, and 4.8).

SKIN TESTING

Reactions of the skin to small amounts of substances injected intracutaneously can help to determine the source of allergy or infection. Skin tests are discussed in Chapter 10.

Methods of Treatment

The treatment or therapy of a patient includes measures used to aid in recovery. It also includes measures to make the sick person comfortable and to prevent complications that can result from disease. As the leader of the health team, the physican plans medical treatment for the individual patient. Then other members of the health team implement parts of the treatment plan according to their area of expertise. For example, the physician might prescribe a special diet that would be arranged and taught by the dietitians. Another example is the doctor's order for a certain drug to be given by mouth. The pharmacist prepares and dispenses the drug to the nurse, who administers it to the patient. As an important member of the health team, the nurse needs an understanding of the types of therapy the doctor may prescribe.

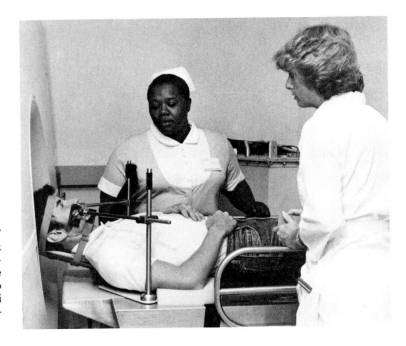

FIGURE 4.5 The practical/vocational nursing student is helping to position the patient for a CAT scan of the head. (Courtesy of Shapero School of Nursing, Sinai Hospital of Detroit, Detroit, Michigan.)

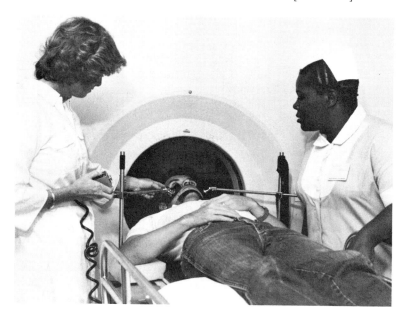

FIGURE 4.6 The patient's head is being placed in the CAT scan chamber. (Courtesy of Shapero School of Nursing, Sinai Hospital of Detroit, Detroit, Michigan.)

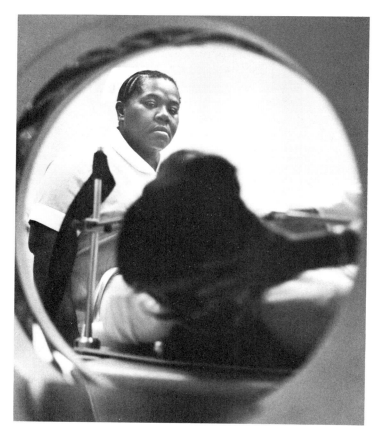

FIGURE 4.7 The patient's view from inside the chamber of the CAT scanner. (Courtesy of Shapero School of Nursing, Sinai Hospital of Detroit, Detroit, Michigan.)

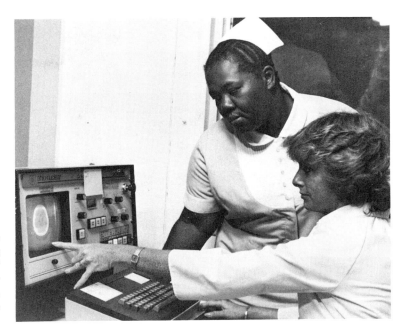

FIGURE 4.8 One of many views of the skull appears on the screen of the CAT scanner. (Courtesy of Shapero School of Nursing, Sinai Hospital of Detroit, Detroit, Michigan.)

DIET THERAPY

Diet therapy is the treatment of a patient by food (see Figure 4.9). The normal diet is modified to meet the requirements of an individual during illness. The physician prescribes the diet, and the dietitian arranges for it in the hospital. The *dietitian* is a person specially prepared in the scientific regulation of diet for healthful nutrition as well as for therapeutic reasons. Patients having certain diseases are treated primarily by diet. For example, one of the main treatments of a person with diabetes mellitus is diet.

The nurse is frequently responsible for some phase of diet therapy, such as preparing and serving food to the patient. For example, the nurse caring for a diabetic patient in the home would have the responsibility for either preparing the special diet or supervising its preparation. The nurse would also serve it and encourage the patient to eat. The nurse caring for a hospitalized diabetic patient might be responsible for serving the tray and feeding the patient. The nurse reports the amount eaten to the team leader or head nurse and records the amount in the nurses' notes. In order to assist properly in diet therapy, the nurse

needs to remember that the doctor's plan of treatment may fail in some cases if the dietary regimen is not followed accurately.

DRUG THERAPY

Drug therapy is the treatment of a person by the use of a substance that prevents, cures, treats, or relieves the symptoms of disease (see Figure 4.10). *Pharmacology* is the study of these substances, which are known as *drugs* or *medicines*. The scientific knowledge of drugs, such as the source, name, characteristics, and actions, is included in pharmacology.

The physician prescribes the drug. The *pharmacist* prepares, compounds, and dispenses the medicine. The nurse generally is responsible for its proper administration to the patient. In selected agencies where a unit dose system is used, the pharmacist or pharmacy technician sometimes administers medication. In some cases, the doctor administers the drug with the nurse's assistance. For instance, the nurse would assist in injecting medication intrathecally (into the spinal canal).

In general, qualified members of the nursing staff administer drugs orally (by mouth), subcutaneously (into the tissue im-

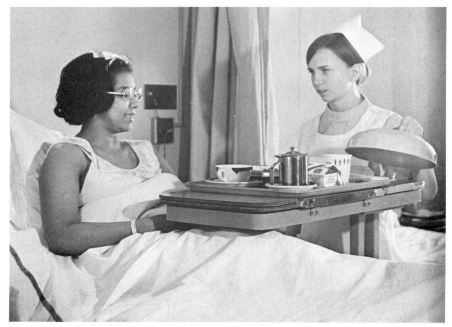

FIGURE 4.9   Diet therapy is the treatment of a patient by food. The licensed practical/vocational nurse plays an important role in this therapy. (Courtesy of Roanoke City Schools and Burrell Memorial Hospital School of Practical Nursing, Roanoke, Virginia.)

mediately under the skin), intramuscularly (into the muscle), rectally, and vaginally. Nurses also give medicine by local applications, sublingualy (under the tongue), and by inhalation. Professional nurses may give certain intravenous medications. In some hospitals and self-care units, patients are permitted to assume the responsibility for administering some of their own medications.

The number of drugs available is multiplying rapidly. Most patients are receiving more than one drug concurrently. An increasing problem for patients on drug therapy is unfavorable drug interaction. A *drug interaction* occurs when a person taking more than one drug experiences effects that could not have been predicted on the basis of what is known about each drug alone.

A wide variety of physical and mental disturbances have been experienced by patients during a drug interaction. Nightmares, nausea and vomiting, and bleeding are examples of clues that may indicate a possible interaction. Physicians and pharmacists often have difficulty determining whether the patient's symptoms and signs result from the disease or drug therapy.

Drug interactions may have unpleasant or even fatal consequences if undetected. Thus, the nurse's observations, reports, and records are extremely important. For example, Mrs. Price is an 86-year-old woman who has been hospitalized for a fractured right radius and is in a cast. Mrs. Price told the nurse about waking up on the floor after a nightmare at home. In further conversation, the nurse learned that Mrs. Price had taken three different medications just before bedtime and that each drug had been prescribed by a different physician. The nurse reported these facts to the physican and pharmacist who determined that a drug interaction had caused the nightmare and indirectly the fracture. The consequences might have been even more drastic if the fracture had required Mrs. Price to move to a nursing home temporarily or permanently for assistance with daily activities. The nurse's observations and reporting enable the physician to discover the drug interaction.

The *drug profile* is a special individual

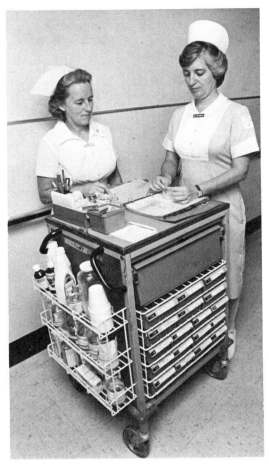

FIGURE 4.10 Drug therapy is the treatment of a person by the use of a plant, animal, or mineral substance. The practical/vocational nursing student is learning to administer medications. (Courtesy of Fredericksburg Area School of Practical Nursing, Fredericksburg, Virginia.)

patient record developed by the pharmacist for the purpose of anticipating and preventing potential drug interactions. The profile, which is usually located in the pharmacy, contains patient information such as age, diagnosis, body weight, and drug allergies as well as specific drugs and dosages, and laboratory values. The information is updated regularly. Computers are tools used in some hospital pharmacies to maintain a drug profile.

Because nonprescribed drugs also may be involved in drug interactions, it is very important for the nurse to ask the patient specifically about the use of laxatives, sleeping aids, painkillers, and cold remedies. Often patients do not mention these medications when providing information for the nursing history. Nonprescribed drugs also are recorded on the drug profile when known.

Recent studies indicate that food and fluids consumed by the patient exert a greater influence on drug activity than was previously realized. The student nurse learning about a particular drug should include information about the effect of food or fluid on that drug. It is especially important for patients to know about specific foods or fluids that should be avoided when taking a drug.

In some hospitals and agencies, the nurse instructs the patient and/or family about drugs the patient is taking. Instructions about medications should be given to the patient and/or family orally and in writing. Guidelines for the nurse in providing complete and accurate information are summarized below. Before using these guidelines, the nurse should check the hospital or agency policy.

- Name of the drug. Example: digoxin.
- General purpose for which the drug is prescribed. Example: to strengthen the heart's pumping action.
- Dosage information—how much, how to measure, when to be taken, how long to be taken. Example: .125 mg, that is one tablet every morning at the same hour, indefinitely. The physician has prescribed refills when you use up this container.
- What are warning signals and what to do if they occur. Example: blurred vision, nausea, lack of appetite, diarrhea, a change noticed in the heartbeat. If these occur, notify your doctor at once.
- Food, beverages, activities, to be included or avoided. Example: a balanced diet, but avoid other drugs unless specifically prescribed by the physician. Tell a new physician you are on this drug.
- Storage information. Example: keep in cabinet away from children.
- Special information. Example: suggest you carry information at all times that indicates that you are on this drug in case of accident or emergency.

NURSING AS THERAPY

Nursing provides substantial therapeutic benefits for the patient. Although this is not widely recognized as specific therapy, the nurse should consider carefully how nursing activities contribute to the patient's comfort and recovery.

As mentioned previously, nurses carry out many parts of the patient's medical treatment plan. Nurses observe, report, and record on a continuous basis the patient's response to illness and medical therapies.

In addition, the nursing care plan includes measures designed to assist the individual with the impact of illness. The common nursing practices described in Chapter 1 are tools the nurse uses. The nursing process described in Chapter 1 is the method the nurse uses. The student may want to review those sections at this time. As a result of nursing care, the patient experiences increased feelings of well-being that have a positive effect on the response to illness and treatment. Generally, it is the patient's requirement for continuous nursing care before, during, and/or after diagnosis and treatment that indicates the need for hospitalization.

PHYSICAL THERAPY

Physical therapy is the use of physical agents and special procedures, such as massage and exercise. Heat, cold, electricity, water, and rays, such as infrared and ultraviolet, are examples of physical agents. These agents may involve the use of very simple methods or the use of highly technical machines. Physical therapy is used in the treatment of a patient with signs and symptoms affecting the muscles, joints, or nerves responsible for movement. The *physical therapist* is a person specially prepared in the use of these physical agents and special procedures. The *physiatrist* is a physician who specializes in diagnosis and treatment using physical agents.

The doctor prescribing physical therapy works with the physical therapist to determine the amount of disability and plan the course of treatment. Members of the nursing staff frequently are asked to assist in physical therapy. For example, the physical therapist may ask the nursing staff to observe the patient who is practicing a new method of getting out of bed. Another kind of assistance from the nurse is not to perform a particular activity which the patient needs to practice in order to recover strength, function, and flexibility. Assisting and encouraging the patient with a passive or active exercise program are other ways the nurse participates in physical therapy.

OCCUPATIONAL THERAPY

Occupational therapy uses creative and manual arts and techniques found in recreation and industry to assist the patient to improve self-care skills. The treatment is through purposeful activities designed to be consistent with the patient's needs and interests. The patient actively participates in activities that aid and contribute to recovery from disease and injury. The *occupational therapist* is a person specially prepared to design, initiate, and teach these activities.

Occupational therapy benefits the patient in many ways. Substituting activity for inactivity often reduces or prevents regression and depression. Arts and crafts projects are used to create opportunities for a patient to participate in a project and experience a feeling of productivity. The emphasis is not on the craft being done or the object being made but on the activity of the body and mind. Self-care training in activities of daily living such as dressing, eating, and manipulating doors, telephone dials, and light switches is another benefit of occupational therapy.

Activities are designed for the specific patient. For example, activity designed for a disabled person who can no longer work is likely to be different from that designed for a person whose disability requires new skills for a change of employment.

Physical and occupational therapy are often thought to be closely related. Both types of therapists may work with the same handicapped patients. However, the tools of each type of therapy are different. As previously mentioned, the physical therapist applies physical agents and special procedures to the patient. These agents and procedures are usually controlled by the physical therapist. The activities of occupational therapy are those in which the patient is participating. The patient's interest motivates activity.

PSYCHOTHERAPY

Psychotherapy means treatment of the mind through a direct relationship between a patient or a group of patients and a therapist. The *psychiatrist* is a physican specializing in this type of therapy. The *psychologist* is another specialist who practices psychotherapy.

During psychotherapy, the patient is helped to explore aspects of thinking, emotions, and behavior as they relate to illness. In addition, the patient is assisted to develop new ways of thinking, feeling, and behaving that are consistent with healthier living.

SURGERY

Surgery is a branch of medicine dealing with the treatment of disease by operation and by manipulation, which means skillful use of the hands. For example, the physician treats a patient with a stone (calculus) in the common bile duct by operating to remove the stone. A stone can obstruct the flow of bile from the gallbaldder and cause a disturbance in fat digestion. The surgeon treats a patient with a dislocated shoulder by skillfully using the hands to manipulate and place the bone back in the joint. The *surgeon* is a physician who has specialized in this type of therapy. The responsibilities of the nurse in caring for a patient treated with surgery are discussed in Chapter 6.

RESPIRATORY THERAPY

Respiratory therapy is the use of gases, humidity, and medication inhaled by the patient to treat disease (Figure 4.11). Oxygen and carbon dioxide are examples of gases commonly inhaled by patients during respiratory therapy. The respiratory therapist and technician are persons with special education who administer this therapy and maintain the equipment.

The nurse at times assists the therapist or technician and may administer types of therapy when supervised by the respiratory therapist or professional nurse. Oxygen

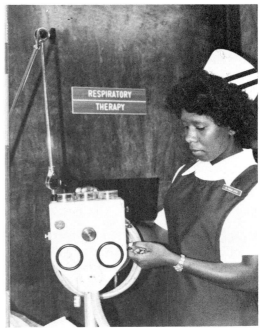

FIGURE 4.11 An intermittent positive pressure breathing machine (IPPB) is one form of respiratory therapy. (Courtesy of Washington County School of Practical Nursing, Neff Vocational Center, Abingdon, Virginia.)

therapy and humidity are two examples of respiratory therapy frequently administered by the nurse.

RADIOTHERAPY

Radiotherapy uses x-rays, radium, and artificial radioactive isotopes to destroy cells, especially malignant ones. The radioactivity for radiotherapy results from the release of parts of the atom from the unstable artificial isotypes and radium as well as radioactive rays produced by x-ray machines. The rays from these sources are capable of destroying malignant cells. These malignant cells are more sensitive to radiotherapy than are normal ones. A *radiologist* is a specially trained physician who prescribes and supervises radiotherapy.

Patients are often upset when the physician tells them they should have treatment by radiotherapy. This type of treatment may establish the diagnosis of a malignancy in a person's mind. The nurse assists the patient receiving radiotherapy by active listening as described in Chapter one, by referring specific questions to the physician, and by helping to prevent and/or minimize undesirable side effects. Additional information on the use of radiotherapy and related nursing measures can be found in Chapter 9.

PARENTERAL FLUID AND ELECTROLYTE THERAPY

When a patient is unable to drink a sufficient quantity of fluids or loses an excessive amount of body fluid, the necessary fluids have to be replaced or supplied by means other than the oral route. The most common way for these fluids to be administered is *parenterally*, which means that the fluid is given by a route other than the alimentary tract. The most common way is the intravenous (into the vein) route (see Figure 4.12). Fluids also may be given into subcutaneous tissue; this method is called hypodermoclysis. The physician orders fluid therapy and specifies the type of fluids to be used, the amount, the route, and the rate of flow. The most common fluid given is glucose—5 percent in distilled water or normal saline. Other solutions also may be ordered for specific conditions.

All body fluids contain chemicals called electrolytes. *Electrolytes* are electrically charged particles that play vital roles in cell functioning. They are essential for maintaining the health of the body. The most common electrolytes are sodium (Na), potassium (K), chloride (CI), and bicarbonate (HCO_3). These particles are normally lost through the kidneys, skin, and lungs. A person who eats a general diet normally replaces those electrolytes by the food and beverages consumed.

However, almost all medical and surgical conditions disrupt normal electrolyte balance. When large amounts of body fluids are lost through excessive perspiration, severe wounds, or extensive burns, the electrolytes contained in those fluids are lost as well. These electrolytes may be replaced either orally or parenterally. When the need for electrolyte replacement is extensive or urgent, the intravenous route is usually used. Fluids containing electrolytes are not given

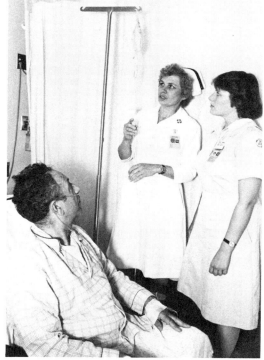

FIGURE 4.12 The licensed practical/vocational nursing student caring for the patient receiving parenteral fluid and electrolyte therapy. (Courtesy of Bergen Pines County Hospital School of Practical Nursing, Paramus, New Jersey.)

by hypodermoclysis for they can cause damage to the subcutaneous tissue.

The practical nurse plays a vital role in determining the patient's fluid and electrolyte balance. In order to prescribe the appropriate therapy, the physician needs an accurate record of the patient's intake and output. The nursing staff is responsible for maintaining that accurate and current record. All fluids consumed by the patient both orally and parenterally are measured and recorded. Likewise, all output is measured and recorded. The output includes not only urine, but also vomitus, wound drainage, and fluid from various body cavities being drained by tubes. In addition, a record is kept describing the number and consistency of stools. This enables the physician to estimate fluid lost through the gastrointestinal tract.

The record of daily weight aids in determining dehydration or the accumulation of fluid in the tissues or body cavities. The nurse should weight the patient at the same time each day, in the same amount of clothing, and using the same scales.

The practical nurse also is often asked to assist in the replacement of fluids and electrolytes. For example, the nurse may help the physician or professional nurse to start an intravenous infusion. When parenteral fluids are running, the nurse may be asked to check the rate of flow. This means that the number of drops per minutes must be counted and reported. The flow rate may require adjustment when it is faster or slower than the rate prescribed by the physician.

The intravenous site is also observed frequently for infiltration. An infiltration occurs when an intravenous needle or catheter becomes dislodged from the vein and fluids flow into the tissue instead of the vein. Swelling around the needle, a slowing of the flow rate, and the patient's report of a burning, stinging sensation at the needle site are indications of an infiltration. The head nurse or team leader should be notified immediately (Figure 4.13).

The patient receiving intravenous fluids is observed frequently for signs of overload. Fluid overload occurs when a patient receives more fluids than the circulatory and renal system can manage. Elderly patients and those with heart and/or kidney disease are more likely to develop fluid overload. A potentially fatal condition which may develop from fluid overload is pulmonary edema. Symptoms of pulmonary edema include restless behavior, difficult breathing (dyspnea), cough, and irregular pulse. If these symptoms appear while a patient is receiving intravenous therapy, the patient's head should be elevated and the head nurse or team leader notified immediately.

REHABILITATION

Rehabilitation may be defined as helping the patient to regain the greatest amount of usefulness and the maximum degree of func-

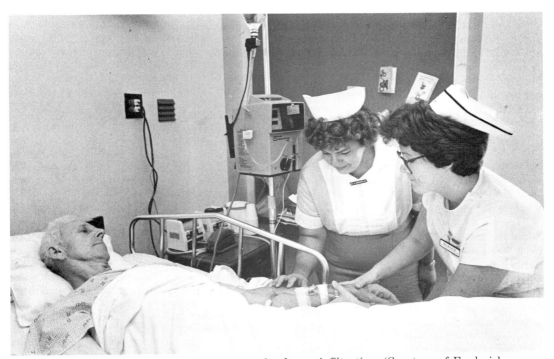

FIGURE 4.13 Checking the intravenous site for an infiltration. (Courtesy of Fredericksburg Area School of Practical Nursing, Fredericksburg, Virginia.)

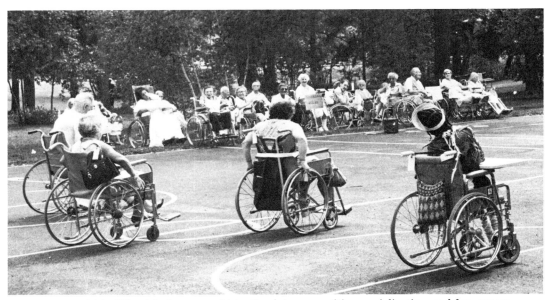

FIGURE 4.14 Wheelchair races, which stimulate competition, socialization, and fun, are arranged by recreational therapists. (Courtesy of Bergen Pines County Hospital School of Practical Nursing, Paramus, New Jersey.)

tion possible within the limitations of a handicap.

A full rehabilitation program includes all aspects of the person (Figure 4.14). Mental, physical, social, vocational, and economic factors are considered in relation to a particular individual. After studying the individual, a rehabilitation plan is designed.

Various professionals provide their expertise to the patient as needed. For example, a speech therapist teaches the patient to talk if that is needed. A physical therapist develops an exercise plan in preparation for walking if that is indicated. The occupational therapist teaches the patient new ways to dress and eat in light of the disease.

The social worker may visit the family at home to assist with preparations for the patient's discharge. The vocational counselor helps the patient to explore and develop new work goals, skills, and opportunities in light of the handicap. The nurse supervises, encourages, and gives feedback to the patient practicing new skills on the nursing unit.

Members of the rehabilitation team meet regularly to communicate, cooperate, and coordinate the plan so that the patient receives maximum benefit from the help available.

Case Study Involving Causes of Disease and Methods of Treatment

Miss Smith is a 19-year-old college student who was admitted to the hospital with fever, cough, and malaise that had persisted for three weeks. The physician ordered blood studies, collections of urine and sputum for laboratory analysis, and a chest x-ray (roentgenogram). The combined results of these studies indicated pneumonia in the right lung caused by bacteria. An appropriate antibiotic was administered intravenously. Inhalation therapy was ordered also. The patient was instructed to increase her intake of oral fluids. After one week of treatment, Miss Smith was discharged from the hospital on oral antibiotic therapy.

QUESTIONS

1. What are the responsibilities of nursing personnel concerning the collection of specimens?
2. What is the role of the licensed practical/vocational nurse in intravenous fluid and drug therapy in your agency?
3. What other factors might have influenced the development of pneumonia in Miss Smith?
4. Describe three nursing actions related to diet therapy.
5. What observations and recordings should the nurse make?

Suggestions for Further Study

1. What bodily symptoms have you experienced because of emotions?
2. Is there an inhalation therapy department in your hospital? If so, try to make arrangements for a visit.
3. Discuss the use of a drug profile with the hospital pharmacist in regard to its advantages.
4. Mason, Mildred A.; Bates, Grace F; and Smola, Bonnie K.: *Workbook in Basic Medical-Surgical Nursing*, 3rd ed. Macmillan Publishing Company, New York, 1984, Exercise 4.

Additional Readings

Carbary, Lorraine Judson, and Carbary, Clinton: "Positive Identification of Patients." *Journal of Nursing Care*, 14:18–21 (Feb.), 1981.

Deni, Laura: "The Nightmare of Sleep Problems." *Journal of Nursing Care,* 13:8–9 and 27 (May), 1980.

Haughey, Cynthia Weidman: "What to Say and Do When Your Patient Asks About CT Scans." *Nursing 81*, 11:72–77 (Dec.), 1981.

Herzoff, Nancy, E.; Stoklosa, Jean M.; and Tierney, Mary Jo: "Therapeutic Nursing: Practical Principles for the Medical/Surgical Nurse." *Journal of Practical Nursing*, 31:22–25 (Nov.–Dec.), 1981.

Lee, Margaret M.: "Stress: How to Manage It Yourself." *Journal of Nursing Care* 14:22–25 (June), 1981.

McConnell, Edwinna: "Urinalysis: A Common Test, But Never Routine." *Nursing 82*, 12:108–11 (Feb.), 1982.

McHugh, Norma G.; Christman, Norma J.; and Johnson, Jean E.: "Preparatory Information: What Helps and Why." *American Journal of Nursing*, 82:780–82 (May), 1982.

Rambo, Beverly J., and Wood, Lucile A. (eds.): *Nursing Skills for Clinical Practice*, 3rd ed. W.B. Saunders Co., Philadelphia, 1982, pp. 259-71, 463-84, and 661-79.

Robinson, Corinne H.: *Basic Nutrition and Diet Therapy*, 4th ed. Macmillan Publishing Co., Inc., New York, 1980, pp. 91–100 and 191–97.

Sackheim, George I., and Lehman, Dennis D.: *Chemistry for the Health Sciences*, 4th ed. Macmillan Publishing Co., Inc., New York, 1981, pp. 480–96.

Smith, Marcy J. T., and Selyé, Hans: "Stress—Reducing the Negative Effects of Stress." *American Journal of Nursing*, 79:1953-55 (Nov.), 1979.

"Test Yourself: Diagnostic Scanning Procedure and Ultrasonography." *American Journal of Nursing*, 80:2005, 2105 (Nov.), 1980.

Tobiason, Sarah Jane Bradford: "Touching Is for Everyone." *American Journal of Nursing*, 81:728-30 (Apr.), 1981.

Chapter 5

The Patient with an Inflammation*

Expected Behavioral Outcomes	Nursing Observations
Vocabulary Development	Nursing Interventions
Inflammatory Process	Case Study Involving Inflammation
Inflammation and Infection	Suggestions for Further Study
Assisting with Diagnostic Tests	Additional Readings

Expected Behavioral Outcomes

Minimum objectives referred to as expected behavioral outcomes have been designed for the practical/vocational nursing student to use as guides in studying this chapter. The student should read these expected outcomes before studying the chapter.

The objectives can be used as guides for study.

Using the content of this chapter, the student should return to the objectives and evaluate the ability to:

1. *Discuss with a classmate a personal experience with inflammation as a result of each injury discussed in the chapter.*
2. *Prepare an outline comparing (a) the body defenses that come into play when no pathogens are introduced with injury with (b) the body defenses that come into play when pathogens are associated with an injury.*
3. *Tell whether an immunity is active or passive when given a hypothetic situation.*
4. *Indicate whether the symptoms are local or general when given a list of symptoms.*

5. *Outline the correct nursing care when given a hypothetic situation in which the patient has general and local symptoms of inflammation.*
6. *State the effects of heat and the precautions associated with its application.*
7. *List at least two therapeutic effects and two toxic effects relevant to nursing care when given the names of several drugs.*

Vocabulary Development

The following prefixes, suffixes, and combining forms pertain to this chapter. By learning and/or reviewing their meanings, the practical/vocational nursing student will have the keys needed to unlock many exciting new medical terms.

Discover the meaning of these keys in a medical dictionary or in the content of this chapter. How does each key pertain to this chapter? In your notebook write the correct meaning of each prefix, suffix, or combining form listed below. Illustrate each key with an example.

bacill—rod, small staff. Ex. *bacillary*—a rod-shaped organism.

anti-	erythro-
bacill-	exo-
bacter-	febr-
cocc-	-form
endo-	gest-

*Revised by the authors and Portia E. Richardson, R.N., M.A., who is Department Chairman of the Central School of Practical Nursing and Staff Nurse at Norfolk Community Hospital in Norfolk, Virginia.

-itis	pur-	sit-	therm-
micr-	py-	spectr-	tox-
-myces	rub(r)-	spor-	traumat-
path-	sep-	staphyl-	vacc-
phag-	sept-	tect-	

The Inflammatory Process

The individual with an inflammation has a defensive reaction of the body to an injury. The suffix *-itis* means "inflammation of." The hundreds of medical terms ending with *-itis* indicate the frequency with which a nurse is called upon to care for a patient with an inflammation. Appendicitis, tonsilitis, colitis, and sinusitis are only a few examples. The first part of these words indicates the part of the body that is inflamed. Since inflammations occur so often, the nurse must have a basic understanding of the changes that occur in the patient's body.

The process of inflammation involves the blood vessels, fluid, and cellular components of the blood and the connective tissue surrounding the damaged area. Inflammation is an important defensive reaction to injury because its main function is to destroy or neutralize the injurious agent and to prepare the involved tissue for repair.

CAUSES

Injury to the body tissue is produced by the surgeon's scalpel, a blow, a foreign body, a chemical; also by electricity, heat, cold, or a pathogenic microorganism (pathogen). A microorganism is a tiny living body that is visible only through a microscope. Disease-producing microorganisms are called *pathogens*. The inflammatory process produced by a pathogen is called an *infection*.

BODY DEFENSES

The human body is surrounded by environmental forces that are constantly threatening the individual as a whole. The body responds to these threats through many forms of adaptation. These mechanisms of adaptation are designed to protect the body from both external and internal harmful agents.

The range of body defenses that have been adapted to protect the human body is both exciting and complex. For our purpose these body defenses will be divided on the basis of where the line of defense is formed, that is external nonspecific and internal nonspecific defenses. The nonspecific mechanism means that these defenses are directed against any foreign substance or invader.

EXTERNAL NONSPECIFIC BODY DEFENSES. The skin and the mucous membrane make up the body's first line of defense against penetration by foreign materials, including pathogenic microorganisms. When the skin is unbroken, it provides a physical barrier to undesirable environmental forces such as heat, cold, and trauma. The skin responds to undesirable invaders by a process call *keratinization*. During the process of keratinization, the skin becomes hard and tough and develops a so-called waterproof covering.

Ordinarily, the skin does permit the growth of microorganisms on the upper, outermost layers and within hair follicles and sweat glands. These microorganisms normally live on the skin and are grouped as nonpathogenic microbes.

The skin and mucous membrane surfaces are good surfaces for the growth and multiplication of certain microbes. The microbes that normally grow in these areas are called normal microbic flora and do not pose a threat to the human body. The presence of normal microbic flora makes it difficult for pathogenic organisms to grow on body surfaces since transient microbes have to compete for nutrients and space that would be essential for growth. If these nonpathogenic microbes enter the tissue of a person with lowered resistance, they may cause significant problems.

The integrity of the skin is broken during surgical operations, arterial catheterization procedures, physical irritation, or trauma. The likelihood that microorganisms will gain entrance to the body increases tremendously as a result of these causes. The skin must be kept relatively dry since continued moisture tends to cause damage to the skin. Essential skin oils should be supplemented through the use of lotions since dry, cracked skin is an entrance for microbes.

Mucous membranes line all body orifices that have external openings and the eyes. When intact, the mucous membranes, like skin, do not allow foreign materials or microorganisms to invade. The mucous membranes increase the secretion of mucus when attacked by invading microorganisms. Cilia also help to protect the body. These are hairlike projections of mucous membrane in various parts of the body. For example, the cilia lining the nose, trachea, and bronchi remove excess mucus and foreign bodies from the upper respiratory tract by their wavelike motion. Hair lining the margins of the nostrils helps to remove foreign material from the air we breathe.

Other structures and functions of the body serve an important role in body defense. The blinking and sneezing reflexes guard the eyes and upper respiratory tract against irritants. Foreign material that does gain entrance to the eye tends to be washed out by tears. The flushing action of saliva and urine prevents the buildup of microorganisms. Vomiting and diarrhea are body defenses which remove harmful products from the gastrointestinal tract.

Many areas of the body are protected by the presence of antimicrobial chemicals that provide protection. The acid and salt concentrations of perspiration provide an unfavorable environment for the growth of some microorganisms. The acid-alkaline balance of certain body fluids such as gastrointestinal juices and vaginal secretions inhibits the growth or kills many organisms.

Vaginal secretions are an acid medium. When either the amount or the acidity of the vaginal secretions is reduced, the chances of a vaginal infection increase. Since vaginal secretions are not present prior to puberty and are greatly reduced after menopause, both young girls and older women are more susceptible to vaginitis.

Lysozmye is an antimicrobial factor in the body. Lysozmye is an enzyme present in mucus, tears, saliva, and skin secretions and also is found in many of the internal fluids and cells of the body. It is capable of destroying many gram-positive organisms. As an internal antimicrobial factor, it works with certain blood factors to destroy bacteria.

INTERNAL NONSPECIFIC DEFENSES. When a foreign invader penetrates the external body defenses and invades the internal environment of the body, it is met by more complex defenses. The physiologic reactions that occur to inhibit the growth of and/or kill the invading agent involve the interactions of cells of the blood, reticuloendothelial system, vascular system, and body tissues.

The blood plays an essential role in providing protection against foreign agents. The blood transports necessary materials to the site of injury or invasion. Because of specific vascular changes, the blood concentrates these materials at the site of invasion. The cellular materials that provide nonspecific defenses include different types of white blood cells. Some of the white blood cells or leukocytes are more important than others because of their phagocytic activity.

The fluid portion of unclotted blood, which is called plasma, also provides nonspecific body defenses. Plasma transports antibodies that aid the white blood cells in engulfing foreign invaders. Plasma contains another substance called fibrin. *Fibrin* causes a meshwork to form, thereby sealing off the injured part and trapping the phagocytic cells within the area.

The reticuloendothelial system is a widespread system of phagocytic cells scattered throughout various body tissues. The role of these cells is to ingest and digest foreign invaders that are causing damage to human tissues. Some phagocytic cells are found in such tissues as lymphoid tissue, liver, spleen, bone marrow, lungs, and blood vessels.

Interferon is a protein substance produced by certain virally infected cells. The protein is released into the blood and, when taken up by uninfected cells, it can protect those cells from the virus. Interferon plays a significant role in the recovery from viral infections; however, it has never been shown conclusively that it is a necessary part of defense against viral infection.

INFLAMMATORY RESPONSE

First, let us examine a simple inflammatory process that is not caused by a pathogen, as in the case of the incision made by the surgeon's sterile scalpel. Tissues surrounding the incision respond immediately to the injury by starting a mild inflammatory process. The cells damaged by the scalpel release a chemical, *histamine*, which is picked up by the blood. The first reaction to this release of histamine is an increased blood supply to the area. Blood vessels dilate, and the flow of blood within this area is slower. The walls of the blood vessels adapt themselves to allow white blood cells and serum to leave the bloodstream and go directly to the injured part. The increased blood supply is spoken of as *congestion*. Since no pathogens are present because the incision was made with a sterile instrument, the inflammation begins to subside. The white blood cells or leukocytes take up the dead cells and return to the bloodstream. This process is called *phagocytosis*. The excess fluid is reabsorbed into the blood. The wound edges grow together, and the area soon heals.

When inflammation is caused by, or complicated by, pathogenic microorganisms, the body's defensive reaction starts in the same manner as described in the simple inflammatory process. After leaving the bloodstream, the leukocytes try to kill the invading organisms. Antitoxins and antibodies are two important immune substances that are carried to the area by blood serum. They act against the invader and counteract the toxins excreted by the pathogens. The battle between the defensive army and the invader has begun. If the immune substances and leukocytes are strong enough to kill the invader, inflammation begins to disappear.

External and internal body defenses are summarized in Table 5.1 and a summary of steps of the inflammatory response is in Table 5.2.

TISSUE REPAIR

Repair of the patient's tissue begins when the inflammatory process has subsided and pus and dead tissue have been removed.

TABLE 5.1
NONSPECIFIC BODY DEFENSES

EXTERNAL DEFENSES

A. Physical factors
   1. Skin
   2. Mucous membrane
   3. Specialized structures or materials
      a. Nasal hairs   e. Saliva
      b. Cilia   f. Urine
      c. Eyelids and eyelashes g. Vomiting
      d. Tears   h. Diarrhea

B. Chemical factors
   1. Body secretions
      a. Perspiration
      b. Gastric juices
      c. Vaginal secretions
   2. pH
   3. Lysozyme

C. Normal microbial flora

INTERNAL DEFENSES

A. Phagocytic cells

B. Blood
   1. White blood cells
   2. Antibodies
   3. Fibrin

C. Interferon

D. Inflammatory response

Pus is a local collection of dead tissue cells, bacteria, and dead white blood cells. Pus also may be referred to as exudate.

After the infected area is clean, new cells are produced to fill in the space left by the injury. The tissue may be repaired with (1) identical tissue or (2) scar tissue or fibrotic tissue.

When the patient has undergone a surgical procedure in which no pathogenic microorganisms or undue stress has been involved, healing takes place with identical tissue, and a small amount of scar tissue is formed. Almost always, unless there is need for drainage, the physician lines up the surfaces of the identical tissue to reestablish the formation of identical cells in the affected area. Identical tissue is sutured. This type of repair is referred to as *healing by first intention*. As the wound increases in

TABLE 5.2
SUMMARY OF STEPS OF THE INFLAMMATORY RESPONSE

STEPS	CAUSE	OUTCOME
1. Injury	Heat, cold, chemicals, trauma, infection	Cell and tissue damage

2. Vascular response
   a. Vessels dilate
   b. Fibrin clot formation
	Histamine and other chemicals released by injured tissue
	Clotting proteins in blood are activated due to injury
		Dilation of vessels causes stasis of blood and leukocytes
		Irritants or foreign invaders trapped in area

3. Fluid congestion	Histamine and other chemicals cause vessels in area to enlarge	Increased amount of white blood cells, blood serum, and 0_2 into tissue
4. Phagocytosis	Antibodies, fibrin, white blood cells, phagocytes	Accumulation of leukocytes and other substances in area Removal and digestion of foreign particles and damaged tissues
5. Healing	New tissue formation	Inflammatory process subsides Formation of identical tissue or scar tissue

size, healing in this manner is less likely to take place.

Healing of a wound that has been infected or traumatized is not likely to have the tissue replaced by identical cells. Highly specialized cells do not generally replace themselves with identical cells following an injury. The student will recall from the study of anatomy and physiology that cells of the central nervous system do not replace themselves.

In some cases, the edges of a wound are so far apart following an injury that it is not possible to pull them into proper alignment. Also, waste products of infection may separate the edges of the wound. The opening in skin provides an avenue for waste products and other dead cells to escape from the healing area. The surgeon may find it necessary to pack the wound to prevent it from healing at the top first. As the wound heals from the bottom, it has scar tissue to replace previous cells. When scar tissue has filled the defect associated with the wound, the skin may be sutured by the surgeon or it may be allowed to grow over the healed area. This process is referred to as *healing by second intention*. This process is also called *healing by granulation*.

Healing by third intention occurs in wounds that are large and gaping, such as a decubitus ulcer. Granulation tissue fills the gaps. Granulation tissue is formed from new connective tissue cells called fibroblasts in which capillaries from surrounding normal tissue extend to provide nourishment. The tissue is delicate and highly vascular. The nurse should avoid damaging this newly formed, delicate tissue when changing the dressing. Nonadherent dressings may be applied over the wound. Gauze that adheres to the tissue should be moistened with sterile normal saline before it is removed to avoid damaging the delicate granulation tissue. Healing by third intention results in a wider and deeper scar than that in second intention.

Inflammation and Infection

Many inflammations result from disease-producing microorganisms such as those that cause tuberculosis, typhoid fever, or pneumonia. Also, the inflammatory reaction of the body to other injuries is often complicated by pathogens, as in an infected burn or laceration. Since inflammation is so frequently associated with pathogenic organisms, this chapter deals primarily with inflammation resulting from infection or associated with an infection.

MICROORGANISMS

All microorganisms do not produce disease. Those that do not cause disease are referred to as nonpathogenic microorganisms. Many are beneficial to man, such as the yeast that causes bread to rise or the mold from which penicillin may be derived. These live minute particles may be compared with the families in your community. Members of certain groups have similar characteristics, just like the family who lives next door to you. They have group names. For example, the bacterium responsible for tuberculosis is *Mycobacterium tuberculosis.* The bacterium that causes leprosy is *Mycobacterium leprae.* Notice that the generic, or group, name for both is *Mycobacterium.* Members of the animal kingdom called protozoa cause malaria and amebic dysentery.

Viruses are infectious agents that are so small that they are visible only with the highpower electron microscope. Since viruses can reproduce only when they are within another living cell, they are known as intracellar parasites. Influenza, measles, and mumps are caused by different members of the virus group. Yeast and molds are fungi that belong to the plant kingdom. One member of this group causes athlete's foot and another causes thrush. Members of an-

other group of simple microorganisms in the plant kingdom are called bacteria. Typhoid fever and tuberculosis are produced by bacteria. Since bacteria produce most of the infectious diseases, it is necessary to learn more about them.

A common classification of bacteria is based upon their shapes (see Figure 5.1). (1) Those that are rod shaped are called "bacilli." Tuberculosis is an infection resulting from the tubercle bacillus. (2) Bacteria in the form of a corkscrew are refered to as "spirilla" or "spirochetes." Syphilis is caused by a spirochete. (3) Bacteria having round forms are referred to as "cocci." This group is further classified according to the way cocci grow in groups. (a) The oval-shaped bacteria that grow alone or in pairs are diplococci; a disease resulting from diplococci is pneumococcal pneumonia. (b) Streptococci grow in chain formation; scarlet fever is one of the many infections caused by streptococci. (c) Other members of the cocci group grow in clusters and are called staphylococci; an infection produced frequently by members of this group is a skin abscess or boil.

BACTERIA

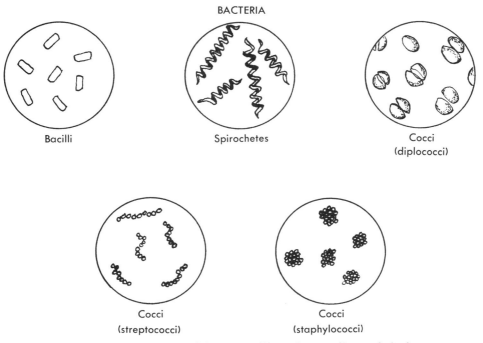

Bacilli

Spirochetes

Cocci
(diplococci)

Cocci
(streptococci)

Cocci
(staphylococci)

FIGURE 5.1 An illustration of the types of bacteria according to their shape.

Some bacteria produce toxins, which are poisonous substances. Toxins secreted by the living microorganisms are referred to as *exotoxins*. Poisons stored within the organism and given off after the bacterium's (singular for bacteria) death are *endotoxins*. Production of toxins by bacteria within the patient's body accounts for much of the general malaise.

A bacterium may go into a period of rest. During this time the protoplasm is concentrated into a small, round body and is covered with a tough membrane. Such a microorganism is spoken of as a spore. Spore-forming bacteria are difficult to kill during this resting stage. Thus, longer exposure to heat or to a disinfectant is required to kill them. A spore is resistant to excessive humidity, temperature, and drying and is capable of living for long periods of time in dust and soil. The autoclave, equipment used to sterilize with steam under pressure, is used frequently to kill spores. The bacillus causing tetanus or lockjaw is spore forming.

Bacteria are referred to as being gram negative or gram positive. This method of grouping bacteria is based upon their reaction to Gram's stain. This specially prepared blue stain is used in the laboratory to aid the medical technologist in identifying the microorganism. The gram-positive bacterium retains the blue color of the stain, and the gram-negative bacterium does not retain the blue color. For example, *Escherichia coli* is a species of gram-negative microorganism commonly called *E. coli*. The *E. coli* normally are found in the intestines of man, but when they enter the urinary tract, infection generally follows. The nurse may see a report of a urine culture that indicates that *E. coli* are present.

Microorganisms enter the body in the food we eat, the water we drink, and the air we inhale. Also, they may enter through a break in either the mucous membrane or the skin. However, a few pathogens can pass through the unbroken skin. Amebic dysentery is caused by the ameba that enters the mouth and continues down the gastrointestinal tract, which is lined with mucous membrane. The virus of the common cold and the tubercle bacillus may produce an infection after entering the body through inhaled air.

The *Anopheles* mosquito punctures the person's skin and deposits the microorganism responsible for malaria. Staphylococci sometimes pass through the hair follicles of the unbroken skin and cause a boil. Some microorganisms, such as *Treponema pallidum*, which causes syphilis, pass through the placenta and infect the fetus.

PREDISPOSING FACTORS TO INFECTION

After the pathogenic microorganism enters the body through the skin or mucous membrane, it may be carried to another part of the body by circulating body fluids, or it may remain at the point of entry. The pathogenicity of microorganisms to a given individual is determined by certain factors. Some of these factors are listed below.

- The *number* of invading microorganisms. A greater number of microorganisms invading the body increases the possibility of infection.
- The *virulence*—the ability to produce disease—of the invading microorganism. A more *virulent* pathogen is likely to produce a more serious disease.
- The presence of *conditions* necessary for reproduction of microorganisms, such as warmth, moisture, food, oxygen, and light.
- The effectiveness of the *defensive powers of the host*.
- Familiarity of the host with the *pathogen* (disease-causing microorganism). An individual who has not been in contact with the invading microorganism previously, is more likely to develop a disease from the unfamiliar pathogen.

NOSOCOMIAL INFECTIONS

Nosocomial infections are those infections acquired during hospitalization which were not present at the time of admission to the hospital. Some factors that predispose individual patients to hospital-acquired infections cannot be controlled by the nurses or other hospital workers. These factors may include the patient's age, the extent of the disease process, the type and number of invasive procedures administered, the therapy received, and the length of hospitalization.

The most common body sites affected by nosocomial infections are the urinary tract, surgical wounds, respiratory tract, and the bloodstream. The most recent organisms identified as causing nosocomial infections are *Pseudomonas* and *Serratia*. These organisms are identified as serious endemic hospital pathogens because they are transmitted from sources other than the patient and are frequently resistant to antibiotic therapy.

Patients are in contact with pathogenic microorganisms on a continuous basis. Exposure to these organisms may be through various sources. Some of these sources are hospital personnel, visitors, various organisms in the hospital environment, patient-to-patient use of various hospital equipment such as wheelchairs, physical therapy tanks, IPPB machines, and bathtub facilities. (Figure 5.2.)

ALTERATIONS OF INFLAMMATORY RESPONSE WITH INFECTION

In spite of the body defenses, some microorganisms will be successful in penetrating the barriers and they will invade the surrounding tissue causing cellulitis. When the body's resistance is too weak or the pathogens too strong, many tissue cells and leukocytes are killed. A collection of dead tissue cells, bacteria, and dead white blood cells is called *pus* or *exudate*. This process of pus formation is called *suppuration*. Infected particles that escape the area of battle are picked up by the lymph-vascular system. When these invaders reach the lymph nodes, specialized cells within the nodes try to render the bacteria harmless. Activity within the lymph nodes frequently causes them to enlarge. At the same time the body attempts to build a wall of white blood cells and tissue around the collection of pus. This collection of pus surrounded by a wall is known as an *abscess* or a *boil*. The abscess tends to enlarge as more pus is added and likewise tends to spread into the tissue that offers least resistance. If the abscess spreads toward a surface, it eventually ruptures. (Figures 5.3, 5.4, 5.5, and 5.6.) The physi-

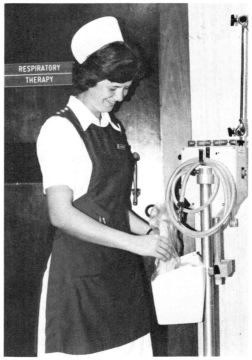

FIGURE 5.2   Proper handling of equipment helps to prevent nosocomial infection. (Courtesy of Washington County School of Practical Nursing, Neff Vocational Center, Abingdon, Virginia.)

cian may have to incise the area to let it drain. Another possible way in which the infection may terminate is for the abscess to be absorbed gradually into the lymph stream. The defenses of the body have successfully overcome the invader.

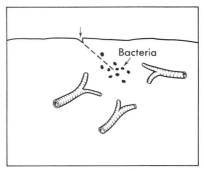

FIGURE 5.3   A break in the skin, allowing bacteria to enter.

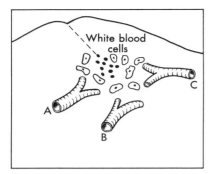

FIGURE 5.4   Blood vessels, *A, B,* and *C,* dilate after an injury. White blood cells and serum containing antitoxins and antibodies go to the injured part. The increased blood supply causes the area to swell.

When the breakdown of local barriers occurs and the specialized cells within the lymph and blood channels are unsuccessful in rendering the invading organism harmless, the organism colonizes in the bloodstream. After colonization, the pathogenic microorganism may cause a condition known as *septicemia* or pyemia and may also set up distant sites of infection throughout the body.

IMMUNE REACTION

Another type of response to infection is the immune reaction. This is a specific response against specific pathogens. The process by which the body has to overcome certain pathogens is also called the antigen-antibody response. An *antigen* is a foreign substance that causes the formation of antibodies in the body. Antigens are discussed further in Chapter 10 in relation to the patient with an allergy. The antibodies, which are formed as a result of the body's reaction to an antigen, and antitoxins are the important immune substances that are carried to the area of infection by blood serum. These antibodies and antitoxins act against the invader (antigen) and/or counteract the toxins excreted by the pathogens. The development of immunity depends on the ability of the body to recognize antigens as being foreign and to form antibodies that can assist in neutralizing or destroying the antigen. A person who is immune to a certain pathogen is protected against it.

There are five major classes of antibodies which are known as immunoglobulins. They are called IgG, IgA, IgM, IgD, and IgE and can be remembered by the acronym GAMDE. IgG, the most prevalent immunoglobulin, helps to fight toxins, viruses, and gram-positive bacteria. IgM is active against substances such as endotoxins of gram-negative bacteria. IgA is found in most secretions and body fluids such as tears, saliva, bile, and perspiration. It provides protection against viruses and bacteria which might enter the body via secretions and body fluids. IgE is associated with allergic reactions. The function of IgD is not yet known.

Other specialized cells that are an important part of the immune response are called *lymphocytes.* These specialized cells rapidly migrate to the site of injury. Once there, lymphocytes stimulate an increase in the production of immunoglobulins and influence the formation of other important substances such as interferon and certain toxins.

NATURAL AND ACQUIRED IMMUNITY

Immunity is classified as either natural or acquired, or active or passive. Natural immunity is defined as a natural resistance to specific pathogenic microorganisms that a person has at birth. The person inherits certain antibodies although no previous contact

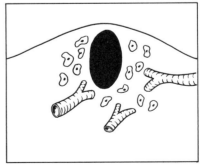

FIGURE 5.5   Pus forms when tissue cells, white blood cells, and bacteria are killed. White blood cells form a wall around the collection of pus, which is called an abscess. It spreads into the tissue that offers the least resistance.

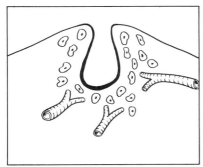

FIGURE 5.6 The abscess ruptures when it reaches the surface. The defenses of the body overcome the infection, and the wound heals.

with the infectious agent has occurred. A person's natural resistance to infectious diseases may be controlled or altered by such factors as diet, environment, or the virulence of the invading microorganism.

Although persons may inherit a natural resistance to certain infectious organisms, natural immunity also may be specific to a race, species, or individual. A comparison of natural and acquired immunity is given in Table. 5.3.

Species immunity is a type of natural immunity in which members of one species are resistant to infectious agents that cause disease in another species. For example, plant diseases rarely infect human beings.

Racial immunity is another type of natural immunity in which some families and races appear to be resistant to infectious agents that cause disease in other groups. For example, the effects of smallpox and tuberculosis vary widely between races and cultures.

Individual immunity is a third type of natural immunity in which an individual is highly resistant to an organism that normally causes disease. For example, one individual may have a high natural resistance throughout life to colds and flu, whereas another person becomes ill with colds and/or flu every winter.

ACQUIRED IMMUNITY. Acquired immunity is defined as a resistance to a specific pathogenic organism either by the individual actively producing antibodies or by the individual receiving antibodies from another person.

Acquired immunity may be either natural or artificial. Natural acquired immunity results from a disease process in the body. A person acquires immunity by producing antibodies in response to an antigen. Antibody production occurs when a person recovers from disease. For example, a child develops active acquired immunity to chickenpox by having the disease and recovering from it.

Artificial acquired immunity develops as a result of the individual receiving a vaccine. A *vaccine* is a preparation containing either the weakened or killed infectious agent causing a disease or a substance produced by the pathogenic microorganisms such as a toxin. After being administered, generally by injection, the vaccine causes the body to form antibodies that render the individual immune to that specific microorganism. Natural acquired or artificial acquired immunity usually makes the person permanently immune.

The person with passive, acquired immunity has received antibodies from another person or animal by injection or by transfer from the mother through the placenta during pregnancy. For example, when an individual is given an antitoxin or gamma globulin that contains antibodies from another source, human or animal, temporary immunity to that specific disease occurs. Since these antibodies were not developed by the person who received them, they do not remain in the blood serum. An example of this is seen in the individual who is injured with an object suspected of carrying tetanus organisms and has not been actively immunized against tetanus. That person may be temporarily protected by being given tetanus immune globulin or tetanus antitoxin.

Antibodies transmitted from a mother to her child through placenta circulation may last less than one year. Passive acquired immunity is a temporary immunity giving the individual immediate protection for a short period of time.

Assisting with Diagnostic Tests

The diagnostic evaluation may include culture and sensitivity tests, hematology studies, x-ray evaluations, and incision and drainage of abcess.

TABLE 5.3
COMPARISON OF NATURAL AND ACQUIRED IMMUNITY

TYPES OF IMMUNITY		
Natural Immunity	**Acquired Immunity**	
Immunity or resistance to specific pathogenic microorganisms or substances present at birth, may be species, racial, or individual	Immunity or resistance to specific microorganisms or substances which a person develops actively or passively during one's lifetime	
Natural Immunity	**Acquired Immunity**	
Influenced by diet, environment, and virulence of organism	Either natural or artificial	
Natural Acquired Immunity	**Artificial Acquired Immunity**	
Occurs in response to having a disease; individual develops own antibodies	Result of receiving injection of antibodies or vaccines; either active or passive	
Active Natural Immunity	**Active Immunity**	**Passive Immunity**
Usually permanent	Result of vaccines or toxoids	By immune serum or from mother through placenta circulation
	Active immunity takes a long time to develop but is usually permanent	Passive immunity is immediate but temporary

Culture and Sensitivity Test. The culture test confirms that infection is present and the specific organism responsible for the infection. The sensitivity test determines the chemotherapeutic agent most effective against the pathogenic agent. The data are a guide to diagnosis, treatment, and care of clients. An awareness of routine laboratory procedure is important. Prompt, accurate laboratory reports are possible only if specimens are properly collected and if they are accompanied by specific client data on laboratory requisitions. The specific client data should include information about medica-tions and the source and purpose of the specimen.

Specimens for culture and sensitivity that have been poorly collected may be rejected by the medical laboratory technologist. Poorly collected specimens yield unreliable results. In collecting specimens for culture and sensitivity tests, the following guidelines should be adhered to:

• collect fresh material
• avoid contamination from surrounding areas
• obtain cultures with sterile equipment

- place the culture in the appropriate container
- secure lids to avoid spillage and contamination
- collect the specimen before starting antimicrobial drug therapy
- label the specimen immediately after collection

HEMATOLOGY STUDIES

Diagnosis is also made by the examination of certain specific blood elements. These studies may include blood cultures, erythrocyte sedimentation rate (ESR), and a complete blood count (CBC) (See Tables 5.4 and 5.5). Blood samples for hematology studies may be collected by the laboratory technician at any time. No specific preparation is necessary; however, the client must be told that it involves having a venipuncture. The nurse should assist and provide emotional support to the client during the procedure.

X-RAY STUDIES

X-ray studies will determine the presence and extent of inflammation and infection in certain body areas. For instance, infection in bone tissue may be denoted as decreased density of bone; lung infection will be seen as increased density of lung tissue. Inflammation of the sinuses (sinusitis)

TABLE 5.4
SELECTED HEMATOLOGY LABORATORY TESTS PERTINENT TO INFLAMMATION

TESTS	NORMAL VALUE	PURPOSE
1. Blood culture	Absence of bacteria	To determine presence of bacteria in bloodstream
2. Complete blood count	Each of these is discussed separately in this summary	To obtain the values of the following formed parts of the patient's blood 1. Red blood cells 2. Hemoglobin 3. Hematocrit 4. White blood cells 5. Platelet count
3. Erythrocyte sedimentation rate (ESR)	Westergren method Men: 1–10 mm in 1 hr Women: 1–20 mm in 1 hr. Wintrobe method Men: 0–9 mm in 1 hr Women: 0–20 mm in 1 hr	To evaluate the body's response to inflammation, infarction, neoplasm, collagen diseases, nephritis, and tuberculosis
4. Hematocrit (packed cell volume)	Men: 40–54 volumes % Women: 37–47 volumes %	To indicate the percentage volume of erythrocytes of whole blood
5. Hemoglobin	Men: 14–18 gm/100 ml Women: 12–16 gm/100 ml	To determine the amount of hemoglobin in red blood cells that enables these cells to transport oxygen to cells and carbon dioxide from cells
6. Platelet count (thrombocytes)	150,000–450,000/cu mm	To evaluate the ability of the blood to coagulate
7. Red blood cell count (erythrocyte count)	Men: 4.6–6.2 million/cu mm Women: 4.2–5.4 million/cu mm	To determine the ability of the blood to carry oxygen to cells, carry carbon dioxide from cells, and maintain normal acid-base balance
8. White cell count (leukocyte count)	5,000–10,000/cu mm	To indicate the body's response to infection and other diseases

Table 5.5
Normal Leukocyte Count in Adults (Differential)

Type of White Cell	Range (per cu mm)	Relative Percentage	What May Variations Indicate?
1. Neutrophils	2500–7500	(40–75)	An increase may indicate such conditions as convulsions, strenuous exercise, acute infections, myocardial infarction, neoplasms, hemorrhage, uremia, diabetic coma, certain drugs, and collagen diseases. A decrease may indicate such conditions as drug poisoning, a deficiency of vitamin B_{12}, acute virus infections, malaria, typhoid fever, an overwhelming infection, lupus erythematosus, and anaphylactic shock
2. Eosinophils	100–300	(0–5)	An increase may be associated with such conditions as allergic reactions, certain malignancies, Addison's desease, and infections caused by parasites. A decrease may indicate acute bacterial infections
3. Basophils	0–100	(<1)	An increase is not common; a decrease may be associated with steroid therapy
4. Lymphocytes	1500–3500	(20–45)	An increase may be associated with such conditions as an acute infection, recovering from viral or bacterial infections, tuberculosis, syphilis, hepatitis, myasthenia gravis, and leukemia
5. Monocytes	200–800	(2–10)	An increase of monocytes may be associated with such conditions as tuberculosis, subacute bacterial endocarditis, malaria, Hodgkin's disease, and leukemia
	Total 4000–11,000		

may be seen as increased fluid level in the sinuses. Thrombophlebitis can be detected by a type of x-ray called a venogram.

Soft tissue infection or inflammation may not be detected on x-ray examination. For example, an infection of the tissue of the forearm which has not penetrated the bone will not present abnormal findings on the x-ray film.

INCISION AND DRAINAGE

Incision and drainage of an abscess is a procedure that may be done for both diagnostic and therapeutic purposes. An abscess is a zone of inflammation containing dead cells and living and dead leukocytes and bacteria. The abscess may rupture spontaneously or be incised (opened) and drained. Drainage of the abscess enables the exudate to flow to the outside. Healing is facilitated because materials within the abscess escape. This avoids a lengthy process of reabsorp-

tion and digestion of infectious material that must precede healing.

An abscess is also incised and drained to obtain a specimen for diagnostic purposes. The specimen may be sent to the laboratory for culture and sensitivity tests.

An abscess is not incised and drained until the walling-off process is completed. Some persons may refer to walling-off as the abscess "coming to a head." If the walling-off process is interrupted, bacteria and other material can spread into the surrounding tissue an spread to other parts of the body. Contents of an inflamed area will spread by the way of the lymph system or bloodstream.

Nursing Observations

The nurse can assist the client with an inflammation or infection by making careful observations of the client's signs and symptoms. Signs and symptoms of an infectious disease may be described as general or localized.

GENERAL SIGNS AND SYMPTOMS

Many early symptoms of infection are nonspecific or general. General signs and symptoms result when the entire body feels the results of infection. Severity of general symptoms depends upon the ability of the body to combat the pathogen and the amount of toxins that are absorbed into the bloodstream. Fever and the signs and symptoms that commonly accompany fever may be present. Headache, flushed cheeks and dry skin, tender, swollen lymph nodes, increased pulse and respiratory rates, and chills are usually present. Malaise, a general and indefinite feeling of discomfort or illness, and weakness are common. Anorexia, or loss of appetite is frequent; nausea accompanied by vomiting or diarrhea and generalized aching are not uncommon. Leukocytosis and an increase in the erythrocyte sedimentation rate may occur in acute conditions with or without infection.

The elevated temperature is another defense mechanism of the body to aid in combating infection. Chills may be associated with the elevation of body temperature. As the temperature rises, the pulse and respiratory rate are also increased. The patient's headache can be associated with the fever or with the toxins in his bloodstream. Dry skin and red cheeks are also associated with temperature elevation. General malaise results from the fever as well as the toxins. The body produces more leukocytes since they are the fighting cells of the blood. A complete blood count, including a differential count, helps the physician to determine the body's reaction (see Tables 5.4 and 5.5).

LOCAL SIGNS AND SYMPTOMS

The symptoms that the patient with a local inflammation experiences are redness, swelling, heat, pain, and loss of function. The extent to which these symptoms are noticed depends upon the virulence of the microorganism, the body's resistance, and the part of the body affected. Redness, swelling, and heat can be noticed by the observer when the battle site is on the body surface. The area is red, swollen, and warm because of increased blood to the injured part and an increased amount of fluid in the tissues. This increased amount of fluid presses on the sensitive nerve endings and produces pain. The inflamed part loses its ability to function efficiently because the increased fluid makes it difficult to move, and the movement increases the pain.

A culture may be made from a localized infection, and the ability of pathogens to grow in the presence of certain chemotherapeutic agents is checked in a sensitivity test (see Figure 5.7). Examples of some chemotherapeutic agents used by the medical tech-

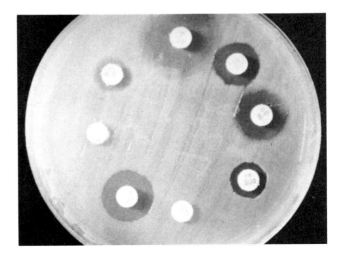

FIGURE 5.7 An agar plate on which microorganisms have grown. Each disk contains an antibiotic. The clear areas around some of the disks indicate that the microorganisms are susceptible to the antibiotic in those disks. The disks without a clear area contain an antibiotic that is not effective against these microorganisms. (Reproduced from Wilson, Marion E., and Mizer, Helen Eckel: *Microbiology in Patient Care,* 2nd ed. Macmillan Publishing Co., Inc., New York, 1974.)

nologist when performing sensitivity testing are in Table 5.6. The culture should be taken before an antibiotic is given.

Nursing Interventions

The nurse's role in helping the person who has suffered cell injury and an accompanying inflammatory response will depend on the nature of the causative agent, the degree of the injury and its location, and also the ability of the person to overcome the insult. Nursing interventions should be designed to (1) provide general and physical rest for the client, (2) provide relief of discomfort, (3) provide adequate nutrition, (4) provide adequate fluid intake, (5) control the infection in the client with drug therapy, (6) prevent the spread of the infection to others, (7) provide client and family education, and (8) provide psychosocial support.

GENERAL NURSING MEASURES

Elevation, rest, and the application of heat or cold are the three main local treatments of an inflamed area. The patient with an acute localized infection or one with a generalized inflammation needs more than these treatments to aid nature in the healing process. Special laboratory studies are done to aid the physician in treatment (see Tables 5.4 and 5.5).

REST. The patient needs mental and physical rest. This enables the body's energies to be directed toward combating the infection. Avoiding unnecessary stimulation and interruptions is a method of conserving the patient's energy. Simple nursing measures, such as a bath, back rub, and change of position, can increase a patient's comfort.

RELIEF OF DISCOMFORT. In addition to measures already discussed—elevation, rest, and application of heat or cold—the patient may have an analgesic prescribed. Analgesics are discussed in Chapter 7 and later in this chapter when commonly used drugs are considered.

The patient with an inflammation caused by microorganisms generally has fever and frequently has chills. An individual having a chill experiences a feeling of being cold and shivering. Shivering is the body's natural response to an excessive loss of heat and its effort to increase the temperature. The patient should be covered with additional blankets.

However, excessive external heat should be avoided because of the possibility of producing excessive perspiration. Excessive perspiration can result in a loss of body fluid, heat, and sodium. The patient's temperature should be taken 20 to 30 minutes after the chill has ended. It is believed that an individual's temperature has reached its peak within a period of 20 to 30 minutes after having a chill. The additional covering should be removed after shivering has stopped and the patient begins to feel warm. This is important to prevent the loss of excessive fluid, as mentioned earlier. The individual with a fever has an elevation of body temperature above normal. Fever associated with an infection may be continuous or intermittent over a period of time. The patient with an infection that causes a fever can be expected to excrete more toxins through the kidneys and lose more fluid by evaporation from the skin. Increased respirations serve similar purposes. For these reasons, the intake of fluids should be increased. Fluids high in calories, vitamin C, sodium, potassium, and protein generally are indicated for the patient with an infection. Such fluids help to supply the patient's need for extra calories, electrolytes, and nutrients. These may be given orally or parenterally.

Sponge baths with tepid water may be given for comfort, to remove waste products

TABLE 5.6
EXAMPLES OF CHEMOTHERAPEUTIC AGENTS
USED IN LABORATORY SENSITIVITY TESTING

Ampicillin	Nalidixic acid
Bacitracin	Neomycin
Cephalothin	Novobiocin
Chloramphenicol	Oleandomycin
Chlortetracycline	Polymyxin B
Clindamycin	Sulfisoxazole
Demeclocycline	(GANTRISIN)
Dihydrostreptomycin	Sulfonamides
Erythromycin	Tetracycline
Gentamicin	Vancomycin
Kanamycin	

from the skin, and to lower the patient's temperature. Care should be taken by the nurse to avoid chilling the patient.

The patient with an elevated temperature is encouraged to stay in bed and generally is allowed to go to the bathroom as needed. The environment should be quiet and conducive to rest because of the tendency toward irritability and sometimes a headache. Dryness of the lips and around the nose can be relieved by the application of a lubricant.

The temperature, pulse, and respiration of the patient with a fever should be checked every two to four hours (Figure 5.8). A high fever increases the pulse rate of the individual and causes the metabolism to increase. Fluid, sodium, and other waste products are lost through excessive perspiration. In some cases, the patient, especially in a debilitated condition, cannot tolerate a high fever. The doctor may order the use of a hypothermia blanket for the patient with a dangerously high fever. Use of hypothermia equipment

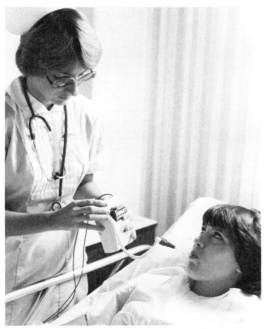

FIGURE 5.8 Using the electronic thermometer to check for a temperature elevation. (Courtesy of Henrico County–St. Mary's Hospital School of Practical Nursing, Richmond, Virginia.)

decreases the metabolic needs of the body and inhibits the multiplication of infecting microorganisms. After having a high or a prolonged fever, the patient can be expected to feel weak, perspire upon exertion, and tire easily. The nurse will need to take these factors into consideration when planning nursing care.

ADEQUATE NUTRITION. The diet indicated is one that is easily digested and assimilated. Liquid and soft foods are usually given to the patient with a high fever. The physician may order a diet higher in calories, vitamins, minerals, and protein, since the metabolic needs of the body are increased. This need may be compared with that of a furnace. As the furnace gives off more heat, it needs more fuel. When the body uses more energy and gives off more heat, it needs more food. In order to obtain adequate nutrition without overtaxing the gastrointestinal system, the patient will need frequent small feedings at two- or three-hour intervals until improvement occurs.

The physician may request a calorie count on the patient's intake. A calorie count would assist the nurses and the physician in determining if the patient's intake of food is sufficient to supply the body's needs.

Periodic weight measurements should be recorded to determine loss of weight or body fluids. It is preferable that the client is weighed at the same time of day, on the same scale, in the same amount of clothing.

INCREASE FLUID INTAKE. The fluid intake of the patient should be increased to 3000 ml (3 qt) or more during a 24-hour period. Forcing fluids increases production and excretion of urine. Since the kidneys are responsible for ridding the body of many bacterial toxins, an increased fluid intake aids in eliminating the toxins. A greater intake of fluid also aids in counteracting the dehydrating effects of fever.

A minimum of 1000 ml of urine in 24 hours is desirable in order to promote excretion of wastes such as toxins and bacteria. If the nurse notices the output to be less than 1000 ml in 24 hours, the nurse in charge or the physician should be notified.

Careful monitoring of the client's fluid intake and output is important in maintaining water and electrolyte balance. The severity of some client's disease process may require fluid replacement therapy by the intravenous route. When a client receives intravenous fluids, nursing intervention includes careful observation of the following: (1) the rate and flow of the prescribed fluid, (2) the site of injection for redness, swelling, and blanching of skin, (3) position of the part supporting the infusion, and (4) aseptic technique at the injection site.

DRUG THERAPY. Drugs frequently used to assist the body's defenses in combating infection are the sulfonamides and antibiotics. After determining the cause of infection, the physician selects the antibiotic or the sulfa drug that is known to be most effective against the particular microorganism. Certain pathogens are killed by a specific drug, whereas other microorganisms are not affected by that drug. For example, penicillin is more effective against the bacteria causing a "strep throat" than it is against the virus that produces the common cold or a type of pneumonia. The physician has a long list of drugs from which to select for a specific pathogen or group of pathogens.

The sulfonamides are a group of chemical compounds used to combat infections. Individual sulfonamides have been found to be more effective in certain types of infections. One may be effective against a urinary tract infection, whereas another may be more effective against gastrointestinal infections. For example, sulfisoxazole (GANTRISIN) may be ordered by the physician when treating the patient with a genitourinary infection, phthalylsulfathiazole (SULFATHALADINE) for a gastrointestinal tract infection, and silver sulfadiazine (SILVADENE) for wound sepsis in a burned patient.

An *antibiotic* is a chemical substance that checks the growth of bacteria or destroys them. Penicillin, the first antibiotic to be discovered, is effective mainly against certain gram-positive microorganisms, such as the pneumococcus. It is effective against some gram-negative microorganisms such as the gonococcus. Streptomycin is an anti-biotic that is effective against a wide variety of gram-negative microorganisms.

Antibiotics that are effective against more types of infections than is penicillin are referred to as broad-spectrum antibiotics. In other words, these antibiotics are effective against a wide range of infections. Chloramphenicol (CHLOROMYCETIN), chlortetracycline (AUREOMYCIN), oxytetracycline (TERRAMYCIN), demeclocycline (DECLOMYCIN), ampicillin (POLYCILLIN), and tetracycline (ACHROMYCIN) are examples of broad-spectrum antibiotics. They are effective against many gram-negative and gram-positive bacteria. A summary of the antibiotics and sulfonamides is provided as a reference in Tables. 5.7 and 5.8.

Analgesics, drugs that relieve pain, may be prescribed by the physician. Members of the salicylate family, such as aspirin, are widely used as pain relievers. Opiate derivatives are used for more severe pain. Morphine, PANTOPON, codeine, and dihydromorphinone (DILAUDID) are members of the opiate family. Synthetic chemical agents that relieve pain offer the physician other choices. Meperidine (DEMEROL), alphaprodine (NISENTIL), and pentazocine (TALWIN) are examples of these analgesics.

Anti-inflammatory drugs (steroid or nonsteroid type) might be prescribed for a patient with an inflammation that is caused by some agent other than a pathogen. The actions of the steroid drugs in lessening the symptoms of the inflammatory reaction appear to be complex. It is felt that these drugs modify the body's immune responses to a large number of stimuli, thereby altering the normal inflammatory response. As the result of altering the normal inflammatory response, the inflamed tissues return to a normal condition more rapidly. Because these drugs do slow down the inflammatory reaction, the patient receiving these drugs should be protected against infections. These drugs may be given orally, parenterally, or injected into a specific inflamed joint or area of inflammation. For example, a person with bursitis of the shoulder might be treated with an injection of hydrocortisone into the affected bursa (see Table 17.6).

Some of the more common side effects
[*Text continued on page 103.*]

TABLE 5.7
ANTIBIOTICS*

NONPROPRIETARY NAME	TRADE NAME	AVERAGE DOSE	NURSING IMPLICATIONS
1. Penicillins			
Amoxicillin	AMOXIL LAROTID	250–500 mg/oral	Hypersensitivity may develop with any method of administration and with any dosage of penicillin. Urticaria, skin rashes, inflammation of mucous membrane of mouth, fever, angioedema, serum sickness, anaphylaxis, and inflammatory reactions at site of injection are examples of allergic reactions that may occur
Ampicillin	AMCILL OMNIPEN PENBRITIN POLYCILLIN	0.5 gm/oral 0.5 gm–1 gm/injection	Allergic reaction may be life threatening and necessitate discontinuing the drug. The nurse should ask the patient about any previous reaction to penicillin and, if so, should not administer until the physician has been informed
Carbenicillin	GEOPEN PYOPEN	1–10 gm/injection every 2 hr or daily	Check with patient to determine allergy to penicillin before giving first dose in series. Rotate injection sites
Carbenicillin indanyl sodium	GEOCILLIN	500 mg/orally every 6 hr	Frequently used in urinary tract infections
Cloxacillin sodium	TEGOPEN	125–250 mg/orally	
Dicloxacillin sodium	DYNAPEN PATHOCIL VERACILLIN	125–250 mg/orally	Administer 1 to 2 hr before meals
Methicillin Nafcillin	STAPHCILLIN UNIPEN	1–6 gm every 2 to 3 hr 250 mg/orally 500 mg–1 gm injection	Injections more painful than some other types of penicillin
Oxacillin	BACTOCILL PROSTAPHLIN	250–500-mg tablets for oral use 250-, 500-mg, and 1-gm vials for injection	Administer 1 to 2 hr before meals to improve absorption Injections every 5 to 6 hr
Penicillin G benzathine	BICILLIN PERMAPEN	300,000–600,000 units for injection 50,000 to 1 million units in tablet for oral use	Benzathine has local anesthetic effect and relieves discomfort of injection. Give ½ to 2 hr before meals to improve absorption

TABLE 5.7 (Continued)
ANTIBIOTICS*

Nonproprietary Name	Trade Name	Average Dose	Nursing Implications
Penicillin G potassium (tablets)		50,000 to 1 million units in tablet for oral use	Give ½ to 2 hr before meals
Penicillin G procaine	CRYSTICILLIN DIURNAL-PENICILLIN DURACILLIN A.S. WYCILLIN	300,000–600,000 units	Procaine makes injection less painful. Notify physician if patient reports allergy to procaine
Phenethicillin	MAXIPEN SYNCILLIN	250-mg tablets for oral use	
II. Tetracyclines			The patient receiving one of the tetracyclines may develop hypersensitivity
Chlortetracycline	AUREOMYCIN	150–300 mg every 6 hr	Reactions, such as rash, urticaria, dermatitis, angioedema, anaphylaxis, burning of the eyes, brownish coating of tongue, vaginitis, irritation around anus, and fever. Gastrointestinal irritation may be relieved or prevented by giving oral drug with food. Do not give milk or antacids containing aluminum, calcium, or magnesium. Intravenous injection of tetracyclines may be complicated by thrombophlebitis. Check expiration date of tetracyclines. Have patient avoid exposure to sun. Skin of patient receiving demeclocycline may react to sunlight. Normal functioning of the kidneys and liver may be affected. Children receiving demeclocycline may develop discolorations of the teeth with long-term therapy with tetracyclines. Infections with fungi and yeasts may occur
Demeclocycline	DECLOMYCIN	150–300 mg every 6 hr	
Doxycycline	VIBRAMYCIN	100 mg every 12 hr, then every 24 hr	
Methacycline	RONDOMYCIN	150 mg every 6 hr	
Minocycline	MINOCIN VECTRIN	500 mg to 1 gm IV 2 times daily	
Oxytetracycline	TERRAMYCIN	50–300 mg every 6 hr	
Rolitetracycline	SYNTETRIN	150–300 mg	
Tetracycline	ACHROMYCIN PANMYCIN POLYCYCLINE STECLIN SUMYCIN	150–300 mg every 6 hr	
III. Cephalosporins			
Cefazolin	ANCEF KEFZOL	250–500 mg every 8 hr by injection	Hypersensitivity reactions to cephalosporins may occur. Serum sickness, fever, urticaria, rash, and thrombophlebitis are examples. Local irritation around site of injection may develop. Kidney damage may occur
Cephalexin	KEFLEX	250–500 mg every 6 hr orally	May be associated with cephalosporins. Rotate site of injection. Used with caution in persons allergic to penicillin

100

Generic Name	Brand Name	Dosage	Side Effects/Comments
Cephaloglycin	KAFOCIN	250–500 mg	Not used often
Cephaloridine	LORIDINE		Not used often
Cephalothin	KEFLIN	1 gm every 6 hr by injection	
Cephapirin	CEFADYL	500 mg to 1 gm every 4 to 6 hr by injection	
Cephradine		250–500 mg every 6 hr by mouth	

IV. Aminoglycosides

Generic Name	Brand Name	Dosage	Side Effects/Comments
Gentamicin	GARAMYCIN	3–5 mg/kg body weight/day	May affect 8th cranial nerve, which involves hearing. Hearing tests may be done. Dizziness, nausea, vomiting, and skin eruptions may occur
Kanamycin	KANTREX	Maximum of 8 gm per day/orally, 15 mg/kg body weight parenterally	Frequent WBC may be done to determine elevated count. Causes pain at injection site. Symptoms of toxicity to ear and kidneys should be observed and reported. Patient may be restless, have a headache, and experience blurred vision. All symptoms of side effects should be noted and reported
Neomycin	MYCIFRADIN, NEOBIOTIC	250 mg IM (intramuscular) every 6 hr; 4–8 gm daily (orally in divided doses); Available in creams, ointments, and sprays	Skin rash, kidney damage, and nerve deafness may occur. Patient may develop inability to absorb food properly during treatment
Streptomycin		1–2 gm/day IM	Hypersensitivity reactions such as dermatitis, anaphylactic shock, stomatitis, angioedema, and fever. Symptoms of toxic effects related to dose such as deafness, dizziness, dysfunction of optic nerve, peripheral neuritis, kidney damage, and local irritation at site of injection should be observed and promptly reported. Symptoms of other infections may develop

V. Others

Generic Name	Brand Name	Dosage	Side Effects/Comments
Bacitracin	BACIQUENT	For topical application	Rarely causes local irritation
Chloramphenicol	CHLOROMYCETIN	2–4 gm/day orally or IV	Blood dyscrasias, GI disturbances, skin rash, hypersensitivity reactions, and bleeding tendency may occur
Clindamycin	CLEOCIN	150–300 mg q6h orally; 600 mg–3.2 gm/day IM or IV	Diarrhea, skin rashes, and ulcerative colitis

TABLE 5.7 (*Continued*)
ANTIBIOTICS*

NONPROPRIETARY NAME	TRADE NAME	AVERAGE DOSE	NURSING IMPLICATIONS
Colistin	COLY-MYCIN	2.5–5 mg/kg body weight orally or by injection, tid	Pruritus, dizziness, visual and speech disturbances, and gastrointestinal disturbances may occur
Erythromycin	ILOTYCIN E-MYCIN ERYTHROCIN BRISTAMYCIN ILOSONE	1–4 gm/day orally or parenterally in divided doses	Fever, elevated white blood cell count, skin eruptions, and epigastric distress may develop. IM injections are painful
Lincomycin	LINCOCIN	500 mg q 6–8 hr	Patient may experience nausea, vomiting, diarrhea, skin rash, and urticaria
Polymyxin B	AEROSPORIN	750,000–1 million units tid parenterally or orally	Fever, urticaria, nausea, vomiting, diarrhea, dizziness, double vision, and slurred speech may complicate parenteral injection
Spectinomycin	TROBICIN	2–4 gm IM	Skin rash, vertigo, nausea, chills, fever, and insomnia may appear as untoward effects requiring nursing observations and appropriate actions
Tyrothricin		For topical application	Do not use on fresh wound or injury because it may increase bleeding
Vancomycin	VANCOCIN	500 mg q6h orally or parenterally	Ear and kidney damage may result. Skin rash and anaphylaxis may also occur

* An antibiotic is a chemical substance produced by microorganisms that have the ability to either destroy other microorganisms or inhibit their growth.

TABLE 5.8
SULFONAMIDES*

NONPROPRIETARY NAME	TRADE NAME	AVERAGE DOSE	NURSING IMPLICATIONS
			The nurse should know that sulfonamide therapy is potentially dangerous. Drug fever, anemia, and disturbances of the urinary tract may occur. The fluid intake of a patient receiving sulfonamides should produce an output of 1200 ml per 24 hr to reduce kidney complications. Nausea, vomiting, liver damage, and dermatitis are additional untoward reactions to sulfonamide therapy. Record intake and output.
Mafenide	SULFAMYLON CREAM	Topical use esp. for burns	Patient may experience pain at site of application and allergic responses. May produce metabolic acidosis
Silver sulfadiazine	SILVADENE	Topically in burn therapy	
Sulfacetamide	SULAMYD BLEPH ISOPTO CETAMIDE	Topical application for eye	Not used for systemic infections
Sulfadiazine		2–4 gm initially, then 1 gm every hr orally	
Sulfamethoxazole	GANTANOL	2 gm initially, then 1 gm every 8–12 hr orally	Encourage adequate intake of fluids to prevent crystalluria
Sulfasalazine	AZULFIDINE	4–8 gm/day	May cause patient to have anemia, nausea, vomiting, and rash
Sulfisoxazole	GANTRISIN SK-SOXAZOLE	2–4 gm initially, then 1 gm every 4–6 hr	Encourage adequate intake of water
Sulfisoxazole and phenazopyridine hydrochloride	AZO GANTRISIN	1 gm 4 times a day	Causes urine to have orange-red color

* The sulfonamides have a bacteriostatic effect on susceptible microorganisms. In other words, this group of drugs inhibits the growth of bacteria but does not kill them. By inhibiting the growth of bacteria, sulfonamides enable the body to overcome the infection.

that occur when these steroid drugs are given systemically (orally or parenterally) are fluid retention causing electrolyte changes and imbalances, the characteristic moonface, hypertension (increased blood pressure), acne, hirsutism (excessive growth of facial hair in women), muscle weakness, hyperglycemia, glycosuria, and occasional personality changes.

The nurse should also be aware of the symptoms of a sudden withdrawal of a steroid drug that has been given systemically over a long period of time. Some of the symptoms might be hypotension (low blood pressure), restlessness, anorexia, malaise, and fatigue.

Some of the more commonly used cortisone preparations are hydrocortisone (COR-

TEF), prednisone (DELTAZONE, METICOR-TEN), prednisolone (DELTA CORTEF), dexamethasone (DECADRON), and triamcinolone (KENACORT).

ACTH (ADRENOCORTICOTROPIC HORMONE) also may be used in steroid therapy. This hormone is normally secreted by the pituitary gland and stimulates the adrenal cortex to secrete cortisone. If ACTH is given parenterally, which is the only route of administration, the patient's adrenal cortex will secrete an increased amount of cortisone.

The nonsteroid type anti-inflammatory drugs have an antiprostaglandin action. These drugs inhibit the production of prostaglandin E. Prostaglandins are described as modified unsaturated fatty acids that are made in the body in almost every tissue in small to moderate amounts. These substances are released into the local tissue fluids and into the circulating blood under both physiologic and pathologic conditions. These chemical substances act as vasodilators, vasoconstrictors, or gastric acid inhibitors. They can also stimulate or inhibit muscular or nervous system functions depending on the quantity of the substance released.

Some of the more commonly used nonsteroid anti-inflammatory preparations are indomethacin (INDOCIN), fenoprofen (NALFON), ibuprofen (MOTRIN), naproxen (NAPROSYN), sulindac (CLINORIL), tolmetin (TOLECTIN), phenylbutazone (BUTAZOLIDIN), and oxyphenbutazone (TANDEARIL). Some of the more common side effects that occur when these nonsteroid drugs are given are dizziness and lightheadedness, gastrointestinal disturbance such as nausea, vomiting, epigastric distress, abdominal pain, and diarrhea, and edema (see Table 17.6).

LOCAL CARE

Treatment and nursing care of the patient with an inflammation are designed to support the body's defense mechanisms. Such measures as local elevation, rest, warm or cold applications, adequate fluid intake, and nutritious diet are some of the factors to be considered.

ELEVATION OF THE AFFECTED PART. The person who has had an infected finger remembers the relief obtained when the finger was elevated. The throbbing pain was eased almost immediately. Elevating the inflamed part also relieves swelling. Drainage from the dilated blood vessels is increased by the force of gravity. As the unoxygenated blood is carried away, fresh blood with an increased amount of immune substances and leukocytes is brought to the site. The extremities, head, and neck are parts of the body that are most easily elevated. In raising an extremity, the entire part should be raised. For example, in elevating the foot, the entire leg should be raised with the foot higher than the knee, and the knee higher than the hip. Plastic-covered pillows should be arranged under the extremity for support. An ambulatory patient can have an infected arm elevated in a sling. In this case, the patient's hand should be approximately 10 to 12.5 cm (4 to 5 in.) higher than the level of the elbow.

REST OF THE AFFECTED PART. Nature causes the patient to rest the infected area because of the pain involved when moving it. Additional rest aids in the healing process. It allows more of the body's defenses to be directed into the battle zone. Delayed healing of a cracked lip illustrates how movement of an inflamed part slows down the process of recuperation.

HEAT. Local applications of heat are prescribed by the physician to dilate blood vessels, thereby increasing the amount of blood to the inflamed area, to relax the muscles, or to relieve pain. The nurse should remember that some patients are more sensitive to heat than are others. Extreme caution is necessary when applying heat to infants, aged persons, patients with diabetes and arteriosclerosis, and unconscious patients. Dry or moist heat may be ordered by the doctor.

Dry Heat: Hot Water Bag. The hot water bag, electric heating pad, and heat cradle are three common methods of applying dry heat. The nurse often hears the patient complain that the hot water bag is not warm enough when it is applied. However, the water must not be too hot, as it may burn the patient. The area beneath the hot water bag should be observed frequently for symptoms of burning, such as increased redness and warmth. These should be reported promptly to the team leader or head nurse.

In order to prevent burning the patient, the nurse should check the temperature of the water to be used in the hot water bag with a thermometer. In general, the temperature of the water should not be higher than 48.9° C (120°F) for an adult. The temperature should be 43.3° to 46.1°C (110° to 115°F) for a child. The hot water bag should be warmed first by filling it with hot water and then emptying it. This simple measure helps to prevent cooling the water when it is poured into the hot water bag, which is then suitably covered. The nurse should remember that some body areas, such as the inner aspect of the arms and thighs, are more sensitive to heat than other body parts.

The hot water bag should be filled one-third to one-half full, depending on the site of application. When a half-filled bag is too much for the inflamed area because of increased weight, the bag should be one-third full. Removal of excess air, also, decreases the weight and makes the hot water bag more manageable.

The aquamatic pad is used to apply constant heat to a part of the patient's body. This piece of equipment enables the patient to have a constant temperature at a level prescribed by the doctor (Figure 5.9).

Dry Heat: Electric Heating Pad. An electric heating pad is prescribed when the physician wants the dry heat applied over a larger area for a longer period of time. Using moisture with an electric heating pad is a dangerous practice, as fluid may cause a short circuit. It is necessary for the pad to be covered with waterproof material. Putting a pin through the pad is another hazardous practice. If a safety pin is used to secure a flannel cover over the pad, care should be used to avoid puncturing the heating pad. It is important to observe the patient frequently to avoid a burn from an overheated pad.

Dry Heat: Heat Cradle. A heat cradle is another method of applying dry heat to an inflamed area. The warmth is often produced by electric bulbs in the ceiling of the cradle. This treatment is frequently used for patients with chronic inflammatory conditions of the muscles and the bones, such as

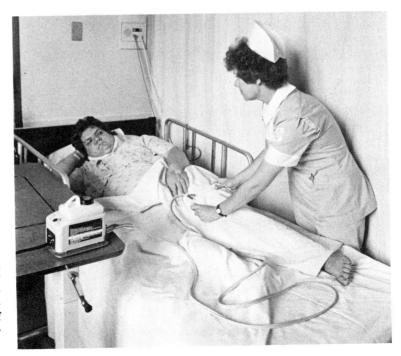

FIGURE 5.9 An aquamatic pad may be used to apply heat at a constant temperature. (Courtesy of Fredericksburg Area School of Practical Nursing, Fredericksburg, Virginia.)

arthritis. A heat cradle may be used to increase the blood supply to the area of a decubitus ulcer and thus promote healing. The actual technique for using a heat cradle varies with the type of equipment available; there are innumerable sizes and shapes. The nurse should seek specific instructions regarding the number of bulbs, the wattage to be used, the distance of the heat cradle from the inflamed area, and the length of time the cradle is to be used. A thermometer may be suspended inside the cradle as a guide for regulating the temperature. The nursing staff should maintain the temperature of air within the cradle as prescribed by the doctor. As with other methods of applying heat, the danger of burning the patient is present. The patient should be observed frequently for increased redness and warmth of the part being treated.

Moist Heat: General Considerations. Moist heat produces effects similar to those of dry heat. Although the results are similar, moisture increases the effect of heat. Why does a humid hot day cause you to feel the effects of heat more than a dry hot day? Moisture is a conductor of warmth. Also, the increased amount of water in the air slows down the evaporation of perspiration from a person's body. Therefore, it is essential to remember that moist heat burns more quickly than dry heat. A warm solution applied to a dressing burns more quickly than if the same solution is placed on the skin, because the rate of evaporation is slower and the moisture increases the effect of heat.

Moist Heat: Hot Wet Dressings or Hot Compresses. Hot wet dressings or hot compresses may be applied by putting warm solution on the part that is already bandaged or by applying compresses saturated with a heated solution and then wrung out. Moisture is retained in these dressings by wrapping the area with a thin piece of rubber or plastic material. Warmth is maintained by applying a hot water bag, an aquamatic pad, or covering the part with a heat cradle. It is necessary to use sterile technique when the inflamed part has an open lesion.

When a continuous hot wet dressing is prescribed, the dressing needs to be

changed when it starts to dry. If a hot water bag is the method used to supply warmth, it should be changed as it begins to cool. The inflamed part of a patient receiving continuous moist heat should be examined frequently for early symptoms of injury by heat.

Moist Heat: Sitz Bath. Having the patient sit in a bath of warm water from 5 to 30 minutes is known as a sitz bath. A temperature of 40.6° to 43.3°C (105° to 110°F) is recommended. This type of moist heat provides much relief to patients following rectal and perineal surgery. It is also used in the treatment of patients with an acute inflammatory disease of the pelvic region. A special appliance that fits onto the toilet seat is available for a sitz bath (Figure 5.10). Regu-

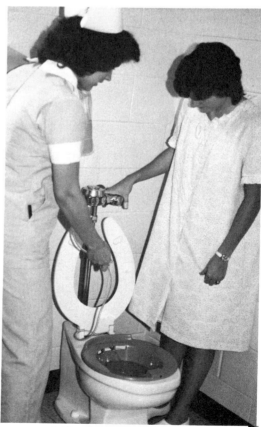

FIGURE 5.10 Sitz bath. (Courtesy of Loudoun County School of Practical Nursing, Leesburg, Virginia.)

lar bathtubs are not as satisfactory for a sitz bath because heat is applied not only to the desired area but also to the lower extremities. This alters the desired effects in the pelvic region.

It is important to observe the patient for signs of exhaustion during this treatment. Remembering that a hot bath for a well person may cause temporary weakness will help the nurse in realizing the effect that a sick person may experience from a sitz bath. The bath should be discontinued if the patient shows signs of weakness. For example, the patient may have an increased pulse rate, perspire excessively, or complain of feeling weak.

Moist Heat: Local Soaks. Immersion of an infected extremity is often indicated. The type of solution, temperature, and length of time are ordered by the doctor. Sterile solution and a sterile basin are used when there is an open lesion on the infected part.

COLD. Local application of cold constricts blood vessels. Because of its constricting action on blood vessels, it reduces the amount of blood in the inflamed area. Cold relieves pain caused by the pressure of increased fluid on the delicate nerve endings. Since the blood vessels become smaller, hemorrhage and the inflammatory process are checked. The effects of moist cold are greater than those of dry cold.

Prolonged application of cold can endanger the life of the area, just as a person's life is endangered during a long period of time in an extremely cold temperature. The site of application should be examined frequently by the nurse for danger signals of tissue damage. The area becoming endangered by cold is bluish purple, has a mottled appearance, and feels numb and stiff. These symptoms should be reported immediately.

The ice bag or ice cap is used to apply dry cold to an area. Moist cold is frequently applied by use of moist gauze. The gauze is dipped into a cold solution, wrung out, and applied to the inflamed area. It is necessary to replace the compress with another cold, moist one every few minutes. This procedure is often used in applying moist cold to the eyes.

PREVENT SPREAD OF INFECTION. An individual with certain infectious diseases is separated from others by a procedure called *isolation*. The purpose of isolation is to protect the patient from superimposed infections and to protect other individuals from the condition currently affecting the patient. In other words, an attempt is made to prevent the spread of pathogenic microorganisms. A patient requiring isolation should be placed in a private room or a separate cubicle. The isolation procedure and its purpose should be explained fully to the patient. Hospital personnel with any type of skin lesions should report them and refrain from patient contact. Hospital policy should be followed strictly when caring for the patient in isolation.

The type of isolation is determined by the purpose of isolation and the mode of transmission of the infecting organism. Respiratory, wound and skin, protective, strict, and enteric isolation are five common examples. The patient in respiratory isolation is considered to have an infection in which the microorganism is airborne. Wound and skin isolation is essential when the infection is in a wound and can be transmitted by direct contact with the area. Protective or reverse isolation is used to protect the patient from other persons in an effort to prevent superimposed infection (Figure 5.11). The patient in protective isolation may suffer from a burn or may have a condition in which defense mechanism have been decreased. Protective isolation is used also when an organ has been transplanted into the patient. Strict isolation is required for highly communicable diseases that may be transmitted by airborne routes and by contact (Figure 5.12). Enteric isolation is indicated when the pathogen is transmitted through the waste products of the gastrointestinal system.

Meticulous handwashing is an important factor in the prevention of infection and in all types of isolation. When possible, a sink with an knee or foot pedal, hot and cold running water, paper towels, and an antimicrobial soap should be used. The nurse's hands should be washed before care is given to the patient, after care to the patient, and before leaving an isolation unit.

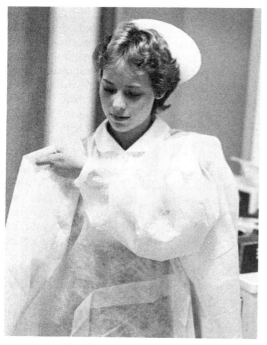

FIGURE 5.11   Wearing a gown prevents transmission of organisms from the nurse's uiform to the patient in protective isolation. (Courtesy of Henrico County–St. Mary's Hospital School of Practical Nursing, Richmond, Virginia.)

CLIENT AND FAMILY EDUCATION. To prevent and control infections, efforts must be made to increase the patient's resistance and provide a hygienic environment. The client and family should be instructed that cleanliness and good hygienic practices help prevent the spread of infection from one person to another. Awareness of the manner in which the specific infectious disease spreads and measures necessary to prevent the spread are essential information that must be imparted to those persons involved.

The client and family should be made aware of the availability of vaccines to prevent disease, the necessity of adequate housing, and nutrition where applicable, and other reservoirs of human infections.

PSYCHOSOCIAL ASPECTS. An inflammation or an infection may cause the individual to experience such reactions as anxiety, disgust, frustration, hostility, and/or apprehension. These reactions may occur whether the patient enters the hospital with the infection or whether the infection is nosocomial, originating in the hospital. The impact of the patient's illness is often felt by the family as well as the patient. The thought of infecting others may be foremost in the individual's mind. Also, the patient who develops a noso-

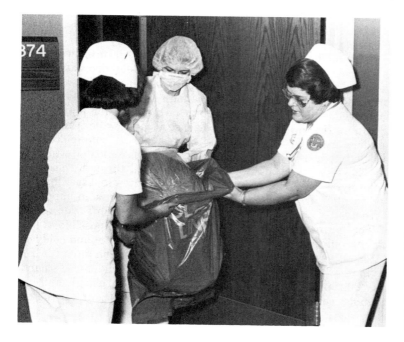

FIGURE 5.12   Using the double-bag technique to remove contaminated supplies. (Courtesy of Tri-County Area Vocational-Technical School and Jane Phillips Episcopal Memorial Medical Center, Bartlesville, Oklahoma.)

comial infection may experience other inconveniences, such as loss of work, additional hospital confinement, additional cost, and prolonged separation from loved ones.

Measures should be taken to help alleviate the patient's psychologic discomfort and concern. For example, the patient should feel accepted by members of the nursing staff and should be helped to realize that self-worth continues although the individual may not perceive self to be valuable at this time.

The client needs to know that members of the health team are doing everything possible to hasten convalescence. Representatives of the clergy and other members of the health team may intervene when indicated. An empathetic, understanding nurse plays a major role in alleviating the emotional impact of an illness, especially one associated with an infection.

When taking care of a patient with an infection, the nurse should know the cause of the infection, the method of transmission, and the nature of the infection. An awareness of the communicability of the infection and how immunity is acquired is important for the nurse. Answering the patient's questions and teaching the patient how to avoid or prevent further infection help to alleviate concern and anxiety.

Case Study Involving Inflammation

Mrs. Eure, a 49-year-old housewife, was admitted to a medical unit with the chief complaint of a sore on the bottom of her right foot. Mrs. Eure stated that she had stepped on a broken bottle in the yard two weeks previously and that the wound had not healed. At the time of the injury she was treated in the emergency department of the same hospital and was given tetanus toxoid and tetanus antitoxin. Upon admission her temperature was 39°C (102.2°F). The nurse observed a moderate amount of purulent drainage from a wound approximately 5 cm (2 in.) on the bottom part of the heel of the right foot. The foot appeared to be moderately edematous, reddened, and felt warm to touch. Mrs. Eure indicated that her foot hurt.

Mrs. Eure is a diabetic and has been taking NPH insulin for 30 years. She has mild hypertension and indicated that she had been told by her physician that the circulation in her lower extremities was poor. She takes methyldopa (ALDO-

MET), 250 mg twice a day, for hypertension. Mrs. Eure administers 50 units of U100 NPH insulin to herself before breakfast each day. In talking with her, the nurse learned that Mrs. Eure also takes isoxsuprine (VASODILAN), 20 mg four times a day, to improve her circulation. Mrs. Eure smokes approximately one pack of cigarettes each day. She indicated that her mother also had diabetes mellitus. Mrs. Eure does not drink alcoholic beverages, attends church regularly, enjoys sewing, and spends much of her time in her garden.

Laboratory findings indicate a white blood cell count of 12,000, blood sugar 300 mg. and a 3 + sugar in her urine with no acetone.

The physician's orders were:

- Bed rest
- Elevate right foot above knee
- Vital signs q4h
- NPH insulin, 60 units before breakfast
- Check urine for sugar and acetone qid
- 1800-calorie diet
- Intake and output
- TYLENOL, 650 mg q4h for temperature above 38.5°C (101.3°F)
- DARVON (plain), 65 mg q4h, prn for pain
- Warm BETADINE soaks to right foot for 20 minutes bid
- Obtain specimen from wound drainage for culture and sensitivity
- Ampicillin, 1 gm q6h, IV in 200 ml of saline initially after obtaining wound drainage for culture and sensitivity
- ALDOMET, 250 mg bid

QUESTIONS

1. Compare the local symptoms included in the case study with those in the textbook and discuss the body changes causing Mrs. Eure to have these symptoms.
2. Differentiate between local and general symptoms of infection exhibited by Mrs. Eure. Describe the nursing care related to these symptoms.
3. The physician ordered ampicillin to be given intravenously after the wound culture had been obtained. Discuss the rationale for this order to be carried out after the wound culture has been obtained.
4. Describe the actions of the drugs prescribed for Mrs. Eure and discuss the nursing implications of each.
5. Mrs. Eure received tetanus antitoxin when she was first injured. What type of immunity would she receive from this injection?
6. Describe the defenses of the body that came into play when Mrs. Eure first stepped on the broken bottle.

7. Mrs. Eure is to receive warm BETADINE soaks to her right foot for 20 minutes bid. What precautions should you take when caring for this patient?

Suggestions for Further Study

1. What inflammations have you experienced that were associated with pathogens?
2. List the diseases to which you have an acquired immunity, a natural immunity.
3. Does dry heat burn more quickly than moist heat? What is the reason for your answer?
4. Mason, Mildred A.; Bates, Grace F.; and Smola, Bonnie K.: *Workbook in Basic Medical-Surgical Nursing*, 3rd ed. Macmillan Publishing Company, New York, 1984, Exercise 5.

Additional Readings

Bond, Gregory B.: "Infection Control: *Serratia—* An Endemic Hospital Resident." *American Journal of Nursing*, 81:2183–86 (Dec.), 1981.

Griffiths, Mary: *Human Physiology*, 2nd ed. Macmillan Publishing Co., Inc., New York, 1981, pp. 332–53.

Hargiss, Clarice O., and Larson, Elaine: "Infection Control: How to Collect Specimens and Evaluate Results." *American Journal of Nursing*, 81:2166–74 (Dec.), 1981.

Pilgrim, Margaret C.: "Are You Infecting Your Patients?" *Journal of Practical Nursing*, 31:18–21 and 41 (Apr.), 1981.

Rambo, Beverly J., and Wood, Lucile A. (eds.): *Nursing Skills for Clinical Practice*, 3rd ed. W. B. Saunders Co., Philadelphia, 1982, pp. 115–29, 708–33, and 752–76.

Robinson, Corinne H.: *Basic Nutrition and Diet Therapy*, 4th ed. Macmillan Publishing Co., Inc., New York, 1980, pp. 155–65.

Robinson, Corinne H., and Lawler, Marilyn R.: *Normal and Therapeutic Nutrition*, 16th ed. Macmillan Publishing Co., Inc., New York, 1982, pp. 284–98 and 419.

Chapter 6

The Surgical Patient

Expected Behavioral Outcomes

Minimum objectives referred to as expected behavioral outcomes have been designed for the practical/vocational nursing student to use as guides in studying this chapter. The student should read these expected outcomes before studying the chapter.

The objectives can be used as guides for study. Using the content of this chapter, the student should return to the objectives and evaluate the ability to:

1. *Select the nursing measures discussed in the text that will help to relieve and/ or prevent abdominal distention, urinary retention, hemorrhage, shock, respiratory complications, vascular complications, and wound infection.*

2. *Restate the symptoms of shock in the sequence that you would observe them. In other words, if you entered the unit of a patient in shock, what would you observe first, second, third, and so forth?*

3. *Compare the nursing care needed by the patient with an inflammation with that indicated for the surgical patient.*

4. *Describe at least three nursing measures related to safety for the patient who is sedated before, during, and after surgery.*

5. *Relate at least four activities of the nurse that help to reduce fear and anxiety of the patient and family who face surgery.*

Vocabulary Development

The following prefixes, suffixes, and combining forms pertain to this chapter. By learning and/or reviewing their meanings, the practical/vocational nursing student will have the keys needed to unlock many exciting new medical terms.

Discover the meaning of these keys in a medical dictionary or in the content of this chapter. How does each key pertain to this chapter? In your notebook write the correct meaning of each prefix, suffix, or combining form listed below. Illustrate each key with an example.

e—out from. Ex. emission—a discharge.

-cis	phylac-
ec-	plas-
ect-	post-
em-	pre-
esthe-	rhag-
hypo-	rhaph-
pec-	sect-
pex-	tom-

Introduction

The surgical patient is a person whose illness or disease is diagnosed and/or treated using a planned anatomic alteration by a specially trained physician, the surgeon. Surgery may be performed for a variety of reasons including to diagnose and/or determine the extent of disease, to cure disease, or to alleviate symptoms. Surgery that is done to relieve symptoms is known as palliative surgery. At times, surgery may accomplish more than one purpose. For example, the surgeon may perform an operation to diagnose disease. When the cause has been identified and can be cured surgically, the diseased organ or part may be removed or repaired during the same operation.

Major surgery is a term used to describe lengthy, complex operations that generally involve large body areas and pose an increased risk to the patient. Minor surgery, by comparison, generally describes shorter, simpler procedures involving smaller body areas and less risk to the patient. Surgical risk is a prediction about the outcome of an operation. An increased risk indicates that unfavorable outcomes such as death, disability, or complications are more likely. An important fact to remember is that these terms describe only the surgical procedure, not the patient's experience. The person facing surgery usually experiences it as a major event which involves considerable risk. A variety of factors are known to affect surgical risk. Beside the disease and type of surgery planned, age, nutritional status, mental health, general health, hydration, and lifestyle are additional influences.

Elective surgery generally means that the operation is not required to preserve life and limb. Emergency surgery indicates that an operation is needed immediately within minutes or as soon as possible to preserve life, limb, or vital organ. Nonelective surgery means that an operation is needed but not urgently.

Preoperative nursing care includes those observations and interventions that are used before surgery. Intraoperative refers to events that occur during surgery. Postoperative care includes nursing observations and interventions after surgery.

Surgical procedures may be done in hospitals, doctor's offices, and ambulatory surgical centers. Major surgery which carries an increased risk to the patient requires hospital admission. Some minor surgery can be done in the doctor's office or ambulatory surgical centers. The duration, intensity, and kind of nursing care required by the surgical patient are critical factors in determining where the surgery occurs.

Most surgical procedures have three characteristics: an intentional break in the skin barrier, a disruption to blood vessels, and a manipulation of one or more body organs. These characteristics mean that whenever a patient experiences surgery, the nurse can anticipate the activation of three important mechanisms: the stress response, psychological and body defenses, and body image.

Preoperative Care

The purpose of preoperative care is to ensure that the patient is in the best possible emotional and physical condition for surgery. This phase usually begins when the patient is admitted to the hospital prior to surgery. The duration of the preoperative period as well as activities in this phase vary considerably, depending on the patient, the disease, and the surgery. For example, when surgery is elective and has been planned for weeks, the patient may enter the hospital the evening before surgery with most of the preoperative preparation completed before admission. However, another patient who enters the hospital for diagnosis and later requires surgery may need days or weeks of preoperative care. The elderly patient generally needs more elaborate preoperative care. The patient who requires emergency surgery may have only a few minutes of preoperative care.

The needs of the individual patient determine which members of the health team participate in preoperative care. The surgeon is the leader of the team and directs the course of preoperative care, beginning with a history and physical examination. The nurse has a key part to play during this period. Typical nursing observations and interventions at this time include:

- Observe and report unusual information that might influence the surgery.
- Assist the patient to identify and cope with common concerns related to surgery.
- Teach the patient what to expect and what is expected before, during, and after surgery.
- Carry out specific tasks related to the patient's physical preparation for surgery.
- Assist with relevant aspects of diagnosis as described in Chapter 4.
- Coordinate related aspects of preoperative care.

Other members of the team contribute their special expertise also. Examinations of the patient's urine and blood are made by the laboratory technician. Services of the dietitian are needed for the patient's diet. A social worker may be asked to help the patient with home problems or financial worries. A rabbi, priest, or minister serves as the patient's spiritual adviser. A technician in the x-ray department takes x-rays requested by the doctor.

PREOPERATIVE NURSING OBSERVATIONS

The head-to-toe guide in Table 1.1 (p. 12) provides the nurse with preliminary information about the patient's physical char-

acteristics that influences preoperative care. For example, the patient who wears dentures usually requires a denture cup, a safe storage area, and removal prior to surgery. The life-style guide in Table 1.2 (p. 13) enables the nurse to identify patterns of living that influence surgery such as allergies, a current list of prescribed and nonprescribed medication, smoking, alcohol consumption, and exercise patterns. The life-style guide also helps the nurse to anticipate how the patient's life style might be altered by surgery.

The patient's height, weight, and vital signs are included in the initial observations. Vital signs are taken regularly during the preoperative period to form the bases for detecting and evaluating the significance of changes that occur postoperatively.

ASSISTING WITH COMMON CONCERNS

A very important nursing activity during the preoperative period is identifying, evaluating, and helping with the patient's concerns about surgery (Figure 6.1). Emotional factors in the preoperative period are known to affect the amount of vomiting, the level of pain medication needed, speed of recovery from anesthesia, and extent of the patient's participation postoperatively.

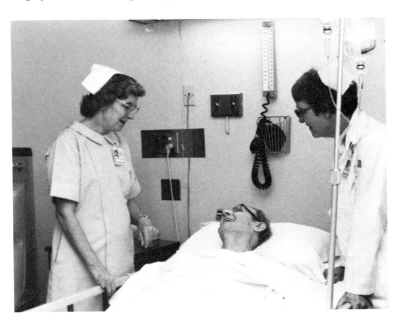

FIGURE 6.1 The nurses are helping the patient with preoperative concerns. (Courtesy of Suffolk City Schools and Louise Obici Memorial Hospital School of Practical Nursing, Suffolk, Virginia.)

In some cases, the patient is aware of specific concerns. In other cases, the patient may experience general feelings of anxiety related to the surgery but may not be aware of specific concerns. Concerns that most surgical patients have include fears of death, pain, or disfigurement. Some persons are concerned about waking up before the operation is completed, not waking up after anesthesia, or telling secrets under anesthesia. Studies show that considerable numbers of patients facing surgery are concerned about the possibilities of cancer or loss of sexual powers. Even when the patient's condition and the surgical procedure do not involve cancer or sexuality, the patient may have these fears. The patient who knows these possibilities are unlikely but has fears anyway may not volunteer this information without help from the nurse.

Because of the continuous mind-body interaction, persistent intense feelings of fear, panic, dread, and doom act as powerful unfavorable stressors. When combined with surgery, the patient's defenses can be overwhelmed, causing serious or fatal complications. Thus, the nurse encourages the person to verbalize concerns so that unfavorable emotional stressors can be identified and minimized. When this is not possible, surgery may be postponed while the patient is helped with these feelings.

One way to encourage the surgical patient to verbalize concerns is to describe common concerns of most surgical patients in a matter-of-fact way. Some patients are reassured and encouraged to learn that these concerns are common experiences which the nurse has anticipated. For example, the patient may be reassured to learn from the nurse that fearing cancer or loss of sexual powers is not uncommon. Sometimes just hearing the feeling expressed in words is reassuring. Other patients are reassured by information from the nurse that addresses each concern. For example, describing the nurse's close observation with highly sophisticated equipment in the recovery room may alleviate fears about anesthesia. The nurse may relieve apprehension about divulging private information under anesthesia by explaining that this almost never happens. Occasionally, a person mumbles while recovering from anesthesia but it is rarely understandable. Also, physicians and nurses who work with patients under anesthesia do not discuss, disclose, or repeat what is said.

In addition to concern regarding the operation, the patient is in strange surroundings, away from family and home, and meting new people. Pausing for a moment to consider the probable feelings of the patient, the nurse sees many ways in which to help a person feel more comfortable. Greeting the new patient in a warm and friendly manner, showing how a nurse can be signaled, showing where to unpack and keep clothes and personal belongings, and introducing a roommate are only a few examples of seemingly small acts the thoughtful nurse can perform to make the patient feel more at ease and help to relieve anxiety. The nurse can contribute further to the patient's feeling of confidence by explaining what to expect in regard to the routine of the nursing unit.

Calling the patient by name and explaining diagnostic tests and procedures in advance convey acknowledgment of the patient as an individual. Questions about the patient's preferences, opinions, and reactions to hospitalization, nursing care, and surgery are interventions that favor an increase in personal autonomy as described in Chapter 1.

Information collected by the nurse, the patient's history and physical examination, and laboratory data form the basis of the nursing care plan.

ASSISTING WITH DIAGNOSTIC STUDIES

The nurse can anticipate that most preoperative patients follow a general protocol of x-ray and laboratory studies. A complete blood count (CBC) gives information about the patient's blood volume, bleeding tendency, and body defenses. A urinalysis is done to identify potential kidney problems. A nursing responsibility is to collect a clean, freshly voided urine specimen, label it correctly, and transport it to the laboratory while it is still fresh. A chest x-ray is taken to identify unsuspected respiratory problems that could affect the patient. When the patient is in middle or later years or has a family history of diabetes, a fasting blood sugar (FBS) is done to rule out diabetes. An electrocardiogram (ECG) is taken on middle-aged and elderly surgical patients as well as those with known or suspected cardiovascular disease. In addition to the general protocol, specific diagnostic studies are ordered related to the diseased organ or system.

When surgery is elective, diagnostic studies may be completed before the patient arrives on the nursing unit. In some hospitals, it is the responsibility of nursing personnel to make certain that written reports of all diagnostic studies are on the chart prior to surgery.

An abnormal laboratory finding or x-ray report may cause the surgeon to delay surgery until the underlying condition is identified and corrected. When surgery cannot be postponed, an abnormal laboratory report alerts the surgeon and nurses to expect possible complications.

ASSISTING WITH PATIENT TEACHING

Preoperative teaching is a very important nursing activity. Studies show that the patient who has received preoperative instruction generally recovers faster with fewer complications. The registered nurse usually plans patient teaching and the LPN/LVN assists the patient by explaining, demonstrating and/or supervising the patient's practice sessions. Some hospitals sponsor regular classes which all surgical patients attend. In other hospitals, preoperative teaching is done by the nurses caring for the patient.

In general, patient teaching includes two basic topics: teaching what to expect before, during, and after surgery; and teaching what is expected from the patient before, during, and after surgery. Topics may include local skin preparation, general hygiene measures, intravenous (IV) therapy, pain medication, recovery room practices, and dressings. A helpful way to teach the patient what to expect is to describe a typical day before surgery, the day of surgery, and the first several days following surgery.

These subjects are described later in the chapter.

Teaching the patient what is expected includes topics such as smoking, diet, exercises, deep breathing and coughing, positioning and turning, and ambulating. It often surprises the patient to learn that extensive patient participation is expected and needed in order to prevent complications. Some patients mistakenly assume that they will lie in bed resting undisturbed and heavily sedated for several days following surgery. This false belief is very difficult to correct after surgery when the patient feels sleepy and uncomfortable. Thus, it is very important that the patient understand that good postoperative care requires periods of activity and stirring up interspersed with rest periods.

PREOPERATIVE ORDERS

The nurses's guide to specific preoperative care includes the preoperative orders written by the surgeon or an assistant. The orders usually are easy to find on the patient's chart because the surgeon writes PREOPERATIVE ORDERS in large letters above them. Components of typical preoperative orders include:

- Name of surgical procedure and time scheduled
- Laboratory work and x-rays
- Specific hour after which the patient is no longer permitted food and fluids
- Local skin preparation
- Preoperative medications
- Instructions about the operative permit

DIET AND FLUIDS

After determining the nourishment needed by the patient, the physician prescribes the diet. The undernourished and dehydrated patient receives a special diet to improve those conditions before surgery. When a patient is unable to take an adequate amount of food and fluids by mouth, intravenous therapy may be prescribed. Supplemental vitamins, minerals, and electrolytes may be administered by mouth or added to intravenous fluids.

Oral food, fluids, and medication are not given for 6 to 12 hours prior to surgery in order to make sure that the patient's stomach is empty. This is especially important when the patient is given a general anesthetic. The reason for having the stomach empty is to prevent vomiting while the general anesthetic is being given. The patient who vomits while unconscious is likely to aspirate some of the food and fluid into the lungs. Vomitus in the lungs causes serious complications such as aspiration pneumonia and lung abscess.

Usually the last meal eaten by the patient before the operation consists of easily digested food. In some types of surgery, this kind of food is given for several days before the operation. When surgery is planned for the next morning, the patient should eat no food after the evening meal. Most surgeons permit drinking liquids until either bedtime or midnight of the night before surgery.

When the order written states NPO after midnight tonight, the following activities are avoided after midnight: eating drinking, smoking, chewing tobacco, chewing gum, and taking medication by mouth. Oral hygiene is encouraged but the patient is cautioned not to swallow the water or mouthwash. It is important to inform the patient about these restrictions well in advance so that accidents do not happen from lack of information or a misunderstanding.

Occasionally, a patient eats or drinks after the specified time. When the nurse becomes aware that this has occurred, the head nurse or team leader is notified. If the amount consumed is small, no action may be needed. If the amount is large, surgery may be postponed until the stomach is emptied naturally or by mechanical methods.

ELIMINATION

The lower intestine should be as empty as possible before surgery in order to prevent fecal incontinence during the operation and postoperative discomfort from gas in the intestines. Enemas may be ordered the evening before or the day of surgery to remove feces from the colon. It is important for the nurse giving the enema to be certain that all of the solution has been expelled.

When abdominal surgery is planned, a more extensive bowel preparation may be needed. A full colon interferes with surgical procedure, and there is additional danger of spillage of intestinal contents into the abdominal cavity causing peritonitis. Components of this preparation may include a low-residue diet for several days before surgery, a clear liquid diet on the day immediately preceding surgery, and a cathartic such as castor oil or magnesium citrate to remove gastrointestinal contents.

When intestinal surgery is planned, a complete bowel preparation is usually ordered. This includes antibiotics to reduce the number of microorganisms present in the intestine at the time of surgery, and special diets, laxatives, and enemas already discussed.

A partial or complete bowel preparation can be tiring and dehydrating to the patient. Considerable amounts of fluids and electrolytes can be lost through the bowel following repeated laxatives and/or enemas. Remembering that undernutrition and dehydration are factors that increase surgical risk enables the nurse to observe and report any imbalances between intake and output. Very young patients and elderly patients develop imbalances more quickly.

GENERAL HYGIENE

An important part of preoperative care is a thorough cleansing bath and good oral hygiene. Cleanliness helps to prevent postoperative infections. When permitted by the physician, the nurse can assist the patient with a shower, tub bath, or bed bath. Hair and nails should be clean and nails free from polish. Oral hygiene is very important prior to surgery because this practice reduces the number of normal bacteria in the mouth. Artificial airways and anesthesia during surgery favor the movement of bacteria from the mouth to lower parts of the respiratory tract where they can cause infection. Toothbrushes and toothpaste are preferred since the friction of brushing helps to cleanse bacteria away. When this is not possible, gauze wrapped around a tongue depressor can be substituted. Lemon and glycerine swabs are not recommended as the only agent for

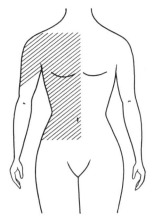 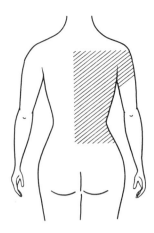

FIGURE 6.2   Area to be prepared for chest surgery.

mouth care because most persons using them do not use enough friction to remove bacteria.

LOCAL SKIN PREPARATION

The purpose of skin care of the operative field is to make it as clean and free of bacteria as possible without harming the skin. A large area around the future wound is cleaned thoroughly and shaved (Figures 6.2, 6.3, 6.4, 6.5 and 6.6). The exact procedure varies according to local custom and the surgeon's preference. The nurse needs to be familiar with institutional procedures.

Generally, soap and water are used to clean the skin first. Sometimes special soaps are used because of bacteriostatic action on skin microorganisms. Oily dirt and adhesive may be removed with benzene, ether, or acetone if the patient does not object to the odor. Next, the operative area is shaved completely. Strong, well-focused light, a sterile razor with a new blade, and shaving *against* the direction of hair growth are factors that improve hair removal. Nicking and scratching of the skin during the shave are avoided because bacteria grow very rapidly in nicks and scratches and secondary infection may occur as a result. The nurse records and reports all nicks, scratches, skin eruptions, and rashes. An antiseptic may be applied to the skin after it has been shaved.

It is desirable to do local skin preparation as close to the time of surgery as possible because bacteria have less time to multiply. Bone, brain, spinal surgeries, and plastic reconstruction are examples of procedures in which local skin preparation may be done in the operating room. In other cases, skin preparation is done the day of surgery or the evening before surgery.

In some institutions, a *depilatory cream,* which is a substance that removes hair, is used for selected cases. When using a depilatory cream, the nurse should remove long hairs by cutting before applying the cream. The nurse should test the patient's skin with the cream to be used 24 hours before actually using it to see if the patient is allergic to the cream. The depilatory cream can be

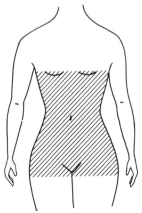

FIGURE 6.3   Area to be prepared for abdominal surgery.

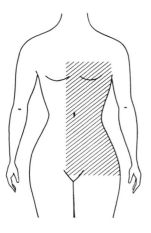 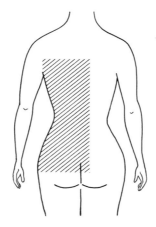

FIGURE 6.4 Area to be prepared for kidney surgery.

spread gently over the entire area to be prepared for surgery with a wooden tongue blade or a gloved hand. The cream containing the hair is removed gently with moistened gauze sponges and the tongue blade. After removing all cream and hair, the practical nurse should wash the area with soap and water and pat dry. The area should be observed for sensitivity reactions.

Many hospitals have a special team from the operating room that is assigned to do each surgical patient's skin preparation the evening prior to surgery or in the operating room holding area. The nurse should be absolutely sure that the patient understands why the skin preparation is done and who will be responsible for doing it.

In some agencies the patient must sign a special consent form giving the nurse permission to remove hair from special parts of the body such as the head. An example of hair that is not removed is eyebrows.

Some recent studies have questioned the value of hair removal in preventing postoperative infection. Injured tissue which can result from shaving and depilatory creams may permit normal skin bacteria to enter the surgical field. Researchers found that postoperative infection occurred more often in patients whose hair was removed prior to surgery. Removal of hair may still be needed for access to a hairy area of the body or to keep hair from acting as a foreign body in the incision. However, research findings may eventually result in changes in the existing procedures. The nursing student can look for new developments in this area in the future.

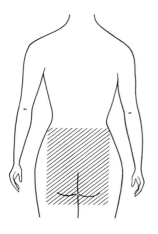 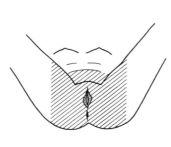

FIGURE 6.5 Area to be prepared for perineal surgery.

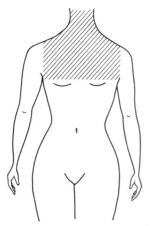

FIGURE 6.6   Area to be prepared for neck surgery.

OPERATIVE PERMIT

The operative permit is a legal document which the patient or the patient's legal representative must sign giving consent for surgery. Since the permit is a legal document, it is very important that hospital policy be followed exactly. Usually, the surgeon explains the surgical procedure in ordinary language first. After the patient understands the surgical procedure, the permit is signed and witnessed. As mentioned earlier, the nurse's responsibility related to the operative permit varies according to hospital policy. Generally, the LPN/LVN may be asked to witness the permit the patient is signing and check the permit to be certain that it is signed before administering the preoperation medication. In addition, the patient may ask the LPN/LVN some questions about the surgery or anesthesia. Since it is very important that the patient be fully informed about the surgery, these questions are usually referred directly to the surgeon. Some patients are helped to ask questions by the nurse's presence during the surgeon's visit.

Rarely, the patient who has already signed the operative permit decides not to have surgery. When the LPN/LVN becomes aware of this, the head nurse or team leader is notified at once. The surgeon and operating room team are also notified.

EXERCISES

An exercise program is taught, demonstrated, and supervised for the patient prior to surgery. The first set of exercises is deep breathing and coughing. Deep breathing and coughing are done five or more times per hour postoperatively to get air to deeper recesses of the lung and to improve venous return to the heart. The patient who is at risk to develop atelectasis and pneumonia following surgery may be instructed to increase the number of exercises per hour or to do them more frequently. Elderly patients, smokers, patients with chest or abdominal incisions, those with an underlying respiratory condition, and those who will be immobilized following surgery are at increased risk for postoperative atelectasis and pneumonia.

The sitting position is preferred during deep-breathing exercises. An alternate position is lying on the back (supine) with the knees slightly flexed. The patient inhales slowly through the nose and holds the breath for 3 seconds at the end of inspiration. Then the patient exhales slowly through the mouth. An alternate method is to instruct the patient to yawn. The abdomen should rise during inspiration and fall during expiration. The patient's hands may be placed on the abdomen as a check to see that exercises are done correctly.

Coughing exercises are done to clear the tracheobronchial tree of retained secretions which have collected during anesthesia. Several types of cough can be taught to the patient. Cascade coughing, huff coughing, and augmented coughing are described in detail in Chapter 14. Patients with chest or abdominal incisions are taught to splint them during deep breathing, coughing, and turning. Splinting means placing the hands, a small pillow, or towel over the incision to minimize movement. At times, the nurse's hands are used for splinting. Incentive spirometry and blow bottles are devices used to promote deep breathing and coughing. The nurse should follow the manufacturer's instructions for using these devices because incorrect use reduces effectiveness. Intermittent positive pressure breathing (IPPB) may benefit selected surgical patients. IPPB is described later in this chapter.

Turning exercises are done hourly in the postoperative period because they improve circulation and move respiratory secretions. Splinting the incision and a pillow between the legs are measures that reduce pain when a patient turns from side to side. The patient may practice turning before surgery.

Leg exercises are taught to the patient because they improve circulation after surgery. The joints of the hips, knees, and ankles of each leg are alternately extended and flexed. The ankle is rotated as though tracing a large circle with the toes. Then, the patient moves the legs as if riding a bicycle. The patient may do similar exercises with the shoulder, elbow, and wrist of each arm. Immediately following surgery, the nurse may assist with these exercises. Within a day or so, the patient does the exercises alone with the nurse observing, encouraging, and minimally assisting if needed.

EQUIPMENT

Equipment that is expected to be used postoperatively should be explained to the patient and demonstrated if possible before surgery. When it is not possible to get the equipment preoperatively, pictures may be shown to the patient instead. All needed equipment should be at the bedside before the patient returns from surgery.

Special areas such as the intensive care unit and recovery room should also be explained. Many hospitals have preoperative teams from the operating room and the recovery room to visit patients and describe the areas they represent. In some cases, the patient is able to visit the operating room or special care unit prior to surgery.

Some hospitals have special waiting rooms where families of surgical patients remain in order to talk to the surgeon after the operation. The nurse can anticipate that the family is interested in knowing when the operation is completed and that the patient has been transferred to the recovery room.

PREANESTHETIC MEDICATIONS

Medication given prior to surgery (preanesthetic medication) enhances the induction of anesthesia. Preoperative medication is the phrase that is most often used to describe one or more drugs given to produce sleep and certain amounts of amnesia, decrease secretions of mucus and saliva, and promote muscular relaxation. The specific drugs administered are usually ordered by the anesthesiologist who visits the patient prior to surgery. In some cases, the surgeon or an assistant orders preoperative medication.

Preanesthesia medication may begin with a sedative-hypnotic given the night before surgery to produce a sound sleep. On the day of surgery, additional medication is administered at a time specifically chosen so that maximum benefit is attained at the time of anesthesia induction. Typical preoperative medication includes a narcotic analgesic, a sedative, or tranquilizer, such as those in Tables 6.1 and 6.2, and a vagolytic drying agent.

It is important to administer preanesthetic medication at the time indicated on the preoperative orders. Medication given too early may peak before the patient is ready for anesthesia. Medication given too late may peak after the patient is under general anesthesia causing severe respiratory depression and/or hypotension. Usually, the nurse administering the preoperative medication checks to make sure the operative permit has been signed before giving the drug. This is important because the patient cannot give legal consent for surgery while sedated. If the LPN/LVN discovers that the operative permit has not been signed, the medication is withheld and the team leader or head nurse is notified at once. Usually, the surgeon and the operating room are notified, and surgery is postponed until the permit is signed and the patient is premedicated.

After the preanesthetic medication is administered, the nurse raises the bedrails, places the call bell within easy reach, instructs the patient to remain in bed, and reduces lighting in the environment. A family member may remain at the bedside at this time. Usually, the nurse asks the family member not to initiate conversation.

A special hazard exists when a patient receives pain medication several hours before

TABLE 6.1
SEDATIVE-HYPNOTICS

NONPROPRIETARY NAME	TRADE NAME	AVERAGE DOSE FOR ADULTS	NURSING IMPLICATIONS
I. Barbiturates			
Amobarbital	AMYTAL	20–200 mg	Barbiturates produce hypnosis and sedation and relieve convulsions. Some are short, long, or intermediate acting
Butabarbital	BUTISOL	30–200 mg	
Mephobarbital	MEBARAL	30–200 mg	
Pentobarbital*	NEMBUTAL	30–100 mg	Therapeutic doses may cause patient to feel listless and depressed, have a skin rash or urticaria, and become restless
Phenobarbital*	LUMINAL	15–100 mg	
Secobarbital*	SECONAL	32–100 mg	
			Large doses are poison and may cause death
			Drug dependence may develop
			Subject to abuse
			May cause paradoxical excitement in elderly individuals
			Alterations in sleep patterns which continue for a time after the drug is discontinued
II. Nonbarbiturate Hypnotics			
Bromisolvalum	BROMURAL	300–900 mg	Nonbarbiturate hypnotics
Chloral hydrate*	NOCTEC	250–500 mg	Habit-forming and may result in physical dependence
	LORINOL		
	SOMNOS		Subject to abuse
Chlorobutanol	CHLORETONE	0.3–1.0 gm	Skin rash and nausea may occur
Ethchlorvynol	PLACIDYL	100–500 mg	Some nonbarbiturate hypnotics are not as predictable in effects as the barbiturates
Ethinamate	VALMID	500 mg	
Flurazepam*	DALMANE	15–30 mg	
Glutethimide*	DORIDEN	0.125–0.25 mg	
Methaqualone	QUAALUDE	150–300 mg	
Paraldehyde		5–10 ml	

* Sedatives and/or hypnotics often used for surgical patients.

a preanesthetic medication. This increases the possibility of dangerous respiratory depression or hypotension. A typical situation occurs when the patient requires a narcotic for pain during the night and preanesthetic medication has been ordered early the next morning. Most hospitals have policies that guide the nurse in this situation. Usually the surgeon and/or anesthesiologist is notified before the preanesthetic medication is administered. The dosage may be reduced, the drug changed, or the preanesthetic medication omitted entirely.

Immediate Preoperative Care

The care of the patient immediately before surgery should be arranged so that last-minute rushing is avoided and the patient does not feel hurried. After personal and oral hygiene is completed, the patient wears a cotton hospital gown. The hair is combed and hairpins are removed. Long hair can be braided to avoid tangles. Many hospitals provide a cotton cap to cover the hair during surgery.

A systematic head-to-toe observation of the patient enables the nurse to detect and report abnormal situations that require a delay or postponement of surgery. For example, sneezing, coughing, hoarseness, and sniffling indicate possible upper respiratory infection. The surgeon usually postpones elective surgery when the patient has these symptoms.

The patient's vital signs are taken and recorded also at this time. Abnormalities are reported to the surgeon immediately. For

TABLE 6.2
TRANQUILIZERS

NONPROPRIETARY NAME	TRADE NAME	AVERAGE DOSE FOR ADULTS	NURSING IMPLICATIONS
Chlordiazepoxide	LIBRIUM	5–25 mg	Frequently used for treatment of anxiety and to promote a change in behavior toward tranquility
Chlorpromazine	THORAZINE	10–50 mg*	Some have antiemetic effect
Diazepam†	VALIUM	2–10 mg	Sedation, loss of muscular coordination, dry mouth, dermatitis, hypotension, blurred vision, jaundice, and blood dyscrasias are examples of some of the side effects of many tranquilizers
Fluphenazine	PERMITIL PROLIXIN	0.25–10 mg	
Hydroxyzine†	VISTARIL	25–100 mg	
Meprobamate	MILTOWN EQUANIL	200–400 mg	Before giving a specific tranquilizer, the nurse should review the literature and become familiar with the possible therapeutic and side effects to be observed in the patient
Perphenazine	TRILAFON	2–8 mg	
Prochlorperazine†	COMPAZINE	5–25 mg	
Promazine†	SPARINE	10–100 mg	
Thioridazine	MELLARIL	10–200 mg	
Trifluoperazine	STELAZINE	1–10 mg	
Triflupromazine*	VESPRIN	10–50 mg	

* Dose varies according to effect desired.
† Tranquilizers often used for preoperative and postoperative patients.

example, an elevated temperature and pulse indicate possible infection which could delay surgery.

Observations that indicate panic, dread, or doom are also reported. Usually the nurse uses an open-ended question to ask how the patient is feeling about the impending surgery. The patient can be expected to verbalize some apprehension or nervousness. However, reports of a "bad feeling about this whole thing," "dreading it," "scared to death" indicate more serious fears which should be reported to the head nurse or team leader.

The hospital procedure manual will specify whether dentures are to remain in the patient's mouth or be removed before the patient goes to surgery. However, the anesthesiologist may request that the dentures be left in the patient's mouth. This may help the anesthetist to apply the mask more securely during anesthesia. When dentures are removed, they should be placed in a container, clearly labeled, which is then put in a safe place, such as the drawer of the bedside table. Jewelry and other valuables and prostheses should be handled according to hospital procedure for safekeeping. A ring may be secured with either adhesive tape or bandage if the patient does not want to remove

it if allowed by the hospital. Usually, the nurse checks the patient's identification bracelet at this time to be sure that it is present, accurate, and complete.

Just before the preoperative medication is administered, the patient is asked to urinate. The time and amount of urine are recorded. Inability to urinate at this time is reported and recorded.

The preoperative checklist is a tool used in many hospitals to assure complete and accurate preoperative patient care. In general, the checklist consists of observations to be made and procedures to be followed before the patient is transferred to the operating room. Generally, the LPN/LVN reviews the checklist to be sure it is complete before giving the preoperative medication. Typical items on the checklist include the signed operative permit, location and care of dentures and/or prostheses, location of jewelry, presence of identification bracelet, completion of local skin preparation, last vital signs taken, time and amount of last voiding, blood work, urinalysis, chest x-ray, ECG reports. Figure 6.7 illustrates a checklist.

Proper identification of the patient is essential before a transfer to the operating pavilion. In addition to checking this verbally, the practical nurse should confirm the pa-

THE QUEEN'S MEDICAL CENTER
HONOLULU, HAWAII

PREOPERATIVE CHECKLIST

	YES/INITIALS	COMMENTS/INITIALS
1. PREOPERATIVE INSTRUCTIONS:		
A. ROUTINE PRE & POST OPERATIVE ACTIVITIES		
B. DEEP BREATHING, COUGHING AND LEG EXERCISES (UNLESS CONTRAINDICATED)		
2. ABLE TO DEMONSTRATE PROPER DEEP BREATHING, COUGHING, & LEG EXERCISES		
3. DIETARY RESTRICTIONS MAINTAINED AS ORDERED		
4. 10 MINUTE BATH OR SHOWER WITH ANTIBACTERIAL SOAP COMPLETED		
5. PREP ORDER SHEET COMPLETED BY M.D.		
6. IDENT-A-BAND ON ____ (LEFT WRIST SHOULD BE USED UNLESS CONTRAINDICATED BY SURGERY)		
7. REMOVE THE FOLLOWING:		
A. PERSONAL CLOTHING (INCLUDING UNDERWEAR)		
B. JEWELRY (IF TAPED, LIST)		
C. HAIRPINS, HAIRPIECES, LIPSTICK, FALSE EYELASHES		
D. FALSE TEETH, PARTIAL PLATES, BRIDGES		
E. PROSTHESIS (ARTIFICIAL EYES, LIMBS, CONTACT LENSES)		
F. NAIL POLISH		
8. TO BE ON PATIENT'S CHART:		
A. MORNING TPR-BP		
B. CURRENT HEIGHT & WEIGHT (CHARTED ON GRAPHIC)		
*C. CONSENT TO OPERATION (PROPERLY COMPLETED)		
D. CONSULTATIONS		
*E. SPECIAL PERMITS		
*F. CBC OR Hgb & Hct REPORT		
*G. URINALYSIS REPORT		
*H. HISTORY & PHYSICAL OR HEART & LUNG CLEARANCE		
I. VOIDED OR CATHETERIZED @ ____ ☐ AM ☐ PM		
J. PRE-OP MEDICINE GIVEN & CHARTED		
K. PREP ORDER SHEET		
L. MEDICATION SHEET REMOVED FROM MED BOOK & PLACED IN CHART		
M. PROGRESS NOTES COMPLETED		
N. ADDRESSOGRAPH PLATE		
9. X-RAYS ON UNIT SENT TO SURGERY		
10. SPECIAL REMARKS (REQUEST OF PATIENT'S MEDS TO O.R., ETC.)		
11. ALLERGY NOTATION TAPED ON FRONT OF CHART		
12. PATIENT INSTRUCTED TO REMAIN IN BED AFTER PRE-OP MEDICINE GIVEN		
13. SIDE RAILS UP, CALL LIGHT IN PLACE, BED IN LOW POSITION AFTER PRE-OP MEDICINE GIVEN		

* MUST BE COMPLETED BEFORE ADMINISTERING PRE-OP MEDICATIONS

TO O.R. @ ____   ☐ A.M.   ☐ P.M.

INITIAL	SIGNATURE

THE ABOVE ACTIVITIES HAVE BEEN COMPLETED AS STATED. PATIENT IS "READY" FOR SURGERY.

SIGNATURE ____

DATE ____

FIGURE 6.7   Preoperative checklist. (Courtesy of The Queen's Medical Center, Honolulu, Hawaii.)

THE QUEEN'S MEDICAL CENTER

NURSING SERVICE DEPARTMENT

RECORDS 502-103-2
PATIENT CONSENT FORMS

103-2-1 (3) Guidelines for Preoperative Checklist

Purpose: To provide a reference list and a place for the documentation of activities necessary in the preparation of a patient for surgery. To provide a direct means of communication between the nursing unit and the Operating Room.

Procedure:

1. ALL patients entering the Operating Room must have a Preoperative Checklist at the front of the chart.

2. All items on the list must be initialed by a nurse. When the activity has been completed, initial "yes" column. If activity has not been done, indicate reason and initial "comment" column.

3. All items with asterisk <u>must</u> be completed prior to administering the preoperative medications.

4. Pajama bottoms must be removed for all cases. Patient is to wear white gown with ties at neck.

5. Jewelry is to be removed, however if a piece of jewelry cannot be removed such as a wedding ring it is to be covered with a piece of tape. List on check list.

6. Nail polish is to be removed on at least one hand.

7. Consultations must be obtained for enuclerations and major amputations.

8. If the history and physical has been dictated but is not in the chart, the physician must record on the Progress Notes "heart and lungs okay for surgery."

9. Signature of nurse and date is to be entered in appropriate area at bottom of page when patient is ready to be sent to surgery. "Ready" means that all activities have been completed.

10. Enter time patient leaves unit for O.R. in appropriate box at bottom of page.

11. Initial/signature - Each initial is to be identified by a signature and status in box at bottom of page.

FIGURE 6.7A   Instructions for the Preoperative Checklist (Courtesy of The Queen's Medical Center, Honolulu, Hawaii)

tient's identity by reading the bed tag and identification bracelet and comparing them with the patient's chart. The chart is transferred to the operating suite with the patient.

The patient is transferred to the operating room on a stretcher or in bed (Figure 6.8). Adequate covering is needed to prevent chilling. The nurse may be asked to accompany the patient to surgery (see Figure 6.9). Having a familiar and interested person nearby reassures the patient. The patient should not be left unattended while on a stretcher. A strap should be placed across the patient and secured to the stretcher as a safety measure.

In many hospitals, the patient may be accompanied to the entrance of the operating room suite by members of the immediate family. The family is then instructed to wait in an area which has been designated in advance.

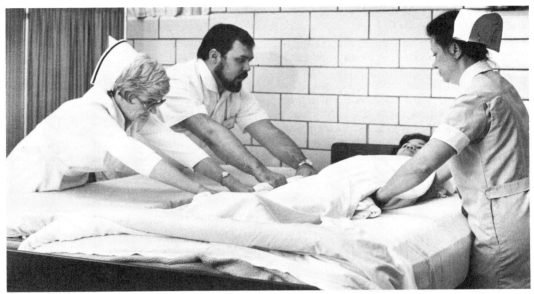

FIGURE 6.8   Transferring the preoperative patient to a stretcher. (Courtesy of Shapero School of Nursing, Sinai Hospital of Detroit, Detroit, Michigan.)

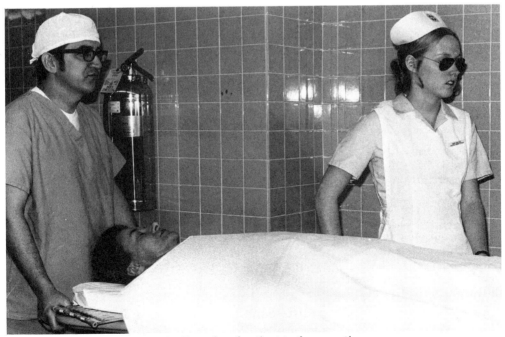

FIGURE 6.9   Transfer of patient to the operating room.

Intraoperative Care

Upon arrival in the operating room or holding area, the patient is greeted by name by the anesthesiologist or a nurse who will remain present throughout the surgery. The patient is placed in a quiet environment with constant observation while the safety strap remains across the legs. Even though resting or sleeping, the patient is not left alone at this time.

The patient can be reassured by the facial expression, the greeting by the individual nurse or surgeon, and the actual touch of someone who communicates a feeling of caring. The patient can be further comforted and reassured by attention to physical needs such as adding an additional blanket if necessary or placing a small pillow under the head. The patient's name should be used by members of the operating room team during each contact.

The patient is usually drowsy but awake when brought from the holding area to the operating room. Therefore, other members of the surgical team are identified and introduced.

THE SURGICAL TEAM

Successful surgery requires a coordinated effort of the operating room team. The *anesthesiologist* or *nurse anesthetist* concentrates on the patient's overall well-being which enables the surgeon to concentrate on the surgical procedure. Activities of the anesthesiologist or nurse anesthetist include:

- Anesthetize the patient for surgery.
- Administer drugs during surgery.
- Administer intravenous fluids and blood as indicated.
- Monitor the patient's respiratory and circulatory status during surgery.
- Alert the surgeon immediately of changes in the patient's condition.
- Initiate, monitor, and supervise the patient's recovery from anesthesia (includes the recovery room period).

The *circulating nurse* is a registered nurse who is the manager of the operating room in which a particular surgery takes place. This position is similar to the head nurse on a nursing unit. Activities of the circulating nurse include:

- Observe the operating room for cleanliness and orderliness.
- Ensure that equipment needed during a particular surgery is available, sterilized if appropriate, and in working order.
- Receive and identify patient.
- Check that preoperative care has been completed and that x-rays, laboratory reports, blood products needed during surgery are available and present.
- Assist in transferring patient to operating table, positioning and draping, and skin preparation.
- Assist members of the operating team to gown and glove.
- Monitor surgical asepsis during operation—report breaks in technique and obtain new sterile equipment when indicated.
- Supervise scrub nurses, surgical technicians, and all students present in the operating room.
- Supervise sponge, needle, and instrument counts during surgery.
- Obtain all additional equipment, drugs, and supplies needed during surgery.
- Call other health team members when needed (x-ray technician, pathologist, laboratory technician).
- Receive, correctly label, and send all specimens collected during surgery.
- Assist with transfer of patient to recovery room following surgery.
- Supervise cleanup of operating room following surgery.

The *scrub nurse* is a specially trained person whose primary responsibility is to provide the surgeon and assistants with the specific equipment needed on a moment-by-moment basis during the surgery. The scrub nurse may be a registered nurse, an LPN/LVN, or a surgical technician. Activities of the scrub nurse include:

- Set up trays of instruments that will be used for surgery.
- Assist surgeon and assistants to gown and glove.
- Hand instruments, suture material,

sponges, and other sterile equipment to the surgeon and assistants during surgery.
- Anticipate the need for additional supplies and report to circulating nurse.
- Participate in sponge, needle, and instrument counts during surgery.
- Observe and report breaks in aseptic technique.

The *surgeon* is the physician who actually performs the surgery. At times, the surgeon has *assistants* whose primary job is to make the operative site as clear and visible as possible. For example, the assistant may retract tissues away from the operative site, sponge or suction blood and fluids which flow into the operative site, and control bleeding using hemostats or suture material. Usually, the assistant is a physician in training to become a surgeon. When there is no assistant, a scrub nurse performs selected activities such as a retraction of tissues and sponging or suctioning of blood from the operative area.

POSITIONING THE PATIENT

The patient may be positioned for surgery either before or after anesthesia. The anesthetized patient does not experience the warning sensations of poor positioning (pain, ache, stiffness, numbness and tingling, burning). Therefore, it is extremely important that positioning during the intraoperative period does not cause damage to tissue.

Factors important to patient positioning at this time include appropriate padding over bony prominences, avoiding pressure on body that could impair circulation, avoiding excessive strain on muscles, avoiding dangling extremities, providing for adequate respiration and circulation. Remembering that the anesthetized patient may be immobilized for hours during surgery enables the nurse to explain the reasons for stiffness and soreness postoperatively. Knowing that hyperextending the neck is important to maintain a patent airway during certain types of anesthesia helps the nurse to understand and explain the patient's stiff neck postoperatively.

THE ANESTHETIZED PATIENT

The anesthetized patient experiences a loss of sensation and motor function because of one or more drugs, known as anesthetics, that have been given. The purposes of anesthesia are to eradicate pain, to relax the tissue, and allay anxiety. A variety of agents and methods may be used for these purposes.

General anesthesia affects the patient's entire body and involves a loss of consciousness. Nitrous oxide, halothane, and cycloproprane are examples of drugs that produce general anesthesia by inhalation. General anesthetic agents that are inhaled are given by way of a face mask, nasal cannula, or a tube (endotracheal tube) inserted into the trachea. Thiopental sodium (PENTOTHAL) is given intravenously to produce general anesthesia. Intravenous anesthesia is used most often for short minor surgical procedures and to induce sleep before inhalation anesthesia is administered. Inhalation anesthesia generally is used for major procedures involving the head, neck, chest, and abdomen as well as selected other procedures. The complications of general anesthesia include cardiac arrhythmias and cardiac arrest, spasm of airways, vomiting and aspiration, hypotension and shock, renal and gastrointestinal complications, cerebral complications, damage and injury to eyes, teeth, tongue, lips, and vocal cords.

Regional anesthesia involves injecting an anesthetic into large nerve bundles at a certain certain distance from the operative site. The area supplied by these nerves becomes anesthetized. In a *spinal anesthetic*, the drug is introduced into the spinal canal (see Figure 6.10). This causes paralysis of the nerves as they leave the spinal cord. When using *epidural anesthesia*, the physician injects an anesthetic solution into the space immediately outside the spinal dura (outermost membrane covering the spine). The selected spinal nerves are blocked before they enter the bony part of the vertebral column. The area of the body supplied by these nerves becomes anesthetized. Epidural anesthesia is known also as *peridural* or *extradural*. Other regions commonly anesthetized include the hand and arm. The drugs

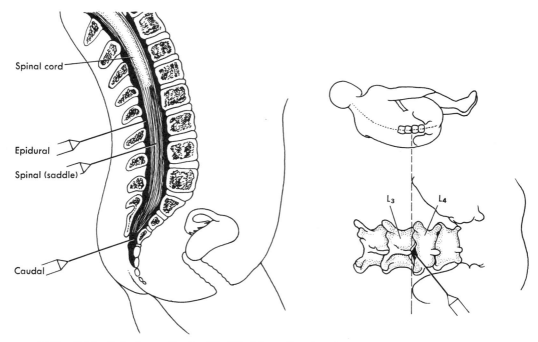

FIGURE 6.10 Spinal anesthesia. (Modified from Pansky, Ben, and House, Earl Lawrence: *Review of Gross Anatomy,* 3rd ed. Macmillan Publishing Co., Inc., New York, 1975.)

most often used are lidocaine hydrochloride (XYLOCAINE) and bupivacaine (MARCAINE). The duration of regional anesthesia is usually short, from 30 to 60 minutes. Unless an additional drug is used, the patient does not lose consciousness or go to sleep. Surgical procedures that may be performed while the patient is under regional anesthesia include some orthopedic repairs to the extremities, herniorrhaphy, removing moles and cysts, diagnostic procedures including biopsy and endoscopy. Possible complications of regional blocks include drug allergy, accidental injury to surrounding tissues, and accidental drug injection into the bloodstream.

Local anesthesia involves applying the anesthetic drug on top of the skin or mucous membrane (topical anesthesia) or injecting the drug into subcutaneous tissue (local infiltration). This method blocks nerve impulses at the site of the surgical procedure. It does not cause the patient to lose consciousness and does not relax tissues or allay anxiety. The duration of anesthesia is usually short, no more than five or ten minutes. Lidocaine hydrochloride (XYLOCAINE) or procaine (NOVOCAIN) is a drug commonly used. Minor

surgical procedures that are done under a local anesthesia include dental extractions, suturing of lacerations, laryngoscopy, rectal examination. Complications are rare but serious because they usually relate to anaphylaxis from hypersensitivity. Anaphylactic shock is discussed in Chapter 10. Important preventive measures include asking the patient about specific allergies, and having emergency drugs and equipment nearby when local anesthesia is used.

Hypothermia, which means lowered body temperature, may be used locally or generally. In local hypothermia, the patient's extremity such as a leg is packed in ice or a special hypothermia unit. Hypothermia may be used for its local effect for the patient whose general condition is poor, for the elderly patient, and to create an unfavorable environment for bacterial growth such as in orthopedic surgery. General hypothermia may be used in connection with other anesthesia for the patient undergoing surgery of the heart or blood vessels. Certain types of neurosurgery are done with hypothermia. Reduction of the patient's body temperatures decreases the activity of the body tissues, which results in a reduced need for oxygen and nourishment circulated by the blood. *Hypothermia blankets* are rubber cooling blankets in which a cooling substance (*refrigerant*) is circulated through coils or channels. The patient may be placed on one hypothermia blanket or between two (Figure 6.11). The thermostat on the blanket is set at the temperature prescribed by the doctor. The patient's temperature can be determined at any time using a special type of rectal thermometer, which is operated by a battery and connected to a probe inserted in the rectum or other body orifice. The patient is warmed by reversing the procedure when hypothermia blankets are used.

Acupuncture is a type of anesthesia which has been used for centuries in Asian countries and recently has been introduced in the United States. Generally, this method involves applying needles or similar mechanical devices to carefully selected anatomic sites. Very few physicians are trained in this method. However, the practical nursing student can watch for future developments in this field.

The method of anesthesia is selected by the anesthesiologist after examining and talking with the patient. Factors that are considered include the type of surgery, the patient's condition, the patient's anxiety level, the situation at the time of surgery. The anesthesiologist and/or surgeon explains the choice of anesthetic to the patient. The operative permit the patient signs prior to surgery usually includes the type of anesthesia to be used.

Postoperative Care

RECOVERY ROOM

Immediately following surgery, the patient is transferred from the operating room to a recovery room which is adjacent or nearby (see Figure 6.12). The purpose of the recovery room is to help the patient reacting from anesthesia, to provide continuous observation, early detection, and treatment of postoperative complications while the patient's condition is relatively unstable. Nurses in the recovery room have additional

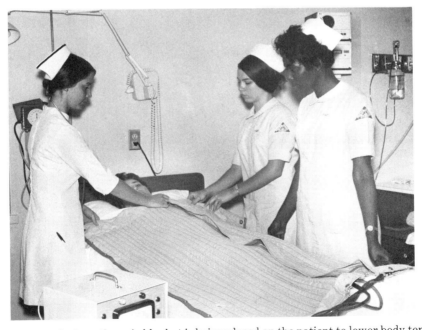

FIGURE 6.11   The hypothermia blanket is being placed on the patient to lower body temperature. (Courtesy of Suffolk City Schools and Louise Obici Memorial Hospital School of Practical Nursing, Suffolk, Virginia.)

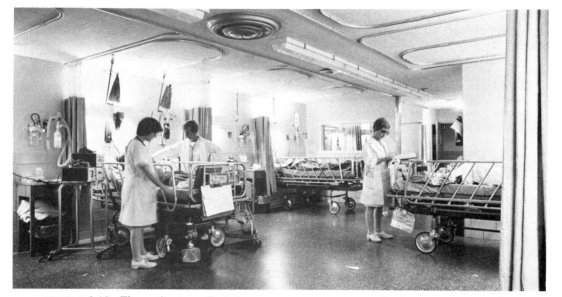

FIGURE 6.12   The patient usually is transferred to the postanesthesia recovery room after surgery. The trend of moving patients to a postoperative recovery room after surgery was started in 1947 at the Ochsner Foundation Hospital in New Orleans. (Courtesy of Alton Ochsner Medical Foundation, New Orleans, Louisiana.)

classes and experience in caring for the patient at this time.

When the patient arrives in the recovery room, the nurse collects information about the surgical experience to anticipate and prevent complications and plan care. Typical information includes the name of the surgical procedure, the type of anesthesia, the duration of surgery, the presence and location of drains and catheters, drugs, fluids, and blood products administered during surgery, output and estimated blood loss during surgery, difficulties that arose during surgery, and the presence of underlying conditions that could affect recovery such as diabetes or heart disease.

The nurse's guide to specific interventions is the postoperative orders written by the surgeon. These are easy to recognize because the surgeon writes POSTOPERATIVE ORDERS at the top of the page. In addition to specific care that relates to the patient's surgery and type of anesthesia, general activities of the nurse in the recovery room include:

• Positioning the patient appropriately.
• Maintaining safety precautions that protect the patient from injury.

• Keeping the patient warm and dry.
• Taking vital signs frequently and evaluating changes.
• Observing, maintaining, recording intake and output including drainage.
• Promoting adequate ventilation and gas exchange.
• Observing and reporting early signs of postoperative complications.
• Assessing the patient's recovery from anesthesia.

As mentioned earlier, specific aspects of the patient's care in the recovery room depend upon the surgical procedure and type of anesthesia used. For example, the patient who is recovering from spinal anesthesia usually remains flat in bed for six to eight hours or longer. Keeping the patient flat in bed reduces the possibility of headache. This headache, which is throbbing in nature and increased when the patient sits up, is thought to be due to the leakage of sinal fluid around the needle puncture. The nurse should not suggest that a headache may occur if the patient sits up before the prescribed time. The nurse should observe the return of movement and feeling in the patient's legs and feet. The patient is considered recovered from the spinal anesthetic when there is a complete return of movement and feeling in the toes. Hypotension may occur with spinal anesthesia; therefore, the patient's vital signs are checked frequently in the recovery room. Even after sensation and movement have returned to the lower extremities, hypotension is a hazard.

The patient who has had a general anesthetic usually is transferred to the recovery room in a special bed (Figure 6.12). Siderails on both sides of the bed should be raised as a safety measure. Usually, the patient is placed on one side to aid the drainage of vomitus and mucus from the mouth and to reduce the range of aspiration. Unless contraindicated, the patient's head is elevated about 30 degrees. An endotracheal tube or artificial airway may be in place. Promoting adequate ventilation and gas exchange is especially important when the patient has received a general anesthesia.

Respiratory difficulty is a dangerous complication that occurs frequently while the patient is reacting from general anesthesia. Depression of the respiratory center in the brain, the falling back of the tongue into the throat, and the collecting of mucus or vomitus in the throat are examples of common causes of respiratory difficulty. The rate of breathing is decreased when the respiratory center is depressed. The physician prescribes a respiratory stimulant when marked depression is present. Keeping the patient's head in good position often keeps the tongue from falling back in the throat. Also, leaving the airway in the mouth and throat until the patient reacts sufficiently to push it out prevents the tongue from falling back. When the tongue slips back into the throat, the nurse can pull it into normal position after protecting the hand with gauze or a piece of clean cloth. The nurse could pull the patient's mandible or chin forward and flex the neck, which forces the tongue forward. Turning the patient's head to the side and gently swabbing the patient's mouth helps to rid the patient of excess mucus. Usually recovery rooms have standing orders for patients to be suctioned as necessary following general anesthesia. Oxygen may also be prescribed for this patient. Because of the danger of respiratory difficulty,

the patient is never left alone at this time. Vital signs are measured and recorded every 15 minutes or as ordered. Deep breathing and frequent turning begin in the recovery room. The patient's dressing is checked frequently for bleeding and drainage.

The nurse can expect changes in behavior as the patient reacts from general anesthesia. Restlessness and incoherent mumbling are not unusual at this time. The patient is not aware of the restless behavior, cannot control it, and needs protection from injury. Repeated explanations that the operation is over, the patient is in the recovery room, and calling the patient by name are nursing interventions that may have a calming effect. The patient's privacy is protected by not disclosing or discussing recovery room behavior or mumblings.

The patient who is fully reacted from general anesthesia is able to respond appropriately to questions asked by the nurse. The patient who is fully reacted from anesthesia, has stable vital signs, and shows no signs of complications is transferred from the recovery room to the nursing unit. Usually, the anesthesiologist and/or surgeon examines the patient before transfer from the recovery room. In some hospitals, preparation for transfer from the recovery room includes gently washing the face and hands, oral hygiene, and a clean gown.

NURSING OBSERVATIONS AND INTERVENTIONS

After the patient has been transferred from the recovery room to a bed on the surgical nursing unit, the nurse first makes certain that the patient is positioned to maintain an airway and prevent aspiration, that siderails are up and the call bell can be easily obtained, and that all tubings and drains are patent, connected, and not twisted or kinked.

Next, the nurse receives a detailed report from the recovery room nurse. In addition to details of the surgery presented upon the patient's arrival in the recovery room, the LPN/LVN is interested in what happened in the recovery room. Information collected includes:

• Time of arrival in recovery room
• Pattern of vital signs

- Intake and output
- Drugs administered
- Problems identified and treated in the recovery room

After receiving this report, the nurse makes a complete head-to-toe observation of the patient using the guide provided in Table 6.3. The patient's wound is observed, the presence, location, and condition of intravenous sites, drains, and catheters are included as the nurse systematically observes the patient from head to toe. Vital signs complete the observations which are then recorded. Unless there are other actions indicated as a result of the observations, the nurse begins the first sequence of deep breathing, coughing, turning, and leg exercises which were described earlier in the chapter.

ASSISTING WITH POSTOPERATIVE EXERCISES

Deep breathing, coughing, turning, and leg exercises were described earlier in the chapter. The practical nursing student may want to review that section on pages 119–20 at this time. As mentioned earlier, exercises usually are done hourly at first and less often as the postoperative period progresses satisfactorily. The drowsy patient may be encouraged by the nurse's frequent reminders of preoperative teaching.

A sample hourly exercise program for the postoperative patient includes the following sequence of activities:

- Exercise the arm and leg on the side opposite to the one the patient is lying on.
- Sit patient at the side of the bed for deep breathing and coughing exercise.
- Turn to opposite side—exercise extremities not previously exercised.
- The patient should rest for an hour and repeat.

ASSISTING WITH HYGIENE

In some hospitals, an immediate postoperative bath is given to remove perspiration, blood, drainage, and antiseptic solutions from the skin. It is important to protect the patient from chilling and drafts at this time because temperature-regulating mechanisms are altered by general anesthesia and surgery. Oral hygiene is given at this time and repeated as often as necessary to prevent overgrowth of bacteria in the mouth.

ASSISTING WITH FOOD AND FLUIDS

Depending upon the type of surgery and anesthesia, food and fluids may be prohib-

TABLE 6.3
GUIDE TO POSTOPERATIVE NURSING OBSERVATIONS AND INTERVENTIONS

WHAT TO OBSERVE	OBSERVATIONS AND INTERVENTIONS
Head and neck	Turn head to one side at first to maintain airway, prevent aspiration
	Check oxygen equipment for proper functioning
	Check mouth for color of mucous membranes, need for oral hygiene
	Ask about possible stiff neck
Chest	Check breathing pattern and rate
	Look for restricted breathing with chest or abdominal incisions, abdominal distention, severe pain, tight dressings and binders, poor sedation
Abdomen	Look for abdominal distention
	Look above symphysis pubis for distended bladder
Back	Check for presence of undetected drainage that has collected underneath patient
	Ask about possible backache
Extremities	Check IV sites for erythema, tenderness, warmth, swelling, twisted tubing
	Check each leg for warmth, erythema, tenderness, swelling in calf and thigh
Urinary function	Ask about pain, burning, itching, or fullness after urinating
	Observe Foley catheter tubing and drainage for patency
Bowel function	Ask if patient has had bowel movement or is passing flatus
Dressing and/or incision	Observe incision for drainage, discoloration, erythema, warmth, tenderness
	Check drains for twisting, kinking

ited for hours or days following surgery. The surgeon's postoperative orders guide the nurse's actions. Intravenous fluids may be given until the patient is able to take adequate liquids by mouth. Some surgeons order ice chips by mouth after surgery. Other surgeons prefer small amounts of tap water instead. It has been suggested that ice and ice water may increase postoperative discomfort from gas. The absence of nausea and vomiting, bowel sounds which can be heard through a stethoscope which the surgeon places on the abdomen, and the patient's report of passing flatus are signs that indicate that the patient can tolerate solid food.

A nourishing diet is important to successful, speedy wound healing. The patient may start with a liquid diet and progress gradually to solid food over a period of days or weeks, depending on the type of surgery.

ASSISTING WITH ELIMINATION

Anesthesia affects the patient's ability to urinate and may cause urinary retention. Bladder walls easily can be damaged by the pressure of too much urine. Therefore, the nurse measures and records the volume and appearance of urine the patient voids after surgery as output. Generally, the nurse can expect a minimum of 30 ml of output per hour following surgery. Urine volume that falls below that level should be reported to the head nurse, or team leader. The patient may be dehydrated and require increased fluids, or there may be other complications. If the patient is unable to urinate in the first 8 to 12 hours after surgery, the surgeon may order catheterization. In some cases, the patient returns from surgery with an indwelling catheter. Knowing that catheters enable bacteria to travel from outside the body to inside the body enables the nurse to take actions that maintain the free flow of urine through the tubing, prevent tension on the tubing, prevent urine from back-flowing from the tubing into the bladder, and promote meticulous cleansing of the genital area.

ASSISTING WITH AMBULATION

In general, the nurse can expect to encourage and assist with early ambulation. Within hours after most surgery, the patient is assisted to dangle the feet over the side of the bed for deep-breathing and coughing exercise described earlier in this chapter. Changes of position are made gradually to prevent dizziness. Within 24 hours after most surgery, the patient is helped to walk a short distance (Figure 6.13). Walking rather than sitting is encouraged at first. Blood pooling in the lower extremities and pressure on the walls of the blood vessels when the patient sits may increase the possibility of thrombophlebitis.

The patient is encouraged to stand up straight and look ahead while walking. Analgesic medication administered about 30 minutes before ambulation and splinting the incision help to reduce pain during ambulation. The nurse uses observations of the patient's skin color, pulse, and respiration as guides to the distance and duration of ambulation. Short, frequent walks interspersed with rest periods generally are encouraged.

The nurse can expect a temporary slight increase in drainage of certain wounds after ambulation. This category includes wounds with catheters and drains and those that have been draining. Wounds that have not been draining usually do not begin to drain during ambulation. Large amounts of drainage in draining wounds or sudden drainage of a nondraining wound during ambulation should be reported after the patient has been returned safely to bed.

The patient should wear a short robe and appropriate footwear when ambulating in order to prevent accidents. Another safety measure is to caution the patient not to use rolling movable objects such as intravenous poles and wheelchairs for support when walking.

ASSISTING WITH POSTOPERATIVE DISCOMFORTS
PAIN

Pain is often the first experience remembered by the postoperative patient. Pain that is expected is acute pain in the area of the operation and incision. Acute pain in other areas not located close to the operative site is not expected, may indicate a complication, and should be reported to the head nurse or team leader. The most appropriate nursing intervention for the patient with acute operative pain is prompt administra-

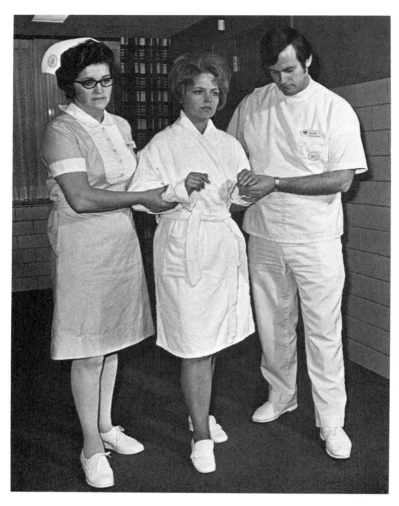

FIGURE 6.13 Early ambu-lation after surgery is an important factor in pre-venting postoperative com-plications. (Courtesy of Shapero School of Nursing, a Program in Practical Nursing of Sinai Hospital, Detroit, Michigan.)

tion of analgesia. Other nursing interven-tions that may be combined with analgesia to relieve postoperative pain include reposi-tioning the patient, exercises, and relaxa-tion exercises.

Most experts on pain agree that relief is more effective when the patient is medicated before the pain becomes severe. In addition, the dosage of analgesia required to prevent severe pain is much smaller than that needed to relieve severe pain after it has occurred. These facts guide the nurse to medicate some postoperative patients on the basis of nurs-ing observations made before the patient ac-tually requests medication. For example, the patient who has received general anesthesia may not be aware of pain until it becomes

quite severe and much more difficult to re-lieve. Nursing observations that influence the nurse to medicate this patient could in-clude restlessness, incoherent mumblings, inability to deep breathe and cough, and stiff-ening of posture when touched or turned.

Hypodermic injections of drugs such as morphine, meperidine (DEMEROL), and PAN-TOPON are given to relieve the pain. Table 7.2 (p. 159) contains a list of analgesics com-monly prescribed for postoperative pain. In some cases, the surgeon prescribes a range of dosages which enables the nurse to select the amount most appropriate for a particu-lar patient. Generally, the analgesic can be repeated every three to four hours as needed. After administering an analgesia, the nurse raises the siderails and places the call bell within the patient's reach. the patient should be instructed not to smoke.

Pain that is not relieved in 30 to 40 minutes should be reported to the head nurse or team leader. The dosage may need to be increased or the interval between dosages shortened in order to relieve the patient's pain.

A few drugs used during surgery exert such powerful effects on respiration that the usual dosage of narcotic analgesia is cut in half for 12 to 24 hours following surgery. Droperidol (INAPSINE) and fenatanyl citrate (INNOVAR) are the most common drugs that make a dosage reduction necessary. This is so important that special notations usually are placed in the postoperative orders so that all persons caring for the patient are alerted for possible respiratory depression.

Perhaps because of increased awareness of problems of drug abuse, an unfortunate trend of undermedication of postoperative pain has caused many patients to suffer more pain than is necessary. In some cases, the patient thinks it is more beneficial to "tough it out" until the pain is very severe in order to prevent possible problems with drugs. In other cases, nurses, not wanting to contribute to a potential for drug abuse, use too small a dosage or administer analgesics too infrequently to provide adequate pain relief. It is important that both the patient and the nurse understand the benefits of adequate pain relief during the postoperative period. Unrelieved pain may act as an unfavorable stressor which delays wound healing. The patient who is relatively pain-free participates much more actively in exercises and ambulation that prevent complications and relieve other postoperative discomforts. The patient who participates actively in care often feels less helpless, afraid, and anxious. This, in turn, reduces the pain and suffering components as described in Chapter 7, and thus, the need for analgesia.

Patient education prior to surgery, knowledge and self-awareness on the nurse's part are keys to preventing undermedication. Facts about the beneficial effects of pain relief are related to the patient before surgery. An important fact to include is the need to prevent severe pain by medicating early when the pain first begins. The nurse can avoid the practice of undermedication by including factors such as the patient's age and nursing observations to select the appropriate dosage of analgesia following surgery. In general, larger dosages are needed in the first 24 to 48 hours after surgery. A practice to be avoided is responding slowly to the patient's request for pain medication. Unavoidable delays should be explained immediately to the patient together with what specific actions are currently being taken to solve the problem. The nurse can expect a loss of trust in the nurse-patient relationship when the patient's need for pain relief is not met promptly.

In addition to acute operative pain, the postoperative patient frequently experiences *joint stiffness, muscle soreness,* and/or a *sore throat.* These symptoms usually result from positioning during surgery and irritation of the throat from an endotracheal tube used for inhalation anesthesia. Nursing interventions that help to relieve stiffness and soreness include range-of-motion exercises, massage (never massage the patient's legs), and low heat to the sore area. A good oral fluid intake when permitted by the surgeon helps to relieve the patient's sore throat. In some cases, lozenges are prescribed. Most patients are relieved by the nurse's explanation of the causes of these postoperative symptoms.

NAUSEA AND VOMITING

Nausea and vomiting are common discomforts after surgery. Anesthesia, pain, manipulation of body organs, and narcotic analgesics are factors associated with nausea and vomiting after surgery. Usually, the nurse places an emesis basin in a convenient place before the patient returns from the recovery room. When the patient vomits, the first action the nurse takes is to turn the patient's head to the side to prevent aspiration of stomach contents into the lungs. Splinting the incision during vomiting may relieve some of the pain, and good oral hygiene increases the patient's comfort. The time, amount, and description of the material vomited are recorded. An antiemetic such as those listed in Table 15.8 (p. 472) may be prescribed for relief of symptoms. Pain is a much more common cause of postoperative nausea and vomiting than previously realized. In addition, the amount of nausea caused by administration of pain medication is much lower than previously realized. These facts should cause the nurse to observe the vomiting patient carefully for unrelieved pain. The nurse reports frequent and persistent nausea and vomiting because these are unusual occurrences that indicate possible complications.

ABDOMINAL DISTENTION

Abdominal distention, a common discomfort following surgery, occurs more frequently after an abdominal operation. The patient who has received a general anesthetic has a gradual return of peristalsis. This allows fluids and gases to collect in the gastrointestinal tract, causing an enlargement of the stomach and intestines called distention. Abdominal distention causes the patient to experience a feeling of abdominal fullness with cramping pain in the abdomen. Nausea and vomiting may occur. The abdomen is so swollen that it may restrict adequate breathing by pressure on the diaphragm above it.

Nursing interventions that are most helpful in relieving abdominal distention include frequent changes of position and early, frequent ambulation. When the flatus is in the lower colon, the insertion of a rectal tube helps the patient expel the flatus. The outer end of the rectal tube can be placed in either a small basin, a urinal, a urine specimen bottle, or a disposable bag to prevent the patient's bed from becoming soiled by the fecal material that is likely to be expelled with the flatus.

Some surgeons prescribe tap water, warm fluids, and crushed ice instead of ice water and other cold fluids. The basis for this request is the belief that warm fluids stimulate the return of peristalsis better than cold liquids and that crushed ice when it reaches the stomach is the temperature of the body.

Occasionally, an enema may be prescribed to stimulate the return of peristalsis. Very rarely, gastrointestinal suction is ordered to relieve abdominal distention. A tube is inserted into the upper gastrointestinal tract and attached to an apparatus that produces suction. Thus, gas and fluid are removed from the upper gastrointestinal tract. Gastrointestinal suction is discussed in detail in Chapter 15. Neostigmine (PROSTIGMIN) is a drug that may be prescribed to prevent and treat abdominal distention.

Generally, the patient with abdominal distention is encouraged to increase the frequency and duration of ambulation in order to move gases and fluids lower into the gastrointestinal tract where they can be expelled. A practice to be avoided is substituting narcotic analgesics for increased ambulation when the patient has colicky gas pains.

Persistent or continuing abdominal distention should be reported to the physician, as it may indicate a serious condition. Acute gastric dilatation can occur and is considered a medical emergency since the patient may go into shock. Abdominal distention is also a symptom of paralytic ileus (adynamic ileus).

ASSISTING WITH WOUND CARE

The nurse can expect that most patients will return from the recovery room with a sterile gauze dressing which covers the incision and is secured by tape. An alternate, relatively new dressing used by some surgeons is called OP-SITE. This is a clear, thin elastic membrane type of dressing which adheres to the skin. The dressing permits easy inspection of the wound and is believed to contribute to faster wound healing and reduced scarring.

A dressing protects the new incision from trauma and contamination, supports the injured tissues by splinting, and can provide pressure to minimize bleeding and edema. The nurse inspects the dressing during the initial postoperative observation for drainage and hourly in the early postoperative period when assisting the patient to exercise or taking vital sighs. In nondraining wounds, minor oozing of the skin edges is expected during the first few hours after surgery. Skin discoloration around the incision that gets larger in the first few hours after surgery and is accompanied by unstable vital signs should be reported to the head nurse or team leader. When observing the patient for signs of bleeding at the operative site, the gauze dressing may have to be lifted at one corner in order to see the incision. In addition, the nurse should check the linens beneath the patient for blood which may have drained undetected from the wound.

In nondraining incisions, the surgical dressing is usually removed within 24 hours. By this time, a seal of fibrin and epithelial cells has formed a protective barrier along the suture line, preventing bacteria from entering the wound. An exposed incision is easier to examine and, some surgeons believe, less likely to become infected. After the fibrin epithelial seal has formed over the suture line, the incision may be palpated (felt with the hands) by the nurse according to the surgeon's postoperative orders related to wound care. When palpating the patient's wound, the nurse looks for local areas that are warmer, more tender, and/or more swollen than the rest of the incision. Within five to seven days after surgery, a hard, blunt elevation of tissue develops along the entire length of the incision. This is called the healing ridge, and it can be seen and felt by the nurse during wound care. When a healing ridge does not occur, the nurse may anticipate complications and delayed wound healing.

When a wound has a catheter or drain, the nurse can expect considerable drainage and the need for dressing changes (Figure 6.14). The number and type of drains used are usually listed and located in the operative note written by the surgeon. Surgical conditions in which wound drains and catheters can be anticipated include operations where large amounts of tissue are removed, leaving a space where fluids can collect, when leakage is expected because of the organ involved, when there is preoperative infection in the operative area, and when there is preoperative trauma to the operative area. The surgeon may select from a variety of available drains such as cigarette drain, Penrose drain, sump catheter, or T tube. The drain usually is not placed in the incision but in a separate incision nearby. The drain may be buried in the surgical dressing, connected to gravity drainage, or

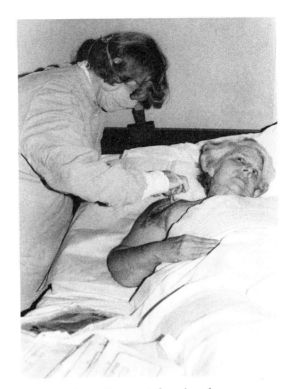

FIGURE 6.14 Frequent dressing changes may be needed when a drain is present. (Courtesy of Southside School of Practical Nursing at Southside Community Hospital, Farmville, Virginia.)

attached to low suction. HEMOVAC suction is an example of a low suction used frequently in wound drainage. When caring for a patient with wound drainage, the nurse inspects the drainage system to see if it is functioning properly. Because drainage is expected, a lack of drainage causes the nurse to examine the complete drain system to see if it is twisted, kinked, or dislodged. Gradual changes in the type and amount of drainage are expected. However, a marked change in the type of drainage or the volume should be reported. For example, Mrs. Slate, an LPN/LVN, observed a 150-ml decrease of drainage during the eight-hour shift in which she cared for Ms. Gorami. This is a marked change that should be reported. When the catheter or drain site is observed, an absent or nonsecured drain is a complication that is reported immediately. A drain that has fallen back into the body requires additional surgery to retrieve it. A drain that falls out or is pulled out by a restless or disoriented patient should be reported and recorded also. As mentioned previously, the nurse observes, records, and reports a description of the drain site, a description of the color, odor, and consistency of drainage, and the volume of drainage. In most cases, drains are removed within two or three days after surgery. After the drain has been removed, usually no dressing is needed.

Dressing changes vary with hospital policy and the surgeon's preference. The postoperative orders guide specific nursing interventions. General principles that guide the nurse who is reinforcing or changing the patient's dressing include:

- Use aseptic technique.
- Use small rather than bulky dressings which can mask considerable bleeding before being noticed.
- Change dressings when wet with drainage to prevent a favorable environment for bacterial growth.
- Unless specifically ordered by the surgeon, avoid removing dressings adhering to the skin due to dried drainage; this can damage the epithelial fibrin seal which has formed over the suture line.
- Cleanse drainage fluids from skin to prevent deterioration of the suture line.
- Unless specifically ordered by the surgeon, avoid tight dressings which can constrict local blood vessels and reduce blood supply to the incision.

The patient's response to the operative would provides the nurse with information about changes in body image which occur as a result of surgery. The incision often represents the most visible sign of the many changes that have occurred because of surgery. Questions that guide the nurse in understanding the information collected about body image include:

- What area(s) of body image is affected (appearance, function, personality)?
- How important is the affected area to the patient?
- Where is the patient in the grieving process?

As mentioned in previous chapters, a person who loses a body part can be expected to show signs of grieving described in Chapter 1. For example, a person who refuses to look at the operative incision may be experiencing denial of the loss. The nurse who makes that observation does not assume that the patient is denying. Instead, the nurse uses this information to open the topic for further discussion. A sample of the nurse's planned response to this observation is an open-ended question that invites a response: "I notice you are not looking at your incision. . . ." During wound care, the nurse's planned communication can help the patient who is adjusting to an altered body image. Reporting positive and neutral features of the incision helps the patient look objectively at this visible change in body image. A sample report is described below:

Well, Mr. Smart, your incision looks clean and dry today. The stitches are holding the skin edges together nicely. There's no obvious bleeding. There is some redness and warmth which is expected at this time. What do you think about it?

When planning this communication, an important precaution is to avoid reporting signs that indicate possible complication. These signs are reported to the surgeon, who investigates further and then discusses them with the patient. This very important precaution protects the patient from needless anxiety and worry.

Other nursing interventions that favor acceptance of a changed body image include:

- Appropriate touching of the patient during care.
- Teaching the patient how to participate in care.
- Encouraging and praising every effort made by the patient to participate in care.
- Suggesting ways to minimize disfiguration which results from surgery (wigs, new hair styles or clothing styles).
- Verbal reassurance that it is normal to feel different after surgery—that temporary feelings of fear, unreality, anger, and depression are expected even when surgery has been successful.

Postoperative Complications

URINARY RETENTION

The patient with urinary retention is unable to urinate despite having sufficient urine in the bladder. Normal mechanisms of urination are disturbed by anesthesia or surgical procedures causing pressure on back or abdominal muscles. The bladder becomes distended by urine, and there is increased pressure on the bladder wall. The increased pressure causes constriction of blood vessels within the wall and deprives its tissue of adequate circulation.

The patient with urinary retention may feel the need to urinate but is not successful. In some cases, the patient does not experience a voiding sensation. As the bladder becomes more distended, enlargement can be seen and palpated (felt) above the symphysis pubis. In addition to these observations, the nurse measures and records the amount of urine each time the patient voids postoperatively for at least 24 to 48 hours.

The patient who has urinary retention may need a catheterization to remove the urine from the bladder. The amount of urine removed during a catheterization varies, but it may be as much as 600 to 900 ml (20 to 30 oz). The nurse should not remove more than 800 to 1000 ml because of the danger of causing hemorrhage of the bladder wall and resulting shock. A bladder that is overly distended causes pressure on the bladder wall and blood vessels of the wall. As the distention is relieved, these blood vessels fill. When the patient's bladder is emptied too rapidly, a rapid filling of the blood vessels can result in rupture. The ruptured blood vessels, of course, cause hemorrhage. The nurse should stop the flow of urine through the catheter or remove the catheter before draining more than 800 to 1000 ml. The situation should be reported to the nurse in charge. The nursing action to be followed after this generally is drainage of the bladder at one-half-hour intervals until the bladder is empty.

The passage of 30 to 60 ml of urine every 20 to 30 minutes indicates an overdistended bladder that is not being emptied when the patient voids. This condition is known as retention with overflow. In this case, the patient voids first and is catheterized immediately afterward. The principles that guide the amount of urine drained are the same.

HEMORRHAGE

The hemorrhaging patient is losing blood from blood vessels. During an external hemorrhage, blood escapes from the body. Blood that spurts with each heartbeat indicates the blood is coming from an artery. Dark-red blood that flows in a continuous stream indicates that the blood is coming from a vein. Blood coming from capillaries flows slowly and steadily. During an internal hemorrhage, blood escapes from the blood vessels but remains within the body. Some hemorrhages are visible by inspecting the skin for evidence of discoloration. *Petechiae* are tiny hemorrhages that appear as pinprick-sized spots on the skin. *Purpura* are larger (up to 1 cm), purplish bruises. *Ecchymoses* are larger bruises commonly known as "black and blue marks." A *hematoma* forms from a massive accumulation of blood within a tissue.

At first, the postoperative patient who is hemorrhaging may show only subtle changes indicating blood loss. Increased restlessness or a change in behavior, an increase in pulse and respiratory rates, a slight elevation of blood pressure, and a slowing of urine output are early signs of adaptive mechanisms that control the hemorrhage and maintain adequate blood volume. These early signs may be present even though there is no obvious increase in bloody drainage on the dressing, cast, or in drainage tubing. Therefore, the nurse reports these early signs to the head nurse or team leader and continues to observe closely for excess bleeding.

In addition to frequent inspection of the dressing, the nurse checks all drainage tubing for evidence of bloody drainage. The nurse should observe and report whether the blood is bright red, which indicates fresh bleeding, or dark brown, which indicates old bleeding.

As hemorrhage continues, the patient may show signs of shock described in the next section. The patient who is bleeding internally may not show any early signs of bleeding until signs of shock appear.

The nurse who finds a patient hemorrhaging summons help immediately but remains with the patient while doing so. When hemorrhage is located at the operative site, pressure may be applied to slow the bleeding. Once help has arrived, the nurse can anticipate one or more of the following physician's orders:

- Start intravenous fluids or increase the flow rate if fluids are already running.
- Emergency laboratory tests to determine the patient's blood volume (CBC or hematocrit and hemoglobin).
- Type and crossmatch for possible transfusion.
- Frequent vital signs.
- Foley catheterization to monitor urine output more closely.
- Temporary pressure dressing over the operative site (pressure dressings can diminish blood flow to the suture line if left on too long.
- Possible emergency surgery to locate and control bleeding.
- Possible oxygen therapy to saturate all available red blood cells with oxygen for tissues.

SHOCK

The patient in shock has an inadequate supply of blood reaching the body's tissues. In order for the tissues to be properly supplied with sufficient food and oxygen, the following three factors must be working in harmony: (1) a sufficient amount of circulating blood is needed, (2) the blood vessels must be normal, and (3) the heart must be pumping adequately.

An insufficient blood volume can occur as a result of hemorrhage or loss of plasma in a severely burned patient. A rapid loss of blood or fluid does not have to exit the body in order to cause shock. Large amounts of fluid that move from within the blood vessels to injured tissue may seriously reduce the patient's circulating blood volume. Vital tissues may be deprived of oxygen and nutrition when needed blood and fluid are present outside the circulatory system. In some conditions, the patient's blood vessels are so dilated (widened) that even the normal amount of circulating blood cannot fill them. This abnormal dilatation causes blood to move so slowly that body cells do not receive sufficient nutrients and oxygen. A person whose heart does not pump adequately likewise cannot get blood containing nutrients and oxygen to cells. Because of the balance that exists between the heart, the blood vessels, and blood and fluid, a change in any one of these organs causes changes in the others.

The four types of shock are (1) hematogenic, (2) vasogenic, (3) neurogenic, and (4) cardiogenic. *Hematogenic* shock is caused by an actual loss of while blood or plasma. In other words, the blood volume is decreased such as in hemorrhage, severe burn when the patient has lost plasma and electrolytes, and marked dehydration associated with diabetic acidosis. The patient with *vasogenic* shock has a marked dilation of blood vessels, which results in the blood moving so slowly that it becomes pooled in the larger vessels. Vasogenic shock usually is caused by toxic substances affecting the tone of the blood vessels. *Anaphylactic* shock (discussed in Chapter 10) is an example of vasogenic shock. Allergic reaction to drugs such as penicillin can result in anaphylactic shock. The patient with neurogenic shock has a marked dilatation of blood vessels as does the patient with vasogenic shock. However, the cause is different. In neurogenic shock, the dilatation of the patient's blood vessels is caused by a diminished tone of the blood vessels resulting from some condition of the nervous system that controls the blood vessels. Deep general anesthesia, brain damage, emotional upsets, spinal anesthesia, and certain drugs such as insulin are examples of such influences on the nervous system that can cause dilatation of the blood vessels. The patient has *cardiogenic* shock when the heart fails to pump a sufficient amount of blood to the tissues. Traumatic injury to the heart, myocardial infarction, and heart failure can result in cardiogenic shock.

Body defenses activated during shock include a release of hormones that support vital functions. Mineralocorticoids and glucocorticoids, norepinephrine and epinephrine, and antidiuretic hormone (ADH) are examples of hormones that act to produce compensatory vasoconstriction and a shift of blood volume from peripheral spaces to internal deep vessels that supply vital organs.

Shock is believed to develop through three interrelated stages. Early detection and treatment are essential to prevent deterioration to the progressive and/or irreversible stages.

NURSING OBSERVATIONS OF THE PATIENT IN SHOCK. Although a variety of conditions may cause shock, the end result is inadequate blood flow through the tissue, also known as diminished tissue perfusion. Nursing observations are related to inadequate tissue perfusion, the activation of body defenses, and the specific underlying condition. As mentioned earlier, early detection and treatment are important to prevent an irreversible state that results in the patient's death. Nursing observations that may indicate that the patient is in shock are listed in Table 6.4.

TREATMENT AND NURSING INTERVENTIONS. The patient in shock is not left alone. For this reason, the patient may be transferred to an intensive care unit after initial lifesaving measures have been started. The nurse who finds a patient in shock summons help immediately while remaining at the bedside. While waiting for the physician to arrive, the nurse covers the patient with a light blanket, monitors vital signs, and reassures the patient. If there is visible external bleeding, a sterile dressing may be applied with pressure to slow the blood flow. Other nurses anticipate the need for supplies by bringing the emergency cart to the bedside. Practices that are avoided include piling blankets on the patient and placing the patient in Trendelenburg position. These interventions are contraindicated in certain types of shock.

TABLE 6.4
GUIDE TO NURSING OBSERVATIONS FOR THE PATIENT IN SHOCK

WHAT TO OBSERVE	OBSERVATIONS
Eyes	Expressionless or staring
	Dilated pupils
Mouth	Pallor or cyanosis of lips and mucous membranes
	Mouth breathing
	Dry mouth
Chest	Rapid shallow respirations
	Uses accessory muscles of respiration
Abdomen	Nausea and vomiting
Extremities	Cool to touch
	Nailbeds pale or cyanotic
	Slow capillary filling
Skin	Moist, cool, clammy to touch
	Color pale or ashen
	Diaphoresis and cyanosis in later stages
Urinary function	Diminishing output, scanty output, or no output
Behavioral changes	Restlessness, irritability, apprehension, weakness in early stages
	Listlessness, drowsiness, loss of consciousness in later stages
	Verbalizes feelings of dread, fear, feeling cold
Vital signs	
Temperature	May fall below normal
Pulse	Weak, rapid, thready in early stages
	May be too weak to count in later stages
	Rate very slow in irreversible shock
Blood pressure	Usually low
	Systolic drops more than diastolic
	Rapid fall of blood pressure when moving from supine to sitting or standing position
	May be too low to measure in later stages
	Pulse pressure narrows

Medical and nursing interventions are directed toward continuous patient monitoring, improving tissue perfusion, and identifying and treating the underlying cause. Monitoring interventions include:

- Continuous head-to-toe nursing observations
- Frequent vital signs, as often as every 15 minutes
- Insertion of a central venous line to monitor central venous pressure, a function of blood volume (see Chapter 12 for additional details)
- Frequent arterial blood gas determinations to monitor arterial oxygen–carbon dioxide levels as well as acid-base balance (see Chapter 14 for additional details)
- Frequent determinations of hematocrit and hemoglobin when blood loss is the underlying cause
- Insertion of an indwelling catheter to monitor urine output frequently
- Specific studies as indicated by the type of shock (for example, blood cultures are ordered when bacteria in the blood are causing shock)

In some hospitals, a special flow sheet is used to record all observations and interventions while the patient is in shock.

Interventions that are directed toward improved tissue perfusion include:

- Fluid replacement with electrolyte solutions, blood, and/or blood products
- Respiratory support using ventilators and supplemental oxygen as described in Chapter 14
- Restoration of normal urinary output using osmotic diuretics such as urea and mannitol (see Table 11.7 for additional information)
- Nasogastric suction to empty stomach and prevent aspiration
- Drug therapy (described later in this section) via the intravenous route since poor tissue perfusion interferes with parenteral absorption
- Frequent changes of position to prevent stasis and pooling of blood
- Meticulous attention to all practices that prevent the spread of infection (the patient in shock has a greatly increased susceptibility to infection)
- Attention to skin care to prevent skin breakdown from poor tissue perfusion

Drug therapy in shock is currently the subject of intense investigation. The practical nursing student will need to update the information provided here with new facts as they become available through continuing research.

Adrenocortical hormones are powerful chemical messengers associated with activation of the stress mechanism. Large doses of glucocorticoid hormones (cortisone and hydrocortisone) are often administered to the patient in shock.

Vasoconstricting drugs may be prescribed as short-term therapy to improve circulation to the brain, heart, and certain other vital organs. These drugs are used less often than they once were because recent studies show that they reduce renal blood flow, can cause cardiac arrhythmias, and can result in fluid overload. Metaraminol (ARAMINE), and norepinephrine (LEVOPHED) are examples of powerful vasoconstrictor drugs given in intravenous fluid. When norepinephrine is given, the blood pressure is taken frequently and the site of the infusion must be observed closely for signs of infiltration. Epinephrine causes a severe local vasoconstriction, which can cause necrosis and sloughing of the tissue.

Vasodilators may be prescribed for some patients whose blood vessels are so constricted that blood becomes trapped in the peripheral blood vessels and is not available to nourish vital organs. Drugs used to dilate blood vessels during shock include dopamine (INTROPIN) and sodium nitroprusside (NIPRIDE). Knowing that drug therapy during shock is administered intravenously enables the nurse to take all necessary actions to observe and maintain functioning intravenous lines. These include.:

- Frequent inspection of all intravenous sites for erythema (redness), edema (swelling), tenderness
- Careful repositioning of the patient to avoid twisting, kinking, or lying on intravenous tubings

- Frequent checking of the flow rate by counting the number of drops per minute of each bottle of fluid the patient is receiving
- Prompt reporting and accurate recording of any signs that indicate a poorly functioning intravenous line
- Application of mitten dressings or other similar protective devices to prevent the disoriented patient from pulling on intravenous tubings

In addition to the drugs already discussed, others are prescribed to treat the specific underlying condition. These drugs may include antibiotics, cardiotonics, and insulin. Narcotics are prescribed with extreme caution for the patient in shock because of the effect on blood pressure and respiratory centers. As mentioned earlier, most drugs are administered intravenously to the patient in shock because poor tissue perfusion results in uncertain and uneven absorption by intramuscular and subcutaneous routes.

RESPIRATORY COMPLICATIONS

Respiratory complications are both frequent and serious in the surgical patient. Obstruction of air passages, atelectasis (collapse of alveoli), and infection are common and serious conditions that can develop after surgery. Anesthesia that affects respiratory centers and muscles, the surgical incision that can distort normal breathing, and pain that restricts normal ventilation are three common surgical events that favor the development of respiratory complications. Factors that increase the risk that a surgical patient will develop a respiratory condition include smoking, advanced age, preexisting respiratory infection, obesity, hypertension, chronic lung disease, prolonged general anesthesia, and chest or high abdominal incisions.

A striking feature of respiratory complications is that most are preventable by the nurse's careful attention to preoperative and postoperative care. Preoperative prevention already discussed in this chapter includes:

- Instruct, demonstrate, and supervise patient practice sessions in turning, coughing, deep-breathing exercises, and breathing devices such as blow bottles and Triflo.
- Observe and promptly report symptoms of respiratory infection in the patient who is being prepared for surgery. The surgeon will usually postpone the operation, if possible.
- Meticulous oral hygiene to reduce bacteria in the mouth before surgery.
- Instruct the patient about the surgeon's orders to withhold food and fluids to prevent vomiting and aspiration.
- Instruct and encourage the patient to avoid or minimize cigarette smoking.

Postoperative interventions that prevent respiratory complications include:

- Carefully position the patient as described earlier in the chapter to maintain an open airway and prevent aspiration.
- Observe and report the patient's temperature since elevations within the first 24 hours after surgery almost always relate to retained secretions in the tracheobronchial tree.
- Assist and encourage the patient to do the exercise program as described earlier in the chapter. Increase the number and frequency of exercises when the patient's temperature is elevated.
- Encourage and assist the patient to use blow bottles, TRIFLO, or other devices according to the manufacturer's instruction.
- Continue careful oral hygiene as described.
- Provide adequate pain relief so that pain does not restrict the patient's breathing.
- Assist and encourage the patient to alternate ambulation with rest periods. This helps to move secretions in the respiratory system and prevents abdominal distention which can restrict breathing.
- Praise every effort the smoking patient makes to reduce or avoid smoking.
- Avoid tight constricting dressings and binders which can restrict breathing.

The practical nursing student can locate additional information about nursing observations and interventions related to the patient with a respiratory condition in Chapter 14.

POSTOPERATIVE ATELECTASIS. The patient with postoperative atelectasis has a portion of unexpanded lung tissue caused by alveoli that become airless, collapse, and shrink. Mucus plugs, retained secretions following anesthesia, inadequate ventilation (breathing), and immobility are common causes of postoperative atelectasis. If untreated, the tissues of the involved alveoli deteriorate and become infected due to poor circulation in the area. The patient with early atelectasis develops difficult breathing (dyspnea) and weakness. As more alveoli become involved, these symptoms increase, and the patient develops fever, tachycardia, and pain in the affected area. A chest x-ray shows the collapsed area.

As mentioned previously, prevention of postoperative atelectsis is desirable using nursing interventions already described. After the physician diagnoses postoperative atelectasis, measures which may be prescribed include inhalation therapy with oxygen, and intermittent positive pressure breathing (IPPB), and aerosols, positioning the patient on the unaffected side to promote drainage, drug therapy to stimulate coughing and liquefy secretions, and antibiotics to prevent or treat infection. In addition, postoperative nursing interventions discussed earlier in this section are increased in order to help the patient reexpand collapsed alveoli.

POSTOPERATIVE PNEUMONIA. The patient with postoperative pneumonia has an acute inflammation of lung tissue which causes alveoli to fill with cells and fluid. The patient who is elderly and whose preoperative condition was poor is more likely to develop pneumonia. Immobility associated with surgery may result in *hypostatic pneumonia*. Overgrowth of normal bacteria in the mouth can migrate to the lungs during general anesthesia and cause infection. Minor respiratory infections such as the common cold may result in pneumonia following surgery. Untreated atelectasis may cause pneumonia when alveoli deteriorate and become infected. Aspiration of vomitus during or after surgery can cause a life-threatening

postoperative pneumonia. Nursing observations and interventions appropriate in caring for the patient with pneumonia are discussed in detail in Chapter 14. Pre- and postoperative preventions discussed earlier apply to this patient as well.

PULMONARY EMBOLISM. An embolus is a foreign body in the bloodstream. It is usually a blood clot or part of a blood clot that is carried by the bloodstream to another part of the body. When the embolus reaches a blood vessel that is too small for it to pass through, it lodges there and causes an obstruction in that vessel. If the embolus lodges in an artery in the lungs, it is called *pulmonary embolism*. As a result, the lung tissue supplied by the affected artery has an insufficient blood supply. The most common source of blood clots after surgery is deep veins in the legs.

Pulmonary embolism is a grave postoperative complication which occurs most often when the patient is convalescing. If a large pulmonary artery is closed by embolus, death results in a very short time. When small branches are obstructed, the patient may recover.

The patient with a postoperative pulmonary embolism may develop sudden, sharp chest pain, dyspnea, and cyanosis which occurs when getting out of bed or while sitting on the toilet. In some cases, the patient experiences a more gradual onset of dyspnea, cough with bloody mucus, and fatigue. The nurse who is present when the patient first develops these symptoms remains with the patient while calling for help immediately. Lung scan, arterial blood gases, electrocardiogram, and chest x-ray are done on an emergency basis for diagnosis. Medical therapy which may be prescribed includes narcotics to control pain and anxiety, oxygen therapy, and anticoagulant therapy. Nursing observations and interventions related to respiratory and vascular complications apply to this patient. Additional information related to caring for the patient with a pulmonary embolism can be located in Chapter 12.

VASCULAR COMPLICATIONS

Postoperative complications that involve the patient's blood vessels generally occur within one to two weeks after surgery. The three most common complications caused by the blood flowing more slowly than normal through the blood vessels because of inactivity are (1) phlebitis, (2) thrombophlebitis, and (3) phlebothrombosis. The patient with *phlebitis* has an inflammation of a vein. In *thrombophlebitis*, the vein is inflamed and a blood clot has developed. The blood clot has formed on the wall of the vein and may occlude the blood vessel. The patient with *phlebothrombosis* has a slight formation of clots that do not adhere to the wall of the blood vessel. These clots travel through the veins and become lodged in a smaller vessel that does not permit the clots to pass through. The clots can stop the blood flow to a vital organ, such as the heart or the lungs. As mentioned earlier, a blood clot that becomes lodged in the lungs is called a pulmonary embolus. Factors that favor the development of vascular complications following surgery include smoking, obesity, prolonged immobility before surgery, pelvic surgery, and oral contraceptives.

The patient with a vascular complication usually experiences tenderness, pain, and warmth along the involved veins. The patient's extremity may be red or pink and swollen. In some cases, the patient does not experience symptoms until embolism occurs. A Doppler flowmeter is a machine that transmits sounds made by blood flowing through blood vessels. Changes in normal sounds of blood flow in deep veins indicate vascular complications. The nurse may also measure the calf and thigh circumference for swelling.

As with other complications, meticulous pre- and postoperative nursing care may prevent their occurrence. Preoperative preventive nursing measures include:

- Instruct, demonstrate, and supervise patient practice sessions in leg exercises described earlier in the chapter.
- Collect, report, and record facts about the patient which increase the risk of vascular complications (smoking, use of oral contraceptive, weight).
- Encourage frequent exercise and ambulation before surgery.
- Instruct the patient to avoid constricting girdles and garters, and knee stockings.
- Record calf and thigh measurements on the preoperative patient at increased risk for vascular complications.
- Explain and encourage the patient not to smoke.
- Apply antiembolism stockings correctly (after elevating the legs) (Figures 6.15, 6.16, 6.17, and 6.18).
- Explain the preferred positions of standing, walking, or lying rather than sitting to the patient.

Postoperative preventive nursing measures include:

- Regularly inspect the legs during the head-to-toe observation for erythema (redness), warmth, tenderness, swelling.
- Passively exercise the patient's legs in the early postoperative period—gradually

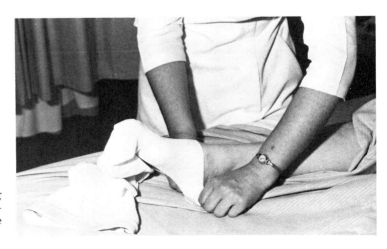

FIGURE 6.15 When applying an antiembolic (elastic) stocking, the nurse turns the inside of the stocking outward.

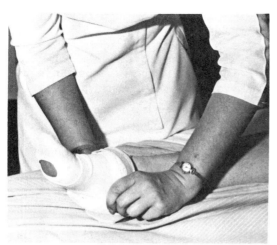

FIGURE 6.16 The antiembolic stocking is worked over the foot and heel.

progress to assisted and unassisted exercises.
- Avoid gatching the knee of the bed postoperatively.
- Assist the patient with ambulation and rest periods that minimize sitting.
- Help the patient to remove and correctly reapply antiembolism stockings at least every 24 hours.

The patient who develops vascular complications may have one or more medical and nursing interventions which include bedrest with elevation of the affected extremity, antiembolism stockings, moist heat to the affected area, anticoagulant therapy, drug therapy with ne fibrinolytic drugs, surgery. Additional information about caring for the patient with thrombophlebitis can be located in Chapter 12 and applies to this patient.

WOUND INFECTION

Wound healing may be interrupted after surgery by microorganisms which enter the operative area and cause a wound infection. Factors that are known to contribute to wound infection include the patient's condition, the type of surgical procedure, and the skill of health team members in preventing and minimizing contamination. The patient with anemia, obesity, cardiovascular disease, or diabetes is more likely to develop a wound infection. Surgical procedures that involve the respiratory, gastrointestinal, and urinary systems are associated with increased infection. Poor local skin preparation and personnel with upper respiratory infections are examples of health team practices that increase the likelihood of wound infection. A *stitch abscess* occurs when the area around one or more skin sutures becomes infected.

The patient with a wound infection often experiences more tenderness in a particular area of the wound than another. Warmth limited to a particular area of the incision is another indicator of possible infection. Redness along the suture line and a delay in the development of a healing ridge also indicate

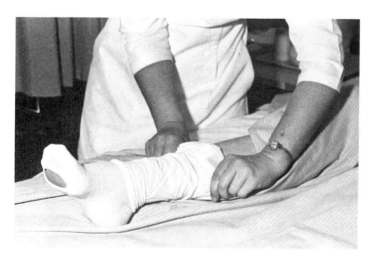

FIGURE 6.17 The antiembolic stocking is worked up the leg.

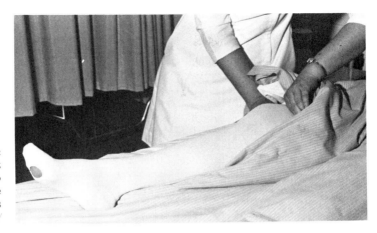

FIGURE 6.18 The antiembolic stocking is applied to prevent thrombophlebitis. Notice that no wrinkles have been left in the hose to irritate the patient's skin.

possible infection. As mentioned earlier, fever in the first 24 hours usually indicates retained secretions in the tracheobronchial tree. Fever after 72 hours may signal wound infection in the absence of respiratory signs and symptoms. Draingage of purulent material in a previously nondraining wound is another signal.

When infection is suspected, the surgeon usually requests a wound culture to identify the pathogen. The correct procedure for collecting this specimen is first to wipe away existing purulent drainage using sterile technique. Next, the nurse rolls a sterile swab against the wound to collect new fresh drainage. The infecting microorganism is most likely to live and grow on a culture when obtained in this manner. A practice that is avoided is collecting material that has drained out of the wound onto the skin. As mentioned in Chapter 1, the specimen is labeled correctly and sent to the laboratory while still fresh. Correct labeling information includes the exact anatomic site from which drainage was collected rather than just the word "wound." For example, abdominal incision is a more descriptive term. This practice is especially important when the patient has multiple incisions or drain sites. Medical and nursing interventions related to the patient with a wound infection include:

- Drainage of the infected area using packing, irrigations, and special antiseptic agents to keep the wound open
- Antibiotic therapy

- Strict aseptic techniques to avoid introducing additional microorganisms into the wound
- Careful handling of soiled dressings to prevent the spread of infection
- Special precautions according to hospital policy to prevent the spread of infection. Precautions may include isolation of the patient, special handling of dressings, linens, and clothing that has come in contact with the patient's wound and skin
- Meticulous handwashing after every contact with the patient
- Assisting the patient to eat a nourishing diet and drink sufficient fluids
- Continuous observation and accurate recording of the patient's wound and drainage including appearance, odor, volume

DEHISCENCE AND EVISCERATION

The patient with wound *dehiscence* has either a partial or complete separation of the edges of the incision. In other words, the wound splits open. The patient with a wound *evisceration* has a protrusion of abdominal organs through the incision. For example, part of the intestine may slip through the opening in the peritoneum, fascia, muscle, and skin and be found on the outside of the patient's body.

Dehiscence and evisceration may occur during the first two weeks after surgery in patients with an impaired healing process. For example, the patient with malnutrition, obesity, debilitation, marked postoperative intestinal distention, or prolonged coughing, vomiting, and sneezing may be prone to eviscerate.

Early warning signs of possible dehiscence include low-grade fever and tachycardia which cannot be explained, increasing wound pain instead of gradually decreasing pain, and prolonged paralytic ileus.

The patient with a wound dehiscence may tell the nurse that something has come loose in the incision or that the dressing or clothing is suddenly wet. When the dressing is removed, separation of wound edges can be seen. The nurse's first action is to return the patient to bed and summon help without leaving the patient. A heavy dressing or binder is applied, and the patient is instructed to remain quiet and avoid coughing or sneezing. This is to prevent evisceration of abdominal organs. It even may be necessary for the nurse to support the wound edges with the hands. While waiting for the surgeon, the patient's vital signs are taken, an intravenous line is prepared if the patient does not have one already, and the operating room is notified to prepare for additional surgery.

When evisceration occurs, a sterile towel or dressing moistened with sterile saline is placed over the wound and abdominal contents to prevent further contamination. This is a surgical emergency which is life-threatening. While one nurse remains with the patient at all times, others anticipate possible shock and the need for additional surgery by obtaining emergency supplies and notifying the surgeon and operating room.

Wound failure is a terrifying experience for the patient. Remaining calm while taking necessary actions and explaining to the patient that help is coming and that he or she will not be left alone are nursing actions that provide some reassurance.

PARALYTIC ILEUS

The patient with a paralytic or adynamic ileus has a temporary loss of peristalsis because of paralyzed intentines or uncoordinated ineffective peristalsis. Surgical factors associated with this condition include anesthesia, electrolyte imbalance, wound infection, wound dehiscence, and abdominal surgery.

As fluids and gases collect in the gastrointestinal system, the patient may have nausea, vomiting, hiccoughing, belching, and pain. The abdomen becomes increasingly distended, and no bowel sounds are heard when a stethoscope is placed on the patient's abdomen. The patient does not pass any gas or feces by rectum. If usual measures to relieve abdominal distention are unsuccessful, the surgeon may order a flat-plate abdominal x-ray to diagnose paralytic ileus. When the diagnosis is confirmed, measures to treat this complication usually include insertion of a long nasogastric tube to decompress the intestines (described in Chapter 15), intravenous fluid therapy, and nothing by mouth.

Discharge Teaching

The postoperative patient needs specific written instructions in understandable language before discharge. In some cases, several practice sessions may be needed for the patient to learn a new skill. The instruction needed varies with the patient and the surgery. General topics usually included are late complications, resumption of usual activities, medications to be taken, and wound care.

Fever, unusual pain, persistent nausea and vomiting, and dysuria indicate possible complications that should cause the patient to notify the surgeon. The patient should be specifically cautioned about the hazards of inactivity as they relate to vascular complications. Periods of activity interspersed with rest periods are generally recommended after discharge. Resumption of usual activities includes showering, stair climbing, lifting, driving, and sexual activities. Usually, the surgeon discusses when these activities may be resumed. The medications the patient is to take after discharge are fully discussed, including possible side effects. Instructions related to wound care are also provided.

Following surgery, the patient's body image continues to change for months. Many patients report feelings of unreality or occasional feelings of depression. Patients usually are reassured to learn that these are normal feelings even after discharge.

Case Study Involving a Surgical Patient

Mr. Martin Jackson, a 68-year-old male, was admitted for a transurethral resection of the prostate gland to be done two days after admission. Mr. Jackson was a thin, but apparently healthy, widower who lived alone. He displayed enthusiasm as he told the nurses of his activities with the Golden Age Club.

Routine preoperative examination included a chest x-ray, ECG, CBC, hemoglobin, hematocrit, routine urinalysis, and urine culture with sensitivity. The results were within normal limits, with the exception of a hemoglobin of 11 gm.

Mr. Jackson asked the nurses many questions as they took his blood pressure, pulse, respiration, and temperature. He appeared to be concerned about his heart and blood pressure. The evening before surgery the surgeon ordered the following:

- Saline enema hs
- Clear liquids for supper
- NPO after midnight
- DEMEROL 75 mg with atropine 0.5 mg IM, on call to the operating room

Postoperatively, Mr. Jackson had an indwelling catheter for three days. He ambulated the evening after surgery and tolerated a regular diet the next morning after his intravenous was discontinued. The catheter was removed the third day following surgery. Mr. Jackson began to run an elevated temperature, which reached 39.5°C (103.1°F) at times, and he developed a productive cough. Following treatment with an antibiotic, Mr. Jackson became afebrile and was discharged seven days postoperatively.

QUESTIONS

1. List the psychologic aspects to be considered when the preoperative and postoperative nursing care are planned for Mr. Jackson.
2. In reading the history of Mr. Jackson, the nurse noted that his low hemoglobin probably was related to a dietary deficiency. What measures can the nurse suggest to Mr. Jackson to remedy the dietary deficiency responsible for his low hemoglobin?
3. Outline the preoperative teaching Mr. Jackson should have based on the information you have been given.
4. Outline the immediate postoperative observations necessary for Mr. Jackson.
5. What discharge instructions should be given Mr. Jackson?

Suggestions for Further Study

1. What fears may be common in patients before surgery?
2. What drugs are ordered frequently by the surgeons in your hospital as preoperative medications? What effects can be expected from these drugs?
3. Why should the patient's bladder and stomach be empty before surgery? What is the nurse's role in accomplishing this?
4. Mason, Mildred A.; Bates, Grace F.; and Smola, Bonnie K.: *Workbook in Basic Medical-Surgical Nursing*, 3rd ed. Macmillan Publishing Company, New York, 1984, Exercise 6.

Additional Readings

Greenwood, Barbara S.: "Check Out Your Patient's Presurgery Fears." *Nursing 80*, 12:34–35 (July), 1982.

Harris, Elizabeth: "Sedative-Hypnotic Drugs." *American Journal of Nursing*, 81:1329–34 (July), 1981.

Hudelson, Evelyn: "Getting the Patient Out of Bed." *Journal of Nursing Care*, 14:24–26 (Mar.), 1981.

Rambo, Beverly J., and Wood, Lucile A. (eds.): *Nursing Skills for Clinical Practice*, 3rd ed. W. B. Saunders Co., Philadelphia, 1982.

Robinson, Corinne H.: *Basic Nutrition and Diet Therapy*, 4th ed. Macmillan Publishing Co., Inc., New York, 1980, pp. 305–13.

Chapter 7

The Patient in Pain

Expected Behavioral Outcomes

Minimum objectives referred to as expected behavioral outcomes have been designed for the practical/vocational nursing student to use as guides in studying this chapter. The student should read these expected outcomes before studying the chapter. The objectives can be used as guides for study.

Using the content of this chapter, the student should return to the objectives and evaluate the ability to:

1. *Distinguish between acute and chronic pain using guidelines of duration, onset, associated emotions, common nursing observations, and effectiveness of pain-relieving interventions.*
2. *Identify the expert on the pain experience and the expert in relieving pain when given an hypothetical situation.*
3. *Compare nursing observations for a patient experiencing postoperative pain with those for a patient with chronic low back pain.*
4. *Describe at least three aspects of communication that are helpful to the patient in pain.*
5. *Compare the nursing interventions indicated for a patient with acute pain to those that might be helpful for a patient with chronic pain.*
6. *Describe how the nurse's attitudes influence the care of a patient in pain.*

Vocabulary Development

The following prefixes, suffixes, and combining forms pertain to this chapter. By learning and/or reviewing their meanings, the practical/vocational nursing student will have the keys needed to unlock many exciting new medical terms.

Discover the meaning of these keys in a medical dictionary or in the content of this chapter. How does each key pertain to this chapter? In your notebook write the correct meaning of each prefix, suffix, or combining form listed below. Illustrate each key with an example.

endo—within. Ex. *endorphins*—chemical substances within the body that block the transmission of pain impulses.

acu-	hypno-
alges-	-ic
an-	neuro-
bio-	-ose
chrono-	psycho-
cut-	spas-
dia-	splanchn-
dis-	therm-
gen-	viscero-

Introduction

Pain is a complex personal experience of hurt that affects the whole person. Because there is continuous mind-body interaction, the person in pain experiences physical sensation, feelings and thoughts about the pain, and a behavioral response to pain. Because each person is unique, each person's pain experience is different.

A complete explanation or understanding of the pain mechanism is not known at this time. It is known that pain can be a harmful stimulus that signals tissue damage or a protective mechanism that protects a person from harm. Within the past 15 years, research has resulted in a wealth of fascinating new information about how the pain mechanism operates and what can be done to relieve pain. This information has special significance for patients and nurses. Nearly every patient the nurse cares for experiences some kind of pain. Both nurses and patients agree that relieving pain and suffering is a very important nursing function.

In order to choose nursing interventions that are effective in relieving pain, the nurse needs information about the pain mechanism as it operates in the individual experiencing pain. In other words, because pain is a uniquely personal experience, the patient is considered the expert on pain. The nursing student studies pain and the patient in order to become expert in relieving pain.

Since exact pain mechanisms remain unknown and pain research is rapidly expanding, the nurse should revise the information presented in this chapter with new knowledge as it becomes available.

Structure and Function

The nervous system is responsible for receiving, transmitting, interpreting, and acting on pain. When pain receptors located in the skin and other tissues are stimulated, impulses travel via large (A delta) and small (C) nerve fibers to an area in the spinal cord known as the *substantia gelatinosa*. According to current pain theory, the substantia gelatinosa acts as a "gating mechanism" for transmitting pain impulses. When the gate is closed, no impulses are transmitted beyond it. Increased activity of large fibers (A delta) is one event known to close the gate. When the gate is open, pain impulses are transmitted to other special neurons in the spinal cord called *T cells*. Activation of T cells to a critical level results in pain awareness and pain response. Increased activity of small nerve fibers (C fibers) is known to open the gate permitting transmission of pain impulses to T cells.

Dorsal column fibers are a special collection of nerve fibers, also located in the spinal cord, which carry patterns of pain impulses up to the brain where certain brain processes are activated. Other special columns of nerves may participate as well, but the dorsal column is believed to act as a central control trigger. Activation of brain processes includes the transmission of pain messages to many areas of the brain through a complex network of neurons. The central control processes are so rapid that impulses can be transmitted back down the spinal cord to influence the gating mechanism before T cells are even activated.

Nerve impulses are transmitted from one neuron to another by chemical substances known as neurotransmitters which are released from one nerve ending and bind to a receptor site on the next neuron. Recently, a group of naturally occurring compounds known as *endorphins* has been identified as neurotransmitters that block the transmission of pain impulses. Receptor sites specific to this chemical have been located in many areas of the body but are more abundant in areas of the central nervous system known to transmit pain impulses. Research shows that endorphins affect pain perception and produce analgesia. Other powerful effects of these substances also have been suggested, including mood alteration and behavior modification. Research stimulated by this important discovery may eventually produce valuable additional information about pain, drug addiction, drug therapy for pain, and certain mental diseases. Other neurotransmitters that appear to be important in pain include dopamine, serotonin, norepinephrine, substance P, and a chemical known as GABA. These powerful chemical substances act in different areas of the brain and spinal cord to enhance or inhibit the transmission of pain impulses.

A variety of stimuli may initiate the transmission of pain impulses. Stretching or contracting beyond normal limits for that tissue may stimulate pain. Pressure caused by swelling or forces outside the body may stimulate receptors. Ischemia (diminished blood flow) to the tissue may initiate pain. Irritation from physical or chemical agents may start pain.

Types of Pain

There are many different kinds of pain. Understanding as much as possible about the patient's pain enables the nurse to select interventions most likely to be effective in relieving pain. Acute pain generally has an immediate onset, is temporary, frequently related to known cause, and associated with anxiety. Some conditions associated with acute pain include fracture, surgery, and renal colic (kidney stone). Chronic pain may develop gradually and persist or recur for months or years. The cause may or may not be known. Depression is the emotion most often associated with chronic pain. Some conditions associated with chronic pain include rheumatoid arthritis, tic douloureux, and low back pain. *Intractable pain* is the term used when persistent pain cannot be relieved.

Cutaneous pain arises from the skin and subcutaneous tissue. Sources of *deep somatic pain* include tendons, ligaments, bones, blood vessels, and nerves. *Visceral pain*, also known as *splanchnic pain*, comes from large organs inside body cavities such as the heart, liver, and kidney.

Pain may be described according to its location. *Localized pain* remains at the site of origin. *Projected pain* occurs along the path of a nerve. For example, back pain may be projected along the pathway of the sciatic nerve. *Radiated pain* extends from the point of origin. For example, chest pain often radiates to the shoulder and arm. *Referred pain* occurs at a place other than the original source. For example, pain originating from the liver may be referred to the right shoulder.

Psychogenic pain is the term used to describe pain that occurs either without known stimulation or when the stimulation results from emotional factors. For example, emotions may result in muscle tension to the point of pain.

Pretended pain describes the situation in which pain is not present, but the person pretends to be in pain in order to get something.

Factors that Influence the Pain Experience

A number of factors are known to influence a person's pain experience. Cultural background may influence why a person might be having pain, what things are painful, how a person in pain should act, and what might relieve a person's pain.

Emotions strongly influence the pain experience. The influence may be positive or negative, depending on the individual. For example, the person who is worried or frightened generally can be expected to have more pain. As mentioned earlier, the person with chronic pain often feels depressed. In some cases, pain may be associated with happiness or joy. For example, pain may signal a return of function in a part of the body.

A person's previous experience with pain is another important factor, although the exact relationship is not known. The person may use previous experience as a kind of measuring stick against which present pain can be measured.

Age is usually associated with increased pain threshold. Pain threshold is the intensity of pain which is present when the patient first becomes aware of it.

The relationship of gender to pain experience is unclear. Studies indicate that pain threshold is similar for men and women. Pain tolerance may be higher in men than in women. Pain tolerance is the length of time a patient is aware of pain before making an obvious response.

Fatigue, suffering, and physical debility are associated with reduced pain tolerance. Level of consciousness also influences a person's pain experience. It is not known if diminished levels of consciousness affect a person's awareness of pain. However, certain comatose conditions are associated with heightened, slower, diminished, or absent responses to painful stimuli. The patient who is less alert may experience pain but be unable to communicate this to the nurse.

The personal significance attached to pain also influences the patient's experience. The kind of pain expected, the amount of pain the patient is willing to have, and the influence of pain on the patient's life-style are factors which contribute to personal significance. For example, a preoperative patient may wonder about the type of pain that can be expected after surgery. Another patient may relate pain to a fear of cancer. Still another patient may have concerns that pain will result in a loss of occupation and income.

Nursing Observations

Because each person's pain experience is different, the patient's report of pain is the single most important nursing observation. The nurse may ask questions that help the patient to provide a complete description of pain so that the most effective method of relief can be chosen. Typical questions the nurse may ask include:

- Where is your pain—can you point to it?
- Is your pain mild, moderate, severe, unbearable?
- What does your pain feel like? (Examples: achy, burning, gnawing, squeezing)
- What usually makes your pain better or worse?

Some patients have pain but do not report it voluntarily. The reasons for this are varied. In some cases, the patient may not associate a present experience with the word pain. When the nurse substitutes words such as hurt, ache, sore, or discomfort for the word pain, the patient is able to provide more information. Some patients do not like to discuss their pain because they do not want to burden others with their problems or because they do not want sympathy. Some patients do not report pain because they are waiting for the nurse or doctor to ask them about it. Therefore, in collecting information for a nursing history, it is important to ask the patient about any aches, pains, stiffness, soreness, or discomforts. Unfortunately, many patients do not report pain because of an erroneous belief that taking an analgesic will cause them to become addicted. Addiction to narcotic analgesics that have been prescribed for the hospitalized patient is extremely rare. When the nurse reports this fact to a patient who appears to be in pain, the patient often provides a more complete report of severe pain.

When making a head-to-toe observation, the nursing student may see evidence that the patient is in pain. Table 7.1 describes observations that may indicate pain when the patient is not alert or is otherwise unable to report pain. It is important to remember, however, that some patients may experience and report severe pain without showing any of the characteristics listed in Table 7.1. For example, patients with chronic pain generally show fewer signs than those with acute pain.

Nursing Interventions

Once the patient's pain has been identified and described, the nurse may select one or more interventions to relieve pain. Generally, effective pain relief is more likely when the following principles are used to guide the nurse's interventions:

- Pain relief is more likely when interventions are started before the pain becomes severe.
- Because the pain experience contains many aspects, relief is more likely from a combination of interventions rather than a single intervention.
- Interventions selected on the basis of the patient's pain experience and the specific type of pain are more likely to be effective.
- Interventions that encourage the patient's participation and control are more likely to be effective.

THERAPEUTIC RELATIONSHIP

A nurse-patient relationship that is perceived by the patient as being helpful is a very important part of relieving pain. The patient who feels cared for and cared about

TABLE 7.1
GUIDE TO NURSING OBSERVATIONS FOR THE PATIENT IN PAIN*

HEAD TO TOE	OBSERVED BEHAVIOR
Eyes	Dilated pupils Rapid blinking of eyes Knotted eyebrows Evident suffering during eye contact Crying
Mouth	Dryness Grimaces around lips Vomiting Verbal expressions of pain Moaning, sighing, screaming
Chest	Respiratory rate may be increased or decreased
Extremities	Clenched fist Wringing of hands Blood pressure and pulse rate may be increased or decreased Legs may be drawn up or flexed at knees Muscle twitching
Skin	Pallor Diaphoresis
Behavior changes	Anorexia Activity level increased or decreased Avoidance of activities associated with pain Rubbing, supporting, splinting of painful area Frequent changes of position when in bed Pacing back and forth when ambulatory Loss of consciousness or diminished level of consciousness Withdrawal from nurse's touch

* Some individuals in pain may exhibit *none* of the described behaviors.

may experience less severe pain from a reduction of fear and anxiety. In addition, a therapeutic relationship may enhance the effectiveness of other interventions.

The nurse's attitudes are crucial to developing a relationship helpful in relieving pain. The nurse's warmth, acceptance, empathy, and compassion encourage the patient to trust pain-relieving measures. Another important attitude is the nurse's confidence that the patient can be helped to feel better. The nurse's willingness and persistence in trying to relieve the patient's pain communicate that the patient's comfort is very important. In addition, the patient becomes aware that he/she is not alone with the pain.

Self-awareness is important to the nursing student who wishes to become expert in relieving pain. The nurse's beliefs, attitudes and previous experience with pain may be quite different from the patient's. Aware-

ness of one's own beliefs and attitudes about pain enables the nurse to select interventions based on the patient's report of pain rather than the nurse's pain experience. Active listening is indispensable to the nurse who wants to help relieve the patient's pain. Listening enables the nurse to obtain more complete and accurate information and communicates the nurse's regard and respect for the patient's report.

Two specific types of verbal communication that help to relieve pain are giving information and interpreting sensation in a positive or neutral way. The patient who has facts about pain and pain relief is less likely to experience anxiety about the unknown. The patient who has a positive or neutral perspective about pain generally experiences fewer feelings of helplessness. For example, Mrs. Green, a student nurse, provides Mr. Fox, a preoperative patient, with information about pain which includes the following topics:

- Sources and causes of pain and discomfort after surgery
- The type and duration of pain that can be anticipated
- Pain after surgery can be thought of as related to a healing process
- Specific pain-relieving measures that are planned after surgery
- Pain-relieving measures are more effective when started before the pain becomes severe

TOUCH

Touch is the use of the hands or other devices to stimulate the skin. The mechanisms by which touch may relieve pain include:

- Stimulation of large nerve fibers closes the gate mechanism and interrupts transmission of pain impulses
- Improvement of blood flow to the painful area
- Reduction of swelling in a painful area
- Relaxation of muscle tension
- Reduction of anxiety

Pressure is one kind of touch that may be applied to the painful area using the fingertips, fingers, or the heel or palm of the hand. Pressure may be applied directly to the painful area, along known nerve pathways, or to special related local areas called trigger points.

Massage is another form of touch the nurse may use to relieve pain. Long, slow handstrokes or rapid circular hand movement may be used to produce muscle relaxation and improved blood flow to the painful area. A variety of creams and lotions is available for lubrication and/or to enhance the pain-relieving effect of massage. Menthol, herb, and peppermint oils are examples of substances that some patients have used successfully. Certain lotions and oils produce sensations of heat or cold. Using a lotion or cream that the patient previously has found helpful increases the likelihood of effective pain relief. Precautions that should be followed when using a lotion or cream include following hospital policy related to substances applied to the skin and asking the patient about allergies.

DISTRACTION

Distraction is a nursing intervention in which the patient is helped to concentrate on something other than pain. Many hospitalized patients develop distracting activities to relieve pain, fatigue, anxiety, and boredom. Counting dots on the ceiling or flowers on the wallpaper, talking on the telephone, and watching television are examples of of distraction commonly reported by patients.

Planned distraction can be effective for short periods of acute and chronic pain. For example, a distracting activity may be used during a painful procedure such as an injection, a lumbar puncture, or bone marrow aspiration. Some patients with chronic pain use distraction for several hours each day. Relief is more likely when the patient actively participates in distraction and when this method is combined with others to relieve pain.

A good distraction avoids anything that might cause the patient to sense, feel, think about or act on pain. In addition, the activity planned should involved more than one sense, if possible, and should emphasize rhythm and breathing. Humor is a good distractor for many patients. Some patients have reported better pain relief when humor produces actual laughing. Examples of this planned distraction include asking the patient to relate the funniest thing that ever happened, singing a song with the patient, or asking the patient to tell a favorite joke. When the nurse holds the patient's hand or touches the patient's arm during the activity, the sense of touch is added. Another example of distraction is to ask the patient to concentrate attention on a particular spot on the ceiling or wall. While the patient is concentrating, the nurse rubs a small area on the skin using a circular motion. The area of massage may or may not be the painful area. A distraction that involves breathing may be done by instructing the patient to breathe in slowly while the nurse counts to three. Then the patient exhales slowly while the nurse counts to four. The number of breaths per minute varies from six to nine using this method.

One disadvantage of using distraction is that relief is usually short term. Also, the patient may not believe that this method can help. Sometimes others believe that the patient who can use distraction is not really having severe pain.

BREATHING EXERCISES

Breathing exercises may help to relieve pain by promoting relaxation and concentrating attention on nonpainful activities. Some breathing exercises increase oxygen delivery to the tissues. This intervention may be helpful for most kinds of pain. Slow rhythmic breathing has already been described in the previous section.

Panting exercises may be more helpful for severe pain. The patient is instructed to pant four times and then blow while the nurse counts one-two-three-four-five. Breathing is shallow, and short breaths are taken through the mouth. Breathing begins slowly at first and gradually becomes faster. Although the rate may be varied according to the severity of pain, the rate should not exceed 60 breaths per minute. Usually the patient breathes faster when the pain is more severe and slower as the pain diminishes. The exercise is continued until the pain stops or is reduced to more comfortable level. Disadvantages of rapid-breathing exercises include fatigue, dry mouth, and possible hyperventilation (excessively rapid breathing). The nurse should consult the physician before using this method for a patient with a respiratory disease. A variation of panting is called *he-who breathing*. The patient inhales quickly and says "he" while exhaling, then inhales quickly again and says "who" during the next exhalation. This process is repeated rhythmically while the rate of breathing gradually increases as previously described.

Massage to the skin while the patient is breathing is a variation which adds the sensation of touch. Visual stimulation may be added by asking the patient, while breathing, to imagine the second hand moving around the clockface or the wheels of a car rotating.

REPOSITIONING

Changing the patient's position can relieve pain associated with muscle spasm and strain, edema (swelling), joint stiffness, and reduction of blood flow to a body part (Figure 7.1). A variety of repositioning interventions is available. For example, the patient's swollen extremity may be elevated to relieve pain. The patient with stiffness in a joint

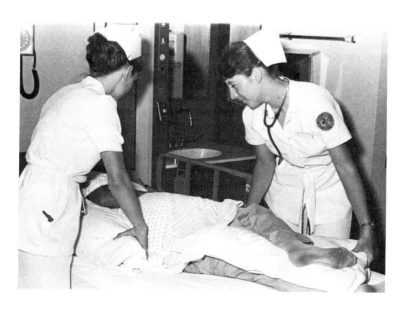

FIGURE 7.1 Changing the patient's position. (Courtesy of Washington County School of Practical Nursing, Neff Vocational Center, Abingdon, Virginia.)

may experience relief when the nurse places the joint in a position of semiflexion. In some cases, the patient's pain is relieved by splinting and immobilizing a painful body part. Turning to a position of correct body alignment may reduce muscle spasm and improve blood flow.

Repositioning may increase the patient's pain if done incorrectly, without preparation, and without appropriate information from the patient. The following guidelines assist the nurse using repositioning to provide effective pain relief:

- Obtain information from the patient about which positions are more comfortable.
- Ask the patient about techniques that reduce pain associated with moving.
- Medicate the patient with an analgesic first if moving is expected to cause pain.
- Have the number of persons on hand needed to move the patient with minimum pain.
- Obtain equipment such as pillows and repositioning devices and place at the bedside before moving the patient.
- Support injured tissue or painful areas while repositioning.
- Watch oxygen tubing, intravenous tubing, and drainage tubings to be sure they do not become kinked, twisted, dislodged, or disconnected during repositioning.
- Ensure that the patient's position does not restrict adequate breathing.
- Develop a schedule with the patient that includes timing of repositioning, diagrams of positions to be used, and special instructions.
- Combine repositioning with other interventions such as analgesic medication, massage, and breathing exercises.

HEAT AND COLD APPLICATIONS

Applying heat or cold to painful areas helps to relieve pain by producing changes in the transmission of pain impulses, blood flow to the tissues, and accumulation of fluid in tissues. Incorrect use of either heat or cold may result in injury to the patient. In many hospitals, a physician's order may be needed before using heat or cold.

Heat may be supplied by warm water during a bath or shower, by special heat lamps, heating pads and moist packs, and also from the sun while sunbathing. Generally, heat is not used when trauma, bleeding, or malignancy is present. Cold may be supplied by immersing a body part in cold water, an ice bag, cold towels, cold packs, or ice massage using ice cubes. Cold is helpful in relieving pain associated with muscle spasm or swelling. In addition, numbness on the skin may be produced by applying an ice cube for several minutes. Cold is generally avoided when the patient's pain is due to ischemia (reduced blood flow), when the patient has an allergy to cold, or when heart disease is present. Applications of cold are usually stopped if the patient starts to shiver.

RELAXATION TECHNIQUES

Relaxation techniques may help to relieve pain by reducing skeletal muscle tension and mental worry. Because there is continuous mind-body interaction, relaxation which starts in one area generally spreads to other areas. For example, relaxation of skeletal muscle may result in less anxiety. Relaxation may be used when muscle tension or contraction is causing the patient's pain, or when fatigue and sleeplessness are influencing increased pain. Relaxation also may improve the effectiveness of other interventions such as drug therapy. An additional benefit of this intervention is that the patient may practice it alone and thus have considerable control. In order to use a relaxation technique, the patient needs a quiet place, a comfortable position, and a passive attitude. Instructions for one relaxation exercise can be located on page 64. When muscle tension is severe, a variation of the relaxation exercise which may help is to contract small muscle groups and relax them in a systematic manner. For example, the person using this method may start by concentrating attention on breathing. Next, the person contracts foot muscles as tightly as possible to the count of three, then releases the contraction. The process is repeated, moving slowly up the trunk until all muscle groups have been contracted and relaxed.

Another variation of relaxation is *guided imagery*. Guided imagery is a process of identifying and using mental pictures to achieve a particular goal such as pain relief. This process may help to relieve pain by promoting relaxation, reducing anxiety, encouraging rest and sleep, and providing distraction. For example, guided imagery was used to help Mr. Smith who reported severe neck pain which felt like knots of rope. During a relaxation exercise involving muscle contraction and relaxation, the nurse suggested that Mr. Smith picture the knot gradually becoming looser with each muscle relaxation until the rope finally untied. At the end of the exercise, Mr. Smith's neck pain was decreased.

Some patients experience side effects during relaxation exercises. Tingling and twitching are common sensations. Occasionally, the patient may experience disturbing feelings of sadness or anxiety during relaxation. When such feelings persist, the exercise is discontinued and other interventions are used.

ASSISTING WITH DRUG THERAPY

Drugs are a very important part of relieving pain. Although the physician prescribes the particular medications to be administered, the nurse's role in drug therapy is vital. For example, after observing the patient in pain, the nurse may decide whether an analgesic is indicated. When several drugs are prescribed for the patient's pain, the nurse may select the particular drug to be used. When the physician prescribes a range of dosage, the nurse may decide the particular dosage. In addition, the nurse frequently observes the patient to determine if the medication has relieved the pain and the presence of side effects. The nurse records and reports these observations to the physician, head nurse, or team leader. Finally, the nurse teaches the patient how to use the medication safely and correctly.

Analgesics are drugs that are prescribed to produce pain relief without a loss of consciousness. Narcotic analgesics such as those listed in Table 7.2 are generally prescribed for patients with either severe acute pain of short duration or severe progressive pain associated with certain fatal types of cancer, nervous system diseases, and heart diseases. Narcotic analgesics provide excellent pain relief but may also produce serious adverse effects such as depressed respirations, suppressed cough reflex, nausea and vomiting, hypotension (lowered blood pressure), and constipation. In addition, physical dependence and drug tolerance may develop with long-term use of narcotics, although this is much rarer than previously believed.

Nonnarcotics such as those listed in Table 7.2 may be prescribed instead of narcotics or combined with them for pain relief. These drugs are generally indicated for the patient with mild to moderate pain. Anti-inflammatory drugs, such as those listed in Table 17.6, are often prescribed for patients with pain in the musculoskeletal system. Psychotropic drugs may be prescribed when the patient's pain is associated with high levels of anxiety or depression. Tranquilizers such as chlorpromazine (THORAZINE), promazine (SPARINE), and hydroxyzine (ATARAX, VISTARIL) are examples of psychotropic drugs that may provide pain relief. Antidepressants such as amitriptyline (ELAVIL), imipramine (TOFRANIL), or haloperidol (HALDOL) may be helpful for the patient with chronic pain.

Placebos are inactive substances which can relieve pain. The exact mechanism is not known. Some experts believe that placebos are effective when the patient, the nurse, and the physician expect and anticipate pain relief. Normal saline, vitamins, and lactose capsules are examples of placebos that have resulted in pain relief. Placebos can produce changes in pupil size, blood pressure, heart and respiratory rates, peristalsis, and hormone levels. Side effects include dry mouth, rash, headache, drowsiness and sleep disturbances. In some cases, placebos must be discontinued due to severe side effects. Nursing responsiblities related to administering placebo include:

- Follow hospital policy (some hospitals and state laws require written consent from the patient).
- Administer a placebo according to the physician's exact prescription.
- Carefully observe the patient for desired and undesired effects.
- Develop a therapeutic relationship that enhances drug therapy.
- Report and record observations related to the effect of the placebo.

TABLE 7.2
ANALGESICS

NONPROPRIETARY NAME	TRADE NAME	AVERAGE DOSE FOR ADULTS	NURSING IMPLICATIONS
I. Narcotic			
Alphaprodine	NISENTIL	40–60 mg	Narcotics produce analgesia, mood changes, mental cloudiness, drowsiness, and depress respiration
Anileridine	LERITINE	30–40 mg	
Codeine		8–120 mg	
Dihydrocodeine	PARACODIN	60 mg	
Hydrocodone* (dihydrocodeinone)	HYCODAN	5–10 mg	Tolerance, physical dependence, and abuse liability can occur if narcotics are not controlled properly
Hydromorphone (dihydromorphinone)	DILAUDID	1.5 mg	
Levorphanol	LEVO-DROMORAN	2–3 mg	Nausea, vomiting, constipation, and behavioral changes may develop
Meperidine	DEMEROL	80–100 mg	
Methadone	DOLOPHINE	7.5–10 mg	
Metopon (methydihydromorphinone)		3.5 mg	
Morphine		10 mg	
Oxycodone dihydrohydroxycodeinone)	PERCODAN	10–15 mg	
Oxymorphone (dihydrohydroximorphinone)	NUMORPHAN	1.0–1.5 mg	
Phenazocine	PRINADOL	3 mg	
Piminodine	ALVODINE	7.5–10 mg	
II. Nonnarcotic			
Acetaminophen	TEMPRA TYLENOL	600 mg	Skin rash and other allergic reactions may occur. Relatively well tolerated, but acute overdosage can cause fatal liver disease
Aspirin		600 mg	Overdose can cause death. Skin rash, irritation of gastrointestinal tract, ringing in the ears, dizziness, and bleeding tendency may occur
Pentazocine	TALWIN	600 mg	Infection may be irritating. Can cause physical dependence
Phenacetin		120–300 mg	Prolonged use can cause anemia
Propoxyphene	DARVON DOLENE	32–65 mg 32–65 mg	Used to relieve mild to moderate pain. Some patients may be hypersensitive

* Antitussive mainly.

159

An erroneous belief is that the patient whose pain is relieved by a placebo is not having real pain. In some cases, this error has resulted in a problem of undermedication and treatment of the patient in pain. Fortunately, pain research has provided new information about the powerful effects of a placebo. For example, patients with acute postoperative pain and progressive chronic pain from cancer have experienced pain relief from a placebo. Currently, placebos are used primarily in research related to experimental drugs and pain clinics for the patient with chronic pain.

An analgesic is generally more effective if administered within 30 minutes after pain starts or returns. The intramuscular route (Figure 7.2) is preferred for severe pain, while the oral route is indicated for mild or moderate pain. In very severe intolerable pain, the physician or registered nurse may administer small amounts of narcotic analgesia intravenously while the patient is continuously observed for adverse side effects.

Factors to consider in selecting from a range of dosage include the severity of pain reported by the patient and age. Elderly patients generally experience pain relief with lower dosages. Body weight is less important a consideration in adults than was once believed. The patient is observed closely after the first dosage so that adjustments can be made in later dosages if necessary. When the patient's pain is not relieved sufficiently, the nurse may increase the dosage and/or decrease the time interval between dosages if the physician's order permits. If these measures are not possible or do not relieve the patient's pain, the physician should be notified at once. A practice to be avoided is keeping the patient waiting until the next dose of pain medication is due. When the patient's pain returns before the time interval specified, pain relief has been insufficient. Waiting until the next medication dosage is due may cause the patient's pain to become much more intense. As mentioned earlier in this chapter, all interventions related to pain relief are more effective when started early, before pain becomes severe.

Administering a nonnarcotic analgesic by mouth may enhance the pain-relieving effect of parenteral narcotics. For example, the physician prescribed aspirin, 625 mg PO q4h, in addition to meperidine (DEMEROL), 75 mg IM q4h prn for Ms. Payne. Other

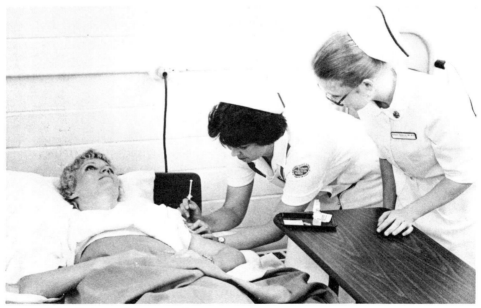

FIGURE 7.2 Giving an intramuscular analgesic. (Courtesy of North Dakota State School of Science—Practical Nursing Program, Wahpeton, North Dakota.)

drugs that may be prescribed to enhance the effects of narcotic analgesics include hydroxyzine hydrochloride (VISTARIL, ATARAX) and chlorpromazine (THORAZINE).

After administering an analgesic, the nurse should return to the patient to ask if pain has been relieved. The patient who has received an analgesic by mouth should experience relief within 30 to 60 minutes. The patient who has received an intramuscular injection should experience relief within 20 to 30 minutes. The patient who is sleeping or drowsy is not necessarily pain-free. Therefore, the nurse should specifically ask the patient if the medication has relieved pain.

Other Therapies

PHYSICAL THERAPY

Physical therapy may be prescribed for the patient with acute or chronic pain in the musculoskeletal or nervous systems. Forms of physical therapy which may be prescribed include active and passive exercise, traction, whirlpool baths, diathermy, and ultrasound.

RADIOTHERAPY

Radiotherapy uses radioactive rays to shrink tumors that are compressing nerves and causing pain. Information related to caring for a patient receiving radiotherapy can be located in Chapter 9.

BEHAVIORAL THERAPIES

Behavioral therapies are prescribed primarily for the patient with chronic pain. The basis of these therapies is that behavior related to pain is learned by positive reinforcement and/or avoiding unpleasant consequences. Pain behavior that consistently results in favorable rewards is likely to occur more frequently. Therapy includes measures to learn what factors influence the ptient's pain behavior and to modify the patient's pain experience. Specific interventions may include analgesics, exercise and activity, and family teaching related to pain behavior.

BIOFEEDBACK

This therapy uses machines to provide information about physiologic processes which enables some patients to learn to control them. Patients with pain due to migraine headache and Raynaud's disease have been helped by biofeedback.

HYPNOSIS

Hypnosis is a state of heightened mental awareness during which the person is more receptive to suggestions. Hypnosis has been used for patients with acute or chronic pain to alter pain awareness and/or pain behavior.

ACUPUNCTURE AND ACUPRESSURE

Acupuncture is a method that uses needles inserted into specific anatomic sites and at a variety of angles and depths. Site selection is based on meridians (circular lines) associated with particular body organs. Acupuncture has been used to treat acute and chronic pain.

Acupressure is a process of applying pressure along certain carefully selected anatomic sites on the skin. This method requires special training not widely available in the United States at this time. Acupressure is commonly used in Asian countries.

ELECTRICAL STIMULATION

Electrical stimulation uses electrodes placed on the skin or implanted in tissue and attached to a power supply. Several types of electrical stimulation are available. *Transcutaneous electrical nerve stimulation (TENS)* is a method in which electrodes are placed on the skin over an involved nerve, a painful area, or at places along the nerve pathway. Electrodes are attached to a battery-operated power supply which delivers electricity according to a preset voltage, frequency, and time interval. Patients with acute and chronic pain have obtained pain relief using TENS. *Permanent implant peripheral nerve stimulation* is a method in which electrodes are surgically implanted around a nerve. Electrodes are attached to a receiver, also implanted surgically in the subcutaneous tissue, and connected to an external battery-driven transmitter. This method has helped to suppress pain perception in patients with chronic pain. *Percuta-*

neous epidural column stimulation uses local anesthesia while inserting two electrodes through the skin into the epidural space. The electrodes are attached either to an external power supply or to one implanted in subcutaneous tissue. The dorsal column of the spinal cord is the area electrically stimulated by this method. *Dorsal column spinal cord stimulation* involves surgically implanting electrodes between the dura (covering) of the spinal cord near the dorsal column. A laminectomy (removal of posterior arch of a vertebrae) is usually done at the same time. A receiver is implanted in subcutaneous tissue and connected to an external power source.

PSYCHOTHERAPY

This therapy may be indicated when pain is associated with emotional conflict. The patient is helped by the therapist to identify unhealthy thoughts and feelings that influence pain.

SURGERY

A number of surgical procedures is available to help the patient in pain. A *nerve block* involves injecting a local anesthetic or other substance close to a nerve to prevent transmission of pain impulses. A *rhizotomy* interferes with the transmission of pain impulses at the nerve root close to the spinal cord. A *chordotomy* interferes with the transmission of pain impulses within the spinal cord. A *craniotomy* is an incision into the cranium to enable the surgeon to interrupt pain pathways. The specific name of the surgery depends upon the area of brain tissue involved.

PAIN CLINICS

The patient with chronic pain who has not been helped by other methods may be referred to a pain clinic. Specialists in all areas work together with the patient and family to develop a comprehensive treatment program which usually includes a combination of interventions already described elsewhere in this chapter.

Case Study Involving Pain

Ms. Beale is a 47-year-old nurse who returned from the recovery room following a cholycystectomy. She was helped to transfer from the stretcher to a side-lying position in bed by two student nurses.

Fifteen minutes later, the nurse, responding to Ms. Beale's call light, found the patient with her eyes closed moving restlessly about in bed. Mr. Beale said "she wants something for pain."

Postoperative orders included:

- NPO
- Continuous intravenous fluids at 100 ml/hr
- D5.45 normal saline
- Turn, cough, deep-breathe q2h
- Vital signs q1h until stable
- DEMEROL, 50–75 mg IM q3–4h prn pain
- TIGAN, 200 mg IM q6h prn nausea or vomiting
- If unable to void by 7 P.M., catheterize for urinary retension.

QUESTIONS

1. Who is the expert on pain experience in the case study?
2. Who is the expert on pain relief in the case study?
3. What type of pain is expected following a cholycystectomy?
4. What factors influence a person's pain experience?
5. What additional information do you need before selecting a pain-relieving intervention?
6. What principles should you consider when selecting a pain-relieving intervention?
7. What decisions can you make related to drug therapy for Ms. Beale?
8. What factors do you consider when selecting the dosage of meperidine (DEMEROL)?
9. What actions should you take if Ms. Beale's pain returns before the next dose of meperidine (DEMEROL) can be given?
10. What other nursing interventions can be undertaken to help relieve Ms. Beale's pain?

Suggestions for Further Study

1. Is there a pain clinic in your area? If so, talk with your instructor about plans to visit it.
2. How would the characteristics of the six cultural groups discussed in Chapter 2 influence their response to pain?
3. What personal feelings about how one should respond to pain will you have to consider in preparing to nurse the patient in pain?
4. Mason, Mildred A.; Bates, Grace F.; and Smola Bonnie K.: *Workbook in Basic Medical-Surgical Nursing*, 3rd ed. Macmillan Publishing Company, New York, 1984, Exercise 7.

Additional Readings

Beyerman, Kristine: "Flawed Perceptions About Pain." *American Journal of Nursing*, 82:302–304 (Feb.), 1982.

Booker, Jack E.: "Pain: It's All in Your Patient's Head (Or Is It?)." *Nursing 82,* 12:46–51 (Mar.), 1982.

Boyer, Marjorie Wenger: "Continuous Drip Morphine." *American Journal of Nursing,* 82:602–604 (Apr.), 1982.

Cummings, Dana: "Stopping Chronic Pain Before It Starts," *Nursing 81,* 11:60–62 (Jan.), 1981.

Fagerbaugh, Shizuko Y., and Strauss, Anselm: "How to Manage Your Patient's Pain . . . and How Not to." *Nursing 80,* 10:44–47 (Feb.), 1980.

Holderby, Robert A.: "Conscious Suggestion: Using Talk to Manage Pain." *Nursing 81,* 11:44–46 (May), 1981.

Knowles, Ruth Dailey: "Managing Anxiety." *American Journal of Nursing,* 81:110–11 (Jan.), 1981.

McCaffery, Margo: *Nursing Management of the Patient with Pain,* 2nd ed. J. B. Lippincott Co., New York, 1979.

_____: "Patients Shouldn't Have to Suffer: How to Relieve Pain with Injectable Narcotics." *Nursing 80,* 10:34–39 (Oct.), 1980.

_____: "Relieving Pain with Noninvasive Techniques." *Nursing 80,* 10:54–57 (Dec.), 1980.

_____: "Would You Administer Placebos for Pain?" *Nursing 82,* 12:80–85 (Feb.), 1982.

_____: "Understanding Your Patient's Pain." *Nursing 80,* 10:26–31 (Sept.), 1980. Pepmiller, Earl G.: "The Patient in Chronic Pain: A Challenge to Nursing Care." *Journal of Practical Nursing,* 32:17–20 and 41 (Jan.), 1982.

Perry, Samuel W., and Heidrich, George: "Placebo Response: Myth and Matter." *American Journal of Nursing,* 81:720–25 (Apr.), 1981.

Rambo, Beverly J., and Wood, Lucile A. (eds.): *Nursing Skills for Clinical Practice,* 3rd ed. W.B. Saunders Co., Philadelphia, 1982, pp. 708–33.

Richter, Judith M., and Sloan, Rebecca: "Stress—A Relaxation Technique." *American Journal of Nursing,* 79:1960–64 (Nov.), 1979.

Wilson, Ronald W., and Elmassian, Bonnie J.: "Endorphins." *American Journal of Nursing,* 81:722–25 (Apr.), 1981.

Chapter 8

The Emergency Patient*

Expected Behavioral Outcomes

Minimum objectives referred to as expected behavioral outcomes have been developed for the practical/vocational nursing student to use as guides in studying this chapter. The student should read these expected outcomes before studying the chapter. The objectives can be used as guides for study.

Using the content of this chapter, the student should return to the objectives and evaluate the ability to:

1. *Describe three nursing interventions appropriate for the patient in crisis.*
2. *List, in sequence, the priorities established for emergency care.*
3. *Describe at least two aspects of patient teaching in the emergency room.*
4. *Recommend and demonstrate appropriate action to be taken by a neighbor whose family member has a foreign body in the eye, ear, or nose.*

5. *Recommend and demonstrate appropriate action to be taken for animal, insect, and snake bites.*
6. *Differentiate between heat exhaustion, heat stroke, and heat cramps as a basis for initiating the proper action to be taken in each case.*
7. *Enumerate the common errors made when caring for victims of frostbite.*
8. *Assess a patient with multiple injuries and initiate proper action to support life.*
9. *Discuss the value of nurse interaction with a rape victim.*
10. *Discuss the value of nurse interaction with an alcoholic patient.*
11. *Describe the characteristics of a victim of child abuse.*

Vocabulary Development

The following prefixes, suffixes, and combining forms pertain to this chapter. By learning and/or reviewing their meanings, the practical/vocational nursing student will have the keys needed to unlock many exciting new medical terms.

*Revised by Alice Z. Welch, R.N., M.S.N. and the authors. Ms. Welch is Assistant Professor of Nursing, University of Utah, in Salt Lake City, Utah. Ms. Welch also provided the clinical photographs for this chapter.

Discover the meaning of these keys in a medical dictionary or in the content of this chapter. How does each key pertain to this chapter? In your notebook write the correct meaning of each prefix, suffix, or combining form listed below. Illustrate each key with an example.

carbo(n)—coal, charcoal. Ex. *charcoal*—carbon made by charring organic material.

cardi-
electr-
hema(at)-
pulmo(n)-
punct-

re-
sens-
therm-
traumat-
vuls-

Description

An *emergency* is considered to be an unexpected or sudden occasion frequently associated with an accident. The person in an emergency situation has a pressing or urgent need. *First aid* is the immediate care given to the person with a pressing or urgent need until more specific medical assistance can be given. The purpose of first aid is to protect the person from further injury and to maintain life when possible. First aid is often given at the scene of an accident. Emergency care includes first aid measures, evaluation of illness or injuries that are life-threatening, and prompt interventions to prevent loss of life, limb, or further deterioration of the patient's condition.

Accidents occur in any environment in which human activity is found: homes, areas of work, highways, schools, and hospital. Accidents are one of the major causes of death in the United States along with cancer and diseases of the cardiovascular system. Automobile accidents lead the cause of accidental deaths, and many of these accidents are related to alcohol. During the past few years, however, a declining death rate from automobile accidents has been observed. This decline is attributed to enforcement of the 55-mile-per-hour speed limit.

This chapter will focus on the nurse's role during common emergencies encountered in the home, community, and emergency department of hospitals. The emergency measures outlined in the chapter include basic first aid and basic life support, which can be administered on the scene. Some sections include the care rendered in the emergency department and special care units of the hospital. Methods of prevention are included in each section.

Prevention is the key to a reduction in the number of accidents. Some of the methods recommended for reduction of accidents are listed below:

- Continued enforcement of the 55-mile-per hour speed limit
- Measures against driving under the influence of alcohol
- Increased use of seat belts and other automobile safety devices
- Safety-oriented programs to correct dangerous intersections and curves; traffic lights for busy intersections; improved street lighting; and elimination of roadside hazards
- Periodic inspection of automobiles
- Knowledge of the hazards of and precautions for motorcycle riding as well as mandatory use of safety goggles and helmets
- Gun control
- Increased emphasis on prevention of accidents in classes for all age groups

Prevention is also a key to reducing nonaccident emergencies. Some practices known to have a positive effect on health include:

- Development and maintenance of habits that promote well-being such as good nutrition, regular exercise, and a balance of work and play
- Avoidance of cigarette smoking
- Maintenance of proper weight
- Periodic medical checkups for early detection of disease
- Written instructions of all recommendations made by the physician
- Regular self breast examination by women and self testicular examination by men

The Emergency Patient

The person in an emergency situation can be viewed by the nurse as having a crisis. Such a person is unable to resolve the event, problem, or situation in the usual way. Several kinds of crises have been identified. *Developmental crises* are associated with the transition periods of the life cycle: prenatal to birth, infancy to childhood, childhood to puberty and adolescence, adolescence to adulthood, maturity to middle age, middle age to old age, and finally old age to death. Changes that occur at these times can precipitate anxiety and internal strife in susceptible individuals. Successful transition from one stage to the next is dependent upon support and nurturance from significant others. Crises may result when individuals are fearful and suspicious of the phases of human development.

Situational crises are usually associated with a traumatic unexpected event which immobilizes the individual's problem-solving abilities. Examples of situations that may precipitate a crisis are natural disasters, diagnosis of fatal illness, loss of job or spouse, or serious accident. An individual's response to a situational crisis depends upon age (phase of life cycle), personal and social support, and success of previous coping patterns.

The crisis situation is usually temporary—lasting from a few days up to six weeks. Crisis provides an opportunity for personal growth and development of additional coping skills. An unfavorable outcome also may result from crisis. For example, a person may find the crisis so overpowering that withdrawal, neurotic, or psychotic behavior develops.

The person in crisis experiences a change in usual thoughts, feelings, and actions. If the event or situation is perceived as life-threatening, the individual may respond with acute anxiety. Events that are perceived as loss may trigger a response of depression. The person in crisis may experience intense feelings of shame, guilt, self-blame, ambivalence, helplessness, loss of control, embarrassment, fear, anger, pain, tension, and acute anxiety.

The individual who is experiencing crisis has difficulty reasoning (thinking) and solving problems. Thought processes may be illogical, nondiscriminating, and memory may be affected. In a severe crisis reaction, the individual may become confused, dazed, or disoriented.

Behavior of individuals in crisis ranges from asking numerous questions to uncontrollable, hysterical crying to violent behavior to severe, nonresponsive, mute behavior.

Recognizing the emergency patient as a person in crisis enables the nurse to alter nursing interventions in ways that decrease anxiety and encourage effective coping. Tables 8.1, 8.2, and 8.3 contain summaries of nursing interventions that promote these goals.

It is important to remember that clients are members of families who are committed to the protection of their members during crisis. A visit to the emergency room because of a serious illness affects the entire family. Successful resolution of the crisis will require the interaction of the family, client, and health care workers. Research has shown that cooperation and support of family and friends strongly influence the client in following instructions from physicians and nurses.

Role of the Nurse

OBSERVATIONS

When providing emergency care for a patient, the nurse needs skills related to rapid, accurate observation and setting priorities as a basis for taking action (Figure 8.1).

TABLE 8.1
SUMMARY OF NURSING INTERVENTIONS FOR
THE PERSON IN CRISIS

- Look for evidence of anxiety in the person.
- Move the client and/or family to a quiet environment.
- Offer the client and/or family warm beverages to increase comfort (if not contraindicated).
- Speak slowly and distinctly using short sentences initially.
- Do not call attention to unusual behavior the patient is using to reduce tension.
- Offer facts and information in small amounts.
- Help client formulate a list of individuals, groups or facilities that can provide support at this time (friends, church, Red Cross, Salvation Army, Meals-on-Wheels, child care services, etc.).
- Provide written instructions for the client.

TABLE 8.2
GUIDELINES TO NURSING INTERVENTIONS
FOR THE HOSTILE CLIENT

1. Recognize your own fear and anxiety concerning personal harm and unpredictability of angry, hostile client.
2. Personal space and body language are crucial when dealing with hostile, angry individuals. Provide maximum personal and physical space. Do not block the exit. Sit, do not stand. Sit at a 45-degree angle to the client. Standing and facing the client with direct eye contact and hands on hips represents aggressive body language. Appear relaxed; lean back in chair.
3. Avoid taking verbal comments personally. The nurse should remember that anger can be a response to illness, and aggression and hostility are the client's way of coping with helplessness and anxiety.
4. Keep your voice low. Speak slowly, clearly, and deliberately. Keep your emotions under control.
5. Ascertain the cause of the client's anger. The nurse may begin by saying, "I can see you are very upset and angry, but I am not sure I understand why."
6. Allow the patient to express feelings without losing face. Avoid belittling comments, e.g., "Adults don't act that way."
7. Listen to the patient, avoid smiling or laughing at client's comments or behavior. Smiling can be interpreted as making fun of, insincerity.
8. Avoid hurrying the client. Use open-ended responses that allow the client to set the pace.
9. If all of the above fails, client may be asked to leave the emergency department.

A patent airway, breathing, and circulation are the basic priorities for preservation of life and are known as the ABC of emergency care. These three vital functions can be assessed simultaneously by placing your ear to the patient's mouth, eyes toward the patient's chest to check for expansion, and fingertips on the carotid artery to assess circulation.

1. Establishment of an airway
   • Remove mucus, blood clots, vomitus, false teeth, or other objects with your finger.
   • Gently tilt head, pull chin forward, and insert oropharyngeal or nasopharyngeal airway.
   • Suction and administer oxygen by mask.
2. Breathing
   • If victim is unconscious, endotracheal tube should be inserted.
   • Positive pressure ventilation.
3. Circulation
   • CPR for cardiopulmonary arrest.
   • Apply direct pressure to control external hemorrhage.
   • Manage shock, administer intravenous fluids, insert central/venous pressure catheter if necessary, insert a Foley catheter if necessary, and monitor vital signs. Blood should be drawn for blood gases, electrolytes, complete blood count, glucose level, BUN, and other tests that may be ordered for baseline monitoring of therapy.
   • A nasogastric tube may be inserted to assess gastrointestinal bleeding and to empty contents of the stomach to prevent vomiting.

Once the ABCs are established, the nurse should make a systematic assessment beginning with the upper part of the patient.

Head and Cervical Neck
• Note level of consciousness.
• Check the skull for deformities.

TABLE 8.3
GUIDELINES FOR RESTRAINING THE VIOLENT
CLIENT

1. Four or five strong individuals are needed to encircle the client.
2. After the arms have been restrained in the back, the client is lowered to the floor in a backward motion.
3. Ankle and wrist restraints are applied together.
4. After restraints have been applied across chest, waist, and thighs, check to ascertain that breathing is not restricted and circulation is adequate.
5. Be sure to tell clients that restraints are temporary measures for self-protection and prevention of injury to emergency room personnel until self-control can be reestablished.
6. Chemical restraints in the form of drug therapy also may be used to help the client achieve self-control.

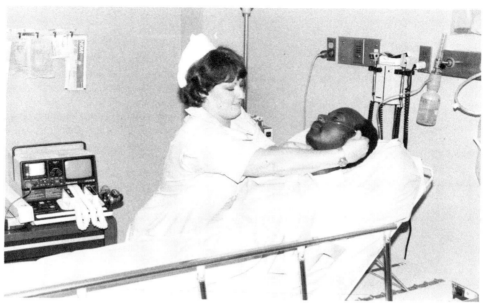

FIGURE 8.1　Rapid assessment in the emergency room. (Courtesy of Halifax School of Practical Nursing, Halifax–South Boston Community Hospital, South Boston, Virginia.)

- Check pupils for size, reaction to light, and location.
- Check ears and nose for spinal fluid, blood, or foreign objects.
- Check jaw for fracture.
- Palpate neck and cervical spine for tenderness, swelling, etc. Immobilize the area if positive signs are observed.

Chest and Thoracic Spine
- Observe for bilateral movement of the chest.
- Palpate the anterior chest wall for crepitus or puncture wounds. Circle the area on the skin if crepitus is noted.
- Observe for a sucking chest wound. If observed, apply petroleum gauze squares to seal the opening or cover the area with several layers of gauze squares and secure with strips of adhesive tape extending 4 in. on both sides of the puncture wound.
- Prepare for thoracotomy if a sucking wound is present.
- Place patient on injured side or immobilize with sand bags if the chest appears flaccid.
- Immobilize upper torso on firm board and

secure to board if thoracic spine injuries are observed.
- Record change in motor or sensory function.

Abdomen, Lumbar Spine, and Pelvis
- Check for evisceration, abrasion, or contusion.
- Apply moist sterile dressing over eviscerated organs. Nasogastric tube may be inserted to check for bleeding.
- Check for abnormal respiratory movement in the abdomen during respiration and peristaltic movement in the chest during respiration. Both are indications of a ruptured diaphragm.
- Check for muscular rigidity and rebound tenderness of the abdomen.
- Check for masses and tenderness in the area above the pubis.
- Check for tenderness when the pelvis is compressed.

Pelvic Injury
- Shock treatment is usually indicated.
- Foley catheter may be inserted unless there is a possibility of urethral laceration.

- Imobilize if lumbar spine injury appears to be a possibility.

Arms and Legs
- Check for deformities, swelling, pain, and discoloration.
- Check distal pulses.
- Check for voluntary movement and responses to painful stimuli.
- Splint fractured area.
- Treatment for shock will be initiated if patient has a long-bone fracture such as humerus or femur.

COMMUNICATION

Communication is a major role of the nurse in the emergency department. It is a basic prerequisite to the development of the therapeutic nurse-patient relationship. Effective communication is crucial to lowering of the client/family anxiety levels in stressful situations. A warm greeting, introduction of self, simple concise explanation before initiation of treatment, and an unhurried approach are all keys to placing a client at ease and development of trust.

Communication must also be tailored to the age and social-cultural background. Clichés should be avoided. Nonmedical vocabulary, with terms pertinent to the age and culture of the client, is used instead. Communicating with non-English-speaking clients may be a frustrating experience for nurses and clients in the emergency room. Often non-English-speaking clients are accompanied by an English-speaking teenage member of the family. The teenager acts as the translator for the client. If a hospital translator is selected, better information can be obtained by one who is the same sex and age as the client.

Written communication on the client's emergency medical record is another important role of the nurse. This document contains legal evidence of the health team's assessment, communication interventions, treatment, and evaluation of patient care. It also provides a record of care omitted and the rationale behind the decision. In the eyes of the law, if you did not record it, it was not done. If the documentation is illegible and not signed, it also was not done.

PATIENT TEACHING

Patient teaching is an essential part of emergency care. The focus of patient teaching includes (1) instruction regarding follow-up care, (2) instruction regarding general health care, and (3) anticipatory guidance. Although patient teaching is most effective when the client's anxiety is low, clients are usually more receptive to new information following life-threatening events.

A first step in patient teaching is to determine if discharge instructions can be followed at home. This can often be verified by asking the patient to describe what is to be done at home and how it is to be done. Written discharge instructions such as those in Figure 8.2 are provided to each client. In addition, a copy of the emergency room record should be given to each client.

Electrical Safety

Electricity is a form of energy caused by electrons flowing through a *conductor*. A conductor usually is metal. However, a conductor may be a solution containing electrolytes. The rate of flow of electrons through a conductor is known as *current*. Current may flow in one direction or in alternate directions. Current that flows in one direction is known as *direct current. Alternating current* is the reversal of the direction of the flow of current and voltage. Homes in the United States utilize alternating current. The current changes direction 60 times per second. The voltage at the wall outlet remains at 115 volts. *Amperes* are the number of electrons passing a specific point per second. *Voltage* is the driving force causing the electrons to flow in one direction through a substance. *Resistance* is the degree of difficulty encountered by electrons in flowing through a material.

Electricity exists in two forms: static and dynamic. *Static* electricity is the buildup of nonmoving electrical charges on the surface of nonconductors. Static electricity occurs when an individual walks over a carpet and receives a shock, pulls a sheet away from a blanket and hears a crackling noise, or combs the hair and notices that the hair

THE QUEEN'S MEDICAL CENTER
HONOLULU, HAWAII

Emergency Department

PATIENT'S NAME _____

DISCHARGE INSTRUCTIONS

ED # _____ DATE _____

The examination and treatment you have received in the Emergency Department have been rendered on an emergency basis only. You should contact a physician of your choice for follow-up care and for any further problems.

☐   **INSTRUCTIONS:** Please follow the written instruction(s) on _____ that is given to you today.

☐   **TETANUS IMMUNIZATION:** You have received ☐ Tetanus Toxoid   ☐ Tetanus Immune Globin

☐   **X-RAYS:** Please advise your follow-up physician that x-rays were taken of the: _____
_____

Your initial x-ray report is a preliminary interpretation. A radiologist, an x-ray specialist, will review your x-rays and give a complete report to the Emergency Department or your follow-up physician.

☐   **MEDICATION(S):** The following medication(s) are prescribed for you. Please take them as instructed.

_____   _____

_____   _____

☐   This drug may cause drowsiness and impair your coordination and judgement. Use CAUTION when operating an automobile or other dangerous machinery. DO NOT perform any hazardous tasks until you have seen what effects the medication has on yourself. Please follow the written instructions on _____

_____   _____

☐   **OTHER INSTRUCTIONS:**
_____
_____
_____

This sheet is evidence that you were in our Emergency Department today. If your employer should require a "Back to Work" slip, please consult your physician of choice or company physician.
_____

I have received a copy of these instructions. I understand these instructions and have had an opportunity to ask questions and have no further questions.

I authorize the Queen's Medical Center to release medical information regarding this emergency care to the physician to whom I will go for follow-up care.

_____

Signature of Patient or Responsible Person

Relationship to Patient

_____

Signature of Nursing Personnel

DISTRIBUTION: White - Emergency Dept. Copy   Yellow - Patient's Copy

Form No. 888150 (11/77)

FIGURE 8.2   Written discharge instructions from emergency room. (Courtesy of The Queen's Medical Center, Honolulu, Hawaii.)

stands out in the direction of the comb. Static electricity is prevalent, especially since the discovery of such synthetic materials as polyester, nylon, and plastic. Static electricity can be reduced by adding an anti-static compound to the final rinse water when washing a garment. A metal surface can be wiped with an antistatic compound to reduce static electricity since moisture in the air carries the electrical charge away.

Dynamic electricity refers to moving electrons along a conductor. Motors, generators, and batteries are examples of dynamic electricity.

EFFECTS OF ELECTRICITY ON THE BODY

The body has been compared with an electrical machine. Electrical activity is constantly being conducted between the brain and the muscles and organs by way of the nerves. An electrical impulse from outside the body can excite the nerve endings, interfere with the permeability of the nerve membrane, and cause the charges to neutralize each other.

An electrical shock occurs when current passes through an individual's body. The shock experienced by the individual may range from a mild tingling to a severe muscular contraction. The size of the body surface involved will determine whether the shock is micro or macro in nature.

The victim of a macroshock has a flow of electrical current through a large area of the body. For example, the electrical current may flow from one arm to the other arm through the chest. Another example of macroshock is seen when the flow of current comes from the bed control through the patient's hand and is transmitted throughout the entire body because the body surface is saturated with urine and/or perspiration. The victim of a microshock experiences the passing of electrical current through a small area of the body as a tingling sensation. An individual may transmit a microshock to another person without feeling it. An example of this is seen when an individual touches another person during cold weather and the second person receives a shock. Another example is evident when a bottle of parenteral solution is being changed and the patient feels a shock at the site of insertion of the needle.

In dealing with electricity, the nurse needs to know that electrical energy seeks to ground itself. Electricity will use an individual's body or any object on its way to the ground.

The amount of injury caused to the human body by electrical energy will depend on the voltage (intensity of the current), the length of exposure, the part of the body involved, and the individual's susceptibility at that time. Electrical energy passing through the body can cause severe muscular contractions and convulsions resulting in bruises and fractures, burns at the point of entry and exit, cardiac fibrillation, cardiac arrest, respiratory arrest, and death.

FIRST AID

The nurse needs to know what to do for a victim or for him-or herself in the event of a macroshock. When observing a victim who is unable to let go of an electrical wire or piece of equipment that is causing severe muscular contractions, the rescuer should remove the plug from the outlet immediately. In the event that a plug is not visible, the rescuer should use the force of the body to hurl the victim away from the electrical contact. The momentum of the rescuer's body must be sufficient to clear the victim away from the electrical contact. The rescuer may also use an insulating material such as a rope, a folded blanket, a stick, or a broom to shove the victim away from the electrical source. The rescuer should remember not to touch the victim with bare hands. If the nurse is a victim of macroshock, the same principle of breaking contact with the electrical equipment should be utilized. For example, if the nurse reaches to remove a plug from an outlet and the plug separates from the electric wire and the hand will not release the live wire, the legs can be kicked and the weight of the body will cause a fall and separation from the source of electricity.

FREQUENT CAUSES OF ELECTRICAL INJURIES IN THE HOSPITAL

Some of the more frequent electrical injuries in the hospital are caused by the following:

1. Light bulbs in the overbed light, which can cause fire or burns to the patient, especially if the bulb wattage is larger than that specified by the manufacturer
2. Tripping over electrical cords strung across halls or corridors possibly causing a short circuit and a burn to the victim

3. Frayed wires and broken plugs
4. Jerking or pulling an electrical plug from the outlet and breaking off the ground prong or wire in the outlet
5. Dust and dirt on motors
6. Electric heating pads

All hospital employees must remember that the hospital is legally responsible for the safety of the patient. The hospital may be responsible if the patient is injured by personal equipment brought into the hospital. For this reason, all such electrical equipment—electric razors, television sets, or radios—should be checked by the hospital engineer before being used on or by the patient.

PREVENTION OF ELECTRICAL INJURIES

Members of the health team should handle all electrical equipment safely. Before using a piece of electrical equipment, the nurse and other members of the health team should ask the following questions:

1. Do I know the proper way to use this equipment?
2. Do I know if this equipment is functioning properly?
3. Do I know if this equipment is safe to use on this patient?

If the nurse or other health professional has any doubt about the answers to these three questions, help or assistance should be obtained *before* using the equipment.

Observing the rules listed in Tables 8.4 8.5, and 8.6 can provide an electrically safe environment for the nurse, the patient, and the family.

Injuries Caused By Lightning

A flash of light produced by the discharge of atmospheric electricity from one cloud to another or from a cloud to the ground is known as *lightning*. Lightning travels at a speed of 1/100th to 1/1000th of a second with a voltage of 12,000 to 200,000 amperes. When lightning strikes a person who is not grounded, he or she becomes

TABLE 8.4
ELECTRICAL SAFETY AT HOME

- Check the cords on all electrical equipment for frayed wires and broken ground plugs before use. Wrapping an electrical cord with tape is not safe.
- Check the electric plug for a tight or secure fit into the wall socket. Do not tape the plug in place because of the danger of leakage.
- Do not cut hedges or lawns with electrical equipment when the hedge or lawn is damp or wet with dew or rain.
- Do not permit electrical cords to drag through water or other liquids while working outside in the yard.
- Use only electrical cords labeled for outside use when utilizing electricity outside the house.
- Do not leave cords dangling from ironing boards when small children are around.
- Do not permit children to bite or chew on cords or to insert them into outlets.
- Do not allow a pet such as a dog to chew on an electrical plug. Young animals under two years of age have a natural instinct to gnaw on objects. Electric plugs and electric wires sometimes are inviting to young animals.
- Do not clean the electric stove, oven, or other electrical equipment while the equipment is plugged into the outlet.

highly charged and the charge is dissipated very slowly. Death may result from the current passing through vital organs such as the heart and brain. In some cases, lightning passes through one victim's body and jumps 10 to 100 yd and passes through a second individual's body. It is for this reason that people are warned to avoid crowds during a thunderstorm.

Approximately 44,000 electrical storms occur a day throughout the world with only a small number of individuals dying from lightning. A majority of those hit survive the experience, primarily because of the skills of the rescue worker.

When the electrical current passes through a victim's body, the current causes severe muscular contractions and causes the individual to be hurled many feet into the air. Breathing and heartbeat cease. The patient may lose consciousness. The person has a burn at the point of entry and exit of the current.

TABLE 8.5
ELECTRICAL SAFETY FOR THE
HOSPITALIZED PATIENT

- The patient should be instructed not to depress the call button when one of the hands is in a basin of water or in a wet soak.
- The nurse's hand should be dry and she or he should not be standing in water when operating electrical equipment or appliances.
- A safety pin should not be used on an electric heating pad.
- Bed controls on a semielectric bed or an all-electric bed should be checked to determine if the wires are frayed or if the controls are cracked. Urine, saline, and perspiration are good conductors of electricity, especially when faulty equipment is present.
- The frame of a bed that is operated by electricity should not be allowed to touch the radiator or other metals.
- Extension cords should be avoided because of the danger of breakage. A cord of sufficient length should be installed on the equipment.
- Do not use two-prong extension cords or "cheater plugs" on electric plugs with a ground wire. Using such an extension cord is comparable to removing the ground wire.
- Do not permit the patient to bring personal electrical equipment into the hospital without having it checked by the hospital engineer.
- When a piece of electrical equipment causes the patient or the nurse to receive even a tiny shock, the equipment should be removed from the area, labeled, and routed to the appropriate department for repair.
- Ether, cyclopropane, and nitrous oxide are potentially explosive and dangerous anesthetics. They should be labeled as such and care should be used in handling them. These gases frequently are found in the operating and delivery room suites.
- Electrical plugs should not be removed from an outlet within 2 to 6 ft of an anesthesia machine when a flammable anesthetic is in use.
- Soap should be rinsed well from conductive floors, and wax should not be applied when an anesthetic is used.
- A nurse entering the operating room or the delivery room should be checked for conductivity prior to entering the suite.
- Tables, pillows, and pads used in the operating room and delivery room should be tested to determine if static electricity is being drained from the equipment safely.
- Flash bulbs, cautery machines, and diathermy machines should not be used in the presence of flammable anesthesia.

FIRST AID

The objective of first aid is to restore cardiac action and breathing. Cardiopulmonary resuscitation should be initiated immediately. Resuscitation may be required for at least 30 minutes before response is evident. The victim may be moved after the heart starts beating and breathing has been established. The patient should be moved to the nearest medical facility. The patient continues to need careful observation. When a person is struck by lightning and does not lose consciousness, evaluation by a physician is needed, especially in regard to cardiac status.

In the event an individual is struck by a falling live electrical wire, the following points should be remembered:

- The victim is electrically charged.
- Do not touch the victim until the wire has been moved.

TABLE 8.6
ELECTRICAL SAFETY FOR THE PATIENT ON A
MONITOR

- A patient attached to a monitor should not be touched by a person who has one hand on another piece of electrical equipment, a siderail, or a metal surface.
- Do not allow water or other liquid on the floor near the patient's bed while he or she is being monitored. The nurse, standing in the water, can become a return path for electric current.
- Do not permit the patient on a monitor to use an electric razor.
- When using several monitors or pieces of electrical equipment on a patient, the nurse should make certain that the outlets are on the same wall cluster.
- When defibrillating a victim, the nurse should not touch the bed, cart, or any portion of the patient's body.
- When the defibrillator is being tested, the nurse should not depress the button to discharge the current while holding the paddles slightly apart because of the possibility of flashover to the hands. The paddles should not be held close together while the equipment is being tested.
- Monitors and defibrillators with ground plugs should be checked monthly by an engineer for leakage and labeled with the date of inspection. The inspector will determine whether current is escaping from the ground plugs.

- The rescuer should stand on a dry surface or a rubber mat.
- The rescuer should use gloves to cover the hands or a newspaper to hold the stick or weighted rope to separate the wire from the victim.
- First aid treatment of the individual struck by a live electrical wire should be the same as for the person struck by lightning.

EFFECTS OF LIGHTNING

Any organ caught in the path of current associated with lightning may lose its function. Renal damage may occur as a result of current passing through the kidney area. This is manifested by oliguria. Some authorities recommend the use of Ringer's lactate and a diuretic.

A person who survives being struck by lightning may have paralysis. Vasoconstriction may occur in the extremities and cause the individual to experience a feeling of coldness in the feet and hands. Tremors, difficulty in using one's hands, depression, emotional instability, cataracts, and optic atrophy may develop, especially in an elderly person. Head injury such as concussion or fracture may occur when the person is being hurled or thrown to the ground.

PREVENTION

In an effort to avoid being struck by lightning, an individual should remain indoors during a thunderstorm. Windows should be closed. Individuals should not sit near fireplaces, main electrical switches, electrical boxes, or any electrical wires. An individual caught in a thunderstorm outdoors should take refuge in a closed car if possible. Lakes, ponds, wire fences, walls, and solitary trees should be avoided. In the event that an individual is on the golf course, the golf club bag should be removed from the back. It is important to keep moving because a warm column of air rises from a stationary body and acts as a conductor of electricity. Therefore, movement is better than remaining in one position. When caught in a thunderstorm, the individual is safer if thoroughly soaked than dry. Wet clothes reduce the flow of current through the body.

Fire

Three basic components are essential for fire: fuel, heat, and oxygen. The point at which heat becomes so intense that the fuel ignites is known as the ignition temperature. Fire will burn as long as there are fuel, proper temperature, and oxygen. The nurse needs to know the chemical basis of fire as a foundation for preventing and extinguishing fire. The chemical reaction can be stopped by the prevention of rapid oxygenation of the fuel. Heat can be removed by cooling, and oxygen can be taken away by excluding air by using such methods as covering the fire with a wet blanket, sand, dirt, or a chemical foam.

An increasing number of Americans die each year because of hospital fires. In 1975, fires took the lives of 11,800 Americans. The United States has the highest hospital fire death rate in the world. Canada has the second highest death rate from hospital fires. Fires in hospitals in the United States have

TABLE 8.7
WHAT TO DO IN A HOSPITAL FIRE

1. Patients should be removed from the immediate area of the fire.
2. The hospital operator should be notified of the location of the fire, the type of fire, and the equipment involved. If a fire alarm box is available, it should be stimulated by either pulling the alarm or breaking the glass, as indicated on the box.
3. Oxygen valves, gas outlets, electrical equipment, and ventilating equipment should be discontinued. Windows and doors should be closed.
4. A fire extinguisher should be obtained.
5. The nurse should pause outside the door for 15 seconds before entering the room.
6. A cloth should be used to protect the nurse's hand when opening a door leading to or from the fire. The hospital employee should first crack open the door instead of opening it rapidly.
7. The fire extinguisher should be used according to the instructions. A wet blanket or wet linen can be used in addition to the fire extinguisher to aid in putting out the fire.
8. Ambulatory, wheelchair, and bedridden patients should be evacuated.
9. Staff should be evacuated from the area.

increased more than 100 percent. In 1970, there were 7800 hospital fires, and by 1974, the number had increased to 15,600. This figure represents approximately 40 hospital fires per day.

A hospital fire represents a true emergency. It is important for the nurse as well as other members of the health team to know what to do in case of fire and how to do it. Table 8.7 contains a summary of information needed in case of a hospital fire. Table 8.8 provides guidelines for the prevention of fire in a hospital.

TABLE 8.8
PREVENTION OF FIRE IN THE HOSPITAL

- Caution the patient against smoking in bed or in an area in which oxygen is used.
- The patient should not smoke unattended after receiving a sedative or an analgesic.
- Workers, visitors, and patients may need to be cautioned against placing ashes or cigarette butts in trash cans. Often these trash cans are lined with plastic liners. Ash trays must be used.
- Employees should not smoke in utility rooms, linen closets, storage areas, or other areas containing flammable material.
- The smallest sign of smoke or the slightest odor of fire should be investigated.
- Trash should not be allowed to collect or pile up in an area.
- Exits and corridors should remain clear and uncluttered at all times.
- Paint cans, aerosol cans, and ether cans should be discarded in a metal can with a top. The can should contain a label indicating that the contents are combustible.
- Oxygen cylinders and cyclopropane cylinders should not be stored in the same location.
- Combustible material should not be allowed to accumulate.
- The patient's gowns, curtains, rugs, drapes, and bed linen should be flame resistant.
- Check all electrical equipment and appliances brought into the patient unit before they are used. The check should include an examination for frayed wires and defective plugs.
- Know the location of all fire extinguishers, fire alarm boxes, fire doors, and exit routes.
- Remain calm. Do not shout *fire*. Use the hospital's code to announce a fire.
- Each worker should know his or her assignment. Team effort is vital in evacuating patients to preserve life.

EVACUATION OF PATIENTS

Four basic types of evacuations are used in a hospital setting. These are partial, horizontal, vertical, and total evacuation. When helping with partial evacuation, the nursing personnel assume responsibility for removing patients from the immediate area of the fire. When assisting with horizontal evacuation, the nurse moves patients to the opposite end of the floor. In vertical evacuation, the nurse moves the patient to a lower floor or to the basement of the hospital. Total evacuation indicates that patients are moved to the outside of the building.

When bedridden patients are evacuated by the staff from the area, three groups of workers are needed. Loaders are needed to place patients in wheelchairs, stretchers, or blankets. Movers are used to transport patients to stairways or exits. Carriers actually transport patients downstairs to another floor or out of the building.

Patients may be carried to safety by utilizing one of six basic types of patient carries. When selecting the appropriate type of patient carry, the nurse should consider the patient's size and physique, the rescuer's strength, and the condition of the patient. Good body mechanics is essential in the use of each type of patient carry. The most versatile item used in the evacuation of patients is the sheet. Examples of this and other types of carries to be used in evacuating patients are shown in the accompanying pictures (see Figures 8.3 to 8.8).

After the patients have been evacuated from the area, the nurse should account for each patient; look in closets and under the beds; and check the floor, bathrooms, and other rooms before closing the doors and sealing off the area. If smoke is intense, the nurse should crawl or remain close to the floor to avoid becoming asphyxiated.

Choking

An individual who is *choking* is unable to breathe or swallow because of an obstruction within the throat or respiratory passage.

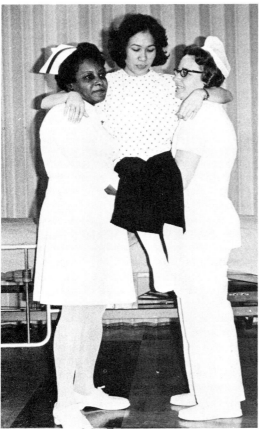

FIGURE 8.3 Two-person seat carry.

CAUSE

A common cause of choking is laryngo-tracheobronchitis. An individual may have a foreign body in the throat, may experience a swelling because of an allergic reaction, or may be a victim of injury to the head, neck, throat, or chest as a result of an accident. A convulsive seizure can cause choking. Large polyps in the nose may protrude downward into the back of an individual's throat and cause spells of choking. Tonsillitis and peritonsillar abscess are also causes of choking.

SYMPTOMS

An individual whose airway suddenly becomes obstructed becomes apprehensive, has distention of the eyes and bulging of the lips, and immediately grabs the throat. Excessive salivation may be present. The per-

son is unable to breathe or speak. The color of the skin rapidly becomes cyanotic (blue). The skin of a black person appears ashen and gray. The individual collapses and will die if the obstruction is not removed.

FIRST AID

A foreign body lodged in the throat constitutes an acute emergency in which the victim may die within four minutes if emergency treatment is not promptly initiated. Children and older adults seem to be more prone to aspirate or choke when eating. With a child, the common cause of acute airway obstruction is tossing a peanut or piece of candy into the air and catching it in the mouth. A child may be treated by reassurance and turning him or her upside down at the same time. The child's feet should be held by the nurse's right hand while the shoulder should be supported with the elbow of the nurse's left arm. The fist should be placed forcefully upward on the child's abdomen between the umbilicus and below the rib cage. This position usually causes the object to be dislodged by gravity. The child

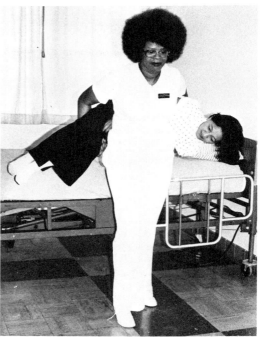

FIGURE 8.4 Saddleback carry.

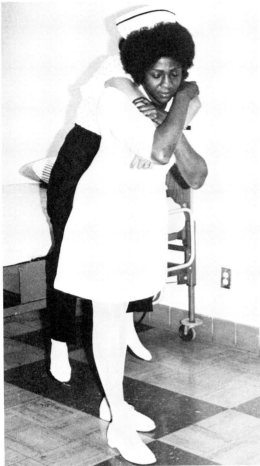

FIGURE 8.5 Packstrap carry. Patient's arms are over the rescuer's shoulders and crossed over the chest. The patient's armpits should be directly over the rescuer's shoulders.

and using the Heimlich maneuver (described below) may not be effective. Emergency treatment for the child who has aspirated a bean or other similar object usually consists of immediate laryngoscopy and bronchoscopy. In doing a laryngoscopy, the physician inserts a laryngoscope into the larynx and removes the object. A similar procedure is followed with a bronchoscopy except that a bronchoscope is used.

Adults also may choke on food. This occurs frequently in restaurants or in hospitals or nursing homes in the case of older patients. The nurse may use a combination of back blows and chest or abdominal thrusts to help dislodge the foreign body. The recommended sequence of activities is four back blows followed by four abdominal or chest thrusts. The abdominal thrust is done when the rescuer grasps one's own fist with the other hand and positions them slightly above the victim's umbilicus (navel) and just below the rib cage. The fist should be thrust forcefully into the victim's abdomen with an upward movement. This action should be repeated several times. By doing this, the rescuer forces the diaphragm upward and compresses the lung, thereby increasing the pressure within the thorax (Figures 8.9 and 8.10).

When an individual gets a chicken or fish bone embedded in the esophagus, this is a frightening experience. Therefore, first aid in this situation consists of reassurance while seeking medical intervention. Bones usually are removed by esophagoscopy. In this procedure, a special instrument called an esophagoscope is inserted into the esophagus to permit visualization and removal of the foreign body. While waiting to have the bone removed, the patient should be cautioned against eating crackers or drinking substances such as vinegar, medicine, cough syrups, and other irritating substances since these aggravate the situation and cause deeper penetration of the bone into the esophagus.

Syncope

The individual with syncope (fainting) has a transient loss of consciousness due to a decreased supply of oxygen to the brain.

should not be slapped or hit on the back as this may cause gasping and aspiration of the foreign body deeper into the respiratory system. The rescuer may be able to put a finger into the back of the throat of the child and remove the food or object that has become lodged there.

Beans, peas, and seeds present a different problem when lodged in a child's throat. These objects are the most life-threatening of the foreign objects frequently aspirated by children. The high humidity of the respiratory tract causes the foreign body to swell, become larger, and produce greater obstruction. Turning the child upside down

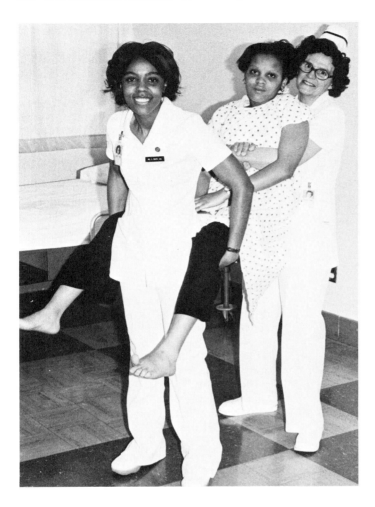

FIGURE 8.6 Two-person extremities carry.

This is a common medical emergency. The loss of consciousness may be complete or incomplete, and recovery of consciousness usually occurs when the individual assumes a recumbent or reclining position. This position facilitates an increase in the circulation to the client's brain and other vital organs.

Fainting frequently is caused by anxiety. Anxiety associated with gruesome sights, bad news, or thoughts of previously traumatic experiences may result in fainting. Orthostatic hypotension (lowered blood pressure associated with body position) may cause an individual to faint. Thus, when an individual assumes an erect position suddenly and has a rapid drop of blood pressure, syncope may occur. Orthostatic hypotension may be associated with either drug therapy or disease conditions such as parkinsonism, inner ear disturbances, diabetes, and neuritis. Conditions causing a reduction in cardiac output with a subsequent decrease of circulating blood to the brain may also produce fainting. Bradycardia, an abnormally slow pulse rate, heart failure, hemorrhage, and peripheral vasodilatation are examples of conditions that might produce a decreased flow of blood to the brain. Some individuals respond to crowded, warm environments or severe pain by fainting. Anemia, which is a decrease in the oxygen-carrying ability of the blood, may cause an individual to faint. The patient with anemia will suffer from an inadequate supply of oxygen to the brain. The patient generally is pallid, short of breath, and chronically fa-

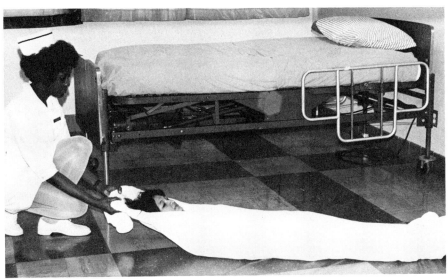

FIGURE 8.7 Blanket or sheet drag when patient must be moved close to the floor or ground. The patient's body should be kept in a straight line.

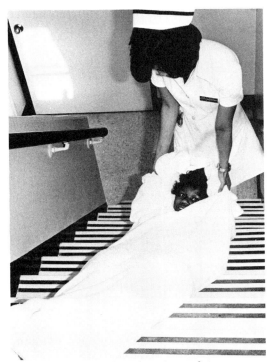

FIGURE 8.8 Blanket drag is used to move a patient down a flight of stairs. Patient's head should be lowered first without bumping it or causing injury.

tigued. Another cause of fainting is hypoglycemia (low blood sugar). The individual with low blood sugar may faint when the blood sugar drops abruptly below the normal value. This may occur just prior to meals, but it can be prevented by eating a high-protein, low-carbohydrate, and low-fat diet.

SYMPTOMS

The onset of symptoms experienced by the individual who faints varies. In general, the individual may experience dizziness or a feeling of being lightheaded; coldness of lips, fingers, and toes; numbness and tingling of the feet and hands; profuse perspiration; visual disturbances; and nausea. The person may appear pale or ashen. The individual may also have rapid, prolonged, and deep breathing. This type of breathing is referred to as hyperventilation. The patient's skin feels cool to the touch, and the pupils become dilated. The pulse may be slow or rapid. In either case, the pulse is thready.

TREATMENT AND NURSING CARE

An individual who indicates that fainting is imminent should be instructed to sit down and place the head between the knees. An-

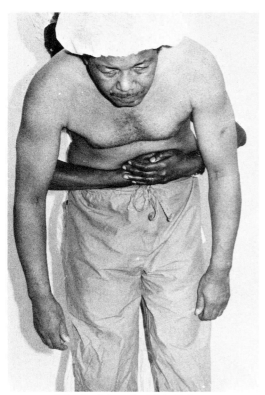

FIGURE 8.9 In doing the Heimlich maneuver, the rescuer stands behind the victim, wraps the arms around the victim's waist, and grasps the fist. After placing the fist above umbilicus and below rib cage, the rescuer should push the fist firmly upward. This forces the diaphragm upward, compresses the lungs, causes food to be expelled.

other position is having the patient lie flat without a pillow. Any clothing that is tight or constricting should be loosened. The patient's head should turned to one side if vomiting develops in order to clear the airway. Another possibility that should be considered for the individual who has fainted or is vomiting is placing the person in a prone position. When the patient is placed in this position, the head should be resting on one hand and turned to the side to prevent the tongue from blocking the airway and aspiration of vomitus. The victim's face may be bathed gently with cool water, but water should not be poured over the face because this practice may result in aspiration of liquid. A cotton ball moistened with aromatic

spirits of ammonia may be held near the patient's nostrils. Ammonia stimulates the medulla by irritating the sensory nerve endings in the upper respiratory tract.

If the individual has sustained a fall, a careful examination is indicated to determine the extent of injury. Following syncope, the patient should be encouraged to lie quietly for a period of time and be carefully observed. While the patient is resting, the muscles of the calves of the legs can be tightened and relaxed and the feet can be flexed and extended. The patient may then gradually assume a sitting position. A combination of these exercises and gradual assumption of an erect position usually will prevent postural hypotension. Fitted antiembolic stockings and abdominal support may be utilized to prevent postural hypotension.

The individual who has fainted recently should be cautioned against operating a motor vehicle or other hazardous equipment or ascending to heights until medical evaluation has been obtained.

Hemorrhage

Hemorrhage is frightening as well as life-threatening. The loss of 1 to 6 pt blood in the average adult may cause shock and possibly death. External hemorrhage is bleeding that can be observed. Bleeding from wounds, open fractures, and other injured areas and nosebleeds are examples of external hemorrhage.

Five methods of controlling external hemorrhage are (1) direct pressure, (2) elevation, (3) cold applications, (4) digital pressure, and (5) tourniquet.

Most cases of external bleeding can be controlled by direct pressure that causes the flow of blood to decrease and allows normal coagulation to occur. A sterile dressing, sanitary napkin, or clean cloth can be placed over the wound. Pressure by hand or with a bandage can be used.

Elevation of the part above the level of the heart when an extremity is wounded helps to check bleeding. Pressure and elevation may be used together.

The application of cold compresses will help to check capillary bleeding. Discoloration associated with contusions can be re-

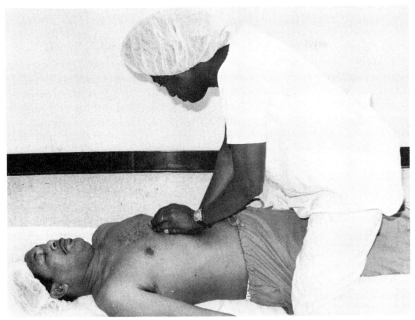

FIGURE 8.10   The Heimlich maneuver can be performed if the patient is in a dorsal recumbent position.

duced by the use of cold applications. Prolonged use of cold packs without specific orders from the physician should be avoided because of the danger of tissue damage.

When using digital pressure or pressure point control, the rescuer applies pressure to the artery to check arterial bleeding in the area supplied by that artery. By recalling basic anatomy, the nurse should be able to apply pressure to arteries close to the surface or those that can be compressed against the surface of an adjacent bone. Although pressure point control of bleeding is used less often than direct pressure, the nurse should know the common pressure point sites, which are the temporal, facial, carotid, brachial, radial, and femoral arteries. Using a tourniquet should be a measure of last resort to control external bleeding. For example, if the victim's limb has been destroyed or amputated, use of a tourniquet may be the only way to control severe bleeding and save a life. Other methods to check the bleeding should be tried first. A tourniquet can be made by folding a triangular bandage several inches wide and six to eight layers thick; a blood pressure cuff, a rubber tube,

or a long, wide piece of cloth may be used. The tourniquet should be placed between the wound and the heart. After wrapping the bandage around the extremity twice, the rescuer should tie a half-knot and place a small stick or comparable object in the knot. The stick can be twisted to tighten the tourniquet after the knot has been securely tied. The tourniquet should be tightened only to the point that bleeding stops. *Do not cover the tourniquet.* Mark the victim's forehead with the letters *TK* to indicate to the medical staff that a tourniquet has been applied. The tourniquet should be released by the physician.

Although internal bleeding usually is not visible, it can be as serious as external bleeding. The patient who is experiencing internal bleeding has a weak or rapid pulse, the skin is cold or clammy, the eyes are dull, and the pupils are slow to respond to light. Blood pressure is low. A person who has internal bleeding will be anxious, restless, and thirsty and may feel nauseated.

Internal bleeding can occur from a closed fracture of any bone, from a perforated peptic ulcer, or from trauma to the internal organs. For example, a ruptured spleen or lacerated liver will result in internal bleeding.

The person suspected of having internal bleeding should be transported to a medical facility immediately. The patient should be lying down and, if possible, on one side in case of vomiting. If the patient has internal bleeding into the tissues of an extremity, external pressure and a splint may be applied. The administration of oxygen during the period of transportation will help the patient since tissues are being deprived of blood containing oxygen because of the hemorrhage.

Epistaxis

Epistaxis, or nosebleed, may occur in normal individuals. It may be due to an injury of the nose or to the rupture of a blood vessel in patients with high blood pressure. Nose picking, especially in children, is a common cause of nosebleed. Epistaxis may also be a symptom of certain diseases, such as rheumatic fever, measles, influenza, or a disease of the blood in which the clotting time is longer than normal. Epistaxis may be due to excessive use of some drugs such as aspirin, or may be due to injury. In addition, irritation of the nasal mucosa from such factors as chronic localized infections, drying of the membrane because of low humidity, and prolonged use of nosedrops can cause epistaxis.

FIRST AID

The patient who is bleeding from the nose should be placed at rest in a sitting position in order to promote drainage. The nostrils may be pinched together with the tips of the fingers for six minutes. The patient should be instructed to breathe through the mouth during this time. The patient should be cautioned against blowing the nose. A gauze pad or folded tissue can be placed between the front teeth and the upper lip to provide pressure. The patient should be instructed to expectorate blood into a paper cup or emesis basin if the blood flows into the throat. Cold compresses may be placed over the bridge of the nose. Because applications of cold cause blood vessels to constrict,

this simple remedy often is effective in relieving a nosebleed.

EMERGENCY CARE

The patient who comes to the emergency room for treatment because of a nosebleed generally is apprehensive and needs reassurance. If the patient's bleeding has been profuse, tachycardia and a lowered blood pressure can be expected. For these reasons, the patient's vital signs should be taken and recorded. A history should include whether or not the patient is receiving anticoagulant therapy. In the event that a drug is being taken to reduce the clotting time of blood, laboratory work such as platelet count, prothrombin time, and complete blood count is done.

The patient generally is examined in a special chair designed with a fixed headrest to prevent movement of the head during the examination. The chair also facilitates easy expectoration of blood.

In 85 percent of the cases, the site of bleeding is the anterior portion of the nasal cavity. Therefore, pinching the nostrils together generally controls bleeding. Bleeding from the anterior portion of the nostrils usually drains forward out of the nose. Posterior bleeding results in a flow of blood into the pharynx and mouth and may be profuse. An individual with posterior bleeding may vomit or may become nauseated if the blood is swallowed. An emesis basin and tissues should be placed within the patient's reach.

If pinching the nostrils does not control bleeding, other measures must be taken. The physician probably will insert a cotton pledget saturated with epinephrine into the nasal cavity. Cauterization with a silver nitrate stick may be necessary to control bleeding in some cases. The patient with a history of hypertension generally will not have epinephrine applied to the mucous membrane.

If the individual is a child, the nostrils should inspected carefully for the presence of a foreign body. Epistaxis may be controlled in children by saturating a cotton ball with hydrogen peroxide and loosely packing the nostril with the saturated cotton ball. The nostrils are pinched and held together gently for 3 to 5 minutes.

The patient with severe hemorrhage may require nasal packing. Having the nostril packed is usually uncomfortable and traumatic to the patient. In packing the patient's nose, the physician passes a small rubber catheter through each nostril until the catheter is visible in the oropharynx. The catheter is pulled through the mouth and a piece of gauze is tied to the catheter with umbilical tape. The catheter with the tape and packing on the other end is gently pulled back through the nose until the packing is secure behind the patient's soft palate. The umbilical tape is then tied and anchored to the external portion of the patient's face. The packing is left in place 48 to 72 hours. An analgesic may be necessary to relieve the patient's discomfort.

Nasal packing generally is avoided if the individual is suspected of having any injury involving the central nervous system in which the cerebrospinal fluid may leak or if the nosebleed is associated with previous trauma. Packing generally is not used on toddlers and small children.

Poisoning

A *poison* is any substance that causes damage to the body or alters the function of a part of the body as a result of chemical action. Poison may be ingested, inhaled, absorbed, or injected.

Poisoning is one of the major causes of accidents in the homes of people of all ages. Drugs account for more than 50 percent of the poison ingested. Pesticides are also major poisons.

Poisoning should be suspected when the victim has unexplained severe illness. Some common symptoms of poisoning are vomiting, convulsions, diarrhea, unconsciousness, depressed respirations, cyanosis, and inflamed eyes. Poisoning should be suspected also when the smell of gas is on the victim's breath or open bottles or containers are found near the unconscious person.

Treatment of poisoning involves three basic steps:

1. Removal of the poison before it can damage tissues
2. Administration of an antidote that combines with the poison
3. Utilization of supportive measures to maintain vital functions

REMOVAL OF POISONS

POISONING THROUGH THE SKIN. The victim with surface poisoning has an irritation of the skin and/or mucous membranes caused by certain chemicals. The skin should be flooded with copious amounts of water for several minutes. Time should not be wasted removing clothes initially. The skin is again flushed with water after the clothes have been removed. Soap may be used also. If they are immediately available, gloves should be used to protect the individual giving first aid. The contaminated area of the rescuer's skin should be washed after having been in contact with the victim.

INGESTION OF POISONS. Vomiting is the most rapid and effective means of removing poison from the stomach if that poison is not alcohol or corrosive and if the victim is conscious. However, the victim should not be forced to vomit if signs of impending convulsions or seizures are present.

Vomiting may be initiated by having the victim drink one or two glasses of water or milk and then touching the back of the throat with the finger or handle of a spoon or other blunt object. Syrup of ipecac may be given to induce vomiting. This drug is commonly found in home medicine cabinets. However, ipecac is not recommended for children under one year of age. The dose to be given is 15 to 20 ml in one or two glasses of water. The dose may be repeated if vomiting does not occur after 20 to 30 minutes.

If the victim does not vomit after a repeated dose of syrup of ipecac, a gastric lavage is needed to remove the poison and syrup of ipecac. Normal saline, tap water, or fluids containing a chemical antidote may be utilized for gastric lavage. This procedure generally is done in the emergency department of a hospital.

The physician may order apomorphine. The average dose of apomorphine is 0.1 mg/kg body weight given subcutaneously. Apomorphine is an alkaloid of opium and a rapid-acting emetic. Apomorphine usually clears the stomach of the poison and sometimes unabsorbed materials from the upper portion of the small intestine. This drug is not used when the victim is stuporous because apomorphine is a central nervous system depressant. In some cases, the physician may order a narcotic antagonist to counteract the depressive effect. Naloxone (NARCAN) and levallorphan (LORFAN) are examples of narcotic antagonists that may be used.

INHALED POISONS. *Carbon monoxide poisoning* occurs as a result of inadequate ventilation at home or at work or in an attempted suicide. Carbon monoxide is a colorless, odorless, tasteless, nonirritating gas produced by incomplete oxygenation of carbon materials.

Common sources of carbon monoxide gas poisoning are faulty heating furnaces, cooking stoves with insufficient drafts, cigarette smoke, exhaust from automobiles, and burning charcoal on a grill indoors. Carbon monoxide has a 200 to 250 times greater affinity or attraction for hemoglobin than does oxygen. Carbon monoxide combines with hemoglobin to form carboxyhemoglobin, which is unable to carry oxygen. The extent to which hemoglobin combines will depend on the concentration of carbon monoxide inhaled, the duration of exposure, and the ventilating rate.

The symptoms displayed by the victim are directly related to hypoxia and anoxia. The victim may experience a headache, lassitude, drowsiness, a cherry-red color to the skin, or a cyanotic pallor of the skin. Another symptom is cerebral edema with increased cranial pressure, as described in Chapter 21, caused by increased capillary permeability. Abnormalities in the victim's electrocardiogram such as atrial arrhythmias and conduction disturbances may be evident. An individual affected by carbon monoxide poisoning also may have hyperglycemia, albuminuria, a tendency toward bleeding, excessive perspiration and skin lesions. No immediate laboratory procedure is available to confirm the possible diagnosis of carbon monoxide poisoning. For this reason it is imperative that individuals concerned with the emergency care of victims be knowledgeable regarding the symptoms.

Emergency treatment consists of:

• Administering artificial respiration.

• Administering 100 percent oxygen. Hyperbaric oxygenation is the treatment of choice. The purposes of hyperbaric oxygenation are to supply adequate oxygen in spite of little or perhaps nonfunctioning hemoglobin and to hasten dissociation and elimination of carbon monoxide from the blood and treatment of cerebral edema.

• Restricting fluids to reduce cerebral edema. Mannitol (OSMITROL) or steroids may be prescribed for the same purpose.

• Keeping the victim cool and quiet to reduce metabolic rate. Extreme hypothermia is contraindicated because carbon monoxide has a grater affinity for hemoglobin when the temperature is reduced.

• Controlling convulsive seizures with the intravenous administration of drugs such as diazepam (VALIUM).

• Observing the victim for seizures, spastic paralysis, visual disturbances, and mental disorders. Mental disturbances may range from a mild personality change to an irreversible psychosis. Parkinsonism is a frequent effect of carbon monoxide poisoning. Parkinsonism is characterized by decreased motor function, muscular rigidity, and tremor.

ADMINISTRATION OF ANTIDOTES

Chemical antidotes are placed in the stomach to neutralize the poison and to prevent further absorption of the poison. *Activated charcoal* is the most effective material for inactivation of poison that is still present in the gastrointestinal tract. Activated charcoal is a fine black powder with no taste or odor. In an emergency, the usual dose of activated charcoal of 10 gm can be approximated by mixing an adequate amount of activated charcoal in water to produce a thick soup. Approximately two tablespoons of activated charcoal can be mixed with enough water to form a paste. This paste can then be diluted in a glass of water and swallowed.

Chelates or *chelating agents* are chemical compounds that combine with metal and are used in the treatment of metal poisoning. These agents contain molecules that have the ability to bind heavy molecules of metals, prevent damage to the tissue, and excrete the new compound in a form that is not toxic to the kidneys. One example of a chelate is dimercaprol, which is effective in emergency treatment of poisoning from arsenic, gold, mercury, and other metallic salts. Calcium disodium edetate (CALCIUM DISODIUM VERSENATE) is used for lead poisoning. Penicillamine is used also for lead poisoning.

SUPPORT OF VITAL FUNCTIONS

RESPIRATION. The airway must be cleared and respiration maintained by every available means. Mouth-to-mouth resuscitation and endotracheal intubation may be used. Mechanical respirators may be necessary also.

The rate, depth, and difficulty of the victim's respiration should be observed. Signs of pulmonary edema such as rales (abnormal sound in air passages in the thoracic cavity) should be noted. The victim's position should be changed at least every two hours to prevent hypostatic pneumonia and atelectasis. The conscious patient is encouraged and assisted to cough and deep-breathe hourly.

CIRCULATORY FUNCTION. Circulation may be maintained by the intravenous administration of blood, plasma expanders, and saline solution to replace blood as well as fluid loss. The administration of intravenous fluids will also help to maintain the individual's blood pressure. Central venous pressure monitoring may be done while the patient is receiving intravenous fluids to detect early signs of heart failure.

The patient who does not respond to blood and fluid therapy generally is placed in the intensive care unit or cardiac care unit. Continuous monitoring of vital signs and cardiac patterns can be carried out in these units. This information will be utilized in planning further therapy for the patient.

KIDNEY FUNCTION. Kidney damage may occur because of damage to the renal tubules by poisons or a prolonged decrease in the circulation to the kidney. The nurse is responsible for measuring the patient's intake and output and giving the patient the prescribed amount of fluids and electrolytes. The patient who develops renal failure may be placed on hemodialysis or peritoneal dialysis. This type of treatment helps to rid the body of high concentration of the poison and other waste products until the kidneys are able to function normally.

PREVENTION OF POISONING

The nurse can play an important role in helping to prevent an accident by poisoning. A well-informed nurse can present pertinent information to interested groups, talk with patients and families at appropriate times regarding safety measures, and practice personal safety measures. Drugs should be handled, stored, and administered with consistent safety.

Families with small children should be urged to keep a poison kit on hand. The kit should contain a bottle of syrup of ipecac and bottle of activated charcoal powder. Each bottle should be clearly labeled with the name of the drug and instructions for use. Tables 8.9 and 8.10 contain a summary of information related to patient teaching and poison prevention.

FOOD POISONING

Food poisoning represents a group of acute illnesses that may be caused by the ingestion of food or drink contaminated by toxins, bacteria, protozoa, parasites, poisonous plants, poisonous animals, or chemicals. The victim of food poisoning generally has vomiting, diarrhea, enteritis, and prostration. Microorganisms most commonly causing food poisoning are *Salmonella, Staphylococcus*, and *Clostridium perfringens*.

PATIENT HISTORY. When food poisoning is suspected, an adequate history is crucial. When possible, a sample of the ingested food should be saved. The nurse should obtain a specimen of the vomitus and stool.

TABLE 8.9
PATIENT TEACHING—COMMON HOUSEHOLD POISONS

1. Baking soda
2. Laundry detergents and bleaches
3. Drain cleaners, lye
4. Mothballs
5. Aspirin
6. Furniture polish
7. Gasoline
8. Insecticides

TABLE 8.10
PATIENT TEACHING—POISON PREVENTION

- Drugs and household chemicals should be stored in locked cabinets out of the reach of children.
- All drugs and chemicals should be retained in the original container. Most containers now have a special closing feature.
- The label of any bottle should be read at least three times before using the contents.
- Medication should be taken under safe conditions. For example, medicine should not be left at the bedside to be taken during the night. Children should be supervised when taking medication.
- Old medication should be destroyed by flushing in in the toilet or washing it down the sink. Old medication should not be discarded in the trash.
- A poison antidote chart with telephone numbers of the Poison Control Center, hospital, physician, police, and ambulance should be posted in the kitchen and bathrooms.

The following information from the patient or accompanying individual is needed.

- How soon after eating did the symptoms occur?
- What food was eaten?
- Did the food have a distinguishing taste or odor?
- Did the patient vomit?
- Did the vomitus contain blood or mucus?
- Did the patient have diarrhea accompanied by pain?
- Has the patient had a fever?
- Has the patient had any neurologic disturbances such as headache, disturbed vision, breathing difficulty, excessive lacrimation, or excessive salivation?

In addition to obtaining the history as indicated above, the nurse should check the patient's temperature, pulse, respiration, and blood pressure. The color and condition of the patient's skin should be observed also. The nurse should document observations by preparing a written report.

SALMONELLOSIS. *Salmonella* food poisoning is caused by the ingestion of food previously contaminated with a large number of organisms of the *Salmonella* group. Examples are *Salmonella paratyphi, Salmonella typhimurium, Salmonella enteritidis,* and *Salmonella choleraesuis*. The *Salmonella* microorganisms are gram-negative rods that usually enter the body by way of the mouth through food or drink. Infected meats, poultry, dried eggs, milk, pet turtles, Easter chickens, pet dogs, and cats may be the source of the microorganisms. Large numbers must be ingested to produce infection because the high acidity of the stomach caused by the hydrochloric acid kills the microorganisms. Individuals with pernicious anemia, partial resection of the stomach, and other conditions causing a decrease in hydrochloric acid content of the stomach may have an increased susceptibility to salmonellosis. Salmonellosis occurs more commonly during the summer months. Nursing care of the patient with salmonellosis is discussed in Chapter 15.

STAPHYLOCOCCAL ENTEROTOXIN POISONING. Acute food poisoning due to the ingestion of food contaminated by the preformed staphylococcal toxin causes an irritation of the gastrointestinal tract. Symptoms of the irritation generally begin within one to six hours after the individual has eaten the contaminated food. The individual affected with food poisoning caused by a staphylococcal enterotoxin generally has an abrupt onset of excessive salivation, nausea, abdominal cramps, vomiting, headache, rapid pulse, and profuse sweating.

Fever usually is not present. Although onset is abrupt, the illness is usually of rather short duration. Usually within a day or two, the patient has eliminated the toxin and has recovered from the food poisoning.

Staphylococcal enterotoxin poisoning usually is spread by contaminated hands or nasal droplets of workers or by improperly cleaned mixers, choppers, cutting boards, or other kitchen utensils. The foods involved generally have been refrigerated improperly. Some of the more common foods are custard, cottage cheese, cream pies, salad dressings, stuffing for poultry, chopped eggs, chicken salad, and tuna salad.

Treatment of the patient with staphylococcal enterotoxin poisoning generally involves the administration of fluids, rest, and sedation as necessary.

Staphylococcal food poisoning can be prevented by individuals handling food. Scrupulous handwashing, clean working areas in which to prepare food, and proper refrigeration of food are necessary in the prevention of food poisoning. Any individual with a minor infection of the hands and arms should not prepare food.

MUSHROOM POISONING.   Mushroom poisoning is referred to as mycetismus. *Amanita verna, Amanita phalloides, Amanita muscaria,* and *Amanita pantherina* are the mushrooms most likely to cause mushroom poisoning in North America.

The onset of symptoms may begin as quickly as 30 minutes after the individual has consumed mushrooms or it may not begin for 24 hours. The victim usually experiences nausea, vomiting, abdominal pain, diarrhea, and prostration. Symptoms, which occur after six hours or more, generally consist of abrupt, severe abdominal pain and nausea. The vomitus may be bloody. The victim may have diarrhea with bloody stools. Extreme thirst, weakness, and dehydration occur. The patient may experience an improvement in the symptoms only to be followed by symptoms of circulatory collapse such as cyanosis and coldness. Renal and hepatic damage may develop. The individual's central nervous system may be involved also. Death may occur within 48 to 72 hours after ingestion of the poisonous mushrooms.

Immediate treatment consists of the induction of vomiting. Apomorphine may be given subcutaneously to induce vomiting. Magnesium sulfate may be given by mouth or by enema to facilitate removal of a poison from the gastrointestinal tract. Medication such as morphine may be given for severe pain and apprehension. Intravenous administration of fluids and electrolytes generally is indicated.

Continuous nursing care is essential since the patient suffering from mushroom poisoning can be expected to be extremely frightened and afraid of possible death. Efforts should be made to prevent and/or combat shock. The individual should be protected by the use of padded siderails to prevent injury if convulsions occur. A padded tongue blade should be easily available along with a suction machine for maintaining a patent airway. Moist compresses may be applied to the eyes for excessive lacrimation.

The prevention of mushroom poisoning is extremely important since it is the most common cause of food poisoning. It can be prevented if individuals avoid eating mushrooms in the free or wild state. They should eat only those grown on mushroom farms or cultivated under controlled conditions. There is no sure way to tell if a wild mushroom is safe to eat.

BOTULISM.   Botulism is an acute and frequently fatal disease caused by the ingestion of a toxin formed in foods by an anaerobic bacterium called *Clostridium botulinum* This microorganism produces neurotoxins A, B, E, and F. Type B is found east of the Mississippi River; type A is found west of the Mississippi River; and type E is found in the Great Lakes area and Alaska. This pathogentic microorganism produces a toxin that is poisonous when released in nitrogenous foods.

Botulism is a form of food poisoning seen primarily as a result of ingestion of poorly processed foods. The toxins associated with home canning are types A and B. Foods that have been contaminated with the organism appear soft and contain gas bubbles. These foods generally have an odor of decay. Some of the common foods associated with botulism are home-canned vegetables, mushrooms, corn, spinach, string beans, olives, pepper, asparagus, fish, meat, beets, and okra.

The victim of botulism generally develops symptoms of this disease within 12 to 48 hours following the ingestion of contaminated food. The toxins gain entrance to the body through the gastrointestinal system and produce early symptoms of nausea, vomiting, and diarrhea. The victim generally experiences malaise, constipation, subnormal temperature, dizziness, headache, and visual disturbance. Eye signs are important in the diagnosis of botulism and appear early. They include photophobia, diplopia (double vision), and blindness because of cranial nerve damage. Other symptoms are general muscular weakness, incontinence, rapid pulse, cyanosis, and difficulty in swallowing and in speaking. Respiratory failure, coma, and death may occur as a result of asphyxia. The prognosis for a victim of botulism depends on the amount of toxin ingested in proportion to body weight.

The four main objectives in treating an individual with botulism are (1) prevention of respiratory failure, (2) neutralization of toxins, (3) removal of toxins from the gastrointestinal tract, and (4) supportive care. The patient generally is placed in a special care unit where maximum ventilation can be maintained. A ventilator, tracheostomy, and suctioning may be necessary to prevent aspiration with resulting pneumonia. Isolation of the patient is not required.

The Center for Disease Control in Atlanta, Georgia, may be contacted for the exact location of polyvalent botulism antitoxin and appropriate dosage. The antitoxin may be given to neutralize toxin, but it cannot reverse the damage that has already occurred. It is used to prevent further damage. Skin testing for sensitivity before administering polyvalent botulism antitoxin is required because the antitoxin is derived from horse serum. Cathartics and a cleansing enema may be used in an attempt to remove toxins that have not been absorbed by the gastrointestinal tract. The prevention of botulism is extremely important. Botulism can be prevented by heating canned products to a temperature of 82.2°C (180°F) for 10 to 20 minutes prior to serving. The food should be stirred often during the heating process. Canned foods should be inspected for gas bubbles and the odor of decay prior to use.

The prevention of food poisoning is summarized in Table 8.11.

Bites and Stings

ANIMAL BITES

The most prevalent animal bites are from dogs, cats, and rats. Approximately 33,000 dog bites occur yearly in the United States, constituting the most prevalent animal bite treated in emergency rooms in the United States. Most of the dog bites that occur in cities are the result of bites by dogs owned by individuals. The dogs generally have been

TABLE 8.11
PATIENT TEACHING—PREVENTION OF FOOD POISONING

1. Do not pick wild mushrooms.
2. Inspect home-canned foods for bubbles and foul odor.
3. Heat canned products, especially home-canned products, for 10 to 20 minutes before serving.
4. Place seafood and salads prepared with mayonnaise on ice to prevent spoiling.
5. Keep milk, dairy products, and mayonnaise in refrigerator until used.
6. Cover all foods at picnics and outings to protect from flies and pets.

inoculated against rabies. Stray dogs within the city usually have little contact with wild animals. For this reason, the number of persons treated with antirabies prophylaxis has been drastically reduced. It is interesting to note that not a single case of rabies has been reported within 100 miles of the city of New York within ten years.

Cat bites often become infected because of cats' long teeth, which make deep puncture wounds. The puncture wounds tend to seal and heal slowly. The mouth of a cat is a focal point of many bacteria, which makes the likelihood of infection very great. Human bites also may become infected because of the high bacteria count of the mouth.

FIRST AID. The victim of an animal bite should have the area washed thoroughly with soap and water for 5 to 10 minutes to remove the saliva and bacteria. Running hot water is best. When deep puncture wounds are present, the area should be squeezed to cause bleeding. Alcohol or some other antiseptic should be used to cleanse the wound. The area should be covered with sterile gauze, and the victim should be taken to the nearest medical facility.

RABIES. Rabies (hydrophobia) is an ancient disease. Strict regulations were recorded concerning mad dogs before the period of Christ. Rabies is an acute viral infection of the central nervous system. The disease is transmitted to man from the saliva of an infected animal. Animals that nurse their young can be a carrier of the virus causing rabies. Rabies has been reported in dogs, cats, bats, squirrels, skunks, foxes, raccoons, and coyotes. Rabies occurs also in cows and horses but does not infect man.

The incubation period is from ten days to a year in man. The incubation period depends on the severity and location of the bite. An individual suffering from a bite around the face, head, or neck usually has symptoms within ten days. The disease is confirmed by the presence of Negri bodies in samples of the brain tissue of the infecting animal or the presence of rabies antibodies in the victim's blood. The disease is usually fatal once it has been established.

The disease has been divided into three stages: prodromal, excitement, and paralytic. Symptoms of the prodromal stage experienced by the patient are headache, nausea, fever, malaise, loss of appetite, sore throat, unusual sensitivity to sound, light, and changes in temperature. The patient's eyes may be dilated and he may have an increased amount of salivation.

The excitement stage is characterized by alternating periods of excitement and calmness, convulsions, and spasm of the throat when the patient attempts to swallow.

Paralysis is the final stage. Death usually occurs as a result respiratory and cardiac failure.

Treatment and Nursing Care. The most important treatment is prevention. After the individual has been bitten, the wound should be cleansed with soap and water and he should receive an injection of one of the two approved vaccines and an injection of the antirabies serum. The two vaccines available are duck embryo vaccine and nervous tissue vaccine. Duck embryo vaccine is the preferred vaccine because of a lower incidence of nervous system reaction. Human rabies globulin is given for possible immunization. The vaccine contains duck egg protein. Individuals sensitive to chicken eggs may be sensitive to this vaccine. The victim should be skin tested with a separate disposable syringe and needle. A separate syringe and needle should be used for each injection to prevent cross-contamination. The patient should be observed for erythema, induration, chills, fever, and malaise, especially beginning on the sixth day.

An individual with rabies is placed in strict isolation, which includes use of gown, rubber gloves, cap, and mask. The room must be darkened and kept a constant temperature, and the environment should be a quiet one because of the patient's hypersensitivity. The light must be reduced for the same reason. Siderails should be padded and in place to prevent injury during hyperactivity and convulsions. The patient generally experiences uncontrollable fear, mania, irritability, and, at times, calmness. Intravenous anesthetics or sedatives such as barbiturates, chloral hydrate, and morphine may be used to calm the patient and control the central nervous system symptoms.

The nurse should bandage the arm securely to the arm board when an intravenous injection is to be given. This is done to prevent injury during convulsion. The patient should not be encouraged to talk as talking may trigger a muscle spasm of the throat. The patient may need to be suctioned. Lowering the patient's head will facilitate drainage of secretions. Death usually occurs in three to four days if the symptoms are acute.

Rabies Control. All animals suspected of having rabies must be reported to the police and health departments. Most states require annual vaccination of pets. Immunization is thought to be effective for 39 months for animals.

HUMAN BITES

An individual suffering from a bite from another human is highly susceptible to infection as is the person who has been bitten by an animal. The high bacteria count increases the possibility of infection. The area should be cultured and cleansed thoroughly with soap and water. The physician will debride excess tissue and repair the area as needed. Antibiotics generally are prescribed.

INSECT BITES AND STINGS

BEES, HORNETS, WASPS, AND YELLOW JACKETS. Insects are prevalent during the summer months especially in the month of August. The environment usually is congested with flies, mosquitoes, bees, hornets, wasps, and yellow jackets. Insects belonging to the *Hymenoptera* order (bees, yellow jackets, wasps, hornets, and ants) usually are the culprits in generalized and systemic reactions. This group causes more fatalities than snakebites. First aid for local reaction consists of the application of a weak solution of household ammonia to decrease the pain. Application of a poultice of sodium bicarbonate and water may be helpful also. The sodium bicarbonate and ammonia neutralize the acid injected by the insect.

Moderate to severe systemic reactions experienced by the victim constitute a medical emergency. The victim may have symptoms such as a feeling of tightness in his throat and chest, wheezing, dizziness, abdominal pain, nausea and vomiting, and generalized edema. As the reaction increases in severity, the victim may have difficulty breathing, hoarseness, weakness, confusion, and a feeling of impending doom. Shock, collapse, incontinence, and unconsciousness may develop.

Treatment and First Aid. Emergency treatment for severe reactions consists of the injection of epinephrine subcutaneously. A tourniquet should be placed above and below the site of the sting or bite to decrease the rate of absorption of the venom. Diphenhydramine (BENADRYL) may be given. Cortisone may also be prescribed. Oxygen and cardiopulmonary resuscitation may be necessary.

The victim must be protected against future attacks. A desensitization procedure, described in the chapter pertaining to allergy, may be prescribed. Some physicians recommend that the patient carry an insect sting kit when hunting, camping, or in a dangerous environment. The sensitive person should also be encouraged to wear a Medic-Alert bracelet. The insect kit contains a preloaded syringe of epinephrine, a tourniquet, an antihistamine tablet, and a phenobarbital tablet. The kit comes complete with very simple, concise instructions. The client must be instructed to check the syringe and replace it if the liquid turns brown.

Prevention. To prevent insect attack, beehives, hornets' nests, and wasps' nests should be removed from the immediate environment. The individual should not go without shoes or wear sandals in the spring and summer. Bright colors such as yellow and orange and flowerly prints attract bees and should not be worn. Khaki, tan, white, and green should be used for the clothing of the individual when camping. The individual should avoid using perfumed lotion, soap, powder, or shampoos. Long pants, long-sleeved shirts, and gloves should be worn when working among fruits and flowers or camping. Shiny jewelry and buckles attract bees and should not be worn. If a member of the *Hymenoptera* family lights on the susceptible individual, the insect should be removed calmly without swatting. If an attack from the insect seems imminent, a susceptible individual should lie face down and protect and face and head with the arms. Table 8.12 contains a summary of additional emergency interventions if anaphylaxis develops.

TICKS. Ticks are small brown, flat parasites with eight legs. Ticks burrow their heads under the skin and suck the blood from the host. Ticks transmit the disease they are carrying at that time. For example, ticks can transmit typhus (Rocky Mountain spotted fever) and babesisis. These diseases are transmitted when the host is bitten or the skin comes in contact with the feces from the crushed tissues and hemolymph. The dog tick is the main vector of the tickborne typhus in the southern and eastern areas of the United States. The disease is transmitted by the wood tick in the Rockies and western part of the United States.

Tick bites are more prevalent in the spring and summer. The incidences of tickborne typhus have increased in the past five years.

Ticks may be removed by covering them with heavy oil such as mineral oil, kerosene oil, or motor oil, which should be left on the tick and the area around the tick for approximately 30 minutes. Oil suffocates the ticks by interfering with their ability to breathe. The tick can then be removed with tweezers, which should be applied to the neck or head of the tick. The area infected by the tick should be cleaned and an antiseptic solution should be applied. Another method of removing the tick is to grasp the tick near the

TABLE 8.12
ANAPHYLAXIS

I. *Common Causes*

Second exposure to
  Hormones
  Horse serum
  Insect stings
  IV contrast media
  Organ extracts
  Penicillin
  Pollen extracts

II. *Symptoms*

Circulatory	Gastrointestinal	Respiratory	Skin
Bradycardia	Diarrhea	Sneezing	Pruritus
Tachycardia	Vomiting	Coughing	Rash
Collapse of peripheral circulation (lowered BP, pale skin, no pulse, cold skin)	Nausea	Tightness of chest	Urticaria
	Cramping (abd.)	Wheezing	Angioedema
		Dyspnea	
		Cyanosis	

III. *Equipment and Supplies Needed*

Equipment
  Stethoscope
  Sphygmomanometer
  Syringes and needles
  IV setup
  Airways
  Laryngoscope
  Endotracheal tube
  Tracheostomy setup
  Oxygen
  Tourniquets

Drugs for injection
  Epinephrine (aqueous), 1:1000
  Antihistamine
  Vasopressor, e.g., metaraminol (ARAMINE)
  Corticosteroid
  Barbiturate
  Intravenous fluids
  Calcium gluconate

IV. *What to Do*

- Position victim in dorsal recumbent position and extend neck to open airway
- Epinephrine 0.3–0.5 ml may be injected into base of tongue
- Apply tourniquet above and below site of insect sting. Leave in place for 20 minutes, release for 5, and reapply
Remove false teeth and other objects from mouth.
- Airway or endotracheal tube may be inserted if necessary
- Tracheostomy may be necessary
- CPR if needed
- Combat shock with IV fluids, and vasopressor drugs, and position
- Barbiturates may be used for convulsion
- Cortisone may be used, especially for bronchospasm

V. *Prevention*

- Encourage allergic person to wear Medic-Alert bracelet or necklace
- Ask patient about allergy to food, drugs, and pollen
- Skin tests are used before foreign proteins are given
- Person going on outings where insects are plentiful should cover skin and carry anaphylactic kit

mouth with tweezers. Using a needle in the other hand, pry the head of the tick out of the tissue with the needle. Remember, do not touch the tick with bare hands. Also, do not mash the body or rub the bite with bare hands.

SPIDERS AND SCORPIONS. The black widow spider, brown recluse spider, and tarantula are three of the main spiders feared by man. The black widow spider is the best-known poisonous spider. It may be called hourglass, shoe button, or "cul rouge." These names are taken from the appearance of the spider's body. The body is jet black, resembling a shoe button, and the abdomen has a crimson hourglass marking. The black widow spider usually is found in dark, quiet places such as cellars, garages, barns, wood piles, tree stumps, and rat holes.

Black Widow Spider. The female black widow spider will bite when she is hungry or disturbed, or if an insect or person becomes entangled in her web and the egg sac is threatened. The venom of the black widow spider is a neurotoxin and death may occur within a short time because of respiratory failure.

After the bite from the spider, the victim will notice two small red spots on the skin followed by swelling, intense pain in the area of the bite, profuse sweating, shock, and nausea. Abdominal muscles become rigid and painful, blood pressure is elevated, and fever with chills develops. Respiratory distress and death follow.

Brown Recluse Spider. The brown recluse spider has dark marks on his back which look like a fiddle. Both the male and female are capable of biting and injecting a lethal dose of venom into the victim. The brown recluse spider hides from people and will bite only when provoked. Usually, this spider is found in folded clothing or in packed, stored materials such as papers, blankets, newspapers, and packing boxes.

The bite of this spider is not as painful as that of the black widow spider but the after-effects are very serious. The venom of this spider destroys red cells in the blood and destroys the body tissue in the immediate area of the bite. The victim experiences painful joints, severe local reaction with the formation of an ulcer within a week or two, chills, fever, nausea, and vomiting. Death has been reported in children.

Tarantula. The tarantula is a hairy spider found in South America as well as the central and western parts of the United States. Most of the reported bites have occurred in fruit packers and handlers of fruit being shipped from South America. The bite is very painful with severe local damage. Symptoms of shock generally appear.

Scorpion. The scorpion belongs to the spider and mite family. The scorpion's body is covered by a shield. The tail has a gland found in the tip that contains a poison. This poison flows through a sharp appendage. Scorpions usually strike at night, preying on other spiders and insects, which they sting. They suck their victim's blood for nourishment.

Intense pain at the point of the sting generally is experienced by the victim. Abdominal pain, nausea, and vomiting occur. One or two hours following the sting the victim experiences shock, convulsions, and unconsciousness. Death can occur if treatment is not properly and quickly initiated.

First Aid. First aid for bites and stings caused by spiders and scorpions consists of:

- Applying a rubber band above and below the site of the sting
- Applying crushed ice in a bag to the site
- Keeping the victim quiet, positioned so that the area of the bite or sting is below the level of the heart
- Maintaining a patent airway
- CPR if necessary
- Transporting to the nearest medical facility with 30 minutes.

SNAKEBITES

The individual who has been bitten by a poisonous snake is indeed in an emergency situation. As a licensed member of the health team in the community, the nurse frequently is called on for health information as well as first aid. Basic information regarding snakes may be beneficial in combating some of the myths regarding them. The four families of poisonous snakes in the world are (1) cobras, (2) coral snakes, (3) vipers, and (4) pit vipers (Table 8.13). Snakes bite primarily to obtain food. They will also strike in self-defense. The venom contains both a hemotoxin and a neurotoxin. The hemotoxin contains clotting and anticoagulating factors. It

TABLE 8.13
POISONOUS SNAKES

NAME	DESCRIPTION	WHERE FOUND	STRIKE OR BITE
Rattlesnake Pit viper	Elliptic pupils, rattles on tail, long, folding, hollow hypodermic fangs, body pattern varies	Every state in U.S. except Maine, Delaware, Hawaii, and Alaska	For food
Cottonmouth Moccasin Pit viper	White mouth Heavy brown body	Swampy areas of southern coastal regions and Mississippi Delta, usually found sunning themselves on branches, rocks near edge of water	When touched
Coral snake	Small blunt head and body—brown, red, and black bands separated by yellow bands, 57.5–117.5 cm (23–47 in.) in length	Coastal areas of North Carolina, south to Florida, Gulf states, Southwest desert area, Mexico, and South America	When stepped on or touched
Copperhead Pit viper	Coppery brown, dark, hour-glass-shaped markings, 75 cm (30 in.) in length	Massachusetts, south to Florida, Texas, and Illinois Prefers dry upland woods, in spring and fall found on hillside and mountain—in summer found in lowlands	When stepped on or touched

causes destruction of red blood cells as well as a lowering of blood pressure. The neurotoxin blocks impulses in the synapses of the nerves. Although snake venom generally contains both hemotoxin and neurotoxin, usually one is dominant over the other.

Snakes seldom come out in the heat of the day as they will die if they become too warm. They usually come out in the evening and night. Humans generally are bitten during the late evening and early night between 5 P.M. and midnight. Although snakebites are more prevalent during the spring and fall, snakes may bite any month of the year. Bites from rattlesnakes are the most common in North America. The second most common is the bite from the water moccasin. Coral snakes account for a small percentage of the snakebites in the United States. The lower legs, feet, hands, and arms are the areas of the body most frequently bitten.

OBSERVING THE VICTIM

The bite of a pit viper has fang marks consisting of two to four puncture wounds. The area around the marks usually is bruised with blood oozing or squirting from the wound. The blood generally does not clot. The victim experiences burning pain at the site of the bite. Swelling occurs in all directions and spreads rapidly in 15 to 30 minutes. If venom is injected into the muscles, it will spread more rapidly and the symptoms mentioned previously will not occur. Instead, the victim will experience nausea, vomiting, tachycardia or bradycardia, low blood pressure, shock, oliguria, unconsciousness, and possibly death.

The severity of the bite is directly related to the size of the snake, the location of the bite, and the amount of venom injected by the snake. Another factor is the relationship of the site of the bite to the trunk of the body. A big snake has large fangs and injects more venom with each bite than a small one. For example, a small child approximately two years of age bitten by a 6-ft rattlesnake will die promptly if adequate treatment is not received immediately. A large dose of rattlesnake venom can kill a man weighing 200 lb in one hour if proper treatment is not started.

FIRST AID. The basic purpose of first aid following a snakebite is to reduce the spread of venom, retard the absorption of venom, reduce the effects of venom, and prevent complications. In order to accomplish these goals, the individual rendering first aid should place the involved part at rest at a level below the heart of the victim and apply a rubber band or light tourniquet above and below the fang marks and area of swelling. The pulse should not be obliterated. Ice should be applied to the affected area in a bag or container. The victim should be carried to a medical facility in a rapid and safe manner. Table 8.14 contains a summary of first aid measures for the victim of snakebite.

EMERGENCY CARE

Once the victim has reached a medical facility, intravenous injection of 5 percent Ringer's lactate solution may be started. Hydrocortisone may be given in the intravenous solution. Although the victim may develop arrhythmia, (irregular heartbeat), lidocaine is usually not prescribed as this drug may precipitate a convulsion in the case of severe snakebite.

Other emergency interventions may include blood transfusion, oxygen therapy, and tetanus prophylaxis. Tracheostomy, assisted ventilation, and similar life-support measures may be needed in some cases.

Snake antivenin is available for certain patients following snakebite. However, anaphylaxis may result following this therapy. The antivenin currently available is pre-

pared from horse serum to which many persons are allergic. A search is currently under way for safer, more effective antivenin.

PREVENTION OF SNAKEBITE

The following measures will help to prevent snakebites:

• Heavy leather boots should be worn when camping. The legs should be protected up to 55 cm (22 in.) above the ground.
• A light should be carried when going outside at night.
• Shorts and halters should not be worn as they leave the legs and body unprotected. The legs, arms, and body should be covered with material of sufficient thickness to protect the individual. Remembering that the snake fangs are comparable to hypodermic needles will enable the nurse to recall the importance of covering the body.
• An individual should not stick hands or feet into places that cannot be visualized such as around rock ledges or holes. The camper should be alert in snake-infested areas for possible danger.
• Snakes roam on sunny autumn days and chilly nights between 5 P.M. and midnight hunting for food.
• Campers should avoid sleeping on the ground as snakes are attracted by the warmth of their bodies.
• The rattlesnake does not always rattle before striking the victim.
• A snakebite kit should be carried by the camper when going on a trip if the distance will not enable a medical facility to be reached in a short period of time. Generally, the kit contains two chemical cold packs, two tourniquets, 70 percent alcohol, an injection of cortisone, syringes, needles, lidocaine (XYLOCAINE) with epinephrine, an elasticized bandage, and sterile dressings.

TABLE 8.14
SUMMARY OF FIRST AID MEASURES FOR THE SNAKEBITE VICTIM

1. Place the involved part below heart level.
2. Apply ice in bags, chemical ice cooler packs, or cold cans of beer or soda.
3. Apply a tourniquet above and below the fang marks and area of swelling.
4. Transport the victim to a medical facility in a safe, rapid manner.

One should be certain not to undertake or allow the following:

1. Do *not* allow water from the ice to contact the skin. Do not apply freon or ethyl chloride.
2. Do *not* suck the poison from the area with the mouth or apply cross cuts. Do *not* give antivenom. Do *not* obstruct the flow of blood with tight tourniquets.
3. Do *not* give alcohol. Do *not* apply tobacco juice, spider webs, or kerosene to the area of the snakebite.

Injuries of the Eyes, Ears, and/or Nose

EYE

An individual who has sustained an eye injury usually is apprehensive, frightened, and in pain. The fear of blindness often is uppermost in the mind of the patient. This fear may be aggravated when body defenses prevent opening the eye.

The person giving first aid must be calm, gentle, and reassuring. The objective of first aid and/or emergency care is to prevent further damage or permanent damage to the eye. Table 8.15 contains a summary of first aid measures for common eye injuries.

The nurse should approach the patient with an eye injury with the possibility in mind that the injury might be penetrating until proven otherwise. An individual may have a foreign body, laceration of the eyelid or the eyeball, a chemical burn, radiation burn, heat burn, or an impacted protruding foreign body in the eye.

FOREIGN BODIES. The most common eye injury is caused by a foreign body. Generally, the foreign body is the result of a flying particle that lodges under the upper lid of the eye.

When rendering first aid to an individual with a foreign body in the eye, the nurse should pull the upper lid down over the lower lash after having thoroughly washed the hands. Pulling the upper lid down over the lower lash stimulates tearing, and tears may dislodge the foreign body and take care of the emergency. In the event that tearing does not wash the particle away, the particle may be washed away with an irrigation of tap water or normal saline that is at room temperature. An alternate method for removal of a foreign body is the use of a sterile cotton-tip applicator or the corner of a clean handkerchief that has been moistened in normal saline.

Technique for Removing a Foreign Body from the Eye. The technique is as follows:

- Stand behind the patient and approach from the right or left side. This position is favored because it decreases the change of the patient jerking the head and causing further damage. Ask the patient to look toward the feet.
- Grasp the upper lashes between your thumb and forefinger.
- Fold the lash up over an applicator swab.
- Instruct the individual to look down. Inspect the upper part of the eye and invert the lid.
- If the particle is seen, stroke it lightly with a moistened swab or irrigate it with tap water.
- An eye cup, rubber bulb syringe, medicine dropper, intravenous setup, or a water pick may be used to irrigate the eye.
- Following the irrigation, release the lash, ask the patient to look up, and the lid will return to its normal position.

If an object is embedded in the eye, the first-aider should apply an eye patch, secure it with cellophane tape to the side of the eye, not to the eyebrow, and instruct the patient

TABLE 8.15
FIRST AID FOR COMMON EYE INJURIES

INJURY	TREATMENT
Foreign bodies	Irrigate with normal saline, sterile or tap water; or invert lid with applicator stick, moisten swab, and remove foreign body
Laceration of lid	Apply direct pressure—gauze square
Laceration of globe	Cover with loose dressing; transport to nearest medical facility
Impaled object	Cut an opening in several gauze squares comparable to size of eye; place hole of dressing over impaled object; crush paper cup and position over eye; use two layers of roller bandage to secure cup; wrap bandage loosely around head covering uninvolved eye
Chemical burns	Irrigate with tap water or normal saline for 5–10 minutes
Heat burns	Apply moist dressing
Light burns	Apply dark patches to both eyes
To remove contact lenses	
Hard	Use suction cup
Soft	Irrigate with normal saline, slide off corner of cornea, squeeze lens, and remove

to see an ophthalmologist immediately. *Never attempt to remove an embedded object in the eye.*

The ophthalmologist may stain the cornea with a dye, fluorescein, that enables visualization of the foreign body. The foreign body is then removed by the physician.

LACERATION. The client with a laceration of the eyelid generally has a marked amount of bleeding. The eyelid has a rich blood supply, which causes profuse bleeding when the lid is injured.

After inspecting the eye to determine if the globe of the eye is injured, the nurse can check the bleeding by applying a pressure dressing directly over the hemorrhaging area. If the globe is lacerated, the nurse should not apply direct pressure. The lid should be covered with a loose gauze dressing to absorb the blood and to aid in the clotting process. Both eyes should be covered with a loose dressing before the patient is transported to a medical facility. The nurse should remember that pressure to a lacerated globe will cause the vitreous fluid to escape from the eyeball. Vitreous humor cannot be replaced or restored by the body. Loss of this vital fluid results in blindness. Remembering this should enable the nurse to bear in mind the importance of not applying direct pressure when the globe of the eye is lacerated (see Table 8.15).

BURNS. *Chemical Burn.* An individual who has received a chemical burn of the eye generally is very frightened. Prompt action by the nurse or one applying first aid is necessary to prevent irreversible damage to the eye. Battery acid, lime, lye, and ammonia are examples of chemicals that may be involved in a burn of the eye.

A burn of the eye requires immediate irrigation with a copious amount of tap water for 5 to 10 minutes every 20 minutes until the victim is seen by an ophthalmologist. When the eye is irrigated, the patient's head should be positioned to prevent the irrigation fluid from running from the affected eye to the unaffected eye. Points to be remembered during an eye irrigation are listed below.

- Reassure the patient.

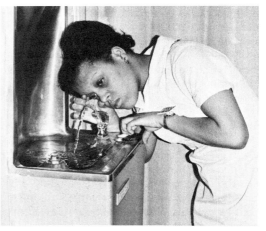

FIGURE 8.11 The victim of a chemical eye burn can dilute the irritant with a copious amount of water from a water fountain.

- Dilute the chemical with copious amounts of tap water or normal saline.
- Hold the patient's eye open with a gauze square. Generally the patient cannot keep the eye open because of pain.
- The affected eye should be placed toward the floor to prevent the return flow of the irrigation solution from draining over the unaffected eye.
- Running water is preferable. If running water is not available, the person giving first aid should pour water over the victim's eye.
- Possible irrigation devices are an intravenous setup or a WATER PIC.
- Water may be obtained from the water fountain (Figure 8.11), water faucet, shower, or a bucket of water. Beer may be used if water is not available. Continue irrigation for 5 to 10 minutes every 15 to 20 minutes until medical help is obtained.
- Transport the patient to the nearest medical facility immediately following irrigation.

After the irrigation has been completed, the physician may prescribe an ophthalmic antibiotic ointment and binocular eyepatch to be used until the cornea heals. The eyepatch is ordered to keep the eyes immobilized and promote rest. Medication may be prescribed for rest and pain. Generally, the physician will examine the eye again in 24 hours.

Radiation Burn. A radiation burn or a light burn of the eye may be caused by gazing directly into the sun during an eclipse. Sunlight reflected by sand, snow, or white linen may produce a burn of the eye. The welding arc flash or overexposure to a sun lamp may also produce a radiation burn. The victim experiences severe pain of the affected eye or both eyes, spasm of the eyelid, and sensitivity to light. The symptoms generally occur 6 to 8 hours after exposure.

Light Burn. First aid usually consists of application of dark eyepatches and rest for 24 hours. The physician will want to rule out the possibility of a foreign body in the eye. A careful history is indicated to assist in this. An ophthalmic topical ointment may be prescribed by the physician to be instilled in the eye for the relief of spasms of the eyelid. Usually 30 to 60 seconds are required after administration of the ointment to relieve spasms of the eyelid and permit the physician to visualize the eyelid and the eye. Following an examination of the eye or eyes, the doctor may order dark patches (Table 8.15) and prescribe an appropriate analgesic. A sedative may be indicated. The client generally is instructed to rest for 24 hours.

Heat Burn. The victim suffering from a heat burn of the face and neck usually has an involvement of the eyelids. The lids become edematous and may not be opened. This is a protective mechanism for the eye. The lids may be covered with steriled moist dressings. The client should be transported to the nearest medical facility (see Table 18.5).

Contact Lens Injury. The nurse should consider the patient with an eye injury as a possible contact lens wearer. The conscious patient is asked about the presence of contact lenses and requested to remove them, if possible. If this is not possible, it may be necessary to check the wallet or look for a Medic-Alert bracelet. If the nurse is not familiar with the proper technique for removing contact lenses, no attempt should be made to remove them. Instead, a label is attached indicating that contact lenses are in place before the patient is transported.

The patient may have one of the two types of contact lenses—hard or soft. If the patient has a soft lens, colored drops or drugs containing such drops should not be instilled in the eye. Normal saline should be used for first aid. The eye may also be irrigated with a copious amount of normal saline. The contact lens may be slid gently off the cornea. After the lens has been moved to the sclera toward the fornix, the nurse should use the index finger and thumb to squeeze the lens and pick it out of the eye. Another irrigation may be used if the lens does not slide easily. Irrigation is necessary to prevent injury to the cornea.

When removing a hard lens, the nurse should use a small, hard suction cup. The suction cup should be placed toward the edge of the lens, which can be elevated in order to break surface tension and facilitate removal.

EAR

FOREIGN BODY. An individual suspected of having a foreign body in the external auditory canal should be questioned carefully regarding the possible type of foreign body. Beans, peas, candy, and other small objects may be placed in the ear by children during experimentation with body orifices. Roaches and other insects may crawl into the ear during sleeping hours, especially in a crowded dwelling. Foreign bodies such as insects can be painful and cause marked discomfort, especially if they are live, buzzing, and crawling around within the external auditory canal. Insects may also be destructive. When possible, direct visualization of the foreign body should be made.

First Aid. The aim of treatment for the victim with a bug or other insect in the is to immobilize the insect by suffocation. This may be accomplished by placing one or two drops of mineral oil or alcohol into the ear canal. The insect also may be paralyzed by placing a cotton ball previously soaked with ether into the opening of the ear (Figure 8.12). Either of these methods relieves the pain and facilitates removal of the insect quickly and easily by the physician. It is important to remember not to put water in the

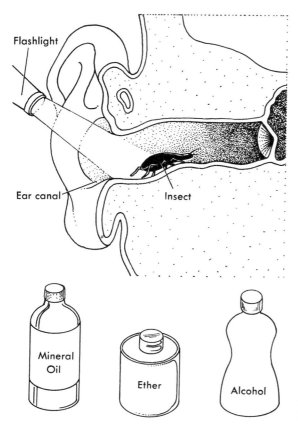

FIGURE 8.12 First aid for a patient with a live insect in the ear.

ear as this causes the insect to become more active and increases the pain and discomfort to the patient.

When the victim with a foreign body lodged in the ear is in the woods or away from a source of mineral oil, alcohol, or ether, first aid may be rendered in another manner. A flashlight or a pen light placed at the external opening of the ear generally attracts insects to it. When the insect crawls toward the light and out of the ear, it then can be removed easily. Do not use an open flame such as a cigarette lighter, candle, or matches because of the danger of burning the victim from hot wax and possibly causing the clothing and tissue to burn. When straightening the external auditory canal, the nurse should pull the earlobe upward and outward on an adult. When straightening the external auditory canal of a child, the nurse should pull the earlobe downward and outward.

The use of hairpins and other sharp instruments that may puncture the eardrum or push the object further back into the auditory canal is dangerous and should be avoided. If an object such as a bean, pea, or other vegetable that swells when placed in water is lodged in the external auditory canal, the client should be instructed to go immediately to the physician's office or to an emergency room. The canal should *not* be irrigated with liquids as this will cause the vegetable to expand. Expansion of a foreign body in the external auditory canal makes the object much more difficult to remove. Careful questioning of the client in order to determine the object that may be in the ear and actual visualization of the object when possible are important.

NOSE

FOREIGN BODY. A foreign body may be inserted into the nostril by a child who is experimenting with body orifices. Foreign bodies such as marbles, peas, and small pebbles may be found in the nares.

First Aid. A foreign object in the nose may be expelled by sneezing. The nurse can make the victim sneeze by covering the mouth and having a puff of cigarette smoke blown against the nose. Visualization of the foreign object in the nostril may be accomplished by shining a light into the nares while retracting the flared cartilaginous expansion forming the outer side of the nostril (*ala*). If the object is near the surface, it can be removed with a pair of tweezers or a blunt object. When the object is firmly lodged in the nose or seems to be pushed backward into the nostril, it should not be removed by the individual giving first aid. Instead, medical advice should be obtained.

In some instances, the physician is unable to obtain the cooperation of the individual, especially an infant or child. In this case, sedation may be necessary in order to facilitate removal of the object with forceps. In the event that sedation is not adequate for the child, a general anesthetic may be needed in order to have the foreign object removed.

Burns

An individual suffering from a burn in a disaster situation or seen in the emergency department of a hospital must be assessed quickly and classified according to (1) cause, (2) degree of burn, especially in regard to the damage of underlying tissues, and (3) the area of body surface involved.

An individual with a burn has an injury to the skin and other parts of the body caused by heat, electricity, chemicals, and/or radiation. Burns are classified according to the damage caused to the layers of the skin and underlying tissues. Burns are classified in Chapter 24, but a brief classification will be reviewed here. A first-degree burn causes redness, discoloration, mild edema, and pain involving the skin. A second-degree burn causes blisters, which contain electrolytes and water. A third-degree burn causes an actual destruction of skin and results in scarring. A fourth-degree burn causes an actual destruction of skin and varying degrees of tissue damage beneath the skin. Fat, muscle, bone, tendon, fascia, and nerve tissue may be involved.

The emergency care of a burn victim has four objectives: (1) maintenance of a patent airway and circulation, (2) prevention of extension of the injury to underlying tissues, (3) prevention and treatment of shock, and (4) prevention of infection.

FIRST AID

First aid for the victim suffering from first- and second-degree burns should include:

- Removing burned clothing and immersion of the burned part in cold water when a small part is involved. Leaving the part of the body that has been burned in cold water for 2 to 5 minutes prevents the formation of blisters, edema, and further tissue damage due to capillary permeability.
- Covering the affected area with a clean cloth or sterile dressing to prevent infection.
- Reapplying a cold dressing when pain recurs.
- Transporting the victim to the nearest medical facility for further treatment.

First aid for the individual suffering from third-degree burns and extensive second- and first-degree burns should consist of:

- Positioning the victim in a dorsal, recumbent position.
- Positioning the victim's head to facilitate an open airway.
- Evaluating the respiratory exchange by listening for mucus and abnormal breathing.
- Checking the victim's mouth and nasal passage for evidence of burns when the face and neck are involved.
- Checking for edema of the neck when the face and neck are burned.
- Removing clothing and checking the body for the extent of surface involved.
- Applying cold compresses if a small area is involved.
- Covering the body with a clean, moist sheet or large burn dressings when a large area is involved.

- Transporting the victim to the nearest medical facility as quickly and safely as possible.

EMERGENCY CARE

Emergency care of the burned patient in an emergency department may include the following measures:

- Oxygen may be administered.
- An 18- or 19-gauge intravenous catheter may be inserted for administration of fluids.
- Intravenous fluid or plasma expander may be started until the hemoglobin, hematocrit, and electrolyte balance have been determined.
- Blood is taken from the patient for such blood work as typing and crossmatching, determining the electrolyte balance, and blood volume.
- A central venous pressure catheter is inserted for monitoring intravenous fluids.
- An indwelling urinary catheter is inserted for hourly output determination.
- Strict record of intake and output is maintained.
- Pain is controlled by adequate doses of narcotics, which may be given intravenously.
- Tetanus toxoid and antibiotics are given for prophylaxis against tetanus and wound infections.
- Vital signs are monitored.
- A nasogastric tube may be inserted to prevent gastric dilatation, vomiting, and aspiration pneumonia especially in the patient with head, neck, and face burns.

CHEMICAL BURNS

Chemical burns are caused by acids and alkalies. Alkali burns are considered more serious than acid burns because alkalies penetrate deeper and burn longer. In general, the first aid treatment for chemical burns consists of flooding the area with water. Exceptions are listed in Table 8.16.

Heat Intolerance

The body's temperature-regulating system is located in the portion of the brain called the hypothalamus. The heat-regulating center is located in the anterior portion of the thalamus. Heat is gained in the body by conduction and radiation. *Conduction* occurs when the air temperature is higher than the body temperature. *Radiation* occurs when objects near the body have a surface temperature greater than the temperature of the body. Heat is lost from the body primarily by radiation, convection, and conduction. Heat also is lost by evaporation of water from the skin, lungs, urine, and feces. Perspiration is the chief means of maintaining normal body temperature, when heat cannot be lost by radiation and conduction. The effectiveness of perspiration in maintaining normal body temperature is proportional to the humidity, temperature, and movement of the air.

When the temperature in the environment rises above 37°C (98.6°F), the body may begin to absorb heat from the environment. The human body makes three physiologic adjustments to a high temperature: (1)

TABLE 8.16
CHEMICAL BURNS*

CHEMICALS	FIRST AID
Strong acids, such as sulfuric acid and nitric acid	Flush with water, remove clothing, pour solution of 1 teaspoon of baking powder in 1 pt of water over area. Place clean cloth or dressing on area. Transport the victim to a medical facility
Lime	Remove the lime by brushing the area, flood with water only if large quantities of water are available for rapid, forceful flushing. Take off all clothing to remove small particles hidden in clothing
Phenol (carbolic acid)	Apply alcohol, 50% (gin or whiskey). Flood area with water. Sodium bicarbonate solution, glycerin, or vegetable oils may be used as a substitute for alcohol

* Do not use these measures for chemical burns of the eye. See the section in this chapter pertaining to eye injuries.

vasodilatation of the blood vessels near the skin, (2) increased heart rate, and (3) increased perspiration. The physiologic adjustments of the body are affected by the amount and type of clothing, obesity of the individual, the individual's age, excessive alcohol intake, drugs, and the body's adjustment to the environment. When an individual's body becomes overheated, peripheral blood vessels dilate. Dilation causes shunting of blood to the skin, resulting in a loss of heat by conduction and convection. Cutaneous vasodilation causes a decrease in peripheral resistance. Therefore, an individual's heartbeat increases to meet the increased circulatory demand. The body's utilization of oxygen is proportionate to the increase in body temperature. Perspiration, which occurs as a result of increased temperature or humidity, contains large amounts of sodium, potassium, and water. The loss of water and sodium causes the extracellular fluid to decrease. Excessive heat may affect the body in a variety of ways causing the onset of several conditions commonly referred to as heat cramps, heat exhaustion, and heat stroke.

HEAT CRAMPS

The victim with heat cramps generally has painful muscle spasms of voluntary muscles of the extremities and abdomen following strenuous exercise in hot weather. The cramps are related to the loss of sodium chloride in excessive perspiration.

First aid measures for the victim affected by heat cramps include:

- Remove the victim to a cool environment.
- Place your hand on the cramped muscle and exert firm pressure and gentle massage to relieve muscle spasm.
- Give the victim one-half glass of salt water every 15 minutes over a period of one hour. The salt solution is made by placing 1 teaspoon of table salt in a quart of water.
- Have the individual rest for a few hours after experiencing heat cramps.

Heat cramps can be prevented by eating foods containing additional salt and drinking more liquids when strenuous exercise is anticipated. Exposure to direct sunlight during periods of high temperature and humidity should be limited.

HEAT EXHAUSTION

The victim with heat exhaustion (heat prostration) has vasomotor collapse characterized by faintness, weakness, headache, nausea, vomiting, dizziness, elevated temperature, pale and clammy skin, and profuse perspiration. Heat exhaustion is caused by loss of fluid and sodium during vigorous exercise in hot weather. First aid consists of the following:

- Give the victim sips of salty water (same as in heat cramps).
- Have the victim lie down in a cool environment with legs elevated or lean forward with the head between the knees.
- Loosen clothing.
- If nausea and vomiting are present, the patient should not receive liquids. In this case, transport the victim to the nearest emergency facility.
- Advise the victim to rest for several hours and prevent exposure during extremely hot weather.

Heat exhaustion can be prevented by decreasing physical activity during the heat of the day, drinking adequate amounts of fluid, and increasing the intake of salt.

HEAT STROKE

Heat stroke (sun stroke) is an immediate life-threatening emergency. Heat is retained by the body and the heat regulation mechanism of the hypothalamus fails. The body temperature may rise to 41°C (105.8°F) or above. The skin is hot, dry, and flushed. Tachycardia may be present. The pulse may be weak and irregular in addition to being rapid. Hypotension, headache, confusion, muscle cramps, and convulsions may occur. Stupor and coma may follow. Elderly persons and those with cardiovascular disease are particularly prone to heat stroke. The victim will die if vigorous and prompt treatment is not initiated.

The first objective of first aid and emergency care is the reduction of body temperature as rapidly as possible to 39° (102.2°F). Persistent elevated temperature can result in permanent brain damage. The victim's temperature may be lowered by removing clothing and spraying with the garden hose. An alternative is to place the victim in a tub of tepid water. Ice should not be placed in the tub bath because ice causes vasoconstriction and decreased heat loss. The surface of the victim's body should be massaged vigorously to encourage the blood to flow to the surface, which will aid in cooling the blood. Ice bags may be placed on the victim's forehead, axilla, or groin. The victim should be transported to the nearest emergency room.

In the emergency department, intravenous fluids are started. A hypothermia blanket may be used for the patient, and a cool saline enema may also be effective in reducing body temperature. A fan aids in increasing heat loss by convection. Diazepam (VALIUM), chlorpromazine (THORAZINE), or antipyretic drugs may be given to aid in controlling shivering and reducing the body temperature.

If the patient is cyanotic, oxygen by nasal catheter or face mask may be started. An endoctracheal tube may be inserted and attached to a ventilator if signs of cardiopulmonary failure appear. A slow infusion of electrolyte solution and careful monitoring of central venous pressure to prevent pulmonary edema may be necessary. If the patient has a convulsion, protective and supportive care is needed.

A flow sheet of the patient's temperature, pulse rate, output of urine, serum electrolytes, and mental status should be maintained. Urinalysis, electrocardiogram, liver function tests, platelet count, and coagulation studies may be performed. The patient may develop severe metabolic acidosis as a result of lactic acid accumulation, and this is treated with sodium bicarbonate. Adequate hydration and restoring electrolyte balance are necessary.

Heat stroke may be prevented by urging elderly persons and cardiac patients to remain inside in a cool environment on hot, humid days. Individuals who are highly sensitive to heat should avoid undue exposure to heat and excessive exercise during hot weather.

SUNBURN

Sunburn can occur when the sun is not visible as well as by exposure to direct sun rays. Sunburns are frequent during the summer when individuals lay on beaches and around pools in an effort to obtain a suntan.

First aid consists of:

- Application of cool compresses to affected area
- Application of bland creams or ointment
- Contact a physician if blisters occur

Prevention is the best treatment of sunburn.

Cold Injuries

Cold injuries are similar to burn injuries in that they cause damage and death of tissue. An individual subjected to freezing temperatures can develop ice crystals in the cells since a large portion of the body cell consists of water. Cold injuries affect capillary blood vessels as well as deep tissue.

The four most important causative factors associated with cold injuries are (1) temperature, (2) moisture, (3) wind velocity, and (4) length of exposure. The temperature and moisture will dictate the type of lesion. The length of exposure and wind velocity determine the severity and speed of development of the lesion.

The effect of cold on the body may be divided into two types: (1) general cooling of the entire body, and (2) local cooling of a portion of the body.

GENERAL COOLING

General cooling of an individual's body usually occurs in connection with a rapidly dropping temperature and cold moisture such as snow or ice. Hunger, fatigue, and exertion are contributing factors in the development of generalized body cooling. Cooling of the body can be described in five stages of progression. The *initial* stage is shivering, which is the body's method of generating heat in an attempt to maintain normal temperature. During the *second* stage, the person appears apathetic, disinterested, and restless. As body temperature continues to decline, the *third* stage develops. The victim becomes sleepy and loses consciousness, the eyes have a glassy stare, and the pulse and respirations are slow. The blood pressure is low, and there is little or no response to pain. During the *fourth* stage, the victim's temperature sinks lower and extremities freeze. In the *final* phase, death occurs.

Emergency treatment consists of immediate transfer to a hospital. A prewarmed blanket or sleeping bag should be placed on the victim immediately. Cardiopulmonary resuscitation should be started when cardiac arrest occurs. If the patient is conscious, warm liquids may be given to drink while being transported to the hospital. The liquid may help to warm the patient. Alcohol and smoking are contraindicated because of their effect on the blood vessels.

LOCAL COOLING

An individual's ears, nose, hands, and feet may be involved when local cooling occurs. Local cooling usually takes place as a result of exposure to extremely cold air or liquid, which causes vasoconstriction and deprives the cells and tissues of warmth and blood supply to prevent freezing. The two phases of local cooling injuries are superficial frostbite and deep freezing. The portion of the body affected by superficial frostbite loses its natural color and has a doughy feeling. The involved part of the victim's body during deep freezing is white but feels hard throughout the area.

Frost nip, superficial frostbite, deep freezing, or frostbite, chillbains, trench foot, and immersion foot are the most frequently seen examples of local cooling of a body part (see Table 8.17).

FROSTBITE. An individual suffering from frostbite has an injury to tissue caused by exposure to low environmental temperature. Frostbite usually occurs when the temperature of a part is lowered to 0°C (32°F). Frostbite may be superficial or deep, depending on the duration of exposure. *Superficial frostbite* involves injury to the skin or tissue immediately beneath the skin. *Deep frostbite* involves skin, subcutaneous tissue, and muscle with gangrene and loss of the part.

Frostbite usually involves the ears, nose, toes, cheeks, and fingers. Alcoholics who sleep in extremely damp, cold areas are much more prone to frostbite than others. Persons who are tired, elderly, easily excited, perspire profusely, have recently recovered from a serious illness, or are affected with peripheral vascular disorders have increased susceptibility to frostbite. The number of individuals suffering from frostbite increases during times of extremes in environmental temperatures. Such conditions as blizzards and winter storms increase the incidence of frostbite.

An individual usually is not aware of having been frostbitten until the affected part feels numb. The symptoms of frostbite usually begin with redness of the skin. Continued exposure to cold causes the skin to lose its natural color and appear waxy.

First aid for an individual with frostbite consists of covering the frozen part with a jacket, blanket, or other piece of protective material. The victim should be brought indoors to a warm environment. Do not place the victim in front of a stove or radiator as this will cause an increased metabolism. The patient may be placed in a tub of water 39°C (102.2°F) to 40.5°C (104.9°F) to rapidly rewarm the part. A bath thermometer should be used in the tub of water and the water should be running to maintain a constant temperature. Once the part has been warmed and becomes flushed, the victim should gently exercise it. Do not permit the individual to bear weight on the extremity once it has been thawed. The involved area should be elevated. Sterile, dry gauze should be placed between affected toes and/or fingers to keep them separated. Aspirin or acetaminophen (TYLENOL) may be given for pain. Pain becomes severe as thawing takes place. Hot coffee and tea may be given to increase the victim's general feeling of warmth. Blisters should not be opened. The patient should be taken to the medical facility for care.

During first aid and treatment of frostbite:

- *Do not* apply snow or thaw the part in cold water.

TABLE 8.17
COMMON COLD INJURIES

CONDITION	FACTORS CAUSING	SYMPTOMS	TREATMENT
Chillblains	Dry, cold weather, temperature 15°C (59°F) to 0°C (32°F) Prolonged, repeated exposure	Pain, redness, swelling; tingling in fingers, toes, knees, and cheeks	1. Apply bland, soothing ointment 2. Dress to prevent exposure
Frost nip	Extreme cold, high winds	Onset—slow, painless, usually unnoticed; whiteness of skin	1. Blow warm breath on affected part 2. Place affected fingers motionless in armpits
Superficial frostbite	Brief exposure to dry, cold temperature below −7°C (19.4°F)	Involved skin is white and waxy—firm to touch; throbbing, aching, and burning for weeks following injury	1. Steady warmth; do not rub 2. Dry covering
Deep frostbite or freezing	Extreme cold, high winds; long exposure	Initially—painless, waxy in appearance; skin will not roll over bony prominences Skin collects moisture "sweat" after victim brought indoors Blisters in 12–36 hours, red-violet discoloration in 1-5 days	1. Take to hospital immediately 2. Keep warm and dry 3. CPR if cardiac arrest occurs
Trench foot and immersion foot	Damp, wet weather, temperature 15.4°C (59.7°F) to 0°C (32°F), duration hours, days	Cold feet, swollen, waxy, mottled, and cyanotic, burgundy to blue splotches; blisters on skin if sodden and very friable; anesthesia and difficulty walking	1. Remove wet boots and socks 2. Improve circulation a. Sympathectomy b. Hydrotherapy c. Vitamin B therapy 3. Prevent infection 4. General supportive therapy—pain medication

- *Do not* rub the part as sharp ice crystals in the cell will cause extreme damage.
- *Do not* apply heat lamps or hot water bottles or place the victim in front of a stove or radiator.
- *Do not* open or puncture blisters.
- *Do not* permit weight-bearing once the part has been thawed.
- *Do not* apply heat directly to the container in which the foot or body is submerged.
- *Do not* permit the patient to smoke as this causes vasoconstriction.

A summary of information about cold injuries is presented in Table 8.17.

During extremely cold weather, the body should be protected from prolonged exposure to cold. This can be achieved first by selecting body garments that are warm and do not constrict. Thermal weight undergarments as well as other garments that repel the wind and water are basic. Special attention should be given to covering the ears, hands, feet, and knees. Extra dry socks and undergarments should be available if the ones being worn become moist. Bathing, shaving the face, smoking, and consuming alcoholic beverages should be avoided prior to going out into the cold, brisk weather. Application of oil and creams to the face is protective on windy, cold days. The time spent out of doors should be limited, and while out of doors, the individual should be constantly moving to aid circulation. Exercising the toes and fingers is also important.

Head Injuries

Head injuries account for two thirds of all deaths from accidents and are a major cause of neurologic disturbances. The outcome of head injuries caused by accidents is determined by two primary factors: (1) the initial damage occurring at the time of impact and (2) the time elasping between impact and initiation of treatment. The high death rate and disability resulting from head injuries are related to the damage from the initial impact. The individual may have injuries from compression caused by a created mass, which can consist of cerebral edema, intracranial hematomas, engorgement of the brain tissue, and contusions. Injury may occur on the opposite side of the brain during the initial impact. This is caused by the force of the brain striking the skull on the opposite side of the impact.

EMERGENCY OBSERVATIONS

Assessment of respiratory exchange is one of the first steps in evaluation of the patient's condition. A lack of oxygen to the brain may lead to retention of carbon dioxide and cerebral edema. The nurse should assess the patient's respiration by observing the rate, presence of cyanosis, and position of the patient's trachea. An endotracheal tube or a tracheostomy may be necessary.

Emergency care of the victim of a head injury requiring assistance in breathing consists of the following:

- Cleaning the mouth of mucus, food, or any foreign body manually or with suction.
- Insertion of an oropharyngeal airway.
- Administration of oxygen by mask.
- Endotracheal intubation, tracheostomy with attachment to a mechanical ventila-

tor. These procedures, of course, must be done by an trained individual.

The individual suffering from head injuries seldom develops hypovolemic shock (see pages 140–41). However, if there are injuries to other organs and related blood loss, shock may develop. Blood may be drawn for complete blood count, for typing and cross-matching for transfusion, and for study of blood gases. A urinary catheter may be inserted and a urine sample sent to the laboratory for analysis.

Scalp wounds bleed profusely because of the abundant supply of blood vessels in the area. Bleeding should be controlled by a light pressure dressing. The physician later may clamp and ligate the bleeding vessel.

The patient's level of consciousness should be noted. The ears and nose should be observed for color and character of drainage. The presence of the halo sign (see page 736) should be reported. Stiffness of the neck or paralysis should be noticed. The patient should be observed for headache, double vision, nausea, vomiting, and ability to see. The pupils should be checked for size and reaction to light, and the patient's vital signs should be monitored. An increased blood pressure, elevated temperature, decreased pulse rate, and decreased rate of respiration are late signs which should be noted and reported promptly. The patient's extremities should be observed for proper position and movement.

EMERGENCY DIAGNOSIS

Diagnostic studies such as an x-ray of the skull, electroencephalogram, echoencephalogram, radioisotope brain scan, pneumoencephalography, computerized transverse axial tomography, and cerebral angiography may be done.

EMERGENCY CARE

As soon as the patient's airway, circulation, and vital functions have been checked, a transfer to the intensive care unit or surgery is arranged. Additional information related to care of the patient with head injury can be located in Chapter 21, pages 748–50. Table 8.18 contains a summary of information related to first aid.

TABLE 8.18
FIRST AID MEASURES FOR THE VICTIM OF
HEAD INJURY

- Maintain a patent airway.
- Check for cervical injuries.
- Stabilize the head if neck injury appears to be present.
- Apply no cover to drainage from the ears, nose, or eyes.
- Apply light pressure dressing for bleeding from the scalp.
- Do not attempt to remove an impaled object.
- Position the patient in a semiprone position and transport to the nearest medical facility.

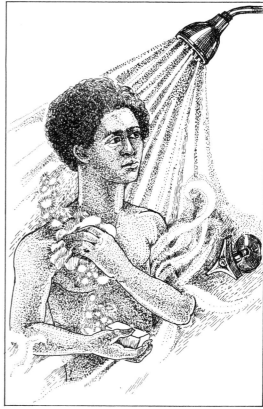

FIGURE 8.13   After a radiation accident, the victim should wash thoroughly in a shower. Hair, pubic area, and folds of skin should be washed thoroughly also.

Radiation Accidents

An individual seen in the emergency situation because of injuries caused by radiation has probably been exposed to radiation falls, spills, or explosion. First aid for radiation accidents, such as vomiting following a dose of radioactive ^{131}I, consists of washing well with soap and water preferably in a shower. All material used should be saved for proper disposal by the radiation safety officer. The victim's skin should be checked with a Geiger counter and washed again if necessary.

If an accident occurs in a public building and a person is exposed to total body radiation and is injured, immediate careful removal is needed. The rescuer must get in and out of the building as rapidly as possible to avoid overexposure to harmful radiation. As soon as the rescuer and the victim are out of the contaminated area, they should remove clothes, shoes, and other attire. The individuals involved should wash and save the water used. Spectators should be kept at a distance to avoid contamination. The hospital should be notified that a person contaminated with radioactive material is being transported. When the individual is received in the emergency room, she or he should be washed in a shower with scrupulous attention to hair and folds of the skin (Figure 8.13). A tub bath is not desirable because particles of radiation are not removed as well. The ambulance and all equipment used on the client must be washed and checked with a Geiger counter. The Atomic Energy Commission must be notified and must check the equipment before it can be used again.

Alcoholism

Alcoholism is a disease, an emotional experience, and a form of drug abuse, but society has been judgmental of alcoholism and slow to accept the concept that alcoholism is a form of drug abuse and a disease. Perhaps this is due to lack of knowledge and insight concerning the nature of the illness. Alcoholism is the fourth major health problem in the United States. Alcoholism is seen in all walks of life including various races, religions, and educational backgrounds. Alcoholism among adolescents is on the increase in the United States.

An alcoholic individual in the emergency department is often hostile, insulting, and verbally abusive. This behavior makes it easy for members of the health team to ignore or neglect the person. An alcoholic generally uses alcohol as a means of escape from life's problems. Such a person may be untruthful about drinking and use mental mechanisms such as denial, rationalization, dependency, and pretense. Abnormal behavior may be caused by hypoglycemia (low blood sugar). The alcoholic may become chronically ill because of dietary deprivation, chronic alcohol poisoning, liver disease, vitamin deficiencies, and disturbances of the central nervous system. An alcoholic is prone to develop infections, especially of the respiratory system.

SYMPTOMS

An individual suffering from alcoholism usually will not admit that; but, a careful history may reveal the following:

- History of blackouts with inability to recall events or actions during periods of drinking
- Acute inflammation of the gastrointestinal system, referred to as alcoholic gastritis, is frequently seen in the emergency department with complaints of burning in the epigastric region, nausea, vomiting, blood in the vomitus, and black, tarry stools
- Inflammation of the pancreas (pancreatitis)
- Ruptured esophageal varicocele, varicose vein of the esophagus
- Cirrhosis of the liver
- Frequent bacterial infections and accidents

The symptoms of an individual with acute alcoholism generally include tachycardia, hypertension, agitation, and a flushed face. Multiple bruises of the body may be observed. Trembling and hyperactive reflexes may also be present. The patient may have an involuntary rapid movement of the eyeballs from side to side (lateral nystagmus).

Symptoms of chronic alcoholism include:

- Decreased tolerance for alcohol
- Symptoms of chronic illness such as cirrhosis, mental disturbances, gastrointestinal bleeding
- Continuous state of inebriation
- Severe withdrawal symptoms when deprived of alcohol (see Delirium Tremens)

TREATMENT AND NURSING CARE

Medical treatment is similar to that needed for the victim who has ingested a poison. Gastric lavage may be needed to remove residual alcohol and prevent vomiting. Support of vital functions is a priority.

The nurse-patient relationship is important in the care of the alcoholic individual. Acceptance of the patient as a person is the first objective in the nurse-patient interaction. Second, the nurse must accept the individual as a patient who is addicted to a drug—alcohol—and third, a genuine caring relationship must be demonstrated in all interactions. The hostile client should be approached in a manner similar to that described in Table 8.2.

Some emergency departments have a counselor available for consultation with the patient and family. Alcoholics Anonymous (AA), which has branches in all states for the patient as well as family members, is a voluntary organization operated by alcoholics who help other alcoholics and in so doing help themselves. AL-ANON is an organization composed of members who interact with alcoholics. Members are helped to understand their own behavior and the behavior of an alcoholic. This understanding leads to improved coping methods when dealing with the alcoholic spouse, friend, relative, co-worker, or client. Adolescent children may find help in the organization ALA-TEEN. This organization is composed of children of alcoholics and is designed to help children in coping with problems of having an alcoholic parent or parents. As a member of the community, the nurse can refer a patient or family to these organizations.

DELIRIUM TREMENS

The individual with delirium tremens is in an acute psychotic state following a prolonged drinking period. The condition is a medical emergency initiated by the abrupt withdrawal of alcohol. Delirium tremens

(DTs) also may occur in spite of continued alcohol intake and is thought to be caused by alterations in the body's metabolic state.

The alcoholic withdrawal syndrome has four stages: acute withdrawal, hallucinations, disorientation, and seizure activity. Stage 1, *acute withdrawal*, is characterized by psychosomatic agitation, tremors, tachycardia, hypertensin, lateral nystagmus mentioned earlier, short attention span, and acute anxiety. During stage 2, the patient has perceptions that have no basis in reality, *hallucinations*. Hallucinations in this stage may be visual, touch, auditory, or a combination of these. The hallucinations may be temporary. Agitation generally is present. In stage 3, the patient becomes disoriented, which implies a loss of proper bearings or a mental state of confusion regarding identity, place, or time. This stage may be complicated by infection, injury, hemorrhage, electrolye imbalance, or multiple drug abuse. The patient experiencing seizure activity is considered to be in stage 4. When caring for the patient in this condition, as with other conditions, the nurse should describe the actual symptoms observed.

The patient with delirium tremens may be brought to the emergency department by a family member, a friend, or a policeman in any stage of withdrawal. The patient usually has severe trembling of the face, tongue, lips, and hands. There may be difficulty in speaking. The pupils usually are dilated and slow to react to light. The patient's face and conjuctiva usually are congested in appearance, and the pulse is rapid, irregular, and weak. Temperature is elevated and the skin is moist due to profuse perspiration. Reflexes are increased and seizures may occur. Delirium tremens may last from three to five days with periods of prolonged sleep followed by a clearing of sensorium, mental clarity, and disappearance of visual hallucinations. The prognosis depends upon the physical health of the patient and the presence of other disease conditions.

NURSING INTERVENTIONS. Good nursing care is the key to emergency care of the patient with delirium tremens. The patient should be placed in a private, well-lighted room to reduce visual hallucinations. A nurse should be present continuously to provide reassurance as well as to observe. The patient may be homicidal or suicidal. The use of restraints should be avoided, if possible, as they seem to agitate the patient. When someone is in attendance on the patient, restraints may not be needed.

The treatment of the patient with DTs usually is geared toward correction of fluid and electrolyte imbalance and improving the body's nutritional state. Parenteral and oral fluids are administered with large doses of vitamins. A high-protein, high-carbohydrate, high-calorie diet generally is indicated.

Sleep and rest may be promoted by the administration of prescribed drugs such as diazepam (VALIUM), chlorpromazine, (THORAZINE), or paraldehyde. Phenytoin (DILANTIN) may be used to control convulsions. The dose of the medication generally is decreased with each use to prevent oversedation. The patient's blood pressure should be taken prior to the administration of chlorpromazine.

Drugs used in the treatment of the alcoholic person experiencing withdrawal symptoms are selected with care. Such drugs should not produce excessive sedation, complicate neurologic symptoms, impair breathing and cardiac function, affect the liver, mask psychosis, influence physiologic recovery, or produce a false sense of wellbeing, which could increase dependency.

Rape

Rape may be defined as forced penetration of the genitalia without the victim's consent. In some states, the legal definition indicates that the assailant need not have an orgasm or an erection, for as long as any portion of the penis enters any portion of the genitalia, rape has occurred. Although state laws differ in their legal definition of rape, they have three common features: (1) the act was done against the person's will, (2) force was used, and (3) penetration of the genitalia occurred.

Extensive interviews with victims of rape and rapists indicate that the personal appearance, dress, and action of the victim have nothing to do with encouraging the assault. The rapist usually is driven to commit the act in an effort to get even with a female figure symbolic of personal hate. The figure usually is someone identified with the rapist's youth. The offender often gets attention from the victim by using one of three methods. The victim may be enticed to take material possessions such as money or candy; position, power, authority, age, or other factors may be used as threats to pressure the victim to accept human contact; or a mentally retarded individual may be pressured to consent by persuasion that sexual contact is the right thing to do and enjoyable. The above usually are hard to prove because the contract between the victim and the rapist carries a pledge of secrecy.

RESPONSES OF THE VICTIM OF SEXUAL ASSAULT

Following a sexual assault, the woman may express emotions by crying and verbally by expressing anger, disbelief, fear, and shock. Certain responses such as smiling, sobbing, restlessness, and tenseness may be considered as inappropriate. In some instances, the woman appears to be calm, composed, and obviously controlling emotions and presenting an outward image of composure and self-control.

Following the initial phase, the victim of rape may experience a disorganized phase, manifested by persistent recurring nightmares, disturbed sleep patterns, tension headaches, fear of crowds, and apprehension when people are walking behind her. Such a person may startle easily at insignificant noises. The woman may experience such feelings as guilt, self-blame, fear, rage, anger, and a desire for revenge.

The individual may experience a feeling of soreness and have bruises. Genitourinary tract disturbances such as burning on urination and vaginal discharge may occur. The woman may develop a chronic vaginal infection.

Following the disorganized phase, the woman may go through a phase of organization. Success of the organized phase is dependent upon the strength of the individual's original self-concept, the support received initially, and the support through-out the experience from her family, friends, and hospital personnel.

EMERGENCY CARE

In rape cases, emotional injury often is greater than physical injury. The victim is usually brought to the emergency department by a police office, family member, or friend. The woman generally is frightened and humiliated. The nurse, doctor, and emergency room staff should be warm, understanding, and portray a sincere empathetic understanding for the victim. A private room should be used for the interview with the clerk, nursing staff, physician, and police officer because questioning at a registration desk only compounds the degradation and humiliation. The nurse's initial contact with the client has three objectives: (1) provide emotional support by being an empathetic, sincere listener, (2) eliminate as much fear as possible by providing pertinent information, and (3) establish a level of trust and confidence that will enable the victim to feel free to ventilate feelings.

The nurse's facial expression, gestures, voice tone, choice of words, body language, and actions such as remaining with the patient throughout the emergency room experience will go a long way toward providing emotional support. Two outstanding fears generally experienced by the patient are of pregnancy and vaginal disease or severe infection. These two fears can be removed by giving the patient information concerning the pill that may be taken the morning after sexual contact and antibiotics for prevention of infection and venereal disease.

Many large emergency departments have teams composed of such persons as a counselor or clinical psychologist available for initial and follow-up care for the raped patient and for the abused child. The counselor listens to the victim and observes for indications of self-destruction or other feelings that need to be handled. The counselor makes telephone calls and visits to answer questions. The counselor also functions in a therapeutic role in handling marital or family problems related to a sexual assault. Continuing support is provided by the counselor by accompanying the client to court in some cases.

A complete physical examination includes careful observation for bruises, marks, lacerations, signs of trauma, and foreign pubic hair. Any foreign pubic hair is saved for the police. If the patient is a minor, the parents must grant permission for a physical and vaginal examination. A culture is taken of the vaginal vault for possible gonorrhea, and a wet-drop specimen is taken of cervical mucus for identification of motile sperm. In some cases, the acid phosphatase level of the vaginal secretions is determined, especially if the attack occurred within a couple of hours prior to examination. Acid phosphatase is high in seminal fluid.

If the female victim was raped during the fertile period of her menstrual cycle, diethylstilbestrol may be prescribed. This drug generally is prescribed within 72 hours following the attack and may be known as the "morning-after pill." The client should be told that diethylstilbestrol may cause nausea and vomiting, but this should not cause her to discontinue taking the medication. The medication should be taken for the prescribed length of time to prevent pregnancy.

The possibility of abortion may be discussed as an alternative for interrupting a pregnancy. This is especially true if the time period has expired during which diethylstilbestrol might be effective or if pregnancy occurs in spite of the medication. The patient may be treated also with an antibiotic as a prophylactic measure against syphilis or gonorrhea.

The nurse must remember that all information included in the emergency room record is a legal document that will probably be used in court. Error on the record will be held against the victim. The patient's statement of what happened should be recorded accurately and in the exact words used in the interview. For instance, if the victim states that the rapist "gagged me and threatened to cut my hand if I screamed," this should be recorded as such. The use of a weapon such as a knife, gun, or other instrument should be reported. When making notations on the victim's chart, the nurse should remember that if the hospital record differs from the statement made by the physician or victim in court, the hospital record will be considered the correct description.

All bruises, scratches, and marks on the victim should be noted in the record. It is a good idea to ask the client to point out areas of soreness, bruises, and marks in an effort to be sure that no areas are overlooked. If a counselor interviews a raped victim, the counselor's written account should be attached to the emergency room record. All individuals making notations on the emergency room record should remember that this document probably will be used by the court as evidence and will affect the verdict.

Child Abuse

Child abuse is a syndrome of altered and abnormal parent-child interaction. The syndrome includes physical abuse, undernutrition, poor physical and medical care, sexual abuse, emotional abuse, and a failure to nurture the child's sense of self.

Child abuse is a growing societal problem, affecting all races, levels of education, and social classes. Physical abuse has been rated from the infectious diseases, malformations, and cancer as a killer of infants between the ages of 6 and 12 months of age. Physical abuse is a second cause of death following true accidents in children one year of age and over.

The magnitude of the problem of child abuse makes it mandatory that every nurse, especially emergency room nurses, become skillful in recognizing the battered or abused child syndrome. There are laws in all 50 states making it mandatory for all professional personnel caring for children suspected of child abuse to report it to the designated agency.

Child abuse appears to be repetitive in nature; the child who was injured once is more likely to be injured again. The abuser usually is the mother, although it can be the father, stepfather, babysitter, or relative. The incidence of child abuse among adopted children and premature children is high.

CHARACTERISTICS OF ABUSER

Abusing parents usually have the following characteristics:

- Immature and self-centered
- Self-concept low, unable to react and

reach out to other people for friendship, and need gratification

- Concerns are strict, puritanical, and distorted
- Were victims of child abuse and/or severe punishment themselves
- No clear concept of how the child feels physically or emotionally
- Criticize the child and have high expectations for the child to behave and act older than his age
- Complain that the newborn or child does not love her or him
- Blame the child for becoming injured, do not feel guilty or responsible for the child's injury
- Appear more concerned about self and what will happen to them than about the extent of the child's injury

NURSING OBSERVATIONS

Careful observations and recording are important when child abuse is suspected. The following signs should alert the nurse to possible child abuse:

- Multiple injuries occurring on different areas of the body and in clusters, such as bruises on the back, cuts on the scalp, and swollen leg lesions
- Lesions that are multiple and in varied stages of healing
- An injury that has the mark of an object used to inflict it, such as a rope, belt, or chain
- An explanation of the cause of the injury by the parent that does not appear to be reasonable in relation to the child's age or to the injury. For example, a child has pulled the pot from the stove and was burned on the bottom of both feet with a clear line of demarcation
- A history of hospital and doctor shopping. For example, each injury of the child was treated by a different physician in a different hospital.

The most frequent sites of physical injury are the soft tissue, bones, head, and abdomen. Soft tissue injuries are most common. They include burns, bruises, and ecchymoses. The lesions may be circular, caused by cigarettes or other hot objects, or they may be bizarre-shaped lesions. Injuries of the buttocks, feet, hands, and perineum usually have a clear line indicating that the child has been hit.

Fractures generally involve the long bones and ribs. There is usually x-ray evidence of numerous fractures, some old and some healed, and evidence of recent fractures. Dislocation usually occurs as a result of the child's being shaken or snatched.

Head injuries cause the highest mortality rate and incidence of permanent injuries. Neurologic injuries include repeated concussions, scalp lacerations, skull fractures, and subdural hematomas.

Abdominal injuries account for a small percentage of the injuries, but the mortality rate can be as high as 50 percent. Frequent abdominal injuries include a ruptured spleen, liver, stomach, and intestine.

Children who have been abused appear passive if under six years of age and very aggressive if older. The child usually does not cry when the parent leaves the emergency room. The child quickly becomes attached to the nurse or doctor and frequently develops a friendship with total strangers quickly. The child generally appears untidy, undernourished, and underdeveloped.

The parent should be observed during the narration of what happened. Usually, the parent is evasive or vague. The parent may blame a neighbor, an unknown person, or another child for the injury. Also, the abuser does not admit responsibility for the injury or show guilt feelings concerning the injury. If both parents accompany the child, they should be interviewed privately and separately.

At the conclusion of the interview, the nurse or counselor should record the observation on a form developed for recording child abuse. The form will help the interviewer to organize observations and conversations in an objective manner. Notations should be made of actual statements or the behavior of parents to validate observations.

NURSING INTERVENTIONS

The nurse who suspects abuse in a child who is three years of age or older should talk privately with the child. Usually, the child will tell whether an adult is responsible for the injury or hurt.

The decision to report child abuse can be very anxiety provoking. The nurse should consult with the supervisor, social worker, and physician. A group decision usually is less stressful. The health professional must be polite and courteous to the parent and remain in control of his or her emotions regardless of the condition of the child. In the final analysis, each member of the health team is responsible for protecting the child from abuse and for channeling the abuser to an agency to receive appropriate help.

Emergency Childbirth

When faced with the possibility of the birth of an infant without medical assistance, the nurse needs to remember that delivery of a baby is a natural process. The function of the nurse or other attendant is merely to guide the infant through the birth canal and to offer psychologic support to the mother. Steps to be followed in a calm and confident manner when birth is imminent without medical assistance are listed below.

1. Position the mother on her back with legs flexed and far apart. Drape the patient for comfort and to avoid overexposure.
2. When the nurse observes that the perineum bulges during the height of a contraction, one hand should be placed below the vaginal opening with her fingers at the perineum to prevent the baby from contacting the anal area.
3. If the membrane is still intact, it will appear at the vulva as a smooth, glistening sac. In this case, the membrane must be ruptured before the head is delivered. In order to rupture the membrane, clip the sac at the nape of the infant's neck to prevent aspiration of the fluid.
4. Instruct the mother to pant during contractions and guide the infant's head from the canal between contractions.
5. As soon as the head is delivered, locate the umbilical cord. If the umbilical cord is around the infant's neck, it should be loosened while the head is supported with one hand. While still supporting the baby's head, the nurse should wipe mucus from the infant's nose and mouth. The head will rotate and the infant will face the mother's thigh usually. The upper shoulder can be delivered by gently guiding the head downward to aid in expulsion of the upper shoulder.
6. Guide the head upward to aid in delivery of the lower shoulder.
7. The infant's body will deliver rapidly as it is more slippery and smaller than the head and shoulders.
8. The infant who does not cry immediately should be supported or held by the ankles and shoulders with the head downward to aid the drainage of fluid and mucus from the mouth and nose by gravity. Traction on the cord should be avoided. Further stimulation can be provided by stroking the infant on the back and by stroking the neck from the throat toward the chin.
9. After breathing has started, place the infant on the left side.
10. If a bulb syringe is available, insert the bulb syringe in the infant's nostrils to use suction to clear the airway.
11. Cutting of the cord is delayed until the physician arrives.
12. Place the infant on the mother's abdomen on the side. The infant's head should be lower than the body to facilitate drainage of mucus. This position enables the mother to touch and feel the infant, provides the warmth from the mother's body for the infant to keep warm, and allows the weight of the infant to be on the mother's abdomen as a stimulus to facilitate contraction of the uterus.
13. As the cord begins to lengthen, this indicates that the placenta is almost ready to be delivered. Instruct the mother to bear down with each contraction in order to deliver the placenta. The fundus of the uterus should be massaged following delivery of the placenta. The fundus of the uterus is felt as a lump below or near the mother's umbilicus (navel). The infant should be wrapped after satisfactory breathing has been established.
14. The sex, time, and place of the delivery of the baby should be noted.

Disaster

During the time of a natural disaster, such as a hurricane, tornado, flood, or earthquake, the nurse will not function in a usual role. This is true also in cases of manmade disaster, such as a plane crash, war, and violent civil disturbances. All members of the nursing team should be familiar with the plan for civil defense of the hospital and the community.

The nurse will probably be working in unfamiliar circumstances with unfamiliar people, directing care and giving first aid. The four priorities of care during a disaster are (1) to save life, (2) to preserve function, (3) to give comfort, and (4) to preserve cosmetic appearance.

The most difficult philosophic adjustment for members of the health team to make at the time of a disaster is triage. *Triage* is the name given to the sorting of casualties so that the greatest number of casualties will receive care. The top triage priority is not the most seriously ill, as is the nurse's usual philosophy. The first priority of a triage is the individual who will most likely benefit from treatment. The nurse will give time to individuals who are most likely to live. The patient who is seriously injured will have lowest priority and will probably die.

Triage sorting includes the *immediate treatment* groups. These are individuals who will respond to treatment. Shock, respiratory problems, hemorrhage, lacerations, fractures, and burns of 15 to 40 percent of the body are included in the immediate treatment group. The *minimal treatment* group is composed of those individuals who can return to assist others following treatment. Persons with simple fractures or burns of less than 10 percent of the body are examples of the minimal treatment group. The *delayed treatment* group includes those who will not die if treatment is delayed. These patients could have long bone fractures, lacerations, and second-degree burns of less than 30 percent of the body. The *expectant group* includes those patients who are so severely injured that their care will be prolonged and complex. They should be made as comfortable as possible. It is impor-

tant for the nurse to realize that the first triage sorting may change as the patient's condition changes.

In a disaster, the nurse should report to either the hospital or another designated area. A cap or laboratory coat should be worn for ease of identification.

All patients should be identified and all treatment recorded. Tags to identify patients are available and should be attached to the patient, not to the bed or cot. The tag may be applied with adhesive tape or a safety pin.

Patients who can care for themselves, but not for others, should be moved away from the casualties who need care. Children should be kept with their parents as much as possible. Older individuals should be placed away from the confusion but given a job to do such as making tags, folding linens, or visiting with less seriously injured people.

After a disaster, many patients will suffer from disaster fatigue. This is a psychologic reaction to the disaster. Some individuals will be depressed. Some may seem stunned and unable to talk or to assume any responsibility for themselves.

All individuals seem to go through a period of slight depression followed by a period in which they are grateful for help but still cannot function very well for themselves. This is followed by a stage of feeling friendliness and brotherhood for all the victims of the disaster. These individuals are enthusiastic about the rebuilding. The final stage is a real sense of the losses suffered and a feeling of dissatisfaction with the handling of the disaster.

Some individuals will become hyperactive and rush from one task to another task. These persons are unable to be of much assistance. Some individuals have an overwhelming desire to get away from the situation. Many individuals have a decreased ability to think clearly and lack the ability to make judgments, similar to the person in crisis described earlier in the chapter. Some persons will develop symptoms of hysterical conversion, as described in Chapter 1. Some of the victims may lose contact with reality.

The nurse should be aware that nonverbal communication may be saying much

TABLE 8.19
OTHER EMERGENCIES

EMERGENCY	DESCRIPTION
Diabetic coma	Included in Chapter 18
Dyspnea	Discussed in Chapters 11 and 14
Epileptic seizure	See Chapter 21
Heart attack	Discussed in Chapter 11
Insulin shock	Included in Chapter 13
Open chest injury	An injury of the chest resulting in an open wound may be called a sucking chest wound since air can enter the lungs through the opening; a sucking sound occurs at site of injury as patient breathes; wound should be covered immediately with the cleanest available dressing to seal the wound
Stroke	Discussed in Chapter 12

more to the victim than what is actually said. All of the victims should be accepted as they are without judgment. Rapid contact should be made with the overactive victim which results in involvement in a useful job. Calm reassurance may be offered, not necessarily that all is going to be all right, but that everything is under control and that the patient will be treated. The first aid the nurse knows can be utilized effectively to treat patients and to direct others in the treatment of victims.

Education and practice are the best methods of ensuring that there will be a minimal loss of life in both natural and man-made disasters. Nurses are in a position to cooperate with an encourage hospitals and communities to be prepared for a disaster.

Case Study Involving a Multiple Injury

An 18-year-old male was admitted following an accident in which he was thrown from his automobile when it struck a guard rail on an interstate highway following a high-speed race with friends. The physical examination of this young man revealed the following:

- Unconscious youth
- Respiration labored, color pale, pulse slow and irregular, blood pressure 60/40

- Steady stream of blood from scalp laceration
- Blood draining from ears and nose; left pupil dilated
- Right kidney area distended and bruised
- Right leg twisted and rotated internally

QUESTIONS
1. List the injuries in the priority necessary for emergency care.
2. Describe the emergency treatment of the various injuries.

Case Study Involving a Choking Victim

The nurse was sitting in the cafeteria having dinner with two nursing aides. The cafeteria had closed 30 minutes before and only a security guard remained. One of the nursing aides suddenly began to choke. Her eyes bulged as she grasped her throat and became cyanotic.

QUESTIONS
1. What action should the nurse take first?
2. What actions, if any, should be delegated to the other nursing aide and the security guard?

Case Study Involving A Hospital Fire

The nurse was working alone in a medical unit at 3 A.M. The nurse in charge of the unit was on a dinner break in the canteen. The nurse on duty in the medical unit noticed an odor of something burning at one end of the hall. She went down the hall and found Mr. Zero asleep in Room 130 in the bed next to the wall. His mattress was smoldering. Mr. Adams was in the best next to Mr. Zero. Mr. Adams was comatose from a cerebrovascular accident and was receiving oxygen. The room had a telephone.

QUESTIONS
1. What action should the nurse take first?
2. What is the role of the nursing stff in reporting and controlling the fire and evacuating the patients?

Suggestions for Further Study

1. What method of communication does your hospital have for contacting other hospitals and the police department to coordinate the handling of a major disaster?
2. Review the emergency nursing actions the nurse may initiate in the emergency department of your agency without immediate supervision.

3. Review the psychiatric emergencies commonly presented in the emergency department of your agency and describe the appropriate nursing actions.
4. How may a counselor, clinical psychologist, or social worker function in the emergency department?
5. Locate the sites of common pressure points to check hemorrhage on a classmate.
6. Mason, Mildred A.; Bates, Grace F.; and Smola, Bonnie K.: *Workbook in Basic Medical-Surgical Nursing*, 3rd ed. Macmillan Publishing Company, New York, 1984. Exercise 8.

Additional Readings

Bailey, Mary: "Emergency! First Aid for Fractures." *Nursing 82*, 12:72–81 (Nov.), 1982.

Ballou, Mary: "Crises: Recognition and Intervention Are Crucial Nursing Roles." *Journal of Practical Nursing*, 31:25–27 and 41 (Mar.), 1981.

Boyd, Linda T., Shurett, Pamela Hastings; and Coburn, Caroline: "Heat and Heat-Related Illnesses." *American Journal of Nursing*, 81:1298–1302 (July), 1981.

Brodsley, Laurel: "Avoiding a Crisis: The Assessment." *American Journal of Nursing*, 82:1865–74 (Dec.), 1982.

Buchanan, Lorraine E.: "Emergency! First Aid for Spinal Cord Injury." *Nursing 82*, 12:68–75 (Aug.), 1982.

Carbary, Lorraine Judson, and Carbary, Clinton N.: "Carbon Monoxide, the Silent Killer." *Journal of Nursing Care*, 14:21–24 (July), 1981.

DeLapp, Tina Davis: "Taking the Bite Out of Frostbite and Other Cold Weather Injuries." *American Journal of Nursing*, 80:56–60 (Jan.), 1980.

Fonger, Linda: "Emergency! First Aid for Burns." *Nursing 82*, 12:70–77 (Sept.), 1982.

Francis, Betty: "Overdose." *Journal of Nursing Care*, 13:12–14 (Aug.), 1980.

Fritz, Carolyn P.: "Emergency! First Aid for Wounds." *Nursing 82*, 12:68–75 (Oct.), 1982.

Gedrose, Judith: "Prevention and Treatment of Hypothermia and Frostbite." *Nursing 80*, 10:34–36 (Feb.), 1980.

Jankowski, Carol B.: "Radiation Emergency." *American Journal of Nursing*, 82:90–97 (Jan.), 1982.

Murphy, Donna: "Iodide—An Rx for Radiation Accident." *American Journal of Nursing*, 82:96–98 (Jan.), 1982.

Sumner, Sara M.: "Emergency! First Aid for Choking." *Nursing 82*, 12:40–49 (July), 1982.

Chapter 9

The Patient with Neoplastic Disease

Expected Behavioral Outcomes

Minimum objectives referred to as expected behavioral outcomes have been designed for the practical/vocational nursing student to use as guides in studying this chapter. The student should read these expected outcomes before studying the chapter. The objectives can be used as guides for study.

Using the content of this chapter, the student should return to the objectives and evaluate the ability to:

1. *Compare the characteristics of a benign and malignant tumor.*
2. *Describe at least three nursing actions that relate to the early detection of cancer.*
3. *List the danger signals of cancer.*
4. *Describe the complications associated with the main forms of cancer treatment.*
5. *Discuss three nursing actions to relieve the discomforts accompanying each of the main treatments of cancer.*
6. *Apply the grieving process to a woman who has had a recent mastectomy.*
7. *Describe personal feelings about a cancer patient and how a nurse should feel about a cancer patient.*
8. *Describe at least three nursing actions related to the rehabilitation of a cancer patient.*

Vocabulary Development

The following prefixes, suffixes, and combining forms pertain to this chapter. By learning and/or reviewing their meanings, the practical/vocational nursing student will have the keys needed to unlock many exciting new medical terms.

Discover the meaning of these keys in a medical dictionary or in the content of this chapter. How does each key pertain to this chapter? In your notebook write the correct meaning of each prefix, suffix, or combining for listed below. Illustrate each key with an example.

anti—against. Ex. *anti*metabolites—substances that act against materials in cells.

cancr-	intra-
caps-	ir-
carcin-	ne-
chemo-	per-
chord-	radi-
-cis	sarc-
cyt-	sect-
dis-	therap-
in-	tme-
inter-	tom-

Tumor

Normally cells of the body grow in an orderly manner and perform certain duties that are dictated by the parent cell. For example, a cell located in the liver duplicates itself during cell division and a cell located in the skin duplicates itself in a similar manner. Each cell has common functions, and each cell has certain duties to perform that are dictated by its parent cell. Each day, millions of cells in a person's body disintegrate and are replaced by new ones having the same shape and function. When these new cells assume a new shape or a different shape, they lose their ability to function properly. New cells having shapes different from their parent cells and contributing nothing to the body in return for the nourishment received are known as either a *neoplasm* or a *tumor*. An individual with a tumor or neoplasm has a *neoplastic disease*. The tumor may be either benign or malignant.

TYPES

A benign or nonmalignant tumor grows slowly, does not spread, and is usually surrounded by a covering or capsule. Such a growth may be referred to as an encapsulated tumor (see Figure 9.1). Looking at the peeling or outer covering of an orange helps one to visualize the covering of a benign tumor. A nonmalignant tumor may have to be removed surgically, especially if it causes pressure on vital organs. In some cases, the physician will remove a benign tumor even though it is not causing the patient any diffi-

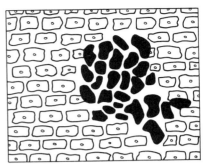

FIGURE 9.2   Malignant tumor: grows rapidly, does spread, not surrounded by covering or capsule.

culty in order not to risk the possibility of the tumor being malignant. The only way a physician can be positive that a tumor is nonmalignant is by removing all or a portion of it and having it analyzed by a pathologist. The physician may also remove a benign tumor if there is a good chance that the benign tumor may become malignant. Moles are good examples of benign tumors. Some moles may later become malignant, especially if they are in a place that is frequently irritated. When a nonmalignant tumor is removed, it is not likely to grow back again.

A malignant tumor is referred to as *cancer* or *malignancy*. It grows rapidly; it is not surrounded by a covering or capsule and spreads to other parts of the body (see Figure 9.2). These abnormal cells invade nearby tissue. They are carried also to other parts of the body by the lymph and blood. This transfer of malignant cells to another part of the body is called *metastasis*. The new growth started from the transported cells is referred to as a *metastatic growth* or *secondary growth*. This spread is often predictable because certain types of tumor spread to certain organs. For example, colon and rectal cancers most commonly metastasize to the liver; Wilms' tumor, a kidney tumor seen mostly in young children, may spread to the lungs and to the lymph nodes in the area of the kidney. A malignant tumor, if not treated, will eventually threaten the individual's life.

Life-threatening conditions associated with malignant neoplasms include anemia, infection, effusion of fluid into an organ or cavity, pain, and/or malnutrition. Death may occur from hemorrhage, kidney failure, ob-

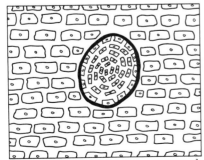

FIGURE 9.1   Benign tumor: grows slowly, does not spread, usually surrounded by covering or capsule.

struction of respiratory passages, destruction of vital centers in the brain, or obstruction of the intestines.

A malignant tumor is classified according to the type of tissue from which it grows. Tissue taken from the suspicious growth is examined by a pathologist under a microscope. The abnormal cells are identified because they differ from the normal cells of that tissue. The two main groups of cancer classified according to the type of tissue from which they grow are *carcinoma* and *sarcoma*. A malignancy of epithelial cells, which are located in the skin, mucous membrane, and serous membrane, is called *carcinoma*. *Sarcoma* is the term used in referring to cancer of connective tissue, such as bone, cartilage, fat, and tendons. These two main classifications are further subdivided according to the particular kind of tissue involved. Two examples of sarcoma are osteosarcoma, which indicates a malignancy of the bone, and liposarcoma, which indicates a malignancy of fatty tissue. *Oncology* is the study of malignant neoplasms.

Cause

The exact cause of cancer is not known. The current concept that cancer is not a single disease but a large group of diseases is causing scientists to look for more than one cause of cancer. One area of research includes studies to determine how healthy cells are transformed into malignant ones. Another research area includes studies to determine if disturbances in the immune system result in a failure to destroy malignant cells once they occur.

Although the cause(s) is not yet known, a number of factors favor the development of malignant neoplasm. Research shows that a malignancy is not inherited. However, an individual may inherit a tendency toward cancer. In other words, the child of parents with cancer is more likely to develop a malignancy than the child of parents without cancer. This does not mean that the child of parents with cancer necessarily will develop a malignancy.

Studies indicate that irritation of a given part of the body over a long period of time may result in the formation of a malignant tumor. For example, irritation of the lip from prolonged pipe smoking may result in cancer. Another example is cancer of the skin resulting from long exposure to the sun. Data suggest that certain physical and/or genetic characteristics may make an individual more susceptible to a particular form of cancer. For example, white persons with red hair are considered to be more likely to develop melanoma (a type of malignant skin cancer) than the rest of the population.

In addition, people who have a low resistance to infection are more likely to develop certain types of cancer. For example, an individual receiving a drug that suppresses body defenses against infection is more likely to develop cancer. For this reason, persons with organ transplants such as kidney transplant are at increased risk for cancer.

The possibility that viruses are related to the development of certain types of cancer is being given serious consideration by research scientists. Some cancer-producing viruses have been found in animals. One virus is closely associated as the agent that causes Burkitt's lymphoma. It is hoped that current research eventually will result in vaccines to prevent certain cancers.

Exposure to high-dose radiation may also predispose an individual to the development of cancer. For example, radiologists who are not extremely cautious have a higher incidence of leukemia than other physicians.

Certain drugs and chemicals have also been linked to cancer. For example, diethylstilbestrol, a hormone formerly taken during pregnancy, is associated with the development of vaginal and cervical carcinoma in female offspring. Cigarette smoking is linked to the development of lung cancer. A higher incidence of lung cancer is found also among workers who deal with asbestos. In addition, persons who work with asphalt have a higher incidence of skin cancer.

Recently, nutritional factors have been associated with the development of certain cancers. For example, a high dietary intake of fat is linked to the development of cancer in the colon. Stomach cancer has been associated with a low dietary intake of fruits and vegetables containing vitamin C. Cancer of the esophagus is associated with a higher alcohol intake.

Prevalence

Cancer is the second leading cause of death in the United States. It affects persons of all age groups but is more common during and after middle age.

Individuals in certain age groups are more likely to develop cancer of specific organs than individuals in other age groups. For example, leukemia, or cancer of the blood, is the most common fatal form of cancer found in children. Malignancy of certain organs is more common in one sex than in the other. An example of this is cancer of the lung, which occurs more often in men than in women. However, this statement may soon become a statistic of the past because cancer of the lung is rising steadily among women. At the present time, the increase of smoking among women is considered the cause of this increased incidence of cancer of the lung. At this time, the most common cancer in women that can result in death is breast cancer. The most common cancer in men that can result in death is lung cancer.

The incidence of cancer is rising. Cancer is presently second only to heart disease as a cause of death in the United States. Although these facts might be depressing, the picture is not as gloomy as one might think. Cancer deaths are decreasing. Another estimate brightens this dark picture; one half of those individuals who develop a malignancy could be cured if the diagnosis were made early and proper treatment started promptly. Right now, one out of every three individuals who develops a malignancy is saved. That statistic could be one out of every two with early recognition of symptoms, early diagnosis, and treatment.

The term *prognosis* refers to the possible course and outcome for the patient with a disease. *Early* is the keyword for improving the prognosis of the patient with a neoplastic disease. Early recognition of the symptoms, an early diagnosis by the doctor, and early treatment are of vital importance in curing the patient.

The Nurse's Role in Early Detection, Treatment, and Prevention

As a member of the health team, the nurse has a vital role in recognizing symptoms, early detection, and treatment of cancer.

Knowing the danger signals of cancer enables the nurse to report them promptly when observed in a patient. For example, Mr. Goodman noted gradual changes in the appearance of a mole on Mr. Law's skin during the daily bath. These changes were reported to the physician and recorded in the patient's chart. A cancer was diagnosed and cured because of the nurse's knowledge and keen observation.

Friends' relatives, and neighbors often consult the nurse about problems related to health and illness. The nurse may provide information about the danger signals of cancer and encourage regular examinations for early detection as listed in Table 9.1. The nurse advises a person who reports a symptom indicating cancer to consult a physician.

The nurse may participate in community programs to educate the public about cancer. The American Cancer Society is an agency with state and local chapters that develops programs to educate the public about the importance of early recognition of symptoms, early diagnosis, and treatment.

The American Cancer Society also helps by emphasizing to members of the medical profession the importance of looking for early signs of cancer, by establishing facilities for early diagnosis and proper treatment, and by doing research in an effort to discover the cause of cancer.

Interested persons may find local chapters listed in the telephone directory. For additional assistance in finding a local chapter, write to:

American Cancer Society
777 Third Avenue
New York, New York 10017

Many individuals are so fearful of developing cancer that they become immobilized when symptoms of cancer appear. Ignoring something will not make it go away. News

TABLE 9.1
RECOMMENDED SCREENING TESTS FOR EARLY DETECTION OF CANCER*

TEST	SEX	AGE	FREQUENCY
Breast self-examination	F	Over 20	Every month
Breast physical examination	F	20–40	Every 3 years
		Over 40	Every year
Chest x-ray			Not recommended unless symptoms are present
Endometrial tissue sample	F	Age of menopause	At menopause, when there are symptoms—
		Any age	infertility, estrogen therapy, obesity, abnormal uterine bleeding, failure of ovulation
Health counseling and cancer checkup (for cancers of skin, oropharynx, lymph nodes, ovaries, prostate, testicles, thyroid)	M & F	Over 20	Every 3 years
	M & F	Over 40	Every year
Mammography	F	35–40	Have baseline test done
		40–50	Consult physician
		Over 50	Every year
Pap test	F	20–65	After two negative exams one year apart, may decrease to every 3 years
		Under 20 if sexually active	
Pelvic examination	F	20–40	Every 3 years
		Over 40	Every year
Rectal examination	M & F	Over 40	Every year
Sigmoidoscopy	M & F	Over 50	After two negative exams one year apart, may decrease to every 3 to 5 years
Sputum examination for malignant cells			Not recommended unless symptoms are present
Stool guaiac examination	M & F	Over 50	Every year

* Adapted from *A Cancer Sourcebook for Nurses*, revised edition. The American Cancer Society, 1981.

coverage of the hospitalization of prominent public figures encourages people to seek a doctor's attention when they think something is wrong. Publicity may also help by providing a more optimistic view about cancer to the person who is very afraid. Television programs regarding cancer of the breast and other organs have been shown, and magazine articles have been published describing how to self-examine the breasts. The nurse may participate in publicity by encouraging others to read, listen, or watch programs related to cancer. Another role of the nurse is to practice and teach others about preventive measures related to cancer.

Because the *specific* cause or causes of a malignancy are not known, it is difficult to prevent an individual from developing cancer. Some factors that predispose to the development of cancer can be avoided. The three main examples are carcinogenic, or cancer-causing substances, constant irritation of any one body area, and prolonged exposure of the skin to the sun. The relationship of cigarette smoking to lung cancer was mentioned earlier in this chapter. Factories should devise safety rules to safeguard workers against prolonged exposure to such substances as radium, asphalt, uranium, and asbestos. The individual with body moles, especially in areas of constant irritation by clothing, shoes, or eyeglasses, should observe these growths for changes. Any apparent difference in the size, color, or appearance of a mole or wart should be brought to the physician's attention promptly. Cancer of the mouth may be aggravated by irritation from improperly fitted dentures, jagged teeth, and possibly the habit of drinking either extremely hot or extremely cold liquids.

Although an individual cannot change fair skin or red hair, prolonged exposure to the sun can be avoided. A sun screen, hats, and protective clothing can be work for trips to the beach or when participating in outdoor activities.

Danger Signals

It is important for the nurse to know the early danger signals commonly associated with cancer. Although these symptoms do not necessarily indicate cancer, the presence of one or more of them should make an individual consult a physicians. The early symptoms can be recalled by remembering the word "trouble":

- *T*hickening or lump, particularly in the breast
- *R*egular color or size or general appearance of a mole or wart changes
- *O*ral sore especially, but for that matter any other sore that does not heal
- *U*nusual change in bowel or bladder habits
- *B*leeding, irregular in nature, or a discharge from a natural body opening
- *L*aryngitis, hoarseness, or a cough that persists
- *E*ating problems, such as indigestion or difficulty in swallowing, that persist.

However, the individual should be encouraged to have physical examinations at least annually and should not wait for these symptoms to occur before going to a doctor.

Since cancer may affect any part of the body, the symptoms vary with the area affected. Later signs of cancer include weakness, anorexia, and loss of weight. The patient should know that the loss of weight generally does not accompany the early signs of cancer. Loss of weight occurs especially in the patient with a malignancy of the digestive system. Anemia, a decrease of the red blood cells or the hemoglobin, is another common symptom. Fever occurs in advanced cases as a result of complicating infections. Pain is usually a late sign.

Rapid growth of the tumor coupled with metastasis causes the patient to become thinner and weaker as time passes. This condition, in which the patient becomes thin and weak because of disease, is known as *cachexia*.

Assisting with Diagnostic Studies

The nurse's role in diagnosis begins with early recognition of danger signals of cancer in self and others. Another important nursing activity is to provide explanation and support to the patient and family since the process of diagnosing cancer may be lengthy, tiring, and frightening. A third important part of assisting with diagnostic studies includes activities directly related to a specific test ordered by the physician such as collecting a urine specimen.

HISTORY AND PHYSICAL EXAMINATION

A thorough history and physical examination are usually the first steps in diagnosing cancer. The physician pays close attention to the presence of factors that favor the development of cancer including smoking, occupational hazards, and family history of cancer. A careful physical examination includes breast, pelvic, and rectal examinations for women and a rectal examination for men. The patient with a danger signal of cancer will have additional tests related to further investigation of that signal. The patient with a disturbance of a body function will have diagnostic tests related to cancer in that area.

LABORATORY STUDIES

Certain laboratory studies are part of a routine physical examination. Abnormal results of common laboratory studies may indicate the presence of cancer. For example, a patient whose hemoglobin is lower than normal may have a tumor of the digestive tract. A urinalysis which contains red blood cells may indicate that the patient has cancer of the bladder. Protein detected in the urine during a urinalysis may cause the physician to suspect cancer of the kidney.

Acid phosphatase is a blood test the physician may order when a patient shows symptoms of cancer of the prostate. Abnormally high levels of this chemical in the blood sample help to confirm the diagnosis. However, normal levels of this chemical do not necessarily mean that the patient does not have cancer of the prostate.

Another blood test called alkaline phosphatase is often elevated when a patient has cancer that has spread to the bones or liver. However, such an elevation occurs when a client has illnesses other than cancer.

A positive stool test for hidden or occult blood can be the first sign of cancer of the digestive tract. However, it may also indicate an ulcer.

The doctor may order a gastric analysis if a patient complains of persistent indigestion. A lack of hydrochloric acid may indicate cancer.

Scientists continue to search for tests to identify primary or recurrent cancer before it damages normal tissue. *Carcinoembryonic antigen* (CEA) is a new blood test based on the discovery that certain tumors produce substances called antigens. For example, it has been shown that the patient with colon cancer has a high level of CEA in the bloodstream. Currently, this test also may be ordered when recurrent cancer is suspected. It is hoped that, in the future, all cancers will be identified at an earlier stage using this and other similar tests.

In addition, cytologic tests may be ordered by the physician. A cytologic test (Pap test) is the microscopic examination of any body fluid that contains cells that have been discarded by the tissue through normal scaling. Malignant cells will scale away from the tissue along with normal cells. Secretions from the uterus, bladder, kidney, bronchi, lungs, and stomach can be examined for malignancy. The cytologic test for cancer is especially beneficial in detecting unsuspected cases of cancer of the female reproductive tract. During a pelvic examination, the doctor obtains a scraping of the cervix, which is placed on a slide. At the same time, a small amount of vaginal secretions is placed on another slide. Abnormal cells in these secretions indicate cancer. A special packet which includes instructions is available to women who wish to collect their own cervical and vaginal secretions. The specimen must then be mailed to the laboratory. Although this method encourages women to have cytology

or Pap smears who might otherwise not do so, it is not a substitute for a pelvic examination. The cytologic test frequently is referred to as the Papanicolaou test in honor of the physician who developed this method of examination.

A histologic test is a microscopic examination of suspected tissue to identify the type of cancer, the degree of malignancy, and the extent of invasion. A biopsy is the special procedure done to obtain an adequate tissue specimen. An *excisional biopsy* includes a surgical incision and removing the entire tumor for a histologic test. *Aspiration biopsy* is removal of a small portion of tumor using a needle and/or syringe. *Frozen section* refers to tissue samples removed during surgery and hardened by freezing. While the patient is still on the operating table, the pathologist examines suspected tissues under the microscope and reports results to the surgeon immediately. The surgeon uses this information to select the appropriate operation for the patient.

X-RAY STUDIES

X-rays of the chest can show lung tumors or lung metastasis. An upper gastrointestinal series and barium enema can be used to diagnose a tumor of the digestive tract. A series of x-rays of the skeleton can show whether a patient's malignancy has spread to the bones.

Radiologists also can use special techniques to help in the diagnosis of cancer. Chest *tomograms* are x-rays done in sections. They have the ability to show more than routine chest x-rays. Mammograms can be ordered if a woman is in a high-risk group for developing breast cancer, or if the doctor feels a lump on examination and wants to double-check its location. A new technique of x-ray examination of the breasts is called xeroradiography, and radiologists believe that more can be seen on these x-rays than on the regular mammograms.

A scan of a part of the body, such as the brain, thyroid, kidney, liver, parathyroid, spleen, and lymph nodes, can be ordered by the physician if a tumor is suspected. During this procedure, a radioactive substance is introduced into the patient's body; then a machine picks up the manner in which this substance is absorbed. If a patient has a tumor, it may show up as a "hot spot" or "cold spot." A "hot spot" means that the tumor has absorbed more of the radioactive substance than the tissue that is in the area of the tumor. A "cold spot" means the tumor has not absorbed as much of the radioactive substance as the normal tissue in the area.

Other special studies use dyes to visualize internal parts of the body. A dye can be injected into a particular artery in order to discover if there is a tumor in a particular organ such as the brain or kidney. A dye can also be injected into the femoral vein (a large vein of the leg), and tumors that are in the area in back of the abdominal cavity can thereby be discovered. The physician also can see if the lymph nodes of the pelvic and groin area have any tumor involvement by ordering a special study called a lymphangiogram. In this study a dye is injected into a lymph vessel in the foot. Dyes also can be introduced into the body in order to visualize other organs, such as the bladder and bronchi. These examinations are a cystogram and bronchogram, respectively.

Another special study that can be ordered by the physician is a thermogram. If a physician suspects that a patient has a breast tumor, a study of the skin temperature of the breast can be done. The area where the tumor is present should have a higher skin temperature than that of the rest of the breast.

One of the newest techniques in radiology is computerized axial tomography (CAT). In this special test, a whole series of x-rays is taken, which are then analyzed by a computer. The eventual result is a three-dimensional picture of the organ.

Ultrasound tests use high-frequency sound waves to locate deep tumors.

ENDOSCOPIC EXAMINATION

Endoscopy is the examination of a hollow body part through the use of an instrument. The instrument enables the physician to see irregularities in the surface of the specific area he is examining. For example, an examination of the sigmoid colon is called sigmoidoscopy, and the instrument is called a sigmoidoscope. This test is recommended for early detection of colon cancer.

DCNB SKIN TEST

A skin test has been developed to estimate the function of a person's immune system related to cancer. A small amount of dinitrochlorobenzene (DCNB) is placed on the skin. A positive response to this test indicates that the patient's immune system is functioning appropriately. A negative response is associated with patients who have malignant tumors and metastatic lesions.

Current Cancer Therapy

The patient with cancer may be treated with surgery, radiation therapy, or chemotherapy, or any combination of them. A new form of treatment, immunotherapy, is now available also for certain cancers. Treatment of the patient with cancer is selected by the physician on the basis of such factors as the type of malignancy, its location, and its extent. For example, if an individual has a solid tumor, such as a breast tumor, that has not metastasized, she would be treated with surgery. An individual with leukemia, which is a disease of the tissues that form blood, probably would be treated with chemotherapy. Current therapies are directed toward removing the tumor, killing the tumor cells, improving body defenses, shrinking the tumor size, and alleviating pain. Two important features of cancer therapy are that they are life-threatening and may harm normal cells as well as malignant ones. Early recognition and reporting of symptoms related to the complications of cancer therapy are part of the nurse's role in helping the patient with cancer.

Because cancer affects the whole person, the patient generally needs the assistance of many members of the health team. Some hospitals have oncology teams composed of health professionals with special interest and skills in helping the cancer patient and family. Members of this team may include the patient's personal physician, the cancer specialist (oncologist), the registered nurse, the dietitian, the social worker, the pharmacist, and the clergyperson. Other specialists may participate, depending on the needs of the patient. Members of the team meet regularly to cooperate, communicate, and coordinate the patient's therapy.

SURGERY

When a malignant solid tumor is diagnosed early, has not metastisized, and is in an operable region, the chances of cure by surgery are good. The surgeon removes the tumor and as much of the surrounding tissue as practical, especially the lymph nodes. This is necessary because cancer cells may have invaded the neighboring tissue. If a malignancy has already metastasized, surgery is sometimes done in an effort to make the patient more comfortable. For example, if a patient has cancer of the bladder that has spread and is causing incontinence, a urinary diversion may be done to make the patient more comfortable. This is called palliative surgery. In addition, if a patient has unbearable pain from cancer, an operation called a *rhizotomy* may be done to sever the nerve that supplies that area.

RADIOTHERAPY

Radiotherapy or radiation therapy is the use of radioactive rays to combat disease. Radiotherapy is used to treat the patient with cancer because certain malignant cells are more sensitive to radiation than are normal cells. In other words, malignant cells can be destroyed more quickly by radiotherapy than can normal cells. Radiation therapy is used to treat the patient with a potentially curable cancer as well as the patient with a poorer prognosis. As mentioned earlier, radiotherapy may be used singly or in combination with other forms of therapy.

The main sources of radioactivity are x-rays, radium, and artificial radioactive isotopes (see Table 9.2). X-rays are produced by the x-ray machine or by a machine that contains a radioactive source such as the linear accelerator or the cobalt 60 (see Figure 9.3). Radium is a metallic element that gives off rays; thus it is naturally radioactive. Radon is the gas given off by radium, which is collected and sealed in tiny glass or gold tubes. These tubes are referred to as seeds or implants. Artificial radioactive isotopes are produced by placing certain nonradioactive elements, such as gold, in an atomic reactor. These previously nonradioactive elements attain a different weight than normal, become radioactive, and are called radioactive isotopes. As the artificially treated isotope gives off the rays, it becomes less radioactive and reverts to its normal state.

The three types of rays involved in radiation are alpha, beta, and gamma (see Figure

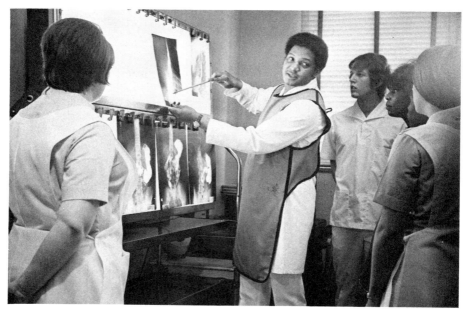

FIGURE 9.3 The radiologist is showing an x-ray of the portion of the patient's body to be treated with cobalt.

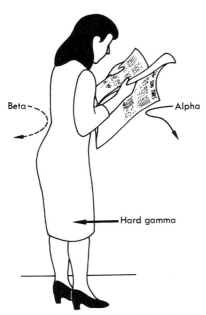

Beta

Alpha

Hard gamma

FIGURE 9.4 An illustration of the three types of rays. Alpha rays penetrate a small portion of the skin and can be stopped by something as simple as a newspaper. Beta rays penetrate a small portion of the skin and can be stopped by clothing. Hard gamma rays penetrate deeply.

9.4). Alpha and beta rays can penetrate only a small portion of the skin. Gamma radiation is further subdivided into soft and hard gamma radiation. Soft gamma radiation has a limited amount of penetration. Hard gamma rays can penetrate deeply into the patient's tissues. Conversely, a radioactive implant that is a hard gamma emmiter sends rays through the patient's body and becomes a hazard to persons nearby. The exact amount of radiation that the well person can tolerate without having any ill effects is not known. In general, members of the health team caring for the patient with a hard gamma emitter implant should have the least amount of exposure possible.

Radiotherapy may be administered in several ways. The rays can be administered externally by having the source of radioactivity directed toward the tumor, as in cobalt therapy. Radiation therapy can be implanting a radioactive substance into or around a tumor, as in radium implantation into the cervix. A radioactive isotope, such

as radioactive iodine, may be given orally. Radioactive iodine may be given to destroy malignant cells of the thyroid gland. Radioactive gold may be injected into body cavities.

Radiotherapy may cause toxic effects including radiation sickness, bone marrow depression, skin reactions, and birth defects. In addition, the risk of developing cancer in the irradiated area is increased. Remembering that radioactive rays may damage normal as well as malignant tissue enables the nurse to understand side effects and toxicity from this therapy.

CHEMOTHERAPY

Chemotherapy is the use of drugs to slow, retard, or stop the process of neoplastic disease. It can be used singly, as in the case of choriocarcinoma, or in combination with other forms of therapy, as in Wilms' tumor. Extensive research is being done in chemotherapy. Certain drugs slow the growth and multiplication of malignant cells. This type of treatment is called palliative. As mentioned earlier, the other forms of therapy can be used as palliative measures as well.

In addition to the radioactive isotopes mentioned earlier, five main classifications of drugs are used in chemotherapy. They are the antimetabolites, alkylating agents, hormones, antibiotics, and a miscellaneous group (see Table 9.3). These may be used in combination with each other or alone.

The antimetabolites slow down the growth of malignant cells by interfering with the cell's reproduction. The alkylating agents slow down the activity, growth, and multiplication of cells. Hormones have a palliative effect on the growth of cancer cells by making their surrounding less favorable. However, malignant cells can grow more rapidly in the presence of certain hormones. When this occurs, the physician may remove the source of the hormone or counteract the hormone by prescribing another one. Antibiotics interfere with the cells' metabolism and resulting growth within the cell. The drugs in the miscellaneous group do not fit into any one of the above classifications.

The drugs used in treating the patient with a malignancy can have severe toxic effects. Generally, the most severe reaction is against the bone marrow cells and the cells lining the gastrointestinal tract. Remembering the functions of bone marrow will help the nurse to understand that the patient can be expected to have a decreased production of red and white blood cells and platelets. This can cause the patient to develop anemia, bleeding tendencies, and a lowered resistance to other diseases. Symptoms commonly associated with damage to the gastrointestinal tract are anorexia, nausea, vomiting, and diarrhea. The patient may develop an ulcer because of destruction of the lining of the gastrointestinal tract.

Special techniques in which the drug is delivered to the tumor by way of its arterial blood supply have been developed. Intra-arterial therapy may be used to treat a tumor in a part of the body that is difficult to reach by surgery or radiation therapy. In intra-arterial therapy, the physician identifies the specific artery that supplies the tumor and injects the drug into that artery. By doing this a high concentration of drug is delivered directly to the tumor before reaching the general circulation. An alkylating agent or an antimetabolite may be used. The patient is said to have an *intra-arterial infusion* when the drug is injected into the artery leading to the tumor and no attempt is made to isolate the return flow of blood and drug for the purpose of redirecting the drug to the tumor. In an *intra-arterial perfusion*, the physician isolates the arterial supply of the tumor as well as the venous flow of blood. The blood is channeled through a closed-circuit pump that enables the doctor to inject the drug into the arterial blood and to redirect the blood containing the medication to the tumor.

Many advances have been made in chemotherapy and more research is continuing. For example, a patient with breast cancer may receive adjuvant chemotherapy postoperatively. *Adjuvant* literally means assisting. In other words, this form of chemotherapy is given to assist another form of treatment. It is hoped that the chemotherapy will destroy any cancer cells that remain. Chemotherapeutic agents are also given in combination. Sometimes a schedule is worked out by a chemotherapist so that

the patient has periods of time in the course of treatments when no drug at all is given. This permits the body to recoup itself. Methotrexate is now given experimentally in very high doses because it is followed by a "rescue agent" that stops the harmful effect of methotrexate.

Two new drugs that show promise for cancer therapy include L-asparaginase and interferon. L-Asparaginase is an enzyme that deprives some tumors of asparagine, a substance needed to make protein. Interferon occurs naturally in the body. This drug is now administered experimentally to patients with certain cancers including breast cancer, melanoma, and osteogenic sarcoma. Scientists are not yet sure how interferon works. It may inhibit tumor growth or affect the patient's immune system.

IMMUNOTHERAPY

The basis of immunotherapy is that the patient with cancer often has a weakened or otherwise impaired immune response. Although immunotherapy is still largely experimental, vaccines and antitumor antiobodies may be given to stimulate or strengthen the patient's immune response to cancer. An ultimate goal is a vaccine that will immunize persons against cancer.

The most common immunotherapy currently in use is BCG, a tuberculosis vaccine consisting of a weakened strain of the bovine tubercle bacillus. The vaccine may be injected intradermally, into a body cavity, or inhaled. Before BCG is used, the patient is skin tested to make sure the immune system is capable of responding. In addition, other therapies usually are used first to reduce the tumor size. Finally, BCG is generally administered as close to the tumor as possible. Serious side effects from this therapy include a wide variety of symptoms related to allergy. Allergic reactions may be life-threatening.

Nursing Care

The patient with cancer needs all the knowledge, skill, and caring the nurse can provide. Understanding the patient's experience enables the nurse to give empathetic, effective nursing care. The nurse's careful observations are needed to identify and report the patient's response to diagnosis and treatment as well as to help with overwhelming concerns related to a life-threatening disease. Nursing interventions help the patient to develop effective coping mechanisms, reduce pain and/or discomforts, and help to prevent complications associated with cancer and/or therapy. In planning nursing care for the patient, the following principles guide the nurse's observations and interventions:

- The patient usually begins treatment while still in denial.
- Nutrition and fluid balance are important influences on therapy.
- A change in body image is less stressful when disfigurement can be reduced or eliminated.
- A reduction or elimination of pain and discomforts improves the quality of the patient's life.
- The family is an important part of the patient's support system.
- The patient's mental outlook can influence the course of cancer and therapy.
- Participating in care may help to increase one's personal autonomy.
- Community resources usually are available for the patient with cancer.
- Complications related to therapy can be fatal.

The nursing care plan is individualized to meet the patient's needs. For example, nursing observations and interventions are slightly different for a patient having surgery than for a patient having chemotherapy.

NURSING OBSERVATIONS
HEAD

Alopecia is a loss of hair which may result from radiotherapy or chemotherapy. While hair loss is not life-threatening, the patient may experience feelings of embarrassment, anger, and shame. Grieving over the loss of valued hair and a changed body image also can be expected. The patient who associates hair with femininity or masculinity may feel less womanly or manly.

Several measures have been tried experimentally to prevent hair loss including applying a scalp tourniquet and/or an ice bag to the head during therapy. These measures may not prevent hair loss but some patients feel better knowing that everything possible is being done to save the hair. Usually, hair regrowth begins after treatment has been completed and continues for months. Wigs, hairpieces, scarves, caps, and hats may be worn until the patient's hair grows back. Some patients use humor to cope with alopecia by selecting outrageous hats or scarves which become a kind of personal trademark.

Mucous membranes of the mouth are inspected closely by the nurse using a tongue depressor and flashlight. Erythema (redness), small blisters, or small ulcers on the lips, gums, and tongue may indicate stomatitis, a complication of chemotherapy. Even before visible signs appear, the patient may report an intolerance for hot, cold, or heavily spiced foods. Burning around the lips in early stages increases to continuous burning pain which increases during swallowing. Alterations in diet and oral hygiene described later in this chapter apply to this patient. In addition, the physician may prescribe rinses and mouthwashes to reduce pain and prevent bacterial overgrowth. Nystatin in oral liquid form is an antibiotic commonly prescribed. The patient is instructed to "swish and swallow." Since stomatitis may signal the beginning of damage involving the entire gastrointestinal system, the nurse closely observes the patient's mouth and reports unfavorable changes to the head nurse or team leader.

Anorexia, nausea, and *vomiting* are common experiences of the patient with cancer. They may be associated with anesthesia during surgery, radiotherapy, chemotherapy, emotional upheaval, or unpleasant odors caused by drainage. Alterations of diet and fluid may be indicated The physician may prescribe an antiemetic or an appetite stimulant. Chemotherapy may be arranged so that the patient is asleep when nausea and vomiting are likely to occur. A careful intake and output record, close observation of weight, and regular observation of the patient's tray are important to prevent undernutrition, weight loss, and dehydration.

CHEST

Observing the patient's chest includes looking for disturbances in respirations. As previously mentioned, the lungs are often the site of metastases from other organs. Dyspnea (difficult breathing) may be the first sign that cancer cells are affecting the respiratory system. In addition, breathing may be restricted by enlargement of diseased abdominal organs or swelling caused by fluid in the abdominal cavity (ascites). In some cases, the patient's breathing may be impaired by fluid which develops in the thoracic cavity. This condition is called *pleural effusion*. *Thoracentesis* is a procedure in which fluid is withdrawn from the thoracic cavity. Additional information about this procedure can be located in Chapter 14.

ABDOMEN

The patient's abdomen may become swollen with fluid, a condition known as *ascites*. This condition may occur when cancer cells spread to the peritoneum or liver. The nurse may monitor an increase or decrease of ascites by measuring the patient's abdominal girth regularly at the same time of day. The girth is measured by placing a tape measure around the patient's abdomen at the level of the umbilicus. A particular hazard of ascites is that it may restrict breathing by pushing upward toward the diaphragm and thoracic cavity. When this happens, fluid may be withdrawn from the peritoneal cavity, a procedure known as *paracentesis*.

EXTREMITIES

In observing the extremities, the nurse looks for skin changes associated with bleeding. Weakness, numbness, tingling, and changes in the patient's gait may occur from damage to the nervous system by chemotherapy. Fractures may occur with tumors of the breast or bone. Edema (swelling) may be present when there is metastases to vital organs.

ELIMINATION

The patient's urine output is observed, measured, and recorded. A fall in output may indicate insufficient fluid intake or kidney damage. Blood in the urine indicates bleeding in the urinary system.

Observing and recording the amount, consistency, appearance, and frequency of bowel movements are important when observing the patient with cancer. Radiotherapy and chemotherapy may cause severe diarrhea by damaging cells in the gastrointestinal system. Blood in the stool may be visible or hidden. When bleeding is suspected but not visible, a specimen of the bowel movement may be analyzed for occult blood in the laboratory. Black, tarry stools may indicate bleeding. Constipation may occur as a result of pain medications, underhydration and nutrition, and immobility. In addition to observing the patient's urine and fecal output, the nurse observes, measures, and records drainage from all body cavities.

SKIN CHANGES

The patient's skin is carefully observed for bleeding. Bleeding may be visible under the skin as petechiae, purpura, or ecchymoses. As previously mentioned, bleeding may be visible from a body cavity, such as the ears, nose, mouth, vagina, or rectum, or in the urine. Bleeding may be prolonged following an intramuscular injection or removal of an intravenous needle or catheter. Pressure to the skin or application of ice to the injection site may reduce bleeding in these situations.

BEHAVIORAL CHANGES

Fatigue is a common experience of the patient with cancer. Fatigue may result from symptoms, diagnostic tests, therapies, emotional turmoil, and/or complications. In some cases, overwhelming fatigue may temporarily interfere with learning new information or skills.

About half of all patients with cancer experience *pain*. When a person with cancer does have pain, it usually occurs late in the disease and is continuous in nature. Pain may be caused by destruction of nerves by invading cancer cells, pressure from a tumor on nerves, organs, or blood and lymph vessels, or inflammation and necrosis of tissue.

Sleep disturbances are often reported by the patient with cancer. Chemotherapy, fatigue, pain, immobility, emotional turmoil, and noise in the environment are factors that contribute to decreased quality of sleep. Measures used to promote sleep include relaxation exercises, warm milk, adequate ventilation, reduction of noise and light in the environment, drug therapy, and back rub.

The patient with cancer can be expected to show changes in behavior consistent with adapting to a life-threatening illness. In addition, the nurse can anticipate that the patient is concerned about the effects of cancer on sexuality, family life, occupation, and income. These concerns are reported to the head nurse or team leader so that appropriate action can be taken.

NURSING INTERVENTIONS
THERAPEUTIC RELATIONSHIP

In developing a therapeutic relationship with a patient who has cancer, the nurse should know that most persons react to illness including cancer in a rather predictable and sequential manner. The five steps in the sequence are (1) denial, (2) anxiety, (3) regression, (4) depression, and then (5) adaptation. At first, the person denies that an illness exists. Fearing the truth, the patient may delay seeing a physician. Even though a person may feel ill, there is a hope that the illness will go away without a doctor's care. After finally accepting the idea of illness, the person may feel anxious. In some cases, feelings of anxiety may be verbalized by the patient. In other cases, the patient may withdraw and become silent. After the anxiety has passed, the patient may regress and become more dependent on others. The patient may seek attention and comfort from friends, family, and the nursing staff. Depression may follow regression. The patient may not be able to make decisions at this time. Finally, there is acceptance of the illness and the changes it has made on the person's life. The patient may pass rapidly or slowly through these stages or return to previous ones. In some cases, the patient remains in one stage without ever going to the next one.

The nurse's attitude toward the patient and about cancer affects the kind of care the patient receives. For example, the nurse with a fatalistic attitude about cancer may inadvertently deprive the patient of hope. One third of all patients with cancer are cured. When cure is not possible, patients can be helped to feel better, live longer, and adapt to a disability. The nurse who is falsely optimistic, however, may prevent the patient from identifying and coping with real concerns and fears. Such a patient may become isolated from those who could help. Most patients with cancer want to meet the future with realistic attitudes and plans as well as a hopeful outlook for a favorable outcome.

In developing a therapeutic relationship with the patients, the nurse sometimes avoids using the word *cancer*. Instead, words such as tumor or abnormal cells are substituted. Some persons do not realize that cancer is curable in many cases. The death of a relative or close friend from cancer may validate the patient's fear that cancer is a death sentence. The loss of hope which may result from such a belief can be as harmful to the patient as the disease process.

Special communication is indicated for the patient with a disfigurement that results from malignancy or therapy. Picture for one moment a person without a chin or tongue, saliva sliding along the neck, a tube through the nose, and a tracheostomy. How would you react upon seeing this person for the first time? If you feel any sense of revulsion, then you can imagine how the patient may feel. Such an individual may feel anger, depression, irritability, and resentment. Active listening on the nurse's part may help the patient to verbalize these feelings. In communicating with such a patient, the nurse carefully controls his or her own facial expressions to avoid showing revulsion. Very slight changes in facial expression can be picked up by a patient who is very sensitive about this change in personal appearance. Any actions of the nurse that reduce disfigurement communicate awareness and concern about the patient's situation. In addition, such actions indicate the nurse's optimism and belief that the patient's appearance can be improved. For example, a malignancy of the face can be covered with a dressing when permitted by the doctor. Arranging the lighting in the room so that a shadow falls on the area is also helpful. A small tumor or the scars of surgery near the hairline can often be covered with a change of hair styling. Many advances have been made in plastic surgery for the permanent removal and correction of disfigurements.

The patient with cancer may be overwhelmed with emotions but afraid to express them to the nurse. Some patients fear rejection by the nurse or doctor if they express rage, resentment, or bitterness. The person who is viewed by the nursing staff as a "good patient" actually may be very angry. In some cases, the nursing staff may inadvertently encourage the patient to be "good" by not expressing feelings such as rage. Such feelings then may be turned inward, causing additional stress and interfering with recovery.

Another special feature of communicating with the patient with cancer develops when the patient is not aware of the diagnosis of cancer. Most physicians tell patients when cancer is found. In some cases, the physician does not tell a patient. This is an individual matter between the doctor and the patient. In gathering information about the patient, it is important to know what the patient has been told about the diagnosis. The patient usually experiences many fears and concerns when seriously ill whether or not a diagnosis of cancer is communicated. Thus, the nurse may use active listening and other skills related to developing a therapeutic relationship. Occasionally, a patient who has not been told the diagnosis asks the nurse directly. In this case, the patient may be told that questions related to the diagnosis must be discussed with the physician.

HYGIENE MEASURES

Some alterations in hygiene may be indicated when the patient has cancer. Assistance in bathing helps the patient who is very tired to conserve energy. During the bath, the nurse has an opportunity to talk with the patient as well as inspect the skin. Touching the patient during care helps with changes of body image which may result from cancer. The patient receiving radiotherapy needs special skin care described later in the chapter.

Alterations in oral hygiene that may be indicated include more frequently oral hygiene and changing from a toothbrush to toothettes to avoid trauma to mucous membranes.

DIET AND FLUIDS

As stated previously, the general nutritional state of the patient with cancer is often affected. The doctor prescribes a diet to meet the needs of each particular patient's body. For example, one patient may need a high-protein diet and another one may need a diet high in vitamins. The patient with a malignancy of the gastrointestinal tract often cannot digest solid food and may be given small liquid feedings. The patient's choice should always be considered as far as possible.

Careful observation of the intake of food and fluids is needed when the patient has a cancer treated by radiotherapy and/or chemotherapy. Anorexia, nausea, and vomiting may result in electrolyte imbalances from reduced intake or increased losses of body fluids. The patient with advanced cancer also is likely to be undernourished. Inspecting the tray after each meal enables the nurse to detect and report inadequate intake in the early stages.

Small, frequent meals constitute one alteration of diet that may be used to encourage intake. Intravenous fluids may be prescribed to prevent or correct fluid and electrolyte imbalances.

Hyperalimentation is a special form of nutrition that helps to correct undernutrition when the patient is unable to eat for prolonged periods. Protein, sugar, vitamins, and other substances are given intravenously through a central line. A central line uses a catheter that is inserted by the doctor into a large vein such as the superior vena cava (Figure 9.5). The patient with major surgery on the digestive tract or extensive weight loss is a candidate for hyperalimentation.

REDUCTION OF PAIN

A variety of pain-relieving measures may be needed when the patient has pain. Interventions which may be used include touch, distraction, relaxation, analgesics, radio-

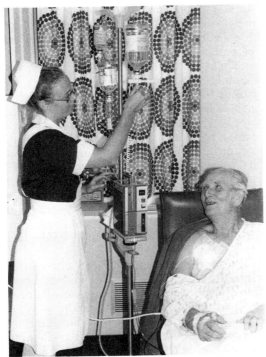

FIGURE 9.5 The patient receiving hyperalimentation to correct undernutrition. (Courtesy of Southside School of Practical Nursing at Southside Community Hospital, Farmville, Virginia.)

therapy, and surgery. These interventions are described in detail in Chapter 7. An important principle related to relieving pain in the patient with cancer is preventing severe pain by administering analgesia regularly rather than when pain become severe. Narcotic analgesics that may be prescribed regularly to prevent pain include levorphanol and methadone by mouth. Combinations of drugs to prevent pain are often prescribed. For example, Brompton's mixture is a solution containing an opiate, cocaine, alcohol, and flavoring syrup. this mixture originated in England and has been adapted for use in the United States. A variation of this mixture is to add prochlorperazine (COMPAZINE).

When pain is not relieved by other methods, surgical procedures may be required to cut the nerves that transmit the pain sensation to the brain. A *chordotomy* is a severing of the pain-conducting pathways in the spinal cord. A *rhizotomy* is a severing of a sensory root as it enters the spinal cord. With these procedures, patients have relief from pain but also may have numbness and possibly some loss of motor function.

PATIENT TEACHING

The patient with cancer may need to learn new skills as a result of therapy. For example, the patient with a colostomy may need to learn how to irrigate the stoma, change the colostomy bag, and alter the diet. The patient receiving radiotherapy or chemotherapy usually needs to learn how to cope with nausea and vomiting, and skin and mucous membrane changes. When possible, family members are included in patient teaching. Guides to patient teaching with a patient has cancer include:

- Demonstrate, whenever possible, the procedure or skill to be learned.
- Plan practice sessions where the patient performs the new skill while the nurse supervises.
- Use encouragement and praise success. Correct errors without criticism.
- Ask the patient to describe and plan how the new learning will fit into a typical day.

REHABILITATION

Not all patients who are diagnosed as having cancer die from that condition. As stated earlier, removal of a neoplastic tumor by surgery or destruction of it by radiotherapy or chemotherapy can cure cancer. Because of improved treatment, there is an improved outlook for patients with cancer. Many services and groups are available to assist patients in coping with necessary changes in daily living. Ostomy clubs are composed of groups of patients who have had colostomies or ileostomies. They can be of great help to a patient who has a colostomy as a result of removal of cancer of the colon. The Lost Cord Club is a group of persons who have had laryngectomies and use esophageal speech and/or mechanical devices to communicate. The nurse should know if these groups exist in the community and be able to work with other nursing personnel and the physician to help the patient adjust to a new way of life.

In the recovery from the treatment of cancer, the patient should be as independent as possible. The patient should be encouraged to look to the future realistically. It is usually helpful to work on short-term goals first and then progress to planning for the future. Public health nurses are available to work with the patient and his family in the home in adapting to his change of life.

SURGICAL PATIENT

The nurse plays an important part in the preoperative and postoperative care of the patient with cancer. As previously mentioned, the patient with cancer may have surgery for diagnosis, cure, or palliation. General principles related to the care of the surgical patient discussed in Chapter 6 apply to this patient. In addition, special situations develop when the diagnosis of cancer is known or suspected. For example, a person may go to surgery not knowing if the operation will be limited to a biopsy or if radical surgery will be performed. Such a person may awaken from anesthesia not knowing, for example, if a breast has been removed. Another person may go to surgery and have to wait days for a diagnosis of cancer because of special laboratory tests needed on the tissue sample. Thus, the nurse can anticipate that patients will experience considerable emotional turmoil before and after surgery.

Since surgery for the treatment of cancer is usually extensive, the patient frequently is admitted to the hospital several days in advance for mental and physical preparation. This period enables the nurse to help the patient with fears about cancer, the loss of a body part, and similar emotions. Overwhelming fear and panic should be reported to the head nurse or team leader since these emotional states may increase the risk of surgery. A longer preoperative period also helps the patient begin the process of adjusting to the loss of a body part. For example, if the patient is to have a colostomy (formation of an artificial anus in the abdominal wall), this extra time provides an opportunity to become oriented to a marked change in the body. Also, it gives the patient an opportunity to develop confidence in members of the nursing team.

Special care is taken in the preoperative period to improve the patient's general health. For example, a special diet containing added protein, vitamins, and calories may be needed. Milkshakes or eggnogs may be encouraged between meals to increase the patient's weight and improve the nutritional status. If a low residue or a clear liquid diet is prescribed in order to prepare the patient for surgery, the reason for the diet should be explained to the patient. Fluid balance is another area of concern in the preoperative period. Diagnostic tests can be very dehydrating. When encouraging the patient to increase fluid intake, the nurse should recommend liquids with nutritional value if possible.

Vitamins, minerals, and antibiotics are examples of drug therapy commonly prescribed to improve the patient's health postoperatively.

Postoperatively, the patient with cancer requires nursing observations and interventions described in Chapter 6. In addition, special consideration is given to the need for helping the patient adjust to a changed body image and teaching self-care skills related to cancer and surgery. For example, the patient with cancer affecting the head and neck may have radical surgery that results in a tracheostomy and feeding tube postoperatively. Early in the postoperative period, the nurse suctions the patient's tracheostomy to clear the airway, cleans the tracheostomy tube, and instills tube feedings according to the physician's orders. However, within the first postoperative week, the nurse teaches the patient how to do these activities alone or with the help of a family member.

In helping a person adjust to a changed body image, the nurse considers the patient, the surgery, and the cancer. The person who must learn to live without a breast, kidney, bladder, arm, or leg may need considerable time and special understanding to appreciate that the choice was made to preserve life. Active listening, touching the patient's body during care, and an accepting attitude are nursing skills that favor a successful change in body image. The nurse also helps the patient adapt to a change in body image by creating opportunities for the patient to participate in care. In some cases, the patient may actually do the care. When this is not possible, the patient may teach a family member while the nurse supervises. The patient with a permanent change in body appearance may lack confidence in facing the world outside the hospital. Such a patient may be reassured by a visit from someone who has had similiar surgery. A patient with a colostomy or ileal conduit may be reassured to learn that these changes are not visible to a stranger. Although the patient may feel like a different person after surgery, the patient actually looks the same to others.

Family members usually need the nurse's support, understanding, and teaching. Many family members experience helplessness, fear, and disbelief similar to the patient's emotional turmoil. In some cases, family members benefit from learning simple comfort measures that can be done for the postoperative patient. Family members may need to learn some or all aspects related to colostomy care, feeding tubes, pain medication, dressing changes, or hand and arm care following mastectomy. Cancer may cause changes in family relationships developed over a lifetime. These changes may strengthen or strain family ties.

PATIENT RECEIVING RADIOTHERAPY

Patients often have a fear of radiotherapy. Knowledge that the rays cause no pain and that the patient feels no heat from them enables the nurse to answer questions more intelligently and allay fear.

The patient may have a reaction to radiotherapy called radiation sickness. Symptoms such as nausea, vomiting, anorexia, malaise, diarrhea, chills, and fever are often associated with radiation sickness. Nursing care is aimed toward relieving these discomforts. The dosage of radiation maybe reduced if these symptoms are marked. The patient may tolerate small, frequent meals better than three large ones. In some cases, the patient will be able to eat a substantial breakfast but become nauseated after external radiotherapy is administered. Such a patient should be given foods and beverages enjoyed and tolerated. Antiemetic drugs, such as dimenhydrinate (DRAMAMINE), prochlorperazine (COMPAZINE), and trimethobenzamide (TIGAN) may be prescribed to relieve nausea.

The patient who becomes dehydrated as a result of vomiting or diarrhea usually will be given supplemental intravenous fluids and electrolytes. In some patients, radiotherapy may have to be discontinued for a period of time to relieve the symptoms of radiation sickness.

Simple and truthful explanations usually help the patient to get through a difficult time. It is probably best to avoid expressions like radiation sickness, which can be fear provoking. However, a patient who is told that there may be some nausea after radiotherapy will be more relaxed than a patient who fears that nausea means something is wrong with the digestive tract. The nurse should not emphasize the possible reactions the patient may experience following radiation therapy. Explanations should be offered even if the patient does not ask for them. The patient's fears may be allayed by simple explanations, but dwelling on the possible nausea, diarrhea, and vomiting associated with the therapy may precipitate thes symptoms in some individuals.

In x-ray therapy, the skin over the treated area is often marked with indelible ink as a guide for the therapist. These marks are referred to as portal-of-entry marks and should not be removed when the patient is bathed. While the patient is receiving x-ray treatment, the skin covering the treated area should be kept dry and free from further irritation, such as the rubbing of bedclothes. Sometimes cornstarch is prescribed by the physician. This powder can be used liberally as long as the patient's skin is in good condition. X-ray therapy may cause the skin to turn pinkish and to have a reaction. Powders and ointments that contain metals should not be used on the site as there increase the dose of x-ray to the skin. For example, zinc oxide is a metallic substance frequently used in many powders and ointments. However, the nurse may be asked to dust the area with powder containing metallic substances, such as zinc oxide, after the radiotherapy has been completed. Since the skin covering the area being treated with x-ray should be kept as dry as possible, it should not be cleaned with soap and water.

When a patient is receiving internal radiotherapy, the source of radiation is within the patient. It may be implanted in a tumor, injected into a cavity, or taken orally. Whether this patient is isolated or not depends on the radioactive material used, its location, and the type of rays it emits. For example, radioactive phosphorus emits only beta rays, which cannot penetrate through the skin. However, if the radioactive phosphorus (^{32}P) should leak out of the cavity where it was injected, there is the hazard of radioactive rays as the liquid saturates linen or dressings. The nurse can easily recognize this leakage if the ^{32}P has been tinted with a blue dye. If a patient has radium implanted in the cervix, this implant emits gamma rays, which can penetrate inches of lead. Therefore, the nurse usually spends less time with this patient than one receiving radiotherapy with radioactive phosphorus.

Other actions that protect the nurse from overexposure to radioactivity include keeping as much distance as possible from the patient with a radioactive implant, especially one emitting hard gamma rays. For example, the nurse avoids leaning over the patient. In addition, the nurse organizes materials, supplies, and activities to minimize time spent at the bedside. For example, when changing a dressing, the nurse should not get tape and place it on the bedside table and then get the gauze dressings because these two trips place her or him next to a source of radioactivity one time more than is necessary.

Usually a patient receiving internal radiotherapy is placed in a private room with a sing on the door restricting visitors (Figure 9.6). It is important that the patient knows why the precautions are being taken to protect nursing personnel and others. The nurse should tell the patient that the isolation is temporary and that the source of radioactivity will be removed at a certain time or that it will eventually lose its potency and no longer emit rays that can be hazardous to nursing personnel.

Care given to the patient should be planned so that rushing and hurrying are avoided. Since the patient's contact with others is limited, the nurse's warmth, friendliness, and understanding are especially important. Listening to the patient enables the nurse to identify and correct er-

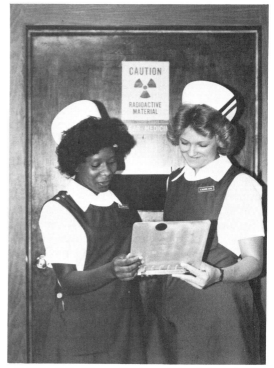

FIGURE 9.6 The patient receiving internal radiotherapy is placed in a private room with a sign on the door. (Courtesy of Washington County School of Practical Nursing, Neff Vocational Center, Abingdon, Virginia.)

rors of knowledge about radiotherapy. Before leaving the patient's room, the nurse should place articles that will be needed with easy reach. If an intercom is used, the patient may need instruction to use it.

Some substances such as vomitus, urine, feces, and perspiration may be radioactive. Therefore, linen and excreta are disposed of according to hospital policy. The nurse caring for a patient receiving any kind of internal radiotherapy should know the source of the radiation, the type of rays emitted, and the precautions necessary to prevent overexposure to harmful radiation (see Table 9.2). All nurses, staff members, family members, and, of course, the patient should be aware of the potential dangers of radiation therapy and how to avoid them.

Should the source of radiation become dislodged from its site of implantation, it should never be handled with bare hands. A

TABLE 9.2
SOME TYPES OF RADIOTHERAPY

SOURCE	FORM	ADMINISTRATION	PRECAUTIONS
I. External Types			
X-ray	Invisible rays	X-ray machine in radiology department	None when patient is on the nursing unit; patient is alone in the special lead-lined room while receiving the therapy
Cobalt^{60} (^{60}Co)	Invisible rays	Cobalt unit in radiology department	
II. Internal Types			
Radium (^{226}Ra)	Needles, plaques, and applicators	Implanted into tumor	Rays are being emitted from the patient; follow instructions as to length of time to remain with patient
Radon	Needles	Implanted into tumor	Rays are being emitted from the patient; follow instructions as to length of time to remain with patient
Cobalt (^{60}Co)	Needles and seeds	Implanted into tumor	Rays are being emitted from the patient; follow instructions as to length of time to remain with patient
Gold (^{198}Au)	Purple liquid	Injected into a cavity	Rays are being emitted from the patient; drainage from the cavity is radioactive
Iodine (^{131}I)	Liquid	By mouth	Same as above plus with large doses; urine, feces, perspiration, and vomitus are also radioactive
Phosphorus (^{32}P)	Liquid	By mouth, intravenously and injected into a cavity	Drainage from the cavity is radioactive (only beta rays are emitted)

pair of long forceps may be in the room in anticipation of such an occurrence. The forceps are used to pick up the material. It is held at arm's length and above waist level. A lead container may be in the room where it is then placed. The radiologist or radiation safety officer should be notified immediately if an implant becomes dislodged or if a radioactive substance leaks from a cavity. The physician or the radiologist accepts the responsibility for removing the implant at a specified time.

PATIENT RECEIVING CHEMOTHERAPY

When assisting in the care of the patient receiving drugs for cancer, the nurse should remember that these drugs can cause severe reactions (see Table 9.3). The drugs are used because they attack rapidly dividing cells. However, the body has cells of its own that normally divide rapidly, such as those of the digestive tract, hair follicles, and bone marrow, and these cells are also attacked by these drugs. Thus, it is easy to understand that toxic reactions most likely to occur include alopecia, gastrointestinal symptoms, and bone marrow depression. A very important nursing responsibility when caring for a patient receiving chemotherapy is to observe, report, and record symptoms that indicate toxicity. Alopecia was described earlier in this chapter. Gastrointestinal symptoms already discussed include stomatitis, nausea, vomiting, diarrhea, and black, tarry stools.

Bone marrow depression results in a decreased production of red and white blood cells. Decreased red cell count usually causes the patient to feel very tired. Platelets (thrombocytes) are cells produced in the bone marrow that are necessary for clotting. A lowered platelet count may cause the patient to have blood in the urine (hematuria),

TABLE 9.3
SELECTED DRUGS USED IN CHEMOTHERAPY OF CANCER

DRUGS	USUAL ROUTE OF ADMINISTRATION	NURSING IMPLICATIONS
I. Antimetabolites		
Cytarabine (CYTOSAR)	Intravenously Intrathecally Subcutaneously	Possible nausea and vomiting, bone marrow depression
Fluorouracil (5-FU)	Intravenously PO	GI ulcerations, bone marrow depression
6-Mercaptopurine	PO	Liver damage, bone marrow depression
Methotrexate	PO IV IM Intrathecally Under investigation—large doses given IV followed by "leucovorin rescue"	GI ulcerations, bone marrow depression
6-Thioguanine (6-TG)	PO Under investigation—IV	Bone marrow depression
II. Alkylating Agents		
Busulfan (MYLERAN)	PO	Pulmonary fibrosis—bone marrow depression
Chlorambucil (LEUKERAN)	PO	Nausea and vomiting, bone marrow depression
Cyclophosphamide (CYTOXAN)	PO IV	Nausea and vomiting, bone marrow depression
Mechlorethamine (nitrogen mustard)	IV Given directly into cavity	Nausea and vomiting, bone marrow depression
Melphalan (ALKERAN)	PO Under investigation—IV	Possible nausea and vomiting, bone marrow depression
Triethylene*thio*phosphoramide (THIOTEPA)	IV Intracavity	Bone marrow depression
III. Antibiotics		
Actinomycin D (dactinomycin)	IV	Nausea and vomiting, GI ulcerations, bone marrow depression
Mithramycin (MITHRACIN)	IV	Nausea and bone marrow depression, GI ulcerations—liver damage
Bleomycin sulfate (BLENOXANE)	IV, IM, SC	Nausea and vomiting, fever, skin changes, pulmonary changes
IV. Hormones		
Androgens	PO IM	Possible nausea and vomiting, masculinization, fluid retention
Corticosteroids	PO IM IV	Fluid retention, hypertension, susceptibility to infections, diabetes, peptic ulcer
Estrogens	PO IV IM	Possible nausea and vomiting, feminization, fluid retention
V. Miscellaneous		
Vinblastine (VELBAN)	IV Under investigation—PO	Some nausea and vomiting, bone marrow depression, loss of reflexes

TABLE 9.3 (*Continued*)

DRUGS	USUAL ROUTE OF ADMINISTRATION	NURSING IMPLICATIONS
Vincristine (ONCOVIN)	IV	GI ulcerations, some bone marrow depression, toxic effects to nervous system
Hydroxyurea (HYDREA)	PO Under investigation—IV	Nausea and vomiting, bone marrow depression, GI ulcerations

vomitus (hematemesis), skin (petechiae, purpura, ecchymoses), and stool, and bleeding from gums, venipuncture, and parenteral injection sites. When the likelihood of bleeding is greatly increased, all interventions that could initiate bleeding are stopped, if possible. These include parenteral injections, using a toothbrush, shaving, and clipping the nails. The patient may be giving blood or blood products and/or platelets intravenously.

The patient receiving chemotherapy may also develop a low white cell count, resulting in an increased susceptibility to infection. The patient's temperature may be taken more frequently, and temperature elevations are reported immediately to the head nurse or team leader. In addition, the temperature is taken any time the patient reports feeling weak, feverish, warm, chilled, or shivery.

The nurse should also watch for any sudden lowering of blood pressure, an increase in respiration called hyperventilation, or confusion because these are some of the signs of shock caused by bacteria in the blood or septic shock. This is a very dangerous condition, and unless medical treatment is promptly initiated, the patient may die. The patient with an extremely low white cell count may be placed in protective isolation. Some hospitals have special rooms with a laminar airflow unit which distributes germ-free air through the room at all times. Visitors stand downwind from the patient. The nurse caring for the patient is protective isolation must use a mask, gloves, and gown. Only sterile items are allowed to come in contact with the patient. The patient in protective isolation usually feels cut off and isolated from others. Feelings of loneliness and despair are also common. The nurse's

warmth, kindness, and support are needed during this time. Transfusions of white blood cells may be prescribed for the patient at this time, also.

The nurse with a calm, reassuring attitude will help the patient through chemotherapy. If a patient is vomiting as a result of receiving a particular drug, the nurse should explain that nausea and vomiting are common side effects of the chemotherapy and will subside. If the nurse knows that the patient will lose hair as a result of the chemotherapy treatments but that it will grow back after the treatments have stopped, the patient should be told this.

PATIENT RECEIVING IMMUNOTHERAPY

The patient receiving BCG (tuberculosis vaccine) is being given this agent in an attempt to stimulate the immune system. If the individual has a melanoma and the nodules caused by this malignancy are injected with BCG, the nurse should observe for signs of infection. The nurse should keep the site of injection clean and dry. The patient should be observed for symptoms of shock associated with an allergic reaction to BCG. Such symptoms should be reported immediately so that prompt treatment can be started.

THE PATIENT WITH TERMINAL CANCER

As the present-day treatment of cancer does not always result in a cure, the nurse frequently is responsible for nursing the patient during a terminal illness. The practical/vocational nurse has a great contribution to make to the patient and the family. The nurse plans care that emphasizes comfort and enjoyment of whatever time is left rather than recovery.

The bedridden patient should be in a clean, pleasant, bright, and cheerful room that is free of unpleasant odors. Since slough or death of tissue produces undesirable odors, the nurse makes every effort to prevent or remove them by keeping the patient and the room clean, maintaining adequate ventilation, changing dressings frequently, and removing soiled materials from the room at once. Deodorizers and commercial products that absorb and remove odors are available in most hospitals.

Measures that enable the patient to remain as active, comfortable, and alert as possible are repeated as often as necessary. For example, narcotic analgesia may be repeated frequently to relieve pain. Intravenous fluids may be prescribed to relieve discomfort associated with dehydration. Oxygen may be prescribed for the patient who has breathing difficulties.

In addition, measures that seem to increase the patient's discomfort generally are avoided. For example, the patient who does not wish to eat, drink, ambulate, or socialize is accepted, cared for, and not pressured to do so.

The nurse's special understanding is needed when dealing with a patient who has developed brain metastasis. This patient often will reject a wife or husband, or children, and other significant individuals. In some cases, the patient may not even recognize loved ones. The nurse must be especially supportive to the patient's family during this stage. Forms of support include listening to the family expressing their anguish and explaining that the patient does not understand or mean to say cruel things. One way to explain is to describe the patient's behavior as resulting from electrical short circuits in the brain caused by tumor cells.

As life ebbs, the inner resources of the nurse are tapped for comfort, understanding, and support needed by the patient and family. The nurse may develop an excellent guide to nursing care needed in this situation by imagining what kind of care would be wanted for the nearest and dearest person in one's own life.

Hospice is a program available to terminally ill patients and their families to control and relieve physical, mental, emotional, and spiritual suffering. This program provides supportive services from a variety of health team members according to the needs of the patient and family. Typical members of a hospice team include the nurse, social worker, physician, and clergyperson. Other members of the health team, such as the pharmacist or dietitian, participate as needed. In addition to relieving suffering, members of the hospice team assist the patient and family with grief work associated with impending death. After the patient's death, the family is helped, when needed, to cope with the loss. Hospice programs may include inpatient and/or outpatient services. Home care is encouraged when possible.

THE GRIEVING NURSE. The grieving process occurs not only in the patient and the family but also in the nurse caring for them. Self-awareness and introspection (looking within oneself) are processes that help the nurse to identify feelings of anger, sadness, and depression that occur when a patient dies. In some cases, persistent unresolved grieving can lead to illness in the nurse or poor care for other patients. Some behaviors that indicate grieving in the nurse include avoidance of other dying patients, withdrawal from other nurses, avoidance of a therapeutic relationship with other patients, fatigue, or recurrent minor illnesses such as the common cold. The nurse who becomes aware that he or she is grieving may be helped by expressing these feelings to a chaplain or trusted friend. Some hospitals have specially trained professional nurses to assist members of the nursing staff, as well as patients and families, with grief work.

Case Study Involving Neoplastic Disease

Mrs. Smith, a 45-year-old married woman, was admitted to the hospital for a workup for breast cancer. She had gone to her gynecologist two weeks previously for an examination, and a small lump in her right breast was found. She has had no breast pain.

Mrs. Smith has been married 20 years to a man she met in college. Mrs. Smith is a high school teacher and a housewife who has spent the majority of her time raising three children, all of whom are now in college.

Mrs. Smith's mother and her maternal grandmother both died of breast cancer. Her grandmother died when she was very young and she doesn't remember very much about it. However, her mother died five years ago and Mrs. Smith remembers her mother's death quite vividly. Her mother first received a diagnosis of metastatic breast cancer seven years ago. Her mother's last months were very painful, and the entire family was left with emotional scars.

Mrs. Smith was admitted to the hospital on Sunday. She appeared very apprehensive and anxious. Monday she received a chest x-ray, had blood drawn for a type and crossmatch for transfusion, CBC and SMA-20. A urinalysis was was done, in addition to an ECG. She signed a permit that stated, "Biopsy with possible right radical mastectomy."

She was scheduled for surgery on Tuesday morning. When the preoperative medication was given, Mrs. Smith started to cry. She was returned to her room late that night. A right modified radical mastectomy had been done. She appeared to be very sleepy. When she awakened, the first thing she said was, "Do I still have it?"

Wednesday morning she got out of bed with assistance. She appeared very withdrawn. When her husband came to visit, Mrs. Smith refused to speak to him.

Thursday morning the nurse found Mrs. Smith staring at her dressing and HEMOVAC and crying.

Saturday morning her dressing was changed. Mrs. Smith took a peek at the incision and cried out, "Oh my God."

The following Thursday she was discharged. Before she was discharged, her doctor told her that her lymph nodes were "negative."

QUESTIONS

1. What do you think was on Mrs. Smith's mind when she was admitted?
2. What in Mrs. Smith's background was making her very apprehensive?
3. What do you think Mr. Smith felt when he found out about his wife's breast lump?
4. What kind of preoperative teaching should be given?
5. Why do you think Mrs. Smith appeared withdrawn after surgery?
6. What could you do to enable Mrs. Smith to start to take an active interest in life again?
7. What is "Reach to Recovery"?
8. What can be done for Mr. Smith?

9. What should you do when you find Mrs. Smith staring at her dressing and crying?
10. Is Mrs. Smith's reaction to her surgery normal?
11. Do you think Mrs. Smith should be forced to look at her incision?
12. What kind of exercises should Mrs. Smith be doing?

Suggestions for Further Study

1. Does your community have a local cancer society? If so, what are its functions?
2. In your opinion, how can the licensed practical/vocational nurse contribute to the early detection of cancer?
3. Mason, Mildred A.; Bates, Grace F.; and Smola, Bonnie K.; *Workbook in Basic Medical-Surgical Nursing*, 3rd ed. Macmillan Publishing Company, New York, 1984, Exercise 9.

Additional Readings

Davis, Anne J.: "To Make Live or Let Die." *American Journal of Nursing*, 81:582 (Mar.), 1981.

Dobihal, Shirley V.: "Hospice: Enabling a Patient to Die at Home." *American Journal of Nursing*, 80:1448–51 (Aug.), 1980.

Hathaway, Donna: "A Cancer Primer." *Journal of Practical Nursing*, 31:20–26 (Oct.), 1981.

Hickman, Robert O., and Bjeletich, Joan: "The Hickman Indwelling Catheter." *American Journal of Nursing*, 80: 62–65 (Jan.), 1980.

Kelly, Patricia Paul, and Tinsley, Cynthia: "Planning Care for the Patient Receiving External Radiation." *American Journal of Nursing*, 81:338–42 (Feb.), 1981.

Koren, Mary Elaine: "Cancer Immuno Therapy: What, Why, When, How?" *Nursing 81*, 11:34–41 (Jan.), 1981.

Maxwell, Mary B.: "Scalp Tourniquets for Chemotherapy-Induced Alopecia." *American Journal of Nursing*, 80:900–902 (May), 1980.

Mondel, Henry R.: "Nurses' Feelings About Working with the Dying." *American Journal of Nursing*, 81:1194–97 (June), 1981.

Moses, Marion: "Cancer and the Workplace." *American Journal of Nursing*, 79:1985–88 (Nov.), 1979.

O'Connell, Anne L.: "Death Sentence: An Invitation to Life." *American Journal of Nursing*, 80:1646–49 (Sept.), 1980.

Paige, Roberta Lyder: "Living and Dying." *American Journal of Nursing*, 79:2171–72 (Dec.), 1979.

Paulen, Ann: "Commit Yourself to Caring." *Journal of Practical Nursing*, 32:26-27 and 40 (Jan.), 1982.

Putnam, Sandra T.; McDonald, Marcia M.; Miller, Margaret M.; Dugan, Sally; and Logue, Gerald: "Home as a Place to Die." *American Journal of Nursing*, 80:1451-53 (Aug.) 1980.

Robinson, Corinne H.: *Basic Nutrition and Diet Therapy*, 4th ed. Macmillan Publishing Co., Inc., New York, 1980, pp. 298-304.

Rose-Williamson, Karla: "Cisplatin: Delivering a Safe Infusion." *American Journal of Nursing*, 81:320-23 (Feb.), 1981.

Sackheim, George I., and Lehman, Dennis D.: *Chemistry of the Health Sciences*, 4th ed. Macmillan Publishing Co., Inc., New York, 1981, pp. 43-66.

Saylor, Rev. Dennis E.: "Nursing Support of the Cancer Patient." *Journal of Practical Nursing*, 32:20-26 (May), 1982.

Strohl, Roberta Anne: "Hospice Care and Professional Coping." *Journal of Nursing Care*, 14:21 and 25 (June), 1981.

Strouth, Sister Clarus: "Radiation: An Invisible Two-Edged Sword." *Journal of Nursing Care*, 14:12-15 (Mar.), 1981.

Taylor, Phyllis B., and Gideon, Marianne D.: "Holding Out Hope to Your Dying Patient— Paradoxical But Possible." *Nursing 82*, 12:42-45 (Feb.), 1982.

Varricchio, Claudette G.: "The Patient on Radiation Therapy." *American Journal of Nursing*, 81:334-37 (Feb.), 1981.

Walker, Marcus L.: "Current Concepts of Hospice Care." *Journal of Nursing Care*, 14:13-15 (June), 1981.

Welch, Deborah, and Lewis, Keith: "Alopecia and Chemotherapy." *American Journal of Nursing*, 80:903-905 (May), 1980.

Chapter 10

The Patient with an Allergy

Expected Behavioral Outcomes
Vocabulary Development
Description of Allergy
Assisting with Diagnostic Studies
Nursing Observations
Nursing Interventions
Respiratory Allergies
Skin and Mucous Membrane Allergies

Gastrointestinal Allergies
Serum and Drug Allergies
Anaphylactic Shock
Autoimmune Diseases
Transplant Rejection
Case Study Involving Bronchial Asthma
Suggestions for Further Study
Additional Readings

Expected Behavioral Outcomes

Minimum objectives referred to as expected behavioral outcomes have been designed for the practical/vocational nursing student to use as guides in studying this chapter. The student should read these expected outcomes before studying the chapter. The objectives can be used as guides for study.

Using the content of this chapter, the study should return to the objectives and evaluate the ability to:

1. *Describe allergy as it relates to the immune reaction discussed in Chapter 5.*
2. *Describe the role of the nurse in each of the diagnostic tests for allergy.*
3. *Describe the role of the nurse in each of the treatments for allergy.*
4. *List the essential nursing observations for a person taking either an antihistamine or a steroid drug.*
5. *Formulate a nursing care plan based on general medical and nursing goals for a person with bronchial asthma.*
6. *List nursing measures that help to relieve some of the discomforts of urticaria, dermatitis, and angioneurotic edema.*
7. *List emergency measures needed for a person who is having an anaphylactic reaction.*
8. *Describe at least six nursing actions that might prevent an allergic reaction.*

Vocabulary Development

The following prefixes, suffixes, and combining forms pertain to this chapter. By learning and/or reviewing their meanings, the practical/vocational nursing student will have the keys needed to unlock many exciting new medical terms.

Discover the meaning of these keys in a medical dictionary or in the content of this chapter. How does each key pertain to this chapter? In your notebook write the correct meaning of each prefix, suffix, or combining form listed below. Illustrate each key with an example.

all—other, different. Ex. *allergy*—a reaction to a substance different from that considered normal.

anti-	hypo-
derm(at)-	ophthalm-
dys-	pne-
ede-	sens-
-gen	

Description of Allergy

The individual with an *allergy* has an overly sensitive reaction to a substance that is normally considered harmless. Another term for allergy is *hypersensitivity*. Allergy develops as a result of a disturbance in the patient's immune response to a foreign substance. Normally, when exposed to a potentially harmful agent, the patient's immune system produces antibodies to destroy or otherwise dispose of that agent. An antigen is the term used to describe those substances capable of stimulating the body to produce antibodies. Inflammation, as described in Chapter 5, is an example of a common antigen-antibody interaction. The patient with an allergy develops a very special antigen-antibody interaction which does not normally occur in nonallergic persons who are exposed to that same substance. The special antigen-antibody interaction that occurs during an allergic reaction does not result in protection but instead causes injury to involved tissues.

The term *antigen* was described earlier as a foreign substance that causes the body to form *antibodies*. An *allergen* is the specific antigen that stimulates the body to defend itself against the normally harmless agent. Allergens are usually natural proteins but can also be complex combinations of proteins, complex carbohydrates known as polysaccharides, lipids, and fats. Eggs, albumins, toxins, bacteria, hormones, viruses, and tissue cells are a few examples of allergens. Allergens are classified by the way they are introduced into the body. Contactants, ingestants, inhalants, injectants, and infectants are the main groups of allergens. Soap is an example of a contactant, foods can be ingestants, pollen can be an inhalant allergen, an insect sting can be an injectant, and certain bacteria can be infectants.

Contact with an allergen is needed for a reaction to occur. In some cases, a reaction occurs on first contact. Usually, repeated contact is needed. The antigen stimulates the body to produce antibodies on first contact. Then, when the allergen is next introduced, an allergic reaction may occur. This process is known as *sensitization*.

There are five major classes of antibodies, or immunoglobulins. They are called IgG, IgA, IgM, IgD, and IgE, which can be remembered by the acronym GAMDE. Although they have basic structural similarities, the antibody classes differ in weight, chemical properties, and what they protect against.

The majority of immunoglobulin, 70 to 80 percent, is comprised of IgG, which helps fight toxins, viruses, and gram-positive pyogenic bacteria.

IgM makes up another 5 to 10 percent and is active against such substances as the endotoxin of gram-negative bacteria.

IgA is found in secretions of the body and helps protect against bacteria and viruses that might try to enter the body through various secretions. Examples of these secretions are saliva, bile, and perspiration.

The function of IgD is not yet known.

IgE, however, is involved in allergic reactions that occur immediately after contact with the allergen. A characteristic of antibodies, or immunoglobulins, is that they are very specific to a particular allergen. When the allergen interacts with IgE, one class of immunoglobulins, the allergic response which usually results is called immediate hypersensitivity. IgE causes the release of histamine. The release of histamine and another substance called serotonin causes constriction of smooth muscle, dilatation of blood vessels, pooling of blood in peripheral blood vessels, and leakage of plasma out of blood vessels into surrounding tissue.

Another type of allergic reaction occurs when special cells called T lymphocytes interact with the allergen to attack, engulf, and destroy it. This can be called *delayed hypersensitivity*. Examples of delayed hypersensitivity are the tuberculosis skin reaction to PPD, contact dermatitis, rejection of kidney transplants, and protection of the body against tumor cells. Scientists believe that T lymphocytes protect by destroying tumor cells when the number is small. Disease results when the number of cells becomes too great.

A third type of allergic reaction, which is currently the subject of considerable research, involves the formation of antibodies against the body's own tissue. Diseases that occur when the body makes antibodies against its own tissues are called autoimmune diseases. Rheumatoid arthritis, systemic lupus erythematosus, and multiple sclerosis are examples of diseases that may be caused by this disturbance in the immune system.

Heredity appears to play an important role in allergy. Persons who have allergies are more likely to come from families who also have allergies. Heredity also may influence the type and severity of allergy a person experiences. The term *atopy* describes allergies that are strongly associated with heredity.

Allergens may be transmitted to the fetus from the mother through the placental circulation. The fetus then develops antibodies and may experience an allergic reaction after birth when exposed to the same allergen. This type of allergy is not inherited, but acquired, and is known as *congenital*.

Other factors known to influence the development of an allergic reaction include infection, hormone disturbances, emotional stress, and weather. The quantity of an allergen and the duration of exposure are influencing factors also.

Assisting with Diagnostic Studies

The diagnosis of allergy can be a long, tiring procedure during which the patient continues to experience unpleasant symptoms. In some cases, the patient may have experienced symptoms for years and been told by others that nothing is wrong before seeing an allergist. Some allergy tests may threaten the patient's life by exposure to an allergen that can result in anaphylaxis (vascular collapse and shock that develop within minutes after contact). The nurse's role in assisting the diagnostic studies related to allergy includes listening, recording, and reporting information from the patient. A second role involves teaching the patient exactly how to participate in diagnostic test. The patient needs explicit instructions so that the allergen can be located as quickly as possible. Some diagnostic tests such as skin tests may be prescribed by the physician and

administered by the nurse. Remembering that diagnostic tests may cause life-threatening reactions enables the nurse to take actions to prevent them or assist when needed. Such actions include locating emergency equipment before diagnostic tests are started and knowing the procedure to be followed when a life-threatening reaction occurs.

HISTORY AND PHYSICAL EXAMINATION

One of the first and most important steps in diagnosing allergy is a careful *history* obtained by the physician. The patient is asked to describe the reaction or illness in detail, including age, onset, activities and diet prior to the attack, exact sequence of symptoms, and frequency of attacks. In addition, a complete health history is obtained including previous illnesses and therapies, and the effects of body changes such as puberty, pregnancy, or menopause. Information about the family is needed to determine if heredity is involved. A social history is needed to determine if a person's life-style has influenced the development of an allergy. An important part of the history includes what the patient believes is causing the allergy and recent stressful life events. During the *physical examination*, the physician carefully examines the area of complaint. Common areas affected by allergy are the nasal mucosa, oral cavity, throat, ears, chest, and skin.

LABORATORY STUDIES

Blood tests may be ordered. The eosinophil count (refer to Table 5.5, page 94) may be helpful in diagnosing an allergy. An elevation of blood eosinophils suggests an allergic condition. Nasal and bronchial secretions also may be examined for eosinophils. Other conditions associated with a rise in eosinophils include parasitic and Hodgkin's diseases. Some physicians order such tests as complete blood count (CBC), blood chemistries, blood serology, and urinalysis. Although these laboratory studies will not detect allergies, they may suggest other conditions requiring treatment. A differential white count, which is done during a complete blood count, includes a measurement of circulating lymphocytes. An additional special test available measures T lymphocytes. IgE levels in the serum also may be measured in some cases. Occasionally, other tests, such as sedimentation rate, cystic fibrosis test, pulmonary function studies, and enzyme studies, may be ordered.

SKIN TESTS

Skin tests may be done to determine the specific allergens. A small amount of a specific allergen is introduced, and the skin is observed for reaction (Figure 10.1). The appearance of a *wheal* (raised, swollen area of skin that itches, burns, or tingles) and an area of redness indicates a positive reaction. The choice of allergens used is based on the client's history. A *scratch* test is a type of skin test in which an allergen is introduced into a superficial scratch and the test site is compared to a control scratch site after 10 to 30 minutes.

An *intracutaneous* test may be used in place of the scratch test. The allergen is diluted in 0.02 ml of sterile liquid and injected between the layers of the skin, *intrader-*

mally. The injection site is compared with the control in 10 minutes.

A *patch* test is used generally to test for allergens causing contact dermatitis. The allergen is placed on the skin and covered with an airtight seal. The site is examined for redness or wheals in 48 to 72 hours.

MUCOUS MEMBRANE TESTS

Mucous membrane tests can be used to pinpoint inhalant allergens that skin tests indicate as doubtful. For example, an *ophthalmic* test may be done by dropping an allergen into the conjunctival sac of the test eye. After 5 to 10 minutes, the two eyes are compared. Redness, tearing, and itching of the test eye indicate a positive reaction. The test eye is immediately flushed with normal saline, and aqueous epinephrine 1:1000 may then be instilled. The *nasal sniff* test is done by introducing the allergen into the test nostril and keeping the other nostril closed. Sneezing, coughing, nasal congestion, and watery nasal discharge indicate a position reaction. This test has more limited use since mildly positive reactions are hard to detect and uncomfortable nasal symptoms

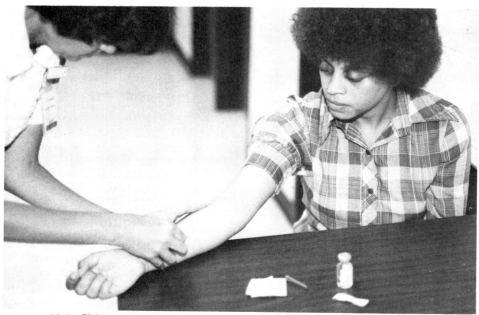

FIGURE 10.1 Skin testing for allergy. (Courtesy of Loudoun County School of Practical Nursing, Leesburg, Virginia.)

may persist after a positive reaction has occurred.

ELIMINATION DIETS

Elimination diets may be prescribed when food is the suspected allergen. The patient may be asked to keep a record of all foods consumed for a certain length of time. Foods likely to act as allergens are eliminated. When all symptoms have disappeared for one week, foods are gradually introduced until symptoms recur. The last food added before recurrence of symptoms may be considered the allergen.

Nursing Observations

Nursing observations of the patient with allergy are usually related to the release of histamine, serotonin, prostaglandins, and other substances that resemble histamine. Histamine has a profound effect on the circulatory system, bronchi of the respiratory system, gastrointestinal system, and skin. Symptoms of allergy are generally the result of histamine and similar substances acting on body tissues. For example, erythema (redness) and edema (swelling) are caused by the dilating effect of histamine on blood vessels. Histamine may cause muscle spasm in the respiratory or gastrointestnal systems, resulting in symptoms such as wheezing or abdominal cramps. Histamine produces skin eruptions that are characteristic of some reactions.

Symptoms may be local or general, immediate or delayed, uncomfortable or life-threatening. An allergy is described as *seasonal* when symptoms occur during a specific time of year or *perennial* if there is no relationship between symptoms and time of year.

The type and amount of allergen exposure, the kind of antibody produced, the nature of affected tissue, and the substances released during the reaction determine symptoms and severity. Table 10.1 provides a guide to nursing observations related to the patient with an allergy.

Nursing Interventions

The patient experiencing an allergy attack needs a quiet, restful environment and an understanding, supportive nurse. Understanding the discomfort, frustration, and fatigue the patient faces enables the nurse to take actions to relieve these conditions. Knowing facts about the client's allergic condition and related therapy enables the nurse to explain and assist in carrying out the doctor's orders. Realizing the influence of emotions and infections on symptoms helps the nurse to teach the patient how to cope with these stressors.

ASSISTING WITH ALLERGY THERAPY

Treatment of an individual with an allergy is determined by symptoms and the type of allergy. The basic methods of treatment include avoidance of allergens, hyposenitization, and drug therapy.

AVOIDANCE OF ALLERGENS

In many instances the food, the inhalant, or the substance can be removed from the person's environment altogether. This eliminates the need for any further therapy. In some cases, the allergen is too vastly distributed to eliminate. The patient may change the place of work or residence in order to avoid exposure. At times, the level of concentration of the allergen can be greatly reduced or eliminate, with careful planning, as with cigarette smoke, house dust, and animal dander.

Avoidance of allergens may cause great inconvenience and unhappiness to the patient and family. Never eating favorite foods, not being able to have a pet, or having to find a new occupation can have an overwhelming psychosocial impact. The person who must change life-style in order to avoid allergens can be expected to show emotions such as fear or anger and to use some of the defense mechanisms described in Chapter 1. Loss of a familiar life-style can cause the person to experience some or all of the phases associated with grieving.

HYPOSENSITIZATION (DESENSITIZATION, HYPERIMMUNIZATION)

Hyposensitization is a treatment that reduces a person's sensitivity to a known allergen by building up tolerance to that aller-

TABLE 10.1
GUIDE TO OBSERVING THE PATIENT WITH AN ALLERGY

WHAT TO OBSERVE	OBSERVATIONS
Eyes	Discolorations under eyes Excessive tearing Redness (erythema) Rubbing the eyes Itching or burning Swelling of eyelids
Nose	Sniffing, sneezing, snorting Changes in sense of smell Nasal congestion Runny nose Twitching of nose
Ears	Decreased hearing Drainage Earache
Mouth	Swelling (edema) of lips, tongue Frequent clearing of throat Erythema (redness) of oropharynx Changes in sense of taste Mouth breathing Nasal sound to voice Vomiting Hoarseness Blisters on mucous membranes
Chest	Wheezing, shortness of breath
Abdomen	Indigestion Colicky, cramping pain
Skin	Dry and scaly Itching Rashes Erythema or pallor
Behavioral changes	Restlessness and other behavior indicating anxiety

gen. An extract of the allergen is injected subcutaneously in minute amounts at intervals. The dose is increased and may reach 100 to 1000 or more times the strength of the initial dose before symptoms subside. The intervals between injections may lengthen and may finally be discontinued by the physician if the person no longer reacts to the allergen. In some cases, a maintenance dose may be needed. The exact action of this therapy is not clearly understood. Repeated exposure to small amounts of the allergen appears to stimulate the formation of *blocking* antibodies, which prevent the allergen from reaching the appropriate antibody to stimulate the allergic response. The nurse often assists with hyposensitization by administering the allergen according to the physician's prescription (Figure 10.2). Table 10.2 contains a summary of nursing actions related to hyposensitization.

Serious local or general reactions can occur during hyposensitization. The patient should be observed carefully in the doctor's office or clinic for 30 minutes following injection. Ice may applied to the injection site in the case of a serious local skin reaction. A general reaction must be treated immediately in order to prevent collapse, shock, and death. A general reaction would include the following symptoms: apprehension, increased respirations, pallor, weakness, and/

nephrine particularly relaxes the smooth muscles of the respiratory tract and dilates the bronchioles, which is effective in relieving asthmatic attacks. Urticaria, hay fever, angioneurotic edema, and serum sickness are allergic conditions discussed later in this chapter that may be helped by epinephrine. Epinephrine may be administered by subcutaneous, intramuscular, and intravenous routes and occasionally by nebulization. The dosage must be adjusted individually but generally is 0.1 to 0.5 ml of 1:1000 aqueous epinephrine. The duration of action is usually short, and repeated injections may be needed to produce the desired effects. Side effects can be extremely serious or fatal and seem to be more common when the drug is administered intravenously. Hypertension, cardiac arrhythmias, tachycardia, apprehension, pulmonary edema, and headache are side effects that the nurse should observe and report.

Epinephrine solution should not be used if it appears brown in color or as sediment.

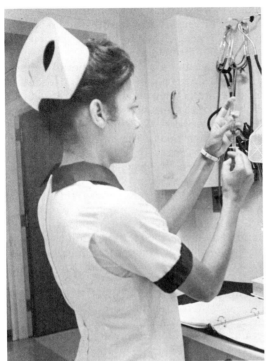

FIGURE 10.2 The nursing student is preparing an allergen to be used for hyposensitization. (Courtesy of Martinsville-Henry County School of Practical Nursing, Martinsville, Virginia.)

or faintness. A tourniquet should be available so that it can be placed above the injection site immediately, if necessary. Emergency drugs such as epinephrine, antihistamines, and steroids should be available for the physician to use if needed.

DRUG THERAPY

Drug therapy may be prescribed by the physician to reverse the reaction, reduce or treat symptoms, prevent complications, or prevent recurrence.

Epinephrine (*adrenaline*) is a hormone, secreted naturally by the adrenal medulla, that apparently counteracts the actions of histamine. Epinephrine is a potent vasoconstrictor that may be prescribed to halt the progress of anaphylactic shock and reduce the harmful changes associated with histamine release. Edema may be reduced by the vasoconstricting action of epinephrine. Epi-

TABLE 10.2
SUMMARY OF NURSING ACTIONS RELATED TO
HYPOSENSITIZATION

1. Before administering an allergen, check emergency equipment to make sure it is complete and in good working order.
2. Store bottles containing allergen in upright position in refrigerator to avoid leakage and contamination of rubber stopper.
3. Before administering an allergen, ask the patient if redness (erythema) and warmth occurred around the site following the last injection. Report the approximate size to the physician since a change in dose may be needed.
4. Before administering an allergen, report to the physician if the patient has missed the previous appointment. A change in dose may be needed.
5. Use an extremity to inject the allergen so that a tourniquet can be applied in case of an anaphylactic reaction.
6. Insure that the needle used to inject an allergen is not in the vein. Accidental injections into a vein may cause anaphylaxis.
7. Observe the patient closely for 30 minutes after hyposensitization for local or general reaction.

The vial should be discarded or returned to the pharmacist.

Ephedrine acts similarly to epinephrine, but it is not nearly so potent. It can be taken orally and in nasal sprays or drops. Ephedrine particularly acts as a nasal decongestant. When such drops or sprays are overused for nasal congestion, rebound congestion may occur when the temporary effects of vasoconstriction wear off. As nasal congestion recurs, the patient uses more drops or spray, congestion follows and a cycle develops of spray-rebound congestion-spray. In order to prevent this cycle, the patient is given information about the cycle and instructed to use sprays according to the physician's prescription.

Antihistamines block the action of histamine on blood vessels and bronchioles. These drugs are especially vital in the treatment of anaphylactic shock, serum sickness, hay fever, and urticaria. Antihistamines also have a drying effect on mucous membranes. They may be prescribed when nasal congestion is a symptom of allergy. The drying effect, however, may actually increase difficulties in asthma by drying bronchial secretions and causing the patient to have much more difficulty in coughing up secretions. For this reason, antihistamines may not be prescribed for a person experiencing an attack of bronchial asthma.

Antihistamine action is generally short, and drowsiness almost always is present as a side effect. Other important side effects include vertigo (dizziness) and visual disturbances. Persons who take antihistamines should be warned of the hazards of driving, performing exacting tasks, or operating dangerous equipment while taking the drug. Hospitalized persons should be protected from accidents by having the siderails up when in bed and by having a nurse or family present when out of bed. Table 10.3 lists commonly prescribed antihistamines.

Steriods are hormones secreted by the pituitary gland and the adrenal cortex. Steroid therapy may be ordered for its anti-inflammatory effects. Table 18.5 (p. 589) lists common steroids the physician may prescribe. A variety of preparations are available for oral, parenteral, or topical use.

Generally, short-term steroid therapy is more desirable in order to avoid serious side effects. When long-term therapy is necessary, certain precautions are taken to pre-

TABLE 10.3
ANTIHISTAMINES

NONPROPRIETARY NAME	TRADE NAME	SINGLE ADULT DOSE	NURSING IMPLICATIONS ASSOCIATED WITH ANTIHISTAMINE THERAPY
Antazoline	ANTISTINE	100 mg	
Carbinoxamine	CLISTIN	4 mg	
Chlorpheniramine	CHLOR-TRIMETON TELDRIN HISTAPAN	2–4 mg	Patient should be warned against hazards of drowsiness
Cromolyn	INTAL	20 mg	Patient should be cautioned to inhale only to prevent asthma. Not effective once symptoms develop.
Brompheniramine	DIMETANE DISOMER	2–4 mg	Patient should be prepared for nuisance of dry mouth and dryness of other mucous membrane surfaces
Dimenhydrinate	DRAMAMINE	50 mg	Drugs have a natural short action
Diphenhydramine	BENADRYL	50 mg	Patient can build up tolerance to antihistamines
Meclizine	BONINE	25–50 mg	
Promethazine	PHENERGAN	25–50 mg	
Pyrilamine	NEO-ANTERGAN PARAMINYL PYRAMAL STAMINE	25–50 mg	May produce changes in sexual interest
Tripelennamine	PYRIBENZAMINE	50 mg	

vent, detect, or treat side effects. Synthetic preparations are used more often because they are less expensive and produce fewer side effects.

The most common side effects of steroid therapy are edema, crampy muscle pains, increased appetite, skin changes, gastric disorders, mental changes, and electrolyte imbalance. A particularly serious side effect is gastrointestinal bleeding. For this reason, antacids or milk may be prescribed for the person on systemic steroid therapy. In addition, frequent examination of the stools for blood may be ordered to detect early signs of gastrointestinal bleeding.

Systemic steroid therapy may cause the patient to experience a feeling of euphoria and psychologic dependence. If this occurs, the patient may not be capable of being concerned about illness. A state of excessive excitement, restlessness, and sleeplessness may occur. The nurse may help the patient to become calmer by reducing and/or removing exciting stimuli from the environment. The patient may experience marked mood swings from agitation to depression. Such extremes in behavior should be reported to the physician. The patient needs support from all members of the health team during this time. The nurse also may help to reorient the patient if necessary. Although such adverse reactions are rare, they do occur, and the nurse should understand that they have little relationship to the length of time the drug has been given. Steroids are tapered when being discontinued to avoid adrenal insufficiency.

A high-protein diet with calcium salt supplements may be prescribed for a patient on long-term systemic steroid therapy. Bone deterioration can result from the metabolic changes that occur during steroid therapy. Antispasmodics such as diphenoxylate and atropine (LOMOTIL) or tincture of belladonna may be prescribed for gastrointestinal symptoms.

Long-term steroid therapy may cause an endocrine disorder as a result of suppression of the pituitary's adrenocorticotropic hormone. This suppression leads to adrenal insufficiency, which leaves the patient unable to withstand any unusual stress. The patient may go into a severe or fatal collapse if steroids are withdrawn abruptly. The likelihood of collapse is increased if there is serious injury, surgery, or other illness. For this reason, the patient on steroid therapy should wear a bracelet or other device that identifies this fact to health personnel in the event of an emergency.

DEVELOPING A THERAPEUTIC RELATIONSHIP

In establishing a therapeutic relationship, the nurse may notice that some patients with an allergy seem irritable, fatigued, and depressed. As previously mentioned, the diagnosis and treatment of allergy may be lengthy, tiring, and expensive for the patient. Active listening is especially important since some patients find it easier to communicate with the nurse than the physician about the effects of symptoms and therapy on everyday life. The nurse's confidence that the patient can be helped often helps the patient to develop a more optimistic outlook. The nurse's interest in the patient may help to uncover new facts important in diagnosis and treatment. In talking with the patient, the nurse may learn of emotional conflicts at home, at work, or in the hospital. This should be reported to the appropriate nurse or physician since such conflicts may start or aggravate symptoms in some people.

The patient with allergies involving skin eruptions can be expected to experience disturbances in body image related to a changed appearance. In some cases, the patient may want to discuss concerns about his or her appearance with the nurse. In other cases, the patient does not wish to discuss concerns but appreciates instead the nurse's warmth, friendliness, and acceptance.

PATIENT TEACHING

Patient teaching for the person with allergy includes general topics as well as those related to the specific allergy and therapy. For example, since colds and respiratory infections may initiate or aggravate an allergic reaction, the patient is taught preventive measures such as avoiding crowds, infected persons, and fatigue. In some cases, patient teaching includes general measures related to health practices such as nutrition and hygiene.

The patient with an allergy is taught to develop a habit of reading labels when purchasing foods, clothing, cosmetics, household products, and other consumer items. Generally, products in spray cans are avoided because the spray may aggravate an allergy. The person with an allergy should report that fact before having a permanent wave or change of hair color. The patient usually is taught to avoid the use of nonprescribed medication as well.

Another topic included in patient teaching is helping the patient find ways to use prescribed therapy at home. For example, the patient may need help in planning when to use prescribed medication, and related foods and fluids to avoid or include. Another patient may need help to avoid certain allergens in the home. Still another patient may need assistance in finding ways to increase fluid intake to 4000 ml per day. In some cases, the patient may be taught how to minimize unpleasant symptoms. For example, some patients obtain partial relief of itching by scratching the bed linens.

Since many persons with an allergy are on drug therapy, an important part of patient teaching includes information about toxic symptoms and side effects as discussed previously in this chapter.

PREVENTING ACUTE ATTACKS

Nursing actions that prevent acute allergy attacks in hospitalized patients may be lifesaving. Table 10.4 summarizes the nurses's activities related to prevention of acute allergic reactions.

Respiratory Allergies

HAY FEVER (ALLERGIC RHINITIS, POLLINOSIS)

This condition affects about 13 million Americans and causes them considerable discomfort. Hay fever is most frequent between the ages of 15 and 40, but occurs in other age groups. The more correct term, *pollinosis*, has not replaced the original misnomer, hay fever, even though hay is not the cause and fever is not a symptom. This is a

TABLE 10.4
GUIDE TO NURSING ACTIONS THAT PREVENT
ACUTE ALLERGY ATTACKS

1. Collect, record, and report information on any allergies reported by a newly admitted patient.
2. When the patient has an allergy, alert other health team members such as the dietitian, pharmacist, and medical laboratory technologist according to hospital policy and procedure.
3. Before administering a new medication or applying a new substance to the skin, ask first if the patient has ever had a reaction. Report reactions to appropriate nurse.
4. Regularly inspect the patient's skin for rashes. Record and report all rashes.
5. Teach the patient to report symptoms of allergy such as itching, burning, and tearing of eyes.
6. Apply the special allergy bracelet to the patient's wrist according to hospital policy.

seasonal allergy induced by airborne pollens of trees, grasses, and weeds. Plant life produces pollen in trees during the spring, in grasses during the summer, and in weeds during the fall, causing three different periods of reactions. An individual may be hypersensitive to pollens in all three groups, producing a nearly continuous reaction. The reaction generally occurs within the same approximate dates each year, frequently producing *rhinitis* (inflammation of the nose).

Pollinosis may also be perennial and may be precipitated by changes in temperature; humidity; atmospheric irritants such as smoke, dust, dander, nasal sprays and drops; or psychosomatic factors. Perennial pollinosis, if untreated, can result in chronic otitis media and loss of hearing. Loss of smell and asthma may occur also. The cause of pollinosis is not known. Heredity appears to be a factor in this type of allergy.

During an acute attack, the person with pollinosis may develop rhinitis. The mucous membrane of the nose may become so edematous that the nostrils close completely. The membrane itches, burns, and secretes a watery, irritating discharge (coryza). Violent parosysms of sneezing occur, and the eyes burn, itch, lacrimate, and appear red. The diagnosis is made by the physician from the history and skin tests.

Since few persons can avoid all pollens, the usual treatment of pollinosis includes hyposensitization and symptomatic relief with an antihistamine such as those listed in Table 10.3. A nasal spray such as dexamethasone (DECADRON) may be prescribed for short periods to relieve nasal congestion. Occasionally, a short course of steroids may be prescribed when the patient's symptoms are especially severe.

BRONCHIAL ASTHMA

The patient with bronchial asthma has recurrent spasms of bronchial airways caused by an allergy. This type of asthma, also known as extrinsic asthma, is frequently associated with a strong family history for asthma and other allergies such as eczema, angioneurotic edema, hay fever, urticaria, and dermatitis, which are discussed in other sections of this chapter. Another type of asthma, known as nonallergic or intrinsic asthma, is seen in clients with emphysema, pneumoconiosis, chronic bronchitis, and cardiac failure and is discussed in other portions of this text.

An acute attack occurs as a result of inhaled allergens which come in contact with IgE antibodies in the tracheobronchial tree. This interaction eventually results in the release of substances such as histamine, serotonin, and prostaglandin which act to produce contraction of smooth muscle, dilatation of blood vessels, swelling, and increased mucous production in the respiratory system. Beside exposure to the allergen, other factors that can contribute to an acute attack include pollutants, laughing, exercise, cold air, nasal polyps, and aspirin sensitivity.

Although most acute attacks are self-limiting regardless of treatment, some patients develop a severe asthma that does not respond to the conventional methods of treatment. Such a continuous condition is called *status asthmaticus* and may be related to overuse of tranquilizers, sedatives, and nebulized isoproterenol (ISUPREL), or respiratory infection. Status asthmaticus is a medical emergency that requires prompt treatment in order to prevent respiratory failure and death. Rarely, a bronchoscopy or tracheostomy (refer to Chapter 14) may be required to save the life of a patient in status asthmaticus. During these procedures, trapped mucus and secretions can be removed, and air passages can be irrigated. Complications such as respiratory failure, cardiac insufficiency, atelectasis, and bronchopneumonia cause most of the deaths associated with asthma. Also, asthma can result in one or more chronic conditions, such as bronchitis or chronic obstructive pulmonary disease (COPD).

ASSISTING WITH DIAGNOSTIC STUDIES

The physician may order a variety of tests to identify the specific type of asthma as well as monitor the patient's response to therapy. During an acute attack, diagnostic tests generally include a history and physical examination, chest x-ray, sputum examination, and frequent measurements of arterial blood gases (see Chapter 14 for additional information). When the patient becomes symptom-free, skin tests and serum Ig levels may be ordered to identify the specific allergen, if possible. Pulmonary function studies such as those described in Chapter 14 also may be ordered to determine if damage to ventilation has occurred.

NURSING OBSERVATIONS

The patient with an acute attack usually notices a nonproductive cough and wheezing at first. Within hours or days, the patient may feel a tightness in the chest and dyspnea. Often, symptoms begin at night while the patient is sleeping. An acute attack may resolve by itself in several hours or may become increasingly severe requiring hospitalization. Table 10.5 contains a guide to nursing observations for the patient during an acute asthma attack. In using this guide, the nurse should remember that signs of other allergies such as those listed in Table 10.1 also may be present.

NURSING INTERVENTIONS

Nursing interventions for the patient with asthma are directed toward relieving

TABLE 10.5
GUIDE TO NURSING OBSERVATIONS FOR THE PATIENT WITH ASTHMA

WHAT TO OBSERVE	OBSERVATIONS
Eyes	May be widened, staring, or show evidence of fear
	Evidences of other allergies from Table 10.1
Nose	Flaring nostrils
	Evidences of other allergies from Table 10.1
Mouth	Mouth breathing
	Dry mouth
	Nausea and vomiting
	Cyanosis about lips in later stages
	Evidences of other allergies from Table 10.1
Cough	Dry at first
	Colorless, thick mucus which gradually becomes thinner
Neck	Neck muscle activity may be visible during dyspnea
Chest	Feeling of tightness
	Accessory muscle activity may be visible during dyspnea
	Shape of chest may be changed by overly inflated lungs
	Pain in chest may be reported
Respirations	Rate is increased
	Expiration longer than inspiration
	Wheezing on inspiration and expiration (Figure 10.3)
Extremities	Cool to touch
	Color pale
	Pulse rapid and weak
Abdomen	Distention may develop from swallowing air
Skin	Diaphoresis (profuse perspiration)
	Cool to touch
	Color pale or ashen
	Cyanosis may develop in later stages

apprehension, making pulmonary secretions thin and more liquid, improving breathing, and monitoring the patient's response to therapy. Most of these interventions are discussed in detail in Chapter 14.

ASSISTING WITH DRUG THERAPY. The nurse can anticipate that a variety of drugs will be prescribed for the patient during an acute attack of asthma. Epinephrine (adrenaline), isoproterenol (ISUPREL or MEDI-HALER ISO) by nebulizer, and ephedrine are examples of drugs used to relax muscle spasm and dilate bronchi.

Epinephrine is such a powerful and rapid-acting drug that it is often the first one prescribed during an acute attack. Unfortunately, tolerance often develops after repeated use.

Another group of drugs commonly prescribed to dilate bronhi is called theophylline preparations. These drugs include aminophylline and theophylline. Specific preparations are available for inhalation, intravenous, oral, or rectal administration. Side effects of theophylline preparations include skeletal muscle twitching, gastrointestinal symptoms such as nausea and vomiting, and tachycardia. Beverages containing caffeine such as coffee, tea, and cola generally are avoided when these drugs are prescribed. Blood levels of theophylline preparations are measured regularly to prevent toxicity.

Steriod therapy may be prescribed to prevent or relieve severe attacks (Table 18.5, page 589). A corticosteroid is usually administered intravenously during an acute attack and orally when longer therapy is

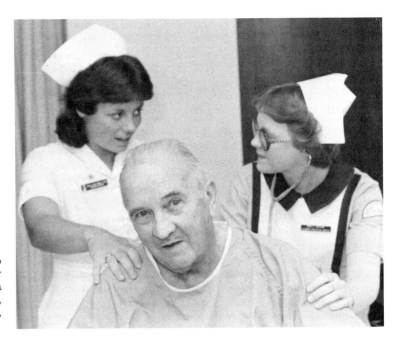

FIGURE 10.3 Listening to the patient's chest. (Courtesy of Crawford County Area Vocational-Technical School, Practical Nursing Program, Meadville, Pennsylvania.)

needed. Long-term steroid therapy has enabled some persons to live a more normal life by reducing the severity and frequency of acute attacks.

A variety of other drugs may also be prescribed. For example, expectorants such as those listed in Table 14.3 may help to loosen retained secretions. Antibiotics may be prescribed to prevent or treat a respiratory infection. Several new drugs are available to prevent acute asthma attacks. Cromolyn sodium (INTAL) comes in powder form encased in a capsule. The medication is inhaled by a special inhaler, usually four times daily. Cromolyn is used to prevent attacks of asthma and has no value in treating the individual who is having an attack of asthma. Metaproterenol and terbutaline are drugs that have actions similar to that epinephrine. They also have the additional advantages of oral administration and longer duration of action without unfavorable side effects on the heart. The physician may prescribe one of these drugs very six hours for relief of bronchospasm. Opiates, sedatives, and tranquilizers are avoided for the patient having an acute asthmatic attack because they cause respiratory depression.

ASSISTING WITH INHALATION THERAPY. Oxygen therapy may be prescribed for the patient having an acute attack of asthma. A nasal cannula may be the preferred route of administratin. When oxygen is ordered as a part of therapy, the dosage is usually low (2 to 3 liters per minute).

Intermittent positive pressure breathing (IPPB) may be prescribed. A machine such as the Bennett ventilator is used for this purpose. The equipment is designed to supply the patient with either air or oxygen under an increased amount of pressure during inspiration. If a medication is prescribed, it is carried into the lungs during inspiration. The patient's inhalation is helped by the increased air pressure, and exhalation takes place without assistance from the machine. Although IPPB therapy may benefit some patients, it cannot be tolerated by others.

Humidification or providing adequate moisture for the mucous membrane of the respiratory tract is essential in relieving and controlling asthmatic attacks. The patient's mucous membrane can become so dry from dyspnea that a condition known as rebound dyspnea may develop. A humidifier can be used in the room to increase the humidity, which in turn would increase the moisture of the patient's mucous membranes. The inhalation of either moisture-laden cool air or steam may be prescribed to soothe irritated mucous membranes. Inhaling moist air may cause the patient's bronchial secretions to become thinner and easier to expectorate.

ASSISTING WITH FOOD AND FLUIDS. The patient usually has no desire to eat or drink because all efforts are directed toward breathing. During an acute attack, more mucous is produced. At the same time, the patient may lose considerable amounts of fluid through perspiration, exhalation, and vomiting. This combination of events leads to thicker, more tenacious secretions in the tracheobronchial tree which cannot be expectorated and may plug small air passages. Therefore, fluid replacement is an important intervention. Intravenous fluids are generally prescribed at the beginning of an acute attack both to dilute intravenous medications and prevent excessive fluid losses. In addition, the physician may prescribe an oral intake of 3000 to 4000 ml per day. Actions the nurse may take to increase the patient's oral intake include setting goals for the amount of liquid to be consumed per hour, offering fluids the patient enjoys, and praising the patient's efforts. The student may locate additional specific information about increasing the patient's fluid intake on page 410.

The patient may be able to tolerate small frequent feedings better than the usual three meals per day. Some patients are too tired from breathing to eat. In this instance, the nurse may feed the patient until the acute attack subsides. Nausea and vomiting may occur as a result of the acute attack or from drug therapy. In some cases, a liquid diet may be prescribed until the patient's symptoms subside.

DEVELOPING A THERAPEUTIC RELATIONSHIP. During an acute asthmatic attack, the patient is generally very frightened. Remaining with the patient and returning as often as possible are nursing interventions that help to reduce fear and prevent panic which can worsen breathing. Other similar interventions include telling the patient when the nurse will return, how to call for help, and placing the call bell within easy reach. Explaining equipment, reasons for certain tests, and therapies also helps to relieve apprehension. Nursing interventions that relieve dyspnea communicate that the patient's well-being and comfort are important to the nurse. For example, helping the patient find a comfortable position, removing constricting clothing, and frequent checking of equipment may be very reassuring to the dyspneic patient.

When talking with the patient, the nurse uses short simple, sentences that do not require responses. The patient generally is not able to participate in conversation when breathing is difficult.

PROMOTING REST AND SLEEP. The person experiencing an attack of bronchial asthma needs mental and physical rest. The increased work of breathing and considerable apprehension which the patient experiences during an acute attack result in overwhelming fatigue. The surroundings should be comfortable, cool, quiet, and unhurried. Generally, the patient will be tired and want to rest after recovering from an acute asthmatic attack. The patient should be allowed to have undisturbed sleep following such an attack.

Medication for sleep generally is avoided because it depresses respiratory centers in the brain. Therefore, nursing measures such as backrubs, hygiene, adequate ventilation, and reduction of noise and light in the environment may be used to help the patient sleep.

HYGIENE. Diaphoresis and humidified air usually cause the patient's clothing and bed linens to become damp within hours. Frequent changes may be indicated during an acute attack. Simple sponging of the patient's face, neck and hands with a cool cloth often provides welcome refreshment and comfort. Frequent oral hygiene is needed when the patient is dyspneic both to keep mucous membranes moist and prevent overgrowth of bacteria in the mouth.

As secretions become more liquid and the patient's cough becomes productive, additional tissues and a paper bag for tissue disposal should be placed at the bedside. The nurse should record characteristics of the patient's sputum in the nurse's notes.

PREVENTING FUTURE ATTACKS. After the acute attack has subsided, the physician and/or clinical nurse specialist usually develops a program to help the patient prevent future attacks. Such a program may include drug therapy, hyposensitization when the specific allergen can be identified, and breathing exercises. For example, exercises for breathing, such as those learned by voice students and musicians playing wind instruments, strengthen the diaphragm and help the patient to expectorate the secretions causing wheezing. Practice in blowing up balloons or blowing into bottles can be helpful if done regularly. Other measures previously discussed in this chapter such as prevention of infection and fatigue and managing emotional upsets apply to this patient. Table 10.6 contains a summary of medical and nursing goals for the patient with asthma.

TABLE 10.6
SUMMARY OF MEDICAL AND NURSING GOALS FOR THE ASTHMATIC PATIENT

I. Acute attacks
  A. Provide a patent airway
  - Administer ordered medications
  - Isoproteronol via nebulizer
  - Aminophylline via slow intravenous drip
  - Epinephrine subcutaneously
  - Corticosteroids for inflammation and edema of respiratory tract
  - Assess effects of drug therapy
  - Check for signs of cardiac involvement with ensuing congestive failure
  - Prepare patient for relief of bronchial obstruction if needed via bronchoscopy
  B. Treat hypoxia
  - Intermittent positive pressure breathing (IPPB) may be used for some patients
  - Use oxygen sparingly
  - Check for buildup of carbon dioxide in bloodstream, called carbon dioxide narcosis
  C. Liquefy secretions
  - Maintain fluid and electrolyte balance

  - Humidify environment
  - Administer drug therapy as prescribed
  - Encourage oral fluid intake
  D. Relieve exhaustion and anxiety
  - Keep the patient comfortable
  - Support patient in chosen position
  - Maintain a quiet, cool environment
  - Hold traffic, talk, and visitors to a minimum
  - Provide opportunity for undisturbed sleep after attack
  - Remain calm; be positive; provide the psychosocial support so necessary to improve the patient's morale and sense of well-being

II. Prevent further attacks with individualized therapy
  A. Discuss precipitating factors to avoid
  B. Determine allergens that must be removed from environment
  C. Encourage and explain desensitization program when indicated
  D. Describe and carry out maintenance therapy
  - Bronchodilators
  - IPPB therapy
  - Cromolyn sodium if prescribed
  - Corticosteroids
  E. Explain the importance of controlling infections
  - Stress need for an early call to the doctor when symptoms of respiratory infection first appear
  - Observe respiratory secretions for change in color and consistency
  - Carry out medical regime for respiratory infections
  - Teach patient to avoid infectious persons
  F. Begin rehabilitation
    1. Teach patient to accept condition and assume responsibility for maintaining good health
    - Avoid irritants
    - Humidify and filter environment air when possible
    - Notify doctor of symptoms
    - Follow planned regime of diet, rest, and exercise that does not increase symptoms
    2. Provide psychosocial support
    - Encourage expression of anxieties
    - Assist patient to see relationship of stress to condition
    - Assist patient to gain insight into situational problems

The patient on drug therapy needs teaching related to toxicity, side effects, and correct usage. For example, cromolyn sodium (INTAL) is not effective once symptoms develop. For this reason, the patient using this drug should be instructed not to take it if symptoms are present.

Skin and Mucous Membrane Allergies

The individual with allergic dermatoses has skin eruptions that are caused by an allergy. Several types of allergic conditions involve the skin.

Urticarial dermatoses include diseases such as urticaria (hives) and angioedema. *Inflammatory* dermatoses include *atopic* (inherited) and *contact* diseases. *Eczema* is a popular term associated with inflammatory disorders. Individuals with allergic dermatoses have certain common symptoms, including *pruritus* (itching) and localization of the eruption to certain body areas.

The diagnosis of these allergic skin conditions is made by the physician, usually on the basis of the patient's history, typical appearance of skin lesions, and skin testing. In addition to measures used to relieve the patient's symptoms, treatment usually includes avoidance of the allergen and/or hyposensitization.

URTICARIA

The individual with urticaria has hives or nettle rash. Many *wheals* (swollen raised areas) appear on the skin, which may itch, tingle, and burn. The wheals vary in size and may come and go quickly. The wheal may be white, pink, or red. Acute attacks may last from several hours to a few days. Also, acute attacks occur more often in summer and usually affect children. Urticaria may be chronic, and this form occurs more frequently in adult women. Urticaria may be caused by allergens such as foods or drugs. In some cases, urticaria is related to systemic disease, particularly infection. Other factors related to the development of urticaria include sunlight, heat and cold, undue fatigue, constipation, and emotional influences. If the specific allergen is identified, the physician may prescribe avoidance or hyposensitization. However, in many individuals, the cause cannot be found. Usually, a simple diet is advised and the patient is instructed to avoid all nonessential medication, especially aspirin and penicillin. Drug therapy such as antihistamines may be prescribed by the physician to clear the wheals. If skin erruptions persist for more than several days, the physician may prescribe short-term drug therapy with a corticosteriod. Local therapy such as calamine lotion, cornstarch, or oatmeal (AVEENO) baths may soothe pruritus. Occasionally, urticaria is so extensive that anaphylactic shock or angieodema occurs. These are life-threatening complications that require prompt medical attention.

ANGIOEDEMA (ANGIOENEUROTIC EDEMA)

The patient with angioedema has diffuse swelling of the deeper layers of the skin and subcutaneous tissue. The skin over the involved area may appear normal or slightly pink. The lips, eyelids, cheeks, hands, feet, genitalia, and tongue are the areas most frequently involved. Mucous membranes of the larynx, bronchi, and gastrointestinal tract also may be affected. The patient often complains of itching and burning before the swelling beings. Swelling may arise in a few seconds or take longer than an hour to reach its maximum size. The patient may find one eye totally closed, or one lip so huge the food cannot be eaten, or one finger so enlarged that the hand cannot be closed. Edema generally subsides in 24 to 36 hours spontaneously. Edema in the gastrointestinal tract causes much pain and in the larynx can cause respiratory distress and asphyxiation.

Since the reaction is precipitated by the same factors as urticaria except for the extent of tissue involvement, the treatment is similar. Epinephrine, antihistamines, or corticosteroids are prescribed by the physician. Close observation for signs of respiratory difficulty from laryngeal edema is needed. The rare individual with hereditary angioedema is more likely to develop sever respiratory symptoms.

Many patients who have experienced angioedema with laryngeal involvement have been taught to administer intramuscular epinephrine to themselves immediately when the characteristic dyspnea, hoarseness, and stridor appear.

ATOPIC DERMATITIS (ALLERGIC ECZEMA, NEURODERMATITIS)

The individual with atopic dermatitis has an acute or chronic inflamed skin condition that is strongly associated with heredity. Asthma and pollinosis (hay fever) are common allergic conditions that occur in families of persons with atopic dermatitis. This allergy frequently begins in infancy and early childhood. At times, the individual with atopic dermatitis will have other allergic reactions, especially if the condition started in childhood.

Symptoms usually occur as a result of an allergen that interacts with IgE. The exact interaction is not yet understood. It is known that patients with this condition often have a depressed function of T lymphocytes as well. This results in increased susceptibility to serious infection, especially from the herpes simplex virus.

NURSING OBSERVATIONS

The patient usually develops papulovesicular lesions (red, raised, blistered) involving skin folds and creases of the wrists, neck, antecubital fossae (bend of the elbows), and popliteal folds (behind the knees). The lesions may ooze and weep at first. Later, the skin becomes dried, thickened, and scaly. There is intense itching (pruritus) which may lead to an itch-scratch-itch cycle causing skin excoriation. Secondary infection with marked thickening and a brownish-gray discoloration may occur.

The nurse may observe behavioral changes in the patient who has repeated attacks of visible lesions. Such a patient may try to hide lesions by wearing long sleeves or other similar clothing even in hot summer weather. The patient may withdraw from close relationships with others or may be very irritable. The patient's appearance may suffer from being unable to use cosmetics.

NURSING INTERVENTIONS

ASSISTING WITH DRUG THERAPY. Antihistamines such as diphenhydramine (BENA-DRYL) and tripelennamine (PYRIBENZAMINE) are the drugs usually prescribed for pruritus (see Table 10.3). At the same time, they may produce needed sedation to the patient, as a side effect. When emotional tension exists, tranquilizers and sedatives may be necessary. Chloral hydrate at bedtime may help the patient to sleep. Hydroxyzine pamoate (VISTARIL) may be prescribed sparingly to allay anxiety and enable the patient to refrain from injuring the skin.

Topical medications which may be prescribed after oozing and crusting subside include corticosteroids such as fluocinolone (SYNALAR) cream, triamcinolone acetonide (ARISTOCORT or KENALOG) cream, and ARISTODERM spray.

Sometimes simple bland, greasy preparations maybe used effectively when expensive steroid preparations need to be avoided in the person with a long-term chronic condition. Such preparations as petrolatum, zinc oxide, and coal tar paste and ointments have been used for years. Menthol and camphor have been added to some preparations. Different combinations of all ingredients are found on the market. These preparations are smelly and messy, and the lesions are frequently covered with a cotton bandage after application. When topical preparations are prescribed, old applications should be removed before a new one is applied.

ASSISTING WITH HYGIENE. The patient usually is advised to avoid soap and water except for unaffected areas. Bland oil, such as olive oil, or cold cream may be used for cleaning. Some patients can tolerate super-fatted soaps or hypoallergenic soaps, but these do tend to be drying. When cornstarch, oatmeal, (AVEENO), or ALPHA-KERI baths are prescribed for very dry skin, the bath tub becomes very slippery and caution is needed to prevent falls. The patient should be protected from chilling during the bath.

The patient's hands should be kept clean and the nails trimmed very short to help prevent infection. The patient may wear gloves or mittens while sleeping to prevent scratching. Children may need cardboard cuffs or splints. Sometimes the patient may find some relief by scratching the bed.

The environment should be kept cool, and clothing and covers should be kept light to minimize itching. Scratchy or irritating materials such as wool and silk should be avoided. Itching is intensified by activities that cause the patient to overheat and perspire.

SPECIAL SKIN CARE. Wet, nonocclusive dressings may be ordered several times per day. Saline or boric acid solution can be used, but the preparation generally prescribed is a dilute solution of aluminum acetate (BUROW'S SOLUTION). About 20 layers of gauze should be used for the compress and it should not be covered with any impervious material that would prevent evaporation. Between changes, the compress must be kept moist, but water rather than the astringent should be added to prevent concentration of the solution. The bed should be protected to prevent soaking and causing discomfort or distress to the patient. If able, the patient may be taught how to remoisten the dressing with a syringe between changes by the nurse.

When the patient's condition is complicated by secondary infection, an antibacterial agent is prescribed by the physician. Such agents as bacitracin, neomycin, and polymixin B may be incorporated into the topical ointment or cream. In such cases, corticosteroid preparations generally are not prescribed because they suppress the patient's immune response.

Other corticosteroid drugs such as those listed in Table 17.6 may be prescribed occasionally when the patient has extensive disabling lesions. Generally, these drugs are avoided because they suppress the patient's immune system at a time when the risk of infection is already increased.

PATIENT TEACHING. Usually, the patient is advised to avoid wool, lanolin, and other irritating substances that may aggravate sensitive skin. Other irritating substances the patient is taught to avoid include dyes, detergents, household chemicals, and cosmetics.

In some cases, the physician may suggest a change in life-style to avoid the influence of sunlight, extremes in temperature, and emotional stress, which are known to precipitate symptoms.

The patient should be protected from contact with a person who has a herpes simplex eruption (cold sore, fever blister caused by a virus) to prevent total body involvement. In addition, the patient should not receive a smallpox vaccination in order to prevent a generalized vaccinia. Generalized reactions can occur from scratching during such an infection and can be very serious, or even fatal. Gamma globulin has been used successfully to prevent reactions in these rare situations.

DEVELOPING A THERAPEUTIC RELATIONSHIP. Understanding the patient's experience enables the nurse to establish a warm, accepting relationship. For example, some patients live with active lesions throughout life. Others live with dread that acute attacks may recur at any time.

If lesions show, the patient may feel shame and withdraw from others. Touch is a very important means of communication. The patient with frequent observable skin reactions feels "untouchable." As symptoms persist or recur, the patient may become very irritable, causing others to withdraw from close relationships.

The influence of severe itching on a person's behavior should not be underestimated. Imagine how you would behave if a large portion of your body itched and you could not scratch. It is not uncommon for a patient to make a statement such as "it's driving me crazy."

The patient needs acceptance and support from members of the nursing staff as well as family. The patient may benefit from activities that temporarily divert attention from the symptoms.

ALLERGIC CONTACT DERMATITIS (ECZEMA)

The patient with allergic contact dermatitis has an acute or chronic inflamed condition of the epidermis caused by external irritants from the animal, vegetable, or mineral realms. *Dermatitis venenata* is an inflammatory reaction to plant resins, such as poison ivy, poison oak, and poison sumac.

Dermatitis medicamentosa is a similar inflammatory reaction caused by sensitivity to certain topical medications such as bichloride of mercury, merthiolate, procaine (NOVOCAIN), phenol, or formaldehyde. Other common agents include chromate, nickel salts, cosmetics, textiles and household cleaning agents. Reactions may occur because the agent is extremely strong, or because sensitivity has developed after repeated contact.

NURSING OBSERVATIONS

Symptoms have a characteristic sequence. The areas involved are generally the exposed portions of the skin, such as the face, neck, hands, and forearms. If the reaction is caused by an item of clothing or jewelry, the area involved is that which is in contact with the offending agent. Initially, there is erythema (redness) and swelling causing a papule. Within the next 24 to 48 hours, vesicles (small blisters) form. If the reaction is severe, these blisters become quite large (bullae). Fluid within the blisters is usually serous, but may show a tinge of blood. The most common an prominent feature is itching or burning, which may range from mild to intense. Pruritus leads to scratching or rubbing, which causes rupture of the vesicles.

Serum oozes from the excoriations and, in a few days, crusting and scaling begin. As the lesions dry up, the crusts or scales gradually fall off or disappear. The entire process usually heals within two weeks, leaving no scarring unless progress is impeded or the acute reaction becomes chronic. The following situations may delay healing:

- Scratching
- Application of irritating medication
- Rubbing or friction from clothing or shoes
- Heat rash from blocked sweat ducts
- Secondary infection

The patient whose reaction becomes chronic usually has less erythema, with some scaling and crusting. The skin becomes thickened (lichenified) and somewhat discolored from constant scratching and frequent excoriation. This condition may persist for years.

TREATMENT AND NURSING INTERVENTIONS

Treatment is effective if the allergen can be isolated. No therapy will prevent frequent reactions if exposure to the offending agent continues. Hyposensitization may be required if the allergen is known and contact is unavoidable. The objectives of treatment are to relieve itching and prevent complications from scratching. Treatment and nursing interventions are similar to those described for the patient with atopic dermatitis.

Gastrointestinal Allergies

The individual with an allergy involving the gastrointestinal tract almost always has had direct contact with an ingested allergen. Eggs, milk, wheat, chocolate, fish and shellfish, cola, corn, legumes, and spices are the most frequent food allergens, although any food may produce a reaction. Research continues into the relationship of allergy to soybean products and food additives.

The diagnosis of gastrointestinal allergies may be a long, tiring, expensive process for the patient. Besides the usual diagnostic tests for allergy described earlier in this chapter, additional tests such as those described in Chapter 15 may be needed to examine disturbances in gastrointestinal structure and function.

Treatment of gastrointestinal allergies includes avoidance, elimination diets, hyposensitization, and measures used to relieve symptoms.

NURSING OBSERVATIONS

Symptoms may be acute, recurrent, or chronic and may involve the entire gastrointestinal tract or any portion of it. Symptoms also can result from allergic responses taking place in other body tissues. Sometimes, it is hard for the physician to diagnose this allergy because an individual can have similar gastrointestinal symptoms with a migraine attack, a pollen injection, or a delayed serum reaction. Generally, symptoms are described according to the portion of gastrointestinal system that is involved.

Buccal and *pharyngeal* symptoms involve the mouth and throat. The patient frequently reports burning, itching, and a puckering sensation, particularly during the hay fever (pollinosis) season. Angioedema, discussed earlier in this chapter, may also affect mucous membranes of the mouth and throat. *Cheilitis* (inflammation of the lips and surrounding tissue) may be caused by the dyes in lipstick or chemicals in toothpaste. Specific foods such as oranges, tomatoes, or carrots may cause cheilitis in infants. If the infant does not have a positive family history for allergy, cheilitis may be due to irritation by the foods rather than true allergy.

Stomatitis is an inflammation of the mucous membrane of the mouth. The patient frequently reports burning and tingling of the tongue. This reaction may be caused by drugs such as sulfonamides or quinines. The reaction resembles contact allergic dermatitis in most respects except that the mucous membrane is involved rather than the skin. Dentures, mouthwash, amalgam fillings, toothpaste, oil of cloves, or troches containing precipitating drugs may cause this reaction. Canker sores (stomatitis aphthous) are vesicles (blisters) that appear inside the mouth. The vesicles rupture within a few hours leaving tiny ulcers. Healing usually occurs in one to two weeks without scarring. Canker sores seem to affect persons from 10 to 30 years old most frequently.

Gastric symptoms include nausea, vomiting, anorexia, and "indigestion" symptoms, such as epigastric discomfort after eating, belching, flatulence, and heartburn. The reaction may be caused by ingestion of a food allergen or may be related to other allergies such as bronchial asthma or migraine. Also, the patient may experience gastric symptoms as a part of a general allergic response. In some cases, the physician may advise the patient to avoid milk, a common cause of recurrent gastric symptoms.

The person with *colonic* symptoms usually has diarrhea. Milk is the most common allergen associated with colonic symptoms. As with other gastrointestinal symptoms, the physician attempts to distinguish between an allergy and food intolerance. The individual with *mucous colitis* (irritable) has

an inflammation of the colon and symptoms of abdominal pain, diarrhea, and mucus in the stools. The person with *ulcerative colitis* has an inflammation of the colon and symptoms of blood and pus in the stools. Ulcers are present on the mucous membrane lining of the colon. These conditions may be associated with food intolerance, food allergy, other allergies such as asthma, and prolonged stress. *Pruritus ani* (rectal itching) may occur alone, with other colonic symptoms, or it may be accompanied by *pruritus vulvae* (perineal itching). Pruritus ani can be caused by the ingestion of elimination of pollens through the digestive tract. The patient may also experience other allergic symptoms such as urticaria (hives) or allergic rhinitis. *Abdominal pain* is frequently associated with a combination of gastrointestinal allergies and is caused by an accumulation of flatus. *Acute abdominal angioedema* is a bowel obstruction caused by excessive swelling of the mucous membranes lining the bowel wall. The patient complains of severe, agonizing pain, and swelling of the bowel wall can be seen by x-rays. Gastrointestinal bleeding may occur as a symptom of allergy.

NURSING INTERVENTIONS

ASSISTING WITH DRUG THERAPY. Drug therapy is used frequently both to relieve unpleasant symptoms and reduce inflammation. For example, antispasmodics such as diphenoxylate and atropine (LOMOTIL), or tincture of belladonna may help to reduce diarrhea and epigastric pain, decreasing gastric motility. Visual disturbances, tachycardia, and excessive dryness of the mouth are important side effects of antispasmodics which the patient and/or the nurse should report.

Antacids such as those listed in Table 15.9 may be prescribed for epigastric distress. Diarrhea is a side effect of antacids that contain magnesium. Constipation is a side effect of antacids containing aluminum. These side effects should be reported so that a change in antacid can be prescribed if needed.

Corticosteroid therapy was described earlier in this chapter. Topical steroids may be prescribed to relieve symptoms in the mouth and throat. Systemic corticosteroids may be prescribed for the patient during an acute inflammatory reaction. Side effects of these drugs were discussed earlier in the chapter.

ASSISTING WITH DIET. The patient may need encouragement, information, and assistance from a dietitian in order to prepare nutritious attractive meals consistent with the prescribed diet. Reading labels on all foods is important to prevent symptoms. In some cases, however, labels may not contain a list of all ingredients. For example, many bread labels do not indicate that milk is an ingredient. Therefore, the patient should have a list of foods allowed and foods to be avoided.

Washing cooking utensils thoroughly is important in order to prevent introducing an allergen from food prepared for nonallergic persons in the family. For example, Mrs. White is preparing corn as a vegetable for dinner as well as string beans for her son, Bill, who is allergic to corn. If Mrs. White stirs the corn first and then stirs the beans, the allergen can be introduced from the corn to the beans for Bill.

As previously mentioned, the patient usually needs special help from the dietitian in order to learn to plan menus, shop, and prepare a special diet. The nurse may help by contacting the dietitian, if needed. In addition, the nurse's knowledge of the patient's life-style may be used to help the dietitian plan appropriate teaching. For example, knowing that the patient frequently eats in a restaurant enables the dietitian to suggest foods to order and avoid when eating away from home.

DEVELOPING A THERAPEUTIC RELATIONSHIP. Food is a very important of everyday life. In addition to providing nutritional value, food and customs related to eating may reflect cultural values, social relationships, economic levels, emotional states, and religious practices.

Food patterns develop early in life, and the patient can be expected to show signs of grieving when allergy requires a change in foods or eating habits. The response of the patient varies according to culture and other factors already mentioned, as well as the number of foods that must be avoided. Avoiding corn is easier than avoiding all corn products. Bill White in the earlier example may not have difficulty avoiding corn. Maria Alvarez, who is Hispanic, will experience a drastic change in her diet because corn is a staple.

The nurse may help the patient with a gastrointestinal allergy by listening with understanding to the patient's concerns, obtaining help from the dietitian when needed, and by expressing confidence in the patient's ability to make necessary adjustments.

Serum and Drug Allergies

The person with a *serum allergy* generally has a hypersensitivity to a foreign serum or serum protein that has been injected. Horse serum is used in the prevention or treatment of diphtheria, rabies, snakebite, botulism and gas gangrene. *Hypersensitivity to drugs* may produce an identical reaction. Drug therapy is a vital tool in the prevention and treatment of disease. As the variety and number of drugs have increased, hypersensitivity reactions have increased also. The most common offenders are listed below.

- Antibiotics—common offenders are penicillin, "mycins," and sulfonamides. Allergy is manifested by urticaria and anaphylaxis.
- Analgesics—the second most common offender of all is aspirin. Allergy is manifested by urticaria and, in atopic individuals, asthma.
- Sedatives—barbiturates particularly. Allergy is manifested by varied skin eruptions.
- Tranquilizers—phenothiazines (PHENERGAN, chlorpromazine, meprobamate). Allergy includes hepatic reactions (jaundice) and central nervous system reactions.
- Anticonvulsants—hydantoins (DILANTIN, MESANTOIN, PEGANONE). Allergy is manifested by marked systemic symptoms (hepatic, hematologic, etc.).

In addition, insect inoculations such as the bee and wasp sting produce a reaction similar to that caused by drugs and horse serum. Reactions of this kind can be fatal in the atopic patient.

Serum reaction may be of three types: (1) serum sickness, (2) anaphylactic, and (3) atopic.

SERUM SICKNESS

The individual with serum sickness has a hypersensitive reaction after receiving a serum or drug for the first time. The patient does not have immune antibodies and is *not* sensitized to this substance. During the next 6 to 12 days, antibodies form against this foreign substance that is still circulating in the system.

NURSING OBSERVATIONS

Symptoms, in the order of their appearance, include fever, skin eruption, enlargement of the lymph glands, polyarthritis, and edema. Symptoms may be mild and last a day or two, or severe and last two or three weeks. They can all exist at once, or only a few may be present.

The patients fever of 37.2° to 39.4°C (99° to 103°F) generally appears a day or two before the skin eruption and may last a week or ten days. The fever is remittent (varying two to three degrees in 24 hours but never returning to normal) and leaves rapidly as the skin erupts. Skin eruptions resemble urticaria. The patient experiences intense pruritus. Eruptions may be more intense at the injection site.

Lymph glands nearest the site of injection are swollen and tender for one or two days prior to eruption (adenopathy) and last two to three days. The spleen may also enlarge. Joint pain and stiffness (polyarthritis) in the knees, ankles, elbows, wrists, hands, and feet are common complaints. At some times there is no organic observable change; at other times the joints are red, hot, swollen, and distended. The joint fluid shows many polymorphonuclear leukocytes (WBCs) upon laboratory examination.

Pain usually follows the skin eruption. Edema generally affects the eyelids, face, and dependent parts. On rare occasions, edema may involve the larynx, and the patient may require emergency measures to prevent asphyxiation. The patient may ex-perience oliguria or show other signs of renal impairment. When the attack is over, the patient's kidney function usually returns to normal immediately.

In some cases, other symptoms such as abdominal pain, vomiting, diarrhea (sometimes bloody), tachycardia, severe purpura, and marked prostration of the neuromuscular system leading to asthenia (debility) may last for days or longer. The reaction generally is nonfatal, in marked contrast to anaphylactic shock.

NURSING INTERVENTIONS

The patient with serum sickness usually receives drug therapy to relieve symptoms. A sample plan for a moderately severe reaction might include:

- ACTH-ACTHAR gel, 40 to 80 U IM every 24 to 48 hours
- Diphenhydramine hydrochloride (BENADRYL)-50 mg PO qid
- Corticoid-triamcinolone, 4 mg, or prednisone, 5 mg qid
- Antipruritic baths (AVEENO or starch) or lotions (calamine)

Severe reactions are treated the same as anaphylaxis, which is described in the next section.

Anaphylactic Shock

The patient experiencing an anaphylactic reaction or anaphylactic shock has a generalized, life-threatening reaction after having received a substance such as a drug, insect sting, or a serum that is an overwhelming allergen. Anaphylaxis is a feared and dramatic allergic response characterized by vascular collapse, shock, and possible death.

NURSING OBSERVATIONS

The patient's symptoms may progress from a hive at the injection site to generalized pruritus and angioedema of the face, hands, and larynx. Wheezing, coughing, and other symptoms of asthma may develop. Circulatory collapse, generalized edema, dilated pupils, incontinence, unconsciousness, and convulsions may lead to death in five to ten minutes from the time of contact!

NURSING INTERVENTIONS

The nurse who suspects that a patient is having an anaphylactic reaction summons emergency assistance while remaining with the patient. If immediately available, a tourniquet may be placed above the injection site to slow absorption of the allergen. Emergency care of the patient in anaphylactic shock was discussed in Chapter 8 and is expanded in this chapter. Providing an adequate supply of oxygen, administering antihistamines, epinephrine, and corticosteroids, and correcting shock are essential emergency measures.

MAINTAINING AN AIRWAY. The patient may be positioned on the back with the neck extended to open the airway. Dentures and other objects must be removed from the mouth. An oral airway, endotracheal tube, or tracheostomy may be needed to open the airway blocked by swollen tissues of the tongue, pharynx, or trachea. If respiratory arrest occurs, the patient will require mouth-to-mouth resuscitation until help arrives. Measures such as intratracheal suction, described in Chapter 14, may be needed to prevent thick, gluey secretions from blocking the patient's air passages. Oxygen therapy, as described in Chapter 14, may also be needed.

EPINEPHRINE. Histamine action is counteracted by epinephrine, and anaphylactic shock can be reversed by the action of epinephrine. For this reason, epinephrine is usually the first drug administered to a patient in anaphylaxis.

ANTIHISTAMINES. Diphenhydramine (BENADRYL) or other similar drugs may be prescribed after emergency care has been given to prevent or reduce skin eruptions which can occur in later stages.

CORTICOSTEROIDS. Corticosteroids are anti-inflammatory drugs used to aid the patient in recovering from anaphylactic shock. Corticosteroids have a slow action and are not effective in aborting the initial attack but are used after the emergency situation has been reversed.

VASOPRESSORS. Vasopressor drugs such as levarterenol (LEVOPHED) or metaraminol (ARAMINE) may be administered intravenously to correct shock. Infiltration of intravenous solutions containing these drugs can cause sloughing of the tissue in that area. Signs of infiltration such as swelling, pain, and induration (hardness) around the intravenous site or a reduction of flow rate should be reported to the physician immediately. The physician may decide to inject phentolamine into affected area to reduce tissue damage.

ASSISTING WITH PREVENTION. When prescribing a potentially dangerous drug for an atopic patient, the physician gives careful consideration to the need for the drug and the possible toxic reactions. The doctor also determines whether the patient has had an allergic response to any drug, especially when penicillin or another parenteral drug is to be prescribed.

The nurse has similar responsibilities before administering potentially dangerous drugs. Specific nursing actions in potentially hazardous situations are listed below:

- Determine if the patient has a personal or family history of allergy. The nurse may need to explain what an allergy is to some persons.
- Do not administer the drug to an atopic patient until the physician has been consulted.
- Determine if the patient has had an allergic response to the drug to be given or to a similar one.

For example, an individual who reports an allergy to penicillin may also be allergic to other penicillin-like drugs such as ampicillin. This phenomenon is known as *cross sensitivity*.

- Do not give medication to which the patient reports a previous allergic response until the physician has been consulted.
- Determine if the patient has received gamma globulin by injection within the last ten days before giving gamma globulin.
- Do not give gamma globulin to a patient who has recently received this serum until the doctor is consulted. A skin test for hypersensitivity is done before a second injection is administered.

- Record information about allergies according to the institution's policy for all personnel to know. For example, the patient may be given a color-coded identification bracelet, a sign may be placed on the bed, and a bright sticker may be placed on the outside of the chart. A list of known allergens can be placed on the general nursing care plan, medication administration record, and patient assessment sheet. Further, the nurse administering medications to the patient with a colored identification bracelet should ask personally about specific allergies and compare this information with the written information with the written information, (Figure 10.4). Sick individuals do not always remember to list everything the first time they are asked.
- Have an emergency kit or box readily available whenever any drug is administered parenterally or when penicillin is administered. The institution probably has such a prepared box in a standard place on each nursing unit, so that all nursing personnel know where to find it. The nurse should know that such a box usually contains epinephrine 1:1000, intravenous antihistamines, intravenous steroid solution, and cardiac stimulants. Appropriate syringes, needles, tourniquets, intravenous tubing and solution bag, intubation equipment, and oxygen equipment should be available also.
- Administer prescribed antihistamine prior to parenteral administration of a drug to which the patient is allergic.
- Carry out prescribed procedure for hyposensitization when giving a drug to which the patient is allergic.

The individual who is highly allergic to insect stings should be taught to prevent them is possible. A summary of the preventive measures discussed in Chapter 8 indicates that the person should be taught to:

- Remove beehives, hornets' nests, and wasps' nests from the immediate environment.
- Wear shoes when outdoors during spring and summer.
- Avoid wearing bright colors when outdoors.

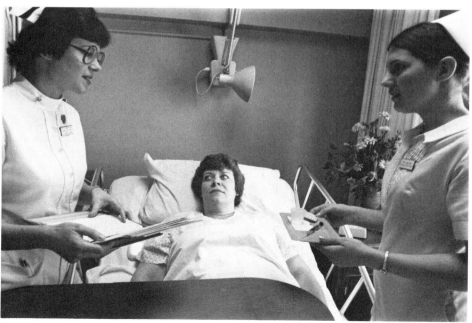

FIGURE 10.4 Discussing possible allergies to medication. (Courtesy of Practical Nursing Program, Fairfax County Public Schools, Falls Church, Virginia.)

- Wear tan, white, khaki, or green clothing when camping.
- Avoid using scented lotion, soap, powder, or shampoo before going outdoors.
- Wear long pants, long-sleeved shirts, and gloves when working among flowers or camping.
- Avoid wearing shiny jewelry and buckles.
- Avoid unnecessary exposure to insects.
- Wear identification indicating specific allergy and immediate care necessary.

Autoimmune Diseases

Extensive research continues in this field. In general, autoimmune disease is believed to occur when a person's body fails to recognize its own substances. For reasons that are not known, the body attempts to protect itself against itself. Some conditions that may be associated with autoimmunity are rheumatoid arthritis and systemic lupus erythematosus. The nursing student will want to be alert for new developments in this field.

Transplant Rejection

When tissues or organs are transplanted from one individual to another, the immune system in the receiver attempts to destroy the foreign substance. If destruction is successful, transplant rejection has occurred. Research efforts are directed toward discovering a method to prevent transplant rejection. At present, the surgeon and immunologist may select one or more of the methods listed below:

- Corticosteroids to suppress the inflammatory reaction at the site of transplant.
- Cytotoxic drugs to destroy or suppress lymphoid tissue.
- Antilymphocyte serum to destroy lymphocytes and decrease antibody production.

Research efforts continue.

Case Study Involving Bronchial Asthma

Mrs. Susan Carlson walked into the emergency department with her husband Jim. Mrs. Carlson appeared pale, diaphoretic, and anxious.

She was wheezing and told the nurse that she was going to die because she could not breathe.

Mrs. Carlson was transported by wheelchair to the treatment room. The physician initiated treatment to relieve an attack of asthma. Mrs. Carlson was given epinephrine 1:1000, 0.3 ml immediately, and administered 30 percent oxygen by mask. Mrs. Carlson did not want to put the mask on at first. After administering the epinephrine, the nurse remained with Mrs. Carlson for approximately five minutes. Mrs. Carlson's symptoms subsided and she asked the nurse to see about her husband.

In talking with Mr. Carlson the nurse learned that they had been married for five years and that nothing like this had ever happened before. He indicted that his wife was allergic to cat hair. They had just bought a home and this was their first night there. He described the trip to the hospital as terrible! He tried to get his wife to lie down on the back seat of the car and relax but she would not.

Mrs. Carlson was released from the emergency department two hours later with a referral to the allergy clinic for the next day.

QUESTIONS
1. What can the nurse tell Mrs. Carlson when leaving her that will help to reassure her?
2. When the nurse leaves Mrs. Carlson, should the door be left open or closed? Explain your answer.
3. What can the nurse tell Mr. Carlson that will relieve some of his anxiety?
4. Considering the information obtained from Mr. and Mrs. Carlson, what factors are important for the physician to know?
5. Describe the beneficial and side effects of epinephrine.
6. Why is bronchial asthma so frightening to the persons involved?
7. What should the nurse tell a patient before applying an oxygen mask?

Suggestions for Further Study

1. Demonstrate to a classmate the symptoms likely to be experienced by a patient with asthma. Following your short demonstration, compare the symptoms that you tried to convey with those observed. Also, discuss the feelings experienced by each of you.
2. Which of the antihistamines, according to their trade names, have you seen advertised on television or in nonnursing magazines? What side effects of antihistamine therapy

could influence a person's ability to drive an automobile?
3. Which of the allergic reactions could result in death?
4. Mason, Mildred A.; Bates, Grace F.; and Smola, Bonnie K.: *Workbook in Basic Medical-Surgical Nursing*, 3rd ed. Macmillan Publishing Company, New York, 1984, Exercise 10.

Additional Readings

Gotch, Pamela Miller: "Teaching Patients About Adrenal Corticosteroids." *American Journal of Nursing*, 81:78–81 (Jan.), 1981.

Griffiths, Mary: *Human Physiology*, 2nd ed. Macmillan Publishing Co., Inc., New York, 1981, pp. 349–53.

Harmon, Annette, and Harmon, David C.: "Anaphylaxis Can Mean Sudden Death Anytime." *Nursing*, 10:40–43 (Oct.), 1980.

Parker, Cherry: "Food Allergies." *American Journal of Nursing*, 80:262–65 (Feb.), 1980.

Robinson, Corinne H.: *Basic Nutrition and Diet Therapy*, 4th ed. Macmillan Publishing Co., Inc., New York, 1980, pp. 314–19.

Robinson, Corinne H., and Lawler, Marilyn R.: *Normal and Therapeutic Nutrition*, 16th ed. Macmillan Publishing Co., Inc., New York, 1982, pp. 691–702.

Chapter 11

The Patient with a Disease of the Heart

Expected Behavioral Outcomes

Minimum objectives referred to as expected behavioral outcomes have been designed for the practical/vocational nurse to use as guides in studying this chapter. The student should read these expected outcomes before studying the chapter. The objectives can be used as guides for study.

Using the content of this chapter, the student should return to the objectives and evaluate the ability to:

1. *Trace a drop of blood through the heart and draw a picture to illustrate normal electrical conduction through the heart.*
2. *Describe the role of the nurse in preventing heart disease.*
3. *Explain at least six diagnostic studies related to heart disease using words appropriate for the patient and family.*
4. *Using a head-to-toe format, list at least six observations which indicate that a person may have heart disease.*
5. *When given a specific heart disease, describe relevant nursing observations and interventions.*
6. *Describe, in sequence, the appropriate actions to be taken when a person reports chest pain.*
7. *Using a head-to-toe method of observation, list signs of digitalis toxicity and related interventions.*
8. *When given a specific cardiac arrhythmia, describe its effect on cardiac output, nursing observations, and nursing interventions.*

Vocabulary Development

The following prefixes, suffixes, and combining forms pertain to this chapter. By learning and/or reviewing their meanings, the practical/vocational nursing student will have the keys needed to unlock many exciting new medical terms.

Discover the meaning of these keys in a medical dictionary or in the content of this chapter. How does each key pertain to this chapter? In your notebook write the correct meaning of each prefix, suffix, or combining form listed below. Illustrate each key with an example.

angi—vessel. Ex. *angi*na pectoris—pain related to the blood vessels of the heart.

arter(i)-	end-	mittent-	sphygm-
bi-	extra-	my-	ster-
brady-	for-	nod-	stol-
cardi-	funct-	per-	super-
corpor-	gest-	pulmo(n)-	thromb-
cycl-	-gram	puls-	tri-
dextro-	graph-	scler-	vas-
elect-	in-	semi-	vers-
em-	lip-	sin-	

Structure and Function

In order to live, all tissues of the body must receive oxygen and food materials. They also must have waste products removed. These essential functions are carried out by the circulatory system. The pumping action of the heart causes the blood to circulate continuously through a closed set of tubes known as blood vessels. This continuous flow of blood picks up oxygen from the lungs, food material from the digestive system, and important secretions produced in certain parts of the body. These substances are then carried to other tissues of the body by the flow of blood. Waste products are removed from the cells and carried to the lungs, kidneys, intestines, and skin to be excreted.

HEART

The heart is the organ that has the vital function of pumping the blood by its rhythmic contractions. This organ is located within the thoracic cavity between the two lungs. The heart is a hollow organ that is divided into a right and left side by a partition called the septum.

The heart is approximately the size of a closed fist. Knowing that the heart accomplishes its function by contracting rhythmically, the nurse can readily understand why it is composed mainly of muscle tissue. This muscle tissue is known as *myocardium*. A membrane called *endocardium* lines the inside of the heart, including the valves. The membranous sac surrounding the heart is the *pericardium*. The innermost layer of the pericardium is the *epicardium*, which covers the outside of the heart.

The two sides of the heart (see Figure 11.1) normally have no direct passageway to each other after birth. Each side is further divided into two cavities. The upper chambers are called atria (auricles), and the lower chambers ventricles. The atria receive blood, and the ventricles force blood from the heart. Openings between the atria and ventricles, and between the ventricles and arteries, are protected by valves. These valves open to permit passage of blood from the atria to the ventricles and from the ventricles to the arteries. They close to prevent the blood from returning. The closing of these valves gives the characteristic heart sound that can be heard with a stethoscope.

The *tricuspid valve* is located between the right atrium and right ventricle. The tricuspid valve is known also as the right atrioventricular valve. The *bicuspid*, or *mitral*, valve is situated between the left atrium and left ventricle. This is the left atrioventricular valve. Both atrioventricular valves are attached by strands of fibrous tissue called *chordae tendineae* to the *papillary muscles* arising from the ventricular walls. These chordae tendineae keep the valve flaps from folding backward into te atria when the ventricles contract. The opening between the right ventricle and the pulmonary artery that carries blood away from the chamber of the heart is protected by the *pulmonary semilunar valve*. The opening between the left ventricle and the *aorta*, the large artery leading from the chamber of the heart, is guarded by the *aortic semilunar valve*. Realizing that the left ventricle must pump with sufficient force to deliver blood to all parts of the body except the lungs, it is easy for the nursing student to conclude that the left ventricle must be thicker than the right ventricle.

Blood vessels supplying the heart with oxygen and nutrients are called the *coro-*

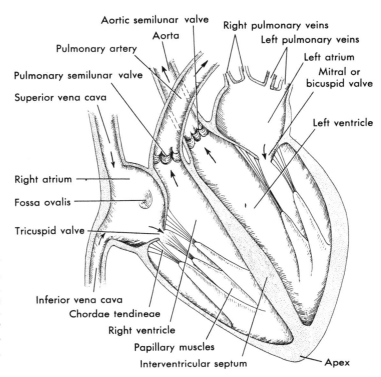

Aortic semilunar valve
Aorta
Right pulmonary veins
Left pulmonary veins
Pulmonary artery
Left atrium
Pulmonary semilunar valve
Mitral or
bicuspid valve
Superior vena cava
Left ventricle
Right atrium
Fossa ovalis
Tricuspid valve
Inferior vena cava
Chordae tendineae
Right ventricle
Papillary muscles
Interventricular septum
Apex

FIGURE 11.1 Longitudinal section of the heart showing chambers and valves. Arrows indicate direction of blood flow. (From Miller, Marjorie A., and Leavell, Lutie C.: *Kimber-Gray-Stackpole's Anatomy and Physiology*, 16th ed. Macmillan Publishing Co., Inc., New York, 1972.)

nary arteries. The coronary arteries arise from the ascending aorta, just above the aortic valve. The right main coronary artery supplies circulation to the right atrium and ventricle, while the left coronary artery and its branches supply the left atrium and ventricle. Coronary veins return blood from the myocardium to the right atrium via the coronary sinus.

CONDUCTION SYSTEM

The conduction system is comprised of a group of specialized cells in myocardial tissue known as pacemaker cells. A unique feature of pacemaker cells is their ability to fire (discharge an electrical impulse) in a rhythmic pattern and at a regular rate. Normally, the primary pacemaker of the heart is the sinoatrial node (SA node), a group of cells located in the wall of the right atrium near the superior vena cava.

After an impulse is discharged from the SA node, it spreads through both atria causing them to contract. The impulse then travels from each atrial wall to the *atrioventric-*

ular node (AV node). The AV node is located in the septum at the lower part of the interatrial septum. Fibers from the atrioventricular node that lie in the interventricular septum are known as the *bundle of His*. Thus, the AV node transmits the impulse from the atria by way of the bundle of His to the ventricle. The bundle of His divides into left and right branches, which further divide into a network of fibers called *Purkinje fibers*. When the nerve impulse reaches these fibers, it causes the ventricles to contract.

The sinoatrial node, atrioventricular node, the bundle of His and its branches, and the Purkinje fibers comprise the *conduction system* of the heart. Although the normal heartbeat is initiated by the sinoatrial node, any portion of the conduction system is capable of starting the impulse.

CARDIAC CYCLE

The term "cardiac cycle" includes two phases: *systole*, during which the heart muscle contracts and squeezes blood out; and *diastole*, during which the heart muscle relaxes and fills with blood. An important event that occurs during diastole is the filling of the coronary arteries with blood.

Both the left and the right atria contract at approximately the same time, forcing blood into the ventricles. Then both ventricles contract, pumping blood into the arteries. The right ventricle forces blood to the lungs, and the left ventricle pumps blood through the aorta into arteries leading to all parts of the body.

CARDIAC OUTPUT

Cardiac output is the volume of blood pumped by the heart per minute. Factors that influence cardiac output include the heart rate, contracting ability of the heart muscle, coordination of heart muscle contraction, the pressure or volume of blood in the heart at the end of diastole (filling), and the resistance against which the heart must pump. Cardiac output is important because it directly affects the volume of circulating blood.

CIRCULATION

Blood that contains a fresh supply of oxygen is brought from the lungs by the pulmonary veins to the left atrium. After passing through the bicuspid valve, blood is pumped from the left ventricle over the aortic semilunar valve into the aorta and then into smaller arteries (see Figure 11.2). These divide into smaller blood vessels called *arterioles*, which connect with even smaller vessels known as *capillaries*. Through the thin walls of tiny capillaries, oxygen and food are exchanged for carbon dioxide and other waste products. The blood that has picked up waste products and given up some of its oxygen flows from the capillaries into small blood vessels called *venules*. These lead to veins. Blood is returned to the right atrium by large veins known as the *superior* and *inferior venae cavae* (see Figure 11.3). It flows through the tricuspid valve into the right ventricle. Contraction of the right ventricle forces blood through the pulmonary semilunar valve into the pulmonary artery and then into the lungs. Here the blood gives up carbon dioxide and receives oxygen. It is then returned to the left atrium through the pulmonary veins.

Pulmonary circulation refers to the flow of the blood from the right side of the heart, through the lungs, to the left side of the heart. *Systemic circulation* refers to the flow of blood from the left ventricle, through arteries, arterioles, venules, veins, and back to the heart again. When blood flows through the various systems of the body, it also goes to the kidneys. These organs act as filters and remove waste products. Blood picks up food substances as it flows through the digestive organs.

The study of the heart is known as *cardiology*, and the physician who specializes in treating patients with heart disease is called a *cardiologist*.

Assisting with Diagnostic Tests

X-RAY AND FLUOROSCOPIC EXAMINATION

X-ray examination of the chest provides a still picture, frequently helpful in the examination of the heart. It may be helpful in determining an enlargement of the heart. In contrast to a still picture, cardiac fluoroscopy is an x-ray examination of the heart in action. There is no special preparation of the patient before or after x-ray or fluoroscopic examination.

ELECTROCARDIOGRAM (ECG OR EKG)

The electrocardiogram is a graphic measurement of electric currents generated by the conduction system within the heart. Connections are made between the patient and the machine by means of electrodes, or leads, that are placed at different sites on the patient's body. The locations generally used are the ankles, wrists, and six positions on the chest. A special conducting jelly is applied between the electrodes and the patient's skin. The machine, called a galvanometer, records the energy wave produced by the action of the heart as the graph paper travels through the machine at a specific rate of speed. Electrical activity of the heart can be measured at various points on the surface of the body. Usually, a 12-lead electrocardiogram is done. The nurse should explain to the patient that the test is not painful and that it simply records the electrical

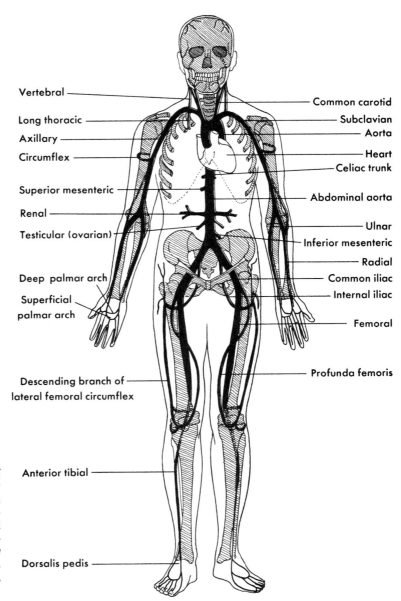

Vertebral

Long thoracic

Axillary

Circumflex

Superior mesenteric

Renal

Testicular (ovarian)

Deep palmar arch

Superficial
palmar arch

Common carotid

Subclavian

Aorta

Heart

Celiac trunk

Abdominal aorta

Ulnar

Inferior mesenteric

Radial

Common iliac

Internal iliac

Femoral

Profunda femoris

Descending branch of
lateral femoral circumflex

Anterior tibial

Dorsalis pedis

FIGURE 11.2 Diagram of arterial circulation. Many arteries are named. (From Miller, Marjorie A.; Drakontides, Anna B.; and Leavell, Lutie C.: *Kimber-Gray-Stackpole's Anatomy and Physiology*, 17th ed. Macmillan Publishing Co., Inc., New York, 1977.)

currents of the heart. After the test is completed, the conducting jelly should be washed off the patient's skin and off the electrodes. The electrocardiogram is done either in the ECG department or at the patient's bedside by a special technician. However, if the patient is located in a special unit for coronary care, the electrocardiogram usually is done by the nursing staff of the

unit in most hospitals. The cardiologist who interprets the electrocardiogram needs to know if the patient is receiving drugs that affect electrical conduction within the heart.

STRESS TESTING

Stress testing consists of taking an ECG during a prescribed amount of exercise. The test is designed specifically to tax the physi-

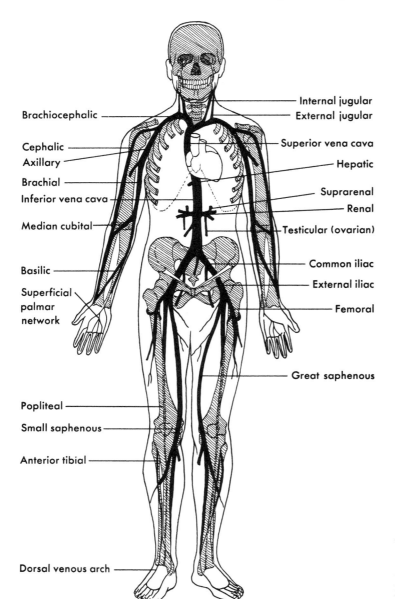

Brachiocephalic

Cephalic
Axillary

Brachial
Inferior vena cava

Median cubital

Basilic

Superficial
palmar
network

Popliteal

Small saphenous

Anterior tibial

Dorsal venous arch

Internal jugular
External jugular

Superior vena cava

Hepatic

Suprarenal
Renal

Testicular (ovarian)

Common iliac

External iliac

Femoral

Great saphenous

FIGURE 11.3 Diagram of venous circulation. Many veins are named. (From Miller, Marjorie A.; Drakontides, Anna B.; and Leavell, Lutie C.: *Kimber-Gray-Stackpole's Anatomy and Physiology*, 17th ed. Macmillan Publishing Co., Inc., New York, 1977.)

cal capability of the patient. If there is myocardial ischemia, or lack of oxygen to the heart muscle, during the test, there will be a change in a specific portion called the S-T segment of the electrocardiogram pattern.

The test can take several forms, including treadmill testing, bicycle testing, and the older Master's test in which the individual makes a specific number of trips up and down a set of steps. A patient scheduled for this diagnostic procedure must be informed of what the test includes because patient participation is essential for a successful test. Undue anxiety may case the patient to hyperventilate or develop arrhythmias, which would cause the test to be canceled or postponed. It is important that each nurse know the stress test procedure used in each particular agency or hospital. In many instances, certain medications that affect the heart should not be taken for a specified period of time before the test. The patient should have nothing by mouth except water for several hours prior to the test and should wear comfortable clothes. The clothing should be suitable for exercise.

VECTORCARDIOGRAM

The vectorcardiogram can be thought of as a stereo version of the electrocardiogram. In a vectorcardiogram, the patient's heart action is recorded in three dimensions in the form of loops.

The patient scheduled for a vectorcardiogram needs to be informed that it is painless and that electrodes are attached to the skin. Relaxation during the test is encouraged. The technician will be photographing the loops as they appear on the screen. The test takes approximately 20 minutes.

ECHOCARDIOGRAM

The echocardiogram uses ultrasound to determine the size, shape, and position of cardiac structures. Vibrating sound waves are aimed at the heart, and the echo that is reflected is recorded. Prior to having an echocardiogram, the patient should know that this test is painless and noninvasive. Noninvasive refers to a procedure in which the circulatory system is not invaded by a foreign object. The patient will be asked to lie still for approximately 20 to 40 minutes.

This test is more accurate and safer than x-ray procedures. An echocardiogram frequently is done before cardiac catherization to determine if a catherization is necessary. An echocardiogram has proven valuable in determining congenital malformations, pericardial effusion, cardiac tumors, and the function of cardiac valves, especially the mitral valve.

PHONOCARDIOGRAM

The patient scheduled for a phonocardiogram will have a permanent written record of the same heart sounds that can be heard with a stethoscope. The individual having a phonocardiogram should be informed that ECG leads are attached to the arms and legs and that a microphone will be strapped to the chest. The patient will be asked to participate by remaining quiet and following any breathing instructions given. The duration of this test usually is 20 to 30 minutes.

CARDIAC CATHETERIZATION

The term "catheterization" describes the passage of a catheter. In a cardiac catheterization, the patient has a small catheter inserted into a vessel in the arm or leg and threaded into the heart. Blood samples for analysis are removed from various parts of the heart, and the pressure within the chambers of the heart is measured. To study the right side of the heart, the physician threads the catheter from a peripheral vein to the vena cava to the right atrium and ventricle. In order to study the left side of the heart, the physician threads the catheter from a peripheral artery to the ascending aorta to the left ventricle and atrium. Common vessels used are the basilic vein and artery in the arm or the femoral vein and artery in the leg if necessary.

Prior to a cardiac catheterization, the patient generally is asked to sign an operative permit. Breakfast is omitted on the morning of the study. Depending upon the procedure used in each clinic or hospital and upon the individual needs of the patient, a sedative and an antihistamine may be administered before the catheterization. The procedure is performed under surgical asepsis in a special catheterization laboratory by a cardiologist. A continuous electrocardiogram is done during the catheterization. Although the procedure generally is not painful, the patient may experience some discomfort when the incision is made in the arm or leg through which the catheter is inserted and when the catheter actually enters the heart. Some patients have expressed a feeling of pain, especially when the catheter passes through an area of difficulty in the cardiovascular tree.

After completing the procedure, the cardiologist removes the catheter, sutures and incision, and places a dressing on it. Nursing care of the patient following a cardiac catheterization includes taking vital signs in the extremity that was not involved during the procedure. The site of the catheter insertion should be inspected for bleeding every 15 minutes for approximately two hours. The chance of bleeding is greatly increased if the arterial approach has been used. The pulse distal to the site of the catheterization also must be evaluated to make sure that occlusion does not occur. The patient's pulse should be checked, especially for rate and irregularity. In addition, the nurse must be alert to any signs of local inflammation and any expression by the patient of numbness or tingling in the extremities. Bed rest generally is prescribed for a specific length of time.

The patient underdoing a cardiac catheterization can be expected to experience fear and anxiety over the procedure itself. The results of the procedure and the eventual outcome of the disease increase the fear and anxiety. Much of the apprehension and anxiety can be relieved by the health team when factual information and appropriate emotional support are provided.

ANGIOCARDIOGRAPHY

The patient having angiocardiography has an x-ray study of the heart and major blood vessels following the injection of an opaque substance. The flow of the radiopaque dye through the heart, and lungs, and major blood vessels is recorded by a series of fast x-ray pictures. This diagnostic test provides a picture of the actual shape and size of the heart chambers and major vessels. An angiocardiogram is done frequently at the same time as a cardiac catheterization in order to provide a more complete basis for diagnosis.

Nursing care before and after the procedure is similar to that for the patient having a cardiac catheterization. In addition, the individual should be observed for any signs of an allergic reaction to the radiopaque substance, such as urticaria, nausea, dropping blood pressure, flushing of the skin, and anaphylactic shock.

CORONARY ARTERIOGRAPHY

Arteriograms of the coronary arteries are performed when the left side of the heart is cateterized. The catheter is threaded from a peripheral artery to the ascending aorta and the openings for the coronary arteries. A dye is injected through the

catheter into the coronary arteries of the heart. A rapid series of films is taken to visualize the flow of the dye through the coronary artiers. This type of study is done to determine the extent of blockage in the coronary arteries and to indicate if surgery might help improve blood flow to the heart muscle (see Figure 11.4).

During and after having an arteriogram, the patient should be observed for symp-

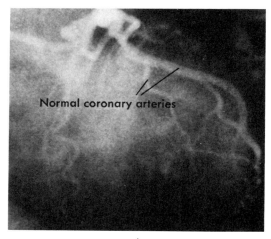

A

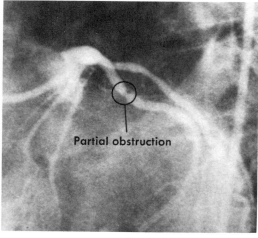

B

FIGURE 11.4 Coronary arteriograms. *A.* Arteriogram showing normal coronary arteries. *B.* Arteriogram showing left coronary artery with partial obstruction (Courtesy of Cardiac Diagnostic Unit, Medical Center Hospitals, Norfolk, Virginia.)

toms of an allergic reaction to the dye such as urticaria, nausea, dropping blood pressure, flushing of the skin, and anaphylactic shock. The care of the patient with an allergic response is discussed in Chapter 10.

A pressure dressing usually is applied over the injection site. This dressing should be checked frequently for bleeding. The pulse distal to the site of injection should be checked frequently also. For example, if the patient's femoral artery was used, the pulse in that vessel below the injection site should be checked. Additional physical and emotional care for the patient would correspond with the nursing care discussed for the patient having a cardiac catheterization.

AORTOGRAPHY

The patient having aortography has an x-ray study of the aorta after an opaque substance has been injected into the appropriate blood vessel (see Figure 11.5). Such a study enables the cardiologist to study the outline of the aorta and other major arterial vessels.

RADIOCARDIOGRAPHY

The patient having radiocardiography has radioactive isotopes injected intravenously. Their arrival in the heart and their flow are measured with a special counter. Certain types of heart disease such as congenital conditions can be detected by measuring the course and timing through the heart.

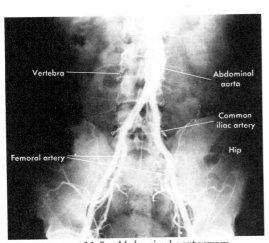

FIGURE 11.5 Abdominal aortogram.

CENTRAL VENOUS PRESSURE (CVP)

The pressure exerted by the blood in the vena cava and right atrium is known as the *central venous pressure*. The central venous pressure is obtained after the physician threads a catheter from a major vein, frequently the subclavian, into the vena cava and right atrium. The catheter is secured in place and the tubing is attached to a measuring device called a *manometer* (see Figure 11.6). The manometer shows the pressure exerted by the blood in the area of the catheter in the right atrium. The central venous pressure measurement is taken and recorded by the nurse at intervals, as indicated by the condition of the patient and according to the physician's directions. The patient having a central venous pressure measurement has intravenous fluids flowing through the catheter except when readings are being taken. Use of the intravenous fluids keeps the central venous pressure line open. A three-way stopcock is placed at the bottom of the manometer to regulate the direction of the flow. Between readings, fluid flows from the bottle to the patient. Immediately prior to taking the reading, the nurse should allow the fluid to flow into the manometer to a level higher than the expected central venous pressure of the patient. The reading is then taken after the flow from the bottle is stopped. The fluid flows from the manometer through the CVP catheter. The level at which the fluid stops falling is read as the central venous pressure. The column of fluid should fluctuate slightly with each respiration. Normal readings are approximately 4 to 10 cm of water pressure, although there is great variation from patient to patient and in different disease conditions.

In order to obtain an accurate CVP reading, the 0 point on the manometer must be level with the right atrium of the heart. In most persons, this level would be at the midaxillary line when the individual is in the supine position. The best reading is obtained when the patient is relaxed and lying completely flat. If the patient cannot tolerate being flat because of the disease condition, the reading may be taken with the head of the bed elevated. The patient's position should

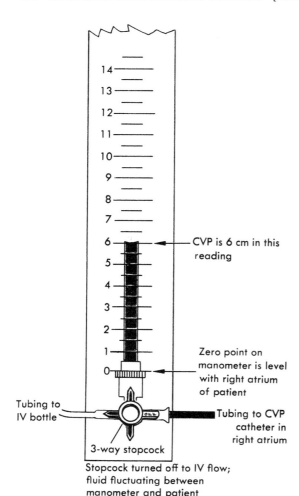

14
13
12
11
10
9
8
7
6 — CVP is 6 cm in this reading
5
4
3
2
1
0 — Zero point on manometer is level with right atrium of patient

Tubing to IV bottle

Tubing to CVP catheter in right atrium

3-way stopcock

Stopcock turned off to IV flow; fluid fluctuating between manometer and patient

FIGURE 11.6 Diagram of central venous pressure manometer during reading of pressure in venae cavae and right atrium.

be recorded at the time of the reading and this information communicated to appropriate members of the nursing staff who care for the patient.

Physical care includes daily changing of the dressing at the site of the catheter entry. The area should be observed for any signs of inflammation or thrombosis.

Central venous pressure redings that are high or are rising usually indicate a decreased effectiveness of the pumping ability of the right side of the heart, as in congestive heart failure. Low readings are usually indicative of decreased circulating blood volume.

CIRCULATION TIME

The circulation time is tested to determine the time it takes a patient to taste a bit-

ter substance, such as sodium dehydrocholate (DECHOLIN SODIUM), after it has been injected intravenously. This test is known also as the arm-to-tongue test since the bitter substance is injected into the vein in the arm and tasted by the tongue. The normal time for the bitter substance to reach the tongue is 12 to 15 seconds. The time usually is prolonged when the patient has congestive heart failure. The test is not used frequently now.

ENZYME TESTS

Certain enzymes are found mainly in the cells of the heart muscle and are released into the bloodstream when a person has an injury to the myocardium. Serum glutamic oxaloacetic transaminase (SGOT), lactic dehydrogenase (LDH), and creatine phosphokinase (CPK) are enzymes found in the heart muscle. Although these enzymes may be found in other parts of the body, they are also released into the bloodstream in connection with a myocardial infarction. For this reason, the physician frequently orders these laboratory studies done when a myocardial infarction is suspected (see Table 11.1 for normal values). Since each enzyme has a particular pattern for the time it is released into the bloodstream and the time the highest amount of enzyme is present in the blood, such studies will be ordered for several days in succession.

Prevalence and Prevention

Diseases of the heart and blood vessels (cardiovascular disease) are the leading cause of death in the United States.

Research has led to identification of major risk factors associated with the development of cardiovascular disease. As the number and severity of risk factors increase, the danger of developing heart disease increases also. Heredity, gender, race, and age are examples of risk factors that cannot be changed. For example, persons whose parents have cardiovascular disease are more likely to develop heart disease. Men are more likely than women to develop cardiovascular disease. The incidence of heart disease rises sharply with age.

Risk factors that can be changed include cigarette smoking, hypertension, elevated serum cholesterol, diabetes, lack of exercise, stress, and abnormalities in the electrocardiogram.

The American Heart Association recommends at least five ways a person may develop a life-style that helps to prevent cardiovascular disease:

1. Avoid cigarette smoking.
2. Reduce saturated fat and cholesterol in the diet by eating more fish and poultry, eating fewer eggs, cook with liquid vegetable oils and polyunsaturated shortenings, and use skimmed-milk products.
3. Exercise regularly or develop a program for regular exercise after consulting a physician.

TABLE 11.1
LABORATORY TESTS FREQUENTLY PERFORMED IN CONNECTION WITH HEART DISEASE

NAME OF TEST	NORMAL VALUE	IMPLICATIONS OF ABNORMAL VALUES
Carbon dioxide (CO_2)	24–30 mm/L	A decrease indicates acidosis; an increase indicates alkalosis
Carbon dioxide pressure (pCO_2)	35–45 mm Hg	An elevation indicates an increased amount of carbonic acid (acidosis); a low pCO_2 indicates a decreased carbonic acid (alkalosis)
Chloride	103 mEq/L	Use of mercurial diuretics may cause excessive loss of chloride, leading to hypochloremic acidosis
Cholesterol	150–250 mg/100 ml	Elevated cholesterol levels are thought to contribute to the progress of atherosclerosis; may be controlled by diet

Coagulation time
  Lee-White method
  Duke method
  Ivy method
	
	5–8 min
	1–6 min
	1–6.5 min
		Patients with prolonged coagulation time should be observed for any signs of external or internal bleeding and protected from injury

Complete blood count	Normal values in Table 5.4 (page 93)	
Erythrocyte sedimentation rate (Westergren)	Men under 50 years 〈15 mm/hr Men over 50 years 〈20 mm/hr Women under 50 years 〈20 mm/hr Women over 50 years 〈30 mm/hr	Elevated when inflammation is present within the body

TABLE 11.1 (*Continued*)
LABORATORY TESTS FREQUENTLY PERFORMED IN CONNECTION WITH HEART DISEASE

NAME OF TEST	NORMAL VALUE	IMPLICATIONS OF ABNORMAL VALUES
Potassium	4–5 mEq/L	Low levels (hypokalemia) may cause anorexia, nausea, vomiting, weakness, drowsiness, and arrhythmias; can be replaced in diet; high levels (hyperkalemia) may cause abdominal cramps, skeletal muscle spasms, nausea, diarrhea, and arrhythmias
Prothrombin time	12–14 sec	Patients with lowered prothrombin time should be observed for any signs of internal or external bleeding and protected from injury
Serum enzyme tests		
Serum alpha-hydroxybutyrate dehydrogenase (SHBD)	15–150 units	Elevated blood enzyme levels indicate damage to the tissue in which the enzyme had been located
Serum creatine phosphokinase (SCPK)	0–4 units	
Serum glutamic oxaloacetic transaminase (SGOT)	8–40 units	
Serum glutamic pyruvic transaminase (SGPT)	5–35 units	
Sodium	138–142 mEq/L	Low levels (hyponatremia) may cause weakness, apathy, and anorexia; high levels (hypernatremia) may cause faintness, muscle twitching, hyperirritability, thirst, hot dry skin with decreased turgor, and lethargy
Urea nitrogen	8–20 mg/100 ml	Elevation may indicate kidney malfunction; levels also may be elevated in dehydration
White cell differential count	Normal values in Table 5.5 (page 94)	

4. Maintain a normal weight for the height, age, and body build.
5. Control high blood pressure (hypertension) by having regular medical checkups and following the treatment plan when hypertension is present.

In addition, the woman planning a pregnancy may prevent certain congenital heart diseases by receiving vaccines for both German measles and rubeola (measles) at least six or more weeks before starting a pregnancy. Measles contracted by the mother during pregnancy is associated with a higher incidence of congenital abnormalities including abnormalities in the heart structure.

Regular use of a relaxation exercise such as the one described on page 64 helps to reduce the harmful effects of accumulated stress.

The informed, alert nurse has a vital role in prevention, early detection, and treatment of heart disease. A very effective way to influence others is to set a good example. The nurse who avoids or stops smoking, reduces saturated fats and cholesterol in the diet, exercises regularly, maintains a normal weight, and practices relaxation techniques is in a better position to understand and assist others to minimize risk factors.

Another way to assist in the prevention of heart disease is to provide information to others about cardiovascular disease, risk factors, and how to minimize or reduce risk factors when possible. The American Heart Association is a community resource which provides information through pamphlets, films, exhibits, and programs for the public, as well as members of the health care team.

Early diagnosis and treatment are important in preventing both heart disease and complications such as kidney failure and cardiac arrhythmias. For example, early diagnosis and treatment of high blood pressure and diabetes are important in preventing heart disease. The nurse who observes a person with signs and symptoms of heart disease such as dyspnea, orthopnea, palpitations, chest pain, fatigue, edema, cough, and cyanosis can help by advising that person to seek medical attention.

Even patients hospitalized for other illnesses may be helped by information related to the prevention of heart diseases. For example, the person hospitalized for hypertension needs an explanation of the relationship of this condition to heart disease.

Because of the nurse's knowledge and skill, family, friends, and neighbors often seek advice when they do not feel well. The person who seeks advice about chest pain needs accurate, complete information as soon as possible. This information can be located on pages 285–86.

Finally, the nurse may encourage the prevention of heart disease by participating as a volunteer in the projects and programs of the American Heart Association.

Nursing Observations

Nursing observations are an important part of caring for the person with heart disease. Direct observations are made by looking, listening, and touching the patient. Indirect observations, such as blood pressure and cardiac monitoring, also are used. For example, taking the patient's blood pressure is an indirect way of observing the resistance in the blood vessels against which the heart must pump. Cardiac monitoring is an indirect method of observing both heart rate and rhythm. A systematic method of observing the patient is needed in order to collect complete and accurate information. Table 11.2 contains a list of pertinent observations, using a head-to-toe format, that may be made in the patient with heart disease.

SKIN CHANGES

Changes in skin color such as cyanosis and/or jaundice may be visible in the patient with heart disease. Such changes may develop from direct or indirect effects of the illness on the circulation. For example, cyanosis may develop when the patient's heart disease deprives affected tissue of adequate circulation. Jaundice may develop if the pa-

tient's heart disease becomes severe enough to disrupt liver activity in processing red blood cells. The patient with heart disease may also have diaphoresis or cool, clammy skin.

CHANGES IN RESPIRATIONS

The patient with heart disease may experience dyspnea, orthopnea, cough, and an increase in the respiratory rate. Dyspnea refers to difficult, labored, or painful breathing. Orthopnea refers to dyspnea that causes a person to sit up to breathe. Nocturnal dyspnea wakes a person at night. The patient may report a smothering feeling. Another type of respiratory change which may develop is wheezing, also known as cardiac asthma. Most changes in respirations during heart disease are associated with inability of the heart to pump all the blood out into the circulatory system. This event results in a backup of blood into the pulmonary circulation, congestion in the lungs, and respiratory symptoms.

When the patient has a cough, the nurse records whether or not there is sputum production. When sputum is present, the nurse observes and records the amount, color, and consistency.

PALPITATIONS

The patient with palpitations has an uncomfortable awareness of the heartbeat, especially a rapid and/or irregular beat. The sensation of a skipped beat is associated with a premature beat.

PAIN

Chest pain is a common experience of patients with heart disease. The quality of pain can vary according to the underlying condition. For example, the patient may report dull, aching pain, sharp, squeezing pain, or crushing, viselike pain. Pain may radiate to the arms, neck, or jaw. Pain may develop while the patient is at rest or may be associated with activity, breathing, or strong emotion. In many cases, the patient with heart disease experiences chest pain because the heart muscle is receiving insufficient blood supply. Chest pain can be a serious warning signal of heart damage. Therefore, whenever the patient reports chest pain, the nurse takes immediate action to collect information about the quality, location, duration, and intensity. The patient's blood pressure and pulse also are taken. This information is reported at once to the appropriate nurse or physician and recorded on the patient's record.

GASTROINTESTINAL SYMPTOMS

The patient with heart disease may report a variety of gastrointestinal symptoms such as nausea, vomiting, indigestion, or abdominal distention. Nausea and vomiting may occur at the same time as chest pain when the patient is having a myocardial infarction.

PULSE CHANGES

The patient with heart disease may have pulse changes as a result of the illness and/or therapy. In measuring the pulse, the nurse observes the rate, rhythm, and amplitude. Usually, the apical pulse is counted for a full minute when the patient has heart disease. This method enables the nurse to detect irregular pulse patterns which may be present. For example, in some patients, every third heartbeat is skipped. This pattern is called *regularly irregular*. In other patients, the heartbeat is irregular but no pattern can be detected. This apical pulse is described as *irregularly irregular*.

When the heartbeat is not strong enough to send blood to the periphery, a *pulse deficit*, or difference between the apical and radial pulse may occur. The exact deficit can be determined when one nurse listens to the patient's apical pulse with a stethoscope while another nurse simultaneously counts the radial pulse. Both the apical and radial pulses are recorded in the patient's chart.

BLOOD PRESSURE

The patient with heart disease may have a blood pressure that is either abnormally high or low. As previously mentioned, hypertension (high blood pressure) is a major risk factor often present in the person with heart disease. Following a myocardial infarction or in certain cardiac arrhythmias, the patient's blood pressure may drop dangerously low. In addition to the patient's

specific heart disorder, medicines prescribed to treat the illness may also affect blood pressure.

Therefore, the nurse carefully measures and records the patient's blood pressure and reports changes to the appropriate nurse or physician. The blood pressure usually is taken in both arms when the patient first visits the clinic, doctor's office, or hospital. In some cases, the physician may request that the patient's blood pressure be taken in the lying, standing, and sitting positions.

TEMPERATURE

The patient with heart disease may develop fever if infection or an inflammatory process is involved. Often, the patient's temperature is taken orally instead of rectally in order to prevent activating certain vagus nerve reflexes that influence heart rate and rhythm.

EDEMA

The patient with heart disease may develop edema, an abnormal collection of fluid in the intracellular tissue spaces. Edema may be observed in the eyelids, wrists, sacrum, buttocks, thighs, ankles, or feet. A number of factors may contribute to edema in the patient with heart disease. These include fluid retention, heart failure, and complications of heart disease such as abnormal kidney function. In addition to observing the patient, two most common methods of estimating edema are measuring the daily weight and recording fluid intake and output.

SYNCOPE

The patient with syncope or fainting has a temporary loss of consciousness caused by a decrease in blood flowing to the brain. The brain receives a large amount of the cardiac output. When disease causes a decrease in cardiac output, the patient may faint.

BEHAVIORAL CHANGES

Fatigue is a common experience of persons with heart disease. In some cases, even a small amount of activity causes the patient to become overly tired and need rest. Other behavioral changes associated with lack of oxygen, such as irritability and mood swings, also may occur.

The patient and/or family members may become depressed or angry about the impact of heart disease on everyday activity such as working, leisure time, sexuality, and community life. In many cases, the patient cannot verbalize these concerns but instead demonstrates other behavior. For example, one patient may appear overly angry about the diet. Another patient may become withdrawn and silent. It is important to observe and record the patient's behavior so that ef-

fective interventions can be made. (see Table 11.2.)

Nursing Interventions

PROMOTING REST AND RELAXATION

An important part of therapy for the patient with heart disease is to reduce the demand on the heart by encouraging the patient to rest and relax. The patient with acute illness is usually placed on some form of bed rest initially. It is important to ex-

TABLE 11.2
OBSERVATION GUIDE FOR THE PATIENT WITH HEART DISEASE

AREA TO BE OBSERVED	OBSERVATIONS
Eyes	Cyanosis may be present in conjunctiva of dark-skinned persons Puffiness of eyelids caused by edema
Mouth	Cyanosis may be present around lips and mucous membranes of mouth Audible wheezes may be heard during breathing Cough with or without sputum may be present Patient may report dyspnea Jaw pain may be present Vomiting may occur
Earlobes	Cyanosis may be present
Neck	Neck veins may become engorged Pain may radiate to or from chest
Chest	Respiratory rate and pattern may change Apical pulse rate and rhythm may change Palpitations may be present Chest pain may be present
Arms	Pulse deficits may be present Pain may radiate from chest to arms Blood pressure may change Hands and wrists may be puffy from edema Cyanosis may be observed in nailbeds Clubbing of fingers indicates long-standing cyanosis
Abdomen	Indigestion, nausea, abdominal distention may develop
Back	Edema may develop over sacrum and buttocks
Legs	Edema may be observed in thighs, tibia, ankles, feet Cyanosis may be observed in nailbeds Clubbing of toes indicates long-standing cyanosis
Skin	Jaundice may occur Diaphoresis may be present Cool, clammy skin may be observed
Behavioral changes	Fatigue Anxiety and concerns related to death, disability, finances, sexuality, occupation, and life-style changes
Other observations	Weight changes reflecting increase or decrease in edema Syncope

plain to the patient which activities are permitted and which are restricted, and how this helps the heart. For example, the physician may prescribe bathroom privileges for bowel movements only. This means that the patient uses the urinal or bedpan to void. It also means that the patient must shave in bed. Some patients find it difficult to understand that additional time and energy spent in going to the bathroom to urinate, shave, or wash up can overtax the heart. Most persons are helped by knowing that activity restrictions are temporary. The patient with heart disease usually needs a restful environment which is free from unfavorable stressors such as noise, bustling activity, and pollution. The nurse may contribute to a restful environment by organizing care, explaining all procedures in advance, and providing uninterrupted rest periods. The patient with acute illness usually is admitted to the coronary care unit in the hospital where specially trained nurses and physicians are available to monitor the patient continuously and take immediate action if life-threatening complications develop.

HYGIENE

The patient with acute illness may be bathed by the nurse in order to reduce the work of the heart. In some cases, the patient is allowed to bathe partially, cleanse the mouth and teeth, and shave. In this instance, the nurse observes the patient carefully for signs of fatigue, tachycardia, and/or dyspnea. If these symptoms occur, the nurse completes the patient's hygiene and grooming. The patient with unstable vital signs may not be permitted any hygiene for several days until vital signs become stable. In some conditions, backrubs are avoided. The nurse should follow hospital policy when assisting the patient with heart disease in bathing, oral hygiene, and grooming.

Elastic stockings usually are prescribed by the physician to prevent venous stasis in the legs. The nurse removes and reapplies the patient's elastic stockings during the bath and every eight hours afterward.

ALTERATIONS IN DIET AND FLUIDS

Most patients with heart disease are placed on a special diet according to the spe-

cific condition (Figure 11.7). A sodium-restricted diet frequently is prescribed. Varying levels of sodium restriction are possible. For example, the patient may be placed on a 250-mg, 500-mg, 1000-mg, or 2000-mg sodium diet. The patient who is used to using salt liberally often finds the sodium-restricted diet tasteless. Flavorings, spices, and herbs may be used to improve the taste of foods. Some patients may be able to use salt substitute only if permitted by the physician. Despite flavorings and substitutes, the patient's perspective often is that dietary restrictions are among the most unpleasant of the changes brought about by heart disease.

As previously mentioned, a reduction of cholesterol and fat intake may be prescribed for the patient with elevated serum cholesterol. Calories may be restricted for the patient who is overweight.

The diet is often planned to include five or six small meals rather than three large ones. Gas-forming foods are generally avoided to prevent abdominal distention.

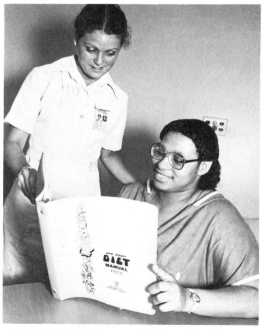

FIGURE 11.7 The practical/vocational nursing student helps the patient to understand her diet. (Courtesy of Bergen Pines County Hospital School of Practical Nursing, Paramus, New Jersey.)

Some persons require more potassium-rich food in the diet in order to replace losses caused by drug therapy with diuretics (see Table 11.7). During an acute illness, very hot and very cold liquids may be avoided. Most patients feed themselves, if able. The earlier practice of feeding patients with certain acute heart ailments has been largely discontinued because being fed often increases anxiety and heart rate.

POSITIONING AND AMBULATION

The patient with heart disease usually is placed in semi-Fowler's position when in bed. This position is preferred because it permits the lungs to expand more fully and reduces venous return to the heart. Even at night, the patient's head may remain elevated in order to prevent nocturnal dyspnea caused by changes in the distribution of body fluids that occur in the suspine position.

Ambulation and exercise usually are increased gradually in a supervised program which begins in the hospital and continues for weeks or months following discharge. Ambulation may begin with a few steps from bed to chair as soon as vital signs are stable. Criteria usually used to adjust activity include pulse rate, level of fatigue, and presence of pain or dyspnea. Any time the patient reports pain, dyspnea, or exhaustion, the activity is stopped at once. For example, the hospitalized patient on a walk in the corridors stops walking and is assisted back to bed in a wheelchair. The nurse may be instructed to check the patient's pulse rate and rhythm during ambulation. The physician may leave orders to stop the activity if the patient's pulse rises past a certain point or if the pulse becomes irregular. In some hospitals, protocols are established that guide the nurse in ambulating the patient with heart disease. The physician selects the protocol and the nurse follows the directions contained in it.

ASSISTING WITH ELIMINATION

The patient's intake and output usually are measured in order to identify and/or prevent complications such as fluid overload, renal failure, and edema. The patient whose vital signs are stable usually is assisted to the bedside commode. Male patients may stand to urinate, if permitted by the physician.

A drastic reduction of usual activities may cause the patient to become constipated if preventive measures are not started early. It is important to prevent the patient from straining to move the bowels since this practice may overtax the heart. The nurse helps to prevent constipation by maintaining the patient's usual routine for bowel movements when possible, providing privacy when the patient is on the bedside commode, and suggesting a natural laxative such as prune juice, if the diet permits. Stool softners and/ or mild laxatives are often prescribed to prevent constipation also.

ASSISTING WITH DRUG THERAPY

A variety of drugs may be prescribed for the patient with heart disease. *Antiarrhythmic drugs* such as those listed in Table 11.3 may be ordered for patients with a disturbance in heart rhythm. These drugs are prescribed to convert an abnormal rhythm either to a normal rhythm or a less harmful one. Often, the patient must take a maintenance dose in order to prevent recurrence of the abnormal rhythm.

Digitalis-related drugs (cardiac glycosides) such as those listed in Table 11.10 are prescribed primarily to improve the contracting ability of the myocardium. A loading dose is usually given in divided doses until the drug reaches therapeutic levels in the bloodstream. This process is known as *digitalization.* After a therapeutic drug level has been reached, the patient receives a maintenance dose. Of special interest to the nurse is the high incidence of digitalis toxicity which can be fatal. It has been estimated that approximately 25 percent of hospitalized patients who receive a digitalis derivative show signs of toxicity. Early signs of toxicity which the nurse should observe and report include anorexia, nausea and vomiting, headache, fatigue, malaise, and disturbances in vision such as blurring, halos, frosted appearance, and disturbances in color vision. Digitalis toxicity may cause a fatal arrhythmia. For this reason, the nurse counts the apical pulse for a full minute before administering a digitalis derivative. If the patient's pulse is below 60, the nurse withholds the drug and contacts the physi-

TABLE 11.3
ANTIARRHYTHMIC DRUGS

NONPROPRIETARY NAME	TRADE NAME	AVERAGE DOSAGE	NURSING IMPLICATIONS
Diphenylhydantoin	DILANTIN	50–100 mg (IV)	Count pulse before administering; if below 60, report immediately
Disopyramide	NORPACE	400–800 mg daily (oral) in divided doses	
Lidocaine	XYLOCAINE	25–50 mg (IV)	
Procainamide	PRONESTYL	100–500 mg	Be alert to any change in the pulse
Propranolol	INDERAL	10–40 mg (oral) 0.5 mg (IV)	Patients should be told to have their blood pressure checked frequently and to report any chest pain
Quinidine		0.2 gm; varies with type of arrhythmia	Patients on antiarrhythmics should learn to count their own pulse

* Antiarrhythmic drugs are used to treat the patient with disorders of heart rate and rhythm. These drugs are also called cardiac depressants.

cian for further instructions. The patient at risk to develop toxicity is one who is elderly, has severe heart disease, and who also takes a diuretic which depletes body potassium (see Table 11.7).

Diuretics such as those listed in Table 11.7 may be prescribed for the patient with heart disease. These drugs help to reduce the work of the heart by decreasing the volume of blood the heart has to pump. As previously mentioned, some diuretics cause a loss of body potassium which makes the patient more susceptible to digitalis toxicity and hypokalemia (abnormally low serum potassium). Potassium supplements may be prescribed either through drug therapy or in the diet.

Drugs used to dilate the coronary arteries are often prescribed for the patient with heart disease. Patients taking coronary artery dilators such as those listed in Table 11.4 may have headache, dizziness, weakness, and postural hypotension.

Anticoagulants such as those listed in Table 11.5 are prescribed for persons with heart disease associated with the formation of clots. The patient who receives an anticoagulant is observed carefully for bleeding. Frequent clotting studies, such as prothrombin activity, usually are ordered to monitor the patient on an anticoagulant. In addition, drug interactions may occur in patients taking anticoagulants. Examples of drugs that may cause an unfavorable drug interaction

in a patient on anticoagulants include salicylates such as aspirin, barbiturates such as phenobarbital and phenylbutazone (BUTAZOLIDIN).

Sedatives and/or tranquilizers, such as those listed in Tables 6.1 and 6.2 may be helpful in providing mental and physical rest for some persons with heart disease. A narcotic analgesic may be ordered to relieve chest pain in an acutely ill patient. Antihypertensive agents may be prescribed for the patient with heart disease and hypertension.

Many drugs are prescribed intravenously for the patient who is acutely ill with heart disease. Thus, an important nursing responsibility is to observe the intravenous site frequently and to report redness, swelling, warmth, or tenderness. When intravenous fluids are running, the nurse monitors the flow rate frequently in order to prevent complications caused by fluid overload. Too much fluid in too short a time may overtax the patient's heart causing symptoms of congestive heart failure, as described on pages 307–312. In some cases, a heparin lock or similar intravenous device is used to maintain a patent intravenous line without the necessity for continuous fluids.

ASSISTING WITH OXYGEN THERAPY

Oxygen frequently is prescribed for the patient with heart disease. Oxygen may help

TABLE 11.4
VASODILATOR DRUGS*

NONPROPRIETARY NAME	TRADE NAME	AVERAGE DOSE AND ROUTE OF ADMINISTRATION (IF NOT ORAL)	NURSING IMPLICATIONS
Amyl nitrite	VAPOROLE	0.1–0.3 ml (inhalation)	The group of vasodilators called the nitrites and nitrates are used primarily for patients with angina. The patient should be observed for signs of hypotension, flushing of the skin, and severe headache. Patients should know that they may feel faint if they stand up immediately after a rapid-acting vasodilator, such as nitroglycerin. These drugs should be used with caution in patients with glaucoma
Cyclendelate	CYCLOSPASMOL	100 mg	
Dioxyline	PAVERIL	100–400 mg	
Dipyridamole	PERSANTINE	25 mg	
Erythrityl tetranitrate	CARDILATE	5–15 mg (sublingual)	
Isosorbide dinitrate	ISORDIL	10–40 mg (sublingual) 20–120 mg	
Mannitol hexanitrate	MAXITATE NITRANITOL	30–60 mg (sublingual or oral)	
Nitroglycerin (glyceryl trinitrate)	NITRO-BID NITROSTAT NITROL	0.2–0.6 mg (sublingual)	Patients taking nitroglycerin should know that the drug deteriorates rapidly. The tablets should be replaced every three months, stored in a dark glass bottle, and refrigerated (except for a few days' supply). The tablet should be taken sublingually and not swallowed. There should be a burning sensation felt under the tongue—this indicates that the tablet has not lost its potency
		2.5–5 cm (1–2 in.) (topical)	Nitroglycerin ointment is squeezed from the tube and spread in a uniform layer on skin. Look for skin rash
Papaverine	PAVABID	100–150 mg	
Pentaerythritol tetranitrate	PENTAFIN PENTRITOL PERITRATE VASODIATOL	10–30 mg	
Propranolol	INDERAL	160–240 mg daily in divided doses	May produce arrhythmias or congestive heart failure. Not a nitrate or nitrite drug

* Vasodilator drugs cause dilation of the blood vessels with an increase of blood flow.

to relieve dyspnea or reduce the work load on the patient's heart. Before placing the patient on oxygen, the nurse explains briefly the need for oxygen and describes the particular equipment to be used. Additional information about oxygen therapy can be located in Chapter 14.

RELIEVING CHEST PAIN

Chest pain is the most significant warning of a heart attack. Pain results from decreased or interrupted blood flow to the myocardium. Persistent pain is associated with continuing damage to the myocardium.

For this reason, immediate action is needed to relieve pain, improve blood flow to the myocardium, and investigate the cause.

Whenever a person reports chest pain, the nurse's first action is to advise the patient to stop all activity and sit or lie down. Constricting clothing may be loosened. Outside the hospital, the nurse activates the local rescue unit if pain persists for longer than two minutes. If a rescue unit is not available, the person should be taken at once to the nearest hospital emergency room. The person with known heart disease may take three nitroglycerin tablets within ten minutes, if they have been prescribed. If

TABLE 11.5
ANTICOAGULANT DRUGS*

NONPROPRIETARY NAME	TRADE NAME	AVERAGE DOSE	NURSING IMPLICATIONS
Acenocoumarol	SINTROM	2–12 mg daily; larger initial dose	The nurse should check the patient's most recent laboratory values before
Anisindione	MIRADON	25–300 mg daily; larger initial dose	administering anticoagulants. Heparin must be given parenterally;
Bishydroxycoumarin Dicumarol		25–150 mg daily; larger initial dose	coumarin is effective orally. Patients should be informed that these drugs
Diphenadione	DIPAXIN	3.5 mg daily; larger initial dose	will prolong their clotting time and that they must be aware of any signs
Ethyl biscoumacetate	TROMEXAN	150–900 mg daily; larger initial dose	of bleeding and protect themselves from injury. These patients should
Phenindione	HEDULIN	25–200 mg daily; larger initial dose	know the importance of reporting for prescribed laboratory tests and al-
Phenprocoumon	LIQUAMAR	1–4 mg daily; larger initial dose	ways carry identification that states the name of their drug, the dosage,
Sodium heparin injection	HEPATHROM LIPO-HEPIN LIQUAEMIN	20,000–30,000 units in infusion over 24-hour period	and their physician. Patients should be informed that many drugs change the effect of their anticoagulant and
Sodium warfarin	COUMADIN PANWARFIN	2–25 mg daily; larger initial dose	should be told not take any other medication without a physician's order

* Anticoagulants prolong the clotting time of the blood and help to prevent further clot formation.

pain persists, the rescue unit is activated or the patient is taken to the nearest emergency room. During this period, the person with chest pain should not eat or drink.

Similar action is taken for the hospitalized patient with chest pain. The patient stops all activity immediately. The ambulatory patient is returned to bed by wheelchair. The nurse takes the patient's vital signs at once and reports the chest pain and vital signs to the appropriate nurse. The patient receives nitroglycerin or a potent analgesic, if prescribed. Oxygen may be administered, if prescribed. The physician is notified if these measures do not relieve the patient's pain.

As previously mentioned, chest pain can be a very frightening experience for the patient and family. While taking the necessary action to relieve the patient's pain, the nurse's calm, organized manner can be very reassuring.

CARDIOVASCULAR RESUSCITATION

Standards for cardiopulmonary resuscitation are set by a special committee of the American Heart Association, and they are updated frequently as more knowledge becomes available from research. Every nurse must keep informed and should be certified to practice basic life support with regular updates and practice.

When an expected cardiac arrest occurs, artificial ventilation and artificial circulation must be employed. Cardiac arrest can be recognized by:

• Lack of pulse in large arteries
• Lack of respiration
• Unconsciousness
• Deathlike appearance
• Dilated pupils

If an unwitnessed arrest occurs, the first person on the scene should establish an airway and ventilate the lungs four times. Next, it must be determined whether there is a carotid pulse or not. If a pulse is absent or questionable, the victim should have external cardiac compression begun immediately. External cardiac compression consists of the rhythmic application of pressure over the lower third of the sternum, avoiding the xiphoid process. An adult should have the sternum compressed at least 3.75 cm (1½ in.) to 5 cm (2 in.). The victim should be in a horizontal position with a firm surface under the body. Establishment of circulation must be accompanied by artificial ventilation to provide the body organs with a minimal amount of oxygenated blood.

When two rescuers are present, one rescuer should compress the heart 60 times per minute and one rescuer should provide one ventilation after each fifth compression of the heart. In other words, the ratio of one ventilation to five compressions of the heart should be carried out when two rescuers are available. When only one rescuer is present, the heart should be compressed 80 times per minute and two ventilations interposed after each fifteenth compression.

Cardiopulmonary resuscitation must be continued until definitive therapy can be instituted by the physician in the form of drug therapy, possibly defibrillation, and mechanical assistance. Improvement will be noted in the patient by occasional respiration, constriction of pupils, presence of a pulse, body movement, and improved color. The ABCDs of CPR are: (A) *Airway*, (B) *Breathing*, (C) *Circulation* (external cardiac compression), and (D) *Definitive therapy* (drugs and defibrillation).

ASSISTING WITH COMMON CONCERNS

In order to assist the patient with concerns that develop from heart disease, the nurse needs a general understanding of what those common concerns are. For example, most persons know that effective heart function is essential to life. The diagnosis of heart disease frequently causes the patient and family to fear death and disability.

As the patient recovers from acute illness, worries and problems associated with chronic illness are often present. These include financial worries, sexual concerns, and job-related anxiety. In addition, concerns often plague the patient at a time when usual coping methods cannot be used. For example, some persons smoke more cigarettes when anxious. Other persons may go to the movies or go for a drive. Still other persons find reassurance from loving sexual activity. These coping methods often cannot be used during the early recovery period because they may overtax the ailing heart. The patient may feel vulnerable, irritable, angry, or depressed.

In some cases, a permanent change in life-style may be needed to prevent additional damage to the heart. For example, the physician may recommend that the patient stop smoking, lose weight, and/or retire early. Such a patient may develop signs of grieving, as described in Chapter 1.

A first step in helping the patient with concerns is observing the behavior and listening carefully to what the patient says. Sometimes, there are no permanent solutions to very difficult problems associated with chronic illness. However, the patient or family may be helped by having an interested, understanding listener.

Another way to assist the patient is to plan communication that encourages the patient to explore concerns. There are several ways to do this. One way is to make a matter-of-fact statement that describes the behavior. For example, the nurse may say, "You seem very sad today." This may encourage the patient to recognize the sadness and explore it further. Another type of planned communication is to make statements which reassure the patient that fears and anxieties are normal and expected. For example, the nurse may say, "Many patients with heart disease wonder if life will ever be the same again. They worry about lots of things like dying, working, or their sex life." Once the nurse knows what the patient's concerns are, additional help may be needed. For example, the clinical nurse specialist may be asked to see the patient and provide more specific information about topics such as medication, exercise, and sexual adjustment. The dietitian may be asked to see the patient and family to help with concerns related to dietary changes. The social worker may be asked to help with financial worries. Thus, the patient and the family benefit from the special knowledges and skills of each member of the health team.

ASSISTING WITH CARDIAC REHABILITATION

Cardiac rehabilitation is a planned program designed to help the patient with heart disease achieve maximum potential for well-being within the limits imposed by illness.

The program is individualized according to the patient and the specific disease process. Sample components of a cardiac rehabilitation program could include:

- Information about how normal heart function is affected by the disease process
- Risk factors present and how to modify those that can be changed (topics could include diet, stress reduction, smoking, obesity)
- A gradual, planned program of carefully supervised exercise to improve fitness
- Sexual adjustment
- What to do about chest pain
- How to take prescribed medications
- How to cope with anxiety, fear, and other common emotions related to heart disease
- Vocational rehabilitation

The nurse participates in cardiac rehabilitation every day by explaining procedures in advance, by explaining the need for increased rest, limited activity, and similar aspects of treatment. In addition, the nurse reports the patient's concerns and problems to the appropriate nurse or physician so that the rehabilitation program is planned to meet the patient's individual needs. Finally, the nurse observes and records the patient's progress in the program. This action could take the form of counting the pulse during a walk or listening to the patient's description of the disease process. The information collected about the patient's progress is reported and recorded appropriately so that the program can be changed, speeded up, or slowed down, if necessary.

Cardiac Arrhythmias

As mentioned earlier in the chapter, the impulse for a normal heartbeat begins with the sinoatrial node, or pacemaker. When the heartbeat follows the normal course of the conductive system, the heart is in *normal sinus rhythm* (NSR).

Although in a strict sense the term *arrhythmia* means the absence of rhythm, in clinical practice *arrhythmia* refers to a disturbance of the rate, rhythm, or conduction of the heartbeat. The patient with a cardiac arrhythmia may or may not have a serious heart disease. A disturbance of either the rate or the rhythm of the heartbeat can, but does not necessarily, indicate the presence of disease. The patient with an arrhythmia may or may not have symptoms, depending upon the effect of the specific disturbance on cardiac output and oxygenation of body tissue.

An arrhythmia is detected by analyzing and measuring the wave forms on an electrocardiogram or the readout of a cardiac monitor. The P wave represents depolarization of the atria. If P waves are present and normal in size and shape, the impulse originated in the sinoatrial node. The QRS complex is a series of waves that represent ventricular depolarization. If the QRS complex is longer than 0.12 second, there is a delay in the ventricular portion of the conduction system. The T wave represents repolarization, or the recovery phase after contraction. By analyzing the size, shape, and interval between wave forms, the specially trained nurse, physician, or technician can detect an arrhythmia.

TACHYCARDIA

The patient with *sinus tachycardia* has a pulse rate of 100 to 150 beats per minute. Tachycardia may be associated with a fever, an overactive thyroid gland, emotional excitement, hemorrhage, congestive heart failure, and exercise. In other words, it occurs when the body has a need for an increased blood supply. Treatment and nursing care are directed toward relieving the underlying cause.

The patient with *paroxysmal atrial tachycardia* has a pulse rate of approximately 150 to 200 beats per minute. The impulse that initiates the heartbeat in paroxysmal atrial tachycardia (PAT) begins in an area of the atrium other than the sinus node. This condition starts suddenly and ends suddenly. Frequently, it will stop without treatment. However, if it does persist, the patient may experience symptoms such as chest discomfort and a pounding sensation in the throat. In order to slow the heart, the physician may try to massage the carotid sinus, which is located below the angle of the jaw. This maneuver slows the heart by stimulating the vagus nerve of the parasympathetic nervous system. Drugs used to treat paroxysmal atrial tachycardia may include digitalis preparations or antiarrhythmic cardiac depressant drugs (see Table 11.10).

The individual with a healthy heart can tolerate a rapid heart rate for a prolonged period, for example, during exercise. However, the person with heart disease may develop insufficient blood supply to the myocardium when tachycardia is prolonged. The blood pressure may fall dangerously. In addition, tachycardia greatly increases the work of the heart.

BRADYCARDIA

The patient with sinus bradycardia has a pulse rate of 60 beats per minute or slower. Bradycardia may occur normally during sleep, in young adult males, and in trained athletes. Bradycardia can also occur in an individual with an underactive thyroid gland, any disorder leading to increased intracranial pressure, and following digitalis therapy. Sinus bradycardia frequently does not require treatment.

Bradycardia also may occur in association with complete heart block, which is discussed later in this chapter.

PREMATURE CONTRACTIONS

Although the heartbeat normally is initiated by the sinoatrial node, the heartbeat can be initiated by an abnormal, or ectopic, focus or site from either the atria or the ventricles. Beats initiated by these foci interrupt the normal sinus rhythm and come before the expected contraction. Therefore, they are called *premature contractions*. A premature atrial contraction is abbreviated PAC or APC. A premature ventricular contraction is abbreviated PVC or VPC. Premature contractions occur occasionally in healthy adults and require no treatment.

Premature contractions in addition to being observed on a cardiac monitor, frequently can be detected by the nurse when taking the patient's pulse. Since these beats interupt the normal sinus rhythm, they will make the pulse slightly irregular. Although premature contractions may be heard when listening to the apical pulse with a stethoscope, these contractions frequently are weak or absent when felt in the radial pulse.

The reason for this is that the beat is not strong enough to send blood throughout the body.

Frequent premature contractions may be a warning of more serious arrhythmias in the patient with heart damage. Occasionally, premature contractions can be alleviated by correcting a low blood level of potassium (hypokalemia), or an acid-base imbalance. Frequently, however, these premature contractions require the use of an antiarrhythmic drug. It is extremely important for the nurse to take an accurate pulse, observe the patient closely to detect any change in appearance or vital signs, and report the findings. The findings should be recorded also.

ATRIAL FIBRILLATION

The patient with *atrial fibrillation* has a pulse that is irregular in both force and rhythm. Atrial fibrillation is known also as *auricular fibrillation*. The atria actually quiver, or fibrillate. The sinoatrial node no longer has the function of regulating the heartbeat, but many areas in the atrium produce a stimulus causing the atrium to contract. As a result, only parts of the atria contract at any one time, and the atrial contraction is uncoordinated and irregular. The atria may have as many as 500 impulses per minute. The ventricles, unfortunately, try to respond to as many impulses as possible. The ventricles frequently contract before they have been filled with blood. The person with this type of arrhythmia will have a grossly irregular pulse with a rate as high as 150 beats per minute. This uncoordinated ventricular response results in a pulse that can be described as irregularly irregular. In other words, there is no regularity to the irregularity of the pulse.

Since the ventricles sometimes can contract before filling with blood, many beats will not be strong enough to send blood to the periphery. The patient may have a *pulse deficit*, or a difference between the apical and the radial pulse. For this reason, apical and radial pulses should be taken at the same time by two nurses for one full minute. When taking the apical-radial pulse, one nurse should listen to the heartbeat with a stethoscope and the other nurse should feel the radial pulse. The beats should be counted simultaneously by both nurses. Both apical and radial pulses should be recorded.

Atrial fibrillation may produce an acute situation in which the arrhythmia occurs suddenly with a significant drop in the patient's blood pressure. In this case, the nurse should have the patient remain in bed and should notify the physician. However, atrial fibrillation can also be a chronic disease condition in which the person may live many years with an irregular pulse. The patient with chronic atrial fibrillation, when treated properly, can tolerate this condition.

Atrial fibrillation usually is associated with congestive heart failure, rheumatic heart disease, or myocardial infarction. The purpose of the medical regime is to reduce the rate of ventricular contractions and to improve the effectiveness of these contractions. This is accomplished by digitalis, a drug that stimulates the vagus nerve and slows the rate of atrioventricular conduction, blocking most of the stimuli that originate in the quivering atria. The physician may also try to restore the heart rhythm to normal by *cardioversion*, that is, by giving a brief electrical shock to the patient's chest. Thereafter, digitalis is often continued, together with such drugs as procainamide (PRONESTYL) or quinidine (see Table 11.3), which reduce the electrical excitability of the heart muscle.

VENTRICULAR FIBRILLATION

The patient with ventricular fibrillation has a rapid, ineffective twitching of the ventricles. Ventricular fibrillation may result from an insufficient blood supply to the heart, which may be caused by electric shock, the use of general anesthesia, or severe coronary artery disease. Since the ventricles are twitching ineffectively, no blood is pumped, the body has no pulse, and oxygen is not being delivered. Ventricular fibrillation, if untreated, will quickly develop into cardiac arrest.

The nurse can easily understand the life-threatening aspect of this arrhythmia by remembering that the right ventricle pumps blood to the lungs for needed oxygen and the left ventricle pumps oxygenated blood to the heart. The person in ventricular fibrillation

has no pulse. In fact, the patient with a cardiac arrest and the patient with ventricular fibrillation cannot be distinguished without the use of the electrocardiogram. Thus, if the nurse were to discover this patient, cardiopulmonary resuscitation would be started.

Ventricular fibrillation can be corrected if treated immediately with defibrillation, which is the delivery of an electrical shock to the heart. Defibrillation will depolarize all the cells at the same time, stop the heart from twitching, and allow the sinoatrial node to take over the function of pacemaker. Defbrillation is done by a physician or an especially trained professional nurse.

VENTRICULAR STANDSTILL

The victim of a ventricular standstill has an arrhythmia that will produce death if not treated immediately. This condition is also called cardiac arrest, cardiac standstill, and ventricular asystole. The patient has no pulse and none of the body organs are receiving oxygen. Irreversible brain damage will occur unless effective heart action is restored within three to five minutes. Effective heat action can be restored through the use of cardiopulmonary resuscitation (CPR).

ATRIOVENTRICULAR BLOCK

The patient with a disturbance in the conduction of the heartbeat has a block. In everyday usage, however, the term *block* generally means atrioventricular block. Atrioventricular block is a delay in the conduction through the atrioventricular node and is classified as first degree, second degree, and third degree or complete.

In first-degree atrioventricular block, all atrial impulses reach the ventricles, but the conduction is delayed through the AV node. Generally, this patient has no symptoms and no treatment is necessary. The condition cannot be detected by counting the pulse but it is apparent on the ECG. This arrhythmia sometimes may be a warning that the block will progress.

In second-degree atrioventricular block, some, but not all, of the atrial impulses are conducted all the way through to the ventricles. In other words, there will be more P waves than QRS complexes on the ECG.

Treatment for this arrhythmia frequently includes the use of a temporary or permanent pacemaker.

In third-degree, or complete, atrioventricular block, none of the atrial impulses reaches the ventricles. In the patient with complete heart block, the atria and ventricles contract without regard to each other. However, with complete heart block, the patient frequently exhibits ventricular arrhythmias. As the ventricles shift from one arrhythmia to another, there may be associated with it a temporary cessation of cardiac output and fall in systolic blood pressure to almost zero. When cardiac output is suddenly reduced, there is also a sudden decrease in the amount of blood supply to the brain. There is, therefore, a decrease in the amount of oxygen supply to the brain and the patient may feel dizzy and weak, lose consciousness, and have a convulsion. Unless the ventricles begin to contract again to increase the cardiac output, death will result. This episode is called Adams-Stokes attack, and recurring attacks are known as Adams-Stokes disease or syndrome.

The physician attempts to treat the cause of heart block, when possible. For example, digitalis toxicity may cause heart block. After removal of the cause, the patient with no symptoms probably will require no additional treatment. Unfortunately, a complete atrioventricular block not is usually cured so easily. In cases of Adams-Stokes attacks, such drugs as isoproterenol and atropine are helpful in increasing the rate and force of ventricular contractions. It is often necessary to supply some other source of stimuli to the ventricles to maintain an adequate heartbeat. The pacemaker supplies artificial electrical impulses to replace those not being received normally by the ventricles.

NURSING THE PATIENT WITH A PACEMAKER

The patient with a pacemaker has an electronic device that generates an electrical impulse to initiate the heartbeat. Pacemakers are classified as external or internal, depending on the location of the pulse generator itself. Pacemakers can be temporary or permanent, although usually external pacemakers are for temporary use. Each pacemaker consists of the pulse generator, which initiates the impulse, and the pacing catheter, which delivers the impulse to the heart.

The most commonly used external pacemaker is the transvenous endocardial. The pacing electrode is introduced into the venous system and threaded into the heart and positioned on the endocardium. The other end of the catheter is attached to the external pulse generator. Frequent insertion sites are the subclavian, the jugular, and the basilic veins.

The patient with a catheter electrode-type pacemaker should be observed for any pain or tenderness or redness or swelling at the site of insertion through the skin. Any elevation of temperature should be reported. Antibiotic ointment applied to the site covered by a sterile dressing usually is ordered by the doctor. The dressing may be changed frequently.

Another type of external temporary pacing is frequently done for patients having open-heart surgery. The pacing electrodes are sutured to the epicardium during the surgery and the wires brought out to the surface through the incision. The wires are available to be attached to the external pulse generator if needed. Occasionally, the patient may develop heart block following cardiac surgery as a result of edema around the conduction system.

Internally implanted pacemakers are used for a permanent conduction problem. Such a pacemaker usually requires a transvenous approach. The catheter is threaded from the subclavian or jugular vein through until it reaches the endocardium. The other end of the catheter is attached to the pulse generator, which is placed under the skin in a subcutaneous pocket. The most common location is beneath the right clavicle. The skin is closed by suturing. This surgical wound should be observed for any sign of inflammation. A sterile dressing is applied and, according to the policy of the hospital or the surgeon's order, an antibiotic ointment may be applied. Aseptic technique, of course, is maintained.

The safest pacemakers are those that do not fire in competition with the normal heartbeat of the patient or with extra heartbeats. The demand pacemaker is set by the doctor to fire an electrical stimulus to the heart only when the heart rate falls below a certain rate, usually 70 per minute.

The synchronous pacemaker picks up the atrial impulses, amplifies them, and delivers them to the ventricles.

The asynchronous pacemaker delivers a periodic electrical impulse to the ventricle regardless of impulse to the ventricle regardless of impulses sent out by the AV node. The batteries need to be changed periodically according to the instructions of the manufacturer, or at any time that mechanical failure occurs. This is a minor procedure requiring local anesthesia.

In addition to postoperative care, other observations and interventions are indicated when the patient has a pacemaker. For example, vital signs are carefully taken and recorded. An elevated temperature is reported at once since infection may develop at the pacemaker site. The apical-radial pulse is counted for a full minute. The pulse rhythm is observed at this time also. The patient with a demand pacemaker is expected to have an irregular pulse. The patient with an asynchronous pacemaker is expected to have a regular pulse. The nurse carefully observed the site of insertion of the transvenous catheter for redness, warmth, tenderness, and swelling which could indicate thrombophlebitis. The involved joint may be immobilized to prevent movement of the catheter. A neurocirculation check of the affected extremity is indicated using the five Ps (*Pain*, *Pallor*, *Pulse*, *Paresthesia*, *Paralysis*). Persistent hiccoughs should be reported to the appropriate nurse or physician since this symptom may indicate malposition of the pacemaker catheter.

Patients being discharged with pacemakers and members of their families should be instructed in the taking of the patient's pulse daily. A pulse rate below the preset rate of a pacemaker could indicate battery failure, and the physician must be notified immediately. At all times these patients should carry identification that states that they have an implanted pacemaker and indicates the manufacturer and rate of heartbeat to be expected. Informative pamphlets are available for patients with pacemakers from local chapters of the American Heart Association.

Coronary Artery Disease

The patient with coronary artery disease has a condition affecting the arteries that supply blood to the heart muscle. Coronary artery disease is usually arteriosclerotic in origin, in which case it is referred to as *arteriosclerotic heart disease*. Over a period of time, deposits, cholesterol, fatty acids, and calcium form on the intima of an artery; calcium deposits form in the media of the artery. (The intima and the media are discussed in the chapter concerned with diseases of the blood vessels [Chapter 12].) The affected artery becomes hard and thick, and loses its elasticity. The passageway within the artery is narrowed, and the heart muscle receives less blood. When the blood supply is temporarily inadequate to the part of the heart being fed by the affected artery, the patient has an attack of *angina pectoris*. Arteriosclerosis may lead to the formation of a blood clot, which is known as a *thrombus*. If the artery channel is completely closed by the blood clot, the patient has a heart attack, which may be called either a *coronary occlusion, coronary thrombosis, myocardial infarction*, or *a coronary*.

Fortunately the network of coronary arteries has an amazing method of compensating for the narrowing of some of its members. While some of the arteries become smaller and less efficient, others feeding the same area get larger so they can carry more blood to the muscle needing it. Small new branches of these healthier arteries are formed. This method of compensation is called *collateral circulation*. Following a heart attack caused by closure of a coronary artery, collateral circulation plays an important part in the recovery of the patient.

ANGINA PECTORIS

CAUSE. The patient with angina pectoris has attacks of chest pain caused by an insufficient blood supply to the heart muscle. The myocardium needs more blood than it is receiving by means of the coronary arteries. When the blood supply to any muscle is inadequate, the muscle begins to ache. For example, if a tourniquet is left on a patient's arm too long, he complains of pain. This discomfort is relieved when the tourniquet is removed and fresh blood flows into the arm.

Attacks of angina pectoris may result from spasm or arteriosclerosis of the coronary arteries. The most common cause is arteriosclerosis. The exact cause of arteriosclerosis is not known. The heart's blood supply may be adequate when it is not working hard, but when the work load is increased by exercise or by emotion, the supply is not sufficient.

SYMPTOMS. Symptoms of this condition occur more often in men over 50 years of age. An attack is usually preceded by physical activity or an emotional upset such as anger or anxiety. The outstanding symptom is a squeezing pain that starts under the sternum (breastbone). It frequently spreads to the left shoulder and down the inner side of the left arm. For some persons, the pain spreads, or radiates, to the right shoulder and down the inner side of the right arm, the neck, the jaw, or even the ear. The pain of angina usually lasts no longer than five minutes in most persons when treated with rest or vasodilators. The severity of the pain ranges from a discomfort to an immobilizing pain. The patient usually feels satisfactory after an acute pain has subsided. However, the outcome may be fatal if a large area of the heart has an inadequate blood supply for too long a period of time. In this case the patient has a myocardial infarction.

DIAGNOSIS. Stress testing is a controlled means of exerting the heart to evaluate the blood supply during exercise while at the same time an electrocardiogram is being performed. Stress testing has been discussed earlier in this chapter. Radiocardiography and coronary arteriography may be done to determine the extent of coronary artery obstruction. These diagnostic procedures were described earlier in this chapter.

TREATMENT. As the pain is caused by an insufficient blood supply to the heart muscle, the aim of the treatment is to increase the blood to the aching muscle. Rest and vasodilators, drugs that cause the blood vessels to dilate, are the two main measures used to accomplish this aim. The amount of work required of the heart is reduced when a person is at complete rest.

Nitroglycerin and amyl nitrite are two examples of drugs commonly used to relieve the pain of an attack of angina pectoris (see Table 11.4). These drugs cause the coronary arteries to dilate, enabling them to carry more blood to the affected area, and thus the pain is relieved. In some cases, the patient is instructed to take the vasodilator drug when an increase in activity is anticipated. This is to prevent pain and ischemia to the heart muscle.

The patient with angina may be placed on a carefully supervised exercise program in order to improve collateral circulation. In addition, the patient is helped to modify or eliminate risk factions such as smoking, obesity, unfavorable stress, and hypertension.

Surgical treatment is sometimes indicated for the relief of angina pectoris. The most common surgical procedure at this time is a coronary artery bypass graft. This technique increases the blood supply to the heart or revascularizes the heart muscle. A vein, usually the saphenous, is removed from the patient and used as a graft between the aorta and the coronary artery beyond the point of the obstruction. Thus, the myocardium will receive more blood, and the patient will experience less pain. Collateral circulation, as explained earlier, will take over the function of the saphenous vein in the leg.

The patient undergoing this surgical procedure will require open-heart surgery with cardiopulmonary bypass, which is discussed later in this chapter. The purpose of the coronary artery bypass graft is to reduce angina and improve the patient's style of life. The surgery is associated with temporary and, in some cases, permanent relief of angina. Often, the patient's disease continues and the angina may recur at a later time as arterioclerosis progresses in the coronary vessels.

Myocardial Infarction

The patient with a myocardial infarction has an obstruction in a coronary artery. The area of the heart fed by the diseased artery suffers from an insufficient blood supply. As previously stated, this disease, which may also be referred to as coronary occlusion, coronary thrombosis, or "a coronary," occurs when an artery is closed. Closure of the artery results in death to tissue supplied by that artery. This type of heart attack is the most common cause of sudden death from cardiac disease. Although myocardial infarction affects both men and women, it seems to be more common in men. However, the occurrence of myocardial infarction in women increases sharply after menopause.

If a small blood vessel is obstructed and the collateral circulation is good, the patient may experience few symptoms, and chances of recovery are excellent. When the obstructed artery is a large one, and the collateral circulation is poor, the patient may die immediately.

SYMPTOMS

The beginning of a myocardial infarction is often sudden, and, unlike an anginal attack, the patient is usually at rest. The patient experiences a severe viselike pain under the lower part of the sternum and shortness of breath. Nausea and vomiting are frequently present. The pulse is rapid and weak, and may be irregular. Symptoms of shock often present are paleness, cyanosis, cold and clammy skin, and a drop in blood pressure. These symptoms occur as a result of the decreased ability of the heart muscle to pump effectively. The cells in the area of infarction are dead and unable to function. One to two days after the attack, the patient may have a low-grade fever, 38.5°C (101°F), and an increase in the white blood cell count. These changes are a response to the inflammatory process.

The doctor makes a diagnosis of myocardial infarction by careful examination of the patient. Electrocardiographic tracings are important aids in helping to confirm the diagnosis. This tracing is a graphic record of the electrical activity of the heart that shows the condition of the heart muscle.

Blood sedimentation rate, complete blood count, and blood enzymes such as glutamic oxaloacetic transaminase (SGOT), lactic dehydrogenase (LDH), and creatine phosphokinase (SCPK) are examples of laboratory studies often ordered by the doctor to aid in diagnosis. See Table 11.1 for normal values.

TREATMENT AND NURSING CARE

Ideally, upon admission to the hospital, the patient is placed in the coronary care unit for four to five days. The most critical period is during the first 48 hours following the attack. Since ventricular fibrillation and cardiac arrest are common causes of sudden death, it is believed that treatment and nursing care in this unit prevent most deaths caused by arrhythmias.

CORONARY CARE UNIT. Over half a million persons die annually in the United States of acute myocardial infarction from coronary artery occlusion. The person may die with little or no advance warning. Mortality is frequently due to the development of serious cardiac arrhythmias, an abnormally fast or slow heart rate, an irregularity in rhythm, or no heartbeat at all. Three techniques developed within the past few years have aided in the survival rate of patients who might otherwise have died. These techniques include cardiopulmonary resuscitation, cardiac pacemaking, and defibrillation, which is the administration of an electrical shock of several hundred watts per second to the chest wall to defibrillate the patient. When these techniques are instituted promptly and appropriately in conjunction with the proper drugs, mortality of hospitalized myocardial infarction patients can be reduced by about one third, approximately 30 to 20 percent. Useful brain function is preserved only if ventilation and circulation are reestablished within four minutes. If these patients are housed all over the hospital, it is difficult to expect specially trained personnel, and the special equipment that is used in such an emergency, to reach the patient to prevent death or brain damage.

The year 1962 saw the beginning of the present-day cardiac care unit. With this unit in operation, all patients with recent myocardial infarctions, special equipment used in coronary care, and specially trained coronary care personnel could be located in one place. Certain members of the specially trained staff are authorized and delegated the responsibility of carrying out the lifesaving techniques. For example, the registered professional nurse who attends classes in how to recognize and interpret certain cardiac arrhythmias observed on the cardiac monitor is then authorized to administer appropriate medications or carry out defibrillation. Careful and continuous monitoring and observation of the cardiac patient are essential. The nurse must be prepared to carry out cardiopulmonary resuscitation at any time. It is also essential to be familiar with the nursing management of congestive heart failure with pulmonary edema and cardiogenic shock.

Inservice educational programs are an integral part of coronary care nursing to teach and maintain the highly advanced skills necessary in a cornonary care unit. The motivated, skilled practical/vocational nurse can be a valuable asset to the staff of the coronary care unit (see Figure 11.8).

ENVIRONMENT. Upon admission, the patient is put to bed, preferably in the coronary care unit in a calm and quiet manner. The confident attitude of the nursing staff enables the patient to feel more secure. Noise should be kept to a minimum and lighting should be subdued. In other words, from a mental and physical point of view, the patient's environment should be conducive to rest.

The patient usually is connected to a monitoring system (Figure 11.9). The purpose of this system is to increase the staff's ability to observe the patient's vital signs and enable the nursing staff to give effective and preventive care. Continuous observation of electrical activity of the patient's heart will reduce the number of crisis situations by the early detection of arrhythmias. As stated earlier, the nursing staff in a coronary care unit is especially trained in recognizing and responding effectively in cardiac emergencies. The patient needs to understand that the purpose of the monitoring system is to enable the staff to give constant attention.

Visitors are restricted to selected members of the immediate family. This is especially true during the early days of the illness. In some cases, the patient is not allowed to have a radio, newspaper, or television. However, selected music is comforting to some patients. Having a clock and a calendar may help the patient feel less isolated.

PAIN AND APPREHENSION. An important goal in the treatment and nursing care of the patient who has had a myocardial infarction is the relief of pain and apprehension. The physician orders drugs to relieve pain as indicated. Either meperidine hydrochloride (DEMEROL) or morphine sulfate (see Table 7.2, p. 159) is frequently selected by the doctor. The practice of taking and recording the patient's pulse, respiration, and blood pressure before giving the narcotic is

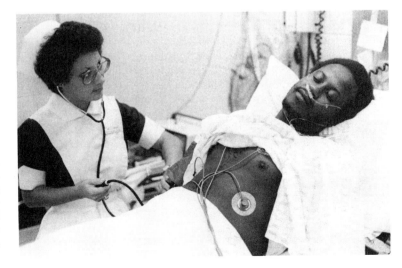

FIGURE 11.8 The practical/vocational nursing student in the coronary care unit. (Courtesy of Southside School of Practical Nursing at Southside Community Hospital, Farmville, Virginia.)

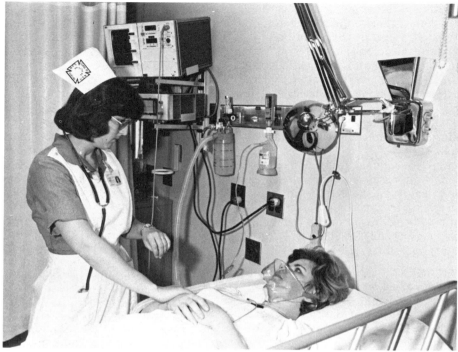

FIGURE 11.9   Patient receiving oxygen and attached to cardiac monitor.

sound. Abnormalities should of course be called to the attention of the nurse or doctor in charge.

A sedative such as phenobarbital (see Table 6.1) or a tranquilizer (see Table 6.2) such as chlordiazepoxide (LIBRIUM) three or four times a day may be prescribed. Apprehension usually decreases as the patient's pain lessens. Sedation helps lessen the body's response to stress, such as the production of epinephrine and norepinephrine. These hormones can produce dangerous arrhythmias. Oxygen therapy usually is ordered via nasal prongs to relieve pain and apprehension associated with hypoxemia (low oxygen in the bloodstream).

Members of the nursing staff must be sensitive to the overwhelming psychologic impact that the pain, environment, and emergency measures have on the patient. What the nurse does and what the nurse says should be in a manner conducive to the patient's feeling of confidence and comfort.

BED REST AND AMBULATION.   Complete bed rest usually is ordered during the early part of the patient's illness. The length of time the patient must remain on strict bed rest depends on the size of the infarction and the patient's response to therapy. As early as 48 hours after the myocardial infarction, the patient may be assisted to an armchair to rest at various times during the day. Armchair care is used by some physicians to decrease the work load of the heart. The work load of the heart is lessened because more of the blood is pooled in the lower extremity, thus reducing the venous return of the blood to the heart. Use of the armchair does not indicate activity on the part of the patient. This is another way of providing rest. The patient is lifted gently to the chair and returned later in a similar manner to the bed. The patient's pulse rate should be taken before the transfer and after placement in a comfortable position in the chair. The patient should be protected from becoming chilled. A footstool is used to elevate the feet slightly. The patient is observed for symptoms of complications such as changes in blood pressure, respiration, and the rate and rhythm of the pulse.

In an effort to prevent the formation of blood clots in the legs, the doctor may have the patient perform simple leg exercises while in bed. Elastic stockings may be applied for the same reason. Use of an anticoagulant drug (see Table 11.5) may help to prevent this complication also.

In an uncomplicated case, after one to two weeks, the patient is allowed to walk. This ambulation is a great boost to the patient's morale as it usually indicates improvement. However, the patient's general condition will guide the doctor in determining at what time ambulation will be permitted. Specific directions will be given by the patient's doctor leading toward a goal of independent activity. The patient usually is conditioned for each new activity. For example, walks that gradually increase in length are usually prescribed. Stair climbing is accomplished a few steps at a time until the full flight can be climbed without fatigue, pain, tachycardia, and dyspnea.

Restricted activity is helpful to the heart in that it decreases the work load. Unfortunately, immobility of the body frequently causes complications such as hypostatic pneumonia and the formation of a thrombus. The physician will consider the advantages and the disadvantages before determining the level of activity to prescribe for an individual patient.

PSYCHOSOCIAL ASPECTS. Psychologic responses frequently exhibited by a patient about a myocardial infarction include anxiety, denial, and anger. The nurse must allow and encourage open expression of the patient in regard to feelings. However, if the patient uses denial, it would be unwise to break down defense unless it interferes with the patient's much-needed rest. In other words, the psychologic responses of an individual to illness and other forms of stress are protective mechanisms. The nurse accepts the patient at a given point without attempting to change these protective mechanisms.

Most patients experience some feeling of depression. The nurse must not attempt to "cheer him up" but instead allow the patient to verbalize feelings. The patient needs to know that these feelings are normal and ex-perienced by most individuals affected by a myocardial infarction.

The patient who develops complications of heart failure such as shock may become confused and restless because of the decreased amount of oxygen reaching the brain. These symptoms should be observed and recorded promptly.

VITAL SIGNS. The patient who has had a myocardial infarction requires constant nursing observation. Blood pressure, pulse, and respiration are determined frequently until they are stable. In addition to taking the patient's pulse in the regular manner and observing the scope of the cardiac monitor, the nurse takes an apical-radial pulse. The quality of the pulse can be determined best by palpation. The purpose of this procedure is to determine if a pulse deficit is present. As stated earlier in this chapter, a pulse deficit occurs when the pulse counted at the radial artery is less than the pulse counted at the apex of the heart. The patient usually will have a low-grade fever one to two days after having a myocardial infarction.

BOWEL FUNCTION. Following a myocardial infarction, especially during the first two weeks, the patient should avoid straining to have a bowel movement. This tends to cause the patient's blood pressure to rise and can be quite hazardous, especially in the patient with hypertension. Straining causes the *Valsalva maneuver*, which involves holding the breath and bearing down. This action is dangerous because it increases the pressure in the thoracic cavity as well as the pressure in the blood vessels. After this maneuver, the patient has a tremendous venous return to the right side of the heart. Stool softeners such as dioctyl sodium sulfosuccinate (COLACE) frequently are prescribed to prevent the patient from straining to have a bowel movement. The patient also may be placed on a bedside commode chair. Studies have shown that less energy is required for the patient to use the bedside commode chair than to use the bedpan while in bed.

DIET. The patient's diet should consist of easily digested foods that do not cause formation of gas. Usually the doctor orders a diet moderately reduced in sodium (1000 mg) (see Table 11.6) for foods high in sodium). In some cases, the physician will allow the patient to use a salt substitute. The nurse should know that many salt substitutes replace the sodium in salt with potassium and would be contraindicated for many patients, depending on the level of potassium in the bloodstream. The calories may be reduced to 1500 to 1800 if the patient is obese. The convalescent period usually is a

Table 11.6
Foods High in Sodium Content*

Almonds, roasted and salted	Liver, beef
Apple brown Betty	Lobster
Asparagus, canned, regular pack	Macaroni and cheese
Bacon	Margarine, salted
Baking powder	Milk, dry, nonfat, instant
Beans, canned, regular pack	Milk, undiluted, evaporated
Beans, green, snap, canned, regular pack	Muffins
Beans, with pork and tomato sauce	Mushrooms, canned
Beans, yellow, canned, regular pack	Mustard, yellow, prepared
Beef, cooked corned	Oatmeal, cooked with salt
Beef, dried	Olives
Beef and vegetable stew, canned	Pancakes
Beef hash, canned	Peanut butter
Beef pot pie	Peanuts, salted
Beets, canned, regular pack	Peas, canned, regular pack
Biscuits	Pickles
Bouillon cube	Piecrust
Bran and bran flakes	Pies
Breads (Boston brown, cracked wheat,	Pizza
French, Italian, raisin, rye, white,	Popcorn
pumpernickel, and whole wheat)	Potato chips
Brownies	Pretzels
Butter	Pudding, bread with raisins
Cakes (all except old-fashioned pound cake)	Pudding, tapioca cream
Candy (caramel and plain fudge)	Rice, cooked with salt
Carrots, canned, regular pack	Rice cereals with salt
Cheese (all types)	Rolls
Chicken pot pie (frozen, commercial)	Rye wafers
Chili con carne, canned with beans	Salad dressings
Chili powder (with seasonings)	Salmon, canned
Clams (hard round meat but not raw, soft meat)	Sardines
Cocoa, processed with alkali	Sauerkraut
Cookies	Sausage
Corn, canned, regular pack	Scallops
Corn cereals	Soups, canned
Cornbread	Spaghetti with meatballs, canned
Cowpeas, canned, regular pack	Spinach, canned, regular pack
Crabmeat, canned	Tomato catsup
Crackers	Tomato juice, canned, regular pack
Cream substitutes	Tuna, canned
Doughnuts	Turnip greens, canned, regular pack
Farina, instant cooking, cooked	Waffles
Haddock, fried	Wheat cereals
Ham	Wheat flour, self-rising
Herring, smoked	White sauce, medium

* Commonly used foods containing more than 150 mg of sodium in 100 gm of the edible portions are included for reference. In other words, the patient on a sodium-restricted diet will have to avoid most of them.

good time for the overweight patient to be started on a weight reduction program.

Many cardiologists prescribe diets low in cholesterol and saturated fats.

OXYGEN THERAPY. The physician may prescribe oxygen therapy for the first few days. A nasal cannual or a face mask with a low flow rate of oxygen and adequate humidification may be ordered.

ANTICOAGULANT THERAPY. The doctor may place the patient on an anticoagulant drug, which prolongs the clotting time of the blood and helps to prevent further clot formation in the coronary arteries. Many physicians, however, believe that the disadvantages of anticoagulants outweigh their advantages.

The two main types of anticoagulants are the coumarin derivatives (dicumarol) and heparin (see Table 11.5). The coumarin derivatives act indirectly and their effect is not realized for approximately 48 hours. Heparin, however, acts immediately.

Blood tests must be done frequently on the patient receiving anticoagulants to keep the clotting mechanism within a safe range. Prothrombin testing will be done for patients receiving coumarin derivatives. Clotting times will be done for the patient receiving heparin. These tests are ordered on a daily basis until the dosage of coumarin and/ or heparin can be stabilized by the physician.

The patient can be expected to bleed longer from minor cuts, such as shaving nicks, and also from venipunctures. When handling the patient receiving anticoagulant therapy, the nurse should avoid any type of injury that could lead to internal hemorrhage. The patient should be observed for bruising, bleeding from the nose, bleeding gums, or bleeding from any body orifice. The patient's urine and feces should be observed for blood also.

COMPLICATIONS OF MYOCARDIAL INFARCTION

Arrhythmia, congestive heart failure, pulmonary edema, and cardiogenic shock are conditions that can complicate a myocardial infarction. Cardiac arrhythmia is discussed in this chapter on pages 288–92 and congestive heart failure is discussed on pages 307–12.

PULMONARY EDEMA. The patient with pulmonary edema has an increased amount of fluid in the lungs. This occurs when the left side of the heart fails to empty properly. This reduced cardiac output on the left side, with a continuous amount of blood getting to the lungs from the right side of the heart, results in an escape of capillary fluid from the bloodstream into the alveoli. This causes congestion of the lungs or pulmonary edema.

Fluid in the alveoli prevents the exchange of oxygen and carbon dioxide. This fluid in the alveoli prevents blood in the pulmonary capillaries from becoming completely oxygenated. The patient's skin and mucous membrane become bluish in color because of the decreased amount of oxygen being delivered. This bluish cast to the skin is called *cyanosis*. Fluid in the lungs also prevents the lungs from completely expanding. *Dyspnea* or shortness of breath occurs because of decreased ventilation.

Symptoms. The patient with pulmonary edema has marked dyspnea and becomes cyanotic. The pulse is rapid and thready, and the blood pressure drops. The collection of fluid in the lungs causes a cough, and frothy blood-tinged sputum may be present. The breathing sounds moist. Frequently, the nurse is able to hear the sounds of the air as it enters and leaves the lungs through the fluid. Moist breath sounds are called *rales* and are caused by the passage of breathed air through the fluid.

Treatment and Nursing Care. The aims of treatment are to improve cardiac function, reduce the amount of fluid in the lungs, and improve the oxygen supply of the blood. The patient is placed in a sitting position to allow the lungs to expand more fully and to pool the circulation in the extremities and away from the heart. Oxygen usually is ordered.

When pulmonary edema is severe, rotating tourniquets may be used to keep a certain portion of the circulating blood volume in the extremities (see Figure 11.10). When placing tourniquets, the nurse applies them

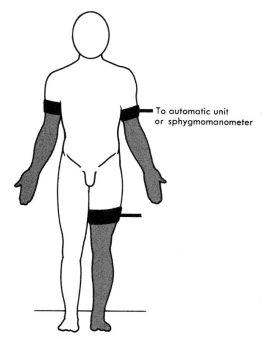

To automatic unit
or sphygmomanometer

FIGURE 11.10 Rotating tourniquets are applied to three limbs for 15 to 20 minutes to keep a certain amount of blood in the extremities. The tourniquets should be rotated in one direction. The arterial flow should not be obliterated in the three limbs.

to three limbs tightly enough to prevent the return of venous blood but not so tightly as to cut off the arterial flow. The pulse in each extremity should be checked frequently. The tourniquets are rotated every 15 to 20 minutes. The tourniquets should be rotated in one direction, such as clockwise. When automatic rotating tourniquets are not available, the nurse may use blood pressure cuffs attached to an anaeroid gauge. The cuff is inflated to the point just above the diastolic pressure. When the treatment is to be discontinued, the nurse should remember that to release all tourniquets at once might cause another attack of pulmonary edema. Specific instructions for gradual removal should be obtained.

Diuretics such as furosemide and ethacrynic acid (see Table 11.7) may be prescribed. These drugs help to reduce the total amount of plasma volume. A phlebotomy to remove 300 to 500 ml of blood is sometimes helpful.

CARDIOGENIC SHOCK. When cardiogenic shock occurs, the patient has a systolic pressure below 90 mm Hg. In addition, the patient is usually restless and may have decreased mental alertness. The urinary

TABLE 11.7
DIURETIC DRUGS*

	NURSING IMPLICATIONS
I. Aldosterone antagonists—substances that reduce the sodium-retaining effect of aldosterone in the kidneys. Aldosterone is a hormone secreted by the adrenal gland which causes the kidneys to excrete less sodium. Thus, a drug that interferes with the normal action of aldosterone causes sodium and water to be excreted	I. May cause potassium to be retained in the body

Nonproprietary Name	*Trade Name*	*Average Daily Dose*
Spironolactone	ALDACTONE	100 mg (divided doses)

II. Benzothiadiazine derivatives (thiazides)—drugs that check the reabsorption of sodium and chloride in the distal convoluted tubules of the kidneys. Water is removed by the extra salt, resulting in diuresis	II. Observe for signs of potassium depletion (drowsy, weak, muscle pain, anorexia); patients who take thiazides and digitalis are more sensitive to digitalis toxicity because of the potassium loss; the diet can supplement potassium loss with foods such as oranges, bananas, meats, and whole

Nonproprietary Name	*Trade Name*	*Average Daily Dose*
Acetazolamide	DIAMOX	250–375 mg
Bendroflumethiazide	BENURON NATURETIN	2–5 mg
Benthiazide	EXNA AQUATAG	25–50 mg
Chlorothiazide	DIURIL	500–2000 mg

TABLE 11.7 (*Continued*)
DIURETIC DRUGS*

			NURSING IMPLICATIONS
Chlorthalidone	HYGROTON	25–100 mg	milk, which are high in po-
Cyclothiazide	ANHYDRON	1–6 mg	tassium
Ethacrynic acid	EDECRIN	50–200 mg	
Flumethiazide		500–2000 mg	
Furosemide	LASIX	40–200 mg	
Hydrochlorothiazide	ESIDREX	25–100 mg	
	HYDRODIURIL		
	ORETIC		
Hydroflumethiazide	SALURON	25–50 mg	
Methylclothiazide	ENDURON	5–10 mg	
Polythiazide	RENESE	4–8 mg	
Quinethazone	HYDROMOX	50–200 mg	
Trichlormethiazide	METAHYDRIN	4–8 mg	
	NAQUA		

III. Inhibitors of carbonic anhydrase—substances that check the enzyme, carbonic anhydrase, that is responsible for the union of water and carbon dioxide to form carbonic acid. These substances also cause sodium and potassium bicarbonate to be excreted along with water from the kidneys

III. This group of diuretics is used infrequently

Nonproprietary Name	*Trade Name*	*Average Daily Dose*	
Acetazolamide	DIAMOX	250–500 mg	Acetazolamide is used in
Dichlorphenamide	DARANIDE	50–200 mg	the treatment of glau-
Ethoxzolamide	CARDRASE	125–1000 mg	coma
	ETHAMIDE		
Methazolamide	NEPTAZANE	100–300 mg	

IV. Mercurial diuretics—decrease the reabsorption of sodium and chloride in the kidney tubules. Water is removed with the extra salt, resulting in diuresis. Most mercurial diuretics must be given by injection unless otherwise indicated below

IV. May produce arrhythmias; may cause excessive loss of chloride

Nonproprietary Name	*Trade Name*	*Average Daily Dose*	
Chlormerodrin	NEOHYDRIN	10–40 mg (oral)	
	MERCLORAN		
Meralluride	MERCUHYDRIN	0.5–2.0 ml	
Mercaptomerin	THIOMERIN	0.2–.0 ml	Mercaptomerin requires
			refrigeration
Mercumatilin	CUMERTILIN	0.5–2.0 ml	
Mercurophylline		0.5–2.0 ml	
Merethoxylline	DICURIN	0.5–2.0 ml	
Mersalyl	SALYRGAN	0.5–2.0 ml	

V. Osmotic diuretics—substances that are filtered through the glomeruli but not readily absorbed in the renal tubules. The presence of these substances disturbs osmosis in the tubules, resulting in diuresis

V. These diuretics are rarely used except in the treatment of cerebral edema

Nonproprietary Name	*Trade Name*	*Average Daily Dose*	
Mannitol	OSMITROL	25% solution in 50 ml ampules (IV)	
Urea	UREAPHIL	1–1.5 gm per kg of body weight (IV)	

VI. Xanthines increase the production of urine resulting in decrease of edema

VI. Observe for signs of gastric discomfort; xanthines will be less effective for

TABLE 11.7 *(Continued)*
DIURETIC DRUGS*

			NURSING IMPLICATIONS
Nonproprietary Name	*Trade Name*	*Average Daily Dose*	patients who have a high intake of coffee or tea
Aminophylline		100–200 mg (oral)	
		250–500 mg (IV)	
		250–500 mg suppositories	
Amisometradine	ROLICTON	0.4–3.2 gm	
Caffeine and sodium benzoate		60 mg (oral) 500 mg (parenteral)	
Dyphylline	LUFYLLIN	100–200 mg	
Oxtriphyllin		100–200 mg	
Choline theophyllimate	CHOLEDYL		
Theobromine calcium salicylate	THEOCALCIN	500 mg	
Theobromine sodium salicylate	DIURETIN	500 mg	
Theophylline	THEOCIN	200–800 mg	
Theophylline sodium acetate	THESODATE	100–200 mg	

VII. Other diuretics

Nonproprietary Name	*Trade Name*	*Average Daily Dose*
Triamterene	DYRENIUM	100 mg

* Diuretic drugs increase the flow of urine, resulting in the reduction of edema. Diuretics cause a lowering of blood pressure and chemical alteration of the blood.
  Diuretics are classified as aldosterone antagonists, benzothiadiazine derivatives (thiazides), inhibitors of carbonic anhydrase, mercurial diuretics, osmotic diuretics, and xanthines. A brief explanation of each and drugs common to that classification are provided as a reference.
  Patients receiving diuretics should be weighed daily to help determine fluid balance. Diuretics should be taken in the morning rather than in the evening. Patients should be observed for signs of dehydration and lowered blood pressure.

output decreases. The patient's skin appears ashen and cyanotic because of the decreased amount of oxygenated blood reaching the periphery.

Efforts are made to reverse the condition. Oxygen, drugs to elevate the blood pressure (see Table 11.8), and digitalis usually are given. The prognosis of the patient with cardiogenic shock is poor. Other methods to reverse cardiogenic shock are being investigated.

Rheumatic Heart Disease

Rheumatic heart disease is a form of rheumatic fever. This is an infection occurring most often in childhood and early adulthood. The patient frequently has an infected throat caused by the hemolytic streptococcus (member of streptococcal family of bacteria) before developing rheumatic fever.

The specific cause of this disease is unknown.

SYMPTOMS AND COMPLICATIONS

The patient has a migrating inflammation of one joint after another; in other words, the inflammation moves from one joint to another. For example, the knee joints may be inflamed first and in a short while an elbow joint becomes inflamed. The inflammation of the first joints to be affected disappears. Symptoms of inflammation, which are discussed in Chapter 5 such as fever, malaise, and local pain and swelling of the joints, are present. Rheumatic infection may affect the endocardium, myocardium, or pericardium. Symptoms vary with the part of the heart inflamed.

The endocardium is most often involved. Since this membrane lines the valves, the patient may develop a heart murmur. The

TABLE 11.8
SYMPATHOMIMETIC DRUGS*

NONPROPRIETARY NAME	TRADE NAME	AVERAGE DOSE	NURSING IMPLICATIONS
Dopamine	INTROPIN	2–5 mcg/kg/ minute (IV)	Frequent readings of blood pressure and pulse will be required during the administration of these drugs; be alert to the development of arrhythmias
Ephedrine		15–20 mg (parenteral)	
Epinephrine Adrenaline		0.5–1.0 mg (subcutaneous)	
Hydroxyamphetamine	PAREDRINE	5–10 mg (IV)	
Isoproterenol	ISUPREL	0.2 mg/ml (injection)	
Levarterenol (norephinephrine)	LEVOPHED	0.002–0.008 mg (IV)	
Metaraminol	ARAMINE	5–10 mg (parenteral)	
Methamphetamine	DESOXYN	10–30 mg (IV, IM)	
Methoxamine	VASOXYL	5–10 mg (IV)	

* Sympathomimetic drugs have their main effect on the circulatory system by stimulating the muscles of blood vessels and causing the heart to beat faster and more forcefully. These drugs have other actions. Also this group of drugs contains other agents not included in this list. Examples of the drugs that have mainly a vasopressor action are included in this list. In other words, they stimulate contractions of the muscle tissue of the arteries and capillaries, increase the heart rate and force, and cause a rise in blood pressure. They are sometimes called vasopressors.

valves, which are normally smooth, become hard and scarred. Blood flowing over a diseased valve makes an abnormal sound called a *murmur*. A diseased valve may be unable to fulfill its function of keeping blood from returning to the cavity that is pumping it on. This valve, which does not close properly, allows blood to flow in the wrong direction, and is referred to as a *leaking valve*. When a valve does not open properly, it is stenosed (narrowed).

The mitral valve between the left atrium and left ventricle is most often involved. Stenosis of this valve is called mitral stenosis. Mitral insufficiency occurs when the mitral valve flaps are so scarred and shrunken that they cannot close the opening. Congestive heart failure may develop during the acute phase, or after many years have passed.

TREATMENT

Treatment is aimed toward relieving the symptoms, preventing permanent heart damage, and preventing another attack. The most important factor during the acute stage is rest. Salicylates, such as aspirin and sodium salicylate, are used to relieve joint pain. Penicillin and cortisone are helpful in some cases.

If the patient's mitral valve becomes inflamed with scarring and degeneration,

symptoms of left-sided heart failure may develop. These symptoms frequently are associated with the arrhythmia of atrial fibrillation. The nursing care of a patient with heart failure is discussed later in this chapter.

The patient with marked mitral stenosis may benefit from a surgical procedure called *commissurotomy*. This procedure usually is done with open-heart surgery to provide direct visualization of the valve by the surgeon. The valve frequently can be repaired or perhaps replaced with an artificial ball valve. The commissurotomy, or breaking apart of the stenosed leaflets of the valve, also can be done without open-heart surgery and the heart-lung machine if the patient cannot physically tolerate the stress associated with this type of surgery. Such a decision is made by the cardiac surgeon and the cardiologist. The primary disadvantage of doing the procedure in the closed method is that symptoms may recur after a few months or years.

Heart Surgery or Cardiovascular Surgery

Surgery of the heart has made great strides in the past few years. Surgical procedures were performed successfully around the heart as early as 1923 but not until 1955 was surgery performed to repair a defect within the heart. This was done with the aid of hypothermia, a technique used to lower body temperature. The amount of anesthetic agent can be reduced and danger of shock is also lessened. In addition, the length of time that oxygen supply to the brain, spinal cord, and other vital organs can be interrupted is increased from four to eight minutes at these lowered body temperatures. However, hypothermia is not used without risk of complications such as ventricular fibrillation, which is more difficult to correct in a cooled heart.

EXTRACORPOREAL CIRCULATION (HEART-LUNG MACHINE)

Almost all open heart surgery is now performed with the aid of the heart-lung machine, a pump-oxygenator. This machine allows the patient more operating time than was possible with hypothermia. Many defects, for example, atrial and ventricular septal defects, aortic aneurysms, patent ductus, as well as leaking and stenosed heart valves, can be repaired with employment of this machine, which has been refined and simplified over the years.

The pump-oxygenator, which takes over the functions of the heart and lungs during heart surgery and surgery of the great vessels, allows the heart to be opened for extended periods of time. Most defects can be repaired in 15 to 20 minutes. Plastic catheters are inserted into the superior and inferior vanae cavae, through which blood is withdrawn into the machine. This diverts venous blood from the heart (right atrium) into the oxygenator. The machine then removes the carbon dioxide from the blood and oxygenates it. The newly oxygenated blood is then pumped back into the body through a catheter that is inserted into the right or left femoral artery in the groin and on up into the iliac artery.

The use of the heart-lung machine makes it possible to replace sections of blood vessels with synthetic grafts made of DACRON or TEFLON. Artificial hearts or heart-assist devices are under experimental investigation and may one day be used with greater success than we can now envision. In December, 1967, the first heart transplant operations were performed in Capetown, South Africa, by Dr. Christian Barnard and in New York by Dr. Adrian Kantrowitz. The procedure, which has passed the experimental stage, is being used for selected patients all over the world.

The major problem, as is true of all transplant operations, is immunologic rejection caused by the body, which sets up a reaction to reject or destroy the new organ. Immunosuppressive therapy with antilymphocytic globulin (ALG) has been used with success, but some patients develop a resistance to the drug. Many problems continue to exist related to heart transplants, including ethical, moral, and economic factors.

Another common heart defect, stenosis or blockage of coronary arteries, which causes angina pectoris and leads to myocardial infarction, has been the subject of much research. Surgical procedures such as the coronary artery bypass graft are being performed to reduce the pain of angina and to improve the patient's life-style (Figure 11.11).

Repair of some types of heart defects can be done without the use of the heart-lung machine. An example is the repair of some types of atrial septal defects.

NURSING CARE

PREOPERATIVE CARE. The patient usually is admitted to the hospital several days in advance for extensive preoperative preparation. In addition to diagnostic studies described earlier in the chapter, the patient participates in a preoperative instruction program which includes information sessions, practice periods, and question-and-answer periods. For example, an information session could include normal heart function, a description of the surgical procedure, and a demonstration of equipment used postoperatively. A practice session could include turning, coughing, and deep-breathing techniques such as those described in Chapter 14. Question-and-answer periods include topics that interest and concern the patient and family. Most patients request additional information about the recovery room and the intensive care unit where they will spend the first postoperative week. In addition, the nurse carefully

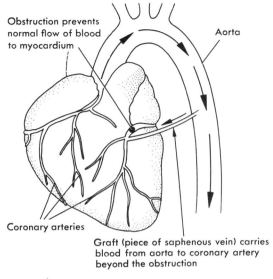

Obstruction prevents
normal flow of blood
to myocardium

Aorta

Coronary arteries

Graft (piece of saphenous vein) carries
blood from aorta to coronary artery
beyond the obstruction

A

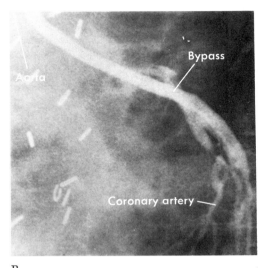

Aorta

Bypass

Coronary artery

B

FIGURE 11.11 *A.* Diagrammatic sketch of coronary artery bypass graft illustrating the direct flow of blood from the aorta to the heart muscle. *B.* Photograph of bypass of left coronary artery using saphenous vein. (Courtesy of Cardiac Diagnostic Unit, Medical Center Hospitals, Norfolk, Virginia.)

observes the patient's behavior and vital signs so that a baseline observation is established against which changes in the postoperative period can be evaluated.

POSTOPERATIVE CARE. Most patients return from surgery with an endotracheal tube in place. Mechanical assistance usually is needed for several hours to ensure that the lungs are properly ventilated. After having the endotracheal tube removed, the patient will receive oxygen, usually by nasal catheter. Intermittent positive pressure breathing (IPPB) or deep-breathing exercises are used to help remove lung secretions and to prevent atelectasis. The patient may have an indwelling or Foley catheter in the urinary bladder. A nasogastric tube may be connected to low suction to prevent gastric dilatation also. Careful and frequent monitoring of vital signs, observation of the color of nailbeds, lips, and skin, and observation of the appearance of the extremities are needed. Numbness, tingling, or mottling of an extremity with pain could indicate formation of a blood clot. Observing and medicating for pain, checking surgical dressings for signs of hemorrhage, positioning, and turn-

ing are extremely important. It is also important for the nurse to remember that both patient and family may be overwhelmed with the equipment. Preoperative instruction of the patient and family can decrease this reaction to the equipment. The patient and his family will need reassurance, honest answers, and accurate explanations.

The patient will have monitoring devices such as the cardiac monitor and a central venous pressure device. In addition, some patients will have pressures of the left atrium and pulmonary vessels measured. It is imperative that the nurse make an accurate reading of the pressure and maintain safe working order of all equipment. It is important for the nurse to remember that air introduced into the arterial or venous system can be disastrous for the patient. Since the chest cavity has been entered, the patient will have chest tubes connected to water-sealed drainage to allow excess air and fluid to drain from the pleural cavity and to restore negative pressure in the pleural cavity. Fluid balance is critical immediately after surgery, and most patients have specific orders to replace fluid loss with intravenous fluids and whole blood.

After the patient is transferred from the intensive care unit to a surgical floor, monitoring may continue while a carefully supervised program of exercise and activity continues. Prior to discharge, patient and family teaching is needed similar to that described earlier in this chapter on pages 287–88.

Endocarditis

Inflammation of the endocardium may be caused by a rheumatic infection or by bacteria; when caused by bacteria, this condition is called *bacterial endocarditis*. When it is caused by bacterial infection, local areas of inflammation result in the formation of tiny masses, called *vegetations*. When these vegetations form on valve flaps, abnormal functioning of the valve occurs. Scar tissue forms in the areas of vegetation after the inflammatory process has subsided. When scar tissue affects the functioning of a valve,

the patient has *valvular heart disease*. A description of other chronic valvular diseases can be located in Table 11.9.

SYMPTOMS

Symptoms usually associated with an inflammation are present: fever, chills, fast pulse rate, increased white blood cell count, and malaise. A murmur is often heard by the physician.

TREATMENT

In addition to bed rest, drugs are used to combat the infection. The physician selects the drug that is most effective against the bacteria causing the infection.Although the infection usually can be cured by drugs, valvular damage is not improved. Heart surgery may be needed to repair damaged valves or replace them. The care of the patient having heart surgery can be located in this chapter on pages 303–306.

TABLE 11.9
CHRONIC VALVULAR HEART DISEASE*

DISORDER	DESCRIPTION
Aortic regurgitation	The pulmonary semilunar valve functions improperly allowing blood to flow back from the aorta to the left ventricle; rheumatic fever, bacterial endocarditis, congenital defects, and syphilis may cause the valve to function poorly; replacement of the valve with a suitable prosthesis is made in some patients
Aortic stenosis	A narrowing at or near the aortic semilunar valve results in varying degrees of obstruction to the flow of blood through the aorta from the left ventricle; this condition may be congenital or develop as a result of rheumatic fever; some cases are treated medically and others surgically
Mitral regurgitation	The mitral valve functions improperly, allowing blood to flow back from the left ventricle to the left atrium; usually follows rheumatic fever; replacement of valve with a prosthetic valve is done in some patients
Mitral stenosis	A condition in which the mitral or bicuspid valve becomes narrowed; usually the patient has had rheumatic fever, which caused scar tissue to form in the valve; surgery generally is indicated if the patient has symptoms of this condition
Tricuspid regurgitation	The tricuspid valve functions improperly, allowing blood to flow back from the right ventricle to the right atrium; rheumatic fever usually precedes this condition; replacement of the valve with a prosthetic valve may be made
Tricuspid stenosis	A narrowing of the tricuspid valve is usually a result of rheumatic fever; frequently the patient has stenosis of the mitral valve also; prosthetic replacement of the diseased valve is of value to certain patients

* Chronic disease of the valves of the heart frequently occurs following rheumatic fever and certain other diseases. In some cases, the condition is congenital. Advances in cardiac surgery are enabling many patients to have the opportunity to be relieved of some of these disabling conditions. A description of the main valvular heart conditions is included for reference.

Myocarditis (Inflammatory or Infective Cardiomyopathy)

Myocarditis (inflammation of the myocardium) may develop as a complication of many different infections of viral, bacterial, protozoal, and rickettsial origin.

Since the major function of the heart is dependent upon muscular activity, an acute inflammation of this muscle is serious. Often the first signs noted are symptoms of rapidly developing heart failure. Measures for the care of a patient with congestive heart failure are employed.

Pericarditis

The patient with pericarditis has an inflammation of the pericardium. It can be caused by a rheumatic infection of the heart or an infection of the lungs, such as tuberculosis or pneumonia, which may spread to the pericardium. This inflammation also may be caused by pathogenic microorganisms brought in by the bloodstream.

Functioning of the heart is affected when fluid collects in the pericardial sac and presses on the heart. The patient usually is admitted to the hospital and placed on bed rest, oxygen therapy, and drug therapy. When heart function is severely compromised by the collection of fluid in the pericardial sac, a procedure known as *pericardiocentesis* or *pericardial tap* may be done to remove excess fluid. The physician uses a long needle to aspirate fluid from the pericardial sac. The patient usually is transferred to the intensive care unit for continuous monitoring.

Congestive Heart Failure

Any of the heart diseases discussed earlier in this chapter may cause the patient to develop congestive heart failure. Heart failure occurs when the heart is unable to perform its pumping function efficiently enough to meet the demand placed on it. This results in a collection of fluid in the tissues, which is referred to as *edema*. Since most of the symptoms of heart failure are caused by congestion, the condition is called *congestive heart failure*. It is also referred to

as *cardiac failure* or *cardiac decompensation*.

The term *heart failure* does not mean necessarily that the patient is doomed to die. Present-day treatment and nursing care are effective in helping many patients return to a compensated condition. The compensated heart has made up for the diesease that produced the failure. For example, the heart may enlarge in an effort to meet the extra demands made upon it by disease. *hypertrophy*

SYMPTOMS

It is important for the nurse to have a basic understanding of symptoms associated with cardiac failure. A majority of patients with heart diesease develop congestive heart failure at some time in the disease process.

FAILURE OF THE LEFT SIDE. When the left side of the heart is not functioning properly, the blood being returned to the left atrium through the pulmonary veins becomes congested in the lungs. The patient whose condition continues is likely to have *pulmonary edema,* which is a collection of fluid in the air sacs and lung tissue, discussed on pages 299–300.

FAILURE OF THE RIGHT SIDE. When the right side of the heart is functioning improperly, the blood being returned to the right atrium backs up into the inferior vena cava. Edema, which is a collection of fluid in the tissues resulting in swelling, develops in the parts of the body drained of its venous flow by this large vein. As the blood backs up in the venous system, pressure builds up in the capillaries. Fluid begins to lead out into the surrounding cells. This excess interstitial fluid is called edema. *Dropsy* and *anasarca* are other names for edema. Thus, the organs below the heart are subject to a collection of fluid in their tissues. This edema develops in the lower area of the body first. Edema progresses from the ankles, to the legs and thighs, and then into the abdomen. A collection of fluid in the peritoneal cavity is called *ascites*.

Edema of the abdominal organs, such as the stomach and intestines, causes loss of appetite, indigestion, and flatus (gas in the gastrointestinal tract). *Oliguria* (a decreased amount of urine) occurs because a decreased amount of blood is pumped through the kidneys. In addition, edema of the kidneys may be present, decreasing their ability to function.

The patient with congestive heart failure usually has a combination of right- and left-sided failure with one side weaker than the other. The severity of symptoms depends upon the degree of cardiac inefficiency. In the early stage of heart failure, or mild cardiac failure, the patient experiences fatigue, dyspnea following slight exertion, and edema of the feet and ankles.

Edema of the feet is referred to as *pedal edema*. The edema usually disappears after a night's rest. A slight cough with a small amount of expectoration may be present. Also, the patient may awaken at night with dyspnea, which is relieved by sitting up. This sudden waking with respiratory difficulty after having been asleep for several hours is known as *paroxysmal nocturnal dyspnea* (cardiac asthma).

The patient in an advanced stage of heart failure has the aforementioned symptoms to a greater degree. Dyspnea is acute even while at rest. Orthopnea may be present, a condition in which there is need to sit up to breathe more easily. The patient coughs and expectorates frothy, blood-tinged sputum. Cyanosis is present. There is marked edema of the feet, legs, back and abdomen. The urinary output is decreased. Mental processes are affected when the blood supply to the brain is inadequate. The patient may have lapse of memory, drowsiness, or restlessness because of this.

TREATMENT AND NURSING CARE

REST. Rest is of vital importance. The heart, which has added strain placed upon it by disease, needs maximum relief from normal demands of body functions. It is the nursing team's responsibility to help the patient obtain the maximum amount of mental and physical rest. Rest lessens the tissue demands for oxygen. Anxiety and restlessness increase the strain placed on the heart. Problems that worry the patient should be reported to the team leader or head nurse.

The patient should be in a quiet, well-ventilated room. The specific amount of rest is prescribed by the doctor. Some physicians order complete bed rest. In this instance, the patient may be bathed, turned, lifted, and fed. The patient should be placed in a comfortable position, which often is semirecumbent. Pillows can be used to support the lower arms and a footboard should be used to prevent footdrop.

The patient with pulmonary edema is often more comfortable in an armchair. Sedatives (drugs having a quieting or soothing effect) are often ordered as an aid in producing rest; phenobarbital and chloral hydrate are two examples. Tranquilizers may be used also. Morphine and other opium derivatives are used because they produce an exaggerated sense of well-being (euphoria) and relieve pain (see Table 7.2, page 159).

Straining when having a bowel movement increases the heart's work load. This should be avoided. It is for this reason that either an enema or a mild laxative is ordered. Of course, the enema must be given with gentleness and skill.

PERSONAL HYGIENE. Oral hygiene is especially important for the mouth-breathing dyspneic patient. Restricted fluids also increase dryness of the mouth. The nurse is responsible for cleaning the mouth if the patient is unable to do so.

The patient in the acute stage of congestive heart failure may be allowed only a partial bath. However, as the condition improves, the patient should have a complete bath. Particular attention must be paid to the patient's skin when edema is present. Edematous tissue is likely to develop decubitus ulcers because the edema limits the flow of blood. The decreased flow of blood reduces the nutrition of the involved area and makes it more susceptible to decubiti. Nursing measure to prevent decubiti are important. Frequent massaging of the skin with an emollient lotion and placing foam rubber pads under bony prominences such as the elbows and heels are helpful. Placing pieces of sheepskin or a newer synthetic substitute under the patient's buttocks and heels helps to prevent irritation. The patient may be placed on an alternating-pressure mattress on an air mattress to prevent decubiti.

DIET.   The physician generally indicates the amount of sodium allowed for the patient. For example, the doctor may order a 500-mg-sodium diet. By ordering a diet with a reduced amount or sodium, the doctor hopes to enable nature to eliminate excess fluid as well as to prevent the collection of more fluid in the edematous patient. Also, the feedings are usually small and served frequently, as it may tire the patient to eat.

The patient with a designated number of milligrams of sodium in the diet can use seasoning aids such as fresh onion, orange extract, oregano, parsley, rosemary, sage, sesame seeds, tarragon, marjoram, mace, lemon juice or extract, garlic, curry, chives, bay leaf, allspice, basil, and dry mustard. The variety of foods allowed on the diet should be emphasized.

Meals must be made as appetizing as possible within the limitations outlined by the physician. For example, a poached egg cooked without salt and not served immediately would not tempt the patient's appetite. Of course, the patient on a low-sodium diet is not allowed to have salt on a poached egg, but it certainly could be served warm. Salt substitutes are frequently ordered by the doctor. However, many of these preparations contain potassium and the cardiac patient frequently has to limit the intake of potassium.

Foods that are more difficult to digest, as well as those that are gas producing, such as cabbage, beans, and peas, should be avoided. Flatus in the stomach causes pressure on the diaphragm, which increases the patient's dyspnea.

Overeating and gaining weight put added strain on the heart. Overweight patients are often placed on a diet low in calories. The practical/vocational nurse is frequently responsible for some aspect of the diet therapy. It may be in the preparation of the food in the home, or in serving and feeding the patient in the hospital. Foods cooked without salt are unappetizing to the average person, who is accustomed to seasoning. Pa-

tients who understand the importance of a restricted diet are more likely to be cooperative.

FLUIDS.   A record of the fluid intake and output is frequently requested by the doctor. An accurate account of the amount of liquids taken into the body, and those excreted from the body, is an important guide for the physician in planning treatment. For example, if the patient's intake for a 24-hour period was 2000 ml (2 qt) and output for the same period was 250 ml (8.3 ox), the doctor might order a diuretic; whereas if the output were 1000 ml (1 qt), this drug probably would not be prescribed. The intake-and-output record and the daily weight and the physician in determining the patient's condition (see Figures 11.12 and 11.13).

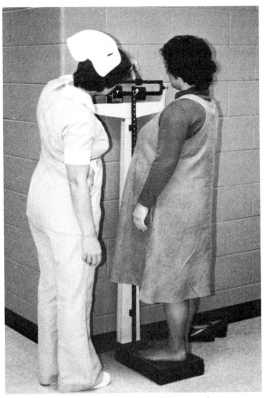

FIGURE 11.12 Daily weights at the same time, on the same scale, and with the same clothing help to determine fluid balance. (Courtesy of Loudoun County School of Practical Nursing, Leesburg, Virginia.)

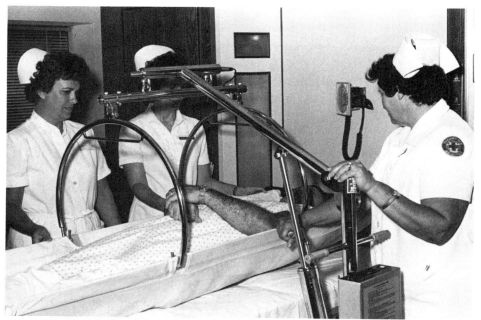

FIGURE 11.13 A bed scale may be used if the patient is unable to stand for the daily weight. (Courtesy of Tri-County Area Vocational-Technical School and Jane Phillips Episcopal Memorial Medical Center, Bartlesville, Oklahoma.)

The fluid intake of the patient may be restricted to a certain number of milliliters or ounces within a 24-hour period. Although the amount of liquids is usually decreased, some doctors increase the intake for patients on a low-sodium diet. It is the nursing team's responsibility to keep the amount of fluids within the range prescribed.

The patient is weighed frequently to determine whether there is an increase or a decrease of edema. For example, a loss of several pounds in a 24-hour period shows a loss of fluid. For accuracy, the patient should be weighed on the same scales, at the same time each day, and have on the same amount of clothing.

DEHYDRATION. Although the patient may experience edema with congestive heart failure, an excessive loss of fluid from the body may also be present. Dehydration occurs when too much fluid is lost from the body (see Figure 11.14 and 11.15).

Water is essential for life. The functions of water in the body are to supply fluid to make secretions, serve as a medium for chemical changes associated with digestion, serve as a vehicle for dissolved products of metabolism to be moved from the body, and help to regulate body temperature by evaporation.

Signs of dehydration include a decreased amount of urine that appears concentrated. The patient will have a warm, dry skin, and the lips will be dry and cracked. Fever may

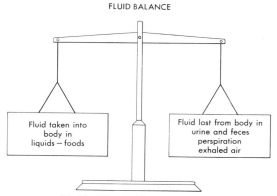

FIGURE 11.14 The fluid balance of the body is maintained by an adequate intake and output of fluids.

DEHYDRATION

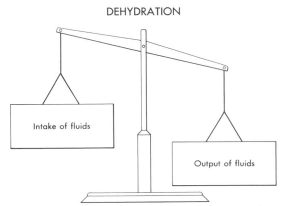

FIGURE 11.15 The fluid balance is disturbed when a person does not take in a sufficient amount of fluid or when a person loses too much fluid. This results in dehydration.

also be present. The tongue will appear dry and coated.

OXYGEN THERAPY. The patient usually receives oxygen therapy by nasal prongs (Figure 11.16). Often, the physician orders intermittent positive pressure breathing

(IPPB) treatments every four hours during the acute phase of illness and less often as the patient's condition improves. Additional information about oxygen therapy can be located in Chapter 16.

DRUG THERAPY. The most frequently ordered drugs for the patient with congestive heart failure are diuretics and digitalis derivatives (see Tables 11.7 and 11.10). As mentioned earlier in the chapter, the nurse carefully observes the patient for signs of digitalis toxicity.

Use of an oral diuretic may necessitate the addition of foods high in potassium, such as bananas, beets, raisins, broccoli spears, raw cabbage, celery, broiled chicken, dried figs, liver, dry nonfat instant milk, dried peaches, peanut butter, baked potatoes, orange juice, and dried uncooked prunes, to the patient's diet as these drugs have a tendency to cause potassium loss. In some cases potassium chloride in either liquid or tablet form may be prescribed.

DIVERSIONS. Helping the patient with diversions during a period of relative inac-

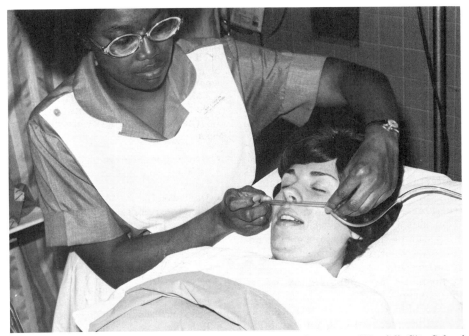

FIGURE 11.16 Patient receiving oxygen by nasal prongs. (Courtesy of Norfolk City Schools and Norfolk General Hospital School of Practical Nursing, Norfolk, Virginia.)

TABLE 11.10
DIGITALIS AND RELATED DRUGS (CARDIAC GLYCOSIDES)*

NONPROPRIETARY NAME	TRADE NAME	AVERAGE DOSE	NURSING IMPLICATIONS
Acetyldigitoxin	ACYLANID	0.1–0.2 mg	Count pulse before administering; if pulse
Deslanoside (desacetyl- lanatoside C)	CEDILANID D	0.2 gm (injection)	is below 60, do not give and report immediately. Note changes in pulse in addition to bradycardia. Be aware that a
Digitalis		1.0 gm (initial) 0.1 gm (maintenance)	loss of potassium from the body that occurs with many diuretics may increase the risk of digitalis toxicity. The patient
Digitoxin	CRYSTODIGIN	1.0 mg (initial) 0.1 mg (maintenance)	should be taught how to count his pulse and to recognize side effects such as nausea, vomiting, anorexia, and vision
Digoxin	LANOXIN	0.5 mg	disturbances
Gitalin (gitaligin)		0.5 mg	
Lanatoside C		0.5 mg	
Ouabain G-Strophanthin		0.25–0.5 mg (injection)	

* Cardiac glycosides are a group of drugs that are plant extracts. These drugs increase the force of the contraction of the myocardium and decrease the rate to some extent.

tivity is indeed a challenge to the nursing team. The nurse with imagination, ingenuity, interest, and enthusiasm can contribute much toward diversional activities.

Factors to consider in selecting diversions for the patient include the amount of activity permitted by the physician, personal preferences of the patient, and available facilities. During the more acute phase of illness, the patient's entertainment may consist mainly of nonexciting radio and television programs, and reading aloud by the nurse. Preparing attractive trays with a miniature vase of flowers or with tray favors give the patient something to anticipate. Arranging get-well cards so that they can be seen gives many hours of pleasure. Watching activities of goldfish and observing the growth of flowers are additional sources of passive entertainment.

As the patient improves and is allowed more freedom of activity, playing cards, working puzzles, collecting articles of interest such as stamps and rocks, observing activities of birds, writing, painting, and knitting may be enjoyed.

Many hospitals have departments of occupational therapy. The occupational therapist helps to plan diversional activities as well as suitable occupations for patients. This member of the health team is of great importance to the person who is a partial invalid because of a heart condition.

Case Study Involving Atrial Fibrillation and Possible Mitral Stenosis

When being admitted to the hospital unit Mrs. Franklin had a rapid and irregular pulse and dyspnea. She indicated that she frequently awakened during the middle of the night and was unable to get her breath. She is more comfortable when sleeping with two pillows.

Mrs. Franklin had rheumatic fever during her childhood and is now 30 years of age.

The following orders were written by her physician:

- Bed rest with bathroom privileges
- 1000-mg-sodium diet (moderate sodium restriction)
- Daily weight
- Electrocardiogram
- Complete blood count and urinalysis
- Digoxin, 0.5 mg PO now
      0.25 mg at 4 P.M.
      0.25 mg at 10 P.M.
      0.25 mg daily
- Oxygen, 4 liters/minute prn for dyspnea
- ESIDRIX, 25 mg qd PO
- Schedule for echocardiogram
- Rule out mitral stenosis and congestive heart failure

QUESTIONS

1. What is the relationship between a history of rheumatic fever and a diagnosis of mitral valve stenosis?
2. Which side of the heart could be causing Mrs. Franklin's symptoms of congestive heart failure? Hint: Failure of which side of the heart could cause congestion in the lungs?
3. What should Mrs. Franklin be told about her low-sodium diet?
4. What should the nurse explain to Mrs. Franklin regarding the echocardiogram?
5. What is the purpose of daily weights for Mrs. Franklin and under what conditions should she be weighed?
6. What specific nursing measures should be taken to improve Mrs. Franklin's rest and sleep?
7. What nursing assistance will Mrs. Franklin need because of diuretic therapy and digitalization?

Case Study Involving Angina Pectoris

Mr. Dozier was admitted to the hospital because of an increase in the sypmtoms of angina pectoris. Although he has never experienced a complete occlusion of a coronary artery, he has angina pectoris. The attacks of pain have become more frequent and more severe during the past month.

Mr. Dozier is 40 years of age and had been in good health until he developed angina several years ago. His brother died suddenly after having a myocardial infarction at the age of 40. Mr. Dozier appears to be anxious and calls the nurse frequently. Mrs. Dozier spends much time with her husband and frequently reminds the nurses of the medication schedule.

The orders written by Mrs. Dozier's physician are as follows.

- Bed rest with bathroom privileges
- ISORDIL, 10 mg PO q6h   vasodilator
- Nitroglycerin, 0.15 mg sublingually as needed Leave tablets at bedside and record number taken by patient every eight hours
- Notify physician if pain is not relieved by nitroglycerin
- Electrocardiogram in A.M.
- Schedule for cardiac catheterization with coronary arteriogram

QUESTIONS

1. Is it possible that Mrs. Dozier is telling the nursing personnel that she is apprehensive about her husband because of her frequent reminders regarding the medication schedule? yes
2. What nursing actions will help to relieve the anxiety of Mr. and Mrs. Dozier? Explain
3. What are the therapeutic and untoward effects of ISORDIL?
4. How should the nursing staff prepare Mr. Dozier for the cardiac catheterization and coronary arteriogram? prep, consent
5. What instructions should the nurse give Mr. Dozier about using nitroglycerin?

Suggestions for Further Study

1. Is there a local heart society in your community? If so, what are its main functions?
2. Visit the diagnostic facilities in your hospital and watch each of the diagnostic procedures described in this chapter.
3. Participate in a drill that simulates the procedure used in your hospital to respond to a cardiac arrest.
4. Interview a patient with heart disease to learn how the illness has affected personal and family life-style.
5. Mason, Mildred A.; Bates, Grace F.; and Smola, Bonnie K.: *Workbook in Basic Medical-Surgical Nursing*, 3rd ed. Macmillan Publishing Company, New York, 1984, Exercise 11.

Additional Readings

Cromwell, Violet; Huey, Ruth; Korn, Ruth; Weiss, June; and Woodley, Rowena: "Understanding the Needs of Your Coronary Bypass Patient." *Nursing*, 10:34–39 (Mar.), 1980.

Dehn, Michael: "Rehabilitation of the Cardiac Patient: The Effects of Exercise." *American Journal of Nursing*, 80:435–40 (Mar.), 1980.

Finesilver, Cynthia: "Reducing Stress in Patients Having Cardiac Catheterization." *American Journal of Nursing*, 80:1805–1807 (Oct.), 1980.

Fuller, Ellen O.: "The Effect of Antianginal Drugs on Myocardial Oxygen Consumption." *American Journal of Nursing*, 80:250–54 (Feb.), 1980.

Hansen, Mary Susan, and Woods, Susan: "Nitroglycerin Ointment—Where and How to Apply It." *American Journal of Nursing*, 80:1122–24 (June), 1980.

Lovvorn, Jo: "Coronary Artery Bypass Surgery: Helping Patients Cope with Postop Problems." *American Journal of Nursing*, 82:1073–75 (July), 1982.

Mar, Dexter D.: "New Topical Nitroglycerin Preparations." *American Journal of Nursing*, 82:462–63 (Mar.), 1982.

O'Flynn-Comiskey, Alice I.: "Stress—The Type A Individual." *American Journal of Nursing*, 79:1956–58 (Nov.), 1979.

Purcell, Julia Ann, and Giffin, Patti: "Percutaneous Transluminal Coronary Angioplasty." *American Journal of Nursing*, 81:1620–26 (Sept.), 1981.

Rambo, Beverly J., and Wood, Lucile A. (eds.): *Nursing Skills for Clinical Practice*, 3rd ed. W. B. Saunders Co., Philadelphia, 1982, pp. 551–56.

Robinson, Corinne H.: *Basic Nutrition and Diet Therapy*, 4th ed. Macmillan Publishing Co., Inc., New York, 1980, pp. 253–62.

Scordo, Kristine Ann: "This Procedure Called PTCA: Your Patient's CABG Substitute?" *Nursing 82*, 12:50–55 (Feb.), 1982.

Sivarajen, Erika S., and Halpenny, C. Jean: "Exercise Testing." *American Journal of Nursing*, 79:2163–70 (Dec.), 1979.

Stanford, Janet L.: "Who Profits from Coronary Artery Bypass Surgery?" *American Journal of Nursing*, 82:1068–72 (July), 1982.

Stanford, Janet L.; Felner, Joel; and Arensberg, Daniel: "Antiarrhythmic Drug Therapy." *American Journal of Nursing*, 80:1288–95 (July), 1980.

Tannenbaum, Renee; Sohn, Catherine A.; Cantwell, Renee; Rogers, Maureen; and Hollis, Rose: "The Pain of Angina Pectoris: How to Recognize It, How to Manage It." *Nursing 81*, 11:44–51 (Sept.), 1981.

Teasley, Barbara: "Don't Let Cardiac Catheterization Strike Fear in Your Patient's Heart." *Nursing 82*, 12:52–55 (Mar.), 1982.

Vaz, Dolores: "Recognizing Common Cardiac Arrhythmias." *American Journal of Nursing*, 79:1971–75 (Nov.), 1979.

Chapter 12

The Patient with a Disease of the Blood Vessels*

Expected Behavioral Outcomes

Minimum objectives referred to as expected behavioral outcomes have been designed for the practical/vocational nursing student to use as guides in studying this chapter. The student should read these expected outcomes before studying the chapter. The objectives can be used as guides for study.

Using the content of this chapter, the student should return to the objectives and evaluate the ability to:

1. *Compare the nursing care needed by a person during the acute phase of cerebrovascular accident with that needed during the convalescent phase.*
2. *Describe nursing responsibilities related to each of the main drugs used to treat hypertension.*
3. *Describe the role of the nurse in the community for early detection of hypertension.*

4. *Compare nursing observations that indicate impaired arterial circulation in an extremity with those that indicate impaired venous circulation.*
5. *List nursing actions that promote venous return to the heart and prevent stasis of blood in the extremities.*
6. *Describe the nursing responsibilities related to anticoagulant therapy.*

Vocabulary Development

The following prefixes, suffixes, and combining forms pertain to this chapter. By learning and/or reviewing their meanings, the practical/vocational nursing student will have the keys needed to unlock many exciting new medical terms.

Discover the meaning of these keys in a medical dictionary or in the content of this chapter. How does each key pertain to this chapter? In your notebook write the correct meaning of each prefix, suffix, or combining form listed below. Illustrate each key with an example.

bol—throw. Ex. em*bol*ism—sudden blocking of a blood vessel by a clot thrown off elsewhere in the body.

*Revised by the authors and Gloria Rudibaugh, R.N., M.S., who is a Practical Nursing Instructor at the Central School of Practical Nursing in Norfolk, Virginia.

hemi-	mot-	plex-	stol-
hyper-	ole-	puls-	strict-
lip-	pher-	scler-	struct-
mittent-	phleb-	sphygm-	thromb-
mon-			

Structure and Function

As described in Chapter 11, the blood vessels are a closed set of tubes through which blood curculates continuously. Pulmonary and systemic circulations were discussed in the same chapter. Arteries, capillaries, and veins form a network through which blood circulates.

ARTERIES

Arteries carry blood away from the heart to the organs and other parts of the body. The arterial system is concerned with supplying food and oxygen to all the tissues of the body. The walls of arteries are thick and strong since the blood within them is under high pressure. An artery is made up of three layers (see Figure 12.1). The inner layer, the intima, is a thin membrane lining of endothelial cells whose surface is suitable for contact with the flowing blood. The middle layer is called the media, which is a thick, strong coat made of smooth muscle, elastic, and some white fibrous tissues. This coat permits constriction and dilation of the artery. The outer coat is the adventitia and is made of white fibrous tissue that allows the artery to stand open instead of collapsing when it is cut. The outer coat also binds the artery to the structures through which it passes.

CAPILLARIES

The vessels that connect the arterial and the venous systems are capillaries. The arteries divide, becoming smaller and smaller in size. The adventitia disappears as the artery becomes smaller, and the media becomes thinner. The tiny artery is called an arteriole. The arterioles become tiny tubes with walls made of a single layer of cells (see Figure 12.2). The tubes, called capillaries, are connected at one end to an arteriole and at the other end to a venule. As the blood from the arteriole, which carries oxygen and

food, passes through the capillary, those materials pass through the one-cell-thick wall of the capillary into tissue fluid. In the opposite direction come the waste products of cell metabolism. These products pass into the capillary through its walls and proceed into the venules.

VEINS

At the distal end of the capillaries, very small veins called venules become progressively larger and larger in size until they are thin-walled veins. A vein is made of three layers or coats, as is an artery. However, the coats ar thinner and less elastic in a vein. Veins carry blood toward the heart (Figure 12.3).

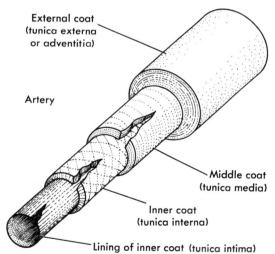

External coat (tunica externa or adventitia)

Artery

Middle coat (tunica media)

Inner coat (tunica interna)

Lining of inner coat (tunica intima)

FIGURE 12.1 Schematic drawing of an artery showing the comparative thickness of the three coats: tunica externa or adventitia, tunica media, and tunica intima. The lining of the internal coat (tunica intima) has been pulled outward in the drawing. Note that the lining of the internal coat differs from the other tissue. This different lining facilitates the smooth flow of blood.

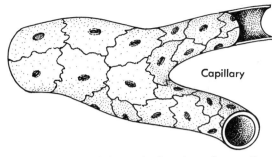

FIGURE 12.2 Schematic drawing of a capillary, which consists of a single layer of endothelial cells. This single layer permits movement of substances between blood and interstitial fluid. The capillary has no muscle coat and no outer coat.

Valves are located at intervals throughout the veins to prevent blood from flowing backward (see Figure 12.4). The venous system is concerned with carrying waste materials from the tissues for disposal from the body.

LYMPH VESSELS

The food and oxygen that pass through the blood capillary walls into the tissue fluid are dissolved in water and leave the blood plasma as a solution; as a result, the volume of tissue fluid is always being added to. Therefore, provision must be made for draining off the excess fluid in order to keep the tissue fluid level the same.

Lymph vessels provide for one-way drainage of excess tissue fluid back into the bloodstream. The lymphatic capillaries are drainpipes which collect some of the cellular waste products that are not carried into the blood capillary. The waste products that pass into the lymphatic capillaries are called lymph. The lymphatic capillaries join to form larger lymphatic vessels. The lymph passes through filters called lymph nodes. Lymph node cells play a primary role in the immune system of the body. In lymph nodes, certain solid waste materials are broken down so that they can be carried by the lymph back to the bloodstream and excreted. The largest lymph vessel, the thoracic duct, carries lymph primarily from the abdomen, trunk of the body, and extremities and empties the filtered lymph into veins.

FACTORS THAT AFFECT BLOOD FLOW

A number of factors affect the flow of blood in the circulatory system by influencing the tension in the smooth muscle of the walls of the arteries. This tension, in turn, can decrease the size of an artery (vasoconstriction) or increase the size or radius of an artery (vasodilation). Nerves, hormones, pressure gradients, and heart muscle action impact on the arteries.

NERVES. Arteries are greatly influenced by the stimulation of the sympathetic nervous system that causes vasoconstriction of arteries. Thus, resistance to blood flow occurs. Sympathectomy or cutting of the sympathetic nerve allows vasodilation to occur. Stimulation of the parasympathetic nervous system usually causes dilation of blood vessels.

HORMONES. Certain hormones also can affect blood flow through blood vessels. One of these hormones is epinephrine or adrenalin, a powerful vasoconstrictor, which is very important in the "fight or flight" reac-

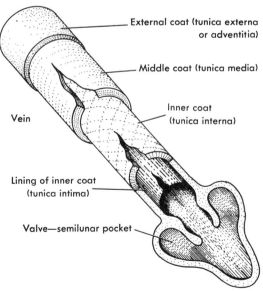

External coat (tunica externa or adventitia)

Middle coat (tunica media)

Inner coat (tunica interna)

Vein

Lining of inner coat (tunica intima)

Valve—semilunar pocket

FIGURE 12.3 Schematic drawing of a vein showing the comparative thickness of the three coats. The outer coat and middle coat are thinner in veins than in arteries. A diagram of a valve is shown also.

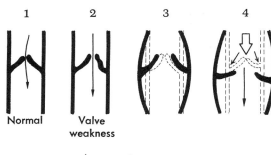

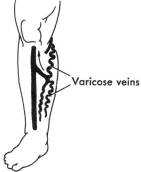

FIGURE 12.4   Diagram of normal vein with functioning valve (1). The valve weakens in 2, causing the vein wall to dilate from increased pressure exerted by venous blood, as illustrated in 3. Increased venous pressure leads to further dilation, as seen in 4 and the diagram of varicose veins. (From Pansky, Ben: *Dynamic Anatomy and Physiology*. Macmillan Publishing Co., Inc., New York, 1975.)

tion of the body to danger. Another hormone, angiotensin, causes vasoconstriction also. When blood pressure to the kidney falls, as occurs during hemorrhage, renin, a hormone released by the kidney, helps to produce angiotensin, which affects arterioles by causing vasoconstriction of blood vessels, thus, raising blood pressure. In this way, blood supply to the kidney is increased.

PRESSURE GRADIENTS.   Within the systemic circulation, blood flows from the left atrium and ventricle to the aorta, to arteries, arterioles, capillaries, venules, veins, inferior and superior venae cavae and returns to the right atrium of the heart. Blood flows in this direction because a pressure gradient exists within the systemic circulation. Fluid always flows from an area of high pressure toward an area of low pressure. The blood pressure within the aorta is higher than that

within arteries. The pressure within arteries is higher than that within veins. Therefore, the flow of blood is always from arteries through capillaries and into veins.

The venous flow of blood toward the heart is against gravity. The flow of blood depends not only on the blood pressure gradient but upon the one-way valves located within the veins and the massaging action of the muscles which surround the veins. The valves and the action of the muscles help to propel blood back toward the right side of the heart.

HEART MUSCLE ACTION.   Blood flow depends upon the continuous and efficient pumping of blood by the heart to all parts of the body. If for any reason the left side of the heart muscle fails as a pump, blood backs up into the lungs, causing congestive heart failure. The decreased cardiac output reduces blood flow to the peripheral blood vessels. When the right side of the heart fails, the patient exhibits edema of the lower extremities and abdomen. As a result of both sides of the heart failing as a pump, the patient, suffering from venous congestion and low cardiac output, dies in shock and circulatory collapse.

Conditions that Compromise Blood Flow to the Tissues

DESCRIPTION

The needs of the tissues of the body for oxygen and nutrients are always changing. Factors that affect these needs are the person's activity, the temperature of the environment, and the person's state of health. For example, when metabolic needs of the body increase due to exercise, more blood flow to tissues is necessary and arteries normally dilate. When the temperature of the surrounding air is low, vasoconstriction of blood vessels normally occurs to conserve body heat. Infections of the body ordinarily lead to dilation of blood vessels supplying the affected tissues so that substances in the bloodstream can be brought to the infected site to aid in the healing process.

Normally, blood vessels dilate and constrict in order to vary the amount of blood that body tissues receive. However, obstructed, narrowed, damaged or sclerosed, inelastic blood vessels are unable to dilate and constrict normally. As a result, these vessels are unable to supply oxygen and nutrients that are requested in varying amounts by the tissues. Any factor that narrows, obstructs, or damages the blood vessels decreases blood flow. When blood flow is decreased, tissue nutrition becomes poor, cellular waste products increase, and tissue damage can develop more easily. Without treatment, tissue damage such as cellulitis, ulcers, and gangrene may occur. If healing does not occur with treatment, limb amputations may be necessary.

ISCHEMIA

To carry blood adequately, arteries must be capable of dilating and constricting normally in response to neural, hormonal, thermal, and chemical stimulation. When arteries become obstructed or damaged, there is a decreased flow of blood which carries oxygen and nutrients to the body tissues. Any tissue, organ, or body part may be affected by ischemia. Deprived of an adequate blood supply, the tissue cannot function satisfactorily. Usually ischemia is temporary. Whether tissue necrosis and gangrene develop depends on the extent of the blockage as well as upon the speed at which the blockage occurs. Many conditions may cause ischemia, but the total or near total blockage of an artery by a thrombus or blood clot is more critical to the functioning of tissue than is the partial narrowing of an artery as a result of atherosclerosis. The gradual development of arterial disease allows time for the growth of new vessels to replace the damaged ones.

Other conditions that may cause ischemia are swelling of tissue against blood vessels, bony prominences, casts, or tight bandages. These conditions reduce the blood flow and result in ischemia.

Symptoms of ischemia vary, depending upon the area of ischemia. One common symptom is pain in the area of ischemia. Ischemia in the tissues of an extremity can be detected by using the five Ps (discussed in Chapter 17) which are pain, pallor, paresthesias, pulse change, and paralysis. These symptoms are also discussed later in this

chapter under the heading Nursing Observations. Myocardial ischemia may result in angina pectoris as described in Chapter 11. Cerebral ischemia may result in memory loss and temporary impairment of speech or vision as described in this chapter (transient ischemic attack).

THROMBOSIS

When an artery is obstructed by a thrombus, blood flow is decreased and the organ or tissue that it nourished is deprived of its blood supply. A thrombus or blood clot usually adheres to the intima of an artery, causing obstruction of blood flow. The greatest danger of arterial thrombi is arterial embolism with total occlusion of a blood vessel occurring.

EMBOLISM

An embolus is a blood clot or other material, not normally present in the bloodstream, that moves along an artery and lodges in a branching artery or arteriole. When either a large thrombus or an arterial embolus occurs, death of tissue may result from lack of oxygen and nutrients.

ARTERIOSCLEROSIS

Arteriosclerosis is a group of disease conditions in which the walls of the arteries become thicker, less elastic, and hardened. Arterial thrombi or aneurysm may occur more readily as a result of this condition. The three main forms of arteriosclerosis are: (1) Mönckeberg's arteriosclerosis, (2) atherosclerosis, and (3) arteriolosclerosis. An individual with Mönckeberg's arteriosclerosis has extensive calcium deposits in the media coat of the arteries. Atherosclerosis is a common form of arteriosclerosis in which cholesterol, lipoid or fatlike material, and cells containing fat are deposited mainly in the intima coat of arteries causing a narrowing of the lumen and critically reducing blood flow. These deposits (see Figures 12.5, 12.6, and 12.7) are yellowish plaques called *atheromas*. Medium-sized and large arteries, such as the aorta and renal artery, are affected mainly in atherosclerosis. An individual with arteriolosclerosis has a rather diffuse or widespread hardening of smaller

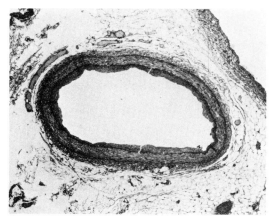

FIGURE 12.5 Normal artery, cross section. (Courtesy of American Heart Association, New York, N.Y.)

arteries and arterioles. An individual may be affected with all three forms of arteriosclerosis and have different vessels involved. As arteries and arterioles undergo changes of arteriosclerosis, their passageway for blood to flow becomes narrower. A thrombus (blood clot) may form and the vessel may rupture. The cells being nourished by the diseased arteries may receive an inadequate supply of oxygen and food. If the cells are deprived of oxygen and food for a period of time sufficient to cause damage, the cells die and may be replaced with fibrous tissue. Areas of fibrous tissue can develop throughout the body and frequently occur in the brain, heart, and kidneys. The extremities and gastrointestinal tract may be involved also.

Although an exact cause of arteriosclerosis is not known at this time, it commonly develops with the aging process and seems to be more common in elderly men than women. An individual having a family history of arteriosclerosis is prone to develop this condition. Arteriosclerosis frequently occurs in persons with either diabetes mellitus or hypertension. Individuals who have a high intake of dietary lipids are prone to develop arterial plaques. A *lipid* is an organic substance that is not soluble in water, is soluble in such substances as ether and alcohol, feels greasy, and serves as a source of fuel. Lipids combined with proteins that are of particular significance in arteriosclerosis are cholesterol and triglycerides. The levels

of both of these lipoproteins are determined by laboratory analysis and frequently are elevated in arteriosclerotic conditions. The normal values of both are given in Table 12.1.

ANEURYSM

An aneurysm is a sac formed by the dilation of an artery as a result of localized weakness and stretching of the arterial wall. The most common cause of aneurysms is arteriosclerosis. Aneurysms may occur anywhere along the aorta. They are found less commonly in the upper extremities than in the lower extremities. Popliteal aneurysms located behind the knee are important causes of ischemic symptoms in the lower limbs. Rest pain, numbness, and coldness may occur as a result of edema behind the knee. Thrombosis and emboli, distal to the aneurysm, may occur as well as bleeding from the aneurysm. Severe ischemia may result with the development of gangrene and loss of the extremity.

INFARCTION

Infarction is an area of dead tissue which results from compromised flow of blood through arteries. Lipid and cholesterol plaques have narrowed the diameter of these arteries, predisposing to the development of thrombi as the flow of blood is slowed. The vessel may be partially or completely occluded by the thrombi that form. The tissue nourished by that particular ar-

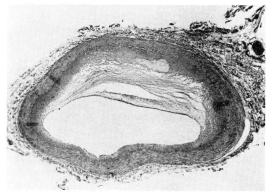

FIGURE 12.6 Atherosclerotic deposits formed in inner lining of artery. (Courtesy of American Heart Association, New York, N.Y.)

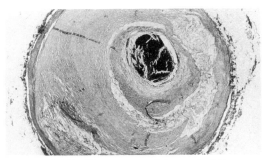

FIGURE 12.7 The narrowed channel of the artery is blocked by a blood clot. (Courtesy of American Heart Association, New York, N.Y.)

tery becomes ischemic and then infarcted as the tissue dies from lack of blood supply.

Assisting with Diagnostic Studies

ANGIOGRAPHY

Angiography is the x-ray visualization of some part of the arteriolar system following injection of a radiopaque substance (see Figure 12.8). An angiogram is done to visualize certain arteries and/or the heart. Abnormal conditions of arteries, such as calcification, aneurysm, occlusion, and cardiac abnormalities may be detected with angiography.

The patient scheduled for an angiogram (arteriogram) generally receives a sedative and nothing by mouth prior to the examination. The site selected may be shaved. For a femoral arteriogram, the groin area is shaved. During the angiogram, the patient usually has to remain in prescribed positions on the x-ray table for one to two hours. This is tiring. Generally, a flushing sensation is experienced when the dye is injected. During the examination and after it has been completed, the individual should be observed for symptoms of reaction to the radiopaque dye. The solution contains iodine, which may cause a severe allergic reaction in some persons. Symptoms of an allergic reaction, such as dyspnea, nausea, vomiting, perspiring, tachycardia, and numbness in the extremities, may occur. Symptoms of anaphylactic shock, as discussed in Chapter 10, sometimes develop and should be reported immediately. The patient may be treated with an antihistamine, epinephrine, and oxygen. After the examination is completed, the pa-

tient will be on bed rest for 24 hours. The site of the injection generally has a pressure bandage and should be checked for bleeding. An ice pack may be ordered to minimize edema and bleeding. The pulse in the distal portion of the involved extremity should be checked at least every 15 minutes for the first hour and then every hour for the first five to seven hours. The extremity also should be observed for coolness and discoloration. These observations regarding coolness and discoloration should be compared with those of the other extremity. A decrease in the warmth of the extremity and beginning cyanosis may indicate an obstruction of the circulation to that extremity. The physician should be notified immediately. The five Ps of impaired circulation to an extremity—(1) pain, (2) pallor, (3) paralysis, (4) paresthesia, and (5) pulse change—as discussed in Chapter 17 are applicable to this patient.

The patient generally is encouraged to have an increased fluid intake to facilitate excretion of the dye by the kidneys. The output of urine should be checked for the first seven to eight hours to determine if the patient has an adequate output.

LUMBAR SYMPATHETIC BLOCK

A lumbar sympathetic block is a test used to determine if a sympathectomy could improve circulation to the extremities. A local anesthetic is injected into the sympathetic ganglia, temporarily blocking the sympathetic vasomotor nerve fibers that supply an ischemic limb. Blocking these nerves causes vasodilation and increased temperature in the legs when the vessels are normal. In limbs diseased by arteriosclerosis, a decrease in limb pain and an increase in skin temperature after the block is done indicate that a sympathectomy (cutting the sympathetic nerve) could improve circulation to the extremities.

DETERMINING SKIN TEMPERATURE

Special thermometers are available to measure the skin temperature, especially of the extremities. However, the specialist of-

[Text continued on page 324.]

TABLE 12.1
LABORATORY TESTS

TEST	NORMAL VALUE	CLINICAL IMPLICATIONS	
		Increase	*Decrease*
Blood			
Blood urea nitrogen	10–15 mg/100 ml	Kidney disease or urinary obstruction from enlarged prostate, shock, dehydration, GI hemorrhage, infection, diabetes	Liver failure, negative nitrogen balance, impaired absorption
Calcium	Total 9.0–10.6 mg/dl 4.5–5.3 mEq/l	Cancer, Addison's disease, hyperparathyroidism, prolonged immobilization, prolonged use of diuretics	Chronic renal failure, hypoparathyroidism, pancreatitis, diarrhea
Chloride	95–105 mEq/l	Dehydration, Cushing's syndrome, anemia, some kidney disorders	Vomiting, diarrhea, Addison's disease, fever, drugs—mercurial and chlorothiazide diuretics
Cholesterol	Total, 400–1000 mg/dl Cholesterol, 150–250 mg/dl Triglycerides, 40–150 mg/dl Phospholipids, 150–380 mg/dl	Cardiovascular disease, hypothyroidism, nephrosis, uncontrolled diabetes	Liver disease, hyperthyroidism, anemia, stress, fat malabsorption syndrome
Creatinine	0.2–0.5 mg/dl	Impaired renal function, chronic nephritis, obstruction of urinary tract	Muscular dystrophy
Glucose	70–110 mg/dl	Diabetes, Cushing's disease, acute stress, pheochromocytoma, chronic liver disease	Overdose of insulin, Addison's disease, bacterial sepsis, hepatic necrosis
Sodium	136–142 mEq/l	Dehydration and insufficient water intake, primary aldosteronism, Cushing's disease	Diarrhea, vomiting, excessive sweating, nephritis
Potassium	3.5–5.0 mEq/l	Addison's disease, renal failure, hypoaldosteronism, diabetes	Diarrhea, primary aldosteronism, renal tubular acidosis, chronic stress
Uric acid	Women—3.0–7.5 mg/100 ml Men—7–8.5 mg/100 ml	Decreased kidney function, gout, leukemia, renal failure	Patients treated with uricosuric drugs

Urine

Test	Value	Clinical significance
		Impaired kidney function
		Renal failure, aldosteronism
		Renal failure, adrenal cortical insufficiency
		Malabsorption syndrome, pyloric obstruction
Creatinine clearance	115–120 ml/min or 0.7–1.5 mg/ml	Impaired kidney function
Protein (albumin)	Negative or 2–8 mg/24 hr	Nephritis, nephrosis, polycystic kidneys
Sodium	130–200 mEq/24 hr	Dehydration, renal failure, mercurial and chlorothiazide diuretics
Potassium	40–80 mEq/24 hr	Renal failure, primary aldosteronism
Chloride	110–250 mEq/24 hr	Addison's disease, dehydration, diuretics
Red blood cell casts	1–2	Pyelonephritis, renal stones
Vanillylmendelic acid	VMA up to 9 mg/24 hr Epinephrine 100–230 mg/24 hr Norepinephrine 100–230 mg/24 hr Metanephrine 24–96 mg/24 hr Normetanephrine 12–288 mg/24 hr	Pheochromocytoma, neuroblastomas, ganglioneuromas
17-Ketosteroids (17KS)	17 Ketosteroids (17KS) Men 8–18 mg/24 hr Women 5–15 mg/24 hr 17 Hydroxycorticosteroids (17OHCS) 10 mg/24 hr 17 Ketogeniosteroids (17KGS) Men 5.5–23 mg/24 hr Women 3–15 mg/24 hr	Hyperplasia of adrenal cortex, tumor, cancer Steroid level in Cushing's syndrome, hypertension

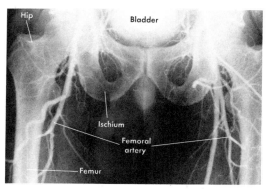

FIGURE 12.8 An angiogram of a femoral artery.

ten can detect a slight difference in the warmth of a patient's extremity by touch. The doctor or nurse may feel and note the temperature of one limb and then contrast it with the temperature of the extremity on the opposite side.

DOPPLER ULTRASOUND FLOW DETECTOR

The Doppler ultrasound flow detector is a noninvasive method of determining blood flow in blood vessels as well as patency of the vessels. Noninvasive methods do not require entering the body or puncturing the skin. The Doppler probe is a small instrument that can transmit and receive sound signals. The probe transmits ultrasound into the patient's tissues. The sound that is transmitted back is from the movement of erythrocytes in the blood vessel. The reflected ultrasound is amplified by the Doppler as an audible sound. Ultrasound reflected off moving blood cells is shifted in frequency by an amount proportional to the speed of blood flow within the vessel. An acoustic gel is placed on the skin where the pulse is expected to be felt. If the Doppler probe is placed over the femoral, popliteal, posterior tibial, or dorsalis pedis arteries, one can hear the flow of blood even when a pulse is not palpable. The sound heard from healthy arteries is a loud swish. In arteries diseased by arteriosclerosis, for example, the sound is reduced to a low, muffled sound. In occluded arteries, blood flow would not be audible. The Doppler may be

used to listen to the flow of blood through veins as well as arteries.

ARM-ANKLE PRESSURES

The Doppler ultrasound flow detector can be used to obtain systolic pressures in the arm, thigh, calf, and ankle. Arm-ankle pressures are commonly done. A pneumatic cuff is placed on the extremity and an acoustic gel is applied to the skin. The cuff is inflated to above systolic pressure. The Doppler probe is placed over the nearest prominent pulse site. The cuff is slowly deflated until the Doppler arterial signal returns at the systolic pressure of the arm or ankle. The ankle pressure is compared to the arm pressure as an ankle-brachial index. The normal ankle pressure is equal to or slightly higher than that of the arm. In arterial occlusive disease, the pressures will be below that of the arm by an amount that is directly proportional to the degree of circulatory impairment. The systolic pressure of the arm or ankle is recorded in millimeters of mercury. The ankle pressure is divided by the highest brachial (arm) pressure obtained. For example:

	Right	Left
Ankle	50 mm Hg	100 mm Hg
Arm	100 mg Hg	120 mm Hg

The ankle-brachial index is found by 50/120 = .41 for the right ankle, and 100/120 = .83 for the left ankle. The following indices represent the normal, asymptomatic, and symptomatic conditions that result from increasingly impaired circulation:

1.0 or greater is normal
.9 asymptomatic condition
.7 claudication
.5 rest pain
    less than .5, ischemia of leg occurs

TREADMILL EXERCISE TEST

Intermittent claudication is a symptom manifested by pain or discomfort in calf muscles after exercise but is relieved by rest. Other signs or symptoms include coldness or numbness of the extremities and absence of pulses in the affected extremities. Most commonly, pain appears in the calf muscles after walking due to the inability of arteries diseased by arteriosclerosis to supply the amount of oxygen needed by muscles during exercise. In the peripheral vascular laboratory, ankle pressures are obtained with the patient in the supine position. Then, how far a patient can walk, for how long, and the rate of walking on the treadmill before experiencing pain in the legs are indications of the adequacy of the arterial circulation. After the exercise test, ankle pressures are again obtained with the patient in the supine position. It is expected that the pressure in an ischemic limb would be lowered by exercise.

PLETHYSMOGRAPHY

Plethysmography is a noninvasive laboratory technique used to measure a change in the size of a limb or other part of the body in response to the volume of blood passing through it or contained in it. Plethysmography can be done to measure changes in venous blood volume such as would be found in deep vein thrombophlebitis. The procedure is also useful in measuring changes in cerebral arterial blood volume attributed to stenosis or occlusion of cerebral arteries which play a major role in transient ischemic attacks (TIA) and cerebrovascular accident (stroke). Plethysmography of digits is also done to determine digital arterial insufficiency and cold sensitivity.

OSCILLOMETRY

Changes in pulse volume can be measured by wrapping a cuff around the extremity and connecting it to an oscillometer. The arterial pressure with each pulsation is recorded as it is transmitted by a diaphragm to a needle which moves across a dial. The reading is helpful in demonstrating differences between deep pulses of two opposite limbs.

TRENDELENBURG TEST

The Trendelenburg test or retrograde filling test is used to diagnose varicose veins of the lower extremities. The effectiveness of the valves in the deep veins as well as their branches is determined. The patient is lying down and the leg is elevated to empty the veins. After having a tourniquet applied around the upper thigh, the patient is asked to stand. Blood flows back into the veins if the valves in the branches are inadequate. A return of blood to the superficial veins after the tourniquet is removed indicates that those valves are probably inadequate also. The same procedure is repeated on the other leg.

PHLEBOGRAPHY

Phlebography (venography) is an x-ray of veins. Contrast media or radiopaque dye is injected into the deep and/or superficial veins. A vein on the dorsum of the foot usually is used. Both normal and abnormal veins can be visualized as well as cusps of the valves. Generally, the patient is permitted nothing by mouth for eight to ten hours prior to the x-ray.

KIDNEY X-RAY

The intravenous pyelogram is an x-ray of kidneys, ureters, and bladder. A radiopaque dye is injected intravenously and as the dye is cleared from the blood and excreted through the urinary tract, the structures can be visualized. This means of evaluating kidney function is often part of the diagnostic studies for hypertension.

The patient is generally asked to restrict fluids and foods for eight to ten hours preceding the x-ray. A laxative may be given the day before. Enemas may be given the night before the x-ray and/or the morning of the examination so that the gastrointestinal tract will be clear of feces and the urinary structures can be visualized on x-ray.

RENAL SCAN

A renal scan is yet another diagnostic test to determine an outline of functioning kidney tissue. A tracer dose of radioactive iodine is given intravenously, after which a probe is passed back and forth over the kidney, and either a record is made or a special electronic photograph is taken. Nonfunctioning areas of the kidney will show no record of radioactivity since that kidney tissue is not filtering wastes containing the radioactive material from the blood.

BRAIN SCAN

A brain scan is a test in which a radioisotope is used to help localize a brain lesion. A radioactive substance is injected intravenously. A few hours later, a scanner is passed over the head. The lesions will pick up an increased amount of the radioactive substance from the blood. These areas of concentration will be recorded by the scanner. No special preparation is necessary. No special observations are required after the procedure.

LUNG SCAN

The flow of blood through the tiny blood vessels within the lung can be demonstrated by injecting radioactive isotopes of certain chemicals into a vein. When the injected isotopes reach the small lung vessels, a scanning device is used to record the concentration and distribution of the radioactive material, making a kind of map. Blood vessels that are obstructed by disease do not permit entry of the radioactive isotope. Thus, an uneven map helps the physician to diagnose respiratory disorders that involve the small lung vessels. No special preparation is needed for a lung scan after the procedure has been explained to the patient.

LUMBAR PUNCTURE

The doctor may do a lumbar puncture, which is known also as a spinal tap, to aid in diagnosis of the stroke patient. In this procedure, a needle is inserted between the vertebrae into the spinal canal. This is known as a lumbar puncture since it is usually done in the lumbar region (lower part of the back) between L4 and L5 or L5 and S1. The needle is inserted below the level of the spinal cord into the area of the cauda equina; hence, there is very little danger of damage to the nerves. The physician usually determines the pressure of the cerebrospinal fluid during a lumbar puncture by attaching a manometer to the hub of the spinal needle. The nurse may need to steady the manometer by holding it lightly well above the area where the physician might have contact with his sterile glove. Usually several specimens of cerebrospinal fluid are sent to the laboratory. These specimens should be labeled accurately. Normal characteristics of cerebrospinal fluid are listed in Table 21.1, page 728.

The nurse is often asked to assist the physician in doing a lumbar puncture. The nurse also will prepare the necessary equipment. In some agencies, the patient must sign a consent form. The nurse may assist the patient to assume a position suitable for the examination, which is on the patient's side and near the edge of the bed or examining table. The patient is usually asked to remain recumbent for 6 to 12 hours following the procedure to avoid a lumbar puncture headache. Headache is caused by leakage of cerebrospinal fluid at the puncture site. As fluid in the cranium decreases, the brain becomes displaced, causing the patient discomfort. The vertical position exerts a greater traction on the brain; therefore, the pain is less when the patient is lying down.

Nursing Observations

The atherosclerotic process, which is a common contributor to peripheral vascular disease, is found primarily in persons over 50 years of age. The age at which the disease begins and the severity of it depend on several factors. Diabetes and hypertension influence the course of the disease, as does heredity, smoking, and diet. Obstruction of the arterial system reduces the supply of oxygen and nutrients to the tissues which produces ischemia and malnutrition of the tissues. This atherosclerotic process can also involve the brain, the heart, and the kidneys. Thus, there are several nursing observations made in general of the patient with peripheral vascular disease.

HEADACHE

Headache is a diffuse pain found in different portions of the head. It may be frontal, temporal, or occipital. There are many reasons why a headache may occur. Abnormalities in blood pressure give rise to headache—both high blood pressure and low blood pressure. Sudden changes in blood pressure can also cause headache. Intracranial vascular diseases such as arteriosclerosis, hemorrhage, thrombosis, embolism, or aneurysm may cause headache.

VISUAL DISTURBANCES

Visual disturbances may be caused by the rupture of capillaries on the retina of the eye such as may occur in hypertensive patients, especially in patients who also have diabetes. Visual disturbances may occur as a result of atherosclerosis which has narrowed carotid arteries or other arteries in the brain. The arteries may become completely occluded by a thrombus or embolus. This condition reduces the blood supply to the brain either temporarily or permanently, leaving the patient with blurred vision or blindness.

DIZZINESS AND BEHAVIORAL CHANGES

Dizziness and behavioral changes may result from narrowed or occluded arteries that reduce the blood supply to the brain. Headache, visual disturbances, dizziness, and behavioral changes frequently precede or accompany a cerebrovascular accident or stroke.

BLOOD PRESSURE

Blood pressure is the pressure exerted by blood against the walls of blood vessels. The systolic blood pressure is arterial pressure exerted against the walls of blood vessels at the time of the contraction of the ventricles or the working phase of the heart. The diastolic blood pressure is the arterial pressure exerted against the walls of blood vessels during diastole or the resting phase of the heart. Several mechanisms serve to increase arteriolar resistance to blood flow in the circulatory system. The nervous system, secretion of hormones of the endocrine glands, and local factors influence the constriction of blood vessels and help to raise blood pressure. For example, stimulation of the sympathetic nervous system, secretion of certain hormones such as epinephrine, and trauma to tissues cause vasoconstriction. Stimulation of the parasympathetic nervous system and certain products of inflammation such as histamine cause vasodilation.

PAIN

Local and temporary lack of blood supply to tissue because of vasoconstriction causes pain to occur. Patients who have diseased arteries in the legs often experience pain in the legs after walking a certain distance. This pain is called intermittent claudication. When arteries are severely diseased with arteriosclerosis, the patient may complain of leg pain even at rest. Rest pain is especially uncomfortable at night. Blockage of the aorta may cause hip and buttock pain also. Tissues that temporarily lack blood supply also are said to be ischemic, and the pain usually is relieved by supplying oxygenated blood to the tissues.

PARESTHESIAS

Paresthesias are abnormal sensations such as numbness, prickling, and tingling. These sensations often accompany a transient ischemic attack or stroke. Temporary blockage or narrowing of a cerebral artery that supplies brain tissue that controls bodily sensation may produce this feeling or sensation in an extremity.

PERIPHERAL PULSE CHANGES

Peripheral pulses are ordinarily palpable at the groin (femoral pulse), behind the knee (popliteal pulse), on the dorsum of the foot (dorsalis pedis pulse), and behind the medial malleolus (posterior tibial pulse). Arteriosclerotic arteries or an arterial thrombus may diminish blood flow in an artery or occlude it altogether. Therefore, an important observation of the patient with peripheral vascular disease of the lower extremeties is the state of pulsations. If the pulsations cannot be palpated with the fingers, the Doppler allows one to hear blood flowing through the arteries. The quality of the pulsations is proportional to the amount of impairment of blood flow through the arteries.

SKIN TEMPERATURE AND COLOR

Circulatory impairment of the extremities produces cool skin temperatures. Even in warm environmental temperatures, the extremities may feel cool to the patient and to the touch. Circulatory impairment also will cause skin to have a pallor or to appear pale when compared to the healthy flesh color. With greater impairment, the skin will appear reddish-blue (rubor) and then become bluish (cyanosis) in color.

EDEMA

Collection of fluid in the tissue spaces occurs when fluid leaves the bloodstream, passing from the capillary into the space between tissue cells, faster than it can be reabsorbed by the capillaries or lymphatics. This condition often occurs when venous circulation is slowed. The patient in congestive heart failure may develop edema of the feet and ankles because the heart is unable to perform its pumping action adequately. The patient with defective valves in the veins of the leg may develop edema because the valves cannot assist adequately to pump blood back toward the heart. Localized inflammation can lead to edema because of increased capillary permeability which occurs locally in response to the inflammatory process.

TROPHIC SKIN CHANGES

Changes in skin and growth of hair and nails may occur in patients who have peripheral vascular disease. Certain nerves control growth and nourishment of the parts they innervate. Because of lack of circulation to the part such as the legs and feet, the skin on the extremities may be devoid of hair and have a shiny appearance. The skin may have a dark, discolored appearance, while the toenails become extremely hard, thick, and brittle.

Nursing Interventions

GENERAL HYGIENE MEASURES WITH FOOT CARE

Foot care is very important to any person who has peripheral vascular disease. The feet should be protected from trauma since preventive measures are easier to carry out than treatment after damage to the skin. Walking barefoot or in stockings should be avoided. The feet should be washed daily with a mild soap and dried thoroughly. Lanolized lotion can be used to help prevent drying and cracking of the skin. Lamb's wool between the toes helps to prevent pressure. A sheepskin pad on the bed under the heels will help prevent friction breakdown of the heels. Proper fitting shoes should be worn to prevent friction and pressure on the feet that predispose to blisters, corns, and calluses. Such trauma requires professional care. Leather-soled shoes provide for ventilation better than rubber-soled shoes. Shoes should be alternated daily so that they can dry thoroughly. New shoes should be broken in gradually. A clean pair of cotton stockings should be worn daily. Nails should be trimmed straight across after a footbath while the nails are soft. Strong antiseptics should be avoided. Minor foot problems easily can become serious.

POSITIONING CHANGES

The legs of the patient with arterial insufficiency should be in the straight position. The patient may be advised to sleep with the head of the bed on blocks so that blood flow by gravity is increased toward the feet. Elevation of the legs may decrease arterial circulation. Changing positions frequently is important to prevent stasis of blood in the extremities. Stasis of blood can lead to dependent edema which can cause pressure on the arterial vessels and decrease arterial circulation, which is already compromised. The nurse needs to know the physician's orders regarding the best position for the patient to maintain.

USE OF HEAT

Heat to extremities should be achieved by warm clothing or blankets rather than by electric heating pads or hot water bottles. Such measures may damage the skin before the patient knows that he or she is being burned. Excessive heat increases metabolism. Increased metabolism requires more oxygenated blood which the diseased arteries are not able to provide. Too much heat injures the tissues. Gangrene may develop if injured tissues cannot heal properly. Shower and bath water should be checked with a bath thermometer or should feel comfortable to the elbow or wrist.

RELIEF OF PAIN AND DISCOMFORT

Any measure that increases circulation to the extremities will help to relieve the pain of ischemia. Providing warmth by proper clothing, such as long underwear and woolen or cotton socks, helps to promote comfort. The room temperature may need to be kept between 75 to 80° F for comfort. Proper positioning, as described above, and moderate exercise will aid circulation to the periphery. If the patient's condition has advanced to the point of pain at rest, the patient should be kept on bed rest to reduce oxygen demands. The use of tobacco, which causes the constriction of peripheral arteries and further decreases already compromised circulation, should be avoided. Vessel spasm contributes to ischemia of tissues. The nurse needs to encourage smokers to abstain from the use of tobacco.

ALTERATIONS IN FOOD AND FLUIDS

A diet that is high in protein is one that helps to prevent tissue breakdown and aids in healing. Obesity should be avoided. Elevation of blood lipids indicates that a low-fat or low-carbohydrate diet may be desirable. A balanced diet with adequate fluid intake is recommended.

EXERCISE

A program of exercise and rest is helpful in increasing the arterial and venous circulation of patients with peripheral vascular disease. Short walks followed by periods of rest help to promote collateral circulation. When patients develop pain in the calf of the leg, they are not receiving enough oxygen to the muscles and tissues of the leg. They, therefore, need to stop and rest. Standing in one place for long periods should be avoided. Walking and sitting will help prevent stasis of the blood. Patients should be instructed not to sit with their legs crossed or wear tight garters or constricting clothing of any kind. When sitting in a chair, pressure on the popliteal vessels in back of the knees is to be avoided. These practices may further decrease already compromised circulation.

PROTECTION FROM INJURY

To prevent injury to the skin, vigorous rubbing should be avoided. The skin should be gently rubbed or patted. Softening lotions and creams are recommended to prevent dryness. Scratching of the skin should be avoided, and measures used to prevent itching or pruritus. Shoes should be worn to prevent injury or trauma to the feet. Patients should be taught to observe for dryness and cracking of the skin on the feet. Any open lesion that does not heal should be brought to the attention of the physician.

USING THE THERAPEUTIC RELATIONSHIP TO ASSIST WITH STRESS

The therapeutic relationship is one perceived by patients as being helpful to them. The nurse helps the patient by meeting those physical needs that have been brought about by illness. The patients know that the nurse cares for them and about them. Acceptance of the patients as worthy human beings is basic to the therapeutic relationship. Helping patients retain their own individuality is also important. Vascular patients are often depressed because their diseases are chronic, painful, and debilitating. The role of the nurse focuses on each patient as an individual with specific needs. Patient and family teaching is an essential component of care.

DRUG THERAPY

There are four general classifications of drugs that are used to treat peripheral vascular diseases. These include vasodilators, anticoagulants, fibrinolytics, and plasma expanders.

Vasodilators may be given when there are spasms of arteries of the extremites. The may also be used when arteries or arterioles are narrowed by arteriosclerosis and atherosclerosis or a thrombus. Vasodilators dilate blood vessels and allow increased circulation of blood to tissues (see Table 12.2).

Anticoagulants are used in the treatment of both arterial and venous thrombosis. They can be used prophylactically to prevent blood clots from occurring. They prolong the

Table 12.2
Medications Used to Treat Peripheral Vascular Disease

Nonproprietary Name	Trade Name	Average Dose	Toxic Reactions
Vasodilators			
Papaverine hydrochloride		30–100 mg PO 3–4 times/day	Flushing, perspiration, tachycardia
Tolazoline hydrochloride	PRISCOLINE	10–50 mg PO, SC, IM, IV 4 times/day	Arrhythmias, angina, tachycardia, palpitations, nausea, vomiting, pruritus
Phenoxybenzamine hydrochloride	DIBENZYLINE	20–60 mg daily	Nasal congestion, miosis, tachycardia, postural hypotension
Isoxsuprine	VASODILAN	10–20 mg PO 3–4 times/day 5–10 mg PO 2–3 times/day	Nervousness, palpitation, nausea, vomiting
Nylidrin	ARLIDIN	3–12 mg PO 3–4 times/day	Nervousness, palpitation, nausea, vomiting
Cyclandelate	CYCLOSPASMOL	400–800 mg PO 2–4 times/day	Dizziness, flushing, nausea, vomiting
Nicotinyl alcohol	RONIACOL	Time span tabs, 150 mg, 1–2 tabs 2 times/day Scored tabs, 50 mg, 1–2 tabs 3 times/day	
Anticoagulants			
Heparin sodium		20,000–40,000 U continuous IV/24 hr	Hemorrhage
Bishydroxycoumarin Dicumarol		8,000–10,000 U sc qgh 50–200 mg qd	Hemorrhage
Warfarin sodium	COUMADIN	Maintenance, 2–10 mg daily	Hemorrhage
Fibrinolytics			
Streptokinase—streptodornase	STREPTASE	Maintenance, 100,000 IU/hr for 24–72/hr IV	Bleeding (internal), allergic reactions, fever
Fibrinolysin and desoxyribonuclease	ELASE	Apply topical ointment	Local hyperemia
Plasma Expanders			
Dextran		In 6–12 % solution 250–500 ml IV	

clotting time of the blood. They will not dissolve blood clots that have already formed but will prevent further clotting from occurring (see Table 12.2).

Fibrinolytics may be used topically or systemically to help dissolve fibrinous and purulent material by enzyme action. They are used topically on leg ulcers, for example, as a form of debridement of necrotic tissue so that healing of tissue may take place.

A plasma expander may be used to help resolve or prevent the extension of thrombi.

It is administered intravenously with caution to prevent circulatory overload (see Table 12.2).

PATIENT AND FAMILY TEACHING

Because peripheral vascular diseases are usually chronic conditions, patients and their families often require much emotional support and teaching from the nurse. The nurse must be able to explain the disease condition to patients in terms they can understand. Patients need to understand the rationale for the treatment; for example, why they should stop smoking, why the prescribed activity is important, or why certain dietary changes are important. Much encouragement and support are needed because, often, changes in life-style are necessary, and those changes must be adhered to for the rest of the person's life.

Many patients will have pain. The nurse must work closely with the patient to determine the cause of the pain and measures that will help relieve it.

Hypertension

DESCRIPTION

An individual with hypertension has high blood pressure. The two main types of hypertension are secondary and essential. When the cause of hypertension is not related to another pathologic process, the individual is said to have essential hypertension. Approximately 90 percent of individuals with hypertension have essential or primary hypertension. When an individual has high blood pressure as a symptom of some other disease condition, that person is said to have secondary hypertension.

Blood pressure is controlled by the nervous, circulatory, urinary, and endocrine systems. The circulatory system was described earlier as a closed network of vessels through which blood is pumped by the heart. Arteries possess the ability to constrict, resulting in increased blood pressure. Constriction of arteries occurs when a center in the medulla of the brain, known as the vasomotor center, is stimulated. In response to the stimulation of the sympathetic nervous system, acetylcholine is released by pregan-

glionic neurons, and the released substance stimulates postganglionic nerve fibers in the blood vessel where the release of catecholamines results in vasoconstriction. Many factors such as stress, anxiety, and fear can affect this vasoconstrictor response. The narrowing of vessels takes place mainly in the peripheral arterioles. The decrease in the size of the arterioles offers resistance to the flow of blood and results in an elevation of blood pressure.

At the same time that the nervous stimulation of the blood vessels is occurring, the adrenal medulla secretes the vasoconstrictor catecholamine hormone consisting of epinephrine and norepinephrine. These substances cause the hypothalamus in the brain to secrete the corticotropin-releasing factor (CRF) which stimulates the anterior pituitary gland to release adrenocorticotropic hormone (ACTH). ACTH stimulates the adrenal cortex to release glucocorticoids such as hydrocortisone, also, mineralocorticoids such as aldosterone. These substances affect the body's electrolyte metabolism by increasing blood sodium and decreasing blood potassium. Vasoconstrictor impulses result in a reduced supply of blood to kidneys, which results in the release of renin, a product of the kidney. Renin is converted to angiotensin, which, in turn, stimulates the adrenal cortex to release the hormone, aldosterone. Aldosterone promotes sodium and water retention in the kidney which increases the electrolyte concentration in the blood vessels to a level that favors the vasoconstrictor response of arterioles. Sustained vasoconstriction of blood vessels, which results in resistance to blood flow through arterioles, is a major factor in essential or primary hypertension.

Arterial blood pressure is measured in two phases, systolic and diastolic. Systolic pressure is a measurement of the force with which blood is pumped from the left ventricle through the aorta and other arteries. Systole, the working phase for the heart, represents pressure at its highest in the arterial system. Diastolic pressure is a measurement of the force of the blood in the arterial system when the ventricles are relaxing and represents pressure at its lowest level. Diastole is the resting period for the heart. Diastolic pressure reflects resistance of the peripheral blood vessels. Some physicians consider the diastolic pressure the more important of the two pressures because it indicates the stress to which the blood vessels and heart are subjected during the relaxing phase. The patient with a persistent systolic pressure above 140 mm of mercury or a diastolic pressure of more than 90 mm of mercury has hypertension.

The seriousness of high blood pressure depends mainly upon the changes resulting in the heart and arteries. Hypertension lasting over a period of time results in enlargement of the heart, especially of the left ventricle. This enlargement is a result of the increased work load placed on the heart as it tries to force the same amount of blood through smaller arteries. When heart disease results from hypertension, it is referred to as *hypertensive heart disease.* An inadequate supply of blood to the heart muscle through the coronary arteries may result in angina pectoris or acute myocardial infarction.

Prolonged elevation of blood pressure eventually damages blood vessels everywhere in the body. The walls become thicker and the size of the passageway becomes smaller. Thus, less blood reaches the body cells. The kidneys, eyes, heart, and brain are most commonly affected, resulting in renal failure, poor vision, congestive heart failure, myocardial infarction, and cerebrovascular accident.

Malignant hypertension is hypertension with an abrupt onset and an accelerated course. The symptoms are severe, and this form of hypertension often resists treatment, threatening to produce death. However, newer forms of drug therapy have improved the prognosis of individuals with this severe form of hypertension.

Another type of hypertension, affecting approximately 10 percent of hypertensive patients, is secondary hypertension. The causes of secondary hypertension are many, including coarctation of the aorta, adrenal causes such as the tumor pheochromocytoma, primary aldosteronism, and Cushing's disease; thyrotoxicosis, brain tumor, anemia, preeclampsia of pregnancy, and renal

stenosis are also causes of secondary hypertension. When the doctor can diagnose the above conditions and effective treatment is provided, the problem of secondary hypertension can be controlled or cured. If the clinical workup produces no evidence of conditions that can cause secondary hypertension, then the doctor diagnoses the condition as essential hypertension.

COMMON DIAGNOSTIC STUDIES

The diagnosis of hypertension is made by history, physical examination, and laboratory tests. A variety of laboratory tests may be done to diagnose hypertension and to determine the extent of damage to organs of the body. To determine the degree of involvement of the kidneys, a BUN (blood urea nitrogen) will be done to indicate the ability of the kidneys to excrete urea, an end product of protein metabolism. The result is dependent on the body's urea production and blood flow through the kidney. BUN may be elevated in hypertension. Creatinine is a test of renal function reflecting the balance between the production and filtration by the glomerulus of the kidney. In the hypertensive patient, an elevated level would indicate the inability to concentrate urine. In the hypertensive patient, the serum sodium may be elevated as well as plasma renin. Urine studies may be done, for example, urinalysis, to check for protein which, if present, can be evidence of renal disease. Twenty-four-hour urine samples may be collected. An elevation of the ketosteroids, hormones, catacholamines, and VMA (vanillylmandelic acid) may indicate the presence of pheochromocytoma, a tumor of the medulla of the adrenal gland. Twenty-four-hour urines for electrolytes may be ordered also.

An electrocardiogram may be done to detect left ventricle enlargement. Special studies, such as the intravenous pyelogram, renal arteriogram, or kidney scan, may be done to diagnose the extent of renovascular disease.

NURSING OBSERVATIONS

The patient with essential hypertension usually has few early symptoms, if any. Thus, it is often referred to as the "silent-killer." However, symptoms may be severe. Headache in the occipital region, especially in the early morning, may be experienced. Fatigue, shortness of breath on exertion, dizziness, nervousness, and visual disturbances are some of the common symptoms that may occur. As hypertension progresses, the individual may develop symptoms of disease in the organs most often affected such as the kidneys. Frequent urination, a sign of not being able to concentrate urine, nocturia, and other signs of renal damage may occur. Symptoms of damage to the brain and central nervous system include transient ischemic attacks. Angina and frequent palpitations and congestive heart failure indicate cardiac involvement. Hemorrhages of blood vessels on the retina of the eye lead to poor vision.

When hypertension occurs as a symptom of another disease, the patient can be expected to have symptoms associated with that condition. For example, the patient with kidney disease has symptoms of that illness. High blood pressure is only one of the symptoms.

COMMON TREATMENT PLANS/ NURSING INTERVENTIONS

Treatment of the specific cause of hypertension is done in the small percentage of cases having a known cause, such as a tumor of the adrenal gland (pheochromocytoma).

Early detection with effective management is the main treatment of an individual with essential hypertension. Effective management includes control of hypertension and prevention of complications, with a lifetime program involving activities of daily life such as diet, exercise, rest, coping with stress, and medication. Modifications in the individual's life-style to provide adequate time for a balance between work, exercise, and rest may be necessary.

A reducing diet is usually prescribed for the overweight patient. The individual may be advised to use a moderate amount of salt in the diet and to avoid adding salt to food. Foods high in salt such as potato chips and pickles should be avoided. A diet low in animal fat may be prescribed to aid in the control of abnormal cholesterol and triglyceride

levels. A low-cholesterol diet may be supplemented with a drug such as clofibrate (ATROMID—S) to aid in lowering blood lipids.

A daily balance of rest, exercise, and relaxation should be planned for the control of hypertension. Bed rest is indicated only when the pressure is extremely high or when treatment is first started. Since emotional stress is considered an important factor, a valuable part of the treatment is the relief and avoidance of worrisome situations. Overuse of stimulants, such as coffee and tea, is discouraged. The patient who smokes is also encouraged to stop.

Remembering that the blood vessels of the brain, heart, eyes, and kidneys may be damaged will enable the nurse to associate complications of high blood pressure with stroke, heart failure, failing vision, and kidney failure. This association also can serve as a framework for helping the patient to follow the prescribed medical regime to prevent such complications. The attitude of the patient toward life, family, and work affects the level of the blood pressure. A factor that is stressful to one person may not be so to another. The nurse is frequently instrumental in helping patients to identify circumstances in life that contribute to hypertension and to gain insight into their behavior. The nurse can also educate patients and their families about the disease process and the importance of remaining under medical care. Sometimes, the patients are taught to measure blood pressure at home. They must be taught to continue to take their medication even though they feel improved and may have no symptoms. They also must understand the importance of continued weight control, reduction of sodium intake, and the need for periods of rest, relaxation, and exercise and for moderation in their activities.

Realizing that blood pressure varies with an individual's posture, emotion, and exercise should serve as a reminder for the nurse to measure blood pressure under controlled or constant conditions (Figure 12.9). For example, blood pressure should not be taken as soon as the individual walks into the doctor's office on one visit and after sitting for 20 minutes the next time. To be more consistent, the nurse should have the patient re-

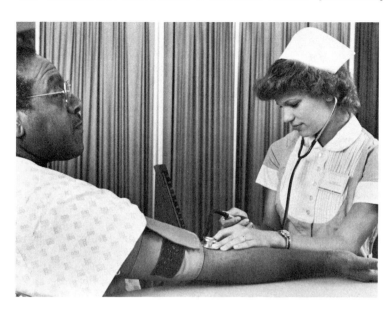

FIGURE 12.9 Measuring the patient's blood pressure. (Courtesy of Shapero School of Nursing, Sinai Hospital of Detroit, Detroit, Michigan.)

main seated for a given period of time, such as 10 minutes, and measure the blood pressure. The blood pressure may be taken in one arm or both. The conditions under which the measurement was made should be noted. For example, position (standing, sitting, lying down) and time of day should be recorded.

A combination of drugs may be used to lower blood pressure. Diuretics, antihypertensive agents, tranquilizers, and/or sedatives may be prescribed. The physician will attempt to select the drugs most appropriate for the individual patient. Antihypertensive drugs and diuretics are listed in Table 12.3. During hospitalization for treatment for hypertension, the patient may need to have the drugs changed and the dosage altered. The nurse should observe the patient for postural hypotension and provide protective measures. For example, siderails may be needed, or the patient may require assistance in assuming an upright position. The patient should be cautioned to arise slowly from a lying or sitting position to a standing one.

Daily weights may be taken to determine weight loss either from a calorie-restricted diet or from the administration of a diuretic. The nurse should know the side effects of the drug or drugs being administered. For example, what reaction would a man be likely to have when he learns that a drug is likely to cause impotence? Which diuretics are likely to cause hypokalemia?

Cerebrovascular Accident

DESCRIPTION

The patient with a cerebrovascular accident (CVA) has a disease of the arteries in the brain. This results in an inadequate blood supply to the part of the brain nourished by the affected blood vessel. Apoplexy, stroke, and cerebrovascular accident are names commonly used in referring to this disease.

Cerebrovascular disease ranks third as the cause of death in the United States. Approximately one third of the patients return to their usual activities, while about one half, although disabled, can carry on activities of daily living. Approximately 15 percent are disabled and totally dependent on others for their care.

The causes of a cerebrovascular accident are hemorrhage, thrombus, embolus, or stenosis of an artery supplying the brain (Figure 12.10). When a stroke results from a hemorrhage, it is referred to as a cerebral hemorrhage. Hemorrhage may occur outside the dura mater (extradural hemor-

TABLE 12.3
MEDICATIONS USED IN THE TREATMENT OF HYPERTENSION (ANTIHYPERTENSIVE DRUGS)

NONPROPRIETARY NAME	TRADE NAME	AVERAGE DOSE	TOXIC REACTIONS
Blocking Agents			
Clonidine hydrochloride	CATAPRES	0.2 mg–0.8 mg/day in divided doses	Dry mouth, drowsiness, sedation, constipation, impotence
Methyldopa	ALDOMET	250 mg 2–3 times/day	Sedation, headache, weakness, dizziness, drowsiness, dry mouth, fluid retention
Guanethidine monosulfate	ISMELIN	25–50 mg/day	Dizziness, weakness, syncope, hypotension, diarrhea
Reserpine	SERPASIL SANDRIL	0.1–.25 mg/daily	Nausea, vomiting, diarrhea, anorexia, depression, hypertension, drowsiness, decreased libido, sodium retention
Propranolol hydrochloride	INDERAL	160–480 mg/day	Lightheadedness, depression, insomnia, fatigue, nausea, congestive heart failure
Trimethaphan camsylate	ARFONAD	IV—500 mg diluted for use during surgery	Urinary retention, angina
Vasodilators			
Hydralazine hydrochloride	APRESOLINE	50 mg 4 times daily	Headache, palpitations, anorexia, vomiting, diarrhea, tachycardia
Sodium nitroprusside	NIPRIDE	3 mcg/kg/minute IV	Nausea, retching, diaphoresis, apprehension, headache
Diazoxide	HYPERSTAT	1–3 mg/kg up to 150 mg. May be repeated at intervals of 5–15 minutes	Sodium and water retention, hypotension, cerebral ischemia, sweating, flushing
Prazosin hydrochloride	MINIPRES	6–15 mg daily in divided doses	Dizziness, headache, drowsiness, weakness, palpitations
Diuretics			
Hydrochlorothiazide	HYDRODIURIL	50–100 mg/day	Anorexia, dizziness, vertigo, nausea, vomiting, cramping, hypokalemia, hyperglycemia, hyperuricemia
Furosemide	LASIX	40 mg twice a day	Anorexia, nausea, vomiting, cramping, dizziness, hypotension, hyperglycemia, electrolyte depletion
Spironolactone	ALDACTONE	50–100 mg/day	Cramping, diarrhea, lethargy, drowsiness, headache
Chlorthalidone	HYGROTON	25–100 mg/day	Cramping, anorexia, nausea, vomiting, dizziness, vertigo, hypokalemia

rhage), beneath the dura mater (subdural hemorrhage), in the subarachnoid space (subarachnoid hemorrhage), or within the brain substance (intracerbral hemorrhage). Cerebral hemorrhages can occur as a result of trauma, cerebral atherosclerosis, cerebral aneurysm, hypertension, or hemorrhagic disorders such as leukemia.

Cerebral thrombosis is the most common cause of cerebrovascular accident and accounts for 90 percent of CVAs in persons over 65 years of age. Cerebral arteriosclerosis is a common cause of cerebral thrombosis. A thrombus or blood clot forms in the diseased artery. Cerebral embolism occurs when a blood clot is formed and moves along an artery until it lodges at a point where it occludes a vessel completely.

Stenosis of an artery supplying the brain results in decreased blood supply to the brain. In all cases where blood supply to the brain is decreased or interrupted, depending

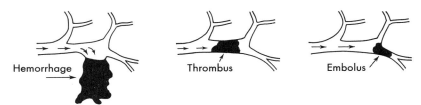

FIGURE 12.10   The three causes of a cerebrovascular accident are a hemorrhage, a thrombus, and an embolus. The portion of the brain nourished by the affected blood vessel has an inadequate supply of blood.

on where in the brain the damage occurs, the patient may have temporary or permanent loss of motor ability, sensation, speech, thought processes, memory, or visual disturbances.

Transient ischemic attacks (TIA) are episodes resulting in temporary neurologic deficits such as temporary loss of motor ability, sensation, speech, thought, or vision. The episode lasts a few seconds or minutes to a few hours, but not more than 24 hours usually. TIA is a warning of impending stroke. The most common cause is arteriosclerosis of the common carotid arteries.

COMMON DIAGNOSTIC STUDIES

Various diagnostic procedures will be done to determine the cause of stroke. Computerized axial tomography (CAT scan) of the head and neck will give information about the number, size, and density of lesions in the head and the extent of edema, if present. A skull x-ray will reveal calcifications of blood vessels, displacement of intracranial structures, and bone destruction. A lumbar puncture to measure the pressure within the spinal column and to analyze cerebrospinal fluid may be done. A cerebral arteriogram provides visualization of cerebral blood vessels. A brain scan may be ordered as well as an electroencephaogram. Possible cerebral hemorrhage must be ruled out before anticoagulant therapy is administered. Anticoagulant therapy is a common drug therapy (Table 12.3) to prevent further blood clotting when thrombus or embolus is the cause of stroke. Anticoagulants would worsen the hemorrhage by preventing clotting.

NURSING OBSERVATIONS

The onset of a cerebrovascular accident is usually sudden. In general, it is more sudden in a patient with a cerebral hemorrhage than in the one with cerebral thrombosis. Some patients experience headache, a feeling of fullness in the head, visual disturbances, sensory loss, and dizziness before other symptoms are evident. The patient who is awake may lapse into a coma or may lose the use of a part of the body without loss of consciousness. The sleeping individual may lapse into unconsciousness without awakening or may fall when getting out of bed. The patient may regain consciousness in a few minutes, hours, or days or may die without regaining consciousness. In some cases, the patient's symptoms develop over a period of minutes or hours. This is referred to as a stroke-in-evolution or a progressive stroke.

The comatose or unconscious patient usually has a flushed face. The breathing is slow, deep, and noisy (stertorous), and the cheek on the paralyzed side flaps out with exhalation and that side of the mouth may droop. The presence of Cheyne-Stokes breathing is considered an ominous sign. The pulse is full and bounding. The patient with hypertension usually has no significant change in blood pressure. Incontinence is often present. Convulsions may occur. The patient may also develop a fever. When the temperature is high and remains so, the patient's prognosis is grave.

The patient most likely to survive this attack regains consciousness within 12 to 48 hours. It is upon the patient's return to consciousness that the presence of *paralysis*, which means loss of function, is most often evident. The amount of paralysis is determined by the location of the diseased cerebral artery and the size of the area involved. For example, the patient with a large thrombus in the left side of the brain is paralyzed on the right side of the body. When the thrombus is small, the patient may have a small amount of paralysis or none at all. When paralysis occurs, it is present on the side opposite the cerebral accident because the fibers of the brain cross over in the medulla to serve the opposite side of the body. Hemiparesis is weakness of one entire side of the body. Hemiplegia, which is paralysis of one entire side of the body, is a frequent result of cerebrovascular accident.

When the lesion is near the speech center in the brain, the patient has aphasia, which is a defect or an actual loss of language ability to communicate by speaking, writing, or other signs. Aphasia is a disturbance of language function resulting from injury or disease of the brain. The speech center is near the left motor center in the left hemisphere of the brain. Therefore, patients who have damage to the brain in the left hemisphere and experience right hemiplegia are often aphasic. For patients with left hemiplegia, aphasia is less common. However, some patients with left hemiplegia may be aphasic if they are a left-handed person whose speech center is located in the right hemisphere of the brain.

The patient with receptive aphasia has difficulty comprehending the spoken word or in silent reading comprehension. Such a person may not recognize people or objects. The patient with expressive aphasia may have difficulty making thoughts or wishes known to others. There are problems with speaking, writing, naming objects, counting, telling time, or gesturing appropriately. The mixed type of aphasia involves loss of voluntary speech, impaired ability to read, and difficulty understanding spoken words.

Following a stroke, there may be impaired sensation in response to urinary bladder filling. Urinary incontinence may develop if control of the sphincter is lost or decreased. Bowel incontinence may develop as a result of loss of sphincter control also.

Impairment of memory and learning capacity may be affected. Limited attention span, lack of motivation, and depression often delay progress later in the plan for rehabilitation.

As the patient's condition improves, there may be a partial or complete return of function of the paralyzed part. However, the patient is usually left with some damage, such as difficulty in walking, impaired function of the hand, or a speech defect. Unfortunately, the patient is likely to have another stroke because the condition, such as hypertension and arteriosclerosis, that caused the accident still exists.

Nursing observations are important in diagnosis and plan of therapy. The observations should be recorded carefully and accurately. A change in the level of consciousness, as evidenced by movement of the patient, resistance to movement, or response to stimulation, should be recorded. The presence or absence of voluntary or involuntary movements should be noted also. Apparent stiffness or flaccidity (relaxation) of the neck should be observed and documented. A nurse should record the reaction of the patient's pupils to light, their size, and equality by using a flashlight. The color, temperature, and moisture of the skin should be noted. The temperature (rectal), pulse, respiration, and blood pressure should be monitored frequently. The patient's temperature may be elevated following a cerebral hemorrhage, especially if the hypothalamus has been affected. A careful record of the patient's intake and output should be maintained.

As previously mentioned, the patient may have convulsions (seizures) following a stroke. In this patient, the nurse should observe and report important points about the seizure. When did it begin? In what part of the body did the muscular contractions start? What part of the body was involved? Did the muscles relax during the attack? Did the patient stop breathing? Was the patient cyanotic? Was the patient incontinent? When did the convulsions or seizure end? It is important for the nurse to observe these factors and give an accurate report. Knowing the answers to these and other questions regarding the seizure may aid the physician in determining the location of the accident in the brain.

The nurse should not assume that the patient cannot hear what is being said because of unconsciousness. A simple explanation of what is going to be done before doing it often seems to comfort and quiet the patient. The nurse should continue to talk with the patient while providing care. The family's questions about the patient should be answered outside of the patient's range of hearing. The family should be told to talk with the patient although he may not appear to hear them.

COMMON TREATMENT PLANS AND NURSING INTERVENTIONS

In patients with cerebral thrombosis or cerebral embolism, anticoagulant therapy may be employed to prevent further clotting. Warfarin (COUMADIN) may be ordered daily in response to the patient's prothrombin time and partial thromboplastin time.

Aspirin may be ordered for patients who have experienced TIAs to decrease the change of cerebral thrombosis occurring. Drugs such as papaverine, which relaxes smooth muscle and dilates blood vessels, may be ordered to increase blood flow to the brain.

In patients with multiple TIAs, carotid endarterectomy may be done to remove atheromatous plaques or thrombi along with a small portion of the carotid artery. Following carotid endarterectomy, the patient is observed closely for signs of stroke. During or after the procedure, material that can become emboli in the carotid artery may cause neurologic deficits. Neurologic assessments, including the reaction of the patient's pupils to light, their size, and equality, should be recorded. A change in the level of consciousness, the presence or absence of involuntary or voluntary movement of extremities, temporal pulse, symmetry of face, and swallowing reflex should be observed. The doctor must be notified of any motor or sensory deficits. Myocardial infarction is another one of the complications of carotid endarterectomy. Another surgical procedure being performed for patients with TIAs is extracranial-intracranial bypass grafting to increase collateral circulation to the brain. The procedure is done to restore adequate blood supply to a portion of the brain. The surgery is similar to the more common coronary bypass procedure, but on a much smaller scale. This procedure diverts a section of a scalp artery and reconnects it inside the skull, bypassing the clogged artery and restoring blood flow. Close nursing observations are required after surgery. The blood pressure is controlled with drug therapy. The graft is kept patent with antiplatelet-aggregation drugs such as aspirin.

The care of this patient is discussed in two phases: (1) the acute phase and (2) the convalescent phase. During the acute phase, the treatment is directed toward saving the patient's life. Following this, treatment is prescribed that should enable the patient to regain the greatest amount of use possible of the affected part. Other members of the health team, such as the physical therapist, speech therapist, and occupational therapist, are often called upon to assist with the patient's rehabilitation. Rehabilitation is aimed at (1) preventing deformities, (2) enabling the patient to regain maximum use of the affected side and of communication skills, and (3) helping the patient to gain independence in activities of daily living.

The welfare of a patient with a cerebrovascular accident is largely dependent upon the nursing care provided. Because of the frequency of strokes and the patient's chronic condition following the accident, the nurse is an important person in the care. The nurse needs a deep understanding and appreciation of the mental and emotional problems of this patient and family, as well as the ability to give the best physical care.

ACUTE PHASE. The patient who has just experienced a life-threatening cerebrovascular accident will require special nursing care. Nursing care is directed toward maintaining a patent airway, assessing the level of responsiveness, evaluating vital signs, and maintaining fluid and electrolyte balance. Supportive care is given as the patient's condition indicates. For care of the unconscious patient, see Chapter 21.

CONVALESCENT PHASE. *Maintaining Safety.* It is the nurse's responsibility to protect the patient from injury. Siderails are used to prevent the patient from rolling out of bed. The convulsing patient needs to be protected from injury. Placing something soft between the patient's teeth prevents injury to the tongue; the nurse needs to protect the fingers when doing so. A wooden or metal object should not be used. Placing the call bell and needed objects within easy reach are safety measures that prevent accidents when the patient is alert.

Fluid and Food. The patient who is unable to swallow is given fluid and nourishment in other ways. A common method of administering liquid nourishment is by gavage. Either the physician or the professional nurse inserts a tube through the nose into the stomach. The prescribed formula at room temperature is poured through the tube following the feeding to rinse the tube. This also gives the patient additional fluid. Intravenous administration of fluids also may be ordered.

When the patient is able to swallow, fluids and foods are given by mouth. When feeding a paralyzed patient, the nurse should turn the patient's head slightly toward the unaffected side. The food should be placed in the side of the mouth that is not paralyzed.

Skin and Mouth Care. The incontinent patient should be kept clean, dry, and free from odor. The skin needs special attention to prevent decubitus ulcers (see Figure 12.11). Oil or lotion may be applied to dry areas after they have been cleaned with warm water and mild soap. Changing the patient's position frequently helps to prevent excess pressure on any one area of the body. Other measures used to prevent pressure sores include an egg-crate mattress, alternating pressure mattress, or a flotation pad (Figure 12.12). If these are not available, the nurse may use a lamb's wool pad under the patient and on the heels and elbows.

The patient's mouth should be kept clean and moist. A lubricating substance, such as glycerin, can be applied to the lips to prevent chapping.

Position. The patient's position should be changed frequently to prevent further

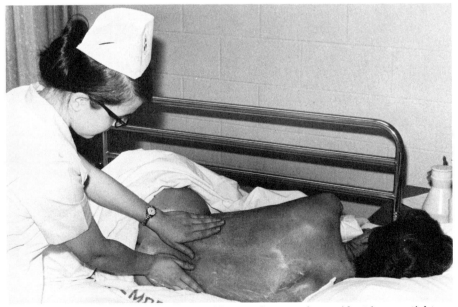

FIGURE 12.11 Back care of the patient with a cerebrovascular accident is essential to prevent decubitus ulcers. (Courtesy of Central School of Practical Nursing, Norfolk, Virginia.)

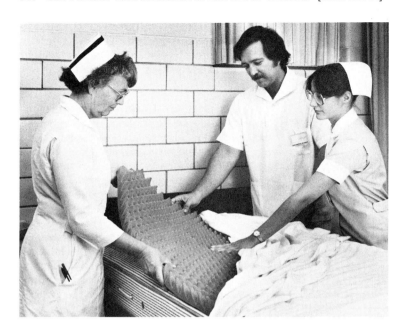

FIGURE 12.12 Using an egg-crate mattress. (Courtesy of Shapero School of Nursing, Sinai Hospital of Detroit, Detroit, Michigan.)

complications such as hypostatic pneumonia and circulatory stasis. It is important to keep the body in good alignment. The prevention of deformities should be started during the acute stage after lifesaving measures have been carried out. A small pillow in the axilla of the paralyzed side aids in preventing adduction of the shoulder. Placing a piece of linen rolled to the appropriate size along the trochanter (trochanter roll) will help to keep the leg from turning outward (external rotation) and to keep the knee from flexing. The arm should be elevated on a pillow to prevent dependent edema. The fingers of the affected hand should be extended to prevent deformity. If the extremity is flaccid, the hand and wrist may be placed in a splint in a functional position. A footboard is helpful in preventing footdrop (plantar flexion) and heel cord shortening as a result of contracture of the gastrocnemious muscle. Special foot devices may be used for the same purpose if a footboard is not desirable. Use of a bed cradle may be an added precaution in protecting the patient's lower extremity from the bedclothing. Maintaining high-Fowler's or low-Fowler's position for long periods of time contributes to hip

flexion contracture. The head of the bed should be flat except for activities of daily living.

When turning the patient to a lateral position, the nurse should place the patient on the unaffected side with a pillow between the legs. The affected thigh should be flexed slightly and the affected arm placed on a pillow with a hand roll in the hand.

Placing the patient on the abdomen, prone position, for 15 to 30 minutes several times a day helps to prevent hip deformity. A small pillow should be placed from the midportion of the abdomen to the midportion of the thigh to help extend the hip joint slightly and increase comfort for the patient.

Elimination. The nurse should check the comatose patient for voiding and defecation. The patient may have. retention of urine, which is the inability to void, incontinence, which is involuntary voiding and defecation. The physician may request that the patient with retention be catheterized.

Absorbent pads are available that can be placed under the incontinent patient to help protect the bed and linen. Placing the urinal in position for male patients helps to keep them dry. Occasionally, a catheter is inserted and left in place to prevent the urine from irritating the skin. This is referred to as an indwelling catheter. It may cause serious irritation to the bladder and urethra. The physician may prescribe an enema for the incontinent patient. Giving a small enema daily helps to relieve rectal incontinence in some patients. Stool softeners may be ordered for the patient with constipation.

Using the Therapeutic Relationship. Upon return to consciousness, the patient becomes aware of disabilities such as paralysis and aphasia. The nurse needs to consider the impact of awakening one morning and not being able to talk or move properly. The nurse can then have a better understanding of the emotional shock experienced by patients. The aphasic patient experiences a great deal of frustration. The nurse should give the patient as much psychologic support as possible by such actions as talking to the patient while giving care, even though the patient is not able to respond verbally. The nurse should use gestures that will help the patient understand what is being said. The nurse should speak slowly and distinctively while facing the patient, but should not shout. Plenty of time should be given to allow the patient to speak or to respond. The patient should be treated as an intelligent adult. The nurse needs to realize that, although the patient cannot talk, the thinking and reasoning process may not have been affected. The family should have this explained to them.

The nurse who knows that these patients are likely to be emotionally unstable at first is more capable of understanding unusual outbursts of emotion.

Rehabilitation to help the patient to communicate and perform other activities of daily living should be started as soon as the stroke is completed. The nurse can expect the patient to experience such behavior as rage, anger, and depression. Frustration caused by having to relearn activities that have been done for years can be expected. The patient is likely to start crying or laughing suddenly. This also may be upsetting to

the patient's family. The nurse can often ease their concern over this unusual reaction by explaining to them that this frequently occurs following a stroke.

The nurse should point out to the patients improvements that are being made. For example, when the patients are first able to do such a minor thing as holding their bread, or helping turn themselves, the nurse should encourage them by calling this to their attention. They need genuine praise from the nurse. Short-term goals, such as accomplishments likely to be made in the near future, should be stressed rather than long-term ones. For example, the goal of being able to feed oneself is much more real and close than the final one of complete or maximal recovering.

Exercise. The patient generally is encouraged to be as active as possible as soon as possible following a stroke unless it was caused by a hemorrhage. In this case, activity may not be permitted for six to eight weeks. Range-of-motion exercises will be started, usually within 48 hours if the patient has not suffered a hemorrhage. The affected extremities should be carried through a normal range of motion several times a day until the patient can begin to participate. Early use of exercise helps to prevent contractures, increase strength, and prevent wasting of affected muscles. Exercises may also encourage the patient.

Directions designed to strengthen the muscles of the individual involved should be obtained by the physical therapy department. Members of the nursing team play an important role in helping the patient with range-of-motion exercises and muscle-strengthening exercises.

The patient is taught a sitting balance while sitting on the side of the lowered bed with feet resting on the floor. This is a good time for the patient to start wearing walking shoes. The nurse should stand in front of the patient and help maintain good posture while in a sitting position. The length of sitting time should be increased until the patient is ready to assume a standing position.

When dressing the patient in a robe, the nurse should put the sleeve on the paralyzed arm first. The nurse can then stand at the patient's unaffected side, provide support, and have the patient stand for a few moments to regain balance. The patient should step forward with the unaffected foot to the chair. The patient's body should be placed in normal alignment in the chair. The degree of paralysis will indicate the necessity for additional persons to help in getting the patient into the chair.

If the patient's arm is completely paralyzed, it may be placed in a sling when the patient is not in bed. The arm is not placed in a sling if any function is present. Any slight use or movement of the arm should prompt sincere encouragement from the nurse. Another source of encouragement for the patient is to give assistance in dressing in street clothes as soon as possible. This practice also helps the patient to learn to dress within the limitations of the disability in preparation for discharge.

Patients should be encouraged to become as active as possible within the framework of their limitations. The goal of helping patients to become as self-sufficient as possible before being discharged is shared by all members of the health team.

Arteriosclerosis Obliterans

DESCRIPTION

An individual with arteriosclerosis obliterans has a narrowing or an obstruction of large and medium-sized arteries. Arteries, such as the abdominal aorta, superficial femoral, and iliac, are vessels commonly affected. The lower extremities are affected more often than the upper ones. Men are more likely to develop arteriosclerosis obliterans than women. In women, the disease is especially evident before menopause. Persons with diabetes mellitus are frequently affected.

COMMON DIAGNOSTIC STUDIES

Diagnosis of arterial insufficiency is made by various noninvasive tests, such as plethysmography, arm-ankle ratios, and Doppler ultrasonic flow studies, as well as the treadmill exercise test.

An angiogram, the x-ray visualization of the blood vessels following the intravascular injection of radiopaque contrast medium, may be done to determine the extent of an occlusion and location of calcified plaques. Arteriography generally is indicated when the patient is a candidate for surgery.

NURSING OBSERVATIONS

The symptoms of an individual with arteriosclerosis obliterans are secondary to the reduced blood supply to the area. The degree of ischemia, interference with the blood-carrying ability of the arteries, is related to the degree of obstruction of the arteries and the size of the involved vessel. The patient generally has intermittent claudication. Intermittent claudication may be described by the patient as an ache, pain, numb feeling, cramp, or sense of fatigue that occurs in certain muscles during exercise and disappears quickly with rest. Intermittent claudication seems to occur most often in the calf muscles of the leg. However, the location of the discomfort gives the physician an idea of the location of the arterial occlusion.

Pain occurs in the extremity during rest when the ischemia is advanced. The patient may notice pain in the toes, foot, and lower part of the leg, especially at night. The pain may be dull, moderately severe, persistent, and interfere with the patient's sleep. The individual may find it necessary to sit up and perhaps rub the foot for hours in order to obtain relief. In some cases, the pain is severe and difficult to control. Increased pain may be related to nerve involvement, local ulceration of the area, and, at times, gangrene. The patient may experience a feeling of coldness, numbness, and paresthesia.

The affected extremity may feel uncomfortably cold to the patient and may feel cool in comparison to the other extremity when touched by the nurse or other members of the health team. The involved extremity is also very susceptible to changes in temperature. Absence of a normally palpable peripheral pulse is a reliable sign of occlusive arterial disease. Comparison of pulses in both extremities should be done. Palpation of pulses at the femoral, popliteal, posterior tibial, and dorsalis pedis arteries is done. Diminished pulsations or absence of pulses indicate impaired blood flow through the arteries. (Sometimes, occlusion of the subclavian artery can lead to absence of pulsations in one or both ulnar or radial arteries.)

Decreased blood supply may result in paleness, abnormal reddish-blue color, and cyanosis. The extremity below the obstruction may vary in the degree of change in color. Impaired circulation causes loss of hair from skin and makes the skin appear smooth, taut, and dry. The skin has reduced resistance to infection. A small injury can lead to an uncontrollable infection, formation of an ulcer, and possibly gangrene. Such an infection frequently starts around a nail. The patient's toenails of the involved extremity become hard and brittle.

COMMON TREATMENT PLANS AND NURSING INTERVENTION

FOOT CARE. The foot should be bathed in water with a soft cloth and mild soap. The temperature of the water used to immerse the foot should be determined by a water thermometer and should not exceed 35°C (95°F). The feet should be observed carefully for bruises, cuts, or irritated areas. After bathing the feet, the nurse should dry them gently but thoroughly.

Soothing lotion or cream can be used on dry feet. Socks or stockings should be clean, nonirritating, and changed daily. Shoes should fit well, feel comfortable, and provide protection to the sensitive feet. The patient should be cautioned against going without shoes because of the possibility of injuring the feet.

Regular trimming of the nails should be done in a manner to avoid injury to the surrounding tissue. Toenail clippers and an emery board may be the best method of clipping the hard, brittle nails. Pointed scissors, a pocketknife, and a razor blade are not safe to use for the patient with peripheral vascular disease. In some cases, the services of a podiatrist are used for the patient with brittle toenails.

AVOIDING BURNS. Although the patient's feet should be kept warm, they should not be exposed to excessive heat. Adding heat to the affected extremity should be done only with a specific order from the physician as the tissues are excep-

tionally susceptible to burns. (Heat usually is not ordered). The danger of injuring the tissue is extremely high. Also, the patient may not be able to detect excessive heat. This increases the susceptibility to burns. Placing an extra blanket at the foot of the patient's bed, providing warm, nonirritating socks, and maintaining a comfortable room temperature should facilitate warmth for the involved extremity.

ULCERS. Ulcers frequently develop on the leg affected by impaired circulation. The nurse caring for the patient should remember that the ulcer is an open lesion and that it has developed in an area having impaired circulation, will heal slowly, and is likely to become infected. These multiple factors emphasize the importance of sterile technique when changing dressings and applying prescribed medication on the leg ulcer.

DIET. Dietary management for the individual who is obese, has diabetes, or has an elevated blood cholesterol level or triglyceride level is increasingly important when complicated by arteriosclerosis obliterans.

IMPROVING CIRCULATION. Elevating the leg of a person with peripheral vascular disease in which arteries are affected by such conditions as arteriosclerosis obliterans does not improve circulation. When the lower extremities are affected, the head of the bed may be elevated on 6-inch shock blocks (reverse Trendelenburg) to allow gravity to help in increasing circulation to the periphery. Elevating the limb decreases the amount of blood reaching the foot. The patient should keep the feet flat on the floor when sitting in a chair. Pressure on the popliteal vessels behind the knees should be avoided. Changing positions frequently is important to prevent stasis of blood in the extremity which leads to edema of tissues. Pedal edema can cause pressure on arterioles and further decrease arterial circulation. The patient should not sit with the legs crossed or wear constricting bands around the extremities. The band may be in the form of the top of a sock that is tight and narrow or, in some women, the band may be a garter. Exercises are sometimes ordered to improve collateral circulation and the flow of blood to the involved part. For example, in Buerger-Allen exercises, the feet are elevated above heart level for two minutes then with the patient sitting on the edge of the bed, the legs are placed in the dependent position for three minutes. The patient lies in the flat or level position for five minutes. The length of time for each cycle and number of times each day that the exercises are done depend on the individual patient and the doctor. Physicians are not in agreement about the benefits of these exercises. One of the best exercises for aiding collateral circulation is walking to the point of pain in the legs several times a day.

The patient who smokes will be advised to stop. Generally, this is a habit perceived to be personally satisfying to the patient and the advice to stop comes at a crucial time in life. The process of stopping the habit of smoking can pose a real problem. The patient will need to perceive the recommendation to stop smoking as important and possible. The patient will need understanding, support, and encouragement from family, friends, and members of the health team. Although it is desirable to stop smoking, the patient may be unable to do so. In this case, feelings of frustration and perhaps guilt may be experienced. The patient needs to be accepted by the health team in either case.

PAIN. A combination of measures is used to control pain. For example, maintenance of a comfortable temperature, special foot care, and proper positioning will facilitate relief of a certain amount of pain in some individuals. An individualized combination of rest with appropriate exercise may be helpful. Analgesics are used in some cases.

SURGERY. In arteriosclerosis obliterans, the blood vessels most commonly affected are the aorta at its bifurcation, the iliac, and the superficial femoral arteries. Other vessels that may be involved are the popliteal, coronary artery, and cerebral vessels.

Arteriosclerosis of these blood vessels may be treated surgically. For example, in some cases, the diseased portion of an artery is cut out and a vascular graft is sutured into place by end-to-end anastomosis.

More commonly, grafts are sutured into place to bypass the obstructed portion of the blood vessel. Either the patient's saphenous or umbilical vein is used or grafts made of synthetic material such as DACRON, TEFLON or GORTEX. The graft is sutured to the artery above the point of obstruction, tunneled between the muscle and the skin, and sutured to the artery below the point of obstruction. The obstructed segment of the artery is not removed. For example, femoral to popliteal, femoral to femoral, or axillary to femoral bypass grafts may be done. Widening the origin of the femoral artery with an autogenous vein patch may be done. This procedure is called *profundoplasty.*

Patch grafts using a vein patch to replace a damaged segment of an arterial wall may be used to increase the size of the lumen of a blood vessel that has been narrowed by arteriosclerosis. The artery is clamped above and below the narrowed section, and a segment in the long axis of the artery is cut out. The patch graft is then sutured into place increasing the diameter of the lumen of the artery. A piece of TEFLON material may be used also.

Postoperatively, the nurse assesses temperature and color changes comparing one leg with the other leg. Capillary refill of digits; and the presence or absence of edema of the leg are noted. Peripheral pulses such as dorsalis pedis, posterior tibial, popliteal, or femoral are palpated and recorded. On occasion, although peripheral pulses are not palpable, they may be audible by a Doppler ultrasonic flow detector. The pulses should be monitored frequently by this method and recorded. A diminished pulse or the absence of pulses may indicate that a thrombus has formed and obstructed the artery or graft. The doctor should be notified immediately. The nurse would note that the leg would feel cooler to touch, and the pale extremity would become dusky and cyanotic in color.

It is most important to maintain adequate circulation through the repaired arteries. The patient should not keep the knees flexed nor cross the legs at the knees or ankles. The legs must not remain in the dependent position. Elastic hose will help to promote venous circulation and prevent edema that may decrease arterial circulation. A foam pad on top of the mattress and a lamb's wool pad under the feet will help to prevent skin breakdown on heels. Skin incisions must be observed for signs of infection.

The two most common complications after surgery are occlusion of the artery or graft by a thrombus or infection at the graft site. The patient will need to undergo further surgery for the removal of the thrombus if one develops and also if infection develops. If circulation cannot be restored or if the patient develops arteriosclerosis gangrene, he may have to undergo amputation of the limb.

PSYCHOSOCIAL ASPECTS. The psychosocial aspects involved in caring for the patient with peripheral vascular disease, such as arteriosclerosis obliterans, are numerous. The condition occurs frequently in older persons and has the tendency to become chronic and progressive with advancing years. Care is directed toward improving circulation, controlling pain, preventing complications, and checking the progress of the disease. Problems associated with a chronic disease that can be debilitating and life-threatening form the framework for this patient's concerns. For example, the person engaged in outdoor work in a cold climate may need to change jobs because of danger to the extremities. This change in occupation may be difficult, if not impossible, for an older worker. Early retirement, reduced income, decreased independence, and possible loss of an extremity are only a few of the problems the patient and family may experience.

As mentioned earlier, the patient may have diabetes mellitus, heart disease, or hypertension. The detailed measures indicated in peripheral vascular disease then must be considered with the overall regime for preexisting conditions. The patient will need to incorporate measures to care for the extremity or extremities into the plan of daily activities, often for the remainder of life instead of a few weeks.

The patient with arteriosclerosis obliterans may become discouraged if leg ulcers occur as the ulcers heal slowly and require meticulous care. The client with an ulcerated area on an extremity may have to stay in bed until healing takes place. This may take weeks and sometimes months. The nurse can readily understand that time will pass slowly for the patient and that the patient will be prone to worry. The patient may worry about security of a job, the family finances, and possible amputation. A feeling of interest in the patient is quickly communicated by the nurse who shows concern when properly caring for an ulcerated area, accurately checking the temperature of bath water, and positioning the extremity for maximum comfort and circulation. The actual touch used to wash and dry the extremity and to apply medication or a soothing lotion communicates the nurse's feeling of concern or lack of concern to the patient.

Thromboangiitis Obliterans (Buerger's Disease)

DESCRIPTION

The patient with thromboangiitis obliterans, or Buerger's disease, has a chronic, recurring condition affecting the peripheral arteries and veins. The condition obliterates the flow of blood through the affected vessel or vessels. Walls of the blood vessels become inflamed, thrombi form, and the arteries and veins may be destroyed. This condition is largely a disease of young persons, especially men between the ages of 20 and 45. Vascular changes may develop in the hands and feet. The cause of inflammation is unknown at this time. Smoking seems to aggravate the condition.

COMMON DIAGNOSTIC STUDIES

Diagnostic studies include peripheral vascular studies such as arm-ankle pressures and index, treadmill exercise test, plethysmography of affected limbs, and leg arteriography.

NURSING OBSERVATIONS

Symptoms result from a deficient blood supply. Intermittent claudication occurs. The patient's feet are cold and may become red when hanging down and pale when elevated. The pulse in the affected extremity may be weak or absent. Thrombophlebitis and/or gangrene is likely to occur.

The nurse notes and records the pulses palpated in the legs. The Doppler ultrasound flow detector may be used to hear pulses audibly that are not palpable.

COMMON TREATMENT PLANS AND NURSING INTERVENTIONS

Measures to improve circulation, such as Buerger's exercises, are often prescribed. In ordering these exercises, the physician designates the specific length of time for the patient to keep the feet and legs in various positions. The use of tobacco is prohibited.

Vasodilators rarely are used because these drugs would dilate healthy blood vessels also; hence, blood may even be diverted away from the partially occluded vessels, which would make the problem worse. Heat should not be applied to the affected extremities. Heat increases metabolism of the tissues and the requirement for oxygenated blood. The diseased arteries would not be able to fulfill the demand. Lumbar sympathectomy may be done in the acute occlusive process. Cutting the sympathetic nerve would permanently dilate the vessels of the lower extremities. Since gangrene is likely to develop, the patient's feet and legs will need to be cared for in a manner similar to those of a diabetic patient, which is discussed in Chapter 16. The care of the feet of a patient with arteriosclerosis obliterans, discussed earlier in this chapter, is also applicable to the person with Buerger's disease. In some cases, amputation is necessary.

Raynaud's Phenomenon

DESCRIPTION

Raynaud's phenomenon is a condition in which the small arteries and arterioles of the digits constrict intermittently, resulting in coldness, pain, pallor, and on occasion ulceration of the fingertips. The condition is most common in women between the ages of 16 and 40. It is seen more frequently in cold climates during the winter months. The cause of primary Raynaud's phenomenon is unknown, but the vasoconstriction of arterioles seems to be influenced by the release of catecholamines at the neuroarteriolar junction. Secondary Raynaud's phenomenon indicates an underlying vascular problem such as collagen vascular disease (scleroderma), Buerger's disease, or emboli, or to certain occupational activities such as typing or piano playing. Raynaud's phenomenon affects hands much more commonly than the feet. It is uncommon for a patient to lose more than digits from gangrene.

The prognosis for primary Raynaud's phenomenon varies. Some patients get better, some get worse, and others stay the same. The prognosis for secondary Raynaud's phenomenon is that of the underlying disease.

COMMON DIAGNOSTIC STUDIES

The noninvasive peripheral vascular studies including the Doppler pressures and plethysmography of the digits may be done.

NURSING OBSERVATIONS

The fingers on both hands blanch when the individual is exposed to cold temperature and stressful situations. They may become cyanotic if vasoconstriction is moderate. If it is severe, the fingers may become very white. The fingers are cold, covered with perspiration, and numb during an attack. After becoming warm again, the patient experiences throbbing pain as the fingers begin to turn bright red. The characteristic color change is blue-white-red. Some fingers may not be involved. At first the attacks occur only in the winter. An attack can end by itself, or it can be stopped by having the patient place the hands in warm water. As the disease continues, the patient's fingers become thin and tapering with shiny skin, which is tightly stretched. The fingernails become ridged or curved. Infections, blisters, and localized areas of gangrene may develop.

COMMON TREATMENT PLANS AND NURSING INTERVENTIONS

The patient with a mild case of Raynaud's disease may be treated with tranquilizers or sedatives and protection from exposure to cold. The use of tobacco should be avoided. Drugs such as reserpine and methyldopa and vasodilators such as priscoline and dibenzylene may be prescribed (see Table 12.2). Surgical resection of some part of the sympathetic nerves of the involved area, *sympathectomy*, may help some patients.

The nurse plays a major role in teaching the patient measures to use in helping to prevent attacks. The two main objectives are to prevent exposure to cold temperatures and to avoid stressful situations. Clothing must be worn to meet the body's demands for heat in relation to the environment.

Aneurysm

DESCRIPTION

An *aneurysm* is an abnormal sac formed by the dilation of the wall of a blood vessel, especially an artery. A *sacciform aneurysm* is one in which only a part of the artery is dilated. It resembles a sac attached to one side of the artery. A *fusiform aneurysm* is one in which the entire circumference of the artery is dilated. A *dissecting aneurysm* is one in which blood from the artery seeps between the layers of the artery.

Atherosclerosis is the most common cause of aneurysm. Injury, syphilis, and congenital malformations also may cause an aneurysm. Although an aneurysm may occur in any artery of the body, it is generally found in the aorta and brain.

COMMON DIAGNOSTIC STUDIES

Diagnosis of aneurysm is done primarily by x-ray of the abdomen and by posterior, anterior, and lateral views of the chest. Ultrasound of the abdomen is more accurate, less expensive, and involves considerably less risk to the patient than angiography. However, angiography is still done to confirm the diagnosis of aneurysm. In abdominal aneurysm, an important diagnostic indication is that the doctor is able to feel a pulsating abdominal mass.

NURSING OBSERVATIONS

Some aneurysms are asymptomatic. Others rupture and the patient dies or is taken to the operating room where surgery is done on an emergency basis. The patient may experience symptoms in the region of the dilation. Pressure on surrounding tissues from the abnormal sac occurs and may cause symptoms such as nausea, vomiting, abdominal pain, and back pain when the aneurysm is one the abdominal aorta. At times, the patient may complain of feeling that the "heart is beating in the abdomen." An aneurysm on the aorta of the thorax may cause dysphagia from pressure on the esophagus or dyspnea from pressure on the trachea. Cough and weakness of the voice or hoarseness may indicate pressure on the laryngeal nerve.

COMMON TREATMENT PLANS AND NURSING INTERVENTIONS

The likelihood of rupture increases as the patient's aneurysm enlarges. Surgery is the treatment of choice for aneurysms that are enlarging and for abdominal aneurysms greater than 5 cm (2 in.) in diameter. Surgery involves cutting out the aneurysm by resecting the aorta above and below the aneurysm and inserting a graft made of synthetic material. The bypass graft is usually made of DACRON or TEFLON. For surgery on the aorta below the renal arteries, the patient's circulation may be interrupted long enough for the surgery to be completed. The cardiopulmonary bypass machine for extracorporeal circulation will not be necessary.

Postoperatively, the patient can be expected to have considerable incisional pain because of the extensive nature of the surgery. Support of the incisional area may enable the patient to cough when instructed to do so. The patient may not want to turn as often as prescribed because of pain. The nurse, of course, should help the patient to change positions and provide support when possible.

After abdominal aortic aneurysm repair, it is important to prevent abdominal distention which may cause pressure on the graft incision. A nasogastric tube or a gastrostomy tube may be inserted and connected to intermittent suction. Gastric decompression will relieve distention and vomiting caused by distention. As soon as peristalsis and bowel sounds resume, the nasogastric tube may be removed and the patient begins to take liquids and progress to a regular diet as tolerated. If a gastrostomy tube has been in place, the tube may be clamped and remain in place until the patient is discharged. In the event that abdominal distention should occur at any time during the hospitalization, the patient's oral intake may be stopped and the gastrostomy tube connected to suction until foods can be tolerated again.

Nursing observations of vital signs are of utmost importance following surgery. Adequacy of blood flow through the affected area should be checked frequently. Often the surgeon marks the location of the pulses distal to the surgical site prior to surgery, for example, the sites where the dorsalis pedis, posterior tibial, and popliteal pulses should be palpated. The pulse may be absent or weak in these distal sites for a few hours after surgery. If, however, the pulses have been present and suddenly are not present, the nurse should report this immediately since this could indicate formation of a thrombus. Coldness, paleness, and cyanosis of the extremity may also indicate a thrombus.

The position of the patient following surgery will depend on the location of the surgical graft. At times, the head of the bed may be elevated on blocks to increase arterial flow. At times, it may be necessary to elevate the foot of the bed to decrease edema of the extremity. If the graft is in the patient's abdominal or thoracic cavity, the patient may have no limitations regarding position. The patient who has a graft located at a flexion point such as the groin or popliteal space, may not be permitted to flex or bend that part of the body for approximately ten days or as ordered by the physician. Flexion would decrease the speed of blood flow through the part.

Sitting for long periods of time should be avoided. Sitting should be alternated with periods of light exercise frequently to prevent stasis of blood and to maintain adequate circulation.

The patient having successful surgery can look forward to relief from the symptoms. The patient's activity will be increased as the condition improves.

Arterial Embolism

DESCRIPTION

The patient with arterial embolism has a clot or other foreign object carried by the bloodstream to an artery that is too small for the embolus to pass. Arterial emboli often occur after myocardial infarction. Occlusion of a coronary artery causes the infarction and oftentimes atrial fibrillation. As a result of atrial fibrillation, thrombi form in the blood leaving the left side of the heart. The thrombi detach and become emboli moving through the aorta into the arterial system where they finally reach an artery that is too small for them to pass. Thrombi and emboli also can occur because of advanced arteriosclerosis of the aorta. These emboli most frequently lodge in an artery where it divides or bifurcates. Cerebral embolism is discussed on page 334 and pulmonary embolism on pages 350-51. Thrombi also may develop in an extremity after arterial bypass surgery such as was discussed on page 347. This discussion of arterial embolism is related mainly to an embolus in an extremity.

COMMON DIAGNOSTIC STUDIES

Noninvasive peripheral vascular studies may be done to determine the extent of occlusion and at what point it is located. The Doppler ultrasonic flow detector may be used, as well as ankle pressures and plethysmography.

NURSING OBSERVATIONS

Generally the patient experiences pain in the area that receives its blood supply from that artery. The location of the pain depends on the location of the embolus. For example, an embolus in the lungs will result in chest pain; an embolus in an artery of the leg results in leg pain. Numbness and tingling may be experienced before the pain. The pain becomes excruciating in most patients, especially if the limb is exercised. The patient may experience nausea, vomiting, and abdominal pain, and faint.

The extremity is pale, cold, and waxy. The patient's arm or leg may have no pulse below the site of the embolus. As the condition continues, the extremity becomes cyanotic in areas. If the patient's collateral circulation can take over the job of nourishing the affected part, symptoms will soon decrease. If collateral circulation is inadequate, the patient will soon develop gangrene.

COMMON TREATMENT PLANS

Medical or surgical management may be the chosen method of treatment. In embolism of small arteries, anticoagulant therapy may be all that is necessary to prevent death of tissue. In embolism of larger arteries, embolectomy is done as an emergency procedure. During this procedure, a special catheter may be introduced into the aorta for removal of embolic material, either proximal to the abdominal aorta or as far away as the ankle. The emboli are extracted with the special catheter. In some cases a bypass graft may be done. Heparin, an anticoagulant, generally is given to prevent further clot formation. The doctor generally orders that the extremity be placed in a dependent position of 15 degrees to increase the flow of arterial blood to the limb. The extremity should be kept comfortably warm. An analgesic is prescribed for pain.

Following surgery, the patient's vital signs and pulse in the extremity distal to the site of embolism should be checked frequently. Absence of the distal pulse, which has already returned, should be reported immediately. The patient's extremity should be placed in the position ordered by the vascular surgeon.

NURSING INTERVENTIONS

It is important that movement of the leg is encouraged by the nurse to prevent stasis of blood and to promote circulation. Anticoagulants are given to prevent blood clots from forming in the operated artery or at the original site of the emboli. The nurse observes for hemorrhage from the incision, as well as making all of the other observations of the patient receiving an anticoagulant. The patient's extremity should be protected from injury during the recovery period. A return to physical activity usually is gradual according to the surgeon's recommended schedule.

Thrombophlebitis— Phlebothrombosis

DESCRIPTION

The patient with thrombophlebitis has a thrombus (clot) along with an inflammation of the vein wall. Phlebothrombosis is a condition in which a clot forms with little or no inflammation. Thrombophlebitis is commonly seen as a result of injury to a vein such as a bruise or perforating wound, infection of tissues surrounding the vessel, pressure against the vein by a tumor or aneurysm, and varicose veins. It is also commonly a complication of bed-rest patients. It is seen in postoperative patients, in the postpartum patient, and in any patient who is ill enough that activity is very minimal. Also at risk are obese patients, elderly patients, and women who take oral contraceptives.

Valves in the veins open and close rhythmically to help propel the blood against gravity to the right side of the heart. Exercises such as walking and active or passive range of motion result in contraction of muscles that press against veins which helps to empty them and promote venous circulation. Stasis of blood in the venous system seems to be a causative factor in the development of thrombophlebitis.

In venous thrombosis, a clot forms in the vein and adheres to its wall. The danger is that the clot will break away from the wall producing an embolus, which is then carried through the right side of the heart to the lungs. This medical emergency is described on pages 350–51. The thrombus is more likely to become an embolus if there is no inflammation (phlebothrombosis). Deep vein thrombosis, which is often secondary to bed rest, results in less inflammation and less pain than some of the other causes of thrombophlebitis, but it is more likely to result in pulmonary emboli. Phlebitis and thrombosis occur most often in the leg veins.

COMMON DIAGNOSTIC STUDIES

Phlebography or venography, x-ray of a vein after the injection of contrast media, is commonly done to diagnose phlebothrombosis. The ultrasonic Doppler flowmeter and plethysmography of a vein are noninvasive peripheral vascular studies often done to diagnose deep vein thrombophlebitis.

NURSING OBSERVATIONS

A patient with thrombophlebitis can have varying degrees of the symptoms associated with inflammation. When the vein affected is in the leg, the patient's extremity is swollen, warm, red, and painful. In deep vein thrombosis, the patient can experience general symptoms of an inflammation, such as fever and malaise, depending on the severity of the condition. Pain in the calf of the leg when the foot is dorsiflexed is called Homan's sign and is present in some patients.

The nurse should question the patients who are at high risk about the presence of leg pain in the calf of the leg or thigh, and observe for edema, especially behind the medial malleolus. The observation of asymmetry of the legs and measurement of calf circumference should be recorded as well as temperature differences between the two extremities.

COMMON TREATMENT PLANS AND NURSING INTERVENTIONS

The patient is treated with bed rest. Warm, moist applications to the affected limb and elevation of the foot of the bed may be prescribed. The anticoagulant, heparin, may be administered by continuous intravenous infusion to regulate the patient's partial thromboplastin time (PTT) to between 50 to 80 seconds (Figure 12.13). Intermittent intravenous injection of heparin every four hours or subcutaneous injections may be ordered. Anticoagulation is later continued with crystalline sodium warfarin (COUMADIN) for a period of approximately 12 to 14 weeks. The patient will have periodic blood tests drawn (prothrombin time and partial thromboplastin time) after discharge from the hospital to determine how the blood is clotting so that the warfarin dosage can be regulated.

Fibrinolytic enzymes such as streptokinase are generally ineffective when the clots have been present for at least four days. Their use also is accompanied by a higher incidence of febrile reaction and

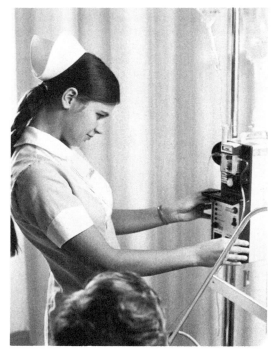

FIGURE 12.13 Using an infusion pump to administer continuous intravenous heparin. (Courtesy of Henrico County–St. Mary's Hospital School of Practical Nursing, Richmond, Virginia.)

bleeding. For these reasons, their use is contraindicated following surgery, childbirth, or trauma. When ordered, they are administered intravenously by infusion pump.

Pulmonary Embolism

DESCRIPTION

The patient with a pulmonary embolism has a clot or other foreign material carried through the great veins and right heart to the pulmonary artery. Thrombi can originate in the pelvic veins and the right atrium of the heart. Stasis of blood or slowing of venous circulation contributes, to the development of thrombi. The thrombus breaks away from the wall of the vein, becoming an embolism. Then, depending on the size of the embolus, it becomes lodged in an artery that is too small for the embolus to pass. Lung tissue nourished by that artery suffers from a lack of blood.

Pulmonary embolism is considered to be a complication instead of a primary disease. In other words, it occurs as a result of some other condition. Blood clots or thrombi in the veins of the lower extremities are a frequent cause. Venous thrombi could be dislodged by any activity of the patient causing a sudden increase in venous return, such as ambulating, transferring from bed to chair, sudden movements of extremities, and straining at stool.

COMMON DIAGNOSTIC STUDIES

A chest x-ray of the patient with suspected pulmonary emboli would be ordered. A radioisotope lung scan and pulmonary angiogram may be done to diagnose defects or obstructions in the pulmonary arteries. (See page 401 for pulmonary angiogram.) Arterial blood gases may be done to determine the respiratory status (Table 14.2, page 401).

NURSING OBSERVATIONS

The patient with a massive pulmonary embolism experiences sudden pain, usually under the sternum, dyspnea, tachycardia, restlessness, anxiety, shock, and syncope. Death may occur suddenly or within a short period of time.

When an embolus or emboli affects smaller blood vessels of the lung, the patient may have periods of dyspnea, pleuritic pain, cough, hemoptysis, fever, tachycardia, and anxiety.

COMMON TREATMENT PLANS AND NURSING INTERVENTION

For the patient with pulmonary embolus, bed rest, an analgesic for pain, and oxygen generally are ordered. Nursing measures for the patient with pain and dyspnea are indicated for this person. An antibiotic may be prescribed to prevent bacterial infection in the lungs.

The patient with a more severe embolus may have continuous oxygen prescribed. The central venous pressure, which is discussed in Chapter 9, may be measured if the patient is given intravenous fluids. The purpose of this is to prevent pulmonary edema by regulating the amount of fluids.

Anticoagulants, such as heparin, generally are given to reduce the possibility of another embolism, which could be fatal. Anticoagulant therapy (see Table 12.2) may be continued for an extended period of time, dependent upon the specific cause of the embolus.

Surgical therapy is indicated in some severe cases. For example, removal of an embolus may be a lifesaving measure in some patients. When this is done the patient is placed on a cardiac bypass machine, which is discussed in Chapter 11.

Varicose Veins

DESCRIPTION

It is necessary to recall certain important points about the veins to have a clear understanding of varicose veins. Blood is returned to the heart through blood vessels called veins. The squeezing action of muscles as well as the valves within the veins aid the blood in its upward climb. The valve flaps close to keep the blood from flowing backward. Stretching of the vein walls causes the valve flaps to close improperly. Therefore, the valve leaks and blood flows backward. This increased amount of blood causes further dilation of the vein. Because of its elasticity, the vein becomes longer as well as larger. The vein appears tortuous, which means that it is twisted, when it can be seen beneath the skin. The nurse may find it helpful to think of a tortuous vein as being similar to a winding stream in appearance. Thus, a person with varicose veins has dilated and tortuous veins.

An individual is most likely to develop varicosities in the saphenous veins of the legs (see Figure 12.14). A tendency toward weakness of the vein walls and valves may be inherited. After the inflammation of thrombophlebitis subsides, scar tissue may affect the vein valves by preventing them from opening and closing properly.

Varicose veins often occur during pregnancy because of pressure from the growing fetus on pelvic veins. They are also likely to develop in obese persons as a result of pressure from pads of fat on vessels in the pelvic area. Varicosities can result from long peri-

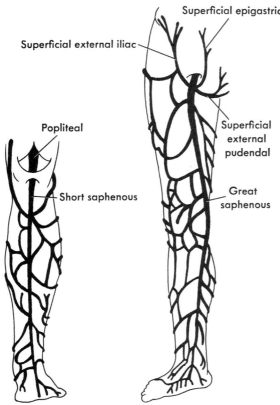

Superficial epigastric

Superficial external iliac

Popliteal

Superficial external pudendal

Short saphenous

Great saphenous

FIGURE 12.14 The veins of the lower extremity. (From Pansky, Ben: *Dynamic Anatomy and Physiology*. Macmillan Publishing Co., Inc., New York, 1975.)

ods of standing and of wearing tight garments. Pressure from close-fitting clothes interferes with the return flow of blood, which causes the vein to dilate.

COMMON DIAGNOSTIC STUDIES

Common diagnostic studies for a patient with suspected varicose veins includes phlebography or venogram. Injection of radiopaque dye into the veins allows the doctor to visualize occluded, tortuous, or twisted veins. Doppler flow studies are done to assess the speed of venous flow of blood, as well as plethysmography to determine the volume of blood found in the leg veins. The Trendelenburg test demonstrates the competence of valves of the superficial veins of the leg. The patient lies with the leg elevated to drain venous blood from the leg. A

tourniquet is applied to the upper thigh. When the patient stands, if blood flows into the superficial veins, the valves of the deep veins are not competent to do their job. When the tourniquet is released, if blood flows rapidly into the superficial veins, they are considered incompetent, also.

NURSING OBSERVATIONS

The person with varicose veins experiences a feeling of heaviness and tiredness in the legs. Aching and muscle cramps often occur. The vein becomes bluish, knotted, and tortuous. Bluish lumps are present, which disappear slightly when the feet are elevated. Blood that should be going back to the lungs for oxygen stays in the vein longer than normal. This slowing down of venous blood interferes with the flow of oxygenated blood through capillaries with resultant secondary edema of the leg. As a result the cells in that area are poorly nourished. This often results in varicose ulcers, which are difficult to heal because of their underlying cause.

COMMON TREATMENT PLANS AND NURSING INTERVENTIONS

An important part of the treatment for varicose veins is *prevention*. Undergarments such as circular garters, tight girdles, and rolled hose should not be worn. It is best to avoid sitting for long periods of time while wearing a girdle. Prolonged sitting should be avoided with periodic plantar flexion and dorsiflexion of the foot, which cause leg muscles to contrast against the deep veins, increasing venous return. Activities that require a great deal of standing should be interrupted by regular rest periods, during which the individual can elevate the feet as well as walk around. The pregnant woman should start her visits to the doctor early in an effort to prevent varicose veins and other complications of pregnancy.

The physician may prescribe an elastic stocking or an elastic bandage to relieve the discomfort from varicose veins. Pressure from these forces the blood into deeper veins that usually have healthier walls and valves. Surgical removal of the affected vein may be necessary. *Vein ligation* is a surgical procedure in which the upper end of the vein is closed by tying; the blood vessel eventually dies. *Stripping* is another surgical procedure, in which a portion of the vein is removed. A skin graft may be needed to help an ulcerated area to heal.

Elastic bandages are applied to the legs after surgery, and the foot of the bed is elevated to prevent venous stasis and formation of thrombi. The legs are checked for evidence of hemorrhage or for impaired circulation from dressings that are too tight.

The patient is ambulated, generally on the first postoperative day. The patient should not sit at any time with the legs in a dependent position. Walking facilitates venous return to the heart.

Sclerotherapy may be employed in some cases rather than surgery. The procedure is generally done in a doctor's office or clinic. A drug, sodium tetradecyl sulfate (SOTRADECAL SODIUM), is injected into the vein. The medication irritates the vein wall and, as the inflammation subsides, the lumen of the superficial vein eventually becomes occluded, forcing the venous blood into deeper veins. A pressure dressing is then applied to the patient's leg. The dressing remains on the leg for a period of three to six weeks at which time it is removed by the physician. Walking is encouraged to force blood into deeper veins. The patient is cautioned about bruising or traumatizing the veins which may lead to ulceration.

Case Study Involving Hypertension

Mr. Marshall, who is 48 years of age, is an automobile parts salesman. His job involves many tension-producing situations. He smokes nearly two packs of cigarettes a day and drinks coffee frequently. He is 167.5 cm (5 ft 7 in.) tall and weighs 440 kg (200 lb). He consulted his physician recently because of severe headaches and shortness of breath. Because his blood pressure was 240/120, he was immediately admitted to the hospital for treatment of essential hypertension. The physician's orders were:

- Complete bed rest
- 1200-calorie diet—low sodium (500 mg) with decaffeinated coffee
- Lying and standing blood pressures in each arm q4h while awake
- Daily weights
- Routine laboratory tests

- Serum cholesterol and triglycerides in A.M.
- LASIX, 40 mg PO qid
- Guanethedine, 25 mg PO daily

The nurse answered Mr. Marshall's call light the morning after his admission. He irritably asked for bacon on his breakfast tray and requested a pot of real coffee.

QUESTIONS
1. What factors in Mr. Marshall's life-style may have contributed to his hypertension?
2. What precautions should the nurse take in measuring Mr. Marshall's weight and standing blood pressure? (*Hint:* Consider the drugs prescribed for Mr. Marshall.)
3. What life-threatening condition can occur from uncontrolled hypertension? What nursing observations would indicate this condition?
4. What items will Mr. Marshall need at the bedside other than those for personal hygiene? (*Hint:* Consider Mr. Marshall's life-style as well as the physician's orders for drug therapy.)
5. When should blood pressures be taken in relation to the drug therapy prescribed for Mr. Marshall?
6. How should the nurse respond to Mr. Marshall's request for bacon and real coffee?
7. What other members of the health team might help Mr. Marshall understand his therapy?
8. What changes of behavior should the nurse anticipate during Mr. Marshall's hospitalization for hypertension? (*Hint:* Consider drug therapy, diet, ambulation, and life-style.)
9. What changes in life-style will be needed if Mr. Marshall's hypertension is to remain controlled following hospitalization?
10. What patient teaching should the nurse anticipate that Mr. Marshall will need prior to discharge?

Case Study Involving Varicose Veins

Mrs. Swope, 44 years old, has four children. She is employed as a sales clerk in a local department store and is on her feet most of the day. Mrs. Swope visited her physician because of fatigue, pain, and swelling in both legs and ankles at the end of the day. The physician told Mrs. Swope that she had varicose veins and measured her for support stockings. The physician asked the nurse to arrange for Mrs. Swope's admission to the local hospital for bilateral vein stripping and ligation.

QUESTIONS

1. What factors in Mrs. Swope's life-style are associated with varicose veins? Which veins are most likely affected?
2. How should the nurse instruct Mrs. Swope to apply support stockings?
3. What activities should the nurse suggest to Mrs. Swope to reduce the pain, fatigue, and swelling associated with varicose veins?
4. What explanation about surgery and postoperative care should the nurse provide for Mrs. Swope prior to hospitalization?
5. What measures should the nurse take to prevent varicose veins in herself or himself?

Suggestions for Further Study

1. Why is it important to prevent a hip flexion contracture in the patient with a stroke?
2. What are the responsibilities of the licensed practical/vocational nurse in your agency in relation to the diagnostic tests mentioned in this chapter?
3. Excessive secretion of which hormone from the adrenal glands contributes to secondary hypertension?
4. How does ambulation help prevent hypostatic pneumonia?
5. Mason, Mildred A.; Bates, Grace F.; and Smola, Bonnie K.: *Workbook in Basic Medical-Surgical Nursing*, 3rd ed. Macmillan Publishing Company, New York, 1984, Exercise 12.

Additional Readings

Ahmed, Mary Cooke: "Op-Site for Decubitus Care." *American Journal of Nursing*, 82:61-64 (Jan.), 1982.

Allan, D.: "Treating Subarachnoid Hemorrhage Using Carotid Ligation." *Nursing Times*, 77:1383-85 (Aug.), 1981.

Allwood, Alinthia C., and Lundy, Carolyn: "Cerebral Artery Bypass Surgery." *American Journal of Nursing*, 80:1284-87 (July), 1980.

Baum, Patricia L.: "Abdominal Aortic Aneurysm? This Patient Takes AAA Care." *Nursing 82*, 12:34-41 (Dec.), 1982.

Blackburn, Donna, and Peterson, Linda K.: Deciphering Diagnostic Studies: Oculoplethysmography." *Nursing 82*, 12:76-78 (Oct.), 1982.

Bramoweth, Ellen: "Acute Aortic Dissection." *American Journal of Nursing*, 80:2010-11 (Nov.), 1980.

Chamberlain, Susan Lee: "Low-Dose Heparin Therapy." *American Journal of Nursing*, 80:1115-17 (June), 1980.

Craven, Ruth F., and Curry, Teri D.: "When the Diagnosis Is Raynaud's." *American Journal of Nursing*, 81:1007-1009 (May), 1981.

Dossey, Barbara, and Passons, Joanne Mary: "Pulmonary Embolism: Preventing It, Treating It." *Nursing 81*, 11:26-32 (Mar.), 1981.

Ekers, Mitzi Andrews: "EAB: A New Route for Vascular Rehabilitation." *Nursing 82*, 12:34-39 (Nov.), 1982.

Hale, Elizabeth: "Deep Vein Thrombosis: Tying the Knot—Venous Ligation." *Nursing Mirror*, 152:42-43 (Feb.), 1981.

Hartshorn, Jeanette Charles: "What to Do When the Patient's in Hypertensive Crisis." *Nursing 80*, 10:37-45 (July), 1980.

Hill, Martha N.: "What Can Go Wrong when You Measure Blood Pressure." *American Journal of Nursing*, 80:942-46 (May), 1980.

Jennings, Susan: "Back to Basics: Communicating with Your Aphasic Patients." *Journal of Practical Nursing*, 31:22-23 and 39 (Apr.), 1981.

Marcinek, Margaret Boyle: "Hypertension: What It Does to the Body." *American Journal of Nursing*, 80:928-32 (May), 1980.

Milem, Margaret M., and Chambers, Jeanette K.: "Decubitus Ulcers." *Journal of Practical Nursing*, 31:17-20 and 41 (May), 1981.

Monahan, Rita Short: "What a Patient Must Know to Control Hypertension." *Journal of Nursing Care*, 14:14-16 (July), 1981.

Moser, Marvin: "How Hypertension Therapy Works." *American Journal of Nursing*, 80:937-41 (May), 1980.

Norman, Susan: "Diagnostic Categories for the Patient with a Right Hemisphere Lesion." *American Journal of Nursing*, 79:2126-30 (Dec.), 1979.

Norman, Susan, and Baratz, Robin: "Understanding Aphasia." *American Journal of Nursing*, 79:2135-38 (Dec.), 1979.

Robinson, Corinne H.: *Basic Nutrition and Diet Therapy*, 4th ed. Macmillan Publishing Co., Inc., New York, 1980, pp. 243-52.

Schoof, Carolyn Sievers: "Hypertension: Common Questions Patients Ask." *American Journal of Nursing*, 80:926-27 (May), 1980.

Sohn, Catherine Angell; Tonnenbaum, Renee Plawner; Cantwell, Renee; and Rogers, Maureen Purcell: "Rescind the Risks in Administering Anticoagulants." *Nursing 81*, 11:34-41 (Oct.), 1981.

"Test Yourself: Cerebrovascular Accident." *American Journal of Nursing*, 81:548, 623 (Mar.), 1981.

Tilton, Colette, and Maloof, Malcom: "Diagnosing the Problems in Stroke." *American Journal of Nursing*, 82:596-601 (Apr.), 1982.

Wallhagen, Margaret Payne: "The Split Brain: Implications for Care and Rehabilitation." *American Journal of Nursing*, 79:2118-25 (Dec.), 1979.

Weinhouse, Iris: "Speaking to the Needs of Your Aphasic Patient." *Nursing 81*, 11:34-36 (Mar.), 1981.

Chapter 13

The Patient with a Disease of the Blood/Lymph*

Expected Behavioral Outcomes

Minimum objectives referred to as expected behavioral outcomes have been designed for the practical/vocational nursing student to use as guides in studying this chapter. The student should read these expected outcomes before studying the chapter. The objectives can be used as guides for study.

Using the content of this chapter, the student should return to the objectives and evaluate the ability to:

1. *Compare the charts of five patients or case histories provided by your instructor in relation to the laboratory findings with those discussed in the text.*

2. *Describe the nursing care indicated for each of the five patients with abnormal laboratory findings reviewed in objective No. 1.*

3. *Compare the nursing care of a patient with cancer to the nursing care of a patient with (a) Hodgkin's disease and (b) leukemia when provided a hypothetic situation.*

4. *Develop a nursing care plan for a patient with a disease of the blood or lymph, with special emphasis on the psychosocial aspects, when given a hypothetic situation.*

5. *Differentiate the nine conditions involving the blood and/or lymph according to red blood cell involvement, white blood cell involvement, bleeding tendencies, and diseases of the lymphatic system. Describe the problems common to all patients with these diseases of the blood and/or lymph.*

Vocabulary Development

The following prefixes, suffixes, and combining forms pertain to this chapter. By learning and/or reviewing their meanings, the practical/vocational nursing student will have the keys needed to unlock many exciting new medical terms.

*Revised by the authors and Gloria Rudibaugh, R.N., M.S., who is a Practical Nursing Instructor at the Central School of Practical Nursing in Norfolk, Virginia.

Discover the meaning of these keys in a medical dictionary or in the content of this chapter. How does each key pertain to this chapter? In your notebook write the correct meaning of each prefix, suffix, or combining form listed below. Illustrate each key with an example.

erythr—red. Ex. *erythro*cyte—red blood cell.

a-	ferr-
act-	haem(at)-
angi-	rhag-
cell-	sanguin-
erythr-	troph-

Structure and Function

Blood is the fluid that flows through the circulatory system. It has the vital task of carrying oxygen and food to all cells of the body. Also, it removes waste material from the cells.

PLASMA

The liquid portion of blood is known as *plasma*. Over one half of the total amount of blood is made of this straw-colored fluid. Body tissues receive waste, food, hormones, and immune substances from plasma. Plasma also contains *fibrinogen*, which is a substance necessary for the clotting of blood. If plasma is allowed to clot, the remaining fluid is called *serum*. It is the plasma without fibrinogen.

Water comprises about 91 to 92 percent of plasma. Plasma consists of 6 to 8 percent proteins. Albumin, the most abundant protein in plasma, is formed in the liver. Albumin helps to regulate the volume of plasma within blood vessels by pulling water from the interstitial fluid. It also binds with essential amino acids, fatty acids, minerals, and hormones to reduce loss of essential nutrients through the urinary system. When whole blood or plasma is not available, albumin may be given intravenously to increase the blood volume after hemorrhage. Fibrinogen, another protein, is made in the liver and, as stated earlier, is useful in the clotting process. The protein, prothrombin, also made in the liver, plays a part in the clotting process of blood.

Nutrients, such as carbohydrate in the form of glucose, amino acids, and lipids, are present in plasma. The nutrients are used by body tissues when needed.

Inorganic salts form about 0.9 percent of the plasma in the form of sodium, potassium, calcium, and magnesium. Iron, copper, iodine, and other elements are also found in plasma. The proper concentration and distribution of these salts are referred to as electrolyte balance. Small amounts of gases such as oxygen, carbon dioxide, and nitrogen are found in plasma. Waste products such as urea, uric acid, lactic acid, and creatinine are metabolic waste products carried to organs of excretion by the plasma.

Hormones from the endocrine glands are carried by the plasma to tissues in all parts of the body.

BLOOD CELLS

Three types of blood cells are found in plasma. Almost one half of the total amount of blood is composed of these cells. Blood cells are formed in the marrow of bones, in the lymph nodes, and in the spleen. The three kinds of cells are (1) red blood cells, which are known as *erythrocytes* or RBCs; (2) white blood cells, which are known as *leukocytes* or WBCs; and (3) platelets, which are known as *thrombocytes*.

RED BLOOD CELLS. Red blood cells, *erythrocytes*, carry oxygen to the body's cells, remove carbon dioxide from the cells, help to maintain normal acid-base balance, and contribute to the specific gravity of blood. Transportation of oxygen and removal of carbon dioxide are made possible by a substance in the erythrocytes called *hemoglobin*. This is the coloring matter of blood and contains oxygen. Since oxygen mixes readily with hemoglobin, it is the substance within the red blood cell that picks up oxygen as blood is pumped through the lungs. After delivering oxygen to the body's tissues, the red blood cells remove carbon dioxide.

Erythropoiesis, formation of red blood

cells, takes place in the red marrow of bone. In the adult, active red marrow is found in the ribs, the vertebrae, the cranial bones, and in the proximal end of the femur and the humerus. The erythrocyte undergoes several phases of development in the bone marrow before being released in the bloodstream. Vitamin B_{12} and an intrinsic factor produced by the mucosa of the stomach are two of the main substances necessary for red cells to mature normally. The intrinsic factor promotes absorption of vitamin B_{12} from food. Vitamin B_{12} is stored in the liver and released to the bone marrow to complete the development of the red blood cell. Folic acid, copper, iron, cobalt, pyridoxine, and protein are essential in the normal development of red blood cells. The mature erythrocyte enters the bloodstream with no nucleus and contains hemoglobin. After spending approximately 120 days in the bloodstream, the red blood cells disintegrate and most of the hemoglobin is reused in other red cells.

The normal red blood cell count ranges from 4½ to 5 million in 1 cu mm of blood. In other words, this is the average number of red blood cells that would be found in a drop of blood the size of a small pinhead. The count is slightly higher in men than in women. The normal amount of hemoglobin is approximately 15 gm per 100 ml of blood, or 80 to 100 percent. Normal values are listed in Table 13.1.

A study of the red cell formation, *erythropoiesis*, may include special examinations such as bone marrow aspiration, which will be discussed later in this chapter. An example of a laboratory test done for this purpose is a reticulocyte count. A *reticulocyte* is a young red blood cell. The patient with a reticulocyte count lower than the normal value of 0.5 to 2.5 percent probably has a slowing down in the process of erythropoiesis. An increase indicates an acceleration of the blood-forming process.

WHITE BLOOD CELLS.   White blood cells (leukocytes), play an important part in protecting the body against inflammation, by phagocytosis. Some white cells are formed in lymphatic tissue, and some are formed in the red marrow of bones. Leukocytes may be classified in a variety of ways, such as ori-

gin, structure of the cell, and reaction to staining dyes in the laboratory. The physician who requests a differential count is asking for information regarding the number of each type of white blood cell. Often this is a valuable aid in diagnosing the patient's illness, as the normal count of different white blood cells varies with certain diseases.

The normal white blood cell count ranges from 5000 to 10,000 in 1 cu mm of blood (tiny drop). The count increases in a patient with an infection. The patient has *leukocytosis* when the white blood cell count is higher than 10,000. When the count is under 5000, he has *leukopenia*.

The blood contains a variety of white blood cells. *Granulocytes* comprise 60 to 70 percent of the total number. *Agranulocytes* or *lymphocytes* make up 20 to 30 percent, and *monocytes* make up 5 to 8 percent of the total number. The granulocytes are formed in the bone marrow and have three main types—the neutrophils, eosinophils, and basophils. The neutrophils, or polymorphonuclear leukocytes, are important in combating infection because they ingest microorganisms. Eosinophils indicate functioning of the adrenal gland and are increased in certain allergic conditions. The basophils help in the healing process. The agranulocytes have two main types—the lymphocytes and the monocytes. Lymphocytes are formed in lymph nodes and the spleen and aid in protecting the body from inflammation. Monocytes are formed mainly in bone marrow. They help to engulf microorganisms and combat infection.

PLATELETS.   Platelets (thrombocytes) are minute particles in the blood and are formed in the red bone marrow. There are approximately 250,000 to 500,000 platelets per 1 cu mm of blood. They play an important part in stopping hemorrhage. Platelets collect in an injured area and give off a substance that is necessary for the clotting of blood. A decrease in the circulating number of platelets (*thrombocytopenia*) can cause bleeding. An increase in platelets is known as *thrombocytosis*, associated with certain disorders.

LYMPHATIC SYSTEM.   The lymphatic or lymph vascular system is a part of the circu-

TABLE 13.1
NORMAL VALUES OF LABORATORY TESTS FREQUENTLY DONE IN CONNECTION
WITH BLOOD STUDIES

TEST	NORMAL VALUE	CLINICAL IMPLICATIONS	
		Increase	*Decrease*
Bleeding time	3–10 minutes Duke method, 1–6 min Ivy method, 2–9.5 min	Thrombocytopenia Leukemia Aplastic anemia Platelet dysfunction	
Calcium	Total, 9.0–10.6 mg/dl Ionized, 4.2–5.2 mg/dl	Cancer Hyperparathyroidism Addison's disease	Hypoparathyroidism Chronic renal failure

Cholesterol	Total, 400–1000 mg/dl
	Cholesterol, 150–250
	  mg/dl
	Triglycerides, 40–150
	  mg/dl
	Phospholipids, 150–380
	  mg/dl
		Cardiovascular disease
		Hypothyroidism
		Uncontrolled diabetes
			Liver disease
			Malabsorption
			Anemia
			Hemolytic jaundice

Complete blood count in Tables 0.0 and 0.0			

Corpuscular values of
  erythrocytes MCH
  (mean cell hemo-
  globin)
	27–32 picograms	Macrocytic anemia	Iron-deficiency anemia

MCV (mean corpuscu-
  lar volume)
	87–103 cubic microns	Liver diseases
		Antimetabolite therapy
		Folate or Vitamin B_{12}
		  deficiency
			Iron-deficiency anemia
			Pernicious anemia
			Anemia of chronic blood
			  loss

MCHC (mean corpus-
  cular hemoglobin
  concentration)
	32–36 gm/100 ml		Iron-deficiency anemia
			Macrocytic anemia
			Hypochromic anemia

Platelet count	15,000–350,000/cu mm	Cancer
		Leukemia
		Splenectomy
		Iron-deficiency anemia
			Pernicious aplastic and
			  hemolytic anemias
			Cancer chemotherapy
			Thrombocytopenia pur-
			  pura

Folic acid	5.9–21.0 ng/ml		Folic acid antagonists Hemolytic anemia Megalobastic anemia Liver disease
Fragility test	Begins, 0.45–0.39 % Complete, 0.33–0.30 %		
Gastric analysis (see Table 0.0)			Gastric carcinoma Pernicious anemia

Heterophil agglutina-
  tion
	Negative	Negative titer of 1:56
		  suspicious
		Titer of 1:2224 is diag-
		  nostic of infectious
		  mononucleosis	

Partial thromboplas- tin time (PTT)	30–45 sec	Coagulation defects	Cancer Acute hemorrhage

Activated partial
  thromboplastin time
  (APTT)
	16–25 sec	Hemophilia
		Vitamin K deficiency
		Liver disease
		Circulating anticoagu-
		  lants	

TABLE 13.1 (*Continued*)
NORMAL VALUES OF LABORATORY TESTS FREQUENTLY DONE IN CONNECTION
WITH BLOOD STUDIES

TEST	NORMAL VALUE	CLINICAL IMPLICATIONS	
Protein electrophoresis	3.2–5.6 gm/100 ml		Malnutrition
			Hemorrhage
Erythrocyte sedimentation rate (ESR)	Westergren method	Collagen diseases	Sickle cell anemia
	Men: 0–15 mm/hr	Carcinoma	Polycythemia vera
	Women: 0–20 mm/hr	Infections	
Schilling test	Excretion of 8% or more of test dose of cobalt-tagged vitamin B_{12} in urine	Absence of intrinsic factor	
		Defective absorption of radioactive vitamin B_{12}	
Bilirubin icterus index	Total, 0.3–1.3 mg/dl	Hepatic or hemolytic causes	
		Hemolytic anemia	
Cold agglutinins	0–8	Hemolytic anemia	
		Leukemia	
		Malaria	
Coombs antiglobulin test	Negative	Transfusion reaction	Negative in nonautoimmune hemolytic anemia
		Autoimmune hemolytic anemia	
Human transferrin test (total ironbinding capacity)	250–450 mg/dl	Iron-deficiency anemia	Pernicious anemia
		Polycythemia	Sickle cell anemia
		Inadequate intake of iron	Chronic infection
Coagulation time (Lee-White clotting)	5–10 min	Marked hyperheparinemia	
Hemoglobin S (sickle cell test)	0		Positive in sickle cell disease and trait
Prothrombin time	11–16 sec or 100 %	Vitamin K deficiency	Circulating anticoagulants
			Hemophilia
			Thrombocytopenia
Reticulocyte count	0.5–1.5 % of total erythrocytes	Hemolytic anemias	Iron-deficiency anemia
		Sickle cell disease	Untreated pernicious anemia
		Leukemia	Radiation therapy
Urobilinogen	Urinary, 1–4 mg/24 hr	Hemolytic anemias	
	Fecal, 50–300 mg/24 hr	Hemolytic anemias	

latory system, consisting of lymph, interstitial or tissue fluid, lymphatics, and lymph nodes. The lymphatic system is the important link or connection between blood and tissue. The lymph vascular system functions in a supplementary manner with the capillaries and veins, returning tissue fluid to the bloodstream. *Lymph* is a clear, slightly yellow fluid derived from tissue fluids and found in lymphatic vessels. Interstitial fluid or tissue fluid is a clear liquid found in tissue spaces. The *lymphatics* are vessels similar to veins (see Figure 13.1). Lymph vessels begin as lymph capillaries in the tissue. Lymphatics are similar to veins in that their walls contain valves. However, the walls of the veins are thicker than those of lymphatics. The lymph vessels unite and form increasingly larger vessels until they unite to form two main channels: (1) the right lymphatic duct and (2) the thoracic duct. The right lymphatic duct receives lymph from the right arm, the right side of the head, and the upper right portion of the trunk. The contents of the right lymphatic duct are returned to the blood through the brachiocephalic vein.

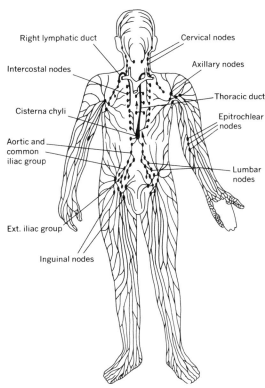

FIGURE 13.1 Lymphatic drainage of the body. (From Pansky, Ben: *Dynamic Anatomy and Physiology*. Macmillan Publishing Co., Inc., New York, 1975.)

The thoracic duct receives lymph from the remainder of the body and drains into the brachiocephalic vein.

Lymph nodes are small, rounded or bean-shaped bodies located along the course of lymphatics. The size of lymph nodes varies from that approximating a pinhead to that approximating the end of one's thumb. Lymph nodes serve as filters for the passing lymph and may combat pathogenic microorganisms draining from an infected part of the body. Lymph nodes may stop the passage of malignant cells to other body parts. Lymphocytes and antibodies are produced by the lymph nodes and added to the passing lymph.

SPLEEN. The spleen is the largest of the lymphatic organs and is located in the left upper quadrant of the abdomen. The spleen enlarges in diseases such as malaria, leukemia, Hodgkin's disease, certain anemias, and some infections.

The spleen is not essential for life despite its several functions. Large quantities of blood can be stored in the spleen and released when required by the body. The spleen is active in producing lymphocytes. It removes aged and damaged red blood cells and platelets from the blood stream. As blood passes through the spleen, microorganisms are destroyed by phagocytosis.

Diagnostic Studies

The blood of an individual suspected of having a blood dyscrasia is obtained from the veins (venipuncture) or from a prick in the end of the finger. Blood can be obtained from a prick of the earlobe. Blood for blood gases is obtained from arteries. The values obtained are then compared with normal values as an aid in diagnosis and treatment. Samples of the blood-forming organs may be obtained from red marrow of bones and lymph nodes.

Many blood studies will be done to diagnose blood disorders (Table 13.1). The tests will be used frequently both for diagnosis and to evaluate the patient's response to prescribed therapy. Having blood taken frequently, whether by venipuncture or finger puncture is unpleasant. Some patients actually believe that they may become anemic from having blood samples taken so frequently. The nurse needs to reassure the patient and explain the purpose of monitoring the blood closely. The nurse may offer encouragement and support to the patient while staying with the patient when the laboratory technician withdraws the blood. Those patients who have a bleeding tendency will appreciate the presence of the nurse who stays in attendance to apply pressure over the venipuncture site until bleeding stops. The nurse's reassurance and support can be a source of comfort to the patient.

SICKLING TESTS

The sickle turbidity tube test (SICKLE-DEX) is a blood test done to determine whether an individual has sickle hemoglobin. In this test, the patient's finger is pricked and the blood is mixed with SICKLE-DEX solution in a tube. Five minutes later, the mixture is observed for cloudiness. The presence of Hb S (sickled hemoglobin) causes the mixture to become cloudy. In the presence of normal hemoglobin, Hb A, the mixture remains clear. Although the test indicates the presence of Hb S, it does not differentiate between sickle cell anemia and sickle cell trait. The test is used frequently as a mass screening test for the detection of sickle cell hemoglobin.

The hemoglobin molecule contains an electrical charge, either positive or negative. This electrical charge of the normal hemoglobin is different from the charge of sickle hemoglobin. If a solution of hemoglobin is placed in an electric field, the hemoglobin molecules tend to move toward the positive or negative pole, depending on their charge. Sickle hemoglobin will move at a different rate from the normal hemoglobin.

If a person carries the sickle trait, blood cells contain both normal hemoglobin, which is known as hemoglobin A, and hemoglobin S. When the blood is electrophoresed, the hemoglobin will show movement typical of sickle cell trait. A person with sickle cell anemia has only sickle hemoglobin; therefore, the hemoglobin will show movement typical of hemoglobin S.

The red blood cell, which normally is round, assumes the shape of a crescent or sickle when the individual has either sickle cell anemia or sickle cell trait. The abnormal type of hemoglobin, hemoglobin S, in the red blood cell causes the erythrocyte to become sickle shaped when deprived of oxygen. The sickle cells are identified under a microscope following deoxygenation treatment of the blood sample.

COMPUTERIZED TOMOGRAPHY

Computerized tomography (CT scan) provides three-dimensional views of different body organs or structures. Total body scanning is helpful in diagnosing Hodgkin's disease and other lymphomas. The detection of abnormal lymph nodes aids the doctor in diagnosis. The advantages of this noninvasive study are that there is less risk to the

patient, and the need for invasive studies such as lymphangiography is decreased.

Although CT scanning is safe for the patient, it can be very frightening because of the complexity of the machine. No special preparation of the patient is necessary. If contrast media is to be given, food or fluids may be withheld for four to six hours prior to the scan because the dye can cause nausea. The patient is made comfortable in a supine position on a table. The patient is required to be very still during the procedure. A small beam of x-ray passes through the organs to be studied. A computer calculates the amount of x-ray absorbed by the various tissues and produces a printout of the information which is reproduced as photographs. The photographs show varying densities of the tissues. The machine rotates around the patient, and the procedure is repeated several times. The contrast media then may be given intravenously, and the complete procedure repeated again.

LYMPHOGRAPHY

X-ray visualization of the lymphatic system from the level of the second lumbar vertebra to the toes following injection of a radiopaque dye is a *lymphogram* (see Figure 13.2). A radiopaque dye injected into the webs of the first several toes makes visualization of the lymphatics possible. After having been located, the lymphatics are isolated surgically by the physician and injected with an appropriate radiopaque dye. This dye reaches the abdominal lymph nodes within a few hours and makes them visible on x-ray. The dye may remain in the nodes for months or years, which makes changes in their size, number, and shape visible by x-ray. Lymphography is helpful to the physician in diagnosing lymphoma and in determining the progress of Hodgkin's disease.

The radiopaque dye not remaining in the lymph nodes reaches the circulation by way of the thoracic duct. After reaching the bloodstream, the dye goes to the lungs. Respiratory symptoms such as cough, dyspnea, chest pain, and hemoptysis may develop. The patient also may have a fever, generalized aching, and malaise. The patient should be observed for such symptoms and have

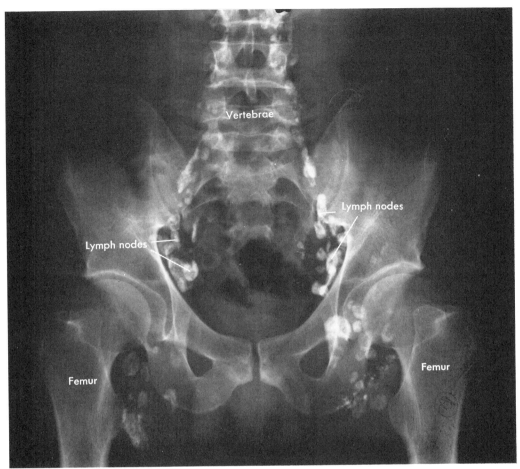

FIGURE 13.2 Lymphangiogram showing lymph nodes in iliac region. (Courtesy of Radiology Department, Eastern Virginia Medical School, Norfolk, Virginia.)

them reported promptly. Symptomatic nursing measures are indicated for this patient. For example, the individual with dyspnea should be placed in a comfortable position and have his restrictive clothing loosened. The room temperature should be comfortable for the patient and air should circulate freely without a draft.

ERYTHROCYTE FRAGILITY TEST

The erythrocyte fragility test is done on a sample of blood in the laboratory. The test measures the rate at which erythrocytes become fragile when placed in hypotonic solutions of saline. The solutions range from 0.85 percent saline to 0.30 percent. Normal values are: hemolysis begins at 0.45 to 0.39 percent saline solution and is completed at 0.33 to 0.30 percent solution. Capillary fragility increases, that is, cells burst at a higher than normal saline (0.9) concentration, in the congenital hemolytic anemias. It is normal in acquired hemolytic anemias.

CAPILLARY FRAGILITY TEST

This test is done to determine how easily capillaries may rupture. The test is performed by the physician. A blood pressure cuff is wrapped around the arm and inflated to cause venous stasis for no longer than five minutes. In some blood diseases, capillary fragility is increased, leading to hemorrhagic spots (petechiae) under the skin. Normally, only one or two petechiae per 6.25 cm (square inch) are noted. If the patient's capillaries are abnormally fragile, there may be additional petechiae. The patient should be told to expect hemorrhagic spots to appear following the test.

ASPIRATION OF BONE MARROW

Bone marrow is obtained in the adult from the sternum, the iliac crest, or the spinous process of the vertebrae. Remembering that many of the blood cells are manufactured in the red marrow of bone will enable the nurse to relate the importance of this test to proper diagnosis.

The physician and nurse should explain the procedure to the patient and provide appropriate explanations as the procedure progresses. The nurse should assist the patient in assuming a comfortable position. The physician selects the site of aspiration, cleanses the area with an antiseptic solution, and drapes the area with sterile towels. A local anesthetic such as lidocaine is injected into the skin at the site of aspiration. After inserting the large aspirating needle in the marrow, the physician aspirates a small amount of blood and marrow.

The patient usually experiences a feeling of pressure when the needle is inserted into the marrow cavity. The patient may also have a sensation of aching at the site of aspiration for a day or two. Specimens should be labeled according to hospital or clinic procedure and sent to the laboratory. A small sterile dressing is placed over the operative site.

LYMPH NODE BIOPSY

Biopsy of the lymph node enables the pathologist to examine the tissues of the lymph node as a basis for possible diagnosis of leukemia or Hodgkin's disease. A lymph node biopsy may enable the physician to identify the typical cell of Hodgkin's disease known as the Reed-Sternberg cell.

One of three methods may be used to obtain a biopsy. Needle aspiration and incisional or excisional biopsy can be done. The excisional biopsy is used most commonly. The whole lymph node is removed and sent

to the laboratory for examination. Lymph node biopsy is usually for cervical, supraclavicular, or axillary lymph node sites.

The patient scheduled for a lymph node biopsy is prepared for surgery in the same manner that one is prepared for other surgical procedures. For example, the patient is given nothing by mouth prior to surgery and usually is given a sedative. In some cases, it may be necessary to biopsy more than one node before a positive diagnosis can be made. A small sterile dressing is placed over the operative site as in other surgical procedures.

The patient is observed for signs of bleeding and infection at the site. The nurse observes for changes in blood pressure, pulse, and respiration until these vital signs have been stabilized.

BLOOD GROUPING

The blood of human beings can be classified in one of four basic blood groups or types. A blood group refers to the type of antigen, a substance that induces the formation of antibodies, or isoagglutinins on an individual's red blood cells. Group A has antigen A on the red cells, group B has antigen B on the red cells, and group AB contains both antigen A and B on the red blood cells. Group O contains neither antigen A nor antigen B on the red cells. The blood serum never contains antibodies against the antigens present on its own red blood cells. Antibodies are agglutinins. *Agglutinins* are chemicals that agglutinate cells or cause them to clump together, thus destroying the red blood cells. In group A blood, antigen A is present on the red cells; therefore, its serum does not contain antigen A antibodies but it does contain anti-B antibodies. In group B, antigen B is present on the red cells; therefore, its serum contains no anti-B antibodies but it does contain anti-A antibodies. In group AB blood, antigens A and B are present on its red cells but the serum contains neither anti-A nor anti-B antibodies. Blood group O contains neither antigen A nor antigen B on its red cells but it does have both anti-A and anti-B antibodies in the serum. As stated in the discussion of nursing care, blood transfusion reactions occur when antibodies present in the serum of the person receiving a transfusion agglutinate and destroy the red blood cells being administered. The clumped cells can cause death in the person receiving the transfusion. For example, if group B blood were administered to a person who had group A blood, the recipient's serum would contain anti-B antibodies and an antigen-antibody reaction would occur. In other words, the red blood cells would agglutinate or clump. Likewise, if group A blood were administered to a person with group B blood, the recipient's serum would contain anti-A antibodies and agglutination of the donor cells would occur. Group O blood is referred to as the universal donor since its red cells contain neither antigen A nor antigen B. Group O blood can be administered to a person with blood of group O, group A, group B, and group AB. Group O blood contains no antigens that can react with the antibodies present in the serum of the remaining blood group.

The universal recipient is one who has group AB because the serum contains neither anti-A nor anti-B antibodies to react with antigens. However, group AB blood donors can give blood only to persons with group AB blood.

Because all persons do not react as expected when receiving a blood transfusion, they must have their blood crossmatched with possible donor blood before it is administered. In crossmatching blood, the red blood cells of donors are exposed to the serum of the recipient and the red cells of the recipient are exposed to the serum of the donor.

Many different agglutinins exist in the blood. The Rh system ranks second to the ABO system in clinical significance. In the United States approximately 80 percent of the white population and 90 percent of the black population possess the Rh antigen and are classified as Rh positive. Those individuals without this antigen are said to be Rh negative. Rh blood group factors are inherited. For practical purposes, all antibodies against the Rh blood group factors result either from incompatible transfusions or from pregnancies. For example, if an Rh-negative individual should receive Rh-positive blood,

he or she will receive the antigen into the blood and become sensitized. After receiving another transfusion of Rh-positive blood, such a person will suffer from an antigen-antibody reaction or agglutination of red cells.

Another way an Rh-negative individual can build up antibodies occurs during pregnancy. If the woman is Rh negative and the father is Rh positive and the fetus is Rh positive, the mother's Rh-negative blood becomes sensitized just as it would if she had received a transfusion of Rh-positive blood. There may be no problems with the first pregnancy, but subsequent pregnancies may increase the number of Rh antibodies circulating in the mother's blood, which may seriously affect the fetus. The condition that occurs when this happens is called erythroblastosis fetalis.

PHERESIS

Blood component transfusions, such as transfusions of leukocytes, platelets, or plasma, have added years to the life of patients of all ages who are stricken by leukemia, cancer, or aplastic anemia and other potentially fatal diseases of the blood. A process called pheresis has been developed to help in the collection of these components which are so crucial to the treatment of these patients.

During the pheresis donation, blood is withdrawn from one arm and passed through a cell-separating machine which can selectively withdraw specific components from the blood. The remaining components, such as the red blood cells and plasma, are returned to the donor through the other arm. The process takes two to three hours but at no time is there more than one unit of blood outside of the donor's body. The body replaces the components within 24 hours.

The advantage of a pheresis donation rather than a whole blood donation is that while a pint of whole blood has enough red cells for a single transfusion, it contains less than an ounce of platelets and a very small portion of white cells. It would take the platelets from six to eight whole blood donations to equal a single donor, platelet-pheresis product. White cells are more difficult to remove from a whole blood donation. Dozens of whole blood donations would be needed to help one patient.

A single donor can give the needed white cells, plasma, or platelets in large enough quantities to help a patient. The donor can give more frequently than every 56 days, the length of time one should wait when donating whole blood.

Just as red blood cells have different ABO and Rh blood types, so white cells and platelets have differences. This white cell and platelet typing is called human leukocyte antigen typing or HLA typing. There are thousands of different combinations of the types, and to find a perfect match can be very difficult. It is sometimes necessary to match tissue. After receiving many transfusions of platelets, for example, some patients become resistant and no longer can make use of these platelets. This is when one must use matched products. The platelets should be of the same type so that they can work effectively and stop the bleeding. Donors who have agreed to participate in the HLA matching program may be called frequently if their cells match those of a patient undergoing intensive treatment. However, at all times, donations are completely voluntary.

BONE MARROW TRANSPLANTATION

Bone marrow transplantation is being used in some medical centers to treat select patients who have aplastic anemia or acute leukemia. Transplants between identical twins are usually always successful as well as sibling transplants. At one time, only identical twins were considered for the procedure. The basic requirement for bone marrow transplantation is the identical match of the blood type and the transplantation antigen. If the donor and the patient are not identical in HLA (transplantation antigen or tissue typing), the patient will need to undergo treatment for immunosuppression so that the graft will take.

After compatibility is determined, the donor must meet all physical examination requirements also, such as being free of infection. The donor is admitted to the hospital. The bone marrow aspiration is done in the operating room. Approximately 500 to 700 ml of marrow is withdrawn from various sites on the pelvic bone. The donor is observed for bleeding from the sites of aspiration. Analgesics for pain are prescribed. Preparation of the recipient for bone marrow transplantation will be given under the discussion of treatment of the aplastic anemia and acute leukemia patients.

Nursing Observations

Blood is a body fluid that nourishes our body cells and tissues and relieves them of their waste products. The blood carries substances that help to protect the body from microorganisms and to help stop bleeding after injury to blood vessels. Blood diseases, therefore, can affect any organ of the body. The three problems that are common to blood diseases are lack of oxygen to the tissues, susceptibility to infection, and hemorrhage. Many symptoms result from these three basic problems. The nurse observes the patient closely for any of the following symptoms and plans nursing care accordingly.

HEADACHE, DIZZINESS, VISUAL DISTURBANCES, SYNCOPE

Insufficient blood supply, hence, insufficient oxygen to tissue cells is common among persons who have severe anemia. Hypoxia of brain tissue may cause the person to have a headache and feel dizzy or lightheaded. This may predispose the patient to falls or make any accident more likely to occur. The person may have syncope and fall, striking the head or fracturing a long bone. Visual disturbances may result from insufficient blood supply also, due to a low red blood cell count, a low hemoglobin, and lack of oxygen to the brain tissue. For patients with these symptoms, the nurse must be in close attendance to the patient if the patient is out of bed for any reason. The bedrails should remain up and the bed in the low position while the patient is in bed.

SKIN COLOR

Insufficient blood supply to tissues may cause the patient's skin color to be very pale.

In severe cases of anemia, the patient may exhibit cyanosis. Pallor in black patients may be assessed by observing the mucous membranes of the conjunctiva or the buccal mucosa.

In blood diseases where hemolysis or excessive obstruction of red blood cells may occur, such as in sickle cell anemia or malaria, jaundice of the skin and sclera of the eye may be evident. When erythrocytes rupture, bilirubin is released from the blood cell into the bloodstream causing skin tissues to become yellow. Itching of the skin may also occur, which causes the patient to be very uncomfortable. A low platelet count is common in some blood diseases. When the platelet count or thrombocytes are low, ecchymosis, purpura, or petechiae may occur. Platelets or thrombocytes are important in the blood-clotting process after injury to blood vessels. Ecchymosis is caused by bleeding into skin or mucous membranes and appears in a large, irregularly formed hemorrhagic area. At first, it is blue-black in color, resolving to a greenish-brown or yellow color. Ecchymosis may be caused by trauma when the platelet count is normal. Purpura is manifested by large areas of bleeding into the skin and mucous membranes, internal organs, and other tissues. The hemorrhage appears red, darkening into purple then brownish-yellow. Thrombocytopenia, a hemorrhagic disorder, is often the cause of purpura. Petechiae are very small, purplish, hemorrhagic spots on the skin due to a blood clotting abnormality. Petechiae may be observed in leukemia patients. The nurse observes, charts, and reports the findings of skin abnormalities.

BREATH—FETID ODOR RELATED TO BLEEDING AND/OR MOUTH BREATHING

Some patients with blood diseases may have an offensive mouth odor because of a bleeding disorder or mouth breathing. Ulcerations on the gums and mucous membranes of the mouth may occur from the use of chemotherapeutic drugs. Bleeding from the ulcerations causes the patient to have a bad taste in the mouth and produces an odor. Patients who are receiving oxygen may have dry mucous membranes of the mouth as well as those patients who are mouth-breathers. The nurse should observe the mouth closely.

DYSPNEA

Insufficient blood supply or a reduced number of circulating erythrocytes and a low hemoglobin may cause a patient to have dyspnea with or without exertion. This condition occurs because the oxygen-carrying capacity of the blood has been reduced. The nurse will observe that the respiratory rate is increased. The extent of breathing difficulty of course, should be observed, charted, and reported.

CHILLS AND FEVER

The patient may have a chill which is characterized by shivering and a feeling of coldness. The increased muscular activity raises body temperature. The nurse should observe and report the time the chill started, its severity, and the ending time. The patient's temperature should be taken 20 to 30 minutes after the chill has ended. The patient can be expected to have an elevated body temperature following a chill. However, a fever can occur without a chill.

PAIN

The patients with blood disorders may experience different kinds of pain. For example, the patient with a hemolytic anemia may experience abdominal pain because of an enlarged spleen. The patient with Hodgkin's disease may experience pain wherever an enlarged lymph node presses against surrounding structures or tissues. The patient with leukemia may suffer skeletal pain. Or the patients who have sickle cell anemia or hemophilia may suffer from joint pain and deformities from bleeding into joints. The nurse should observe the patient closely for signs of pain and discomfort.

FATIGUE

Fatigue is common in patients who have blood disorders when the red blood cell count is low or when the hemoglobin is low. The nurse may observe that the patient is so fatigued that he does not feel like getting out of bed or bathing.

Fatigue may be discouraging to the patient and it may be perceived by the patient as being too minor to bother discussing with the physician. The individual should be encouraged to discuss this and other symptoms with the doctor.

GASTROINTESTINAL SYMPTOMS

Some patients with blood disorders may experience anorexia, nausea, or vomiting. Patients with pernicious anemia also may suffer from indigestion and bloating as a result of lack of free hydrochloric acid in the stomach and lack of functioning of certain cells of the gastric mucosa.

PARESTHESIAS

Paresthesias of extremities may occur in patients with pernicious anemia and other anemias. Because of insufficient nourishment of tissues and nerves, patients may complain of a "pins and needles" sensation of the extremities. With appropriate drug therapy, the symptom usually subsides.

INSPECTION OF URINE AND STOOL FOR BLEEDING

Bleeding from any body orifice is common in patients with blood diseases. The nurse should be especially alert for bleeding from the gastrointestinal tract. Stools should be examined for evidence of fresh bleeding or for tarry color. The tarry appearance is characteristic of bleeding high in the intestinal tract. Stools for occult (hidden) blood are often ordered.

Urine should be observed for blood also. It may not be evident; but, microscopic blood in the urine may be diagnosed in the laboratory. Bright blood in urine is very noticeable but smoky-colored urine, caused by lesser amounts of blood, may not be noticed as readily. The nurse needs to observe the patient closely for these symptoms.

SIGNS OF LOCAL AND/OR SYSTEMIC INFECTION

Patients with diseases involving the white blood cells, such as leukemia, are especially prone to local and systemic infections. When the leukocytes are immature and ineffective in fighting infections, the patient is more likely to develop infections. Also, drugs used in the treatment of other cancers may cause leukopenia and greater susceptibility to systemic infection.

BEHAVIORAL CHANGES

Patients with blood diseases often have psychologic problems. Because their disease conditions are chronic and sometimes fatal, they often become anxious or depressed. They frequently suffer from pain and other discomforts common to their illness. The nurse should observe patients for any change in behavior and report findings to the physician.

Nursing Interventions

GENERAL HYGIENE WITH ORAL CARE

The patient with a disease of the blood or abnormal blood condition has a blood dyscrasia. Patients who have abnormal conditions of the blood share many common problems and require common nursing interventions.

There is a need for good general hygiene to be provided for all patients with blood disorders. Since resistance to local and systemic infection is lowered, good hygienic measures will help to reduce the incidence of infection. The patient who is fatigued and dyspneic may need to be bathed by the nurse to conserve energy or strength. Lanolin lotions or creams may be applied to dry skin. Backrubs to help stimulate circulation to the skin may help to prevent skin breakdown of patients who are bedridden and prone to decubiti. Frequent linen changes are required for the patient who is prone to fever and chills.

Mouth care is an important aspect of nursing care for the patient with a blood disease. The patient's lips, gums, and other parts of the mouth may tend to bleed easily and should be a prime consideration for the nurse. Cleaning the patient's teeth and mouth in a nonirritating manner presents a major nursing challenge. Prevention of further bleeding with gentleness is extremely important. The nurse should swab the patient's teeth and gums with soft cotton applicators. Nonirritating mouthwash can be used on the applicator. The teeth may be cleaned with gauze wrapped around the nurse's fingertips. Several tongue depressors can be placed between the patient's upper and lower teeth to prevent the closing of teeth on the nurse's fingers. A weak solution of hydrogen peroxide, alkaline mouthwash, or water may be used to soften crusts of blood and exudate in the mouth. Mouth care should be given both before and after meals. A nonirritating cream or petrolatum can be applied to the patient's lips and nose for further comfort and protection. Irritating foods and beverages should be avoided.

REST AND POSITIONING

Rest is necessary for lowering the oxygen requirements of patients with blood disorders. Mildly anemic patients are seldom hospitalized, but they should be advised to rest periodically throughout the day or to take naps occasionally. Patients with severe anemia usually are hospitalized and will be placed on bed rest until their red blood cell count and hemoglobin increase. The nurse may need to provide complete care for these patients until they feel like having increased activity. Patients who are dyspneic may need to have the head of the bed elevated to facilitate breathing and allow for better aeration of lung tissue. Other nursing measures include placing the patient in a comfortable position, loosening restricting clothing, and providing adequate ventilation. The nurse should remember that a person with dyspnea frequently finds irritating and unpleasant odors that may otherwise be pleasant. The person may later remark that the nurse's cologne caused a feeling of suffocation. Thus, the presence of odors on the nurse or in the area should be avoided. Nursing care should be planned to minimize the fatigue and to conserve the patient's strength.

If the ambulatory patient experiences dizziness, or lightheadedness, the nurse should have the patient lie flat for a few minutes so that circulation of blood and oxygen to the brain is increased. The symptoms should be relieved within a few minutes after which the patient may sit up slowly.

Frequent turning of the severely anemic patient is necessary to prevent skin breakdown. The tissues are lacking in blood supply and oxygenation, therefore, are more susceptible to pressure sores. Other measures include backrubs and massages to stimulate circulation and the use of devices on the bed to help reduce pressure. Such devices include a sponge rubber pad over the mattress, alternating pressure mattress, flotation pad, and lamb's wool pads.

Providing quietness, reducing the glare from strong lights, decreasing the number of interruptions, and other measures conducive to rest should be utilized. Sleep should be encouraged.

OXYGEN THERAPY

Oxygen may be ordered for severely anemic patients. They need oxygen because their blood is greatly reduced in the capacity to carry oxygen since erythrocytes and hemoglobin are low. The administration of oxygen helps to prevent tissue hypoxia. Oxygen also reduces the work load of the heart as it has been beating faster in order to supply the tissues with an adequate amount of blood and oxygen.

ALTERATIONS IN FLUIDS AND DIET

The dietary intake of the anemic patient should be high in protein, iron, and vitamins such as B_{12}. These substances are essential for the formation of normal erythrocytes. Oftentimes, anemic patients are anorexic, or they may feel too fatigued to feed themselves. Some patients may not want to eat because of ulcerations in the mouth caused by chemotherapy. So that patients will receive as much good nutrition as possible, the nurse should serve six small, easily digested meals a day rather than three. The food should be served attractively after providing mouth care for the patient. The nurse should feed those patients who are too fatigued to feed themselves. A nutritious diet may help to decrease fatigue.

The patient with a blood disease who has frequent chills and fever is losing an increased amount of body fluid through an increased respiratory rate, perspiration, and voiding. This increases the importance of providing an increased intake of fluids for the patient. Fluids high in calories, protein, salt, and potassium should be given to meet the body's increased metabolic and electrolyte needs. The intake and output of fluids should be measured and recorded. If an output of less than 1000 ml in a period of 24 hours is noticed, this should be reported to the charge nurse.

ASSISTING THE PATIENT WITH FEVER

Commonly, patients with malaria or leukemia will have chills and fever. An antipyretic such as acetominophen (TYLENOL) may be administered. While the patient is chilling, blankets should be applied for comfort. The patient may have a warm beverage, if desired and not contraindicated. The nurse should observe and report the time the chill started, its severity, and the ending time. The patient's temperature should be taken 20 to 30 minutes after the chill has ended.

After the patient's chill has ended the extra blankets should be removed. Leaving additional clothing on the patient after the shivering and chilly sensation have ceased will cause excessive perspiration, which can result in a serious loss of sodium and water, especially in an infant or a small child.

A tepid water bath may be indicated if the patient's temperature exceeds 39.5°C (103.1°F). An ice cap generally is placed on the patient's head when fever is extremely high. The patient's temperature, pulse, and respiration should be checked before giving the cooling bath and applying the ice cap, and again 30 minutes after the treatment is ended. After having a high or prolonged fever, the patient can be expected to feel weak, perspire with exertion, and tire easily. These factors must be given careful consideration in planning the nursing care for this patient as the patient is already subject to fatigue. The patient will need additional rest. A diet with an increased amount of protein and calories may be prescribed. An increased fluid intake should be encouraged.

MANAGEMENT OF PAIN AND DISCOMFORT

The patient who has pain will have analgesics prescribed to help provide comfort. The administration of an antipyretic may keep a patient from suffering the effects of fever and chills. Warm clothing and blankets help the anemic patient feel more comfortable. However, hot water bottles or electric heating pads should not be used to help provide warmth. Because their circulation is poor, anemic patients could burn easily. They may not feel a burning sensation since their skin is poorly supplied with blood and oxygen.

The patient should be protected from injury that may cause or increase bleeding. If the patient is disoriented, siderails should be provided. Fingernails should be short to prevent scratching and possible bleeding. Soap should be used sparingly. Emollient lotions used on the skin will help to soothe and make the patient more comfortable. Intramuscular injections are avoided because of the possibility of bleeding into the muscle. The patient's gown or pajamas should be loose and not restricting or irritating. A bed cradle may be used to keep the pressure of bedding off the patient's extremities.

PREVENTION OF INFECTION

Patients with blood disorders should be protected from infection. Patients who are severely anemic are fatigued and debilitated. Their body defenses are low, and they can develop infections easily. Nurses who have a cold or sore throat should not care for these patients. Visitors or other health care workers who have colds should not come into contact with these patients.

Patients who are receiving chemotherapy and have a severe leukopenia may be placed in reverse isolation. Personnel and visitors are required to wear a gown and mask when entering the patient's room so that organisms will not be introduced to the patient. Strict handwashing is necessary to prevent cross-contamination.

ASSISTING WITH TRANSFUSION THERAPY

Whole blood or such blood components as packed red blood cells, frozen red blood cells, platelet concentrates, fresh or fresh frozen plasma, and other plasma products frequently are administered. Hospitals have policies and regulations governing the collection, labeling, transportation, and administration of blood or blood products. Administration of the wrong blood can cause death. Meticulous attention to detail in following the procedure of the hospital is essential to prevent the patient from receiving the wrong blood.

Symptoms of a transfusion reaction usually occur during the infusion of the first 50 to 100 ml of blood. If the transfusion is stopped at the first sign of an untoward symptom, a fatal reaction may be prevented. For this reason, it is advisable for the nurse to stay with the patient for at least 15 minutes after the blood transfusion has been started. The nurse must check frequently to see if the blood is flowing properly and at the prescribed rate.

The patient known to have allergic reactions may have a prophylactic dose of an antihistamine drug such as diphenhydramine (BENADRYL) prescribed. The nurse should observe the patient for such untoward reactions as a sudden onset of fever, chills, itching, erythema, urticaria, nausea, and vomiting. Feelings such as fullness in the head, chilliness, burning of the face, pain in the chest, pain in the back or flank, and symptoms of shock may occur. Bacterial contamination of donor blood can result in the patient having a high fever, flushing, headache, or vomiting. In the event the patient has any of these symptoms, the nurse should stop the transfusion immediately and notify the physician.

The patient's vital signs should be monitored carefully for as long as indicated. Following a transfusion reaction, the nurse can be expected to obtain a specimen of the first voided urine after the reaction and send it to the blood bank for analysis. The remainder of the donor blood should be returned to the blood bank. Generally, a blood culture of the recipient is done following such a reaction. Analysis of the blood can detect incompatibility or bacterial contamination. The urine is analyzed for hemoglobin, which indicates hemolysis of red blood cells. Blood incompatibility results in an antigen-antibody reaction, causing hemolysis of the donor red blood cells.

Administration of an excessive amount of blood or at a rate faster than the heart can accept can result in circulatory overloading.

The nurse must observe the patient receiving a transfusion for symptoms such as distended neck veins, dyspnea, cough, and rales. When observing any of these symptoms, the nurse should immediately stop the flow of blood and contact the charge nurse or physician for further instructions.

In addition to the immediate reaction to a blood transfusion, the patient may develop certain diseases. Although the incidence of transmission of disease by transfusion generally is not high, the possibility does exist. Such diseases as viral hepatitis and malaria are two examples.   AIDS

USING THE THERAPEUTIC RELATIONSHIP TO ASSIST WITH CONCERNS

An individual with a blood dyscrasia generally has long-term therapy combined with an uncertain diagnosis in some cases. These two factors tend to increase the anxiety of the patient and family. When the individual is faced with a chronic illness and a frightening diagnosis, much unnecessary money and time may be spent in searching for other more favorable opinions and hoping to escape the dreaded truth. Patients may fear the necessity of changing their life-styles, losing their jobs, becoming dependent, being abandoned, and possible death. Patients' reactions, of course, will depend on their personal viewpoints, their past experiences, the manner in which they perceive themselves, their relationships with others, the nature of their illness, the extent of their symptoms, and their prognosis.

Individuals may use a variety of coping mechanisms such as denial, anger, bargaining, depression, and acceptance. They may use a combination of these reactions, and they may use them in various sequences. The nurse must allow patients the use of these mechanisms while they are adjusting to their disease. However, the nurse must maintain a positive and realistic attitude toward patients and their conditions. In helping patients and their families to adjust to a given disease, the nurse should be well informed about the disease condition. The nurse can answer the patients' questions or seek the answers from a reliable source. As stated earlier, the nurse should allow patients to use the coping mechanisms most helpful to them during their period of adjustment. The nurse has to be a good listener in order to enable patients to verbalize their feelings, fears, and concerns. At times, feelings of anger and/or hostility appear to be directed toward the nurse from patients or their families. Such feelings should not be taken as personal. The nurse must be aware of the resources available to provide support to patients, such as the hospital chaplain, voluntary organizations concerned with the disease that is affecting the patient, and other community agencies.

The emotional drain on the nurse who supports individuals with blood dyscrasias can be taxing. The nurse can become susceptible to the same feelings that patients experience. For example, helplessness, frustration, anger, and sadness may be experienced by the nurse. The nurse may need to seek help from peers in order to deal more effectively with personal feelings. Clinical conferences and inservice programs can be beneficial to the nurse. They can enable the nurse to put into proper perspective an acceptable attitude toward patients, their illness, their attitudes, and their needs. The nurse may find it helpful to seek assistance from associates in the form of suggestions for providing the quality of emotional support most needed by the individuals and their families.

PATIENT AND FAMILY TEACHING

The nurse can help the patient and family by listening to them as they express their concerns about a chronic disease condition and how they are to deal with it. The nurse can give attention and care to the patient as needed and explain to the patient and family the rationale for the care being given. The nurse should explain to them the reasons why the patient should continue to take prescribed medication and remain under the care of the physician, even though the patient improves and feels better. The condition is probably chronic. Although not curable, the patient can be treated to the extent that symptoms will be fewer and the patient will be more comfortable for a longer period of time if treatment is maintained. The nurse may assist the family in planning the care of the patient at home. For example, the nurse may have the dietitian talk to the patient and family about specific dietary concerns. The nurse may explain the use of medications that are prescribed and the side effects that may be expected from the drugs. The nurse can explain the importance of rest and pacing of activities so that the patient does not become overtired. The patient needs to understand the importance of avoiding infections and that the physician should be contacted whenever necessary.

ANEMIAS

Description

Anemia means a decrease in the number of red blood cells or in the amount of hemoglobin. Usually both are reduced.

An individual develops anemia when (1) there is an impaired production of erythrocytes, (2) red blood cells are destroyed faster than they can be produced, and (3) there is a loss of blood. Failure of the bone marrow to produce sufficient numbers of red blood cells may be caused by a congenital defect or by an injury to the marrow. In the absence of any blood-forming activity, the bone marrow is said to be aplastic. Bone marrow showing evidence of less-than-normal activity is hypoplastic. An inadequate production of red blood cells occurs when the body has an insufficient amount of the substances necessary for blood formation. Vitamin B_{12} and folic acid are necessary for the production of erythrocytes.

A diet deficient in meat and green, leafy vegetables which supply folic acid, iron, and protein can lead to anemia. Poor absorption of vitamin B_{12} and folic acid from the gastrointestinal tract can also lead to anemia. An example of anemia due to increased destruction of red blood cells is seen in the individual with sickle cell anemia. Infections such as malaria also cause a destruction of red cells. Anemia can result from a loss of blood following a large hemorrhage. The loss of small amounts of blood over a period of time can produce anemia also. chronic

Anemia may be classified according to etiology, as described in the preceding paragraph. Morphology, which refers to the size and shape of cells, is another means of classifying anemia. The classification of anemia based on morphology includes (1) macrocytic, (2) normocytic, (3) microcytic, and (4) hypochromic. In *macrocytic* anemia, the patient has abnormally large red blood cells. The patient with *normocytic* anemia has erythrocytes that are normal in size but their number is decreased by such conditions as hemorrhage and conditions affecting the production of an adequate number. *Microcytic* anemia is characterized by an unusually small red blood cell that has normal color. The term *hypochromic* is used to indicate that the erythrocytes have less color than normal.

Anemias Caused by Impaired Production of Erythrocytes

APLASTIC ANEMIA

DESCRIPTION. Aplastic anemia is caused by failure of the bone marrow to manufacture blood cells in adequate numbers. Bone marrow may fail to produce blood cells in the terminal stage of leukemia or as a result of metastasis of cancer from other parts of the body. Chemicals and other agents also may produce aplastic anemia. For example, benzene, anticarcinogenic drugs, anticonvulsants such as mephenytoin (MESANTOIN), certain insecticides, thiazide diuretics, gold, and phenylbutazone (BUTAZOLIDIN) can produce aplastic anemia.

Before prescribing a drug known to produce aplastic anemia, the physician will weigh the risk of adverse effects with the beneficial effects to the patient. For example, the risk of adverse effects from an anticarcinogenic agent may be less than the risk of advancing carcinoma.

COMMON DIAGNOSTIC STUDIES. Many blood studies will be done in the laboratory. A bone marrow aspiration procedure will be done. The patient's symptoms and a careful history of possible exposure to chemicals or other agents that may have been toxic to the bone marrow will be taken. The patient with aplastic anemia will have leukopenia, thrombocytopenia, and a decrease in the formation of red blood cells.

NURSING OBSERVATIONS. The nurse should observe the patient for fatigue, weakness, dyspnea on exertion, lowered resistance to infection, and a bleeding tendency. The patient will appear pale and may complain of anorexia, headache, fever, and bleeding of mucous membranes of the mouth or nose.

COMMON TREATMENT PLANS AND NURSING INTERVENTIONS. Treatment of the individual with aplastic anemia is directed toward removing the causative agent if it is known and possible to do so. Transfusions of red blood cells, platelets, and white blood cells are given as necessary. Bone marrow transplantation is being used in some medical centers. In preparation for the transplant, the patient is given cyclophosphamide (CYTOXAN) to destroy immunity to antigens. The patient must be protected from all sources of infection until the bone marrow transplant takes, which is approximately 10 to 20 days. Protective isolation is necessary to maintain a germ-free environment. The bone marrow is administered intravenously within four hours after being withdrawn from the donor. The new marrow goes to the bone marrow from the bloodstream. The patient is observed for signs of circulatory overload such as distended neck veins or shortness of breath. The patient is also observed for pulmonary emboli. Survival of the patient after bone marrow transplantation may depend on whether or not the bone marrow takes and whether the patient can be protected from infection.

IRON-DEFICIENCY ANEMIA

DESCRIPTION. Iron-deficiency anemia is the most common type of anemia. The erythrocyte count and the hemoglobin are both reduced, with the latter being more reduced. The cause of this deficiency is the failure of the patient to ingest or absorb a sufficient amount of dietary iron needed by the body. Iron deficits can occur due to menstrual bleeding, pregnancy and postpartum bleeding, faulty diet during childhood or adolescence, gastrointestinal disorder leading to malabsorption, and recent or past blood loss.

COMMON DIAGNOSTIC STUDIES. Laboratory tests confirm a decrease in erythrocytes, hematocrit, and hemoglobin. The erythrocytes are microcytic-hypochromic. Iron stores are decreased. X-rays of the gastrointestinal tract and stools for occult blood may be ordered by the physician. Gastroscopy and sigmoidoscopy also may be ordered if the source of bleeding cannot be found.

NURSING OBSERVATIONS. The symptoms of mild iron-deficiency anemia are fatigue, pallor, and dyspnea on exertion. The patient may also have a stomatitis, dry skin, and numbness and tingling of the extremities.

COMMON TREATMENT PLANS AND NURSING INTERVENTIONS. The treatment of iron-deficiency anemia is directed toward determining the cause and correcting the deficiency. In the absence of active bleeding, oral iron preparations such as ferrous sulfate or ferrous gluconate can be prescribed (see Table 13.2).

Parenteral injections such as iron dextran (IMFERON) may be prescribed. IMFERON is administered by the Z-track injection technique. Liquid iron should be given through a straw to prevent deposits on teeth. Oral iron should be given with meals to prevent gastric irritation. Iron preparations will cause the stools to become black in color. The nurse should inform the patient.

Individuals whose food intake is not sufficient in iron should be encouraged to increase their intake of iron-containing foods. Good sources of iron include lean meats, egg yolk, shellfish, and organ meats. Green, leafy vegetables are good sources of iron as well as such fruits as raisins, prunes, peaches, apricots, and grapes.

Iron-deficiency anemia is another example of an anemia resulting from defective formation of red blood cells. In this case, the formation of red blood cells is inadequate because of inadequate amounts of iron.

PERNICIOUS ANEMIA

DESCRIPTION. The patient with pernicious anemia has an inadequate production of red blood cells and hemoglobin caused by a lack of intrinsic factor. The anemia continues to increase unless treated. Persons developing this disease were doomed to die until the treatment was discovered in 1926; now no one should die from it. This is one of the many advances made in medical science during the present century.

Pernicious anemia occurs most often in individuals over 50 years of age and in young black women. Normally, the stomach secretes a substance called intrinsic factor which is necessary for the absorption of oral vitamin B_{12}. This gastric substance is lacking in persons with pernicious anemia. One common cause for the lack of intrinsic factor is atrophy of the gastric mucosa. An individual who has a total gastrectomy also needs treatment to prevent the development of pernicious anemia. The fundus is the portion of the stomach that produces intrinsic factor. When the fundus is surgically removed,

TABLE 13.2
DRUGS USED IN THE TREATMENT OF ANEMIAS

NONPROPRIETARY NAME	TRADE NAME	CLASSIFICATION	AVERAGE DOSE	SIDE EFFECTS
Ferrous gluconate	FERGON NOVOFERROGLUE	Hematinic	300 mg tid	Nausea, constipation, abdominal distress, diarrhea
Ferrous sulfate	FEOSOL FER-IN-SOL	Hematinic	300 mg tid	Nausea, constipation, abdominal distress, diarrhea
Iron-dextran injection	IMFERON	Hematinic	50–250 mg IM (Z track) or IV	Headache, arthralgia, paresthesias, syncope
Vitamin B_{12} (Cyanocobalamin)	REDISOL RUBRAMEN	Hematopoietic vitamin	100–200 mcg monthly	Diarrhea, itching, rash, flushing
Folic acid	FOLVITE	Hematopoietic vitamin	0.1–1 mg daily	Rarely toxic, rash, pruritus

the patient develops pernicious anemia unless treatment is provided. Intrinsic factor is necessary for the absorption of materials necessary in the production of red blood cells.

COMMON DIAGNOSTIC STUDIES. When the contents of the patient's stomach are examined in the test called a gastric analysis, no hydrochloric acid is found due to atrophy of the gastric mucosa. Another diagnostic test, the Schilling test, is used to test for failure of absorption of vitamin B_{12} in the intestine. Radioactive B_{12} is given orally to the patient, and a 24-hour urine collection is started. One hour later, nonradioactive vitamin B_{12} is given intramuscularly to saturate the liver, which stores this vitamin. Therefore, any radioactive vitamin B_{12} that is absorbed from the intestine cannot be stored and will be excreted in the urine. The 24-hour urine sample is analyzed for radioactive vitamin B_{12}. The normal person will excrete 10 to 20 percent of the oral radioactive vitamin B_{12} dose. The individual with a malabsorption defect will excrete less than 10 percent of the oral dose. The validity of the test depends on the nurse's careful collection of the 24-hour urine sample. The Schilling test is the definitive test for pernicious anemia.

Laboratory findings will show a reduced erythrocyte count. The bilirubin is increased because of hemolysis of defective erythrocytes. The serum LDH is elevated and the bone marrow aspiration study shows abnormal erythrocyte formation.

NURSING OBSERVATIONS. The patient with pernicious anemia has symptoms associated with the blood, gastrointestinal system, and nervous system. The patient may complain of tiredness, indigestion, bloating, weakness, shortness of breath, faintness, and appear pale. These symptoms usually progress over a period of several months and possibly years. The patient may experience numbness or tingling in the hands and feet, and walking may be difficult. The senses of taste and smell may be lost. Hypoxia of the brain can result in apathy, dullness, irritability, and decreased ability to concentrate. The patient's tongue may be sore and appear red and smooth. The skin has a yellowish color.

COMMON TREATMENT PLANS AND NURSING INTERVENTIONS. The patient with pernicious anemia can be treated successfully with intramuscular injections of cyanocobalamin (vitamin B_{12}). At first, large doses are given. When the blood picture has returned to normal, vitamin B_{12} is given less often and in smaller doses. Most patients are managed with monthly injections of 100 micrograms. The doctor adjusts the amount of medication needed to keep the red blood cell count normal. It is necessary for the patient to continue this treatment for life. Pernicious anemia is a good example of a chronic disease that cannot be cured but can be controlled.

The patient with pernicious anemia is encouraged to eat a diet high in iron, protein, and vitamins. If the patient has a sore mouth, oral hygiene should be given before and after meals. Foods that are not highly seasoned and are easily digested should be encouraged.

Often, the patient with pernicious anemia will be on bed rest until the blood picture improves. The patient should be turned frequently and given good skin care. The individual who has difficulty walking may need physical therapy before leaving the hospital. The nurse should observe this type of patient when out of bed and give assistance when ambulating to prevent falls and injuries.

FOLIC ACID DEFICIENCY

DESCRIPTION. Folic acid is necessary for normal erythrocyte production. Folic acid deficiency may be found in persons who rarely eat raw fruits and vegetables such as the elderly or alcoholic individual. Patients who are on intravenous therapy for long periods of time may also develop the deficiency. Requirements are increased in pregnancy and in chronic hemolytic anemias.

COMMON DIAGNOSTIC STUDIES. Laboratory tests indicate that anemia is present and the serum folate level is reduced. The patient may have a sore tongue but will be without the neurologic symptoms present in pernicious anemia.

COMMON TREATMENT PLANS AND NURS-
ING INTERVENTIONS. Folic acid, 1 mg a
day, is usually sufficient. Vitamin C may be
given to help promote erythropoiesis. A nutritious diet high in iron, protein, and vitamins should be encouraged.

Hemolytic Anemias

CONGENITAL HEMOLYTIC ANEMIAS

SICKLE CELL ANEMIA

DESCRIPTION. The individual with
sickle cell anemia has an hereditary form of
hemolytic anemia. As discussed earlier in
this chapter, the patient's red blood cells
contain an abnormal type of hemoglobin, hemoglobin S, which reacts to low concentrations of oxygen and causes the red cells to
become shaped like a sickle or a crescent
(see Figure 13.3). This form of anemia primarily affects black individuals from infancy
to adulthood. However, Puerto Ricans and
persons of Italian, Spanish, Greek, Middle
Eastern, and Indian ancestry also may be involved. The incidence of sickle cell anemia is
lower than that of sickle cell trait because of
the high mortality occurring in sickle cell
anemia. Whether a person will have sickle
cell anemia, sickle cell trait, or neither depends upon the genes for hemoglobin the
person has inherited from each parent.

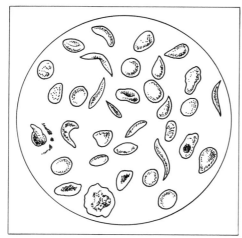

FIGURE 13.3 Drawing of a blood smear from
a patient with sickle cell anemia. Note the
sickle-shaped cells.

The zygote resulting from fertilization
receives half of its genes from the sperm of
the father and half from the ovum of the
mother. Sickle cell anemia is inherited as an
autosomal recessive trait. This means that
in order for an infant to be born with the disease, it must inherit a gene for sickle cell hemoglobin from each parent. If the gene for
normal adult hemoglobin is received from either parent, the child will not have sickle cell
disease.

For simplification, geneticists use letter
symbols as a means of indicating inherited
gene combinations. This is known as the
genotype. As each parent must contribute at
least one gene for each characteristic, the
genotype will consist of a minimum of two
genes.

Normal adult hemoglobin is usually represented by the letter A (Hb A), and it is
dominant over sickle cell hemoglobin, which
is represented by the letter S (Hb S). The
three possible inherited gene combinations
are as follows:

- Hb AA—Each parent has transmitted a
  gene for normal adult hemoglobin. Individuals having this genotype will have
  normal hemoglobin.
- Hb SS—Each parent has transmitted a
  gene for sickle cell hemoglobin. Individuals having this genotype will have sickle
  cell anemia with characteristic clinical
  symptoms.
- Hb SA—One parent has transmitted a
  gene for sickle cell hemoglobin and the
  other the gene for normal hemoglobin. Individuals having this genotype will have
  sickle cell trait. Under normal conditions,
  the individuals with this genotype will not
  display clinical symptoms of the disease.
  However, they do possess the "S" gene
  and are capable of passing the gene on to
  their offspring. Such individuals are
  therefore known as "carriers" of the disease.

WHAT IS THE PROBABILITY OF PARENTS
PRODUCING CHILDREN WITH SICKLE CELL
ANEMIA OR SICKLE CELL TRAIT? This
might best be answered by studying the following theoretic situations in which the parents have different genotypes. The sample

problems are shown in an arrangement called the Punnett square, with the genotypes of the parents along the periphery and the possible genotypes of the offspring shown in the four center squares.

Situation 1. If one parent has normal hemoglobin (Hb AA) and the other parent has sickle cell anemia (Hb SS), with every pregnancy, the probability that the child will be born with sickle cell trait (Hb SA) is 100 percent.

	A	A
S	SA	SA
S	SA	SA

Situation 2. If both parents have sickle cell trait (Hb SA), with every pregnancy, there is a 50 percent chance that the child will have sickle cell trait (Hb SA), a 25 percent chance that the child will have sickle cell anemia (Hb SS), and a 25 percent chance that the child will have normal hemoglobin (Hb AA).

	S	A
S	SS	SA
A	SA	AA

Situation 3. If one parent has sickle cell anemia (Hb SS) and the other parent has sickle cell trait (Hb SA), with each pregnancy, there is a 50 percent chance that the child will be born with sickle cell anemia (Hb SS) and a 50 percent chance the child will have sickle cell trait (Hb SA).

	S	S
S	SS	SS
A	SA	SA

Situation 4. If one parent has sickle cell trait (Hb SA) and the other parent normal hemoglobin (Hb AA), with each pregnancy, there is a 50 percent chance that the child will be born with sickle cell trait (Hb SA) and a 50 percent chance that the child will have normal hemoglobin (Hb AA).

	S	A
A	SA	AA
A	SA	AA

Situation 5. If both parents have sickle cell anemia (Hb SS), they may be unable to have children. However, if a child is born, there is 100 percent probability that it will have sickle cell anemia (Hb SS).

	S	S
S	SS	SS
S	SS	SS

COMMON DIAGNOSTIC STUDIES. The laboratory tests will include the *sickledex* or sickle prep. If either is positive, the hemoglobin electrophoresis will be ordered, which differentiates whether an individual has sickle cell trait or sickle cell anemia.

NURSING OBSERVATIONS. *Sickle Trait.* The person with sickle cell trait will not have the same symptoms as the person with sickle cell anemia. The person with the trait will be protected from crises because the hemoglobin A prevents the erythrocytes from sickling. The person will have no anemia and feels well.

Sickle Cell Anemia. The patient with sickle cell anemia usually displays symptoms of the condition in infancy. The individual may go for months with no apparent symptoms except anemia. However, an infection, exertion, exposure to cold, emotional stress, and any condition that increases the patient's need for oxygen can trigger a sickle cell crisis. The erythrocytes then become sickle shaped and do not flow smoothly through the capillaries. These abnormally shaped cells cause a blockage in the blood vessels. The occlusion may be complete or partial and may affect any organ. The spleen, kidney, heart, lungs, brain, joints, and bones seem to be common areas for occlusion to occur. The patient experiences abdominal, muscular, and joint pains. The patient is prone to chronic ulcers of the legs, particularly over the ankle bone, because of stasis of blood and blockage of blood to the tissue in this area. The patient is likely to develop chronic infections of the urinary system and pneumonia. Jaundice is common.

COMMON TREATMENT PLANS AND NURSING INTERVENTIONS. At the present time there is no cure for sickle cell disease. The main emphasis is directed toward preventing a sickle cell crisis by avoiding infections, stressful situations, excessive exercise, and other conditions that increase the patient's need for oxygen. During an acute crisis the patient generally is placed on bed rest to decrease the body's need for oxygen. Analgesics may be required to relieve pain in the affected part of the body. The patient is encouraged to drink fluids to increase the blood volume and mobilize the sickled cells. Blood transfusions are used only in severe cases of anemia complicated by other conditions. Oxygen and steroid therapy may be used. Good skin care is important because of impaired circulation. The long-term care of the patient with sickle cell anemia includes any measure that will help the venous return of blood to the heart and lungs for oxygenation. Persons with sickle cell anemia should avoid high altitudes or flying in unpressurized planes. Oxygen tension is lowered under these conditions and could precipitate a crisis.

Massive efforts to detect black children with sickle cell trait or sickle cell disease have been conducted in many parts of the United States. Those with either the disease or the trait may receive genetic counseling. Young couples should know their chances for having children with either sickle cell disease or the trait.

G-6-PD DEFICIENCY (GLUCOSE-6-PHOSPHATE DEHYDROGENOSE DEFICIENCY)

DESCRIPTION. The abnormality is the deficiency of or a defect in G-6-PD, an enzyme within the red blood cell that is essential for membrane stability. The deficiency is sex linked and passed from females who are asymptomatic to male offspring. The deficiency occurs in about 15 percent of black males in the United States.

Usually the patient has no symptoms until subjected to a situation that causes hemolysis of the red blood cells. Most frequently, the patient has a viral or bacterial infection which precipitates the hemolysis. Certain drugs may cause hemolysis also, such as sulfonamides, antimalarials, nitrofuratoins, and common coal tar analgesics including acetylsalicylic acid (aspirin), thiazide diruretics, and oral hypoglycemic agents.

COMMON DIAGNOSTIC STUDIES. The doctor will order a screening test or a quantitative assay of G-6-PD.

NURSING OBSERVATIONS. After exposure to the stressor or situation that causes hemolysis of the red cells because of G-6-PD deficiency, the patient develops pallor and jaundice. Hemoglobin in the urine rises, as well as the blood reticulocyte count.

COMMON TREATMENT PLANS AND NURSING INTERVENTIONS. The treatment is removal of the drug that is causing the hemolysis of red cells. The patient should be given a list of medications to avoid such as those mentioned under the heading Description, on page 373.

ACQUIRED HEMOLYTIC ANEMIA

Many factors can cause a hemolytic anemia which are not congenital in nature. These anemias are referred to as acquired hemolytic anemias.

Some examples include anemia caused by hemolysis of red blood cells due to trauma from burns or surgery. Another hemolytic anemia may be caused by a chemical agent such as lead, ingestion of which causes lead poisoning. Certain infections such as infectious hepatitis, bacterial endocarditis, or malaria cause a hemolytic anemia. An isoimmune hemolytic reaction is an antigen-antibody reaction which may occur because of antibodies that have developed in response to an antigen from another person of the same species and cause destruction of red blood cells. Examples of this type of anemia are blood transfusion reactions and erythroblastosis fetalis.

ANEMIAS FROM BLOOD LOSS

ACUTE HEMORRHAGIC ANEMIA (NORMOCYTIC ANEMIA)

DESCRIPTION. The nurse will recognize this type of anemia to be the result of blood loss, as implied in its title. The common causes of acute blood loss are severed blood vessels due to trauma, erosion of a blood vessel by an ulcer, such as might occur with gastric ulcers or a cancerous tumor; and hemorrhagic disorders.

COMMON DIAGNOSTIC STUDIES. The erythrocyte count, hemoglobin, and hematocrit will be decreased. Once bleeding stops, blood restoration begins in about four to five days. The red blood cells and hemoglobin usually return to normal within four to six weeks.

NURSING OBSERVATIONS. The patient's symptoms will depend on the rate of bleeding, where the patient is bleeding from, and how much blood is lost. The nurse will expect the patient with hemorrhage to be restless, dizzy, diaphoretic, and to complain of thirst and faintness. The pulse and respirations will be elevated and the blood pressure decreased. Untreated, shock becomes irreversible and the patient will die.

COMMON TREATMENT PLANS AND NURSING INTERVENTIONS. The patient should be kept quiet and warm. Blood transfusions, human plasma, a plasma expander, or dextrose may be given intravenously. After the hemorrhage and its cause have been controlled, the patient should receive a high-protein diet. Iron may be prescribed. Other nursing measures for the patient in shock

(Chapter 6) are applicable to this patient during the time of shock.

ANEMIA DUE TO CHRONIC BLOOD LOSS

Some of the causes of chronic blood loss are uterine tumors, hemorrhoids, rectal polyps, peptic ulcers, and cancer of the gastrointestinal tract. The patient loses erythrocytes in small numbers, which are usually replaced by the bone marrow. However, continuous loss of iron may result in total depletion of the iron stores. For this reason, laboratory findings and symptoms are the same as for iron-deficiency anemia. The site of bleeding must be identified and treated appropriately. Iron supplements and proper diet are two measures used to treat the iron deficiency.

Malaria

DESCRIPTION

The patient with malaria has an infectious disease which causes damage to erythrocytes and results in anemia. Malaria is a common infectious disease in many parts of the world. It is caused by *protozoa*, which are microorganisms belonging to the animal kingdom. The protozoa causing malaria are introduced into a person's body through the bite of an infected female Anopheles mosquito. As this insect is found more frequently in tropical and subtropical areas, malaria is more common in these regions. Malaria has also been transmitted from infected needles and syringes shared by drug addicts and by blood transfusions.

Protozoa causing malaria are called parasites because it is necessary for them to obtain food from another living organism. After the parasite has been introduced into a person's body by the bite of the Anopheles mosquito, it enters a red blood cell. While there, it grows by dividing and subdividing until the red blood cell is filled with parasites. The wall of the red blood cell ruptures, allowing the young parasites to enter the bloodstream. Hence, malaria is one example of a disease that causes an acquired hemolytic anemia. The patient has shaking chills followed by fever during this time. The protozoa enter more erythrocytes, and the process of growth and rupturing of the red blood cells is repeated.

There are four types of malaria. Each is caused by a different kind of malarial parasite. The time required for each of these four parasites to reproduce and to cause the red blood cells to rupture varies. Thus, the patient who has chills and fever every two days has a type of malaria caused by a parasite that differs from the parasite causing a patient to have chills and fever every three days.

COMMON DIAGNOSTIC STUDIES

Travel to or living in an area where malaria is endemic is a diagnostic clue. The diagnosis is made by examination of the patient's blood in the laboratory. The specific parasite can be identified in the blood.

NURSING OBSERVATIONS

The patient with malaria has attacks of fever. Usually these bouts of fever occur at regular intervals. Frequently, the patient experiences a shaking chill, headache, nausea, and vomiting at the beginning of this acute attack. After the temperature returns to normal, the patient usually feels well until the return of symptoms.

Untreated, the patient's general health becomes affected. Anemia develops because the protozoa are destroying the red blood cells. The spleen may become enlarged, since it is filled with blood pigment and red blood cells containing malarial parasites. The patient may become unconscious and die if prompt and adequate treatment is not received.

COMMON TREATMENT PLANS AND NURSING INTERVENTIONS

Fortunately, drugs that kill the malarial parasite have been discovered. Chloroquine phosphate, hydroxychloroquine sulfate, or amodiaquine hydrochloride are examples of drugs the physician may prescribe for this patient (see Table 13.3).

The administration of antipyretics to control fever as well as cool sponges may be ordered. Analgesics for the treatment of headache and muscular aches may be administered. The care of the patient having anorexia, nausea, and vomiting is applicable.

Malaria can be prevented if the people living in areas where malaria is common avoid coming in contact with Anopheles mosquitoes. This can be done by draining pools of stagnant water where these insects breed. Pouring oil on stagnant water causes the mosquito larvae to die. This seemingly

TABLE 13.3
ANTIMALARIAL DRUGS*

NONPROPRIETARY NAME	TRADE NAME	AVERAGE DOSE	NURSING IMPLICATIONS
Amodiaquine	CAMOQUIN	100–600 mg	Observe patient for nausea, vomiting, diarrhea, and increased salivation
Chloroguanide Proguanil	PALUDRINE	100–200 mg	
Chloroquine	ARALEN AVOCLOR RESOCHIN	125–250 mg	Patient should be observed for headache, itching, and gastrointestinal symptoms
Hydroxychloroquine	PLAQUENIL	200–400 mg	
Primaquine		45 mg	
Pyrimethamine	DARAPRIM	25 mg	
Quinine		600 mg–1 gm	Patient may experience ringing in ears, headache, nausea, dizziness, and visual disturbances. Not often used for malaria now

* Antimalarial drugs are used mainly to treat patients with malaria. All such drugs may produce toxic effects. The dosage for treating an acute attack of malaria differs from the amount used to prevent or to suppress malaria. When administering a specific antimalarial drug, the nurse should review the literature for the toxic effects as a basis for observing such symptoms of toxicity in the patient.

simple measure is effective because the larvae must come to the surface to obtain air, and when the water's surface is covered with oil, the larvae's supply of air is cut off and they die. Houses and beds should be screened in mosquito-infested areas. Area-wide indoor spraying of dwellings with insecticides is useful in the mosquito-eradication program. When it is not possible to avoid exposure to these mosquitoes, the patient may be treated prophylactically with chloroquine phosphate, amodiaquine, or hydroxychloroquine. For example, persons traveling to malaria-prevalent areas may begin taking one of these drugs once a week for two weeks before entering that area and while there. The drug should be taken for six weeks after leaving the area.

Primary Polycythemia (Polycythemia Vera)

DESCRIPTION

Polycythemia is described as an abnormal increase in the production of red blood cells, white blood cells, and platelets. The blood becomes thicker because of the increased numbers of red blood cells, white blood cells, and platelets. The possibility of thrombosis occurring becomes greater as the number of blood cells increases. Excessive bleeding from minor cuts and bruises also may occur. Although the cause of the disease is not known, it is regarded by some experts as being neoplastic in nature.

COMMON DIAGNOSTIC STUDIES

The red blood cell count may rise to 8 to 12 million per cu mm. The white blood cell count may rise beyond 10,000 per cu mm. The hemoglobin may rise to 8 to 25 gm/100 ml.

NURSING OBSERVATIONS

The patient with polycythemia vera may have headache, fatigue, elevated systolic blood pressure, and edema of the feet and legs. Dizziness, dyspnea, numbness and tingling in the extremities, and visual disturbances occur because of diminished blood flow. The person with polycythemia vera generally has a reddish-purple or ruddy, cyanotic complexion.

COMMON TREATMENT PLANS AND NURSING INTERVENTIONS

When the hematocrit rises above 55 to 60 percent, the patient may have a phlebotomy done. Removal of 500 ml of blood every two or three days until the hematocrit reaches the desired level is common. Chemotherapeutic drugs such as chlorambucil (LEUKERAN), busulfan (MYLERAN), and sodium phosphate P32 (PHOSPHOTOPE) may reduce bone marrow activity, resulting in a reduction in red blood cells.

The patient with polycythemia is a prime candidate for the development of thrombi, including deep-vein thrombophlebitis, myocardial infarction, and cerebrovascular accident. Every effort should be made to keep the patient ambulatory and to promote circumstances that will aid in the venous return of blood to the heart. Fluids should be forced and a careful record of intake and output should be maintained.

The average survival of an individual with polycythemia is approximately 10 to 15 years. Some clients develop acute leukemia, myelofibrosis, and myeloid metaplasia.

Leukemia

DESCRIPTION

The individual with leukemia has a neoplastic disease of the blood-forming tissues, spleen, lymphatic system, and bone marrow. Usually, there is an increased number of white blood cells, which are immature, abnormal in appearance, and do not function as normal white blood cells. Also, there is a reduction in the number of red blood cells, hemoglobin, and platelets, which results in anemia, an increased susceptibility to infection, and an increased possibility of hemorrhaging. To date, the exact cause has not been determined. The effects on the bone marrow of ionizing radiation by atomic explosions and radiation therapy have been studied as a possible cause of leukemia. Certain chemicals that are toxic to bone marrow are also being studied as causes. The possibility that leukemia is caused by one or more viruses is being studied carefully by scientists involved in this research.

Leukemia continues to be a fatal disease for which no cure is yet known. The more acute forms affect children and young adults. In some cases, the child with acute leukemia may die in a few weeks. Since chronic leukemia occurs more frequently in adults, they may live 10 to 30 years. At the present time, the highest mortality rate seems to occur in children under five years of age. The rate of incidence in adults past 70 years of age appears to be increasing.

Leukemia may be classified according to the rapidity with which the disease progresses. For example, the physician may refer to the condition as either acute or chronic. In order to better understand that leukemia is classified according to the type of white blood cells involved, the student needs to recall that blood contains two main types of leukocytes: granulocytes and agranulocytes. The lymphocytes and monocytes are agranulocytes. A marked increase in the number of these white blood cells is referred to as lymphocytic leukemia or monocytic leukemia. Neutrophils, eosinophils, and basophils are granulocytes. A marked increase in the number of neutrophils with or without an increase of the other granulocytes is referred to as granulocytic leukemia.

COMMON DIAGNOSTIC STUDIES

The physician makes a definite diagnosis on the basis of blood studies and a biopsy of the patient's bone marrow. The white blood count varies from 10,000 to 100,000 per cu mm. Anemia and a low platelet count are usual. The bone marrow biopsy characteristically yields a large number of immature leukemic cells. Bone x-rays are abnormal in many patients.

NURSING OBSERVATIONS OF THE PATIENT WITH ACUTE LEUKEMIA

Acute leukemia may be lymphocytic, granulocytic (myelocytic), or monocytic. The onset is generally abrupt and begins in most patients as an infection or bleeding tendency. The infection is often a severe upper respiratory one that does not respond to treatment in the usual manner. A bleeding tendency due to the low platelet count usually is manifested by purpura, petechiae, or bleeding from the nose, mouth, stomach, rectum, and urinary tract. Symptoms of anemia develop, such as easy fatigability, dyspnea, and tachycardia. As the disease develops, weight loss and fever may appear. The patient frequently complains of increased sweating and heat intolerance. Because the process of leukemia involves all tissues, the patient's symptoms are complex and varied. Bone and joint pain may develop. The tissue that produces the particular kind of abnormal leukocyte may become enlarged. For example, frequently the spleen is enlarged, causing abdominal pain. In some cases of leukemia the lymph nodes are larger than normal. Pressure from enlarged lymph nodes on adjacent tissue causes pain. Sometimes the liver enlarges. Hemorrhage may occur anywhere in the body. Hemorrhages in the skin, mucous membrane, retina of the eye, and central nervous system may develop. The patient develops infections easily. Without normally functioning neutrophils, the patient's body is unable to wall off an infection. Ulcers frequently form in and around the mouth.

COMMON TREATMENT OF ACUTE LEUKEMIA

As the cure for leukemia has not yet been discovered, the treatment and nursing care of this patient are mainly symptomatic to provide the patient with as long and as normal a life as possible. However, efforts are made to check the growth of malignant cells for as long as possible, to maintain a normal level of red cells, hemoglobin, and platelets, and to provide relief from symptoms common to leukemia patients.

Chemotherapy helps to produce remissions of the disease and to prolong the patient's life. Drugs usually are given in combination to kill tumor cells at different stages of their growth cycle and to produce fewer toxic effects. The dosage of the drug is in a state of change as the research scientists continue to search for the cause and the cure. Some chemotherapeutic drugs such as cytarabine, doxorubicin (ADRIAMYCIN), thioguanine, mercaptopurine, daunorubicin (daunomycin), and methotrexate are given. Also, cyclophosphamide, vincristine, L-asparaginase, hydorxyurea (HYDREA), and the corticosteroids may be used. Table 9.3, page 236, lists some of these drugs found to be effective in the treatment of acute leukemia; the major signs of toxicity and the usual routes of administration are itemized in the table. Such toxic symptoms as nausea, anorexia, vomiting, bone marrow depression, loss of hair, weight loss, and weakness may occur. The nurse should review the literature of the drugs currently being used for the patient and become familiar with toxic symptoms. The destruction of a great number of cancer cells by chemotherapy tends to lead to the formation of uric acid crystals in the urinary tract. The crystals may contribute to the development of a life-threatening uremia. The oral administration of allopurinol (ZYLOPRIM) helps to prevent the formation of these crystals. Proper hydration of the patient to ensure a urine output of 3000 ml or more per day is also helpful in preventing the formation of uric acid crystals.

Platelet transfusions may be necessary to help in controlling bleeding. This is especially true when the bleeding is associated with a lowered number of platelets. Packed red cell transfusions may be used to maintain an adequate hemoglobin level.

Use of laminar airflow rooms, leukocyte transfusions, antibiotics, and antifungal agents are often necessary because of the patient's susceptibility to all types of infections.

BONE MARROW TRANSPLANTATION. Bone marrow transplantation is being done selectively and experimentally in some medical centers for patients with acute leukemia. Prior to the transplant, cyclophosphamide (CYTOXAN) or some antineoplastic agent is given to the patient. Total body irradiation is then done to assure that all leukemic cells are killed. Many side effects may occur as a result of this preparation of the patient for the transplant. Nausea, vomiting, and diarrhea may occur immediately. Later, alopecia, dry skin, and hyperpigmentation with peeling of the skin may occur. Irreversible conditions such as cataracts, ste-

rility, retardation of growth, and liver or kidney damage may also occur. These patients must be protected from all sources of infection until the bone marrow graft takes, which is 20 to 30 days after transplantation. The transplant is administered intravenously 24 hours after total body irradiation. The transplant has to be given to the recipient within four hours after being aspirated from the donor. The new marrow migrates from the blood to the bone marrow.

The greatest complication is graft-versus-host disease (GVHD). The disease affects the liver, gastrointestinal tract, and skin. Infections may occur. Methotrexate may be given to the patient approximately three months after the transplantation to reduce the risk of GVHD.

NURSING OBSERVATIONS OF THE PATIENT WITH CHRONIC LEUKEMIA

Chronic leukemia may be granulocytic (myelocytic) or lymphocytic. Chronic myelocytic leukemia is mainly a disorder of young adults, while the chronic lymphocytic type occurs mostly in persons over 50 years of age.

Chronic leukemia has a gradual onset of symptoms. This type of leukemia is characterized by generalized lymph node involvement, anemia, fever, bleeding tendencies, enlargement of the spleen, weakness, weight loss, and pain in the long bones.

COMMON TREATMENT OF CHRONIC LEUKEMIA

The objective of treatment is to achieve a remission of symptoms. The use of ionizing irradiation to the enlarged lymph nodes and spleen is effective in slowing the growth of abnormal blood cells. Good results have been obtained from internal irradiation with phosphorus, administered intravenously or orally. Radiation of the entire body with supervoltage (for example, with cobalt) is used to achieve remission of symptoms.

Whole blood and packed red blood cells are given to maintain an adequate blood picture. Steroids are given for symptomatic relief to decrease the size of lymph nodes and spleen. Chemotherapeutic drugs used in the treatment of chronic leukemias include chlorambucil (LEUKERAN), busulfan (MYLE-RAN), triethylenemelamine (TEM), cyclophosphamide (CYTOXAN), and melphalan (AL-KERAN).

NURSING INTERVENTIONS

As stated earlier, the objective in caring for the patient with leukemia is directed toward helping to maintain as normal a life as possible, for the patient to be as free of symptoms as possible, and to prolong life with a maximum of comfort.

In caring for the patient with leukemia, the nurse needs to recognize that the individual and the family are likely to be frightened, depressed, concerned, anxious, lonely, and frustrated. Members of the nursing staff need to be informed regarding leukemia, the symptoms of leukemia, the effects of the drugs to be expected, and the side effects that may be evident, and be prepared to answer questions regarding the patient's condition.

PREVENTION OF INFECTION. The patient's resistance to infection is lowered. The body's defense mechanisms are not able to function normally because of the reduced number of normal white blood cells. Special efforts will be made to protect the patient against infections because of lowered resistance. In some cases, the patient is placed in reverse isolation or laminar airflow rooms to prevent infection. Members of the nursing team should be keenly aware that the individual in isolation is likely to feel a sense of rejection. The nurse must be sensitive to this reaction and help the patient through the period of isolation.

Members of the health team responsible for caring for the patient with leukemia should be especially careful in washing their hands between caring for different patients to avoid transferring infection to the patient. Individuals with an infection, such as a common cold, should not enter the patient's room.

The patient's skin should be inspected daily for the appearance of bruised or injured tissue. Any unusual findings should be reported. In some cases an antiseptic solution will be ordered for the patient's bath.

The formation of an abscess in the anorectal area is a real possibility for the person with leukemia. For this reason, the patient's temperature generally is not taken by rectum. An enema is usually avoided also. However, if either of these is necessary, the nurse should be extremely gentle.

Symptoms of inflammation around the site of an intravenous injection should be observed. The patient may receive intravenous therapy for long periods of time and is a prime candidate for phlebitis. When caring for the patient receiving an intravenous injection, the nurse should observe the area and report any unusual signs.

HYGIENE. The patient's skin should be kept clean with baths as necessary. Any symptom of skin irritation should be reported promptly, as mentioned earlier. Pruritus is a common complaint, and efforts to prevent irritation of the skin should be made. The patient's fingernails and toenails should be kept short to prevent scatching and injuring the tissue.

The patient's mouth and gums will need special care because of the likelihood of ulcerations associated with chemotherapy and the patient's general condition. If the patient is unable to use a toothbrush because of bleeding gums, cotton-tipped applicators may be used with a nonirritating mouthwash. The lips and nostrils may need a soothing lubricant to prevent dryness and cracking.

Irritating, sore lesions in the mouth can interfere with the patient's ability to eat. When this occurs, the patient should receive food that seems palatable and nonirritating to the mucous membrane in the mouth. Allowing the patient to rinse the mouth with a bland mouthwash before and after mealtime may improve the ability to eat.

DRUG THERAPY. The patient with leukemia generally will receive a combination of drugs. The nurse needs to know the expected action, method of administration, and toxic effects of the various drugs being given. The patient should be observed for allergic reactions, in addition to toxic reactions, to a drug. Such symptoms should be reported promptly and accurately. The patient can be expected to have frequent blood analysis during the time that chemotherapy is being given.

Some of the chemotherapeutic agents have a tendency to cause alopecia. Some patients prefer using wigs, hairpieces, and scarves. This should be encouraged if it enhances the patient's self image.

The patient receiving chemotherapy may suffer from nausea and anorexia. Antiemetics may alleviate nausea so that nutrition can be improved. Constipation can be prevented by the administration of stool softeners. Constipation may cause bleeding of the rectal mucosa. Diarrhea associated with chemotherapy may be controlled by the administration of antidiarrheal agents such as diphenoxylate hydrochloride (LOMOTIL).

In some types of leukemia, the patient will have an enlargement of lymph nodes. Pressure from the enlarged lymph nodes on adjacent tissue can cause pain. At times, the liver may enlarge. The patient may experience generalized discomfort and pain, and this of course will necessitate gentle handling and analgesic drugs for the relief of pain. The analgesic drugs prescribed generally are of a nonirritating nature. Intramuscular injections of the medication generally are avoided. The possibility of causing bleeding into the muscle tissue is the reason for avoiding intramuscular injections. However, when an intramuscular injection has to be given, firm pressure over the injection site should be used to control bleeding after the needle has been withdrawn.

Antipyretic drugs may be given to control fever. Cool sponges may be given to control fever and to help keep the patient comfortable.

CONTROL OF BLEEDING. The nurse should inspect the skin for bruising and petechiae. Inspection of the urine and stool for the presence of blood should be done. Bleeding from any body orifice should be recorded and reported. All nursing measures that commonly would be given to the anemic patient would be appropriate for the patient with leukemia.

Thrombocytopenia

DESCRIPTION

The individual with thrombocytopenia has a hemorrhagic disease characterized by purpura. *Purpura* refers to areas of bleeding located in the skin and mucous membranes. The bleeding disorder may occur as a result of another condition, such as chronic leukemia, certain infections, and drugs.

An individual with purpura accompanied by a reduction in the number of circulating platelets in his body with an undetermined cause has *idiopathic thrombocytopenic purpura*. The condition may begin suddenly and subside, or it may cause death within three to four months. The chronic form begins gradually and may persist for months or years.

COMMON DIAGNOSTIC STUDIES

Laboratory studies confirm idiopathic thrombocytopenic purpura when the platelet count is below 100,000 per cu mm and when the bleeding time is prolonged but coagulation time is normal. The capillary fragility, as demonstrated by the tourniquet test, is increased.

NURSING OBSERVATIONS

The individual with idiopathic thrombocytopenic purpura has a bleeding disorder characterized by petechiae and *ecchymoses*, the escape of blood into tissues causing a large bruise. These areas of bleeding occur most often over the legs and pressure sites. In some cases, the bleeding is generalized over the entire body. The client may have bleeding from the nose, gums, and other organs. Bleeding from the kidneys and gastrointestinal tract may occur. Bleeding in the brain is a common cause of death. If the blood loss is severe, the patient may experience symptoms of acute hemorrhagic anemia. Chronic blood loss may be responsible for the development of iron-deficiency anemia.

COMMON TREATMENT PLANS AND NURSING INTERVENTIONS

The course of the disease is characterized by remissions and relapses. Corticosteroids help to reduce bleeding. Platelet transfusions may be used to treat certain individuals. Iron therapy is used for the individual with a deficiency of iron. A splenectomy may provide improvement in the individual by causing an elevation of the platelet level.

Nursing care of the patient with idiopathic thrombocytopenic purpura is the same as for the patient with anemia. In addition, unnecessary trauma must be avoided. The patient must be observed for hemorrhage from the nose, gastrointestinal tract, and urinary system. During periods of active bleeding, the patient should be kept quiet and at rest. Cerebral hemorrhage can be a fatal complication. Therefore, constipation should be avoided to prevent straining at stool. Upper respiratory infections, which can cause coughing and sneezing, should be avoided.

Careful handling of the individual is important in order to prevent unnecessary bruising. Frequent and gentle mouth care should be given for oral comfort and hygienic measures.

Hemophilia

DESCRIPTION

Hemophilia is a rare blood disease that is hereditary. The person with hemophilia A has a deficiency of factor VIII, a plasma protein required for clotting of blood, whereas the person with hemophilia B has a deficiency of factor IX. Deficiency of factor VIII is more common.

The gene responsible for causing hemophilia is carried on one of the X chromosomes of the female. The disease appears mainly in males who have the hemophilic gene on their only X chromosome. Since hemophilia is a sex-linked recessive trait disease, with each birth, the woman carrier has a 50 percent chance of producing a son with hemophilia and a 50 percent chance of producing a daughter who is a carrier. The daughters of a man with hemophilia become carriers, while the sons are normal. Spontaneous mutations of genes or chromosomes may cause the condition when the family history is negative for the disease.

COMMON DIAGNOSTIC STUDIES

Hemophilia is seldom diagnosed in infancy unless the baby has excessive bleeding from the umbilical cord or following circumcision. The disease usually is diagnosed after the child begins to crawl and walk, which increases its vulnerability to injury. The blood of a patient with hemophilia takes longer than normal to clot. The partial thromboplastin time, which is a widely used screening test for blood coagulation in general, is prolonged in the person with hemophilia, but bleeding time is normal. Factor VIII is missing from the plasma.

NURSING OBSERVATIONS

The patient with hemophilia bruises easily and bleeds longer than normal following an injury. Prolonged bleeding from the nose, mouth, or lacerations may occur. Internal bleeding and bleeding into the neck or pharynx can cause serious complications. Hematomas may occur anywhere over the body as a result of injury. Hemorrhages into the elbows, knees, and ankles (hemarthrosis) cause pain, swelling, and limitation of movement. Repeated hemorrhages may result in deformity. The prognosis is uncertain and depends on the severity of the disease. Cycles may occur with relatively little bleeding followed by periods of severe bleeding. Death may result from intracranial hemorrhage or from severe bleeding.

COMMON TREATMENT PLANS AND NURSING INTERVENTIONS

The treatment of an individual with hemophilia includes measures to control active bleeding of wounds, such as applying pressure over the area or applying fibrin foam in the wound and keeping the patient quiet. Blood, plasma, or preferably, factor VIII concentrates are given to supply the necessary clotting factor. The most widely used concentrate is cryoprecipitated factor VIII, given to supply the antihemophilic factor or AHF. In cases of hemarthrosis, immobilization of the joint and application of ice packs are used to control the bleeding. Blood and plasma concentrates may be administered.

Often the weight of bed covers is painful to the individual. A bed cradle to hold the linen away from the patient's feet may enhance comfort. Excessive movement is avoided as much as possible. Analgesics may be prescribed for pain. Passive range-of-motion exercises are important to prevent crippling deformities after the bleeding has been controlled. The passive range-of-motion exercises should be carried out in a gentle manner.

The patient with hemophilia should lead as normal a life as possible within the realm of safety. Overprotection because of fear of causing bleeding episodes can produce emotional problems that may be more disabling than the effects of the disease itself. The patient and family need to understand the nature of the illness and to be alert to the signs of bleeding. Early signs of bleeding should cause them to seek medical help. A bracelet or tag indicating the patient's disease condition should be worn.

Hodgkin's Disease

DESCRIPTION

The individual with Hodgkin's disease has a malignant condition that originates in the lymphatic system and primarily involves the lymph nodes. The cause of Hodgkin's disease is not yet known.

The diagnosis of Hodgkin's disease is based on the identification of a malignant cell, which is a giant, atypical tumor cell found in an excised lymph node. The cells are abnormal histiocytes, one category of reticuloendothelial cells, called Reed-Sternberg cells.

COMMON DIAGNOSTIC STUDIES

Many diagnostic tests may be necessary in order for the physician to evaluate the extent of the disease process in the individual's body. An attempt is made to pinpoint the location of the tumor and/or tumors and to exclude the presence of a tumor in organs and tissues not yet involved.

In addition to a lymph node biopsy, to identify the characteristic Reed-Sternberg cell, a complete blood count is done to determine the patient's blood picture. An x-ray of the chest, skeletal x-rays, CT scan, and bone scans can detect the presence of tumor involvement. A bone marrow biopsy may also reveal the typical Reed-Sternberg cell. The lymphangiogram, described earlier in this chapter, is a valuable diagnostic test and reveals the size of lymph nodes in addition to detecting involved lymph nodes that cannot be seen or felt by ordinary means (see Figure 13.4).

Use of the above diagnostic measures allows the physician to determine the extent and activity of Hodgkin's disease. The staging of Hodgkin's disease and other lymphomas is described in Table 13.4. After determining the stage and extent of Hodgkin's disease, the physician can then plan appropriate therapeutic measures. Some doctors state that with early diagnosis and treatment, 90 percent of the patients with localized Hodgkin's disease now can be cured, that is, have a ten-year survival without recurrence.

NURSING OBSERVATIONS

Hodgkin's disease usually begins as a painless enlargement of the lymph nodes on one side of the individual's neck. Generalized itching (pruritus) may be experienced by the patient. Anemia, sweating, weight loss, and fever also may occur. Pain in the lymph nodes may occur after the ingestion of alcohol.

Lymph nodes in other regions may begin to enlarge and cause pain. However, the enlarging lymph nodes may cause no discomfort to the individual. Enlarged lymph nodes along the course of the trachea can cause the patient to experience dyspnea, and enlarged nodes can cause pressure against the esophagus and difficulty in swallowing—dysphagia. Pressure of the enlarged node against the laryngeal nerve can cause laryngeal paralysis. Pressure against nerves in the arm, back, and sacral area may also result in pain. Pressure against veins from enlarged nodes may result in edema of the extremities. Later, the spleen and liver may enlarge. Blood studies may show decreased red blood

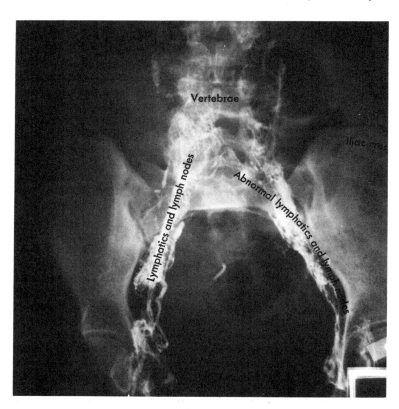

FIGURE 13.4 Lymphangio-gram of patient with Hodgkin's disease. Note fluffy appearance of lymphatics and lymph nodes. (Courtesy of Radiology Department, Eastern Virginia Medical School, Norfolk, Virginia.)

cell counts, white blood cell counts, and platelets.

COMMON TREATMENT PLANS AND NURSING INTERVENTIONS

The patient with Hodgkin's disease generally is treated with radiotherapy. Treatment may be limited to radiation of the involved areas, or it may be extended to include all regions rich with lymph nodes. Ionizing radiation interferes with the production and division of malignant cells. Thus, the progress of the disease is decreased and, in some cases, stopped for long periods of time. Patients in stages I or II of Hodgkin's disease sometimes can be cured.

Radiotherapy is planned carefully to cause as little damage as possible to normal tissue. Chemotherapy is used also in the treatment of Hodgkin's disease. In stages III and IV, radiotherapy and chemotherapy combined are currently being used. The chemotherapy treatment regimen is called the

MOPP program. The MOPP program includes mechlorethamine (MUSTARGEN), vincristine (ONCOVIN), procarbazine (NATULAN or MATULANE), and prednisone.

Nursing measures for the patient receiving radiation therapy and chemotherapy for leukemia, which were discussed earlier in this chapter, are applicable to this patient.

Surgery is a third form of therapy that may be done to remove tumors causing pressure on an adjacent organ or nerve. Fever is controlled with antipyretics and cool water sponges. Anemia is treated with transfusions. Pruritus is sometimes relieved by the administration of either colchicine or chlorpromazine (THORAZINE). Reverse isolation may be necessary to guard against any source of possible infection.

The outlook for the patient with Hodgkin's disease has changed dramatically in the past few years. Although the prognosis depends on many factors, not the least of which is the extent of the disease, greater

TABLE 13.4
STAGING OF HODGKIN'S DISEASE AND OTHER LYMPHOMAS

Stage I:	Disease limited to the region of a single lymph node or lymphatic structure, or to a single organ or site outside the lymph system and on the same side of the diaphragm
Stage II:	Disease limited to two or more lymph node regions or other lymphatic structures. Structures outside the involved area and on the same side of the diaphragm may or may not be affected
Stage III:	Disease involves lymph node regions other than lymphatic structures on both sides of the diaphragm. Other structures may or may not be involved
Stage IV:	Disease involves one or more organs or structures other than the lymphatic system

numbers of patients are remaining free of disease for longer periods of time.

Non-Hodgkin's Lymphoma

DESCRIPTION

An individual with non-Hodgkin's lymphoma has a malignant tumor of the lymphoid tissue involving lymphocytes and/or histiocytes. The nurse may hear this disease referred to as lymphosarcoma, also, as reticulum cell sarcoma.

COMMON DIAGNOSTIC STUDIES

Lymph node biopsy reveals abnormal cells. The physician determines the stage of the disease as a basis for treatment. The staging of the disease is done in a manner similar to that for the patient with Hodgkin's disease.

NURSING OBSERVATIONS

Non-Hodgkin's lymphomas are characterized by painless enlargement of the lymph nodes, fatigue, anorexia, weight loss, fever, sweating, pruritus, and enlargement of the spleen. Pressure on organs and organ obstruction may produce such symptoms as abdominal pain, nerve pain, or paralysis.

COMMON TREATMENT PLANS AND NURSING INTERVENTIONS

Radiotherapy usually is given to the individual with lymphoma. Chemotherapeutic agents used in the treatment of Hodgkin's disease also may be used for this person. The nursing care of the patient with leukemia is applicable to this individual also.

Infectious Mononucleosis

DESCRIPTION

Infectious mononucleosis, also known as "mono," or glandular fever, is a benign, self-limiting condition. It is caused by a herpes-like virus called the Epstein-Barr virus (EBV). The exact mode of transmission remains unknown. The greatest number of cases occurs in the 15- to 30-year age group.

COMMON DIAGNOSTIC STUDIES

Diagnosis is established by means of the heterophil agglutination test. The blood of patients with infectious mononucleosis contains antibodies that clump or agglutinate the red blood cells of sheep. Normal human beings do not produce agglutinins against sheep erythrocytes. The white blood cell count is elevated, including atypical lymphocytes.

NURSING OBSERVATIONS

The disease is characterized by a sore throat, painful enlargement of cervical lymph nodes, fever, and malaise.

Infectious mononucleosis is not a highly contagious disease. Transmission from one family member to another is rare. Hospital patients are not isolated, and other patients and personnel do not seem to acquire the disease. The infection is thought to be transmitted from one person to another by means of the secretions of the mouth and throat. However, repeated efforts to transmit it in this way have failed.

COMMON TREATMENT PLANS AND NURSING INTERVENTIONS

No specific treatment is known at this time. The disease usually is self-limiting. Symptomatic measures such as warm saline gargle for the sore throat and rest may be of

TABLE 13.5
OTHER CONDITIONS AFFECTING THE BLOOD/LYMPH

DISORDER	DESCRIPTION
Agranulocytosis (agranulocytic angina)	An abnormal decrease of the white blood cells, especially the neutrophils; a sensitivity to drugs or chemicals is a common cause; patient has symptoms of an acute bacterial invasion; treatment is directed toward removing the offending drug or chemical
Amyloidosis	Tissues of the liver, spleen, kidneys, and adrenal glands are infiltrated with an abnormal starchlike or proteinlike substance; symptoms depend upon the areas in which these complex substances are deposited; no treatment is known
Anemia associated with infection and chronic systemic diseases (simple chronic anemia)	Anemia in which the red blood cells are normal but are too few in number; occurs frequently during the course of other diseases such as chronic conditions of the kidney and liver, malignancy, arthritis, and leukemia; symptoms usually represent the underlying disease; therapy is directed toward the basic disease
Bacteremia (septicemia)	An infection of the bloodstream caused by bacteria; after determining the causative organism, the physician will order an appropriate antibiotic; bloodstream infections are most likely to be found in the aged person, the newborn, and the person with another serious illness such as leukemia, cirrhosis of the liver, or diabetes mellitus
Fat embolism	Fat globules that are carried by the bloodstream until they lodge in a blood vessel too small for them to pass. The fat globules are formed from liquid fat that is released from fat cells following crushing injuries to soft tissues and long bones; it may also follow closed cardiac massage
Gaucher's disease	A disease occurring in certain families in which abnormal cells are found in the liver, spleen, and bone marrow; pigmentation of the skin occurs and yellowish spots appear on the sclera
Multiple myeloma (plasma cell myeloma, myelomatosis)	Neoplastic disease of the plasma cells in which there is skeletal destruction, anemia, impaired kidney function, and susceptibility to infections; chemotherapy may lengthen patient's life.
Mycosis fungoides	A fatal disorder of reticuloendothelial system that starts first in the skin; eruptions of the skin are followed by plaque formations; as the disease progresses, tumors develop in the skin
Myelofibrosis with myeloid metaplasia	A disease characterized by fibrosis of the marrow that affects development of blood cells; it may occur without known cause or as result of involvement of bone marrow by such conditions as tuberculosis or Hodgkin's disease
Myelophthistic anemias	A group of anemias occurring when some other disease occupies the space in the bone marrow that normally produces erythrocytes; in other words, some other disease has caused its cells to invade the bone marrow; metastatic carcinoma is an example
Secondary polycythemias	Elevated erythrocyte count and level of hemoglobin associated with other conditions that cause an inadequate supply of blood to the tissue; the body reacts to this tissue hypoxia by increasing red blood cells and hemoglobin; chronic disease of the heart or lungs and certain neoplastic diseases are examples of conditions leading to secondary polycythemia
Sideroblastic anemias	A group of anemias characterized by the presence of certain types of cells in the bone marrow called *ringed sideroblasts*; cause is not known

benefit. Mild analgesics may be prescribed for discomfort. Cool water sponges may help to control fever. Fluid intake should be increased. Steroids are sometimes given.

Case Study Involving Anemia

Laura Robinson, a 16-year-old girl, was admitted to the local hospital with the complaints of tiredness and shortness of breath. Upon admission, she appeared pale and stated that she had anorexia. The laboratory report indicated that her erythrocyte count was 2.2 million/cu mm and hemoglobin 6 gm/100 ml. The physician's orders were:

- Complete blood count
- Gynecologic evaluation for menstrual irregularities
- Ferrous gluconate, 300 mg tid

QUESTIONS

1. What implications for nursing actions do Ms. Robinson's shortness of breath and tiredness have?
2. What relationship could shortness of breath and tiredness have to the low hemoglobin and erythrocyte count?
3. What principles should govern the nursing care provided for this patient?
4. What foods should Ms. Robinson be encouraged to eat in an effort to increase her dietary intake of iron?
5. When should ferrous gluconate be given?
6. What nursing implications related to the administration of ferrous gluconate are indicated?

Case Study Involving Leukemia

Mrs. Marilyn Metz, a 27-year-old divorcee and mother of two children, was admitted to the hospital with a diagnosis of acute leukemia. Upon admission, her hemoglobin was 6 gm, white blood count was 30,000, red blood cell count was normal, and platelet count was normal.

Mrs. Metz's two children are 7 and 9 years of age. They are staying with her parents while she is in the hospital.

QUESTIONS

1. Assuming that Mrs. Metz was told by her physician that she has leukemia, identify some of the specific concerns that she can be expected to have.
2. In what ways can the nursing staff help Mrs. Metz with some of her stated concerns?
3. The doctor ordered chemotherapy for Mrs. Metz. One of the drugs is vincristine. For what toxic symptoms should Mrs. Metz be observed? (Hint: See Chapter 9).
4. What nursing actions will help to minimize the toxic effects of vincristine?
5. The physician ordered 1 unit of packed red cells for Mrs. Metz. What are the responsibilities of the LPN/LVN in your agency regarding transfusion therapy?
6. Mrs. Metz had received 100 ml of the transfusion when she complained of itching. What immediate actions should be taken?
7. Describe the nursing measures indicated for Mrs. Metz for the prevention of infection, provision of skin and mouth care, and preservation of strength.

Suggestions for Further Study

1. What are the responsibilities of the LPN/LVN in your agency in relation to the diagnostic tests mentioned in this chapter?
2. What types of anemia have you known someone to have?
3. Why is a patient who is having a massive hemorrhage likely to develop shortness of breath?
4. Does the law allow the LPN/LVN in your state to do a venipuncture?
5. Mason, Mildred A.; Bates, Grace F.; and Smola, Bonnie K.; Workbook in Basic Medical-Surgical Nursing, 3rd ed. Macmillan Publishing Company, New York, 1984, Exercise 13.

Additional Readings

Griffiths, Mary: Human Physiology, 2nd ed. Macmillan Publishing Co., Inc., New York, 1981, pp. 150–57.

Hedlin, Anne: "Hemostasis and the Nature of Its Defect in Hemophilia." Canadian Nurse, 76: 15–17 (Dec.), 1980.

Iveson-Iveson, Joan: "Malaria." Nursing Mirror, 151:43 (Sept.), 1980.

Kenny, M.W.: "Sickle Cell Disease." Nursing Times, 76:1582–84 (Sept.), 1980.

Levitt, Doreen Zeh: "Multiple Myeloma." American Journal of Nursing, 81:1345–47 (July), 1981.

Robinson, Corinne H.: Basic Nutrition and Diet Therapy, 4th ed. Macmillan Publishing Co., Inc., New York, 1980, pp. 84-87.

Robinson, Corinne H., and Lawler, Marilyn R.: Normal and Therapeutic Nutrition, 16th ed. Macmillan Publishing Co., Inc., New York, 1982, pp. 511–19.

Sackheim, George I., and Lehman, Dennis D.:

Chemistry for the Health Sciences, 4th ed. Macmillan Publishing Co., Inc., New York, 1981, pp. 407–35.

Wroblewski, Sandra Sieler, and Wroblewski, Sheila Hainley: "Caring for the Patient with Chemotherapy-Induced Thrombocytopenia." *Journal of Practical Nursing*, 32:22–25 and 39 (Apr.), 1982.

Chapter 14

The Patient with a Disease of the Respiratory System

Expected Behavioral Outcomes

Minimum objectives referred to as expected behavioral outcomes have been designed for the practical/vocational nursing student to use as guides in studying this chapter. The student should read these expected outcomes before studying the chapter. The objectives can be used as guides for study.

Using the content of this chapter, the student should return to the objectives and evaluate the ability to:

1. *Demonstrate the normal pathway of oxygen and carbon dioxide through the respiratory system.*
2. *Describe each of the diagnostic tests as the nurse should explain them to a patient.*
3. *Describe nursing observations and measures that relate to the care of a patient with an infection of the bronchi and lungs.*
4. *Demonstrate at least three nursing interventions that reduce retained secretions in the tracheobronchial tree.*
5. *Describe at least four actions that reduce the spread of infection from infected sputum.*
6. *Compare nursing observations and measures related to the individual having a chest injury with those indicated for a person experiencing chest surgery.*
7. *Compare nursing observations and measures indicated for the individual with a temporary tracheostomy with those needed for a person with a laryngectomy.*

8. *Describe at least six nursing actions that help to allay anxiety for the patient with a respiratory disease.*
9. *Compare the patient teaching needed for a person with pulmonary tuberculosis with that needed by a person with COPD.*

Vocabulary Development

The following prefixes, suffixes, and combining forms pertain to this chapter. By learning and/or reviewing their meanings, the practical/vocational nursing student will have the keys needed to unlock many exciting new medical terms.

Discover the meaning of these keys in a medical dictionary or in the content of this chapter. How does each key pertain to this chapter? In your notebook write the correct meaning of each prefix, suffix, or combining form listed below. Illustrate each key with an example.

alve—trough, cavity. Ex. *alve*olar—a small saclike dilatation.

bronch-	pne-
cost-	pneum(at)-
epi-	pneumo(n)-
lal-	pulmo(n)-
laryng-	punct-
nas-	rhin-
pha-	sial-
pharynx-	sin-
phrag-	spirat-
phys(a)-	thorac-
physe-	trache-
pleur-	tuber-

Structure and Function

The respiratory system is a group of organs that provides for the exchange of gases, regulation of body heat, communication of sounds, and regulation of acid-alkaline balance within the body. All living cells within the body require an effective exchange of oxygen and carbon dioxide. Thus, the functions of the respiratory system are essential to life.

The organs that make respiration possible include the nose, pharynx (throat), larynx (voice box), and trachea (windpipe), which are located in the head and neck (see Figure 14.1). The bronchi and lungs are located in the thorax (chest), and bony protection is provided by the sternum, ribs, and vertebrae (see Figure 14.2). The space between the lungs is known as the mediastinum and contains the heart. The diaphragm is a respiratory muscle that separates the thoracic and abdominal cavities. Other important respiratory muscles are the intercostal muscles located in the chest.

The nose, pharynx, larynx, trachea, and bronchi are lined with mucous membrane and tiny hairlike projections, known as *cilia*, that trap particles and bacteria and sweep them upward, where they can be swallowed or expectorated.

The nose filters, warms, and moistens air entering from outside the body. The nose is divided by a septum (wall), which separates it into two cavities. Coarse hairs located in the nasal cavities help to trap large particles. The nose also contains olfactory organs, which are responsible for the sense of smell.

Four pairs of hollow cavities called sinuses are located in the head and drain mucus directly into the nose. They are the ethmoid, sphenoid, maxillary, and frontal sinuses. Sinuses give resonance to the voice.

After entering the nose, air passes into the *pharynx,* or throat. The pharynx generally is divided into three parts: the nasopharynx, the oropharynx, where the tonsils are located, and the laryngopharynx. The *larynx,* voice box, acts primarily as an airway between the pharynx above it and the *trachea* below it.

Behind the tongue and atop the larynx is a flaplike structure known as the epiglottis, which opens to let air pass through the larynx and into the trachea. The epiglottis closes over the larynx if food or foreign bodies are present, thus helping to prevent choking. Also, the larynx contains two vocal cords (folds), which vibrate as expired air passes over them. The vibrations produce sounds that are formed into words by struc-

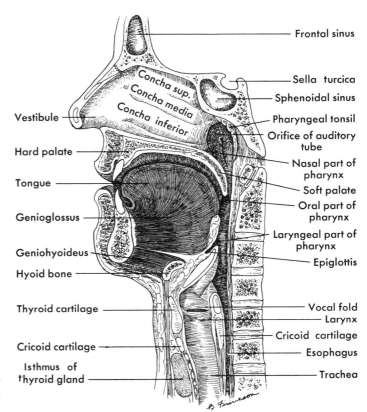

Frontal sinus

Sella turcica

Sphenoidal sinus

Pharyngeal tonsil

Orifice of auditory tube

Nasal part of pharynx

Soft palate

Oral part of pharynx

Laryngeal part of pharynx

Epiglottis

Vocal fold

Larynx

Cricoid cartilage

Esophagus

Trachea

Concha sup.
Concha media
Concha inferior

Vestibule

Hard palate

Tongue

Genioglossus

Geniohyoideus

Hyoid bone

Thyroid cartilage

Cricoid cartilage

Isthmus of thyroid gland

FIGURE 14.1 Sagittal section of the nose, mouth, and pharynx. (From Miller, Marjorie A.; Drakontides, Anna B.; and Leavell, Lutie C.: *Kimber-Gray-Stackpole's Anatomy and Physiology*, 17th ed. Macmillan Publishing Co., Inc., New York, 1977, page 421.)

tures such as the lips, teeth, tongue, and palate. Organs of the upper respiratory tract normally contain considerable *normal flora* such as *Staphylococci, Klebsiella, Pseudomonas, E. coli,* and *Proteus.*

The trachea is a tube about 11.2 cm (4½ in.) long and 2.5 cm (1 in.) wide in adults. Strong rings of highly elastic cartilage support the trachea. At the end of the trachea, the respiratory system divides into the right and left mainstem bronchi. Each structure is known as a bronchus and branches into smaller and smaller components that finally end in bronchioles, which are part of the lung itself. Each bronchiole supplies air to a cluster of tiny, highly elastic sacs known as *alveoli.* Alveoli are the working units of the lung. Oxygen and carbon dioxide are exchanged between the alveoli and the tiny capillaries that surround them. Oxygen-rich blood returns to the heart via the pulmonary veins and is pumped to all parts of the body.

Carbon dioxide and water vapor ascend the respiratory tract and are expired into the atmosphere. The process of gas exchange is known as *respiration.*

The right lung is slightly larger than the left lung and is divided into three lobes. The left lung contains only two lobes. Each lobe is further subdivided into segments. Each lung is covered by a tiny serous membrane called the *visceral pleura.* The thoracic cavity is also lined with a similar membrane called the *parietal pleura* (see Figure 14.3). A lubricating substance separates the two membranes and prevents friction between them. Organs of the lower respiratory tract, as well as the membranes around them, are normally sterile.

Ventilation is the process of taking air into the lungs (inspiration) and out of the lungs (expiration). Inspiration is made possible by the contraction of the muscles of the diaphragm and chest. Expiration is possible

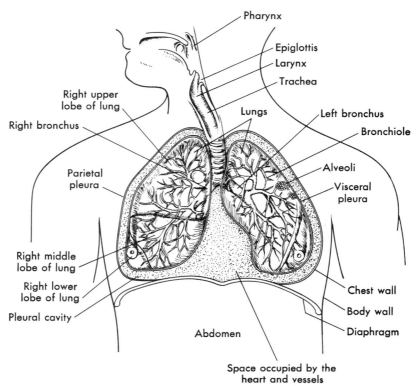

FIGURE 14.2 Lungs, showing the relative position in the chest cavity with the lungs cut away to show the bronchi and the details fo the alveoli.

because of the elastic recoil action of the lungs, which pushes air out. Compliance is a term that describes the elastic properties of lung tissue. Surfactant is a material se-

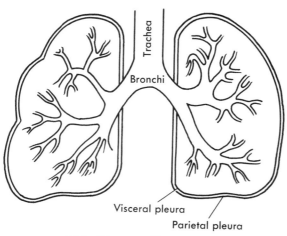

FIGURE 14.3 Diagram illustrating the two layers of pleura.

creted by certain alveoli that maintains surface tension and protects the alveoli from collapse during pressure changes.

The respiratory system has an extensive circulation including bronchial and pulmonary arteries and lymphatic vessels. The lymphatic system within the respiratory tract is believed to play a major role in transporting and removing lung fluid. In addition, certain lymphocytes and macrophages are abundant in the respiratory tract. Thus, the lymph system is important in the lung's immune response.

Several mechanisms control respiration. One is the respiratory center located in the medulla oblongata and lower pons in the brain. Another is chemoreceptor bodies in the aorta and carotid arteries that respond to changes in oxygen, carbon dioxide, and hydrogen ion levels in arterial blood and cerebrospinal fluid. A third mechanism is the phrenic nerves, which innervate the diaphragm, and the branches of the vagus nerve, which innervate much of the tracheo-bronchial tree as well as the larynx. The vagus nerve has three kinds of receptors located in the lung. These are stretch, irritant, and J receptors. The stretch receptors respond to variations in pressure. Irritant receptors are activated by contact with irritating particles. J receptors are stimulated by noxious chemicals, edema in the lungs, and microscopic clots which can clog the tiny lung capillaries.

Body heat and acid-alkaline balance are affected by the amount of water vapor and carbon dioxide that are expired during ventilation. Since respiration is a process that is essential to life, the correction of respiratory disorders is given a very high priority.

Assisting with Diagnostic Studies

PHYSICAL EXAMINATION

Physical examination of the chest and lungs provides the examiner with important information about a person's ability to exchange oxygen and carbon dioxide. The examiner is usually a physician but may be a professional nurse or a physician's assistant who has received special training. Physical examination is accomplished by four methods: inspection, palpation, percussion, and auscultation.

Inspection is the process of looking for abnormalities in the head, neck, and chest. *Palpation* is a method of touching and feeling for abnormalities. *Percussion* is a process of tapping the chest with the fingers, setting up vibrations in the thorax and underlying structures. *Auscultation* is a process of listening to sounds. A stethoscope is used to listen to the sounds of breathing.

Breath sounds are caused by the movement of air within the respiratory passages. *Rales* are abnormal breath sounds caused by the passage of air over fluid. The nurse may see these terms when reading the chart of a patient with a respiratory disorder.

X-RAY AND FLUOROSCOPIC EXAMINATION

The roentgenogram (x-ray) of the chest is a still picture of the lungs (see Figure 14.4). Air in the lungs is visible in the picture and outlines lung tissue. The size of the heart can also be ascertained from the chest x-ray. X-rays may be taken from several different positions in order to get a complete picture of lung tissue.

Fluoroscopic examination allows the roentgenologist (radiologist) to view the thorax and lungs in motion.

X-ray examination of the chest is one of the most frequently ordered x-rays. An x-ray often demonstrates the presence of disease long before a person experiences symptoms. For this reason, some employers require periodic x-rays of the chest for all employees. Hospitals often require a chest x-ray for all newly admitted patients. Some communities have x-ray units located in portable vans that visit neighborhoods and screen residents for respiratory disorders.

For a chest x-ray, the patient wears a loose-fitting drape or gown without pins or metal fasteners since metal is visible in the picture and may obscure lung tissue. The nurse should instruct the person to remove necklaces, brassieres, or slips. The hospitalized patient may need a robe or blanket as protection from drafts in the x-ray department. If the patient cannot be transported to the x-ray department, a portable x-ray machine can be wheeled to the bedside. The nurse may need to assist the x-ray technician to position the patient so that an acceptable picture can be obtained. Usually, the nurse leaves the room while the picture is being taken in order to avoid unnecessary exposure to x-rays. Nurses who must remain at the bedside while roentgenograms are being made should wear protective lead aprons. If the nurse is pregnant and assistance is needed during the x-ray procedure, she should ask another person to remain at the bedside and she should leave the room.

TOMOGRAMS

Body section roentgenograms are special x-ray films taken at different levels or planes of the lungs until the area being studied comes clearly into view from a variety of positions. Depending on the method used to obtain the film, they may be known as *tomograms, laminograms,* or *planigrams.* These special x-rays are particularly helpful in de-

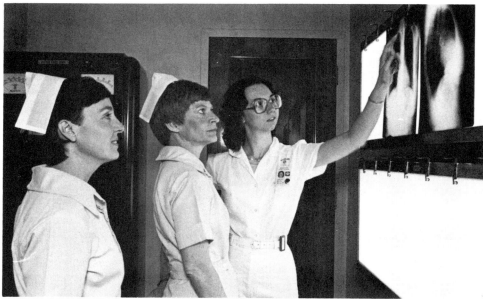

FIGURE 14.4   Looking at x-rays of the lungs. (Courtesy of Bergen Pines County Hospital School of Practical Nursing, Paramus, New Jersey.)

termining the exact location of tumors or other lesions in the lung.

COMPUTED TOMOGRAMS OF THORAX

Computerized tomogram of the thorax (CAT scan, CT scan) is an important new tool whose use is expected to increase in diagnosing diseases in the respiratory system. General information about CT scan can be located in Chapter 4.

A scan may be ordered by the physician to detect or evaluate abnormalities in large blood vessels in the chest, cysts on the pericardium, and lesions in the mediastinum. In addition, the test helps the physician to locate both benign and malignant tumors. Occupational and drug-induced lung diseases may be detected before the patient experiences symptoms. CT scans also may assist the physician in correct needle placement for biopsies and thoracentesis.

When scanning is limited to the thorax, the time needed is generally less than a minute. Most patients are able to hold their breath during the scanning so that the images produced are clear. The need to lie in a supine position may be difficult for a patient who is experiencing dyspnea. In some cases, the head is elevated slightly for the patient's comfort. The patient wears clothing similar to that for a chest x-ray.

The radiologist generally reads and interprets the scan on the same day. This information is then made available to the patient's physician.

SPUTUM EXAMINATION

Sputum is material that is raised from the tracheobronchial tree by coughing. After the nurse assists the person to raise and collect the sputum, the container is correctly labeled and sent to the laboratory. Complete labeling information includes the source of the specimen, the purpose if known, method of collection, and current drug therapy which might affect results. Steroids, immunosuppressives, and antibiotics are examples of drugs that greatly affect results of sputum examination. When sputum has been induced, the method used should be noted on the label. Sputum specimens should be transported to the laboratory promptly after collection.

Trained technicians then examine the sputum for tumor cells (cytology) or pathogenic microorganisms. Some of the common tests ordered to determine the presence of pathogens in the sputum are smear, acid-fast bacilli (AFB), and culture and sensitivities. Sensitivities are usually done when pathogens are found in sputum. This test helps the physician to select the most effective antimicrobial drug. (Refer to Tables 5.7 and 5.8, pages 99 and 103.)

Sputum specimens are usually collected in the early morning, upon arising. Repeated examination on successive or alternate days may be ordered. The nurse should instruct the patient the night before to rinse the mouth with clear water prior to the collection. Patients are advised to raise the sputum from the chest instead of the mouth. A wide-mouth container should be placed at the bedside. If sputum is to be collected for culture, the container must be sterile and no one should touch the inside of the container or its cover.

The patient who is having difficulty raising sputum may find it helpful to take several deep breaths and then try to cough. If this is unsuccessful, the physician may order warmed saline-moistened air from a nebulizer in order to stimulate the production of sputum from the tracheobronchial tree. This method is sometimes referred to as *induced sputum collection*.

Occasionally, the physician may request a quantitative analysis of sputum on the amount of material raised by the patient over a 24-hour period or longer. A covered container is kept at the bedside in a paper bag or other similar wrapper. After the physician visits, the amount, color, odor, and consistency of sputum are recorded, and a new container is placed at the bedside if the collection is to be continued. The nurse instructs the patient to cough all sputum into the container at the bedside.

Persons who are raising sputum need extra tissues at the bedside and a conveniently located bag to discard used tissues. Frequent oral hygiene also is needed, although toothpaste and/or mouthwash should not be used prior to sputum collection for laboratory analysis.

When sputum has been ordered for culture and the physician has also prescribed a new antibiotic, the nurse collects the specimen prior to administering the first dose of the new drug. Even one dose of antibiotic can alter the outcome of laboratory sensitivity tests. If the patient is unable to raise sputum, the nurse should contact the physician before beginning the antibiotic. The physician may wish to induce sputum collection.

GASTRIC WASHINGS

Sometimes a person is unable to raise sputum. Since cells from the respiratory tract may be swallowed, an examination of the stomach contents may show malignant cells or pathogenic microorganisms.

To obtain gastric washings, a nasogastric tube is inserted prior to breakfast after the patient has fasted for eight or more hours. Sterile distilled water is sometimes instilled into the tube to facilitate removal of gastric contents. A sterile syringe is used to gently withdraw gastric fluid. The fluid is placed in a sterile, covered container and sent to the laboratory for examination. The nasogastric tube is then removed, and the patient can eat breakfast. The insertion of a nasogastric tube is generally unpleasant and uncomfortable for the patient. The experience may be made tolerable by the nurse's explanation that the tube remains in place only until the specimen is collected.

Labeling information pertinent to the collection of sputum applies to specimens of gastric washings also.

NOSE AND THROAT CULTURES

The nurse may be asked to obtain material from the nose and/or throat for culture.

Many bacteria are normally present in the nose and throat. They are called *normal flora*. However, some microorganisms, including the ones that cause tuberculosis, diphtheria, and streptococcal pharyngitis, are not normally present. The physician uses the information obtained from the culture to determine if the organisms present are related to the person's illness.

Cultures from the nose and throat are obtained by swabbing the area with a sterile cotton applicator or swab. The nurse should use a tongue depressor when collecting material from the throat in order to be certain that material is being obtained from the posterior pharynx. The swab is then carefully placed in a sterile culture tube. In some cases, it may be necessary to break off the end of the applicator that the nurse has held in order to prevent contamination of the culture tube with the nurse's own microorganisms.

Labeling information appropriate to sputum collection applies also to nose and throat cultures.

PULMONARY FUNCTION TEST (PFT)

Studies can be done to evaluate the ventilation capability of the lungs. Ventilation is the movement of air in and out of the lungs. Table 14.1 contains a list of common measurements of pulmonary function. Other measurements of pulmonary function include pulmonary compliance, timed vital capacity, oxygen uptake, carbon dioxide output, and forced vital capacity. Measurements may be obtained directly or extrapolated mathematically from other measurements.

One of the most common pulmonary function tests is called spirometry. Measurements are obtained by breathing through a mouthpiece into a device called a spirometer, a floating drum that moves up and down with changes in pressure. Pressure changes are recorded on a graph (spirogram). Nose clips may be placed over the patient's nares to ensure that all inspired and expired air passes only through the mouth so that it can be recorded on the spirogram.

Pulmonary function tests are not painful but may be very tiring to a patient with respiratory disease. Some measurements may be taken several times in order to obtain accurate results. Usually, smoking and bronchodilator medications are prohibited before these tests. No other special preparation is needed after the test has been explained.

BLOOD GAS ANALYSIS

An analysis of the important gases in arterial blood is a valuable indicator of respiration. Respiration is the exchange of gases, primarily oxygen and carbon dioxide. Factors influencing respiration that can be measured by this test include the rate of cellular metabolism, ability of hemoglobin to transport oxygen, and acid-base balance.

If an arterial catheter is not already in place, the physician or technologist will obtain the needed blood sample using a needle and a syringe containing a small amount of an anticoagulant, called heparin. After the sample is collected, the syringe is capped and may be placed on ice and sent immediately to the laboratory for analysis. Air bubbles in the blood sample are avoided since they affect the results. Fever and supplemental ogygen also influence results. Therefore the patient's temperature and percentage of inspired oxygen are important parts of complete labeling information.

Common sites for obtaining arterial blood samples include the brachial, radial, and femoral arteries. Following arterial puncture, the nurse may be asked to apply pressure to the arterial site. Continuous pressure is applied for five full minutes in order to prevent bleeding. When the patient is receiving anticoagulant therapy, the time needed for continuous pressure may increase to ten or more minutes.

Analysis of arterial blood gases gives the physician a moment-by-moment picture of the effectiveness of a patient's respiration. Therefore, the nurse can expect that frequent analysis of arterial blood gases will be needed in any conditions where respiration is compromised. Such conditions might include respiratory or cardiac insufficiency or arrest, head injuries, hemorrhage, diabetic acidosis, asthma.

Repeated arterial punctures cause considerable discomfort to the patient. The nurse may prevent some of the discomfort by noting the puncture site so that a subse-

TABLE 14.1
COMMON MEASUREMENTS OF
PULMONARY FUNCTION

Tidal volume—the amount of air expired while breathing normally

Total lung capacity—the amount of air in the lungs at peak inspiration

Residual volume—the amount of air remaining in the lungs following a maximum expiration

Vital capacity—the maximum amount of air that can be expired following a maximum inspiration

quent analysis can be obtained from a different site. When possible, the patient is encouraged and assisted to exercise the extremities so that blood flow is increased. Pulse, skin temperature, and skin color may be observed to detect impaired circulation.

Table 14.2 describes the normal values of blood gas analysis.

LUNG SCAN

The flow of blood through the tiny blood vessels within the lung can be demonstrated by the inhalation and/or injection of radioactive isotopes of certain chemicals. When the injected or inhaled isotopes reach the small lung vessels, a scanning device is used to record the concentration and distribution of the radioactive material, making a kind of map. Blood vessels obstructed by disease do not permit entry of the radioactive isotope. Thus, an uneven map helps the physician to diagnose respiratory disorders that involve the small lung vessels. No special preparation is needed for a lung scan after the procedure has been explained to the patient.

PULMONARY ECHOGRAM

Ultrasound waves are transmitted to the lungs and reflected back to a special receiver, which records the reflected waves or "echoes." By analyzing the waves, an expert can detect abnormal fluid in the lungs that may not be evident in other studies. The test is not painful, and no special preparation is needed after it has been explained to the patient.

PULMONARY ANGIOGRAM

The pulmonary blood vessels can be seen by injecting radiopaque dye into a catheter which has been threaded through a vein into the pulmonary artery via the right and left ventricles. After the catheter is properly positioned, a contrast dye is injected and a series of x-rays is taken. This technique helps to detect structural defects and abnormal lesions including tumors, blebs, and emboli in the lungs.

Pulmonary angiogram involves potential risk to the patient from problems associated with positioning the catheter or using the contrast dye. The patient is monitored continuously for cardiac arrhythmias and closely observed for untoward reactions to the medications used. Patient preparation includes a discussion of the potential risk and a signed consent for the procedure. This is usually the physician's responsibility. The nurse may tell the patient to anticipate a temporary hot flash and a possible cough after the dye has been injected.

Following pulmonary angiogram, the patient is observed for unstable vital signs which may indicate a delayed reaction to the local anesthetic or contrast dye. An irregular pulse may indicate irritability of the myocardium to the catheter. The catheter site is inspected for evidence of bleeding. In addition, skin temperature, pulse, and color of the arm distal to the catheter site are observed for impaired circulation.

BRONCHOSCOPY

Bronchoscopy is the inspection of the bronchial tree using a long, hollow, lighted instrument called a bronchoscope. The bronchoscope is passed through the mouth and into the respiratory passages. By looking through the bronchoscope the physician can examine air passages, remove secretions and tissue specimens for laboratory examination, remove foreign bodies from air passageways, and remove excessive secretions that may be blocking airways. In other words, bronchoscopy may be therapeutic as well as diagnostic. In some cases, bronchoscopy may be done on an emergency basis to clear an obstructed airway.

Food and fluids are withheld for eight or more hours prior to bronchoscopy, and oral hygiene is given as part of the preparation. Dentures are removed and stored safely. The patient usually receives a sedative and atropine before going to the operating room

TABLE 14.2
BLOOD GAS ANALYSIS: NORMAL VALUES

pO_2—the pressure of oxygen	85–100 mm Hg
pCO_2—the pressure of carbon dioxide	38–42 mm Hg
Saturation—percentage of hemoglobin that is carrying oxygen	97%
pH—acidity or alkalinity of blood sample	7.38–7.42

where the bronchoscopy is done. During the procedure, the patient lies on the back with the neck hyperextended to facilitate passing the bronchoscope.

Before introducing the bronchoscope, respiratory passages are sprayed with a topical anesthesia to prevent coughing and gagging. Since some persons are allergic to certain topical anesthetic agents, allergies should be prominently recorded on the patient's chart.

Following bronchoscopy, the patient is allowed to rest. Food and fluids are not given until the gag reflex returns. The patient may have a sore throat and hoarseness for several days after the examination. If a biopsy has been obtained, there may be small amounts of blood in the sputum for several days. Generally, an increase in sputum production can be expected as a result of tissue injury during the procedure.

Symptoms of difficult breathing may indicate excessive swelling or spasm of airways and should be reported immediately. Crackling puffiness (subcutaneous emphysema) visible around the face and neck indicates possible perforation of airways and should be reported immediately.

Nursing measures such as warm, soothing liquids and an ice collar may be used to relieve a sore throat.

BRONCHOGRAM

A bronchogram is an x-ray of the bronchi and bronchioles that is taken after a radiopaque dye has been instilled through a catheter inserted through the nose or mouth. A bronchogram is usually done in the x-ray department. During the bronchogram, the patient's position may be changed several times to let the dye move through the many respiratory passages.

Preparation of the patient for bronchogram is similar to that for bronchoscopy. Some persons have found it helpful to practice breathing through the nose when the catheter is to be inserted by way of the mouth. Practicing breathing through the mouth may be helpful when the catheter is to be inserted through the nose.

Food and fluids are withheld, dentures removed, and oral hygiene administered. After checking to be sure a consent form has

been signed, the nurse administers atropine and a sedative in the dosage prescribed. Air passages are sprayed with topical anesthesia by the physician.

Following bronchogram, food and fluids are withheld until the gag reflex returns. Certain positions may be specified by the physician in order to facilitate drainage of the dye from the bronchial tree. The sputum may look milky or chalky from the dye. Sometimes, follow-up x-rays are taken hours or days later.

Observations and nursing measures appropriate to the care of a patient following bronchoscopy apply to this patient. In addition, the physician may order aerosol therapy to help remove the dye from the lungs.

This procedure also involves risk to the patient from an untoward reaction to the topical anesthesia, spasm of the airways as the bronchoscope is manipulated, and tissue injury during the procedure. These risks are explained to the patient by the physician, and a consent for the procedure is signed.

Since the patient is awake during bronchoscopy, prior instruction and support may reduce the anxiety and discomfort. Some patients have found it helpful to breathe through the nose while the bronchoscope is passed through the mouth. When practiced in advance, the patient actively participates in reducing anxiety and discomfort.

LARYNGOSCOPY

Indirect laryngoscopy is an examination of the larynx using a lighted mirror that is held in the pharynx. Usually, the patient is sitting very erect and the tongue is grasped firmly with a gauze square. The patient may be instructed to pant or breathe normally during the procedure in order to prevent gagging.

Direct laryngoscopy is an examination of the larynx using a hollow lighted instrument called a laryngoscope. In some cases, direct laryngoscopy is an emergency procedure needed to extract a foreign body that is obstructing an airway. In other cases, direct laryngoscopy is needed to insert a special tube through the nose or mouth (nasotracheal and endotracheal tubes) into the trachea to establish or maintain a patent airway, to remove retained secretions from the tracheobronchial tree, or to administer anesthesia. In these cases, the procedure is referred to as *nasotracheal* or *endotracheal intubation.* Since emergency laryngoscopy and intubation may save a person's life, the nurse will find a laryngoscope and a variety of different-sized endotracheal tubes located with other emergency equipment in the hospital. In a nonemergency situation, patient preparation is similar to that for bronchoscopy, including written consent.

Following direct laryngoscopy, the patient should be observed for restlessness, apprehension, swelling of the throat or neck, dyspnea, or stridor. These observations may indicate excessive bleeding, swelling, or spasm of the airways and should be reported promptly.

THORACENTESIS

Thoracenteis is a procedure in which a needle is used to puncture the chest wall and space between the two pleura so that fluid and air can be withdrawn. Fluid withdrawn from the pleural space is sent to the laboratory for examination.

Thoracentesis is also done when breathing has been impaired due to excessive accumulation of fluid in the pleural space. This is a therapeutic use of thoracentesis.

Sometimes, during thoracentesis, a needle biopsy of the pleural tissue is obtained for laboratory examination. This is called a *pleural biopsy.* When a pleural biopsy is planned, a special needle is needed in addition to the usual thoracentesis t-ray.

Prior to thoracentesis, the patient usually has a chest x-ray to determine the exact location of the fluid. Patient preparation includes an explanation of the procedure, a signed consent, and instructions not to move during certain parts of the procedure. Since a local anesthetic is injected under the skin, any allergies should be prominently recorded and reported.

The nurse positions the patient either in a chair or in a sitting position at the side of the bed. Arms are slightly elevated, bent at the elbow, and supported by a pillow on the overbed table. After cleansing the area with an antiseptic solution and asking the patient about allergies, the physician injects a local anesthetic. Some patients report feeling a burning sensation while the anesthetic is being injected. The thoracentesis needle is then inserted between the ribs and fluid is withdrawn using a large syringe and a three-way stopcock. Fluid is removed slowly and gently in order to avoid a rapid shift of fluid in the thoracic cavity. Usually, the physician does not remove more than 1200 to 1500 ml of fluid for the same reason.

During the thoracentesis, the nurse continuously observes the patient's pulse, respirations, and color and reports significant changes to the physician. In addition, the nurse supports the patient by providing a continuous calm commentary about the progress being made and what comes next. This commentary reduces the likelihood that the patient will be surprised and move unexpectedly at the wrong moment.

After the fluid has been removed, a dry sterile dressing is usually placed over the puncture site.

Signs of respiratory distress or leakage of fluid at the puncture site are reported to the physician at once. Usually, a chest x-ray is ordered after a thoracentesis. The amount, color, odor, and consistency of the fluid are recorded on the chart, as well as the patient's response to the procedure.

SKIN TESTS

Skin tests are done by injecting a small amount of a substance intracutaneously and observing subsequent skin reactions to the injection site. Skin tests may help to establish the source of an allergy or respiratory infection such as tuberculosis, diphtheria, or fungi.

When the nurse administers a skin test, a marking pen is used to show the location of skin test sites, and the patient is instructed not to wash the markings off until the test has been read. A raised white wheal that persists for several minutes after the injection means that the substance has been properly injected. The skin reaction is measured in millimeters of induration (hardness) around the injection site.

BLOOD TESTS

In addition to examining certain aspects of arterial blood, described earlier in this chapter, the physician may order a variety of tests on venous blood. A CBC (complete blood count) provides the physician with information about the number of red blood cells available to carry oxygen, as well as the number and differential of white blood cells involved in body defenses. Table 13.1 describes normal values for these tests. Serum electrolytes may become unbalanced during respiratory diseases. The nurse can anticipate that these common blood tests will be ordered frequently both to assist in diagnosis and evaluate the patient's response to therapy.

Nursing Observations

Nursing observations help the patient's recovery, prevent complications, and help the physician to evaluate the patient's response to illness and treatment. In addition, complete and accurate nursing observations form the basis for selecting those nursing interventions most likely to be effective.

Systematic nursing observation is more likely to result in complete and accurate information. A systematic method used in this chapter is to use the guide provided in Table 1.1, page 12. The nurse observes by looking, listening, touching, smelling, and asking questions. An essential component of good observation is recording and reporting.

A special feature of observing the patient with a respiratory disorder is the need for adequate lighting during evening and night hours in order to detect subtle but important changes in the patient's condition.

EYES

The patient with a respiratory disorder may have excessive tearing of the eyes, as in the common cold or an allergic reaction. Cyanosis in dark-skinned persons may be observed in the conjunctiva of the eyes.

NOSE

A person with dyspnea may show flaring of the nostrils with each inspiration. There may be mucus-like drainage from the nose. Epistaxis, or nosebleed, may occur. Nursing measures related to the care of the patient with epistaxis are discussed later in this chapter.

MOUTH

Some persons are mouth breathers; that is, air is inspired and expired through the mouth instead of the nose. Sometimes nasal passages are obstructed by disease, which necessitates breathing through the mouth. The person with difficult breathing may exhibit pursed lip breathing, especially on expiration.

Mucous membranes may be sticky or dry. The mouth is a good place to look for cyanosis or bluish tinge to the skin, which results from inadequate oxygen in the tissues. Mucous membranes inside the mouth look bluish gray when cyanosis is present. This is especially important to look for in a person who has dark skin.

The mouth can also be the source of infection in the lower respiratory tract from overgrowth of normal flora. Erythema (redness), warmth, drainage, and a foul odor in the mouth, gums, or teeth should be recorded and reported.

COUGH

The person with a cough has a forceful involuntary expiration of air following a deep inspiration. This is caused by the buildup of pressure against the closed glottis during expiration. Cough is one of the most common symptoms associated with a respiratory disorder. Coughing generally indicates irritation within the respiratory tract but occasionally may be related to a nervous habit. Irritating substances such as food particles, smoke, dust, or chemicals may cause coughing. Diseases such as bronchitis, lung tumor, or pneumonia can also cause coughing. A cough that persists for longer than two weeks is one of the danger signals of cancer which should cause a person to seek medical attention.

A cough may be productive (sputum is raised) or nonproductive, shallow or deep, and may have a variety of sounds such as dry, rattling, croupy, or hacking. The nurse should record the type of cough, amount, color, consistency, and odor of sputum if present. Usually, coughing is desirable since it rids the respiratory tract of irritating substances and secretions. Efforts are directed toward helping the patient cough more ef-

TABLE 14.3
DRUGS USED TO LIQUEFY BRONCHIAL SECRETIONS AND PROMOTE EXPECTORATION

NONPROPRIETARY NAME	TRADE NAME	AVERAGE DOSE	NURSING IMPLICATIONS
Acetylcysteine, N.F.	MUCOMYST	3–5 ml of 20% solution inhaled	May produce bronchospasm, nausea, and vomiting
Ammonium chloride		500 mg	
Guaifenesin	ROBITUSSIN	5–10 ml	No foods or liquids after swallowing
Hydriodic acid syrup			
Pancreatic dornase	DORNAVAC	200,000 units inhaled	
Potassium iodide		300–mg tablet	Gastric disturbances and diarrhea

fectively. Drugs such as those listed in Table 14.3 may help the patient raise sputum by making it thinner. Proper positioning and other measures to promote effective coughing are described later in the chapter.

Occasionally, it is not desirable to cough. When coughing is related to a nervous habit, hemoptysis (bloody cough), or when the cough center in the brain becomes irritated due to other disease, the physician may prescribe one of the drugs listed in Table 14.4 to suppress the cough.

The person who is coughing should be instructed to cough into several layers of tissue (see Figure 14.5) and dispose of used tissues in a receptacle provided such as a paper bag. When caring for a person who is coughing, the nurse should avoid being in the direct line of cough and practice meticulous hand washing before and after each encounter with the patient.

HICCUP

Hiccup is an involuntary spasm of the muscles of inspiration. The glottis then closes quickly, making the familiar sound. Normal persons sometimes hiccup after eating or drinking. But the hiccup also can be a sign of disease. Some of the conditions that are associated with hiccup are pleurisy, peritonitis, uremia, and brain lesions. Usually, hiccup does not last very long and can be relieved by drinking cold water, holding the breath, or breathing into a paper bag. Occasionally, the hospitalized patient has persistent hiccup due to illness. The physician may prescribe chlorpromazine, 25 to 50 mg intravenously, for relief.

HEMOPTYSIS

Hemoptysis is the expectoration of blood from the respiratory tract. The color of ex-

TABLE 14.4
ANTITUSSIVES

NONPROPRIETARY NAME	TRADE NAME	AVERAGE DOSE	NURSING IMPLICATIONS
I. Narcotic Antitussives with Central Action			
Codeine phosphate		10–30 mg	Nausea and vomiting, sedation
Hydrocodone bitartrate	HYCODAN	5–10 mg	Overuse may result in physical dependence
II. Nonnarcotic Antitussives with Central Action			
Benzonatate	TESSALON	100 mg	May mask cough as a sign of disease
Dextromethorphan hydrobromide	ROMILAR	15–30 mg	
Levopropoxyphrene	NOVRAD	50–100 mg	
Noscapine	NECTADON	15–30 mg	

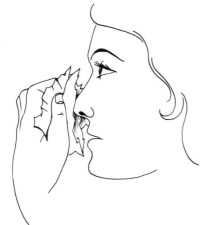

FIGURE 14.5 The patient should cover the mouth with a tissue when coughing.

pectoration may be bright red, brownish, or rusty. The expectoration may also be foamy in appearance. Hemoptysis may occur in pneumonia, lung abcess, tuberculosis, heart failure and lung cancer.

The observation of hemoptysis should be reported to the physician. The patient should also be observed for other signs of excessive bleeding such as pallor, cool and clammy skin, tachycardia, hypotension, restlessness, and apprehension. A complete description of the patient's expectoration is reported and recorded. The patient may be positioned to prevent aspiration of blood to unaffected areas of the lung. As mentioned previously, hemoptysis is one instance in which coughing generally is not desirable since it may increase bleeding. Antitussives may be prescribed to reduce cough. Table 14.4 contains a list of common antitussives that may be prescribed by the physician.

EARLOBES

The earlobes may appear pale, grayish, or bluish if cyanosis is present.

HOARSENESS

A person who has a rough, harsh, grating sound in the voice is said to be hoarse. Upper respiratory infections such as the common cold are sometimes accompanied by hoarseness. Hoarseness also can be a symptom of more serious disease such as cancer. Persist-

ent hoarseness is one of the seven warning signals listed by the American Cancer Society.

RESPIRATIONS

Observation of the client's respiratory rate and pattern is a very important nursing responsibility. Since respiration is essential to life, the respiratory rate is one of the vital signs. Each respiration consists of an inspiration and an expiration. Normally, an adult breathes 16 to 20 times per minute. Many factors can influence the rate of respiration such as exercise, body temperature, emotional state, drugs, and illness. Components of a complete observation of respirations include counting the rate, describing the pattern, and looking for aspects of breathing difficulty.

APNEA. Apnea is a temporary cessation of breathing. The nurse reports periods of apnea and notes the time interval.

BIOT'S BREATHING. This type of abnormal breathing pattern is characterized by uniform deep gasps, followed by a period of apnea, followed by more deep gasps. The patient with lesions in the brain area responsible for regulating the breathing pattern may demonstrate this type of breathing.

CHEYNE-STOKES RESPIRATION. Cheyne-Stokes respiration is an abnormal breathing pattern characterized by gradually increasing snoring respirations—followed by gradually decreasing respirations—followed by a period of apnea before the next cycle begins. This abnormal breathing pattern may be observed in patients with brain injury, kidney failure, heart disease, or other critical conditions. In addition, this breathing pattern may be considered normal for certain patients with chronic lung disease. When Cheyne-Stokes respirations are recognized in a patient, the nurse must count the respiratory rate for a full minute in order to obtain an accurate measurement.

DYSPNEA. The person who has dyspnea has difficult, labored, or painful respirations. The patient is very aware that breathing is difficult and may experience a sensation of smothering and feelings of anxiety and fear.

Dyspnea that wakes a person up at night is called nocturnal dyspnea. Dyspnea that causes a person to sit up to breathe is called *orthopnea*. The patient may experience dyspnea only on exertion or when at rest. It is important to record the characteristics of the patient's dyspnea. Another helpful piece of information is how many words the patient can say without taking a breath.

Dyspnea may be a symptom of obstruction in the respiratory tract, lung disease, heart disease, anemia, or anxiety.

STRIDOR. Stridor is a noisy type of respiration caused by air being forced through an abnormally narrow passage. Partial obstruction of the larynx or trachea by edema or foreign body can cause stridor. The nurse should observe and record whether there is stridor on inspiration, expiration, or both. Stridor may indicate the need for emergency measures to improve the patient's airway.

HYPERVENTILATION. A person who breathes abnormally deep and fast is hyperventilating. The patient may experience dizziness, tingling, lightheadedness, or fainting. Symptoms result from the rapid depletion of carbon dioxide, which is eliminated during expiration. Hyperventilation is sometimes associated with a high level of emotional stress but can also be a sign of more serious conditions such as acidosis or central nervous system disorders. When emotional stress is associated with hyperventilation, the person may be relieved by breathing into a paper bag. In other words, the person is rebreathing expired carbon dioxide from the bag.

HYPOVENTILATION. A person who breathes abnormally slowly is unable to exchange enough oxygen and carbon dioxide to meet normal body demands. This abnormal breathing pattern may result from drugs that depress the respiratory centers in the brain, injuries and diseases affecting the brain, and injuries and diseases that affect the respiratory muscles such as the diaphragm and intercostals. When hypoventilation is observed, the nurse also looks for other evidence of oxygen deprivation. Hypoventilation is reported immediately to the physician so that measures to improve gas exchange can be started promptly.

SKIN AND EXTREMITIES

Observation of nailbeds may reveal peripheral cyanosis. Excessive dryness or moistness of the skin may accompany certain respiratory disorders. Clubbing of the fingers or toes usually indicates that the person has had hypoxia for a long time.

Hairlessness of the skin also may indicate long-term hypoxia. Edema of the legs and feet can indicate impaired cardiac, kidney, or respiratory function. Brown stains on the fingers of the dominant hand may indicate a long-standing cigarette habit. Reddened areas and calluses on the patient's elbows may indicate leaning on the elbows, a characteristic of postural changes associated with chronic impaired breathing conditions. Postural changes are described later in this section.

CHEST

The patient's neck and chest may show evidence of breathing impairment. Retractions occur when muscles are abnormally sucked in during inspiration. The three areas that may retract during difficult breathing can be located above the clavicles (supraclavicular, under the sternum (substernal), and the intercostal muscles. Discoordinated chest movement may be observed.

ABDOMEN

Because the abdominal cavity lies below the thoracic cavity, the patient's abdomen affects and is affected by disturbances in the respiratory system. For example, when a patient breathes abnormally fast, an increased amount of air may be swallowed. Large amounts of swallowed air can result in abdominal distention (enlargement). Abdominal distention exerts pressure on the diaphragm above it and may restrict the patient's inspiration. Fluid in the peritoneal cavity (ascites) and fat can have a similar effect. Severe unrelieved abdominal pain may cause the patient to restrict ventilation voluntarily in order to reduce abdominal movements which aggravate pain. Thus, the nurse observes and records pertinent facts about the patient's abdomen.

SACRUM

Edema in the area just above the sacrum may indicate impaired cardiac, renal, or respiratory function.

POSTURE

The patient with a respiratory condition that has persisted for a long time gradually makes changes in posture in order to improve breathing and reduce the work of breathing. A characteristic posture is elevation of the shoulders and leaning on the elbows while in sitting position.

PAIN

Disorders of the respiratory system often cause pain. The nurse uses listening skills to determine the location, duration, and description of the pain. Some descriptions of pain which patients have reported include knifelike, catch or stitch in the side, deep aching, and raw, burning sensations. The nurse also asks whether the pain is related to an event such as coughing, inspiration, expiration, or turning. Pain in the chest also indicates possible myocardial infarction. Therefore the nurse's observations about the patient's pain are recorded in the patient's own words whenever possible.

The physician prescribes pain medicine cautiously for patients with a respiratory disorder since many analgesics depress the central nervous system and the respiratory centers located in the brain. However, measures to relieve pain are very important in circumstances when the patient's active participation is needed to ambulate or cough up retained secretions.

BEHAVIOR

The brain is very sensitive to the levels of oxygen and carbon dioxide in the bloodstream. Changes in behavior of the person with a respiratory disorder are often the earliest sign that brain tissue is being affected by hypoxia (inadequate oxygen) or hypercapnea (excessive carbon dioxide). When recording behavioral changes in the chart, the nurse should record what the person actually said or did that was unusual. Words such as "confused" have a variety of meanings to the reader. Lethargy, drowsiness, anxiety, fatigue, irritability, and restlessness are behavioral changes associated with impaired respiratory function.

When a change in the patient's behavior is noted, the nurse should listen carefully and ask appropriate questions before deciding that the behavior is unusual. A practice to be avoided is rapidly drawing conclusions about a person's behavior before collecting all the facts. An interaction to obtain facts about the patient's change in behavior can be initiated by the nurse simply by describing the observed behavior to the patient in a matter of fact way, and characterizing the behavior as either unusual or different from the usual. This approach very often encourages the patient to explain the behavior and the important facts can be discovered.

Nursing and Other Therapeutic Interventions

A variety of nursing and other therapeutic interventions is available for the nurse to use in promoting comfort, relieving symptoms, and improving the patient's respiratory function. Knowledge of the individual patient, the disease condition, and available nursing interventions enables the nurse to develop and implement an effective nursing care plan.

HYGIENE

The patient with a respiratory disease generally requires some alterations in usual hygiene practices. Frequent sponge baths may promote comfort for the patient who is diaphoretic. The individual with dyspnea can be expected to require additional help with hygiene in order to conserve energy to breathe. Careful oral hygiene is essential to moisten the mouth and remove unpleasant tastes associated with dyspnea and productive cough.

In addition, meticulous oral hygiene removes overgrowths of bacteria in the mouth which can cause lower respiratory tract infection in certain highly susceptible individuals. A practice to be avoided is using only the lemon and glycerin swabs without prior cleansing of the mouth.

Lubricant may be needed to protect the lips from cracking. Additional tissues and an appropriate receptacle should be provided for the patient who is raising sputum. The call bell should be conveniently located so that the patient may call for assistance when needed. The nurse may need to plan for rest periods during care. The daily bath provides an excellent opportunity for the nurse to observe the color of skin and mucous membranes, changes in behavior, and type of respirations.

AMBULATION AND EXERCISE

Generally ambulation and activity are encouraged for the patient with a respiratory disorder. An exception is the bed rest usually prescribed for a patient with hemoptysis. A carefully supervised exercise program may be prescribed for the patient with chronic obstructive pulmonary disease (COPD). Often, the physician prescribes elastic stockings for the patient with a respiratory disorder. The nurse should follow measurement instructions carefully in order to obtain the correct size.

REST

Rest reduces a person's need for oxygen and frees energy that can be used for breathing. A quiet environment, suitable room temperature, and adequate ventilation may enhance a person's rest. The nurse may need to be especially creative in planning rest periods for the patient with a respiratory disorder. In addition to a myriad of hospital routines, respiratory symptoms such as dyspnea, coughing, restlessness, pain, and associated apprehension may interfere with the patients' rest.

The patient with a respiratory condition usually awakens several times during the night. Retained secretions in air passages as well as a shift in the balance of lung fluid are common events that interrupt sleep. Drug therapy that dilates air passages often produces a side effect of wakefulness and excitement.

Drug therapy and inhalation therapy may be prescribed to relieve dyspnea, pain, and cough. Measures such as backrubs, sponge baths, positioning, and oral hygiene may increase the patient's sense of well-being and promote rest. The nurse may also plan with other departments, such as x-ray, schedules that reduce the waiting time for diagnostic procedures. A trusting relationship between the patient and the nurse may help to decrease apprehension and increase rest.

When the nurse finds the patient awake during the night or when a patient must be awakened, further sleep interruptions may be prevented by making observations, taking vital signs, and implementing appropriate medical treatments at that time.

POSITIONING

Proper positioning of the patient with a respiratory disorder is an essential nursing measure which provides rest, encourages effective coughing, promotes drainage from the tracheobronchial tree, relieves dyspnea, and ensures a patent airway. In some cases, the physician will prescribe positions for the patient. For example, for a patient with hemoptysis, the physician may ask the nurse to position the patient on the affected side to prevent blood from entering the healthy lung. Following bronchogram, the physician may specify certain positions to facilitate drainage of the dye from the tracheobronchial tree.

Generally, the nurse can anticipate that the patient with a respiratory disorder will need additional pillows. The patient with dyspnea may be more comfortable with a pillow placed lengthwise behind the back while sitting up to breathe. At times, for a very weak, dyspneic patient, a pillow can be placed on the overbed table, which has been elevated. Changes in position help to promote drainage from the tracheobronchial tree. For example, the patient with pneumonia in one of the lobes of the right lung should spend some of the time lying on the left side to promote drainage. Postural drainage may be prescribed in some instances to facilitate drainage from the respiratory passages. Generally, the patient is assisted into positions in which the head and chest are lower than the pelvis. This therapy uses gravity to help promote drainage. Postural drainage is explained in greater detail later in this chapter. A patent airway is essential. The patient should be positioned in bed so that the chin does not fall too far forward and reduce the width of the airway.

DIET AND FLUIDS

The physician may prescribe small, frequent meals for the patient with a respiratory disorder. Gastric distention causes pressure on the diaphragm and increases the work of breathing. Oral hygiene, handwashing, and covered sputum containers are nursing measures that increase the chances that the patient will enjoy a meal. Proper positioning also enables the patient to eat.

Generally, an increased fluid intake is needed by a person with a respiratory disorder. Increased fluid intake helps to liquefy secretions in the tracheobronchial tree so that the patient may cough them out. Also, increased fluid intake is needed to make up for losses of water through perspiration and exhaled water vapor when the patient is dyspneic or coughing frequently.

If there are no contraindications, the physician may prescribe a fluid intake of 3000 to 4000 ml per day. The nurse is challenged to help the patient meet this goal. A first step is to calculate the volume of fluid needed per waking hour in order to meet the goal. For example, the physician has prescribed a fluid intake of 4000 ml for Mr. Puffer. The nurse, knowing that Mr. Puffer usually sleeps about eight hours, has divided the total volume needed (4000 ml) by the number of waking hours available (16). The result (250 ml) is the hourly fluid intake needed to meet the goal. The second step is to explain the need for increased liquids to the patient and encourage an intake of 250 ml per waking hour. At this time, the patient's preferences are determined, and the nurse includes information that hot, steamy liquids held in the mouth for a moment before swallowing may help to loosen mucus. The third step is to offer the preferred fluids every hour. At this time, the patient is encouraged to continue by the nurse's words of praise and support. The fourth step is to record the volume consumed each hour on the patient's intake-and-output form.

DRUG THERAPY

The physician may prescribe a variety of drugs for the patient with a respiratory disorder. *Antihistamines,* such as those listed in Table 10.3 (page 248), may be prescribed for disorders related to allergy such as bronchial asthma. *Antibiotics,* such as those listed in Table 5.7 (pages 99–101), may be prescribed when the respiratory disease is associated with infection. Cough medications include *antitussives,* such as those listed in Table 14.4. Many cough preparations are prepared in syrup to reduce local irritation. When administering a syrup preparation, the nurse should give all other medications first. After taking the syrup, the patient should be instructed not to swallow water, food, liquids, or other medications. Occasionally, certain *enzymes* such as trypsin (TRYPTAR) and streptokinase-streptodornase (VARIDASE) may be ordered to help liquefy especially purulent, thick sputum. *Narcotic antagonists* such as nalorphine hydrochloride (NALLINE) or levallorphan tartrate (LORFAN) may be prescribed if respiratory depression has been caused by overuse of narcotic drugs. *Respiratory* stimulants such as ethamivan or doxapram hydrochloride may be ordered for the patient whose respiratory centers are depressed.

The nurse should remember that drugs that are inhaled act very rapidly because of the large surface area of the lungs and the many tiny capillaries. The patient should be observed carefully when receiving drugs by inhalation, and untoward symptoms should be reported at once.

RESPIRATORY THERAPY (INHALATION THERAPY)

Respiratory therapy includes the use of gases, humidity, and medications administered by aerosol to help the patient with a respiratory condition (see Figure 14.6). Specially trained therapists and technicians provide this therapy after it has been prescribed by a physician. When mechanical ventilators (respirators) are needed, respiratory therapists provide the highly specialized knowledge that is needed to set up and maintain this complex equipment. The scope of respiratory therapy is increasing rapidly due to greater knowledge about respiratory diseases and therapies. A visit to the respiratory therapy department in the hospital will

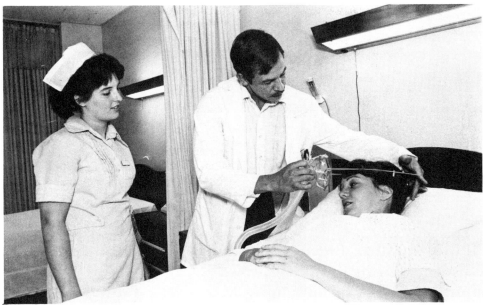

FIGURE 14.6 The patient is receiving respiratory therapy. (Courtesy of Bergen Pines County Hospital School of Practical Nursing, Paramus, New Jersey.)

greatly increase the nurse's appreciation of this very valuable therapy. Nursing responsibilities related to the care of a patient receiving oxygen therapy are discussed on pages 413–15.

Frequently, the physician prescribes humidification of air to help loosen thick secretions and improve breathing. Extra moisture can be added to the patient's room at home by simple methods such as a vaporizer or a steaming kettle of hot water. The nurse should make certain that the flow of steam is far enough away from the patient to prevent burns. The vaporizer or kettle should be checked frequently and refilled as necessary.

In the hospital a special device used to humidify air is *ultrasonic mist*. High-frequency sound waves are transmitted through water or saline, causing the formation of very tiny particles that can reach deeper portions of the respiratory system. Generally, the mist is inhaled by the patient through a mask, hood, or tent. The patient is encouraged to breathe through the mouth because filtering by the nose may break up particles before they reach lower airways.

When ultrasonic mist is used continuously, the tubing must be checked regularly to assure that kinks and pooled fluid do not obstruct the flow of mist to the patient. The nurse should anticipate that the patient may need additional changes of gown and linen when receiving extra humidity.

Another form of respiratory therapy is known as intermittent positive pressure breathing (IPPB). The machine used for this therapy applies positive pressure to the airways during inspiration (Figure 14.7). At the start of expiration, positive pressure stops and the patient exhales normally. A tight-fitting mask or a mouthpiece is used during the treatment which usually lasts ten or more minutes. This treatment promotes an increase in the volume of air inhaled (tidal volume) and may open airways in deeper lung tissue. Oxygen, humidity, and medication also may be delivered to lower airways during an IPPB treatment. In some cases, IPPB treatments may be prescribed to loosen secretions, promote productive coughing, and improve gas exchange in the lungs. Side effects which may occur during an IPPB treatment include changes in the

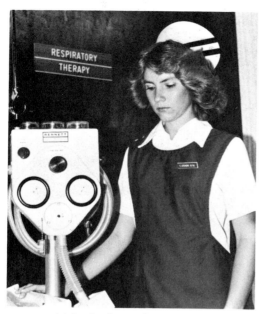

FIGURE 14.7   An intermittent positive pressure breathing (IPPB) machine. (Courtesy of Washington County School of Practical Nursing, Neff Vocational Center, Abingdon, Virginia.)

cardiac output, venous pooling, a change in pulse rate, and overinflation of airways. IPPB treatments are administered by a respiratory therapist or technician. Nurses who have received advanced training in IPPB therapy also may administer this treatment.

When a patient is unable to breathe effectively, a mechanical ventilator (respirator) may be ordered by the physician to inflate the lungs at regular intervals. The patient who needs continuous mechanical ventilation also needs an artificial airway in the trachea to have a relatively tight seal between the patient and the ventilator. One type of artificial airway is an endotracheal tube inserted through either the nose or the mouth into the trachea. The other is a tracheostomy. The care of a patient with a tracheostomy is discussed later in this chapter. There are two main types of ventilators: volume cycled and pressure cycled. Volume-cycled devices such as the Bennett-MA-1 (Figure 14.8) and Ohio respirators inflate the lungs with a specific preset volume. After the specific volume of gas has been delivered to the patient, the cycle allows exhala-

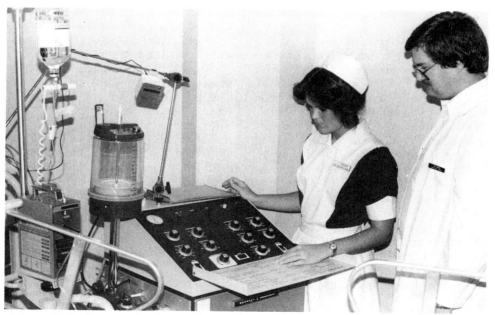

FIGURE 14.8   An example of a ventilator. (Courtesy of Southside School of Practical Nursing at Southside Community Hospital, Farmville, Virginia.)

tion. Pressure-cycled respirators such as the Bird Mark 7 and Bennett machines inflate the lungs with oxygen until a preset pressure has been reached and the patient is then allowed to exhale. The nurse who cares for a patient receiving mechanical ventilation must have additional training in the special nursing observations and interventions that this patient needs.

A general principle which guides the nurse in caring for the patient receiving respiratory therapy is that gases, humidity, and medications administered by aerosol have immediate, potent effects because of the extensive blood supply and large surface area in the lungs. Increasing the oxygen flow by only a few liters per minute may cause patients with certain respiratory disorders to stop breathing. The physician's orders for aerosol therapy should be followed carefully.

As mentioned in a previous section, the lower respiratory tract normally contains no microorganisms. Careless handling of equipment or improper cleaning techniques may cause the introduction of life-threatening pathogens into the patient's lungs.

OXYGEN THERAPY

Oxygen is a gas necessary for life; in fact, it truly can be called the breath of life. Different tissues of the body vary in their reaction to an insufficient amount of oxygen. For example, there is permanent damage of the brain when it is deprived of oxygen for 5 to 7 minutes. When the heart receives no oxygen for a period of 30 to 40 minutes, it, too, has permanent changes. Skeletal muscles can be deprived of this gas for several hours and then regain their function when the supply is reestablished.

Oxygen is prescribed by the physician when the cells of the patient's body do not receive an adequate supply. The physician's order for oxygen therapy includes whether it is to be continuous or intermittent, the method to be used, and the dosage. The nurse's responsibilities may include patient education, setting up the equipment, adjusting the regulator to provide the prescribed dosage, maintaining a safe environment, observing the patient's response to therapy, and preventing certain complications of

therapy. An inhalation therapist and/or technician may have similar responsibilities.

Table 14.5 contains a description of common methods of providing supplemental oxygen. The specific method is selected by the physician on the basis of the patient's underlying condition. No matter what method is prescribed, the nurse can anticipate the need for added moisture and safety precautions (Figure 14.9). Additional moisture is needed because oxygen is drying to the patient's mucous membranes. Humidity is usually supplied by running a tubing from the source of the oxygen (cylinder or wall outlet) through distilled water and then to the patient. Distilled water generally is used to avoid clogging the humidifier with mineral substances normally present in tap water.

Safety precautions are needed because oxygen supports combustion. An important nursing responsibility is to teach the patient, hospital roommates, family members, and visitors about safety measures related to oxygen. These include:

- No smoking of any kind in the room
- No open flames of any kind (such as a candle)
- Avoid using electrical equipment that may produce a spark

In some cases, the patient or roommate may not be able to remember safety precautions because of illness and/or sedation. In this situation, the nurse prevents an accident by removing cigarettes, matches, pipes, cigars, and/or lighters from the room and storing them according to hospital policy. When cylinder oxygen is used (rare, except in homes and agencies without an oxygen-piping system), the tank should be placed in a special holder that maintains an upright position and prevents injury caused by accidental overturning.

Nursing observations for the patient with a respiratory disorder were described earlier in the chapter. Additional observations indicated for the patient receiving oxygen therapy can be located in Table 14.6. After observing the patient, the nurse observes the oxygen equipment starting with the patient and moving systematically back toward the source of the oxygen. As previ-

TABLE 14.5

COMMON METHODS OF OXYGEN THERAPY

METHOD	DESCRIPTION	USUAL DOSAGE PRESCRIBED	NURSING IMPLICATIONS
Cannula	Plastic prongs approximately 1.25 cm (½ in.) long which fit into each nostril	1–6 L/min	Instruct patient to breathe through nose, if possible Concentration of oxygen varies with patient's pattern of ventilation Check skin contact areas for signs of irritation
Face mask	Mask fits over face; room air drawn in around holes in sides of mask	5–8 L/min	Ventilatory pattern affects concentration Check skin contact areas for signs of irritation Check for additional orders for oxygen during meals
Nonrebreathing mask	Contains reservoir bag with one-way valve which collects expired air	Varies, 6–15 L/min; must be high enough to keep reservoir bag partially inflated at all times	Mask must fit snugly Provides higher concentrations of oxygen (60–90 %) Check for additional orders for oxygen during meals
Venturi mask	Designed with special connecting tubing to provide a specific concentration of oxygen	Dosage is prescribed in concentration instead of liter flow. 24 %, 28 %, and 35 % concentrations are commonly prescribed. Liter flows are selected on basis of manufacturer's recommendations for the prescribed concentration	Some manufacturers do not recommend added humidity since it may change oxygen concentration of mask Check for additional orders for oxygen during meals

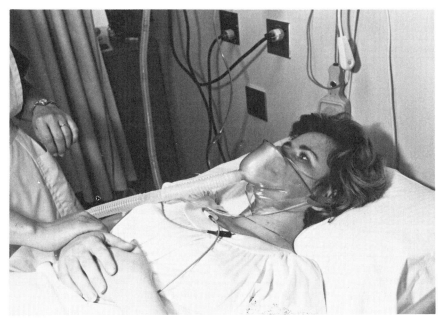

FIGURE 14.9   The patient is receiving exygen by a nasal cannula. The tube leading from the cannula is visible above the face tent. Extra humidity is delivered directly to the patient through the face tent.

ously mentioned, the use of contaminated equipment may introduce pathogens into the patient's respiratory system. To prevent the spread of infection, the patient's mask or cannula, oxygen tubings, and humidifier are changed every 24 hours.

PULMONARY PHYSIOTHERAPY

Pulmonary physiotherapy consists of a number of activities such as breathing, productive coughing, and postural drainage techniques. In larger hospitals and clinics, pulmonary physiotherapy may be performed by inhalation therapists, physical therapists, or nurses with special preparation. In some cases, the nurse may be asked to assist or supervise the patient in one or more of these activities. This type of therapy may be prescribed by the physician for a patient with either acute or chronic pulmonary disease.

Breathing exercises improve the ventilation of the lungs and help the patient to conserve energy. During *abdominal* or belly breathing, the patient is encouraged to use the abdominal muscles to breathe. The patient can check the progress by placing one hand on the chest and one on the abdomen. The abdomen should gently rise during inspiration and fall during expiration. Another breathing exercise that helps the patient prolong expiration is for the nurse to place one hand on the epigastrium. As the patient breathes out, the nurse's hand gradually and gently increases the pressure over the area. An alternate position is to place two hands over the lateral bases of the thorax and gradually increase the pressure while the patient expires.

Postural drainage is a procedure that uses gravity to drain secretions from the tracheobronchial tree. The physician may prescribe postural drainage for the individual with a chronic lung disease such as bronchiectasis and cystic fibrosis or for an acute illness such as lung abscess or pneumonia. In addition, postural drainage may be prescribed to prevent atelectasis or pneumonia in an unconscious patient, in a person needing mechanical ventilation, or following surgery. The physician prescribes the positions or areas of the lung to be drained, and the length and frequency of treatments. In addi-

TABLE 14.6
NURSING OBSERVATIONS AND INTERVENTIONS RELATED TO OXYGEN THERAPY

AREA TO BE OBSERVED	OBSERVATIONS AND INTERVENTIONS
Head	Cannula or mask should fit properly
	Check for irritation where there is skin contact with mask or cannula (face, nares, back of head, and/or ears)
	Pad irritated areas, if possible, without changing the fit of the mask or cannula
Oxygen tubing	Look for disconnection, twisted or kinked tubing
	Make sure tubing is not dragging on floor
	Look for condensed moisture in tubing which should be removed by disconnecting and draining
	Do *not* drain tubing by causing a backflow into humidifier (may contaminate with pathogens)
Humidifier	Check water level and refill, if necessary
Flowmeter	Check to see that correct liter flow is set—report discrepancies to appropriate nurse or physician
Tubing to wall outlet	Check for hissing sound or leaks in tubing—replace or notify respiratory therapy department

tion, deep breathing, intermittent positive pressure breathing (IPPB), or humidity may be ordered prior to each postural drainage session. Postural drainage can be tiring, uncomfortable, and embarrassing to the patient. The nurse should make certain that the patient has an emesis basin or sputum cup, extra tissues, and privacy. Oral hygiene and a rest period will be needed following the treatment. To reduce vomiting, treatments should not be scheduled within an hour after mealtimes. In some cases, suctioning may be needed if the patient is unable to expectorate drainage. Elderly, weak, and debilitated patients should be observed carefully in postural drainage positions where the head and chest are lowered. Dizziness and faintness, tachycardia, and diaphoresis are common during postural drainage. At times, the treatment may have to be shortened. One important event that can occur during postural drainage is the blockage of a larger bronchiole with a mucus plug. The patient becomes dyspneic and cyanotic. If the mucus plug cannot be coughed out, emergency bronchoscopy may be needed. After assuming the prescribed position, the patient is encouraged to deep-breathe and cough. At times, the specially trained nurse or therapist uses additional techniques such as clapping or vibrating the chest wall to help dislodge thick, tenacious secretions. Clapping (also known as cupping, percussion) consists of clapping the chest wall with cupped hands. Vibrating consists of gentle, shaking movements of the therapist's hands and arms that are transmitted to the chest wall during exhalation. These techniques, as well as postural drainage, are generally contraindicated in conditions that involve hemoptysis, extreme pain, seizures, hypertension, and unstable vital signs. Also, positions may have to be modified at times due to the patient's condition. For example, the patient with a tracheostomy would not be placed in the prone position.

The lower lobes of the lungs are the areas that most frequently require drainage of retained secretions. Several positions facilitate drainage from these areas. The patient may lower the head and chest over the bed, resting the arms on a padded footstool. The knee gatch of the bed may be elevated, and the patient may lower the head and chest over the gatch. The patient may be placed prone in Trendelenburg position with a pillow under the hips. The patient also should be placed in the side-lying positions while in the Trendelenburg position.

Effective coughing is valuable to the patient with lung disease as well as to the surgical patient and others who must remain immobilized. An effective cough is one that clears the lower airways of retained secretions which are then expectorated.

Patient teaching is a key to effective coughing. Several types of coughing are believed to be effective. When teaching a cascade cough, the patient is instructed to take a deep breath in and hold it for a moment. The patient is then instructed to cough repeatedly while exhaling until no more air is left. When teaching a huff cough, the patient is instructed to take a deep breath with mouth open and to huff repeatedly during expiration until no air is left. This practice is believed to stimulate natural coughing mechanisms. A third method is to instruct the patient to exhale completely then inhale completely and hold for a moment before coughing forcefully.

A patient also may be helped to cough more effectively by slowly bending forward from a sitting position while slowly exhaling. Have the patient return slowly to a sitting position while slowly inhaling. After repeating this several times, the patient is asked to begin coughing while slowly bending forward. Some patients may be able to cough effectively after taking two or three deep breaths. The surgical patient may be helped to cough by placing a pillow or folded towel over the incisional area and applying gentle pressure during the cough. If pain is associated with cough, the patient should be medicated, if possible, prior to coughing. Effective coughing is more likely if the patient's secretions are thinned by an adequate fluid intake and medication.

In some cases, the physician may use or prescribe methods to stimulate a cough. Suctioning, nebulizers, and direct pressure over the trachea are a few cough stimulators. Occasionally, sterile saline or distilled water is injected into the trachea by the physician using a transcutaneous catheter.

INTRATRACHEAL SUCTION

Intratracheal suctioning (endotracheal suctioning, deep suctioning) is the removal of secretions from the trachea and upper portions of each bronchus using a sterile catheter. This procedure may save a person's life or may take away a life if done improperly. Intratracheal suctioning should be performed only by those who have received training and supervision. Except in extreme emergencies, this type of suctioning requires a physician's order. The nurse should understand the purpose of suctioning and should explain it to the patient. For example, if suctioning is needed to stimulate coughing, the catheter is generally inserted only far enough to stimulate a cough. If tracheobronchial secretions must be removed, intratracheal suctioning may be needed. The nurse should remember that intratracheal suctioning can be hazardous and should strive to help the patient expectorate secretions by coughing, postural drainage, adequate hydration, positioning, and humidification whenever possible.

In order to prevent infection or control existing infection, sterile technique is used whenever suctioning is needed. After each use, the equipment is discarded or returned for sterilization. Separate catheters are used for nasal, oral, or pharyngeal suctioning and tracheobronchial secretions.

Before suctioning begins, the patient's head is elevated above the level of the shoulders, and the head and neck are extended. The patient should be oxygenated before and after intratracheal suctioning. Rolling the catheter between the fingers increases maneuverability. The sterile catheter may be inserted through the mouth, nose, endotracheal tube, or tracheostomy tube after being lubricated with sterile saline or water. The tip of the nose is elevated slightly as the catheter is passed through the nose. In addition, the patient's tongue may be pulled gently forward and held with a gauze pad. Some experts believe that turning the patient's head to one side allows the catheter to enter the opposite bronchus.

The catheter must be inserted approximately 50.8 cm (20 in.) or more in the adult in order to reach lower airways. Suction is never applied while introducing the catheter and only intermittently while withdrawing it in a gently rotating manner. Suctioning should not exceed ten seconds, since large amounts of oxygen are removed along with secretions. Prolonged suctioning may cause hypoxia, cardiac arrhythmias, cardiac arrest, and spasm of the airways.

Following intratracheal suctioning, the nurse should closely observe the patient for bradycardia, cyanosis, and wheezing and should report these symptoms to the physician. Repeat suctioning should not be attempted for at least five minutes. Oral hygiene will be needed following all types of suctioning.

PREVENTING INFECTION

Some patients have an infection as the underlying cause of a respiratory disorder. Other patients do not have an underlying infection but acquire one while hospitalized. Hospital-acquired infection (nosocomial infection) of the respiratory tract is a serious illness with a high mortality rate.

The widespread use of antibiotics in the hospital is believed to promote conditions that favor the growth of more resistant organisms. Currently, gram-negative bacteria such as *Pseudomonas, Klebsiella,* and *Proteus* cause a higher number of nosocomial infections than gram-positive organisms.

The two most frequent sources of nosocomial respiratory infection include equipment used during respiratory therapy and procedures that invade the lower respiratory tract (endotracheal intubation, tracheostomy care, bronchoscopy, bronchogram, and laryngoscopy are discussed elsewhere in this chapter) and bypass normal defenses in the upper respiratory tract.

Nursing practices that prevent nosocomial respiratory infection include:

- Do not come to the hospital with symptoms of a common cold.
- Wash hands frequently when caring for patients.
- Follow hospital policy for draining pooled fluid from the tubes attached to respiratory therapy equipment.
- Request a change of tubing if it falls on the floor.
- Give meticulous oral hygiene to prevent overgrowth of normal flora which can be aspirated into the lower airways.
- Encourage optimum fluid intake and good nutrition.
- Select nursing interventions that prevent aspiration and accumulation of retained secretions.
- Practice flawless aseptic technique when caring for a patient with an artificial airway.
- Use aseptic techniques for all suctioning procedures.

ASSISTING WITH COMMON CONCERNS

Apprehension, fear, and panic are common emotional experiences of the patient with a respiratory disorder who is struggling to breathe. These emotions, when unrelieved and very intense, may worsen breathing. The nurse can expect that most patients with a breathing disorder are afraid that breathing will stop altogether. Therefore, a priority of the nurse is to lessen fear and apprehension and prevent panic.

A trusting relationship develops when the patient feels cared for and cared about. This is accomplished when the nurse meets physical needs promptly and kindly, tells the patient at each interaction when to expect the next interaction and returns promptly. Pinning the call bell to the patient's gown and returning to the bedside during spare moments reassure the patient that the nurse is nearby and can be counted upon to be there when help is needed. Many patients are afraid to be alone when breathing is difficult.

Verbal communication at times is limited to conserve energy for the work of breathing. Thus, the nurse must find other ways of observing and communicating attitudes and feelings. For example, the nurse should not try to engage the patient in lengthy conversations, but the simple act of sponging the face and neck refreshes the patient and communicates a caring attitude.

Fear, hypoxia, and difficult breathing have a way of making a person feel restless and disorganized. The nurse who develops a calm, organized approach to nursing care may find that a trusting relationship can be established more quickly. Anticipating a person's need for extra tissues, a paper bag, additional fluids, or help in bathing also reduces worry and fatigue. The nurse may have to plan care very carefully to conserve energy for breathing, coughing, ambulating, or postural drainage. For example, after consulting the head nurse, the nurse may decide to give the patient a complete bed bath in order to conserve energy for postural drainage treatments.

The patient with a chronic pulmonary disease such as emphysema, tuberculosis, or cancer usually faces a drastic change in life-style, which is permanent. This also requires a change in the family's life-style. Giving up smoking, changing occupations, frequent trips to the doctor, taking one or more medications, and a host of other changes may cause the patient to experience many of the emotions, defense mechanisms, or grieving processes described in Chapter 1. The nurse can anticipate that the patient and his family will need support as they struggle to accept their changed life-style. The nurse should be familiar with community organizations such as the Lost Cord Club, local agencies of the American Lung Association, nonsmokers programs, and other rehabilitation programs. A social worker may be asked to help obtain referrals for special equipment or socioeconomic assistance. The costs of several hospitalizations, medications, oxygen, and other equipment over a period of years can stagger a family's finances.

Patient and family teaching is an important aspect of nursing the patient with a respiratory disorder. This includes explaining diagnostic procedures, medications, and treatments as well as planning for the patient's discharge. Patient teaching may help to allay anxiety, foster a trusting relationship, and increase the likelihood of recovery or control of disease. The nurse may find it helpful in patient teaching to ask the following questions:

1. What does the patient need to know?
2. Who is responsible for explaining?
3. What is the best way to explain?

For example, the patient may need to be told the diagnosis, but that is the physician's responsibility as head of the health team. The patient also may need to know how to cough effectively; the nurse may show how to do this. The patient may need to know that an increased fluid intake is needed; the nurse may explain this and offer appropriate fluids at frequent intervals. The respiratory therapist may explain the precautions of oxygen use when setting up oxygen equipment in the patient's room; the nurse may reinforce this patient teaching while checking the humidifier and replacing the water in it. In other words, patient teaching is a shared responsibility of the health team. Thus, the patient benefits from the special skills of each member of the health team.

Generally, patient teaching includes the following topics in addition to medical therapy:

- Avoiding pulmonary irritants such as cigarette smoke and aerosol spray products
- Balancing a pattern of work, rest, and leisure activities
- Avoiding and preventing respiratory infection
- Maintaining good nutrition and hydration

The nurse can expect that the patient with a breathing disorder has sexual concerns. Some patient's may verbalize these concerns with the nurse or another member of the health team. Other patients are reluctant to discuss sexual concerns but may indicate them indirectly using vague words or behavior. The nurse should report both direct and indirect expressions of the patient's sexual concerns to the head nurse or team leader so that appropriate information can be provided. Adjusting medication, changing positions, and choosing a different time of day may enhance sexual enjoyment, even for a patient with a breathing disorder.

The Common Cold

The common cold is an acute infection that most often affects the upper respiratory system: nose, pharynx, and larynx. It is caused by one or more viruses. Although fatigue, chilling of the body, and wet feet do not cause the common cold, these factors may lower an individual's resistance to the virus. A cold is the most common infection of the respiratory system. The cold and its complications cause the loss of a larger number of working days than any other disease. Most people have one or more attacks of this infection every year. Because of the large number of viruses that can cause a cold, a person may develop another cold within weeks.

The viruses are spread by an individual who is sneezing, coughing, and blowing the nose during the early stage of the cold. They may also be spread by direct contact, such as by kissing.

The mucous membranes lining the nose and throat become inflamed when a person develops a cold. Resistance to secondary invasion by bacteria present in these areas, such as streptococci and pneumococci, is lowered. Thus, colds can be complicated by pneumonia, infections of the ear, sinusitis, and bronchitis. The person who is elderly or has chronic disease is more likely to develop complications from a cold.

NURSING OBSERVATIONS

Usually a person notices a burning or itching feeling in the back of the nose and throat when the cold begins. Within several hours, there is a watery discharge from the nose. The mucous membranes are swollen, and the nasal passage may become closed. In a few days the clear mucous discharge gradually decreases and becomes slightly yellow. The patient with a cold also has general symptoms of inflammation. There are usually malaise, a chilly feeling, a headache, and a burning feeling in the eyes. If the infection spreads into the larynx and bronchi, the patient becomes hoarse and develops a cough. At first, the cough is dry and hacking; then it becomes productive.

TREATMENT AND NURSING CARE

Specific measures to prevent the common cold have not yet proved effective. Vaccines, vitamins, and outdoor exercise have not been successful in preventing a cold. The best safeguards against developing this disease are to avoid contact with persons suffering from a cold and to maintain the best possible health. A person should avoid excessive exposure and becoming overly tired.

After the cold has developed, the treatment is entirely symptomatic. The patient should avoid contact with others whenever possible to prevent spreading the disease. The patient with a temperature of 37.8°C (100°F) or over should rest in bed and increase fluid intake.

Frequently, aspirin and similar drugs are prescribed to relieve the generalized aches and pains. Discomfort from nasal congestion is relieved by nasal spray or nose drops as ordered by the doctor. The inhalation of steam may be used to soothe the irritated mucous membrane. A cough mixture may be ordered to relieve a useless, dry, and irritating cough. Drugs, such as sulfonamides, penicillin, streptomycin, and other antibiotics, do not cure the common cold. They may be effective in treating a bacterial infection, such as sinusitis or pneumonia, when it is a complication of the common cold. Self-medication with numerous widely advertised cold remedies is prevalent. In some persons, repeated use of these remedies can produce serious or even fatal disease. Persons taking medications prescribed by the physician for other disorders should never take any nonprescribed drug without first consulting the physician. Interactions between prescribed and nonprescribed drugs can have dangerous consequences. The nurse, as a health team and community member, has an important responsibility to discourage self-medication.

Persons with chronic disease are usually advised to seek medical attention when symptoms of a cold develop. The cold may seriously worsen usual symptoms in a patient with a chronic respiratory disorder.

Influenza

The person with influenza has an acute, contagious respiratory infection caused by a virus and spread by droplets of virus in the air. Four main groups of viruses (A, B, C, D) can cause influenza. Group D virus is known as a parainfluenza virus since it differs slightly from the other groups. Subgroups of each main group have been identified. An infection caused by one subgroup does not result in immunity to the others. For example, a person who has influenza caused by one of the A subgroup viruses does not become immune to the other subgroups.

Although influenza usually occurs in epidemics, it can affect individuals when an epidemic is not in progress. Subgroups of influenza A have been associated with epidemics more frequently than the others. Examples of these are the Asian and Hong Kong flu epidemics that occurred in recent years.

The mortality rate for all diseases rises during an epidemic of influenza which lasts for several years. Influenza is especially dangerous for the elderly, those with pulmonary or cardiovascular disease, and pregnant women. Persons with these conditions are more likely to develop the complications of influenza such as pneumonia.

NURSING OBSERVATIONS

Influenza has a rather sudden onset with headache, malaise, chilly sensations, weakness, dizziness, and mild, substernal chest pain. Fever is common and usually exceeds 38°C (100.4°F). Fever may reach as high as 41°C (105.8°F) in more severe cases. The person usually has respiratory symptoms such as dry, sore throat, sneezing, and coughing.

TREATMENT AND NURSING CARE

At the present time, no specific antibiotic is effective against influenza. However, an antibiotic may be prescribed in some cases to combat secondary bacterial infections such as bronchitis and pneumonia.

Rest in bed, an increased intake of fluids, and a nourishing diet are recommended. Acetylsalicylic acid (aspirin) may be ordered to relieve aching and reduce fever. Inhalation of steam or cool vapor may soothe the mucous membrane of the upper respiratory system and help to relieve coughing. The physician may prescribe one of the drugs listed in Tables 14.3 and 14.4 for cough.

Nursing measures such as backrubs, sponge baths, and oral hygiene may reduce some of the discomfort associated with influenza. The patient may need assistance to get to the bathroom since weakness and dizziness accompany influenza. The patient with an uncomplicated case of influenza usually is not hospitalized. This reduces the likelihood of spreading the infection as well as of exposing the patient to a secondary bacterial infection.

The patient may gradually resume activities as fever and other symptoms subside. However, normal activity and work are avoided until the patient is symptom-free.

Vaccines are available to protect persons from some of the viruses that cause influenza. Vaccines are especially recommended for high-risk persons, such as those with chronic heart and lung disease and the elderly. The duration of immunity is short, and yearly boosters are needed. The vaccines are made from viruses that have been grown in a chicken embryo. Persons who are allergic to eggs are generally advised not to receive the vaccine.

Sinusitis

The patient with sinusitis has an inflammation of the mucous membrane lining one or more nasal sinuses. The opening that leads from the air-filled cavity to the nose has become narrowed or closed. This can be caused by congestion of the nasal mucosa, by a plug of pus or mucus blocking the tiny passage, or by nasal deformities such as a polyp or deviated nasal septum.

Sinusitis often occurs with infections of the nose such as the common cold. Usually, inflammation of the sinuses disappears when the nasal infection is cured. Also, nasal obstruction caused by an allergy may result in sinusitis (see Chapter 10). The maxillary sinuses of the cheek can become infected from an abscess of an upper tooth.

Acute sinusitis occurs when bacteria growing in nonflowing secretions cause an infection. *Staphylococci* and *Haemophilus influenzae* are the organisms most frequently involved. Chronic sinusitis is associated with repeated infections which lead to a thickening of the mucous membrane lining the sinuses. Other factors associated with chronic sinusitis include underlying disease such as allergy, cigarette smoking, stress, and exposure to irritating dusts and gases. Early treatment of both acute and chronic sinus conditions is important in order to prevent complications. Because the sinuses are near bone and brain tissue, bone and brain infections are particularly feared complications.

Sinusitis that continues over a period of time may cause an inflammation of the lower respiratory tract. Infectious material drains from the sinus into the nose and throat. If it is aspirated into the bronchi and lungs over a period of time, the patient may develop chronic bronchitis.

NURSING OBSERVATIONS

Secretions from the mucous membrane lining the sinus do not drain properly when the opening that leads to the nose is obstructed. This causes pressure on the sinus wall and results in pain. The patient generally complains of a facial headache on the involved side and may have tenderness and swelling over the area. There may be purulent nasal discharge if affected sinuses are draining. Frequently, the person loses the sense of smell when sinuses are obstructed. The drainage of nasal discharge into the nose and throat can cause a cough, sore throat, and a foul breath odor. In addition, there may be general signs of inflammation and infection such as malaise, fever, and anorexia.

ASSISTING WITH DIAGNOSTIC STUDIES

A diagnosis of acute sinusitis generally is made by the physician on the basis of the patient's symptoms and signs. In some cases, purulent drainage is collected and sent to the laboratory for culture and sensitivity. X-rays may be taken when chronic sinusitis is suspected.

TREATMENT AND NURSING INTERVENTIONS

Treatment of a patient with sinusitis is directed toward promoting sinus drainage, combating infection, and relieving symptoms. Underlying conditions such as allergy are also treated.

In addition to antibiotics for infection and analgesics for pain, drug therapy includes nasal sprays or drops to relieve congestion and promote drainage. Epinephrine (adrenaline), ephedrine, and phenylephrine (NEO-SYNEPHRINE) are examples of drugs that constrict blood vessels causing mucous membranes to shrink. If overused, these drugs may also cause excessive drying of the mucous membrane, which the body attempts to correct by secreting more mucus. This, in turn, increases nasal congestion. These facts are related to the patient as a part of patient teaching about drug therapy. Good handwashing and proper disposal of infected secretions are nursing interventions that prevent the spread of infection.

Patients usually benefit from avoiding irritants such as cigarette smoking; having a constant room temperature and humidity; and avoiding cold, dampness, and chills. Patient teaching is directed to these areas.

When medical treatment and nursing care do not cause the diseased sinus to drain, surgery may be needed. Surgical treatment of sinus conditions includes procedures to correct nasal deformities, remove diseased mucous membrane, or enlarge sinus openings to improve drainage. A *nasal polypectomy* is performed under local anesthesia to remove polyps that are blocking nasal passages.

Rhinoplasty is a procedure in which a congenital or acquired nasal deformity is corrected, using tissue from another part of the body or synthetic materials. Rhinoplasty generally is performed under local anesthesia, and the incisions usually are not visible after healing.

A *submucous resection* (SMR) is designed to straighten the septum between the nares in order to improve breathing and drainage. SMR generally is performed under local anesthesia after suitable preoperative sedation.

A *Cadwell-Luc* procedure is performed on the maxillary sinus through an incision made in the gum tissue under the lip. Diseased tissue is removed, and drainage is improved.

Following SMR, Caldwell-Luc, and other sinus surgeries, the nose is packed with gauze or tampons to control bleeding. The physician may order continuous ice packs over the nose during the immediate postoperative period to reduce edema and bleeding. The nurse can expect that the patient will need frequent changes of mustache dressing and gowns. A mustache dressing can be made by rolling several 4″ × 4″ gauze squares. The roll is then placed under the patient's nose and secured by tape. Usually the patient is allowed ice chips or clear liquids while the packing is in place. The patient should be instructed not to blow the nose and to expectorate all drainage into a tissue or emesis basin.

Generally, the patient is placed in Fowler's position to facilitate drainage. Frequent oral hygiene will be needed, and cold cream or petrolatum should be applied to the lips to prevent cracking. Temperature is taken rectally since the patient must breathe through the mouth while the packing is in place. The nurse can expect edema of the nose and under the eyes as well as ecchymotic discoloration of the skin. Although considerable drainage can be expected, increased swallowing, expectoration of bright-red blood, and an increased trickle of blood through the nasal packing, accompanied by a rise in pulse and blood pressure, should be reported to the physician since these signs can indicate hemorrhage. Generally, the packing is removed after about 24 hours, and the patient is encouraged to ambulate and eat a diet as desired. Hematemesis and tarry stools are not uncommon following nasal surgery due to bloody drainage that has been swallowed.

The sense of smell is lost temporarily following some sinus surgeries. Numbness of the upper lip and teeth may persist for several months following a Caldwell-Luc procedure.

Epistaxis

The individual with epistaxis has a nosebleed. Nosebleed may occur in normal individuals because of injury, such as nose picking, or low humidity, which dries the mucous membrane in the nose. However, epistaxis also may occur as a symptom of serious diseases such as hypertension, rheumatic fever, measles, cancer, influenza, or bloodclotting abnormalities. Excessive use of aspirin and nosedrops may also cause nosebleed. The most common source of nosebleed is the rupture of a cluster of blood vessels in the anterior nasal septum located in what is known as Kiesselbach's areas. Measures to control epistaxis are discussed in Chapter 8.

Pharyngitis

The patient with pharyngitis has an inflamed pharynx, or a sore throat. This condition may be caused by either irritation or infection. For example, irritation from excessive smoking, inhaling irritating substances such as dust and chemicals, and talking too much can result in a sore throat. Usually pharyngitis is associated with infections of the upper respiratory tract, such as the common cold and sinusitis. Discharge from the nose and sinuses drains into the throat, causing it to become inflamed. Also, pharyngitis may result from a direct infection by viruses and bacteria such as streptococci.

A sore throat can be a symptom of other diseases, such as poliomyelitis and diphtheria, or it may be followed by rheumatic fever. As these infections occur more frequently in children, it is important to report a child's sore throat to the physician.

NURSING OBSERVATIONS

A patient with pharyngitis can have both local and general symptoms of inflammation, such as redness of the throat and fever. These symptoms vary according to the cause. The person who has been smoking excessively may have only a red or slightly scratchy throat, whereas a patient with an acute infection in the pharynx has an extremely sore throat and discomfort when swallowing. General symptoms of inflammation, such as fever, malaise, and headache are common in the latter situation.

The physician diagnoses pharyngitis on the basis of the patient's symptoms and a visual inspection of the pharynx. When infection is suspected, a throat culture may be obtained in order to identify the specific pathogen. Other diagnostic tests may be ordered to rule out underlying disease such as sinusitis.

TREATMENT AND NURSING INTERVENTIONS

Treatment of pharyngitis is directed toward eliminating the cause and alleviating symptoms. The person whose smoking causes pharyngitis is advised to stop. Voice rest is prescribed when excessive talking has caused pharyngitis.

When infection is the cause of pharyngitis, rest in bed is generally advised. In some cases, the patient may need to be isolated from others in order to prevent the spread of infection. Other interventions discussed earlier that prevent the spread of infection apply to this patient. Antibiotic therapy is prescribed to kill the pathogens.

Application of heat or cold may relieve soreness. Frequently heat is used in the form of gargles. An example of this is warm salt water (saline). The application of an ice collar to the neck is the method commonly used in applying cold to the area.

Although swallowing may be painful, the patient is encouraged to increase the fluid intake. An increased fluid intake, nourishing diet, bed rest, and frequent oral hygiene are nursing interventions that promote comfort and improve the overall condition.

Tonsillitis

Tonsillitis is an inflammation of the lymphatic tissue in the throat known as tonsils. Frequently the adenoids (lymphatic tissue in the nasopharynx) are inflamed also. The patient with tonsillitis has symptoms of pharyngitis. In addition, the tonsils are red and swollen and may have whitish patches on them.

Cervical lymph nodes may become enlarged and the white blood count rises. Complications that may arise from tonsillitis include chronic tonsillitis, abscesses on the tonsils, otitis media, pneumonia, and rheumatic fever.

TREATMENT AND NURSING INTERVENTIONS

The treatment and nursing care of a patient with an acute attack of tonsillitis are the same as those discussed under pharyngitis. The physician may recommend surgery if tonsillitis is chronic with a sore throat that remains between acute infections. Chronic tonsillitis is not as common as was believed, and surgery is performed less often.

TONSILLECTOMY

Surgical removal of the tonsils is known as tonsillectomy. The physician generally removes the adenoids in connection with the tonsillectomy if the patient's adenoids are diseased also. Pieces of lymphatic tissue located in the nasopharynx are known as adenoids. Enlargement of the adenoids is present mainly in childhood and may cause the child to be a mouth breather because the nasopharynx is obstructed. When a patient is scheduled for a tonsillectomy and adenoidectomy, the operation is referred to as a "T and A."

PREOPERATIVE CARE. In addition to the care of a patient before surgery already discussed in Chapter 6 the physician orders the blood to be examined to determine whether or not it clots normally. Normally, it takes the blood from three to ten minutes to clot after being exposed to air. The length of time varies slightly with the technique used to determine the clotting time. The patient with a prolonged clotting time is a poor surgical risk because of the danger of hemorrhage; therefore, this condition is treated before surgery. Sometimes vitamin K is administered to hasten the clotting of blood. Some physicians order this drug for many of their patients posted for a "T and A" to prevent excessive postoperative bleeding. Tonsillectomy is hazardous and contraindicated if a person has an upper respiratory or other infection. Since arrangements for surgery may have been made well in advance, the surgeon may not know that a patient has a cold or other infection prior to admission. The nurse should be especially alert for signs of infection when admitting a patient to the nursing unit. Any sign of infection should be reported promptly to the surgeon. Generally, surgery is canceled, the patient is discharged, and readmitted at a later date. During patient teaching, the nurse emphasizes the importance of an increased fluid intake and avoidance of clearing the throat and coughing postoperatively.

POSTOPERATIVE CARE. The patient who has had a tonsillectomy done under a local anesthetic is awake when returned to bed following surgery. This patient usually is positioned with the head of the bed raised and the knees slightly elevated.

The patient who has had a general anesthetic (put to sleep for the surgery), is placed in bed on the side or the abdomen. The purpose of either of these positions is to allow mucus and blood to drain from the throat. This prevents the fluid from draining into the larynx and trachea. When the patient is turned on one side, a pillow should be placed under the lower chest and the knees should be flexed. If the patient is placed on the abdomen, the head is turned to one side.

The responsibility of the nurse caring for the patient who is still unconscious from the anesthesia is to watch for bleeding and to prevent aspiration of mucus. A small amount of bright-red blood can be expected for a short while after surgery. Excess fluid in the mouth should be removed by frequent wiping and with suction. In using a suction machine the nurse should keep the pressure low. Also, extreme care should be used to prevent the suction tip from injuring the operative area. The patient should be checked frequently for signs of bleeding after anesthesia. The nurse will need a tongue depressor and flashlight when checking the patient's throat. Blood coming from the throat is bright red. If blood has been swallowed, vomitus is brownish. The nurse should report frequent expectoration of bright-red blood and a moderate-to-large amount of brownish vomitus. Symptoms of hemorrhage, such as restlessness, pallor, and a fast pulse, should also be reported. The nurse should save emesis or clots for the physician's inspection when excessive bleeding is suspected.

In the absence of complications, such as bleeding, the patient is given cracked ice, water, and other cold liquids as soon as desired. Popsicles, sherbet, and ice cream may soothe the sore throat as well as provide needed fluids. Generally, red liquids such as strawberry- or raspberry-flavored beverages are avoided since the color may be confused with blood, and assessment of bleeding is more difficult. Adequate fluid intake is important to keep mucous membranes moist. Some experts believe that dry mucous membranes increase the likelihood of postoperative bleeding. No fruit juices should be given because they irritate the throat, and fluids are not given through a straw since sucking may initiate bleeding. Soft foods are given when the patient can tolerate them. Frequent oral hygiene helps to clear mucus from the mouth, refreshes the patient, and increases the likelihood that the patient will drink adequate fluids.

Other measures to prevent or minimize bleeding that should be explained to the patient include use of an ice collar, avoidance of talking, clearing the throat, coughing, nose blowing, and sneezing.

Many physicians prescribe chewing gum the day after surgery to relieve dryness and soreness. ASPERGUM is an example of the gum that may be ordered. Usually the patient is discharged from the hospital the day after the operation.

Patient teaching before discharge includes avoiding coughing, sneezing, and nose blowing, continuing an increased fluid intake, avoiding raw fruits and vegetables, avoiding strenuous exercise, and expecting one or more tarry stools caused by the swallowing of blood during surgery.

Hemorrhage may occur in the immediate postoperative period or between the fifth and tenth postoperative day as the membrane that has formed over the suture line sloughs. The patient should be instructed to contact the physician or come to the emergency room immediately if bleeding does not stop promptly. The physician may need to remove a soft clot that may have formed. Occasionally, hemorrhage continues, and the patient must return to surgery for suturing or cautery of bleeding vessels.

Laryngitis

The patient with laryngitis has an inflammation of the larynx, or voice box. Usually it follows an infection of the upper respiratory tract, such as pharyngitis or the common cold. It may accompany infectious diseases, such as measles, diphtheria, and whooping cough. Laryngitis may result from excessive use of the voice, inhaling irritating fumes and dust, and smoking too much. Tuberculosis, syphilis, and a tumor may cause it. The nurse should remember that persistent hoarseness is the chief symptom of cancer of the larynx. A person who is hoarse for more than a few days should consult a physician.

NURSING OBSERVATIONS

Although hoarseness is the main symptom, some individuals also have aphonia which means inability to speak or loss of voice. A slight elevation of temperature may be present when the laryngitis is a result of infection. The patient may also have a cough and a feeling of tightness in the throat.

TREATMENT

The doctor recommends that the patient with laryngitis avoid use of the voice. Inhalation of steam may be ordered to soothe the irritated mucous membrane. If laryngitis is a result of another disease, such as infection or cancer, the doctor directs treatment toward the underlying cause.

Obstruction of the Pharynx, the Larynx, or the Trachea

An obstruction of the pharynx, larynx, or trachea may be caused by a tumor, inhaling a foreign object such as a pea or a coin, paralysis of the vocal folds, edema, or spasm of the airway. Laryngeal obstruction also may occur during or after an operation on the neck, such as a thyroidectomy.

SYMPTOMS AND DIAGNOSIS

When air passages are obstructed, a person can be expected to show signs of respiratory distress such as dyspnea, diaphoresis, purple flush, rapid pulse, and panic. Other signs that may indicate obstruction include croupy cough, stridor or whistling noises while breathing, hemoptysis, and excessive mucus expectoration. Laryngoscopy or bronchoscopy may be needed to detect the source of obstruction.

TREATMENT AND NURSING INTERVENTIONS

When airway obstruction is sudden and unexpected, emergency procedures must be started quickly to preserve life. Chapter 8 discusses and illustrates maneuvers that may dislodge a foreign body. The nurse should be thoroughly familiar with these procedures. If these actions are unsuccessful, emergency laryngoscopy, bronchoscopy, or tracheotomy may be needed to remove the foreign body or create an adequate airway.

The physician performs a tracheotomy on the patient with an obstruction of the larynx. A tracheotomy (known as a tracheos-

tomy when the opening is to be permanent) is an artificial opening into the trachea that is made below the obstruction so that the patient can breathe. This is a lifesaving operation when the patient has an acute blockage of the larynx.

After making an incision into the trachea, the surgeon inserts a tube into the new artificial opening to prevent the opening from closing over and to facilitate removal of tracheobronchial secretions. The tube is called a tracheostomy tube and may be made of silver, disposable plastic, rubber, or other substances. A variety of tracheostomy tubes is available in different sizes. The physician selects the type and size tube to be used. Tracheostomy tubes may consist of several separate pieces, as illustrated in Figure 14.10. When a tube is selected like the one in Figure 14.10, an obturator fits inside the outer cannula and guides it into the trachea. Then the obturator is removed and the inner cannula is inserted. Tapes are attached to the larger tube, or cannula, and tied around the patient's neck to keep the tube in place.

Many of the tracheostomy tubes that are used today have an inflatable balloon called

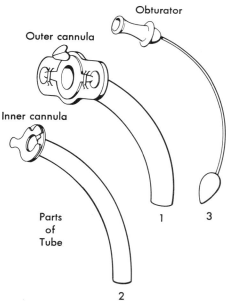

FIGURE 14.10 Parts of a tracheostomy tube. (Adapted from drawings of the American Cancer Society, New York, N. Y.)

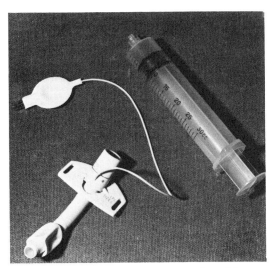

FIGURE 14.11 A tracheostomy tube with an inflatable balloon called a cuff around the end of the tube. The amount of air indicated by the manufacturer is injected with a syringe into the small white bag with a tube leading to the inner cuff.

a cuff around the outside (see Figure 14.11). After the tube is inserted, the cuff is inflated with air in a manner similar to that used to inflate the balloon of a Foley catheter. The inflated cuff makes a seal that prevents the tube from sliding up and down the walls of the trachea, causing damage to mucous membranes. The inflated cuff also prevents

trickling of secretions from upper portions of the trachea to the lower trachea and bronchi (see Figure 14.12). The cuff should not be overinflated since excessive pressure can cause erosion of the mucous membrane lining the tracheal wall and subsequent bleeding. Some cuffed tubes are prestretched in the manufacturing process so that a seal can be obtained without excessive pressure. Other tubes come equipped with two cuffs, which can be alternately inflated, thereby changing sites of pressure while providing a continuous seal.

Postoperatively, the patient with a tracheostomy needs close observation and meticulous nursing care. Frequently, the patient is transferred to the intensive care unit for several days following surgery.

One of the primary nursing responsibilities is to maintain the patency of this artificial airway. This is the patient's only lifeline for air. Equipment is needed at the bedside to prepare for events that may obstruct the patient's airway and threaten life. The nurse may be asked to obtain this equipment, for it should be at the bedside when the patient returns from surgery. A duplicate set of sterile tracheostomy tubes (of the same size and type) should be placed on the bedside stand. Generally, a sterile tracheostomy spreader will be needed also. In addition, suction equipment should be at the bedside when the patient arrives from surgery. The nurse

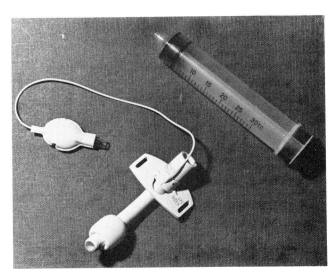

FIGURE 14.12 After the tracheostomy tube has been inserted in the patient's trachea, the tube is held in place by the inflated cuff. Air is injected into the balloon in a manner similar to that used for a Foley catheter. The inflated cuff helps to prevent the tube from sliding.

should check the suction to be sure it is functioning properly prior to the patient's return. A variety of sterile suction catheters and sterile saline also will be needed. Most hospitals now use disposable suction kits. Many kits will be needed, since the patient may require suctioning every 15 to 30 minutes in the immediate postoperative period, and a new kit must be used each time the patient is suctioned. Remembering that upper respiratory passages, which trap and filter particles and bacteria from incoming air, have been bypassed enables the nurse to understand the need for strict aseptic technique in caring for the operative area. No hands but gloved hands, no catheter but a sterile one, and no saline but sterile saline should be in contact with the tracheostomy site. The patient's life is at stake and, although it may have been saved by a tracheostomy, it can be lost to overwhelming infection. Oral hygiene equipment, a self-inflating bag such as an AMBU bag, and pencil and paper will also be needed. If the patient does not require continuous ventilation with one of the ventilators described earlier in this chapter, continuous humidification of air will be needed since the nose and mouth have been bypassed. Special collars are available that are placed around the neck and attached to a hose leading to a nebulizer or humidifier.

Mucus, which is blood tinged at first, should be wiped away gently with a sterile gauze square as soon as it comes from the tube. Facial tissues should not be used for this since lint can be aspirated into the tracheostomy. Generally, the patient should be suctioned as needed to remove secretions. Unless otherwise ordered by the physician, the catheter should not be inserted more than 12.5 cm (5 in.). The technique used is the same as that described for intratracheal suctioning earlier in this chapter.

The inner cannula or tube, if present, is removed and cleaned as often as necessary, using sterile technique and equipment. Usually, cleansing of the inner cannula is needed every one to two hours. Later, cleansing may be scheduled every four to six hours. The inner cannula may be cleaned with a solution of half hydrogen peroxide and half sterile saline. Sterile pipe cleaners, roller gauze, or a stiff brush can be inserted into the inner cannula to scrub any remaining particles. The inner cannula is then rinsed in sterile saline. Disposable tracheostomy care kits are now available that contain the items needed for cannula cleansing. Silver tracheostomy tubes must be polished with silver polish to remove tarnish before the inner cannula is reinserted. After suctioning the outer cannula, the nurse reinserts the inner cannula and securely locks it into place.

When changing the tapes that secure the tracheostomy tube in place, the nurse should remove one side at a time. The tape is generally doubled for added security. Another person holds the tube in place with a gloved hand while the tapes are being changed. The outer cannula is changed by the physician, usually every 24 to 48 hours. The nurse may be asked to assist the physician with changing the outer cannula.

The skin around the tracheostomy site is cleansed and dried as often as necessary. It is important to avoid having the cleansing or rinsing solution enter the trachea. The cleansing solution used varies according to hospital policy; normal saline, hydrogen peroxide, or mild antiseptics are examples of typical solutions.

A tracheostomy dressing is placed between the outer cannula and the skin to collect secretions that can ooze from the site. When special tracheostomy dressings are not available, a 4″ × 4″ gauze square without inner cotton liner may be cut from edge to center to make a dressing that fits. A disadvantage of this dressing is possible loose strings which can be aspirated into the tracheostomy. An alternate method is to unfold the 4″ × 4″, roll it lengthwise, and gently place it around the outer cannula next to the skin.

The patient with a tracheostomy should be turned and repositioned at frequent intervals. This is important for all surgical patients but especially important to the patient with a tracheostomy because coughing is generally less effective following this surgery. Since the glottis lies above the tracheostomy, the patient has difficulty building up enough pressure to produce an effective cough. Thus, secretions tend to remain in the tracheobronchial tree. A more effective cough may be generated by instructing the patient to contract abdominal muscles quickly while exhaling at the same time. An increased fluid intake is generally needed to help thin pulmonary secretions and keep mucous membranes moist. Clear liquids usually are prescribed first.

If a cuffed tracheostomy tube is used, the nurse should make certain that the patient's cuff is properly inflated before drinking. This prevents aspiration of liquids into the tracheobronchial tree. Small sips should be taken at first, and the patient should be observed carefully for evidence of aspiration. If these are tolerated, other liquids may be introduced. The nurse should be prepared to suction the patient when fluids are offered. Swallowed fluids that continue to be expelled through the tracheostomy may indicate that an abnormal channel (fistula) has formed between the trachea and the esophagus located behind it. This is a serious complication that may require additional surgery. In some cases, feedings may be ordered via a nasogastric feeding tube.

Signs of difficult breathing or hemorrhage should also be reported to the physician at once. Rarely, the tracheostomy cannula is expelled accidently. In this event, the nurse should use the tracheostomy spreader located at the bedside to maintain an open tracheostomy site until the physician arrives. The nurse should not attempt to replace the cannula.

The patient with a tracheostomy is a very frightened individual. Since this is frequently an emergency procedure, the patient may return from surgery with no idea of what has happened or why. In addition the patient is unable to talk because air no longer passes over the vocal cords located above the tracheostomy site. The nurse must quickly and calmly explain these facts to the patient, showing the pencil and paper or magic slate provided for communication. Some patients may not be able to write, and the nurse will need to arrange for signals for communication. The arranged signals should be prominently recorded at the bedside and on the Kardex for use by other members of the health team. The nurse should also remember that the patient's family is likely to be terribly anxious too.

Similar explanations of procedures and equipment should be given to the family as well as the arranged communication signals.

The tracheostomy tube is removed before the patient leaves the hospital if the operation was a temporary measure. This removal usually is done gradually. One method that may be used for this purpose is the insertion of a small, sterile cork into the tracheostomy tube. The cork is left in place for short periods of time at first so that the patient becomes adjusted to normal breathing. The length of time is increased gradually. Before plugging a cuffed tracheostomy tube, the nurse must be certain that the cuff is deflated to prevent complete airway obstruction. Another method used is to replace the outer cannula with gradually smaller ones. This, of course, is done by the physician.

The tube is entirely removed by the physician when the patient's breathing pattern and blood gases indicate that it is no longer needed. After the tube has been removed, the nurse should observe the patient closely for signs of respiratory distress. A tracheostomy spreader generally remains at the bedside for several days for emergency use.

If the tracheostomy is permanent, a plan is developed to teach the patient and/or family how to care for it. In addition to cleansing and suctioning, an important feature of the teaching plan is avoiding or modifying activities that increase the danger that water or other substances can be aspirated into the tracheostomy. Careful showering generally is advised, and the patient usually is cautioned against swimming.

Atelectasis

The patient with atelectasis has a portion of the lung that does not expand properly. The affected lung tissue becomes airless, then collapses and shrinks. Atelectasis can occur from a variety of causes and may be partial or complete, acute or chronic. Retained secretions in the alveoli, aspirated foreign bodies, infections such as pneumonia or bronchitis, neoplasm, edema, and pressure on the airways by enlarged lymph nodes are the most common causes of this condition.

NURSING OBSERVATIONS AND MEDICAL DIAGNOSIS

Symptoms of atelectasis vary with the size of the area of the lung that is airless and with the rate of development. For example, the patient who develops atelectasis in a large part of the lung tissue probably will have dyspnea, chest pain, cyanosis, and sweating. The person with atelectasis of a lobe associated with a neoplasm of the lung may have no symptoms, probably because of the slow development of the airlessness.

When the physician listens to the patient's chest, breath sounds in the affected area are diminished or absent. A chest x-ray usually is ordered to locate the involved area more specifically and determine the size. When bronchial obstruction is suspected, a bronchoscopy may be done.

TREATMENT AND NURSING INTERVENTIONS

After the physician confirms the diagnosis with a chest examination and chest x-ray, treatment is directed toward correcting the underlying cause when possible. For example, the patient with bronchitis will be treated for that primary condition. As infection subsides, the patient's atelectasis gradually disappears.

Many occurrences of atelectasis can be prevented, especially by meticulous, conscientious nursing care. For example, postoperative atelectasis may occur as a result of secretions retained during anesthesia. This is more common following chest or high abdominal surgery, when severe pain may interfere with effective coughing. Frequent turning, deep-breathing exercises, and regular coughing are nursing interventions that prevent atelectasis.

These measures are also important for the patient who must remain immobile for long periods. Other measures that prevent atelectasis include early ambulation, avoidance of constricting dressings and restraints, careful use of sedatives and opiates that depress respiratory centers, deep breathing hourly while awake, and maintaining adequate fluid intake. The physician may also order IPPB treatments for prevention or treatment. Preventive measures described above are also part of therapy for a person with atelectasis. Postural drainage, suctioning, oxygen, and drug therapy are additional measures that may be needed.

Pneumonia

A patient with pneumonia has an infection of the lungs. Normal lung tissue is spongy. When an inflammation is present, the tissue becomes more solid. This change in the lung tissue associated with pneumonia can be compared with a sponge. After the sponge is filled with water, it has fewer air spaces and is more solid.

In most cases, pneumonia is caused by a pathogen such as bacteria or viruses. However, *aspiration pneumonia* can follow inhalation of materials such as vomitus into the lung. *Hypostatic pneumonia* may occur in a patient who remains in the same position and does not cough, deep-breathe, or turn. *Chemical pneumonia* may result from inhalation of noxious gases. The nurse may also hear of pneumonia that is described by the part of the lung involved. For example, *lobar pneumonia* means that an entire lobe of the lung is involved. *Bronchopneumonia* means that the infection is distributed in patches around the bronchioles and alveoli.

Pneumonia is more likely to occur in persons who are poorly nourished, who are in a weakened condition from bad health habits, or who are in a debilitated conditions from disease. For example, it may follow some of the communicable diseases, such as whooping cough and scarlet fever. Frequently, it affects infants, aged individuals, alcoholics, and persons who have had a previous attack of pneumonia.

The discovery and use of drugs such as sulfonamides and antibiotics, especially penicillin, have dramatically reduced the death rate from pneumonia.

BACTERIAL PNEUMONIA

SYMPTOMS. As stated previously, bacterial pneumonia is caused by bacteria that invade the lungs. The most common bacteria causing pneumonia are pneumococci. After the lungs have been attacked by the microorganisms, an inflammatory process begins. Because of this, the patient has a fever, malaise, chest pain, and other symptoms of an inflammation. Respiration is rapid, difficult, and painful. Generally, the cough is dry and hacking at first. Later it becomes productive, and the sputum is rusty in color. Cyanosis may be present, and chills are common.

DIAGNOSIS, TREATMENT, AND NURSING CARE. The nurse can expect that the physician will order a white blood count, chest x-ray, and sputum culture to help establish the diagnosis of pneumonia. Additional studies such as arterial blood gases and electrocardiogram may be indicated if the patient's respirations are severely compromised.

Treatment is likely to include an appropriate antibiotic, bed rest or limited ambulation, oxygen and postural drainage, IPPB, and a liquid diet. Generally, aspirin is not ordered for the patient with pneumonia since it may mask fever.

General nursing interventions related to rest, hygiene, positioning, coughing, and deep breathing were discussed earlier in this chapter and apply to the patient with pneumonia.

Measures to prevent the spread of infection are essential. Frequent handwashing and proper collection and disposal of soiled tissues are especially important. A fluid intake of 3000 to 4000 ml per day is generally needed unless contraindicated. Careful observation of the abdomen and elimination patterns is also important. Abdominal distention is a complication of pneumonia. If undetected, abdominal distention may become severe enough to restrict the patient's breathing. Measures such as rectal tubes and repositioning help to prevent distention.

The patient should be observed for symptoms that might indicate an unfavorable change in condition. For example, a sudden elevation of temperature, an increased pulse rate, more difficulty in breathing, cyanosis, and disorientation should be reported promptly.

VIRAL PNEUMONIA

The patient with viral pneumonia has an inflammation in lungs caused by a virus. Most acute pulmonary infections are viral pneumonias. The nurse may hear this disease referred to as either viral pneumonia or primary atypical pneumonia. Young adults seem to be affected most often by this type of pneumonia. Although the convalescent period is frequently prolonged, the outlook is good.

NURSING OBSERVATIONS

The onset of viral pneumonia is usually gradual. The patient complains of general aches and pains, malaise, and a cough. The cough is dry, hacking, and annoying. The patient also has a fever. The symptoms may last from one to six weeks.

TREATMENT AND NURSING INTERVENTIONS

In addition to general respiratory measures such as turning, deep breathing, and IPPB, rest is especially important. The patient is instructed to resume activity very slowly under the physician's supervision. Antibiotics usually are not prescribed since they do not kill viruses. A nourishing diet, increased fluid intake, and nonstrenuous activity are indicated because of the long convalescence.

Pleurisy

The patient with pleurisy has an inflammation of the pleura. The condition is known as dry or fibrinous pleurisy when the inflamed area contains little or no excess fluid. The condition is known as pleurisy with effusion when fluid collects between the two pleural layers (see Figure 14.13). The patient has empyema if the fluid becomes purulent (contains pus). Pleurisy usually is secondary to another disease; that is, it follows or complicates another disease. It may result from bacterial pneumonia, an injury to the chest wall, psittacosis, pulmonary tuberculosis, infarction, lung abscess, or bronchiectasis.

DIAGNOSIS AND NURSING OBSERVATIONS

A person with pleurisy has a sharp pain in the side caused by the two layers of the inflamed pleura rubbing together. The pain is usually more severe when the patient breathes in deeply. Thus, respirations are

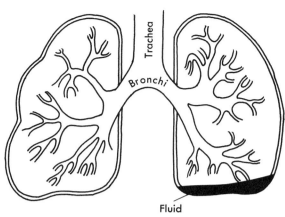

FIGURE 14.13   Diagram illustrating pleurisy with effusion.

shallow and rapid. A dry, painful cough and a fever often occur. The patient's pain decreases if fluid collects in the pleural cavity. This fluid prevents the two layers of the pleura from rubbing together.

When listening to the chest of a patient with dry pleurisy, the physician may hear a harsh, scratchy sound throughout the respiratory cycle. This is known as a pleural friction rub. Chest x-rays are taken. If effusion is suspected, additional studies such as pleural biopsy, ultrasound, and thoracentesis usually are ordered.

TREATMENT AND NURSING INTERVENTIONS

Generally, treatment is directed toward removing the cause of pleurisy if possible and relieving unpleasant symptoms. Rest in bed or limited ambulation usually is ordered. Drug therapy with antitussives, analgesics, and antibiotics may be prescribed. Narcotics generally are used sparingly since they depress respiratory centers. Heat to the painful area may relieve some patients.

A common procedure used not too long ago was to restrict chest movement, using a binder or strapping the chest with adhesive tape, in an effort to reduce pain. Binding and strapping of the chest are rarely used today because this restricts breathing and may promote the development of pneumonia and atelectasis as complications. Other important nursing measures include regular position changes, splinting of the painful

area of the chest while coughing, and deep breathing.

Thoracentesis may be needed to drain excess fluid which interferes with breathing. Very rarely, the patient may require closed chest drainage to prevent excess fluid from collapsing the lung. Caring for the patient with closed chest drainage is described later in this chapter.

Lung Abscess

The person with a lung abscess has a cavity in a lung that is filled with pus and dead lung tissue. Lung abscess may be caused by infection, neoplasm, or aspiration of foreign material such as vomitus. The body attempts to prevent the spread of infectious material to other portions of the lung by forming a wall or capsule around the infection. As infectious material accumulates, a cavity is made within lung tissue.

Aspiration of infectious material frequently takes place when the patient is in a stupor or unconscious. For this reason, the chronic alcoholic is likely to have a lung abscess. Convulsive seizures, anesthesia, and diabetic coma may result in the development of a lung abscess.

DIAGNOSIS AND NURSING OBSERVATIONS

The patient with an abscess of the lung experiences fever, sweating, malaise, loss of weight, anorexia, and a productive cough. The sputum is usually very thick and has a foul odor. Sputum color varies according to the infecting pathogen. Hemoptysis may occur.

A roentgenogram of the chest usually helps the doctor make a diagnosis. Examination of the sputum in the laboratory generally is done to identify the causative organisms as well as the most effective antibiotic.

TREATMENT AND NURSING INTERVENTIONS

On the basis of the culture and sensitivity report from the laboratory, the physician prescribes the most effective antimicrobial agent. Postural drainage may be prescribed to help empty the cavity of pus. The patient usually needs to be treated with an antibiotic for four to six weeks. Surgical resection of the affected portion of the lung may be necessary in some cases.

Care of the patient with chest surgery is described later in this chapter.

Nursing interventions such as frequent oral hygiene and good handwashing are important when caring for the patient with a lung abscess.

Chronic Obstructive Pulmonary Disease (COPD)

Chronic obstructive pulmonary disease is a group of conditions characterized by an obstruction to the normal exchange of gases in the lungs. The term *chronic* implies that the condition has existed for a long time. Frequently, conditions that do obstruct the passage of air in the lungs are referred to as chronic obstructive lung disease or as chronic obstructive pulmonary disease.

Generally, the person with COPD has a progressive disease; that is, the disease tends to worsen with time. Asthma, chronic bronchitis, bronchiectasis, and emphysema are the most common conditions associated with chronic obstructive lung disease. The incidence of COPD appears to be rising at an alarming rate. Factors believed to be associated with this increase include increased cigarette smoking, air pollution, and larger numbers of aged persons in the population. Degenerative changes in the lung that occur during the aging process are strongly associated with COPD. Thus, the nurse can expect to care for an increased number of persons with chronic obstructive pulmonary disease.

Each of the conditions is discussed separately in this text. Bronchial asthma was discussed in Chapter 10. However, a certain sequence of events is likely to occur in a patient with COPD that will help the nurse to understand the crippling nature of this disease.

- Bronchial walls are swollen, and bronchial secretions are thickened from infection or allergy.
- The alveoli may become either distended and/or collapsed because of obstruction in the bronchial tree.

- Bronchial and lung tissue is gradually destroyed and the elasticity of the bronchi and lungs is greatly reduced. Ciliary action is impaired and more secretions are retained.
- Increased work of breathing causes excessive fatigue, hypoxia, hypercapnia, weight loss, and decreased ability to respond to stress such as infection.
- Changes are seen in the heart, blood, and kidneys as they attempt to compensate for impaired lung function.

It is believed that preventive measures can be taken that reduce the likelihood that a person will develop COPD. These measures also apply to the person who already has the disease since they may help to control or slow the progression of destructive changes. Preventive measures include:

- Avoidance of respiratory irritants such as cigarette smoking, industrial irritants, and aerosol sprays used in the home
- Prevention of respiratory infection when possible by immunization and avoidance of contact with infected persons
- Prompt treatment of respiratory infection when it occurs
- Removal or correction of deformities such as nasal polyps or deviated nasal septum
- Promotion of good general health and good dental health

Asthma (Intrinsic)

Bronchial asthma was discussed at length in Chapter 10. Some scientists have observed that a type of asthma exists that is not related to allergy. This type of asthma is referred to as *intrinsic asthma*. The individual with intrinsic asthma usually has a negative family history for allergy and is 40 years of age or older. Symptoms of asthma in this patient generally develop during or after a respiratory infection. Other conditions such as nasal polyps and enlarged adenoids are frequently found by the physician during the physical examination. Usually, skin tests for allergy are negative and IgE (refer to Chapter 10) levels are normal. The symptoms, treatment, and nursing care are similar to those for the patient with bronchial extrinsic (allergic) asthma.

At times, intrinsic asthma is associated with bronchitis, giving rise to the term *asthmatic bronchitis*. At other times, this type of asthma coexists with emphysema.

Chronic Bronchitis

The individual with chronic bronchitis has a persistent or recurrent inflammation of the tracheobronchial tree that causes a productive cough. The incidence of chronic bronchitis is very high in England and appears to be increasing dramatically in the United States. Middle-aged and elderly men are affected more often than others. Heavy cigarette smoking, dusty occupations, air pollution, allergies, and foggy, cold, wet weather are factors strongly associated with chronic bronchitis.

The patient's mucous glands and mucous goblet cells increase in size and number resulting in an increase of sputum. As the disease progresses, cilia are destroyed, scarring occurs in bronchial airways, and muscular layers of the bronchi are deformed. These changes usually result in narrow airways, retained secretions, and frequent infection.

DIAGNOSIS AND NURSING OBSERVATIONS

The physician generally diagnoses this condition on the basis of the patient's history of chronic productive cough. Bronchoscopy, bronchogram, and pulmonary function tests may be ordered to determine the severity of disease. Arterial blood gases also may be done to assess the effectiveness of gas exchange. Other tests may be ordered to rule out tumor, tuberculosis, or bronchiectasis. The person with chronic bronchitis usually begins the day by coughing and expectorating mucus soon after getting out of bed. Some mucoid sputum may be expectorated later during the day.

As the condition progresses purulent sputum is produced continuously or at some time during the day. The nurse may hear this condition referred to as recurrent mucopurulent bronchitis. The condition may be called chronic obstructive bronchitis when the patient develops an obstruction to airflow. Exposure to irritants, such as smog and a common cold, frequently causes the patient to have an acute flareup, which may be life-threatening. Symptoms of fever, wheezing, malaise, paroxysms of coughing, dyspnea, and cyanosis may be present. Respiratory failure may follow, and death can occur.

The patient's appearance during later stages is so characteristic that the term "blue bloater" is used for descriptive purposes. The blue refers to cyanosis which is common. Bloat refers to a distended abdomen and tendency toward overweight which is also common.

TREATMENT AND NURSING INTERVENTIONS

Treatment and nursing care of the patient with chronic bronchitis are directed toward activities that minimize bronchial irritation, improve the raising of sputum, and prevent infection.

Since cigarette smoking is the most common irritant associated with chronic bronchitis, the smoking patient is advised to stop. Some patients are helped to stop smoking by participating in a community program or stop smoking clinic. The patient whose condition is aggravated by occupational hazards is advised to reduce known irritants as much as possible. Changing one's occupation to avoid such irritants is not easy to do. For example, the coal miner who has no other skill and no other possible place of employment in the community is not likely to give up a job. The patient whose condition is associated with allergy is treated as described in Chapter 10.

Drug therapy includes an appropriate antibiotic for the patient with infection and bronchodilators such as aminophylline.

Exercise programs are also an important part of therapy. Walking is the exercise most frequently prescribed. Breathing exercises, IPPB, effective coughing, postural drainage, increased fluids, and air humidification are measures discussed earlier in this chapter that may apply to the patient with chronic bronchitis. The patient's progress and response to treatment are generally monitored by pulmonary function studies, x-rays, and arterial blood gases.

Patient and family teaching is an important aspect of treatment and nursing care. Many of the above activities must be carried on at home. The patient is instructed that increased purulence, thickness, and amount of sputum are early signs of infection which should be reported to the physician at once. In some cases, continuous antibiotic therapy is prescribed during periods of increased susceptibility.

Bronchiectasis

A patient with bronchiectasis has a chronic disease of the bronchial tree in which there is a dilatation of one or more bronchi. This dilatation is accompanied by reduced elasticity of the affected bronchi, increased secretion of mucus, and chronic bronchial infection. As the condition progresses, bronchial walls become weakened by disease. These changes favor the formation of pus in the lower end of the bronchial tree. (See Figure 14.14.)

Bronchiectasis may occur following atelectasis, tuberculosis, aspiration of a foreign object, pulmonary complications after surgery, and pneumonia. Heredity and congenital factors such as cystic fibrosis are associated with bronchiectasis. Immune deficiency disease and atopic asthma also are associated with bronchiectasis.

DIAGNOSIS AND NURSING OBSERVATIONS

The patient with bronchiectasis has a chronic productive cough. The cough is frequently worse following a change in position. For example, going to bed and getting out of bed may cause a coughing spell. A

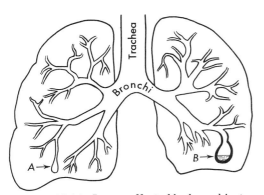

FIGURE 14.14 Lungs affected by bronchiectasis. A small cavity is located at A, and a larger one containing pus is located at B.

large amount of sputum is produced which usually contains pus. Hemoptysis (expectoration of blood) occurs when a blood vessel is involved. After the patient has had this disease for some time, fingertips may become flattened and widened. This is known as clubbing of the fingers. Fever, malaise, and other symptoms of an active infection are present during the acute stage of the disease.

The diagnostic procedures the physician may order include chest x-ray, bronchoscopy, bronchogram, sputum examinations, and pulmonary function tests. These tests, together with the patient's history and symptoms, help to confirm the diagnosis and determine its severity.

TREATMENT AND NURSING INTERVENTIONS

If bronchiectasis is not treated, it develops into an incurable disease that shortens the patient's life. It may be complicated by pneumonia, lung abscess, and hemorrhage.

In treating a patient with bronchiectasis, the physician tries to improve the person's general health and to remove the cause if possible. For example, the patient who has this disease as a result of chronic bronchitis caused by chronic sinusitis is treated for both conditions.

Antibiotics are a very important part of therapy. An increase in the volume and purulence of sputum generally indicates that a specimen should be collected prior to beginning antibiotic therapy.

Bronchoscopy may be needed as a therapeutic measure to aspirate secretions and fluid from the dilated bronchi. Other important measures discussed earlier in this chapter that apply to the patient with bronchiectasis include rest, oral hygiene, postural drainage, breathing and coughing techniques, and increased fluid intake. General preventive measures for chronic obstructive pulmonary disease also apply to this patient. Yearly vaccines for influenza and pneumonia are recommended.

Surgery to remove diseased tissue is much less common than it once was. Pulmonary surgery may be considered in selected patients who have local involvement, whose condition does not respond to medical therapy, and who are severely disabled. Other possible indications for surgery include repeated episodes of hemoptysis and recurrent pneumonia. Information about caring for a patient with chest surgery can be located on pages 441–45.

Emphysema

The individual with emphysema has abnormal enlargement of the alveoli with destruction of alveolar walls. Since tiny capillaries are located in alveolar walls, they too are destroyed and the surface area of the lungs available for gas exchange is greatly reduced. As air spaces lose their elasticity, inhaled air becomes trapped in the dilated, less elastic air passages. In other words, the patient is not able to exhale the usual amount of air from the lungs. There is continued difficulty in deflating lungs adequately. The basic disease process sets the stage for trapping of mucus and bacteria, destruction of cilia, narrowing of airways, and collapse of the bronchi during expiration.

The incidence of emphysema is increasing rapidly along with other chronic respiratory diseases such as chronic bronchitis. Men in the middle or later phases of life seem to be especially prone to developing this disease. Emphysema is increasing, especially in heavily polluted industrial areas. Cigarette smoking is strongly associated with emphysema. The death rate from emphysema also is increasing.

NURSING OBSERVATIONS

Early emphysema causes the patient to experience fatigue, dyspnea on exertion, and persistent productive cough. The neck veins may become visibly distended during expiration. Usually the patient is a mouth-breather. The lips may be pursed during expiration. In observing the patient's breathing, the nurse notices that the normal pattern is reversed, that is, expiration now is longer than inspiration as airways collapse during expiration (due to trapped air), and wheezing may be heard. Inspiration is usually short and rapid. The patient's color may be pale, pink, or ruddy. The patient's appearance is so characteristic that the term "pink puffer" has come to be used for descriptive purposes. As the disease progresses, the patient may be forced to assume a sitting position even at rest. The neck appears shorter and neck muscles are tight and tense. The patient speaks in short, jerky sentences. Gradual changes in the shape and size of the chest may result from overdistention of alveoli and trapped air. The chest becomes barrel shaped. The back becomes more rounded, a condition known as dorsal kyphosis. During ventilation, chest and abdominal muscle movements are visible as they help to push trapped air out. The patient may assume a posture as described earlier in this chapter on page 408. The patient looks thin and wasted. The nurse may observe other signs of hypoxia such as cyanosis and clubbing of the fingertips. The patient experiences more anxiety as breathing difficulties increase.

In the later stages of emphysema, additional symptoms of heart failure, such as tachycardia, edema, and venous distention in the neck, may occur. The patient experiences impaired memory, headache, lethargy, and disorientation.

Death may follow from heart failure, respiratory failure, or collapse of the lung caused by rupture of a highly distended liquid-filled air sac (bulla).

ASSISTING WITH DIAGNOSTIC STUDIES

Some or all of the diagnostic tests described earlier in this chapter may be ordered by the physician to establish the diagnosis or check the progression of disease.

The chest x-ray may seem normal in the early stages of disease. In later stages, the x-ray shows changes in the chest diameter, widening of rib spaces, and lungs enlarged by trapped air. Pulmonary function studies show increased residual volume, reduced expiratory volume, and an increased total lung capacity. Arterial blood gases show reduced gas exchange as the arterial oxygen level falls and arterial carbon dioxide level rises (hypercapnia). Rising carbon dioxide levels result in respiratory acidosis (the pH drops). In some cases, the red blood cell count (RBC) rises because the body has responded to hypoxia by increasing the number of red cells available to carry oxygen. Additional studies such as an electrocardiogram (ECG) and complete blood count (CBC) may be ordered. As mentioned earlier, diagnostic studies can be especially exhausting to the patient with a respiratory disorder.

TREATMENT AND NURSING INTERVENTIONS

Treatment and nursing care of the patient with emphysema are directed toward preserving and improving pulmonary function and preventing complications. Preventive measures discussed earlier apply to the patient with emphysema.

Drug therapy includes bronchodilators and expectorants to reduce retained secretions. Additional drug therapy such as digitalis and diuretics may be indicated in later stages when the heart is affected. Steroid drugs also may be prescribed. A large number of patients with emphysema develop peptic ulcer. The nurse should be especially alert for abdominal soreness, hematemesis, and epigastric pain when a patient receives steroid therapy. When there is infection, an antibiotic is prescribed.

In addition to drug therapy, numerous other interventions help to remove retained secretions. Breathing and coughing techniques, intratracheal suctioning, postural drainage, IPPB (with compressed air), and increasing the fluid intake are vital parts of therapy. These measures are described in earlier sections of this chapter.

Oxygen therapy is prescribed very cautiously for the patient with emphysema. The nurse must be especially observant and careful when oxygen is used for a patient with chronic obstructive lung disease such as emphysema. Remembering that this patient has experienced long-standing hypoxia and hypercapnia enables the nurse to understand that the normal balance between oxygen and carbon dioxide is altered. High-dose oxygen may remove hypoxia, which is the patient's remaining stimulus to breathe. When oxygen is needed, the dosage ordered is usually low—no more than 2 to 3 liters per minute. The nurse should check the liter flow frequently to maintain the desired oxygen level. Special masks, such as Venturi masks, are available that are so constructed that the patient cannot receive too much oxygen.

A practice to be carefully avoided is increasing the flow of oxygen when the patient is dyspneic. This practice may cause the patient to stop breathing because of an oxygen and carbon dioxide imbalance, as described above. Appropriate nursing interventions include elevating the head of the bed, checking to make sure oxygen tubing is not kinked or twisted, assisting the patient with a deep-breathing exercise. If these and similar measures do not help, the head nurse, team leader, or physician should be consulted. These facts are an important part of patient teaching when the patient is to use oxygen at home. The patient and family members are taught about possible hazards of oxygen overdosage.

Rest is an important part of therapy. The nurse is challenged to plan nursing care that includes time for therapy and time for rest. The patient usually does not sleep well due to the combined effects of dyspnea, anxiety, and drug therapy. Usually, frequent brief rest periods between activities are helpful. Rushing the patient is avoided because this worsens breathing.

Occasionally, selected patients may benefit by surgical resection of the lung when large local bullae (blisters) are compressing normal lung tissue. Most patients, however, have widespread disease and cannot be helped by surgery at the present time.

Despite the fact that the patient experiences considerable fear and apprehension, tranquilizers and sedatives are avoided because they depress the respiratory centers. Thus, the nurse must develop highly skilled approaches to help allay anxiety that might further worsen the patient's breathing. The student may refer to earlier sections in this chapter for nursing measures to reduce anxiety.

Patient teaching is also an essential part of therapy. Coughing and breathing exercises, postural drainage, medication, and other measures already discussed are part of a lifelong treatment plan that also may include vocational rehabilitation. The nurse can expect that a variety of health team members may be needed to help the patient and family cope with this serious disease.

Remembering that emphysema is more common among middle- and older-aged men enables the nurse to understand the devastating financial effect of emphysema on the family when the breadwinner is affected or when income is fixed or reduced as in later years.

Local chapters of the American Lung Association help to provide public education, professional training, and rehabilitation. The nurse can contact the local chapter for assistance. For information and assistance in locating a local chapter, interested persons may write to the following address:

American Lung Association
1740 Broadway
New York, New York 10019

Respiratory Failure

The individual with respiratory failure has a life-threatening impairment of oxygen–carbon dioxide exchange. Respiratory failure may result from a variety of conditions, including drug overdose, head injury, chest injury, chronic obstructive pulmonary disease, and renal failure. If not treated, respiratory failure results in respiratory arrest and death.

DIAGNOSIS AND NURSING OBSERVATIONS

The symptoms the patient experiences vary with cause of failure. Therefore, the physician must obtain a careful history. Behavioral changes are the earliest indicators of respiratory failure. Anxiety, lethargy, irritability, restlessness, headache, and dyspnea are early warnings the nurse should observe, report, and record.

Mental confusion and sleepiness are later signs that the patient's brain is not receiving enough oxygen. In some instances, the patient may be comatose, and family or friends must provide needed information. One diagnostic test the nurse may expect to see repeatedly is arterial blood gases. Respiratory failure is considered evident when arterial oxygen pressure (PaO_2) falls below 50 mm Hg or when arterial carbon dioxide pressure ($PaCo_2$) rises above 50 mm Hg. Additional studies include complete blood count (CBC),

blood urea nitrogen (BUN), serum creatinine and electrolytes, electrocardiogram, and chest x-ray. Other studies may be indicated to help the physician locate the underlying cause of respiratory failure.

TREATMENT AND NURSING INTERVENTIONS

Prompt treatment is needed to prevent death. Lifesaving measures to establish an adequate airway and provide adequate ventilation and oxygen are needed. Usually, these include endotracheal intubation or tracheostomy, oxygen, suctioning, and mechanical ventilation with a pressure- or volume-cycled ventilator. The patient is generally transferred to the intensive care unit or respiratory intensive care unit, where specially trained doctors and nurses observe and care for the patient.

In addition to measures to ensure adequate gas exchange, the underlying cause of the patient's respiratory failure is identified and treated.

Adult Respiratory Distress Syndrome (ARDS)

The patient with ARDS has a life-threatening condition associated with fluid and acute injury to lung tissue. A variety of names has been used to describe this condition including *wet lung* and *shock lung*. Massive trauma, drowning, drug overdose, shock, and inhaled toxins are examples of a wide variety of factors associated with this syndrome.

Injury causes the alveoli to collapse and stiffen. The work of breathing increases, and gas exchange is impaired. In some cases permanent scarring results, and elastic recoil is lost from stiffened lungs.

DIAGNOSIS AND NURSING OBSERVATIONS

The patient's symptoms depend on the underlying cause. At the time of the initial injury, there may be no signs or symptoms of this respiratory syndrome. Several hours later, an increase in the respiratory rate can be observed and the patient may complain of dyspnea. The physician may hear fine rales on inspiration when listening to the chest, and the chest x-ray shows some evidence of scattered infiltrate.

As the patient's condition worsens, the respiratory rate increases, dyspnea is more pronounced, tachycardia increases, and the blood pressure may fall. Cyanosis may occur. Oxygen fails to improve the patient's color or vital signs. Arterial oxygen falls dramatically even when the patient is inspiring 100 percent oxygen. Subsequent chest x-ray shows an increase of fluid in the lung tissue. Death results if prompt treatment is not instituted.

TREATMENT AND NURSING INTERVENTIONS

The patient with suspected ARDS is usually transferred promptly to the intensive care unit or respiratory intensive care unit. Usual treatment plans include an artificial airway using an endotracheal tube, mechanical ventilation with a special pressure device, steroid therapy, and treatment of the underlying cause.

Chest Trauma and Surgery: General Considerations

Changes that occur as a result of chest trauma and surgery have some common features, with implications for nursing observations and interventions (Table 14.7). First, normal pressure relationships between air inside and outside the body are changed.

Second, there is interference with normal breathing patterns and protective mechanisms such as cough. Third, there is a disturbance in the large volume of blood that normally passes through the lung. Fourth, usually there is swelling. Last, generally there is pain. These changes which occur as a result of chest trauma or surgery increase the likelihood of air in the pleural space, infection and retained secretions in the tracheobronchial tree, hemorrhage, and abnormal fluid collection in the lung.

FRACTURED RIBS

Fractured ribs constitute a common chest injury which can result from injury to the chest or from bone disease which weakens bone structure. A disturbance in respiratory function may occur from bony fragments which injure pleural or lung tissue or from pain which causes the patient to restrict breathing.

DIAGNOSIS AND NURSING OBSERVATIONS

The patient with fractured ribs generally has pain and tenderness in the affected area. There may be swelling, bruising, or visible bone fragments at the site of injury. Respirations are usually shallow and rapid, and the patient holds the chest during breathing to minimize movement and pain. Bright-red sputum, cyanosis, labored respirations, and symptoms of shock indicate that air and/or blood have entered the pleural space. This is

TABLE 14.7
IMPLICATIONS OF COMMON CHANGES RESULTING FROM CHEST SURGERY OR TRAUMA

CHANGES	IMPLICATIONS
Disturbances of normal pressure relationships between air inside and outside the body	May allow air to enter pleural space May require chest tubes to reestablish normal relationships
Interference with normal breathing patterns and protective mechanisms such as cough	May disturb normal acid-base balance May result in retained secretions in tracheobronchial tree
Disturbance in large blood volume that normally passes through the lung	May result in hemorrhage May allow blood to enter pleural space or alveoli
Swelling (edema)	May allow fluid in pleural space or in alveoli Accumulation of fluid may compress the heart
Pain	May restrict breathing and cause retained secretions in tracheobronchial tree

a serious complication which the nurse reports immediately. The physician diagnoses the patient's condition on the basis of a history, physical examination, and chest x-ray.

TREATMENT AND NURSING INTERVENTIONS

Deep breathing, coughing, and frequent changes in position are nursing interventions that help prevent pulmonary complications of rib fractures.

Local anesthetic or small doses of meperidine (DEMEROL) are prescribed to control pain and to enable the patient to deep-breathe and cough effectively. Large doses of opiates are avoided because they depress respiratory centers in the brain.

The old practice of strapping the chest with adhesive tape or a chest binder is now avoided. Strapping the chest restricts breathing movement and increases the likelihood of pulmonary complications.

Hemothorax, Pneumothorax

The individual with *hemothorax* has a collection of blood in the pleural space. The term *pneumothorax* indicates that the patient has air in the pleural space. Hemothorax may result from lacerated blood vessels or lung tissue and abnormal bleeding following chest surgery. Pneumothorax may be caused from a hole in the chest wall that allows air to enter the pleural space. In some cases, air escapes into the pleural space from a rupture or laceration of the bronchi, bronchioles, or alveoli. As air and/or fluid collects in the pleural space, pressure around the lung increases, causing partial or complete collapse.

Tension pneumothorax is a life-threatening condition in which air leaks into the pleural space as the patient inspires but remains trapped there. With each inspiration, the amount of trapped air increases and finally collapses the patient's lung. This, in turn, causes pressure on the trachea, heart, vena cava, and opposite lung—a condition known as *mediastinal shift*. Unless the patient receives prompt emergency treatment, death may follow.

DIAGNOSIS AND NURSING OBSERVATIONS

The patient with hemothorax or pneumothorax generally has pain and difficult breathing, increased pulse and respirations, and cyanosis. Symptoms of shock may be evident. If the patient has a tension pneumothorax, some of the trapped air may escape into the subcutaneous tissue, causing swelling, a spongy feeling, and a crackling sound when the tissue is palpated. This condition is known as *subcutaneous emphysema*. In addition, the physician or nurse may observe that the patient's trachea is pushed to one side, and that blood pressure is lowered or absent. After listening for breath sounds with a stethoscope, the physician may order a chest x-ray if the patient's condition permits. If this is not possible, the physician may insert an 18-gauge needle into the pleural space. This procedure is both diagnostic and therapeutic. In other words, air or fluid escaping from the pleural space tells the physician that blood or air has caused the lung to collapse. At the same time, pressure around the patient's lung is relieved temporarily. This may be a lifesaving procedure when the patient has tension pneumothorax.

TREATMENT AND NURSING INTERVENTIONS

The patient with a hemothorax or pneumothorax generally requires closed chest drainage, which permits air and fluid to leave the pleural space, prevents air from the atmosphere from entering the pleural space, and allows the lung to reexpand. The care of the patient with closed chest drainage is discussed later in this chapter.

Generally, an antibiotic is prescribed to prevent infection. The patient also may need oxygen. General nursing measures such as coughing, deep breathing, and positioning apply to this patient. In some cases, surgery may be needed to correct the underlying cause of the patient's condition.

Thoracotomy

A thoracotomy is a surgical procedure in which the thoracic cavity is opened to promote free drainage of pus or blood, locate the source of injury or bleeding, or biopsy tumor tissue. The incision is usually large, and postoperative closed chest drainage is usually necessary.

Pulmonary Resection

The patient may require surgery to remove part or all of a lung that has been diseased from cysts, carcinoma, or chronic infection such as bronchiectasis or pulmonary tuberculosis. *Lobectomy* refers to surgical removal of a lobe of the lung. *Segmental resection* refers to surgical removal of one or more segments of diseased lung tissue. *Wedge resection* refers to surgical removal of a small, wedge-shaped portion of diseased lung tissue. Following each of these three procedures, the patient requires closed chest drainage.

Pneumonectomy refers to surgical removal of an entire lung. Following this procedure, the patient generally does not have closed chest drainage because the surgeon wants the fluid to collect and consolidate in the space left by the lung that has been removed. The surgeon may request that the patient be placed on the affected operated side in order to promote collection and consolidation of fluid.

NURSING CARE FOR THE PATIENT WITH CHEST SURGERY

PREOPERATIVE CARE. In addition to the usual preoperative tests described in Chapter 6, the patient usually has a sputum examination, pulmonary function tests, bronchoscopy, bronchogram, x-ray and fluoroscopy, tomograms, and an electrocardiogram.

Frequent oral hygiene with antiseptic mouthwash reduces the number of potential pathogens. Postural drainage, IPPB, deep breathing and coughing, antibiotics, and bronchodilators may be prescribed to ensure that the patient is in optimum condition prior to surgery. The patient is urged to refrain from smoking before and after surgery.

Preoperative teaching is essential for the patient before chest surgery. The nurse may be asked to assist or reinforce this teaching. Generally, the patient is given a complete explanation of equipment such as incentive spirometry (Figure 14.15), closed chest drainage and breathing, turning techniques, and coughing routines. Practice sessions may be scheduled so that the patient can breathe correctly, turn, and cough following surgery. The family also receives explanations so that they will not be frightened by

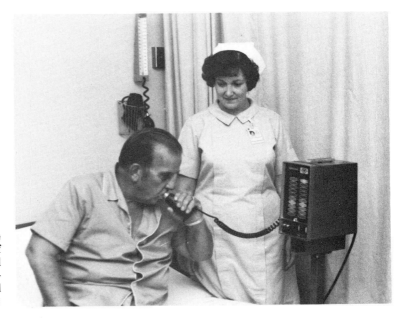

FIGURE 14.15 Incentive spirometry. (Courtesy of Suffolk City Schools and Louise Obici Memorial Hospital School of Practical Nursing, Suffolk, Virginia.)

the variety of equipment when they visit the patient after surgery.

The use of pain medication is discussed with the patient and family prior to surgery. They are told that pain medication is administered to control or diminish pain but that pain is not completely eliminated. The patient and family are encouraged to ask questions and verbalize their feelings about the surgery.

POSTOPERATIVE CARE. Generally, the patient is helped to be as active as possible soon after surgery. During the first 24 hours postoperatively, the patient usually is assisted to turn, cough, and deep-breathe every hour (Figure 14.16). Measures such as suctioning, oxygen, and positioning, as well as the usual postoperative care, apply to this patient. This care is so vital that the patient is awakened as often as necessary to participate. Range-of-motion exercises of the arm and shoulder nearest the incision are important to prevent joint stiffness and contractures. At first, exercises are passive. As the postoperative period progresses, the patient assumes a more active role.

The nurse's skill in relieving the patient's postoperative pain has a direct effect on preventing complications. The patient must be comfortable enough to participate in turning, deep breathing, and coughing exercises. However, overmedication with narcotics depresses brain respiratory centers and may cause the patient to be too sleepy to participate effectively. Meperidine (DEMEROL) is prescribed often following chest surgery because it appears to dilate the bronchi in addition to relieving pain. Postoperative activities are planned so that they occur during the time when the patient is receiving the maximum pain relief. In addition to medication, the nurse selects other pain-relieving interventions such as repositioning, massage, and diversion as described in Chapter 7.

The patient's position is often specified by the surgeon. The position orders are followed carefully by the nurse. Generally, the patient's position is changed frequently to avoid retained secretions and to improve blood flow. It is very important to be aware of and control the movement of chest tubes when the patient has closed chest drainage. Usually this means that two persons are needed to turn the patient. One person assists the patient directly. The other person holds the tubes and manipulates them so

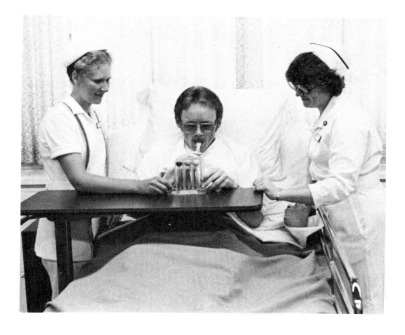

FIGURE 14.16 A spirometer assists the postoperative patient to take deep breaths. (Courtesy of North Dakota State School of Science, Practical Nursing Program, Wahpeton, North Dakota.)

that they do not become dislodged, pulled, twisted, or kinked while the patient is repositioned.

In addition, special nursing observation and interventions are needed to maintain closed chest drainage. As mentioned earlier, closed chest drainage permits air and fluid to drain from the chest through a tube into a drainage bottle and prevents air from the atmosphere from entering the chest (see Figure 14.17). Using sterile equipment, the surgeon inserts as small rubber or plastic tube through an incision into the cavity. This tube is clamped to prevent air from entering the pleural cavity. The tube is then attached to long tubing, which has its open end under water in a sealed drainage bottle. The amount of sterile water used is designated by the doctor. The purpose of the water is to prevent air from entering the pleural cavity through the tubing. Since water makes a seal, this type of drainage is often called water seal drainage. Normally, pressure between the lung and the pleura is less than at-

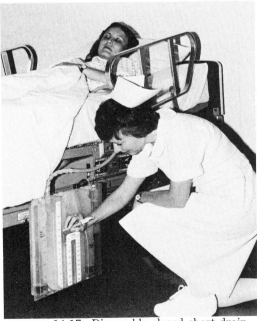

FIGURE 14.17 Disposable closed chest drainage used following chest surgery. (Courtesy of Newport News Public Schools and Riverside Hospital School of Practical Nursing, Newport News, Virginia.)

mospheric pressure. If air enters the chest cavity through the tubing, it will cause the lung to collapse because of the difference in pressure.

When helping to care for the patient with closed drainage of the chest, the nurse needs to remember that the setup is actually closed. In other words, no air should be allowed to enter it. Thus, it is of extreme importance to keep the tubing connected. Usually tube connections are taped. The equipment should be observed frequently for leakage. The open end of the tube in the drainage bottle should be below the water. The drainage bottle must always be kept below the level of the patient's chest. This also should be checked often by members of the nursing staff. Water in the tubing should rise and fall with inspiration and expiration. If it does not, the tubing may be kinked or clogged with drainage. There should be no pressure on the tubing by pillows or the patient's body. The nurse may relieve clogged drainage tubing by manipulating the tubes in a process called *milking* and *stripping*. In a very gentle fashion beginning at the portion of the tube nearest the chest, the nurse grasps the tube in one hand to stabilize it. With the other hand, the tubing is gently squeezed while moving it in a downward direction away from the patient's body and toward the drainage bottle. An alcohol sponge held in the squeezing hand helps to reduce friction and ensure smoother movements. Another method is to gently compress the tube against the palm of the hand while moving in a downward direction. The physician should be notified if these measures do not promote drainage and reestablish fluctuation of water during inspiration and expiration.

Continuous bubbling indicates an air leak in the closed system. The nurse should check for air leaks around the tube insertion site, at connections, and up and down the tubing. The physician should be notified if a leak is present. Evidence of respiratory distress, puffy appearance of the tissue around the tubing, and drainage that exceeds 100 ml per hour should be reported also.

Usually the closed water seal drainage bottle is changed only by the physician or specially trained nurse. Other nurses should not attempt this procedure unless they have been specifically instructed and supervised to do so. Generally, two clamps are applied to the tubing at a point near its insertion in the chest. The new water seal bottle is connected using aseptic technique. A piece of tape is placed on the water seal bottle and drainage levels are marked between bottle changes.

The patient may ambulate, sit in a chair, be transported to x-ray, or be repositioned with this type of drainage so long as the bottle remains below the level of the chest, the tubes are not kinked or otherwise occluded, and the connection remains intact. When drainage is especially thick or copious, or contains many blood clots, gravity alone may not be sufficient to drain material from the pleural space. The physician may attach suction to the drainage apparatus, as shown in Figure 14.17. One or two additional bottles may be used. When this type of suction is used, air and fluid are removed from the pleural space by gravity and suction. The water seal tubing must be under water but will not fluctuate with inspiration and expiration because suction keeps the water level constant. As mentioned previously, continuous bubbling in the water seal bottle indicates an air leak, which should be reported. The second bottle is known as the suction control bottle. A long rod (suction control tube) that is open to the air controls suction by its depth below the water line. Pressure is maintained by this rod by drawing air in from the atmosphere. Air passes through the rod into the water, causing it to

bubble continuously. Absence of bubbling in the suction control bottle indicates that pressure is not being maintained properly. After checking for loose connections, kinked or clogged tubing, and air leaks, the nurse should notify the physician.

As a general rule, chest tubes should not be clamped unless there is a specific order to do so. The nurse can understand the importance of this by knowing that the purpose is drainage of fluid and air. When a chest tube is clamped, air and fluid quickly surround the lung and may cause it to collapse. Table 14.8 contains a list of accidents that may occur together with appropriate nursing actions.

A sterile, disposable plastic unit to provide underwater seal drainage of the pleural cavity, PLEUR-EVAC, is used in some localities. The conventional three-bottle system is incorporated into a single unit having one chamber for suction, one for water seal, and one for collection of drainage. This sterile unit is easy for both the patient and the nurse to handle. Specific instructions from the manufacturer should be followed when handling the Pleur-evac and other commercially prepared units.

When drainage diminishes sufficiently, the surgeon removes the chest tubes. The nurse may be asked to assist. The patient usually receives pain medication about 30 minutes prior to the procedure. The surgeon uses a suture set to remove the stitches holding the tubes in place. The patient is instructed either to take a deep breath in and hold it or to breathe out completely and hold

TABLE 14.8
NURSING ACTIONS RELATED TO COMMON ACCIDENTS WITH CLOSED CHEST DRAINAGE

PROBLEM	NURSING ACTION
Disconnected chest tube	Reconnect the tube and tape it. Check all other connections and tape them. Report to head nurse
Bottle elevated above level of chest	Lower bottle at once and immediately notify physician. Observe patient for signs of difficult breathing
Water seal bottle kicked over	Return bottle to upright position and secure to rack, floor, or bed with tape. Instruct patient to take several deep breaths. Report to head nurse
Water seal bottle broken	Plunge end of tubing into a glass, cup, or basin of water until another bottle is obtained. Notify physician at once and observe patient closely for signs of respiratory distress. Anticipate that contaminated chest tubing may have to be changed by physician

it. The tubes are removed by the surgeon during breath-holding. Usually a petrolatum gauze dressing is applied to the site to seal the wound and prevent air from entering the chest through the wound site. Additional dressing is applied over the petrolatum gauze and secured firmly with wide adhesive. Usually a chest x-ray is taken immediately after the dressing is in place. The patient is observed closely for signs of air leakage. Dyspnea, anxiety, tachycardia, and tachypnea (rapid breathing) are signs of respiratory distress that should be reported immediately. Subcutaneous emphysema (swelling of tissue underneath the skin which crackles when touched) around the dressing also should be reported.

Prior to discharge the patient receives oral and written instructions about activities to be included and avoided, drug therapy, and any alterations of life-style recommended because of the surgery and/or underlying disease condition. Preventive measures described on page 148 apply to the surgical patient as well.

Pulmonary Tuberculosis

Pulmonary tuberculosis is a chronic communicable infection of the lungs caused by a microorganism known as *Mycobacterium tuberculosis*. Tuberculosis infection has been known since biblical times. Early in this century, the patient with tuberculosis had a bleak future of illness, disability, isolation, separation from loved ones, and premature death. Later, antibacterial drugs were developed that enabled many persons with pulmonary tuberculosis to be cured and drastically changed the mode of treatment. Bovine tuberculosis, caused by *Mycobacterium bovis* and spread by cow's milk, has been dramatically reduced by the testing and pasteurization of milk.

Certain social factors have altered the present-day picture of tuberculosis. For example, migration of rural people into large cities has concentrated tuberculosis primarily in large urban areas. In addition, a high rate of pulmonary tuberculosis is seen in the population over 65 years of age.

A person in poor physical condition is more likely to develop tuberculosis than is a healthy neighbor. An inadequate diet, continuous overwork, and poor living conditions, such as overcrowding, can make a person more susceptible. Anemia, diabetes, chronic alcoholism, and other chronic disease can predispose to tuberculosis.

TRANSMISSION

The tubercle bacillus is covered with mucoid material or a capsule, which makes it capable of living for long periods of time. It can live outside the body in both hot and cold weather. However, the bacillus cannot reproduce itself except in the body or in the laboratory. Although this micoorganism can live for months in a dark area, it dies after a few hours of direct sunlight or ultraviolet light. The tubercle bacillus can also be killed by heat, such as burning and boiling, and by certain disinfectants such as coal tar preparations.

The spread of tuberculosis generally is by inhalation. In other words, the tubercle bacilli make their journey from an infected person to another person by air. Minute droplets of moisture containing the bacilli are exhaled by the infected person during coughing, sneezing, and laughing. Air currents then carry the particles and distribute them somewhat like cigarette smoke in the air. In order for a person to become infected, minute particles containing the bacilli must arrive in *susceptible* lung tissue and multiply. Larger particles generally are trapped in the nose and upper respiratory structures and do not cause infection.

Present evidence indicates that objects such as books, linen, and furniture that contain tubercle bacilli generally do not cause infection. Good handwashing after handling such objects is generally sufficient to remove organisms from the hands. Within the hospital, the infected person is generally separated from other patients until becoming noninfectious. This is because sick individuals generally have lowered resistance to infection and are therefore more susceptible to infection caused by *Mycobacterium tuberculosis*. Methods once thought to decrease the transmission of tuberculosis, such as use of cap, gown, and mask as well as boiling of dishes and washing of walls, are now considered unnecessary and ineffective. Occasionally, nursing personnel may mask and gown for close contact with a patient who is just beginning drug therapy and who is unable to cover the nose and mouth when sneezing and coughing. Measures such as teaching the infected individual to cover the mouth with a tissue when coughing or sneezing and meticulous handwashing by the patient and the nurse are generally considered effective in preventing the spread of infection.

DISEASE PROCESS

After the tubercle bacilli reach the lungs, they find a suitable place to live. Then the battle begins between the invading microorganisms and the body's defenses. A wall of fibrous tissue begins to form around the colony of tubercle bacilli. Eventually, the wall surrounds the invaders, forming a tubercle or small nodule. (The bacilli causing this disease are called tubercle bacilli since they cause small nodules of tubercles to form in the tissue.) This wall prevents the blood vessels from nourishing the bacilli. Cutting off the blood supply also causes the body's tissues within the affected area to die. The tissue breaks down into a cheeselike substance. This process is called *caseation*. The tubercle bacilli stop multiplying if the body's defenses are strong. Although the bacilli may remain alive within the wall or capsule for months or years, they eventually die. However, if the patient's resistance is lowered by such factors as overwork and poor health habits before the tubercle bacilli die, the infection may be renewed. If the body continues to win the battle, scar tissue is formed and lime salts are deposited. This area is known as a healed calcified lesion. The patient has recovered.

Unfortunately, the invader is not always killed so easily by the body. If the patient's resistance is not adequate, or if too many tubercle bacilli invade the lungs, the body may be the loser of the battle. Also, tubercle bacilli may penetrate the wall of the tubercle. Once on the outside, they seek other suitable places to live. The bacilli may invade a blood vessel and be carried to a distant part of the body. New infections are started. Ulceration occurs when the spreading infection reaches the surface of a bronchus wall. The cheeselike or caseous material within the infected area empties into the bronchus, leaving a cavity in its place. The patient then expectorates sputum containing tubercle bacilli. If the patient's resistance is improved at this time, the cavity is surrounded by a wall.

DIAGNOSIS/NURSING OBSERVATIONS

Frequently the patient with pulmonary tuberculosis notices no symptoms during the early stage of infection. Periodic chest x-rays and routine use of tuberculin tests are encouraged in an effort to detect cases in the beginning stage. It is important to locate tuberculosis during this stage in order to start early treatment as well as to prevent its spread to other people. The patient generally develops vague symptoms as the tuberculous infection continues. A person may notice fatigue, a poor appetite, and a gradual loss of weight. Indigestion may be present. Women may notice irregular menses. In some cases, the patient awakens during the night and finds the bedclothes soaked with perspiration. This is known as a night sweat. A cough develops which frequently is nonproductive at first. The cough becomes increasingly productive as the disease progresses. Hemoptysis may occur, although this is unusual in the early stages of tuberculosis.

The patient develops a fever. Usually, the temperature is slightly below normal in the morning and goes up in the afternoon. It frequently reaches 37.8° to 38.9°C (100° to 102°F) during the late afternoon.

When the inflammatory process extends to the pleura, the patient is likely to experience pleuritic pain. The condition may be referred to as dry pleurisy in the event that no fluid forms in the irritated area. The condition is called pleurisy with effusion when associated with fluid in the pleural cavity.

In addition to a thorough history and physical examination, the physician generally orders a series of chest x-rays. Repeated chest x-rays assist the physician to diagnose the disease, determine the extent of lung involvement, and evaluate the patient's response to therapy.

Skin testing with minute amounts of tuberculin is used to detect tuberculosis in its early stage when possible. A positive reaction occurs when the skin test area becomes *indurated* (hardened). Not all persons who have positive skin reactions have tuberculosis. Some persons may have infection with other mycobacteria similar to the one that causes tuberculosis. In other cases, the person may have had a tuberculous infection at one time. Or, the person may have active present tuberculosis.

Use of the tuberculin test also helps to identify the person who has had a recent change from negative to positive. For example, the physician who finds a patient with a negative reaction to a tuberculin test last year and a positive reaction this year, will examine that patient for active tuberculosis. The tuberculin test becomes positive approximately two to ten weeks after the patient has the inital infection.

In the Mantoux test, either old tuberculin (OT) or the purified protein derivative (PPD) is injected into the superficial layer of the skin. Occurrence of redness, hardness, and edema at the site of injection after 48 to 72 hours indicates a positive reaction. Although the Vollmer patch test is less accurate, it is used in special cases. A piece of gauze treated with tuberculin is applied to the patient's skin. The area is examined for a reaction in 72 to 96 hours. In the Heaf test, the patient has old tuberculin placed on the skin. A disk with tiny needles is used to puncture small holes in the skin. In the tine test, the tuberculin is applied to small tines or prongs. The tines treated with tuberculin pierce the patient's skin. No syringes or needles are needed for the multiple puncture technique. Various companies produce multiple puncture kits.

When tuberculosis is suspected, the physician usually requests that the patient's sputum be examined for acid-fast bacilli (AFB). Sputum may be examined by smear or culture. Results of the smear are available in a relatively short period of time, whereas a culture for tuberculosis may take four to eight weeks.

The patient may be directed to provide a sputum specimen for a series of times. The nursing student will find it helpful to understand that the reason for this is that the organism may not be present consistently in the patient's sputum.

Other measures that were described earlier in this chapter include induced sputums and gastric washings. As mentioned before, sputum specimens must be properly collected and labeled so that reliable information can be obtained.

TREATMENT AND NURSING INTERVENTIONS

After the diagnosis is made, the physician starts the patient on chemotherapy. This may be initiated during a short stay of several weeks in a general hospital or on an outpatient basis. At the present time, three main principles of drug therapy generally are employed. The first principle is that drug therapy must be continued over a long period of time, which can range from 18 to 24 months or longer. The second principle is that the use of more than one drug seems to prevent the development of an infection resistant to a drug. Consequently, the nurse can expect the patient to receive approximately two drugs for many months. The third principle is that drug therapy appears to be most effective when taken in a single daily dose on an empty stomach rather than in divided daily doses. Drugs used in the treatment of tuberculosis are listed in Table 14.9.

The characteristic of the tubercle bacillus to retreat into a dormant state presents a problem. If the patient does not continue chemotherapy beyond the dormant stage, a cure will not occur. In other words, if the therapy is stopped before all of the tubercle bacilli in the lesion have been killed, the patient may develop active tuberculosis at some later date. Some patients discontinue therapy prematurely because they feel well and think they are cured.

Other patients may discontinue therapy because of financial hardship. Prior to discharge, the nurse should make certain that the patient understands the reason for prolonged chemotherapy and how to obtain prescription refills. The nurse may need to contact the social worker or other health professionals if economic assistance is needed to pay for drug therapy. One helpful question is to ask the patient where refills will be bought and how they will be paid for. A vague answer from the patient may indi-

TABLE 14.9
CHEMOTHERAPY OF TUBERCULOSIS

NONPROPRIETARY NAME	TRADE NAME	AVERAGE DOSE	NURSING IMPLICATIONS
Aminosalicylate sodium (Para-aminosalicylic acid) Aminosalicylic acid	PAMISYL PARASAL REZIPAS	8–12 gm daily	Anorexia, nausea, vomiting, diarrhea—toxic to liver—avoid in peptic ulcer, irritable to bowel
Capreomycin	CAPASTAT	20 mg/kg daily gradually decreased to 3 gm/wk (injection only)	Hearing loss—not given with other "mycins" listed in this table
Cycloserine	OXAMYCIN SEROMYCIN	500 mg daily	Irritability, insomnia, convulsions—sedatives and anticonvulsants may be needed
Ethambutol	MYAMBUTOL	15–25 mg/kg of body weight	Occasional optic neuritis—decreased visual acuity—loss of ability to perceive green color; not recommended during pregnancy
Ethionamide	TRECATOR-SC	125–250 mg, gradually increasing to 1 gm/day	Anorexia, nausea and vomiting, severe postural hypotension, mental depression, drowsiness
Isoniazid (isonicotinic acid hydrazide)	NICONYL, NYDRAZID, RIMIFON, TYVID	3–5 mg/kg of body weight, daily	Aching joints, neuritis, liver damage, urinary retention
Kanamycin sulfate	KANTREX	50 mg/kg of body weight	Toxic to kidneys, ototoxicity
Pyrazinamide	ALDINAMIDE	20–35 mg/kg of body weight	Toxic to liver—increases blood uric acid levels
Rifampin	RIFADIN RIMACTANE	600 mg	Nausea and vomiting—jaundice
Streptomycin sulfate		1–2 gm daily	Ototoxicity, optic nerve damage

cate that help is needed. The patient may be more likely to continue chemotherapy when potential problems have been anticipated and solutions worked out in advance.

While undergoing chemotherapy for tuberculosis, the patient has frequent chest x-rays and sputum examinations to determine progress. A complete blood count, an erythrocyte sedimentation rate, and urinalysis are frequently done also.

BCG vaccine is used in some parts of the United States and other countries to vaccinate tuberculin-negative persons. This is especially true if the population has a high incidence of tuberculosis. Isoniazid is also used prophylactically in similar situations.

While in the hospital, the patient is usually placed in a single room with an ultraviolet light. The nurse can provide for adequate ventilation by keeping the windows open when possible.

Patient teaching is an essential part of therapy. In addition to knowledge about drug therapy, the nurse should instruct the patient to cover the nose and mouth with several layers of disposable tissue when sneezing, coughing, and laughing. The patient is also instructed to expectorate all sputum into a disposable sputum container, which is later burned. The patient should wash the hands after each expectoration. The patient who is unable to cover the nose and mouth may wear a mask when close contact with others is needed. Masks should be discarded according to the hospital policy and should be changed frequently if needed for longer than 20 minutes. The nurse assists to prevent the spread of infection by thorough handwashing before and after caring for the patient.

In the past, surgery was a main part of treatment but is much less common since chemotherapy became effective. Early surgical treatment included collapse of the lung to provide additional rest and resection of the diseased part. Occasionally, surgery is necessary if the disease is far advanced or drug resistant. If needed, a lobectomy or pneumonectomy may be done.

Neoplastic Disease

Cancer may be found in any part of the respiratory tract, but most often it affects the larynx and lungs. Cancers of the upper respiratory tract are considered among the most preventable since many of the factors believed to cause a cancerous lesion are known and symptoms frequently appear early enough to be treated effectively.

In general, cancers of the upper respiratory tract affect men more often than women. Cigarette smoking is the factor most commonly shared by persons who develop cancer of the respiratory tract. Other factors include exposure to industrial carcinogens, such as asbestos, and chronic inflammation and scarring of lung tissue by other diseases such as scleroderma. At present, surgery is the treatment of choice for most neoplasms of the respiratory tract.

LARYNX

The person with cancer of the larynx is usually a male in his middle years (40 to 60 years). The patient frequently has a history of chronic heavy use of alcohol and tobacco and may have a familial predisposition to cancer. Intrinsic cancer is one that develops on the vocal cords. More than half of laryngeal cancers are this type. Extrinsic cancer extends beyond the vocal cords. Early detection and treatment improve the chances of cure as well as retaining the voice.

DIAGNOSIS AND NURSING OBSERVATIONS

An early symptom of intrinsic cancer is hoarseness. As the tumor slowly enlarges, the patient may have difficulty swallowing (dysphagia), dyspnea, cough, and pain. Extrinsic cancer does not produce early symptoms. The person may notice pain or burning when swallowing hot or acid liquids. Enlargement of cervical lymph nodes, weight loss, and general disability may indicate that there is metastasis.

Diagnostic tests that the physician may order include direct and/or indirect laryngoscopy with biopsy, tomograms, and esophagograms.

TREATMENT AND NURSING INTERVENTIONS

The patient with early intrinsic cancer may be treated with radiation or partial laryngectomy or a combination of both. *Partial laryngectomy* enables the patient to retain the voice and a normal airway. When the cancer is more advanced, a *total laryngectomy* may be needed. This procedure results in a permanent loss of voice as well as a permanent tracheostomy. *Radical neck dissection* is done when cancer is believed to have spread to the lymph nodes of the neck. This extensive surgery involves removal of lymph nodes, muscle, fat, and blood vessels in the area near the tumor. A total or partial laryngectomy is done at the same time. This extensive surgery usually requires several surgical procedures involving removal of diseased tissue, reconstruction of remaining tissue, and long-term tube feeding as described in Chapter 15.

A variety of new surgical procedures has been designed to remove diseased tissue and preserve or reconstruct remaining tissues into a functional larynx. *Subtotal laryngectomy and laryngoplasty* are examples of such procedures. The nurse can watch for new and interesting developments in this field.

When the surgeon performs a total laryngectomy, the entire larynx is removed. The trachea is brought out to the skin and a permanent stoma (opening) is created.

Preoperative preparation includes extensive discussions between the surgeon, patient, and family members about the results of the surgery. For example, the patient is told to expect a temporary voice loss, which will result in a need for special training in order to learn a new method of speaking. The patient will not be able to sing or whistle following surgery. The need for a permanent tracheostomy also is explained to the patient.

Another part of preoperative care includes descriptions of what the patient can expect in the recovery and early postoperative periods. This includes descriptions of the laryngectomy tube, suctioning, humidity and oxygen devices, vital signs, intravenous therapy, and tube feedings. At this time, the nurse and the patient develop the communication system that will be used following surgery. It is very important to record and report the system to be used by family members, other health team members, and all persons who will be in contact with the patient following surgery.

Developing a therapeutic relationship with the patient is an important part of preoperative care. The patient facing this surgery has many fears which are easy to anticipate and understand: Will I live? How will I look? Has the cancer spread? Will I be able to breathe? Since the patient must depend on others for maintenance of vital functions after surgery, a trusting relationship is essential. Nursing interventions that build trust include meeting physical needs promptly, giving accurate information, referring the patient to others for information when appropriate, listening with interest to the patient's concerns, performing technical skills skillfully and confidently, and explaining all activities to the patient before beginning them.

Postoperatively, the patient returns with a laryngectomy tube in place. This tube resembles a tracheostomy tube except that it is somewhat shorter and wider. The tube may be cuffed or not cuffed. Nursing care is similar to that described for a patient with a tracheostomy. Deep intratracheal suctioning is avoided unless specifically ordered by the surgeon because there is danger of injuring the suture line. Because nose and mouth structures have been bypassed, humidified air is provided using a special collar which fits over the laryngectomy tube. The patient is carefully observed for signs of respiratory distress.

In addition to intravenous therapy, the patient usually receives tube feedings. A tube is passed through the nose and esophagus into the stomach. After a specially prepared formula has been warmed to body temperature, it is poured through this tube into the patient's stomach. After the operative area has healed, the patient is allowed to eat a regular diet. As mention earlier, in multiple stage surgery, tube feedings may continue for weeks or months.

The patient's head usually is elevated slightly after surgery. When repositioning or moving the patient, the nurse supports the head since neck muscles are weak. Frequent oral hygiene is needed to prevent overgrowth of normal flora in the mouth.

Drainage catheters usually are placed near the operative area at the time of surgery and attached to a suction device such as a HEMOVAC. A dressing also may be in place. Two persons may be needed to turn the patient at first. One person assists the patient to turn while the second person holds the drainage catheters to prevent them from becoming dislodged, kinked, twisted, or disconnected.

Since the patient has sustained numerous losses, the nurse can expect to observe signs of grieving and depression. Losing one's normal voice involves a loss of communication, a loss of part of identity, and possibly a loss of occupation. Other losses that may be important include whistling or blowing out the candles on a birthday cake or singing. The changes in body image that occur after this surgery are so extensive that some experts have suggested that several years are needed to complete the process. The patient needs reassurance, understanding, and kindness. Encouraging, supporting words from the nurse are very much needed and appreciated by the patient at this time.

Patient teaching begins early after surgery in order to encourage independence, self-care, and body-image changes. The patient has many new skills to learn. For example, after the wound edges have healed, the laryngectomy tube may be removed. The patient then learns how to care for the permanent stoma. If tube feedings continue, the patient learns how to prepare and administer them. In addition, the patient learns a new method of speech. *Esophageal speech* is one method during which the patient swallows air and produces sounds by forcing the air back from the stomach. Learning to control the muscles involved is an important part of this method. Another method involves learning to use an electronic larynx. Several devices are on the market. A *speech therapist* is the professional person who assists the patient to learn how to speak. The nurse assists the patient by encouraging and praising every effort and by listening to the patient during practice sessions.

Many parts of the country have Lost Cord Clubs, which are composed of persons who have had a laryngectomy. When the community has such a club, its members are delighted to help new laryngectomized patients. The International Association of Laryngectomees helps provide public education and assists the laryngectomy patient in recovery.

One precaution that may save the life of a laryngectomy patient is always to *check the neck* before beginning mouth-to-mouth resuscitation on an unknown person. The rescuer must place the mouth around the hole in the neck of a laryngectomy patient in order to inflate the lungs. If the rescuer does not see a rise and fall of the chest, one hand is placed over the mouth, the nostrils are pinched with the fingers, and mouth-to-neck breathing is started.

LUNG

Both benign and malignant neoplasms occur in the lung. Most primary neoplasms of the lung occur in the tracheobronchial tree. When lung neoplasms spread, the organs most commonly affected include the scalene lymph nodes, bone, brain, liver, and adrenal glands. In addition, the lung is the frequent site of metastases from another organ. The spread of a malignant neoplasm to the lungs is particularly common from the intestines, kidneys, thyroid gland, breasts, and testes. According to the American Cancer Society, cigarette smoking is the cause of most lung cancers.

DIAGNOSIS AND NURSING OBSERVATIONS

The person with cancer of the lung commonly experiences early symptoms of cough, or change in the pattern of a chronic cough, and wheezing. Later symptoms such as weight loss, malaise, and anorexia usually indicate metastases. In some cases, the patient has no pulmonary symptoms but has one or more syndromes involving other body systems that are associated with occult (hidden) lung malignacy.

Diagnostic studies include chest x-ray, tomograms, Papanicolaou smears and cytologic studies of sputum, bronchoscopy, and biopsies of the scalene lymph node. A complete history and a careful physical examination are important diagnostic measures. After cancer has been detected, the tumor is staged according to size and characteristics, regional lymph nodes involved, and distant metastases.

TREATMENT AND NURSING INTERVENTIONS

Early detection and treatment by surgical resection offer the best hope for cure. In order to conserve lung function, a lobectomy is preferred if the tumor can be removed completely. A pneumonectomy may be needed in some cases. Care of the patient following chest surgery was discussed earlier in the chapter on pages 441–45 and applies to this patient.

About half of the patients with lung cancer are inoperable when first seen by the physician. Radiation therapy is generally used to help these individuals. In some cases, radioisotopes or chemotherapeutic agents are placed between the pleura. Intravenous chemotherapy is also used in some cases.

A therapy which shows promise is adjuvant immunotherapy using BCG, a tuberculosis vaccine to stimulate the patient's immune system. This therapy is still experimental in patients with lung cancer but has been used for patients with other forms of cancer. The nurse can locate additional information about nursing care when radiation, chemotherapy, or immunotherapy is used by reviewing Chapter 9.

The nurse plays an important part in the prevention of lung and other forms of cancer. The nurse's knowledge about health and illness causes friends, family, and neighbors to come for advice about a variety of symptoms and problems. As mentioned previously, one way to influence people to improve health practices is to set a good example. A second way is to provide correct information, and a third way is to participate in community educational projects. It is a fact that people who smoke are more likely to develop lung cancer than those who do not. Smokers need encouragement to stop, a referral to community smoking clinics, and a chest x-ray every six months. Persons with a persistent cough, a change in the usual cough, or frequent respiratory infections are advised to seek medical attention. The nurse may participate directly or indirectly in programs to educate people about cancer, improvement of air quality, and cancer detection screening clinics. (See Table 4.10.)

TABLE 14.10
OTHER DISORDERS

DISORDER	DESCRIPTION
Aspergillosis	A fungal infection that starts in the lungs and may spread to the bones, meninges, heart, and other parts of the body; may coexist with asthma; drug therapy usually includes amphotericin B; lobectomy may be needed
Asthma	Paroxysmal wheezing and dyspnea produced by obstruction of airflow in bronchioles and bronchi. Described in Chapter 10
Blastomycosis (North American)	A chronic fungal infection that starts in the respiratory system and spreads to other organs; caused by inhalation of causative spores; amphotericin B is the antifungal drug currently used
Bronchogenic cysts	Cysts that develop in the bronchi and usually cause no symptoms; may be a congenital defect
Coccidioidomycosis (valley fever)	A fungal infection that starts in the respiratory system and spreads to other parts of the body; caused by inhaling dust-containing spores; current treatment is with amphotericin B. Usually seen in southwestern U.S.
Cryptococcosis (European blastomycosis, torulosis)	A chronic systemic fungal infection that starts in the respiratory tract and spreads to brain and meninges. Drug therapy usually includes flucytosine and amphotericin B
Giant bullous emphysema (vanishing lung)	Abnormal blebs in the lungs containing air; most common in older men. Surgical excision may provide temporary improvement of symptoms
Guillain-Barré-Stohl syndrome	Progressive ascending neuromuscular weakness or paralysis that may affect respiratory tract. May occur following an infection. Spontaneous recovery is usual but intensive respiratory care usually needed in acute phase
Histoplasmosis	A fungal infection that starts in the respiratory system and spreads to other parts of the body; caused by inhaling the fungus from dust contaminated with chicken or bird excreta; current treatment is with amphotericin B. Usually seen in eastern and midwestern U.S.
Lipoid pneumonia	Pneumonia caused by introduction of mineral oil or animal fats into the lungs; may be associated with use of nosedrops with mineral oil base; may also occur in certain patients who take mineral oil habitually and some of it is aspirated into the lungs; in some cases, cholesterol collects in a part of the lung
Psittacosis (ornithosis, parrot fever)	Infection of the lung transmitted by infected parrots, parakeets, finches, turkeys, ducks, and chickens. Can cause death. Tetracyclines are drugs of choice

TABLE 14.10 (*Continued*)
OTHER DISORDERS

DISORDER	DESCRIPTION
Scoliosis	Lateral curvature of the vertebral column that can interfere with pulmonary function
Streptococcal sore throat (hemolytic streptococcal sore throat)	Pharyngitis caused by streptococci; may be followed by rheumatic fever
Tracheobronchitis	An inflammatory condition involving the trachea and bronchi

Case Study Involving Pneumonia

Mrs. Chester, a 48-year-old housewife, was admitted to the medical unit with a diagnosis of right lower lobe pneumonia. On admission, Mrs. Chester's vital signs were temperature 39°C (102.2°F), pulse 116, respirations 28. The physician's orders included:

- Portable chest x-ray upon admission
- Sputum culture and sensitivities stat
- Penicillin, 600,000 units IM q6h
- Force fluids
- Diet as tolerated
- IPPB with normal saline qid
- Vital signs q4h
- O_2 by prongs at 3 liters/minute

QUESTIONS

1. How should the nurse prepare Mrs. Chester for x-ray?
2. What precautions should the nurse take while the technician obtains the portable x-ray?
3. What actions should the nurse take to obtain a suitable sputum specimen?
4. When should the nurse administer the first dose of penicillin and what precautions are needed before the first dose is given?
5. What additional equipment will be needed at the bedside that relates to Mrs. Chester's diagnosis and the physican's orders?
6. What nursing measures should the nurse select to prevent retained secretions in the tracheobronchial tree?
7. What changes in vital signs should be reported to the physician?
8. How should the nurse describe IPPB to Mrs. Chester?
9. What should the nurse tell Mrs. Chester and her family about oxygen?
10. What positions will help Mrs. Chester's breathing?
11. What hygiene measures will help Mrs. Chester to be more comfortable and enable her to drink more fluids?

Case Study Involving Chest Trauma

Mr. James Trask, a 22-year-old male, was admitted to the surgical unit of the hospital following an automobile accident. The physician's diagnosis was left pneumothorax. When entering the patient's room, the nurse observed that a chest tube was coming from Mr. Trask's left anterior chest and was connected to a closed chest gravity drainage system with a water seal bottle. The physician requested the nurse to assist Mr. Trask to the chair today.

QUESTIONS

1. What is the purpose of the chest tube and how should the nurse explain this to Mr. Trask?
2. What is the purpose of the water seal type of drainage bottle?
3. What nursing observations and nursing measures are indicated in order to maintain proper functioning of Mr. Trask's closed chest drainage system?
4. What precautions should the nurse take before assisting Mr. Trask to the chair?
5. What nursing observations would indicate that Mr. Trask is in respiratory distress?
6. What nursing observations would indicate that Mr. Trask's closed chest gravity drainage is not functioning properly?
7. In view of the diagnosis and the cause of the pneumothorax, what should the nurse do if bloody drainage in the water seal bottle is observed?
8. What nursing measures are indicated when Mr. Trask has a portable chest x-ray?
9. What nursing observations and measures are indicated after Mr. Trask receives DEMEROL?
10. What should the nurse know about infection in caring for Mr. Trask while he has a chest tube?

Suggestions for Further Study

1. Visit the respiratory therapy department and observe the variety of equipment available to help persons with respiratory disorders.

2. Locate emergency intubation equipment such as laryngoscope and endotracheal tubes.

3. Take a deep breath. Let about half of the breath out. Continue to breathe that way, each time letting out only half of the air you have taken in. Then describe the sensations and reactions you experienced and relate them to the symptoms of a person with emphysema.

4. Find out what programs exist in your community for early detection and treatment of pulmonary tuberculosis.

5. Ask an individual with a laryngectomy to demonstrate esophageal speech.

6. Practice mouth-to-neck breathing in a simulated classroom respiratory arrest.

7. Develop a skit in which one person plays the role of a person with a new tracheostomy trying to communicate to the nurse and another person plays the nurse. Then exchange information about the feelings each of you experienced while trying to communicate.

8. Mason, Mildred A.; Bates, Grace F.; and Smola, Bonnie K.: *Workbook in Basic Medical-Surgical Nursing*, 3rd ed. Macmillan Publishing Company, New York, 1984, Exercise 14.

Additional Readings

Anderson, Susan Joyce: "Sarcoidosis: A Multisystem Disease." *American Journal of Nursing*, 82:1566–69 (Oct.), 1982.

Broussard, Randy: "Using Relaxation for COPD." *American Journal of Nursing*, 79: 1962–63 (Nov.), 1979.

Cameron, Terrie J.: "Fiberoptic Bronchoscopy." *American Journal of Nursing*, 81:1462–64 (Aug.), 1981.

Cline, Barbara A., and Fisher, Mary L.: "A.R.D.S. Means Emergency." *Nursing 82*, 12:62–67 (Feb.), 1982.

Erickson, Roberta: "Chest Tubes: They're Really Not That Complicated." *Nursing 81*, 11:34–43 (May), 1981.

Francis, Betty: "Respiratory Care." *Journal of Nursing Care*, 14:9–13 (July), 1981.

Greenwood, Barbara S.: "The Before and After of Good Postop Pulmonary Care." *Nursing 81*, 12:68–69 (Dec.), 1982.

Hudgel, David W., and Madsen, Lorie A.: "Acute and Chronic Asthma: A Guide to Intervention." *American Journal of Nursing*, 80: 1791–95 (Oct.), 1980.

"Influenza: Test Yourself." *American Journal of Nursing*, 81:731, 844 (Apr.), 1981.

Kaufman, Jane Steinman, and Woody, Johnsie Whitt: "For Patients with COPD: Better Living Through Teaching." *Nursing 80*, 10:57–61 (Mar.), 1980.

Larsen, George: "Rehabilitation for the Patient with Head and Neck Cancer." *American Journal of Nursing*, 82:119–21 (Jan.), 1982.

Maszkiewicz, Ruth C., and Kirilloff, Leslie H.: "Guide to Respiratory Care in Critically Ill Adults." *American Journal of Nursing*, 79:2005–12 (Nov.), 1979.

McCormick, Glen P., *et al.*: "Artificial Speech Devices." *American Journal of Nursing*, 82: 121–22 (Jan.), 1982.

Rambo, Beverly J., and Wood, Lucile A. (eds.): *Nursing Skills for Clinical Practice*, 3rd ed. W. B. Saunders Co., Philadelphia, 1982, pp. 640–60.

Schumacher, Linda L.: "Common Cold." *Nursing 82*, 12:78–79 (Jan.), 1982.

Sherry, Deborah: "Adult Respiratory Distress Syndrome: A Challenge to Nursing Care." *Journal of Practical Nursing*, 32:21–23 (Feb.), 1982.

Visich, Mary Ann: "Knowing What You Hear: A Guide to Assessing Breath and Heart Sounds." *Nursing 81*, 11:64–79 (Nov.), 1981.

Wehner, Robert J.: "The Nurse's Role in Respiratory Care." *Journal of Practical Nursing*, 32:16–20 (Feb.), 1982.

Woodin, Linda M.: "Your Patient with a Pneumothorax: A Patient in Distress." *Nursing 82*, 12:50–56 (Nov.), 1982.

Chapter 15

The Patient with a Disease of the Gastrointestinal System

Expected Behavioral Outcomes

Minimum objectives referred to as expected behavioral outcomes have been designed for the practical/vocational nursing student to use as guides in studying this chapter. The student should read these expected outcomes before studying the chapter.

The objectives can be used as guides for study. Using the content of the chapter, the student should return to the objectives and evaluate the ability to:

1. Describe the responsibilities of the nurse in your agency when assisting with diagnostic studies discussed in this chapter.

2. Compare nursing observations and actions indicated for patients having each of the tubes used in gastrointestinal decompression.

3. Prepare a table in which the problems of the patient with an ileostomy are compared with those of the patient with a colostomy. The factors to be considered are location, consistency of discharge, frequency of discharge, means of collecting discharge, extent to which patient can control elimination, and diet.

4. Compare the differences in the diet needed by the patient who has an ileostomy and the patient who has a colostomy.

5. List nursing observations and actions related to the care of a person with gastrointestinal bleeding.

6. After reviewing the stages associated with loss discussed in Chapter 1, relate these stages to those likely to be experienced by the patient with a gastrostomy, colostomy, or ileostomy.

7. Relate the preoperative and postoperative nursing care discussed in Chapter

*6 to that needed by the patient having
an appendectomy and/or other surgery
of the gastrointestinal tract.*
8. *Describe community and hospital resources available to help the ostomate.*
9. *Match the appropriate danger signals
of cancer discussed in Chapter 9 to
those of neoplastic diseases of the gastrointestinal system discussed in this
chapter.*

Vocabulary Development

The following prefixes, suffixes, and
combining forms pertain to this chapter. By
learning and/or reviewing their meanings,
the practical/vocational nursing student will
have the keys needed to unlock many exciting new medical terms.

Discover the meaning of these keys in a
medical dictionary or in the content of this
chapter. How does each key pertain to this
chapter? In your notebook write the correct
meaning of each prefix, suffix, or combining
form listed below. Illustrate each key with
an example.

cec—blind. Ex. *cecum*—a blind pouch.

col-	peps-
colon-	pept-
creat-	proct-
duct-	pto-
enter-	rhe-
eso-	scop-
fiss-	-scope
gastr-	sial-
gloss-	stal-
glott-	stear-
ili-	steato-
jejun-	sten-
lapar-	stom(at)-
lingu-	strict-
pend-	struct-

Structure and Function

The gastrointestinal tract may be referred to as the digestive tract, digestive
system, or alimentary canal. Its function is
to change food into simpler substances that
can be carried by the blood to the cells. In order to accomplish this function, the system
must provide digestive juices. Food must
also be transported through the canal. This
movement is accomplished by *peristalsis*,
which is a wormlike contraction of the intestines. After the food has been transformed
into simple substances and absorbed, the
waste products are carried to the lower part
of the canal by peristalsis.

The digestive system consists of a tube
approximately 7.8 to 9.4 meters (25 to 30 ft)
in length. It begins with the mouth and ends
with the anus (see Figure 15.1). The mouth,
the pharynx (throat), the esophagus, the
stomach, the small intestine, and the large
intestine are the organs of this system. The
tongue, the teeth, the salivary glands, the
pancreas, the liver, and the gallbladder aid
the digestive system in its function. They
are known as accessory organs.

The process of chewing food, which takes
place in the mouth, makes digestion easier.

Enzymes in saliva help to break down food.
Swallowing moves food from the mouth
through the pharynx and esophagus into the
stomach. The esophagus is a muscular tube
approximately 22.5 cm (9 in.) in length.

Food remains for a while in the stomach,
which is a dilatation of the alimentary canal
resembling a pouch. The stomach is located
in the upper left portion of the abdomen.
The opening between the esophagus and the
stomach is the *cardiac orifice*. The *pyloric
orifice* is the opening between the stomach
and the small intestine. The food is changed
into a semiliquid condition in the stomach by
its churning motion and by the gastric juice.

The mucous membrane lining the stomach secretes gastric juice, which is a clear
liquid. The function of gastric juice is to
start the digestion of food proteins. Gastric
juice contains pepsin, hydrochloric acid, and
rennin.

Peristalsis forces the partially digested
food through the pylorus (lower part of the
stomach) into the small intestine, where absorption and further digestion take place.
The upper portion of the small intestine is
known as the *duodenum*. Substances to aid
in digestion usually are emptied into the duodenum through a single opening known as

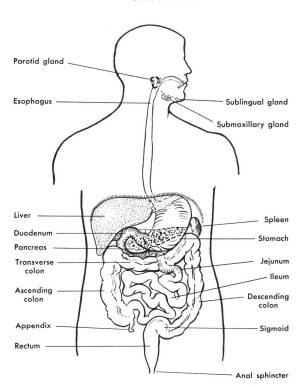

FIGURE 15.1 The gastrointestinal tract. (From Robinson, Corinne H., and Lawler, Marilyn R.: *Normal and Therapeutic Nutrition*, 15th ed. Macmillan Publishing Co., Inc., New York, 1977.)

the *ampulla of Vater*. The pancreatic duct and the common bile duct join to form this short tube. The pancreatic duct brings digestive juice from the pancreas. The common bile duct brings bile from both the liver and the gallbladder. The duodenum connects with the *jejunum*, which is the middle part of the small intestine. The jejunum leads to the *ileum*, which is the last portion of the small intestine. As the digested food is carried through the small intestine, the usable portion is absorbed into the lymph and blood vessels.

The waste products pass from the ileum into the large intestine. The four parts of the large intestine are the cecum, the colon, the rectum, and the anal canal. The first portion of the large intestine, which is the *cecum*, resembles a pouch. The *ileocecal valve* prevents the waste material from going back into the small intestine. The *vermiform appendix* is a small tubular or wormlike projection attached to the cecum. The term *vermiform* means shaped like a worm.

Waste products are carried from the cecum into the colon, which is subdivided into the ascending, transverse, descending, and sigmoid colon. The ascending portion goes upward on the right side, and the transverse goes across the abdomen. The descending colon goes downward on the left side. It leads into the sigmoid colon, which is shaped like the letter S; thus, it is called sigmoid, which refers to the letter "S" in the Greek alphabet.

After waste material has been forced through the colon, it reaches the rectum. The rectum connects with the anal canal, which is the end portion of the large intestine. The anal canal is approximately 2.5 cm (1 in.) in length. It is closed by two sphincters (ringlike muscles) that open during defecation. The external opening is called the *anus*.

The *peritoneum* is a serous membrane that covers the abdominal organs. It consists of two layers in contact with each other. The inner layer of the peritoneum covers the abdominal organs, and the outer layer lines the abdominal wall. A cavity may develop between the two layers when disease is present. This space, which may become a cavity, is referred to as the *perito-neal cavity*. The peritoneum secretes serum, which lubricates the enclosed organs, and it also helps to hold these organs in place.

Assisting with Diagnostic Studies

The nurse's role in assisting with diagnostic studies is important. For example, the nurse is usually the person who explains the test to the patient in understandable language. A feature of many diagnostic studies is special preparation of the gastrointestinal system with laxatives, enemas, and withholding food and fluids to obtain the necessary information. Special preparation is the responsibility of the nursing staff. Incomplete or incorrect preparation may cause the patient to incur a repeat test, more discomfort and fatigue, and additional expense. As previously mentioned, many studies require that the patient refrain from eating and drinking for hours in advance. Bowel cleansing with one or more enemas also may be needed. This increases the likelihood that the patient, who is already ill, may develop dehydration and/or undernutrition. Therefore, during the diagnostic period, the nurse carefully observes and records the foods and fluids the patient is taking in and excreting.

X-RAYS

An abdominal x-ray usually is ordered to identify abnormal shadows, air, and/or fluid that may be present in the patient's abdomen.

GASTROINTESTINAL SERIES

The patient having a gastrointestinal series has x-rays made of the stomach and small intestine after swallowing a radiopaque substance, barium. This series of x-ray pictures of the upper portion of the gastrointestinal tract is used to reveal abnormalities such as tumors, ulcers, inflammations, and strictures.

The patient scheduled for a gastrointestinal series should have nothing by mouth for approximately eight hours before the x-ray examination. The roentgenologist examines the passage of barium from the patient's mouth to the stomach with the fluoroscope. X-ray pictures of the stomach and duode-

num are taken as the barium outlines the walls of these organs. More roentgenograms (x-ray pictures) may be taken four to six hours after the initial x-rays to determine if any barium remains in the stomach.

After a gastrointestinal series, the patient may have a laxative prescribed. The purpose of this is to facilitate rapid elimination of barium. Barium that is retained may become hard and result in constipation, a fecal impaction, or possibly an obstruction. The passage of the barium, which has a chalky appearance, should be observed and reported.

BARIUM ENEMA

The patient having a barium enema has barium instilled into the colon. The barium outlines the walls of the large intestine and makes it visible by x-ray examination. The roentgenologist usually observes the passage of barium into the large intestine with the fluoroscope. X-ray pictures of the colon are made after it has been filled with barium. Additional films are taken after the patient expels the barium. In some cases, the roentgenologist will instill air also into the colon for contrast studies.

A laxative and enemas are prescribed to prepare the patient for a barium enema. The type and amount of laxative, as well as the type and number of enemas, will be specified. These vary with different roentgenologists in various institutions. Cleansing enemas usually are prescribed after a barium enema to remove the radiopaque contrast material from the bowel.

A barium enema is used to aid in diagnosing improper functioning of the large intestine. Polyps, tumors, and other lesions also may be visualized.

After barium x-rays have been taken, a small amount of contrast material remains in the tissue for weeks. This material may interfere with other diagnostic studies. Therefore, barium x-rays usually are scheduled after all other x-rays have been completed satisfactorily.

ENDOSCOPY

The patient having an *endoscopy* has a hollow instrument passed through one of the body openings to enable the physician to examine certain organs. Endoscopes made of flexible fiberglass enable the physician to examine such organs as the stomach and esophagus with less discomfort to the patient and with greater visibility than was possible previously. Endoscopic examinations frequently used in relation to the gastrointestinal tract include examination of the esophagus, stomach, upper part of the duodenum, sigmoid, rectum, and anus.

Esophagoscopy, gastroscopy, and *duodenoscopy* are procedures done by the physician to permit visualization of the mucous membrane of the esophagus, stomach, pylorus, and upper portion of the duodenum. In addition to inspecting the mucosa of the upper gastrointestinal tract, the physician can obtain specimens of tissue for microscopic study and take pictures of abnormalities during the examination.

The patient is not allowed to have anything by mouth for approximately eight hours preceding the esophagoscopy, gastroscopy, and duodenoscopy. The presence of food or fluid could cause the patient to regurgitate while the gastroscope is being passed, as well as prevent the physician from having a clear view of the gastric mucosa.

This procedure may be done in the operating room or endoscopy room, and preparation of the patient is similar to preoperative care. The patient should have a bath and oral hygiene prior to the examination. Written statement of permission is needed before this procedure can be done. A sedative and/or a tranquilizer may be prescribed to relieve apprehension. In some cases, discomfort is lessened if the patient practices breathing through the nose with a closed mouth prior to this examination. The patient's throat will be sprayed with a local anesthetic, such as cocaine or tetracaine (PONTOCAINE), by the doctor prior to passage of the gastroscope, which is illustrated in Figure 15.2. Knowing this will help the nurse to remember the importance of *not* giving the patient anything to swallow until the gag reflex returns. The return of this protective reflex may take three to four hours.

After the patient has been returned to bed, rest generally is encouraged as this procedure usually is tiring. The nurse should ob-

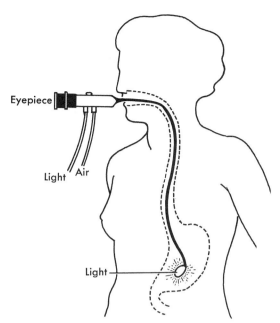

FIGURE 15.2   An illustration of a gastroscope being used by the physician to visualize the esophagus, stomach, and upper portion of the duodenum.

serve, report, and record any vomiting or expectoration of blood. Although the expectoration of a small amount of blood-streaked sputum is not unusual, this, too, should be reported. The patient may experience a slight sore throat for several days following a gastroscopy.

Anoscopy, proctoscopy, and *sigmoidoscopy* are procedures done by the physician to visualize the mucous membrane of the anus, rectum, and sigmoid, respectively. Ulcerations, inflammations, tumors, and polyps can be examined and biopsied if necessary.

The patient is prepared for either of these examinations with cleansing enemas until the returns are clear. The solution to be used is specified by the doctor since irritants, such as soap and glycerin, can cause an abnormal redness that would give a false impression upon examination. The lapse of four to five hours after the last enema is desirable to permit the absorption of excess fluid from the intestine.

The patient usually is placed in the knee-chest position on the treatment table in the doctor's office, clinic, outpatient department, or treatment room in the hospital. The patient should be draped to avoid undue exposure and embarrassment. After doing a rectal examination with the use of rubber gloves and lubricant, the physician inserts the scope. The room is usually darkened to facilitate the ability to see the mucosa through the hollow, lighted instrument. The patient's anal region should be cleansed following the examination.

GASTRIC ANALYSIS

An analysis of the gastric contents may be made. Alcohol, caffeine, histamine phosphate, betazole hydrochloride, or pantagastrin may be used to stimulate the flow of gastric juices. The gastric contents may be collected from vomitus or through a nasogastric tube. The tube is passed into the nose or mouth through the esophagus into the stomach. A syringe is used to aspirate the gastric contents. Generally, the patient is not allowed to have anything by mouth for at least eight hours before having a gastric analysis.

The test usually is done early in the morning. Samples of gastric contents are aspirated at specified time intervals and for a designated number of times. Each sample should be placed in a separate container and labeled with the patient's name and time of collection. The first specimen is labeled 1, the second 2, the third 3, and so on. The end of the nasogastric tube is clamped when a specimen is not being collected.

The patient with a peptic ulcer generally has an acid secretory response similar to or greater than the person without disease. A marked increase in the secretion of hydrochloric acid may suggest to the physician that the patient has a condition other than an ulcer. A complete absence of hydrochloric acid following stimulation with drugs such as histamine rules out hyperacidity. The normal values of a gastric analysis are given in Table 15.1.

In some cases, the use of a nasogastric tube is not possible or desirable but the physician needs to know if hydrochloric acid is present or absent in the gastric juice. Azuresin, a dye called DIAGNEX BLUE, may be prescribed for oral administration. After being acted upon by hydrochloric acid in the stomach, the dye will be eliminated from the body by the kidneys and cause the urine to be blue in color. The lack of blue urine following administration of DIAGNEX BLUE indicates a lack of hydrochloric acid. The presence of blue urine indicates the presence but not the amount of hydrochloric acid in the stomach.

EXFOLIATIVE CYTOLOGY

The patient may have a study made of cells from the mucosa of the upper gastrointestinal tract, to rule out or to identify a malignancy. Such a study is known as exfoliative cytology. The cells that separate (exfoliate) from the tumor are removed through a nasogastric tube and studied under the microscope, a procedure similar to

TABLE 15.1
NORMAL VALUES FOR GASTRIC FLUID

TESTS	NORMAL VALUE	SIGNIFICANCE
Basal acid output (1 hr)	0.6 mEq/hr	An absence of gastric acid generally rules out benign gastric ulcer
Basal acid output/maximal acid output	<0.40	
Fasting residual volume	Up to 50 ml	
Maximum histamine stimulation acid output (1 hr)	Males: 10–40 mEq/hr Females: 5–30 mEq/hr 0.9–1.5	High basal secretion of gastric acid frequently indicates active peptic ulcer
pH	0–0.3 mg/2 hr	
DIAGNEX BLUE		
Anacidity		
Doubtful	0.3–0.6 mg/2 hr	The amount of gastric acid may serve as a guide for the surgeon in determining whether to do a vagotomy or not
Normal	More than 0.6 mg/2 hr	
Volume, fasting stomach content	50–100 ml	
Emptying time	3-6 hr	
Specific gravity	1.006–1.009	

other Papanicolaou smears. In obtaining cells for study, the physician may have the patient's stomach lavaged forcefully with large quantities of saline solution to hasten exfoliation. All of the solution used in the irrigation and any pieces of tissue should be sent to the laboratory for examination. Of course, the specimen and solution should be labeled properly before they are sent to the laboratory.

STOOL SPECIMEN

Accurate observation of the patient's bowel movements supplies valuable information to the doctor in making a diagnosis. The nurse should report stools that are abnormal in odor, amount, color, consistency, and number. A specimen of the abnormal stool should be saved. The doctor may want to have that specimen examined in the laboratory, or additional specimens may be ordered. If the specimen is not needed, it can be discarded later.

The physician may request that the stool be examined for fat, mucus, pus, pathogenic microorganisms, intestinal parasites, and occult blood. *Occult blood* is not observable by the naked eye.

Certain foods and medications cause the patient's stool to vary in color. Examples of this are seen in the milky white stool following a barium x-ray, black associated with the intake of iron, red as a result of eating carrots and beets, green resulting from the ingestion of spinach and other similar green vegetables, and dark brown resulting from the digestion of meat. Orthotolidine (HEMATEST, OCCULTEST) and guaiac filter paper (HEMOCCULT) are substances commonly used to determine the presence of blood in feces. In some cases, the nurse is responsible for testing the stool specimen in the im-

mediate clinical area using one of these substances. Unless otherwise indicated, the specimen should be sent to the laboratory for examination. The normal values of feces are listed in Table 15.2.

A wooden spatula or tongue blade can be used to transfer the stool specimen to a disposable container. The container should then be labeled and sent to the laboratory or taken to the utility area for testing as indicated by the physician's orders. When performing the HEMATEST in the clinical area, the nurse should use the feces from the inner portion of the stool. The outside of the stool specimen may have come in contact with streaks of blood from hemorrhoids or an anal fissure, thereby giving a false-positive reading. The nurse can use a tongue blade to expose the inside portion of the stool for examination. The instructions accompanying the product to be used for testing the stool for blood should be followed carefully.

If the specimen is to be examined for parasites, it should be taken immediately to the laboratory while the feces are still warm. This enables the medical technologist to examine the motion of the parasites under the microscope. In some institutions the standard procedure indicates that a warm water bottle be placed on or around the container for transportation.

A diet containing no red meat may be ordered for the patient who is having stools examined for occult blood. Generally, this type of diet is ordered 24 hours before collection of the specimen. This type of diet helps to prevent a false positive.

COMMON BLOOD TESTS

A variety of blood tests may be ordered to evaluate the patient with a disturbance in

TABLE 15.2
NORMAL VALUES FOR FECES

	NORMAL VALUE	SIGNIFICANCE
Amount	100–200 gm in 24 hr	The amount of feces is increased in certain diseases.
Dry portion	23–32 gm in 24 hr	An increased amount of fecal fat may indicate some
Fat, total amount	Less than 6.0 gm in 24 hr	type of malabsorption. Excess water and electro-
Nitrogen, total	Less than 2.0 gm in 24 hr	lytes are lost in cases of diarrhea
Urobilogen	40–280 mg in 24 hr	
Water	Approximately 65 %	

the gastrointestinal system. For example, a complete blood count (CBC) may be ordered when the physician suspects bleeding. Blood chemistries may be ordered to assess the effect of a gastrointestinal disturbance on the patient's chemical balance. SMA-12 is a term that refers to a specific battery of screening tests (Sequential *M*ultiple *A*nalyzer of 12 laboratory tests) to evaluate body chemistry. Table 15.3 contains a list of normal values for an SMA-12. Serum electrolytes also may be ordered (refer to Table 15.4).

Nursing Observations

The patient with a disturbance in the gastrointestinal system may experience a variety of widespread changes related to the disruption of normal nutrition, fluid balance, and/or elimination. Table 15.5 is a guide to assist the nurse in observing the patient with a disease of the gastrointestinal system.

MOUTH

The nurse observes the patient's mouth carefully for conditions that may either affect nutrition or indicate disease. A flash-light and tongue blade are needed to inspect the inside of the mouth. *Leukoplakia* are abnormal, white, thickened patches which may develop on mucous membranes of the mouth, cheeks, gums, and/or tongue. These lesions do not rub off during oral hygiene, are more common in smokers, and may become malignant. *Cold sores* are vesicles caused by the herpes simplex, type I virus which may be visible on the lips or nares. *Canker sores* are ulcerations inside the mouth and/or around the lips. The medical term for this condition is *aphthous stomatitis*. These abnormal lesions are reported and recorded in the patient's record.

The patient's teeth may be inspected for abnormal drainage, odor, and bleeding at the gums. Missing or obviously diseased teeth may interfere with the patient's ability to eat a nutritious diet. When the patient wears dentures, the nurse may look for signs of improper fit. For example, redness or abrasions in the mouth may indicate poorly fitting dentures. The nurse who finds dentures in a cup or wrapped in tissue instead of in the patient's mouth may suspect poorly fitting dentures, also.

The gums may be observed for changes in color and abnormal bleeding. The lips may

TABLE 15.3
NORMAL VALUES OF SMA-12

Chemistry	Normal Range	Purpose
Albumin	3.5–5.0 g/dL	Four tests help to evaluate patient's nutritional
Cholesterol	140–310 mg/dL	status
Glucose	70–105 mg/dL	
Protein (total)	6.4–8.3 g/dL	
Bilirubin (conjugated)	0–0.2 mg/dL	Evaluates liver function
Blood urea nitrogen (BUN)	8–20 mg/dL	Two tests help to evaluate kidney function
Uric acid	3.0–6.5 mg/dL (F) 4.5–8.2 mg/dL (M)	
Serum glutamic-oxaloacetic transaminase (SGOT)	8–20 U/L	Help to evaluate injury to tissue
Lactic dehydrogenase (LDH)	45–90 U/L	
Alkaline phosphatase Bowers and McComb method	20–70 U/L 25–90 U/L	Helps to evaluate bone tissue
Calcium	8.4–10.2 mg/dL	Evaluate function of parathyroid gland
Phosphates	1.5–2.6 mEq/L	

TABLE 15.4
NORMAL VALUES OF SERUM ELECTROLYTES

Bicarbonate	22–29 mmol/L (venous blood)
Calcium	8.4–10.2 mg/dL
Chloride	96–106 mEq/L
Magnesium	1.3–2.1 mEq/L
Phosphates	1.8–2.6 mEq/L
Potassium	3.5–5.1 mEq/L
Sodium	136–146 mEq/L

be inspected for color and turgor. For example, cracked, dry lips may occur when the patient does not drink enough fluids. The odor of the breath can provide important information. For example, fruity odor of the breath may be noticed when the patient has diabetes with ketoacidosis (refer to Chapter 18). A fecal odor of the breath may be noticed when the patient has an obstruction in the intestines.

DYSPHAGIA

The patient with dysphagia has difficulty swallowing. A variety of disorders may cause a person to develop dysphagia including scarring of the esophagus, tumors, and swelling. Difficulty in swallowing is one of the danger signals of cancer which should cause a person to seek medical attantion.

ANOREXIA

The patient with *anorexia* has a loss of appetite. The anticipatory pleasure of eating contributes markedly to a person's appetite. The individual with a disease of the digestive system, such as peptic ulcer, may have anorexia caused by visceral changes. Visceral changes influence the desire to eat. Factors not necessarily associated with the gastrointestinal system can influence a person's desire to eat. Unpleasant surroundings, unappetizing food, or the absence of a feeling of well-being can produce anorexia also. A decreased desire to eat is evidenced also in the person who has a disease in another part of his body, such as an infection. Emotional tension may produce anorexia.

NAUSEA AND VOMITING

The patient with nausea has a feeling of discomfort in the region of the stomach, anorexia, and a tendency to vomit. When vomit- ing occurs, the contents of the stomach, duodenum, and jejunum are ejected forcefully through the mouth. The ejected contents are referred to as *vomitus*. The actual act of vomiting results from a sudden and strong contraction of the diaphragm and abdominal muscles.

Nausea and vomiting are commonly caused by excessive fatigue, strong emotional reactions, generalized infections, drugs such as opium and general anesthetic agents, the intake of poisons, and many diseases. A peptic ulcer, appendicitis, gall-

TABLE 15.5
GUIDE TO OBSERVING THE PATIENT WITH A
DISEASE OF THE GASTROINTESTINAL SYSTEM

AREA TO BE OBSERVED	WHAT TO OBSERVE
Mouth	Mouth lesions such as leukoplakia, cold sores, canker sores
	Teeth missing or diseased
	Improperly fitting dentures
	Drainage or bleeding from gums. Color of gums
	Abnormal breath odors
	Cracked, dry lips or lesions on lips
	Dysphagia
	Anorexia, nausea, vomiting
	Eructation
Chest	Dyspepsia
	Disturbances in respiratory rate and/or pattern
Abdomen	Abdominal distention
	Presence and location of pain
	Softness or tautness of abdomen
Bowel pattern	Changes in color, frequency, appearance of usual bowel movements
	Constipation
	Diarrhea
	Flatus
Height and weight	Recent losses or gains
Behavioral changes	Signs of grieving
	Patterns of self-medication, especially with laxatives, antacids
	Usual eating patterns
	Hospitalized patient's tray

stones, and a brain tumor are only a few examples of diseases that produce nausea and vomiting. Motion sickness resulting in nausea and vomiting is caused by stimulation of the structures in the inner ear.

The nurse should observe, record, and report the time of vomiting, its nature, odor, amount, and color and whether or not it is associated with a spell of coughing or with the intake of food and drugs. It is also important to report projectile vomiting. In this case the contents of the stomach are expelled with great force. In noting the nature of the vomitus the nurse can ask these questions: Is it clear? Does it appear to contain partially digested food? Does it seem to contain blood or mucus? When the blood has been acted upon by gastric juice, it has the appearance of coffee grounds.

The presence of either a foul or a fecal odor should be reported. It is important to report the approximate amount and color of vomitus. For example, it may be observed that the fluid is colorless, green, yellow, or red. Bright-red vomitus usually indicates recent hemorrhage. *Hematemesis* is the term used in referring to the vomiting of blood. If the vomitus appears unusual or if it is a kind of vomitus that has not been seen in this patient before, it should be saved for either the head nurse/charge nurse or the doctor to see.

DYSPEPSIA

The patient with dyspepsia has epigastric discomfort following meals. The patient may report heartburn (a burning sensation in the region of the esophagus and heart), belching (eructation), and/or pain. The nurse reports and records this information including foods the patient had eaten before dyspepsia occurred.

RESPIRATIONS

The patient with abdominal distention may develop restricted respirations from pressure on the diaphragm which is located just above the abdomen. The respiratory pattern may also be affected by chemical imbalances which can develop from gastrointestinal disease. Additional information about abnormal respirations can be located in Chapter 14.

ABDOMINAL DISTENTION

The patient with abdominal distention has an enlargement of the abdominal cavity caused by the collection of fluids or gases, the presence of tumors or growths, or enlarged organs. Abdominal distention is monitored by measuring the abdominal girth at the level of the umbilicus. In addition, the nurse may observe and record whether the abdomen is soft or hard, the presence or absence of pain, and whether or not the patient is passing flatus (gas) through the rectum. The presence or absence of bowel sounds may be observed by placing a stethoscope over the abdomen.

PAIN

The patient with a disease in the gastrointestinal system frequently reports pain. The nurse collects information about the location of the pain, its relation to food intake or elimination, the type of pain, and the intensity. In order to locate abdominal pain precisely, the nurse draws two imaginary lines that divide the abdomen into four parts known as quadrants. A horizontal line is drawn across the abdomen at the level of the umbilicus. The vertical line is drawn through the umbilicus also. This separates the abdomen into right and left upper quadrants and right and left lower quadrants. The nurse then reports and records the location of the patient's pain according to the quadrant in which it occurs.

OBSERVING THE BOWEL PATTERN

Observing, recording, and reporting information about the patient's bowel movements constitute an important part of nursing observation. For example, a change in bowel habits is one of the danger signals of cancer which should cause a person to seek medical attention. There is a variety of normal bowel patterns among healthy persons. Therefore, the nurse collects information both about the patient's usual pattern and any departures from the usual pattern.

CONSTIPATION

The individual who has fewer stools than usual has constipation. The fecal material is usually hard and dry. Often the patient who reports constipation is actually defecating less frequently than what is normal according to personal beliefs. However, the consistency of the stool is believed to be a more reliable guide than the frequency of stools. Constipation may be a symptom of an organic disease, or it may be functional. In an organic disease, there is a change in the organ or tissue to explain the patient's symptoms. Functional constipation is more common than organic.

Two types of functional constipation are atonic and spastic. An individual who is habitually constipated usually has decreased muscle tone in the colon. This type of constipation is referred to as *atonic*. The colon in some nervous individuals may develop an increase in muscle tone. Parts of the colon become spastic and prevent the normal passage of feces. This is called *spastic* constipation.

Functional constipation results from the individual's habits. The most frequent cause is failure to respond to the desire to have a bowel movement. Other factors such as eating a diet low in roughage, fruit, and vegetables; drinking an insufficient amount of fluids; and lack of exercise may cause constipation. Also, a change of daily habits, such as occurs when taking a trip or being hospitalized, causes many individuals to become constipated.

In severe cases, the rectum may become impacted, filled with masses of hard fecal material. This is referred to as a *fecal impaction*. This condition also may be accompanied by the leakage of liquid stool around the impaction and out of the body.

DIARRHEA

The passage of an increased number of loose stools is known as diarrhea. The number of stools may vary from 1 to 30 or 40 a day. Diarrhea is a symptom of an irritation in the bowel and not a disease. The body tries to rid itself of the irritation by increasing peristalsis, which is the wormlike contraction of the intestines. There is more fluid in the intestinal tract because the rapid passage of its contents does not allow for proper absorption.

Increased peristalsis causes the patient to have intestinal cramps. *Tenesmus*, which is painful straining without having a bowel movement, may be present. Nausea, vomiting, feeling of weakness, and fever are commonly associated with diarrhea. Dehydration occurs in severe cases of diarrhea, resulting in thirst and dryness of the mouth and skin. An excessive loss of fluid is especially dangerous in infants and small children, as it may result in death if allowed to continue.

Diarrhea causes loss of pancreatic juice, which contains more sodium than does plasma. Gastric juices and all other secretions of the intestinal tract are lost when the patient has diarrhea. Thus, both sodium and chloride are lost by the patient with diarrhea. Normally, much of the sodium bicarbonate coming from the pancreas and basic secretions coming from the small intestine are returned to the bloodstream as the fecal material slowly passes through the large intestine. When the patient has diarrhea, passage of feces through the large intestine is so rapid that reabsorption of base fluid cannot take place. This may result in metabolic acidosis (blood pH approximately 7.1). The symptoms of metabolic acidosis are similar to those of diabetic acidosis, which is discussed in Chapter 18.

Irritation of the intestinal tract resulting in diarrhea has many causes. Generally, these causes may be divided into the three following groups: functional disorders, generalized disorders, and intrinsic diseases of the intestine.

Functional disorders involve malfunction of the gastrointestinal tract itself and include food allergies, defective digestion and/ or absorption, vitamin deficiencies, abuse of cathartics, and side effects of drugs.

Generalized disorders causing diarrhea refer to the systemic disease conditions that affect the intestine, such as heavy-metal poisoing, cardiac decompensation, neurologic disease, endocrine imbalance, and uremia.

Intrinsic disorders of the intestine include those conditions that are situated entirely within the gastrointestinal tract. Infections of the gastrointestinal tract caused by viruses, bacteria, fungi, or protozoa frequently result in diarrhea. Alteration of the normal intestinal flora by drugs such as antibiotics can cause diarrhea. Other causes of diarrhea are intestinal stasis, intestinal inflammation such as regional enteritis or ulcerative colitis, and partial intestinal obstruction.

The nurse should report the approximate amount, color, and consistency of feces, and the frequency of diarrhea. The stool should be examined for mucus, blood, pus, and other abnormalities that might aid the doctor in the diagnosis. Also, the presence of tenesmus and intestinal cramps should be reported and recorded in the nurse's notes.

HEIGHT AND WEIGHT

Height and weight are important observations in the patient with a disturbance in the gastrointestinal system. The patient's height and weight usually are measured on admission to the hospital, clinic, or first visit to the doctor's office. Weight may be measured regularly in order to detect changes that are a result of illness or treatment. The patient should be weighed at the same time of day, wearing the same type of clothing, and on the same scale. Recent weight gains or losses that the patient reports are reported to the appropriate nurse or physician and recorded on the chart.

BEHAVIORAL CHANGES

The patient with a disturbance in the gastrointestinal system may experience many behavioral changes. Unpleasant odors and sights associated with illness, marked dietary changes, and changes in taste and smell may cause the patient to experience one or more stages of grieving as described in Chapter 1.

An important observation is the patient's practices of self-medication with antacids, laxatives, and similar drugs that may affect the digestion and absorption of foods. The nurse records all prescribed and nonprescribed drugs the patient uses at home.

The patient's eating behavior is of special interest to the nurse because this information often contains valuable clues to the patient's condition. In addition to asking the patient about the usual eating behavior, the nurse may observe the hospitalized patient's tray to determine how much and what kind of foods were eaten. In some cases, the tray may be returned to the dietitian so that an exact calculation of the food intake can be made.

Nursing Interventions

HYGIENE

The patient should be assisted, if needed, to wash the hands before meals and after elimination. Oral hygiene both helps to prevent bacterial overgrowth in the mouth and removes unpleasant tastes and odors after vomiting. The patient with diarrhea needs perineal care after each stool. A protective ointment may be applied to prevent skin irritation around the anus.

ALTERATIONS OF DIET AND FLUIDS

Dietery therapy is often an important part of medical and surgical treatment for the patient with a disease of the gastrointestinal system. Factors that guide the physician's selection of a specific diet include the patient's nutritional status, the nutritional adequacy of a specific diet, the specific disease, stress factors in the patient's life, and the patient's personal and cultural preferences related to food.

The nurse may be responsible for checking to see that the patient receives the correct diet as well as recording the food and fluid intake. The dietitian should be consulted before any substitutions are made for the patient on a special diet.

Another important nursing intervention related to diet is teaching healthy eating habits. For example, the nurse may encourage the patient to eat slowly in small bites. Some persons with gastrointestinal disorders have developed eating habits that may cause or worsen symptoms. For example, the person with dyspepsia and gas may eat too fast and swallow air in the process. Excessive air may contribute to feelings of fullness, dyspepsia, eructation, and flatulence. Frequent family feuds at mealtimes also may contribute to gastrointestinal symptoms in some persons.

Patients with constipation usually are helped by adding fiber to the diet. This change can be made by using whole-grain breads and cereals, eating at least four servings of fruits and vegetables each day, and eating more raw fruits and vegetables. In addition, the patient is encouraged to drink at least 1200 to 1500 ml of fluid every day, exercise, and develop a regular elimination pattern (discussed later in this chapter).

The patient with diarrhea may temporarily receive no foods by mouth in order to rest the gastrointestinal tract.

As the patient's condition improves, the physician prescribes a nonirritating diet, which progresses from liquids, such as tea, weak broth, buttermilk, and boiled milk, to soft foods. Soft-cooked eggs, toast, custard, plain gelatin desserts, and strained cereals are examples of bland foods often ordered by the doctor. The patient is usually left on a bland diet until the diarrhea has been absent for several days. A return to a regular diet should be gradual.

Since dehydration may be a serious complication of diarrhea, it is of vital importance to replace the fluids lost. The nurse should encourage the patient to drink fluids allowed by the doctor when nausea and vomiting are not present. If the patient cannot take fluids by mouth, fluids may be prescribed intravenously.

The patient with anorexia is not forced to eat but is, instead, encouraged to eat. The nurse is in a key position to help this patient. Surroundings that are clean, neat, orderly, and free from odor help to improve the patient's desire for food. Such objects as a half-filled emesis basin or an empty transfusion bottle can ruin a patient's meal. The patient also should be made as comfortable as possible for his meal. The sight and smell of tempting food served as attractively as possible will aid in stimulating the appetite. The diet should be served in small portions at regular times. If at all possible, the patient's desire for a special food should be fulfilled. Placing a bloom in a small bud vase or other simple favors on the tray adds to its attractiveness. After the patient has finished eating, the tray should be removed. The nurse should observe the type and amount of food eaten by the patient and record this information appropriately.

The patient with an aversion to food caused by profound emotional problems has *anorexia nervosa*. This illness is discussed later on page 507–508.

When feeding a patient, the nurse should endeavor to do so in an unhurried, pleasant manner (Figure 15.3). The nurse should appear relaxed and interested in feeding the patient. The patient should be given time to chew and swallow the food. The desires of the patient in regard to sequence and amount of food to be eaten should be followed, if at all possible.

GAVAGE. Tube feeding or gavage, as it is also known, is a special form of nutritional therapy for the patient who is unable to swallow or chew. A nasogastric feeding tube is inserted through the nose and advanced into the stomach. A liquid diet, commercial

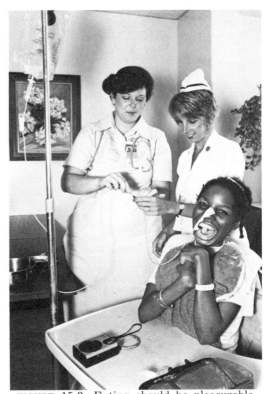

FIGURE 15.3 Eating should be pleasurable. (Courtesy of Bergen Pines County Hospital School of Practical Nursing, Paramus, New Jersey.)

tube feedings, or special prepared formula may be instilled into the feeding tube. Generally, the tube feeding is prepared to provide a total of 2000 kilocalories in 2000 ml of fluid. The feeding may be instilled continuously using a special setup similar to intravenous tubing or intermittently (Figure 15.4). Table 15.6 contains a summary of information that guides the nurse to assist the patient receiving tube feedings.

GASTROSTOMY FEEDINGS. The patient with a gastrostomy has a temporary or permanent surgical opening through the abdomen to the stomach in order to provide nutrition. A gastrostomy may be done when the patient has an obstruction in the esophagus caused by scarring, tumors, and/or swelling. The feeding is administered in a manner similar to tube feedings.

The nurse attaches a funnel or syringe to the rubber tube to feed this patient. Assessing the amount of residual gastric contents is done before feeding the patient through a gastrostomy tube. This is done by aspirating fluid from the stomach prior to feeding. If the nurse obtains 100 ml or more by aspiration prior to feeding, the physician is notified before the feeding is begun. The gastric aspirate should be given back to the patient by way of the tube to prevent loss of electrolytes. After aspiration, the nurse should pour the prescribed fluid slowly into the funnel.

The nurse should notice the character of the gastric aspirate. An abnormal appearance is reported to the nurse in charge or the physician. In the author's own experience, examination of gastric aspirate after noting the fact that it appeared dark black enabled the physician to reach a diagnosis that the patient had an active bleeding ulcer.

The patient with a permanent gastrostomy should see, smell, and, if possible, taste the food before a feeding. In some cases, the patient is advised to chew the food and then place it in the funnel connected to the gastrostomy tube. This procedure is unappealing to many persons and the patient may be one of them. In any case, the patient needs privacy when being fed through the gastrostomy tube.

Nausea and cramps may be prevented by first warming the liquid to body temperature. Water should be allowed to run through the funnel and tube after the feeding. This helps to remove the liquid food from the tube in addition to supplying part of the patient's daily water requirement. The tube should be clamped off after the feeding to prevent the fluid from escaping. The tube may be left in place, or it may be removed after the feeding. The nurse who has any doubt about removing a gastrostomy tube should leave the tube in place.

The patient's dressing needs to be changed frequently because of leakage from the stomach. Gastric juice tends to digest the skin. Because of this, the operative area should be kept clean and dry. The nursing staff should receive instructions for cleaning the area from the doctor. In addition, frequent oral hygiene and rinsing of the mouth are helpful for the patient who is unable to consume oral food and fluids.

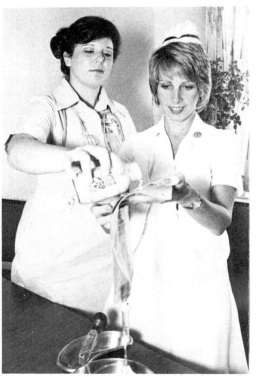

FIGURE 15.4 Preparing a gavage feeding. (Courtesy of Bergen Pines County Hospital School of Practical Nursing, Paramus, New Jersey.)

TABLE 15.6
SUMMARY OF INFORMATION RELATED TO TUBE FEEDINGS

1. Keep the patient's head elevated during tube feedings and for at least one hour after an intermittent feeding.
2. Check the position of the feeding tube before each feeding or at least once per shift.
3. Aspirate the feeding tube before each feeding and return any material collected back into the tube. Report any amount over 100 ml to the appropriate nurse since the feeding may be withheld or postponed.
4. Use gravity to promote the flow of liquid during an intermittent feeding.
5. Flush the feeding tube with water after each feeding.
6. Refrigerate all feedings including commercial preparations after they have been opened. Intermittent tube feeding may be warmed just prior to the feeding.
7. Discard remaining feedings after 24 hours. Change all equipment except the actual feeding tube every 24 hours.
8. Report the patient's feelings of fullness, eructation, flatus, regurgitation, nausea, abdominal cramps, diarrhea.
9. Record the amount of feeding and water instilled.
10. Assist with oral hygiene after each intermittent feeding or every four to six hours during continuous feedings.

TOTAL PARENTERAL NUTRITION (TPN, HYPERALIMENTATION). The patient receiving total parenteral nutrition receives solutions containing glucose, amino acid mixtures, minerals, vitamins, and fats through an indwelling catheter placed in the superior vena cava. Total parenteral nutrition may be prescribed as short- or long-term therapy for the patient with intestinal obstruction, gastrointestinal fistula, uncontrolled malabsorption, extensive burns, or cancer. The patient usually requires nursing observations and interventions similar to those indicated for intravenous therapy, including maintaining sterility of the fluid and administration equipment, monitoring the flow rate of the fluid, recording intake and output, observing and reporting signs of irritation and/or clots along the vein caused by the indwelling catheter, observing and reporting air bubbles which develop in the tubing, and preventing the tubing from becoming twisted, kinked, or disconnected during care. Additional observations and interventions are needed to identify and/or prevent complications which may develop with total parenteral nutrition. For example, infection is a particularly hazardous complication, both because the patient has increased susceptibility and because the nutritional solution contains a high concentration of glucose which favors bacterial growth. To prevent infection, the nutritional solution is usually refrigerated and discarded after 24 hours. A special filter is attached to the intravenous tubing to trap particles and bacteria. The tubing and the dressing over the catheter site are changed every 24 hours using sterile technique.

Abnormalities in glucose metabolism may develop during total parenteral nutrition. In order to identify and/or prevent hyperglycemia and/or hypoglycemia, the nurse checks the patient's urine regularly for sugar and acetone. A mechanical infusion pump is used to provide a steady flow rate of the nutritional solution. The pump prevents abnormalities in glucose metabolism which may develop if the fluid infuses either too fast or too slowly. In addition, the pump has several alarms to notify the nurse of problems such as occlusion of the line or air in the tubing.

Observations that indicate an abnormal response to total parenteral nutrition should be reported such as nausea, headache, fever, lethargy, disorientation, and wide mood swings. The patient's intake and output and daily weight are carefully measured and recorded. In addition, the physician usually orders frequent blood chemistry tests to help evaluate electrolyte imbalance and the patient's response to therapy. The patient who requires long-term therapy may be taught to administer the nutritional solution at home. This situation requires extensive patient and family teaching prior to discharge.

The Hickmann catheter is a relatively new variation currently available, primarily to selected cancer patients who need long-term total parenteral nutrition. The catheter is a silicone rubber tubing approximately 90 cm long which is inserted into the right atrium of the heart via the cephalic or other vein during a minor surgical procedure. Two small incisions usually are made. One incision is made in the anterior chest wall. The catheter is then threaded through a tunnel made in the subcutaneous tissue. A second incision is made in the area of the deltoid pectoral groove to expose the appropriate vein. The catheter actually enters the vein at this point and is sutured in place after the tip reaches the right atrium. The catheter is capped when not in use. The patient may bathe and participate in other daily activities. The catheter is flushed daily with a saline heparin solution to prevent clotting. Regular dressing changes using sterile technique are also needed. Since the parenteral solution used is the same, observations and interventions related to infection, disturbances in glucose metabolism, and untoward reactions already described apply to the patient with a Hickmann catheter.

POSITIONING AND EXERCISE

Certain positions and exercises may be indicated for the patient with a disturbance in the gastrointestinal system. For example, normally the patient is placed in semi-Fowler's position for each meal including tube feedings. This position helps the passage of food and fluids through the digestive tract.

The patient who is vomiting, however, is usually assisted to turn either the head or the whole body to one side so that vomitus is not aspirated (breathed) into the lungs. As mentioned earlier, the patient receiving gastric decompression may be turned to the right side to improve drainage of gastrointestinal contents.

Positioning and exercise also help the patient who has a problem with elimination. For example, the patient who is constipated may be helped by starting or increasing the

exercise program. Walking is an exercise that is especially helpful in promoting peristalsis and relieving gas. Such a patient also may be helped to have a bowel movement by leaning forward while sitting on the bedpan, commode, or toilet seat.

ASSISTING WITH DRUG THERAPY

The patient with a gastrointestinal disorder is likely to receive one or more drugs either to alleviate symptoms and/or treat the underlying condition. In addition, many patients with gastrointestinal symptoms self-medicate with nonprescribed drugs. These two factors increase the likelihood of drug interaction.

The patient with constipation may receive a laxative such as those listed in Table 15.7. Laxatives generally are not prescribed when the patient has abdominal pain, ulcerative conditions of the intestines, appendicitis, an intestinal obstruction, or inflammatory conditions of the intestines. Also, laxatives are prescribed with caution during the late stages of pregnancy.

Drugs that may be prescribed for the patient with diarrhea include preparations containing bismuth, kaolin, atropine, or opium. These drugs may be helpful in relieving cramps, slowing peristalsis, and reducing the number of stools.

An antiemetic from Table 15.8 may be prescribed for the patient who is nauseated or vomiting. An important side effect of many antiemetic drugs is drowsiness. The patient usually is instructed not to drive or operate machinery after taking this drug.

Other drugs that may be prescribed for the patient with a disease in the gastrointestinal system include gastric antacids (Table 15.9) and antimuscarinic agents (Table 15.10).

ASSISTING WITH ELIMINATION

The nurse can take many actions that are helpful to the patient with a problem related to elimination. For example, the patient who must use a bedpan usually has more success when privacy is assured. The nurse may place a sign on the door and/or completely screen the patient to prevent a disruption of privacy during a bowel movement.

TABLE 15.7
CLASSIFICATION OF CATHARTICS AND LAXATIVES*

Stimulant cathartics
  Castor oil
  Bisacodyl (DULCOLAX)
  Phenolphthalein
  Oxyphenisatin acetate (ISOCRIN)
  Cascara sagrada
  Senna
	Stimulant cathartics are absorbed partially from the intestine and may cause the urine to be discolored. They may cause a cramping sensation. Cathartic action usually within 6 to 12 hours

Saline cathartics
  Magnesium sulfate (epsom salt)
  Milk of magnesia
  Magnesium citrate
  Potassium sodium tartrate (Rochelle salt)
	Saline cathartics are absorbed slightly from the gastrointestinal tract. They increase the water content of feces. Peristalsis is enhanced. The increase of fluid in the bowel and peristalsis result in several liquid or semiliquid stools. May be used also to relieve edema

Bulk-forming laxatives
  Methylcellulose
  Psyllium preparations (KONSYL, METAMUCIL)
	Bulk-forming laxatives stimulate peristalsis by increasing the bulk in the gastrointestinal tract. These drugs can cause fecal impaction and obstruction. They do not interfere with absorption of food

Emollient laxatives
  Dioctylsodium sulfosuccinate (COLACE,
    DOXINATE)
  Mineral oil (liquid petrolatum)
	Emollient laxatives are composed of oil, which is not digested. The feces are softened and retain water. Especially useful when the patient's stool should be soft to avoid straining. These laxatives may prevent the absorption of fat-soluble vitamins

* Cathartics cause increased motility of the intestines with a fluid evacuation. Laxatives cause excretion of a soft, formed stool and have a less drastic effect than cathartics.

Most persons benefit from a regular schedule for having a bowel movement. Hospitalization may interfere with usual patterns of exercise, diet, and toileting which have developed over a lifetime.

When possible, the patient should be helped to maintain the usual pattern of elimination. For example, the patient who usually has a daily bowel movement after breakfast may be offered a bedpan or assisted to the commode or bathroom at the usual time during hospitalization. The patient who feels constipated during the hospital stay may be helped by increasing the fluid intake, exercise, and drinking prune juice, if permitted. When possible, the patient's usual home remedies for constipation should be incorporated into the nursing care plan. In some cases, the home remedy may be modified slightly, if necessary. For example, Mr. Lange was accustomed to having a daily bowel movement after consuming two cups of coffee at breakfast. Since Mr. Lange's bland diet did not permit caffeine, the nurse substituted two cups of decaffeinated coffee after checking with the dietitian. This modification of Mr. Lange's usual pattern enabled him to continue the regular pattern of bowel movements.

The patient with persistent constipation may have developed a pattern of ignoring the early urge for a bowel movement. Such a patient often may be helped by setting aside a regular time for elimination as a part of a program that also includes increasing the fluid intake, exercise, and dietary fiber.

In some cases, enemas are prescribed to empty the bowel before or after a diagnostic test, stimulate peristalsis, or relieve constipation. Careful attention to measures already described often prevents the need for enemas to relieve constipation. Oil retention enemas may be prescribed to soften the feces of a patient with a fecal impaction. In some cases, a fecal impaction must be removed with gloved fingers.

Bowel training is a planned program to help a patient achieve control over bowel movements usually without laxatives or enemas. Bowel training includes measures such as adjustment of food and fluids to develop a soft, formed stool, providing the specific equipment needed (toilet, commode, bedpan, raised toilet seat, or incontinent pads), set-

TABLE 15.8
ANTIEMETICS

NONPROPRIETARY NAME	TRADE NAME	AVERAGE DOSE FOR ADULTS	NURSING IMPLICATIONS
Chlorpromazine	THORAZINE	25–100 mg suppository 3–4 times/day	May affect muscle tone and may mask symptoms of acute surgical conditions. Hypotensive reaction and drowsiness may occur. May also be ordered for IM injection
Cyclizine	MAREZINE	50 mg	Low incidence of drowsiness. Dryness of mouth and blurred vision may occur
Dimenhydrinate	DRAMAMINE	50 mg/single dose	May cause drowsiness and sedation. Used for motion sickness also
Meclizine	BONINE	25–50 mg	Dry mouth relieved by oral care
Prochlorperazine	COMPAZINE	25 mg 2 times/day (suppository)	Drowsiness may occur
Promazine	SPARINE	25-50 mg every 4–6 hours	May be prescribed for oral or intramuscular injection. Nasal stuffiness and dry mouth may occur
Promethazine	PHENERGAN	25–50 mg/day	Also used for antihistamine effect. Often used for motion sickness
Thiethylperazine	TORECAN	10–30 mg/day	May be ordered for parenteral, rectal, or oral administration
Triflupromazine	VESPRIN	5-15 mg/day	Oral or parenteral administration may be prescribed. May cause hypotension
Trimethobenzamide	TIGAN	50–200 mg	Vertigo, blurred vision, drowsiness, and headache may occur. Suppository has benzocaine and should not be given if patient is allergic to this or other local anesthetics

ting a specific time for defecation (usually after a meal), and positioning the patient. During the training program, suppositories, laxatives, enemas, or massage of the anal sphincter may be used temporarily to establish a regular bowel movement. An important feature of the training program is the need for consistency. Members of the nursing staff must follow the routine exactly for training to occur. The exact routine varies according to the patient's needs, physician's and nurse's preferences, and local custom.

ASSISTING WITH PATIENT AND FAMILY TEACHING

The nurse has many opportunities and topics for patient and family teaching. Possible topics that may be appropriate for the patient with a disease in the gastrointestinal system include:

- Developing good dental health by brushing the teeth correctly, flossing the teeth, eating a nutritious diet, visiting the dentist regularly, and obtaining dentures that fit correctly
- How to plan, shop, and prepare a nutritious diet
- Developing good eating habits such as eating slowly, chewing thoroughly, avoiding stress at mealtimes
- Developing healthy bowel habits through proper diet, regular exercise, adequate fluid intake, and a schedule for defecating
- The hazards of long-term, regular use of laxatives
- Recognizing and reporting rectal bleeding and changes in bowel patterns as a danger signal of cancer
- The importance of a yearly digital rectal examination after age 40 for early detection of cancer
- The need for regular sigmoidoscopy and stool guaiac slide test after age 50 for early detection of cancer

TABLE 15.9
GASTRIC ANTACIDS*

NONPROPRIETARY NAME	TRADE NAME	AVERAGE DOSE†	NURSING IMPLICATIONS
Aluminum hydroxide gel	ALKAGEL AL-U-CREME AMPHOJEL COLLUMINA CREAMALIN	15 ml	Administer a sip or two of water or milk after giving drug to ensure passage into stomach. Constipation may be problem with aluminum preparations. The
Aluminum phosphate	PHOSPHALJEL	15–45 ml	number and consistency of
Basic aluminum carbonate	BASALJEL	10 ml	stools should be observed by the patient and/or nurse. The pa-
Calcium carbonate	TITRALAC	10 ml	tient may be advised to switch to a magnesium preparation if an aluminum antacid causes constipation. Affects absorption of salicylates, indomethacin, sulfa drugs, anticoagulants, and tetracycline
Cimetidine	TAGAMET	300 mg orally 4/day with meals and at bedtime May also be administered by intramuscular and intravenous routes	Drug interactions possible as described above. Should be withdrawn gradually
Dihydroxyaluminum aminoacetate	ROBALATE	500 mg–1 gm	
Dihydroxyaluminum sodium carbonate	ROLAIDS	660–1320 mg	
Magaldrate	RIOPAN	400–800 mg	
Magnesium and aluminum hydroxide suspension	ALUDROX MAALOX	4–8 ml	Magnesium antacids have a slightly laxative effect. Patients
Magnesium carbonate		0.6–2 gm	should be observed for frequency and consistency of
Magnesium hydroxide (Milk of Magnesia)		5–30 ml	stools. Diarrhea can result in severe dehydration. Diarrhea
Magnesium oxide		250 mg 1 gm	should be reported promptly

* Nonsystemic antacids neutralize the contents of the stomach but do not neutralize other body fluids such as the blood and urine.
† Dosages currently being revised in light of new research.

Additional patient teaching is related to changes caused by the disease condition and therapy.

ASSISTING THE PATIENT WITH GASTROINTESTINAL DECOMPRESSION

The patient with *gastrointestinal decompression* has a tube passed through the nose to the stomach or intestines for the purpose of removing the contents by suction (Figure 15.5). The suction may be provided by an electrical machine, such as the intermittent GOMCO suction machine, by wall suction outlets, or by equipment that creates a vacuum by permitting water to run through a closed system from one bottle to another. Wangensteen suction is an example of the equipment used to create suction with water. Since this was an early type of suction, the term *Wangensteen suction* may be heard used today in reference to other types of equipment used for gastrointestinal suction.

Gastrointestinal decompression may be indicated to obtain specimens of gastric contents for examination, to relieve and/or prevent postoperative distention, to remove a collection of gastrointestinal contents resulting from an obstruction, to empty the

TABLE 15.10
ATROPINIC AND ATROPINIC-LIKE DRUGS (ANTIMUSCARINIC AGENTS)*

NONPROPRIETARY NAME	TRADE NAME	AVERAGE DOSE	NURSING IMPLICATIONS
Belladonna alkaloids (Belladonna tincture)		0.6 ml	The patient's pulse and respiration should be checked to detect toxic effects. The patient's pulse may increase from 4 to 26 beats per minute. Flushing of the face and neck may be noted. Dry mouth and thirst may develop. Oral hygiene and use of mouthwash may relieve these symptoms. Hard candy, if permitted, sometimes will refresh the mouth and increase salivation. The patient may experience dizziness, blurred vision, and difficulty in swallowing. Constipation and urinary retention may develop. The patient should be taught to observe urinary output and notify the physician if symptoms of cystitis develop.
Dicyclomine hydrochloride	BENTYL	20 mg	
Glycopyrrolate	ROBINUL	1–2 mg	
Hexocyclium methylsulfate	TRAL	25 mg	
Isopropamide iodide	DARBID	5 mg	
Mepenzolate methylbromide	CANTIL	25 mg	
Methantheline bromide	BANTHINE	50 mg	
Oxyphenonium bromide	ANTRENYL	5 mg	
Piperidolate hydrochloride	DACTIL	50 mg	
Propantheline bromide	PRO-BANTHINE	15 mg	
Scopolamine methylbromide	PAMINE	2.5 mg	

* Atropinic and atropinic-like drugs are used to lessen peristaltic movement of the stomach and intestines and decrease gastric secretions.

stomach before an emergency operation, and to remove poisons.

When assisting with gastrointestinal decompression, the first step is to obtain the type of nasogastric tube prescribed by the physician and the type of suction apparatus appropriate for the specific tube. Figure 15.6 illustrates several common types of gastrointestinal tubes.

The *Levin tube* is either rubber or plastic and has several holes or openings near the tip to permit aspiration of the stomach contents. The Levin tube is used for gastric suction. Intermittent GOMCO suction at low pressure usually is prescribed when the patient has a Levin tube.

The *Salem sump tube* is similar to the Levin tube except the sump tube has two

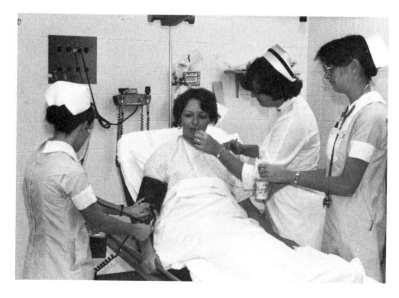

FIGURE 15.5 Inserting a nasogastric tube. (Courtesy of School of Practical Nursing, Twin County Memorial Hospital, Galax, Virginia.)

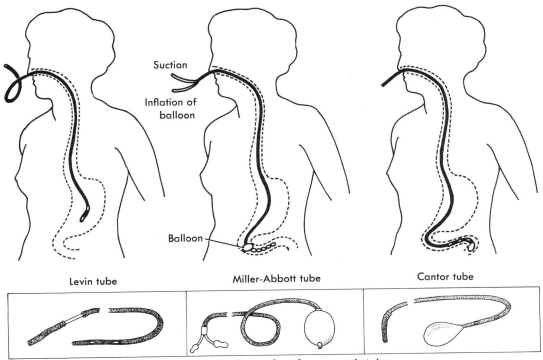

Suction

Inflation of balloon

Balloon

Levin tube   Miller-Abbott tube   Cantor tube

FIGURE 15.6   Examples of nasogastric tubes.

holes in the proximal end. The double open-ing enables the nurse to irrigate the tube while suction is maintained. The suction source is continuous and should not be dis-connected nor should the tubing be aspi-rated. The nurse is able to hear a hissing sound when the tube is functioning properly and the side arm of the tube is held near the ear.

Another example of a nasogastric tube is the *Anderson tube*, which consists of two smaller tubes. The larger of the two tubes is attached to continuous suction and the smaller tube permits air to enter the gastro-intestinal tract. Air can be forced through the smaller airway tube to prevent constant suction on the mucosa from continuous suc-tion. The nurse may be instructed to inject 10 cc of air at specified intervals into the tube serving as an airway to the gastrointes-tinal tract.

The Cantor and Miller-Abbott tubes are used for intestinal suction. Because of this they are longer than the Levin tube and con-tain devices that help the tube to be moved downward. The *Cantor tube* has several openings and a bag on the end that is in-serted into the patient. Mercury is injected directly into the bag. The heavy weight of the mercury helps the tube to be moved along the intestinal tract. The portion of the tube remaining outside the patient's body has only one opening, which is attached to suction.

The *Miller-Abbott* is a tube within a tube, or a double-lumen tube. One tube connects with a balloon near the end of the portion in the patient's body. The physician inflates this balloon with air after it has passed through the pylorus. The inflated tube en-ables the peristalsis to carry the end of the tube along the intestinal tract. The second tube connects the openings (holes) in the portion in the patient's body to outside suc-tion. The openings for suction and to the bal-loon should be marked clearly. Only the suc-tion opening should be attached to suction. Only the suction opening should have pre-scribed irrigating solution instilled into it.

After having the tube for intestinal de-compression inserted by the physician, the patient may be assisted to assume specific positions to facilitate passage of the tube to the proper level in the intestine. Passage of the tube generally is confirmed by fluoroscopic examinations and x-ray. The position of the tube may be checked by x-ray on a daily basis. The nurse should remember that the intestinal tube is not to be secured by taping it to the patient's face or pinning it to the bed linen while it is being advanced. The physician will indicate the exact amount of tubing that is to be advanced and when the tube can be secured with tape to the patient's face.

After inserting the tube to the desired location in the stomach or intestine, the physician indicates the amount of suction to be maintained. The flow of fluid can be observed through the clear plastic adapter and in the drainage bottle or bag. Positioning the patient on the right side at frequent intervals may improve drainage because of the anatomic shape of the stomach. When the flow of fluid from the tube appears to have stopped, it should be checked. The suction equipment can be checked to see if it is working properly by disconnecting the nasogastric tube temporarily and placing the tube leading to the suction in a container of water. Properly functioning equipment will suction the water.

The physician may want the tube irrigated with normal saline solution at specific times. The prescription also may indicate the exact amount to be used and whether it should be aspirated by syringe or by the suction apparatus. In either case, the nurse measures and records the amount and type of fluid instilled and the amount aspirated (see Figure 15.7). In general, no more than 50 ml are instilled at one time. The amount of fluid in the drainage bottle is observed and recorded every eight hours, and the total for 24 hours also is indicated. The doctor uses this information to prescribe fluid and electrolyte replacement for the patient. It is important for all members of the nursing staff to conscientiously measure and record all fluid excreted by the patient and given to the patient. For example, the patient may lose fluid both in urine and in other ways

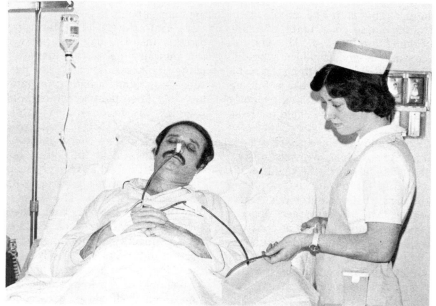

FIGURE 15.7 The patient's nasogastric tube is being irrigated. The amount and type of fluid being instilled and aspirated should be observed and recorded. (Courtesy of Indianapolis Public Schools, School of Practical Nursing, and Indiana University Hospitals, Indianapolis, Indiana.)

such as bleeding. All should be reported. The color and appearance of all drainage should be recorded also.

The patient with gastrointestinal suction generally is bothered by the tube in the nose and frequently has to breathe through the mouth. This, in addition to the lack of fluids by mouth, causes the mouth to be dry. In caring for the patient with gastrointestinal suction, the nurse utilizes measures to keep the mouth clean and moist. Frequent oral hygiene is important. The patient who is able usually feels more comfortable after brushing the teeth and/or using mouthwash. The patient may be instructed not to swallow the water, toothpaste, or mouthwash. In some cases, the patient requires assistance from the nurse for oral hygiene. Gauze, tongue depressors, mouthwash, and lubricants for the lips and nares are needed.

In some cases, the oriented patient may be allowed to chew gum. In addition to the pleasant taste, the chewing of gum stimulates the flow of saliva. The nurse should check with the physician before allowing the patient to chew gum. In some cases the physician orders throat lozenges. Small amounts of cracked ice and sips of water may be given to the patient if permitted by the doctor.

The portion of the nose through which the tube passes should be cleansed gently to prevent the secretions from forming dry crusts. A water-soluble lubricant may be applied to the external portion of the nostril through which the tube passes. Tape used to secure the tubing should be changed when needed and at least daily.

The tube should be clamped prior to removal so that gastric contents do not leak from the tube into the esophagus or pharynx. While the patient is holding his or her breath, the tube should be removed gradually, usually several inches at any one time. After having the tube removed, the patient should have mouth care.

ASSISTING THE PATIENT WITH SURGICAL CARE

The patient having surgery on the gastrointestinal system usually needs special preoperative preparation related to the passage of food through the digestive system. For example, the patient may be placed on a low-residue or liquid diet for one or more days prior to surgery. A complete bowel preparation, as described on page 485, may be indicated. The combination of diagnostic tests that often require the withholding of foods and fluids and a bowel preparation may cause an increase in the risk of surgery from undernutrition and/or dehydration. Imbalances between intake and output are reported to the appropriate nurse or physician so that corrective action can be taken before surgery. Many kinds of gastrointestinal operations require the patient to have a nasogastric tube inserted preoperatively which is attached to suction for several days postoperatively. Many patients report that the nasogastric tube is at least as unpleasant as having surgery. The patient may be helped by knowing approximately how long the tube will be in place.

Following surgery on the gastrointestinal system, food and fluids are usually withheld until peristalsis returns and/or healing occurs. The nurse can check for the return of peristalsis by placing a stethoscope on the patient's abdomen to listen for bowel sounds. When no bowel sounds are present, no sounds are heard through the stethoscope. The patient experiencing a return of peristalsis usually reports passing flatus also. When resuming food and fluids, the diet usually is advanced slowly in several stages from liquids to solids.

The nurse carefully observes and records the first bowel movement following gastrointestinal surgery. Following rectal surgery (described later in the chapter), the patient usually is instructed to ask for an analgesic before the first bowel movement. The analgesic is given by injection since rapid action is desired. Constipation is especially undesirable postoperatively because straining to have a bowel movement may place too much stress on the suture line. Occasionally, a very mild laxative or a low, gentle enema may be prescribed by the surgeon to prevent constipation if a bowel movement does not occur. An important nursing action is to observe and report the presence or absence of bowel movements so that preventive measures can be taken early. When possible, the patient with a regular schedule for bowel movements is assisted to the bathroom at the same time postoperatively to reestablish that previous routine.

Discharge instructions following gastrointestinal surgery usually include topics such as diet, resumption of usual activities including sexual activity, and symptoms of complications such as fever, cough, calf pain, and dysuria. At this time, the nurse often has the opportunity to describe the relationship of dental care, nutrition, exercise, fluid intake, and regular bowel habits to good health.

ASSISTING THE PATIENT WITH AN OSTOMY

The patient with an ostomy has a new anatomic pathway created by a surgical procedure for the elimination of feces through an opening (stoma) on the abdomen. The specific ostomy depends upon the part of the intestine affected. For example, the patient with a *colostomy* has an opening through the abdominal wall to the colon. Fecal material no longer passes through the rectum but is discharged through the portion of the colon that opens on the abdominal wall. A patient may have the colostomy performed on the descending colon, as seen in Figure 15.8. An ostomy at the end of the sigmoid is referred to as an *end* or *sigmoid colostomy* (see Figure 15.9). An ostomy in the cecum is a *cecostomy* (see Figure 15.10). A transverse colostomy is in the transverse colon. The patient with an *ileostomy* has an opening through the abdominal wall into the small intestine (ileum). As with the colostomy, fecal material leaves the body through the artificial opening in the abdominal wall instead of the rectum. The artificial opening called a *stoma* is made when the surgeon brings a part of the intestine through the abdominal wall and secures it.

An ostomy may be temporary or permanent, depending on the underlying disease condition. For example, the patient with ulcerative colitis usually has a permanent ileostomy. The patient with intestinal injury may have a temporary colostomy in order to rest the injured portion of the intestine. After healing occurs, the patient returns to the

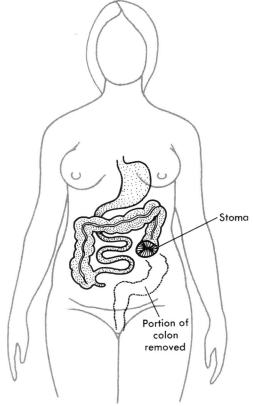

FIGURE 15.8 Diagram of a colostomy performed on the descending colon. The nonshaded portion of the colon has been removed, and the stoma is on the outside of the abdomen.

operating room for another surgical procedure to reconnect the intestine. Other conditions that may result in an ostomy include cancer and intestinal obstruction.

The major changes experienced by the patient who has an ostomy involve a drastic change in body image and the need to learn new skills related to care of the stoma and application of a collecting device. The nurse is likely to be the single most important person in the hospital in helping the patient to make the changes needed.

ADJUSTING TO CHANGE. The nursing student needs to consider the implications of not having a normal bowel movement to a person. For example, in Western culture, many persons associate elimination with sexual and/or reproductive function, per-

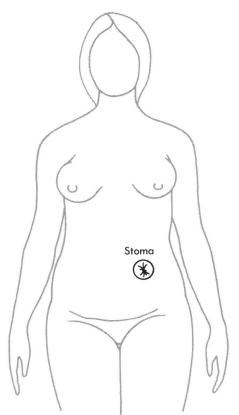

FIGURE 15.9 Diagram of the stoma of a sigmoid colostomy.

ostomy may experience an unfavorable change in the self-concept associated with feeling repulsive to others, fear of rejection by others, and a belief that the ostomy is visible even to strangers.

The nurse can take many actions to help the patient with the initial adjustment in body image. A first step in selecting specific actions is the nurse's self-awareness of personal feelings about an ostomy. The nurse's personal feelings of discomfort, distaste, or repulsion can be conveyed easily to the patient during ostomy care. A positive aspect of self-awareness of such feelings is the ability to understand and accept similar feelings in the patient. For example, the student nurse who becomes aware of personal feelings of discomfort when seeing a colostomy for the first time usually finds it easier to un-

haps because the external body organs are near each other. The nurse can anticipate that most patients with an ostomy experience serious fears and concerns about the impact of surgery on sexuality.

Learning to control elimination usually is associated with a certain period of growing up during childhood. The baby wears diapers which need to be changed by a parent or other adult. As the baby grows, parents and others often encourage toilet training by telling the child that a big girl or boy uses the toilet and diapers are for babies. Thus, the adult patient who requires assistance with an ostomy may experience embarrassment and emotional conflict related to feeling like a baby.

Finally, in Western culture, the sights, sounds, and odors associated with having a bowel movement are generally considered unpleasant and private. The patient with an

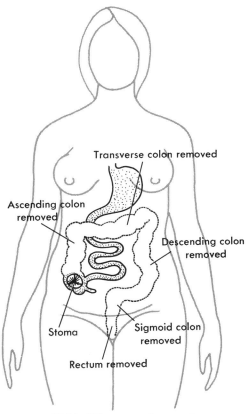

FIGURE 15.10 Diagram of an ostomy performed on the cecum. The ascending, transverse, descending, and sigmoid portions of the colon and the rectum have been removed.

derstand the patient's feelings when seeing a colostomy. The student who explores and discusses these feelings with an instructor, other students, or experienced nurses usually discovers that the feelings are temporary and gradually go away in time and after additional experience in helping the patient with ostomy care. This provides a basis for reassuring the patient that temporary feelings of distaste are normal and gradually diminish with time. Even when experiencing temporary feelings of distaste during ostomy care, the student nurse can take special measures not to convey such feelings to the patient by controlling facial expression, concentrating on the person with the ostomy, talking with the patient, and pointing out positive and neutral aspects of the ostomy such as progress in healing or adequacy of drainage.

Another action that helps the patient to adjust to a changed body image is the nurse's touch during care. Even when no words are spoken, the patient who feels physically repulsive may feel accepted and reassured by the nurse's gentle touch during the bath, backrub, oral hygiene, and other activities.

Teaching the patient new skills related to ostomy care is another important nursing action that favors a successful change in the body image. The patient who learns these skills regains important feelings of independence and personal autonomy. Many patients benefit from associating with other *ostomates* (persons who have had an ostomy).

The United Ostomy Association is a national agency that helps to rehabilitate ostomy patients. Local units of this association can be found in many cities throughout the country. First-hand knowledge of living with an ostomy through visits from ostomates, lectures, exhibits, and literature is invaluable in helping a new ostomate accept and adjust to this change in body image. An *enterostomal therapist* is a person with special knowledges and skills related to helping patients and families with an ostomy. In some cases, the enterostomal therapist is also an ostomate. This person may be available in some hospitals, agencies, or commu-

nity organizations to help the new ostomate both adjust to a change in body image and learn new skills.

When changing the patient's dressing, the nurse should provide privacy. Frequently the patient is concerned that the nurse has to see the stoma and even more distressed if visitors or other patients see it also. The patient's surroundings should be clean and neat. Soiled dressings should be removed from the unit so that the patient's visitors will not be offended by unpleasant odors or dirty dressings.

The nurse who visits and talks with the patient and loved ones about topics other than the ostomy helps to provide a perspective of wholeness. In other words, this action helps the patient and loved ones to put the ostomy experience into a bigger picture of living, working, eating, sleeping, playing, and interacting with others. An important point to remember (and to communicate to the patient and loved ones) is that the process of adjustment is a long one which begins with surgery and continues over a period of months or years.

EARLY POSTOPERATIVE CARE. The ostomy patient usually returns from surgery with a nasogastric tube, intravenous fluids, and bulky dressings that cover the surgical incision. A drain also may be present in or near the incision. The stoma usually is located several inches away from the incision and may be covered either by a dressing or a temporary disposable plastic pouch (see Figure 15.11) which adheres to the skin. In addition to the usual postoperative care described in Chapter 6, the nurse has responsibilities related to the nasogastric tube and gastric suction discussed earlier in the chapter.

Depending on the type of ostomy, there may or may not be drainage of mucus or liquid intestinal contents through the stoma into the plastic pouch or dressing. The nurse observes and records the condition of the stoma as well as a description of any drainage from the stoma. During the first few postoperative days, the stoma appears beefy red and swollen. Gradually, the swelling recedes and the color becomes more pink. The

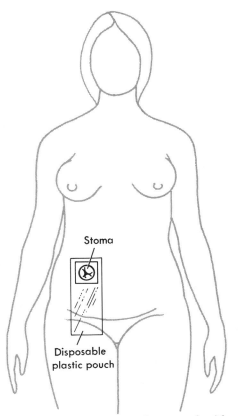

Stoma

Disposable
plastic pouch

FIGURE 15.11 The stoma is covered with a disposable plastic pouch.

surgeon is notified immediately if the stoma looks dark bluish, blackish, or purple. These colors indicate insufficient blood supply to the stoma tissue which must be corrected at once.

The disposable pouch is emptied if it becomes full of fecal drainage and changed if leakage develops around the stoma site. Leakage problems are corrected at once in order to prevent fecal contamination of the surgical incision and skin damage from irritating substances present in the drainage. The specific method used to change the disposable pouch varies according to the manufacturer's direction and local custom. Two important requirements for a secure, leak-free pouch are dry skin around the stoma site and correct sizing of the opening of the new pouch which fits over the stoma. For example, a pouch opening that is too large al-

lows intestinal fluids to come in contact with the skin and eventual leakage through the adhering surface. Wet or damp skin prevents the new pouch from adhering closely.

Incisional dressings may require frequent changes in order to keep them clean and dry. As previously mentioned, it is especially important to prevent fecal drainage from coming in contact with the surgical incision.

During the early postoperative phase, the nurse usually does most of the care. The patient, who is recovering from major surgery, is encouraged to participate in the usual postoperative activities such as coughing, deep breathing, leg exercises, and early ambulation.

ILEOSTOMY CARE. The patient with an ileostomy has an artificial opening of the ileum onto the abdominal wall. Because the colon functions related to water absorption are lost with this surgery, liquid intestinal contents continuously flow from the stoma into a collecting bag.

After the ileostomy stoma has healed and becomes less edematous, the temporary pouch is discontinued and a permanent appliance is used instead. This appliance may be thought of as a prosthesis that enables the patient to continue activities of daily living without leakage or odor. A variety of appliances is available which may consist of one, two, or three pieces. The appliance may be secured to the skin around the stoma by double-faced adhesive disks, a karaya gum ring, or surgical cement. In some cases, a belt is also used to hold the appliance in place.

When removing the ileostomy appliance, the nurse should apply a small amount of the prescribed solvent with a medicine dropper between the skin and appliance. Separate the appliance from the skin *gently* after the solvent has had time to soften the cement. The skin around the stoma should be cleaned with cement solvent as needed to remove the cement. Warm water, mild, nonirritating soap, and a soft cloth can be used. Drainage that continues during the change of bag can be handled by gently holding several rolled gauze squares lengthwise over the stoma so they act as a wick. The substance prescribed by the doctor should be applied to the moist, reddened skin around the stoma. Gum karaya powder may be the physician's choice. Excess powder should be removed. A few drops of the cement are applied with a clean finger to the skin on which the appliance is to be placed. A similar amount of cement is applied to the disk of the appliance before it is placed on the patient. A second coat of cement generally is applied to the patient's skin and the disk, and both are allowed to dry before attaching the appliance to the patient. After placing the appliance in contact with the cement around the stoma, the nurse should hold the two together firmly for several minutes. The patient should be encouraged to remain still for ten minutes to allow the cement to seal.

The patient may be able to wear the ileostomy appliance from two to four days. However, the nurse must remember that the pouch must be emptied at least every four to six hours. The bottom of the appliance has an emptying spout for this purpose. The spout should be closed tightly after having been opened for emptying the contents.

The manufacturer will provide directions for cleaning and airing the appliance. Directions for changing a specific appliance are available from the manufacturer also.

Having an unpleasant odor is usually of great concern to the patient. An odor associated with emptying the ileostomy pouch can be expected. A change in the type of pouch used, more frequent changes of the pouch, avoiding leakage, and avoiding foods likely to cause gas (such as cabbage) may help in reducing odor. Deodorants and deodorizers are available also. Some tablets are available for oral administration, such as chlorophyll, bismuth subcarbonate, and DERIFIL. Of course, these must be prescribed by the doctor. Other tablets and liquids are available for use in the pouch.

Skin irritation is a major nursing problem in caring for the patient with an ileostomy. The fluid from the ileum contains enzymes that cause destruction of the skin. Another source of irritation is the cement used to adhere the ileostomy appliance to the skin. The tissue may be injured by the cement or when it is removed. Substances

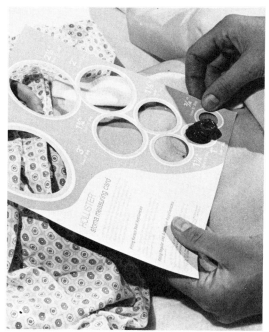

FIGURE 15.12 An applicance is placed over the stoma to prevent digestive enzymes from coming in contact with the skin. Before using an appliance, the nurse or therapist must measure the stoma and cut an appropriate-sized opening in the ostomy pouch. Approximately 0.3 cm should be allowed in the opening of the appliance. (From Lamanske, Jacqueline: "Helping the Ilesotomy Patient to Help Himself." *Nursing 77*, 7:38 [Jan.], 1977.)

such as plain tincture of benzoin, calamine lotion, or milk of magnesia may be applied to the skin and allowed to dry before the cement is applied. Tincture of benzoin should not be used if the patient's skin appears irritated because of the possibility of further irritation. Antacids, such as magnesium and aluminum hydroxides plus simethicone (MAALOX) or karaya powder, may be used on the excoriated skin. COLLYSEAL, a nonirritating type of seal, may be employed with the disposable bag. COLLYSEALS come with varying-size holes to fit the patient's stoma or with no holes so the nurse or patient can cut it for a better fit. Hollister bags with karaya gum rings are used also (see Figures 15.12 to 15.16).

In some cases, the patient cannot have the appliance cemented to the skin. Other

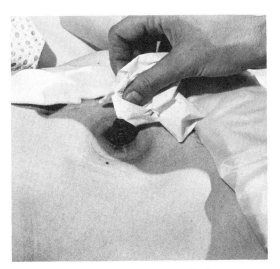

FIGURE 15.13 The skin around the stoma should be cleaned gently with warm water. The cleaned portion of skin should be protected from irritating drainage. Fresh squares of gauze can be used for this. (From Lamanske, Jacqueline: "Helping the Ileostomy Patient to Help Himself." *Nursing 77*, 7:38 [Jan.], 1977.)

types of ostomy appliances are available for such patients.

The diet for the patient following an ileostomy usually is limited to clear fluids at first. A low-residue diet generally is ordered as the patient's condition improves. Some foods such as parsley may be encouraged because they reduce odor. New foods are added slowly. The patient's tolerance of each new food should be noted. For example, if creamed tomato soup causes discomfort, this should be reported and recorded. The diet should be relatively high in protein and calories. Injections of vitamin B_{12} may be ordered to prevent the development of anemia. The patient frequently is started on strained vegetables and fruits as early as possible.

The patient with an ileostomy has an increased risk for developing *hypokalemia* (abnormally low potassium level in the bloodstream) because large amounts of potassium are present in the drainage from the ileostomy stoma. In some cases, the physician may prescribe an increased intake of foods rich in potassium such as bananas, potatoes,

meats, fruits, and vegetables. Occasionally, a potassium supplement may be prescribed. The patient with hypokalemia may experience nausea, vomiting, apprehension, listlessness, muscle weakness, and disturbances in respirations and cardiac rhythm. These observations should be reported to the physician at once. The patient who is also taking a diuretic such as those listed in Table 11.7 or a digitalis derivative has a greatly increased risk for hypokalemia and must be closely observed and carefully taught to report symptoms at once.

COLOSTOMY CARE. The patient with a *colostomy* has an artificial opening of the colon through the abdominal wall (see Figure 15.9). The opening may be temporary or permanent. A colostomy may be performed when the patient has an obstruction in the colon, has some type of injury or congenital malformation that interferes with the passage of feces, or has cancer of the colon. The closer to the rectum that a colostomy is made, the more formation the patient will have in the feces. In other words, the patient

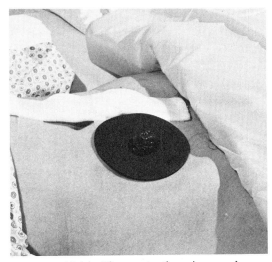

FIGURE 15.14 The protective ring, such as the karaya ring, is moistened to activate cementing action. The ring is placed over the stoma so that it fits securely on the skin around the base. None of the patient's skin should be visible between the inner part of the ring and the stoma. (From Lamanske, Jacqueline: "Helping the Ileostomy Patient to Help Himself." *Nursing 77*, 7:38 [Jan.], 1977.)

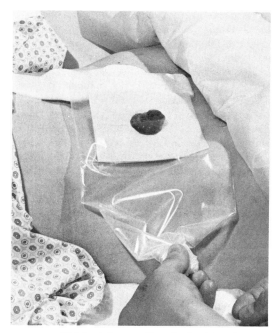

FIGURE 15.15   After peeling the backing from the appliance, the nurse should apply the pouch over the stoma. The pouch and ring should be placed together to facilitate an even sealing around the stoma. Wrinkles should be pressed out to avoid leakage. (From Lamanske, Jacqueline: "Helping the Ileostomy Patient to Help Himself." *Nursing 77,* 7:38 [Jan.], 1977.)

with a colostomy in the ascending colon will probably have more fluid in the feces than will the patient with a colostomy in the descending colon. As the waste products pass through the large intestine, much of the water is reabsorbed and they become more solid. Therefore, the patient with a colostomy will have semiformed stools that are not irritating. The patient with an ileostomy will have liquid discharge that contains irritating enzymes. This does not mean that the skin around the stoma of the colostomy does not need to be cleaned gently and protected also.

The patient may have a *temporary colostomy* done to allow a portion of the colon to heal after surgery or a bowel obstruction. The patient probably will have a *permanent colostomy* if there is a condition that re-

quires removal of the rectum and varying parts of the colon.

The patient with a single-barrel colostomy has one loop of the colon attached to the outside abdominal wall.

The patient with a double-barrel colostomy has two loops of the colon attached to the outside abdominal wall. One loop leads from the upper intestinal tract and is known as the *proximal loop.* The lower loop, the *distal loop,* leads to the rectum. The distal portion of the colon may be removed later when the colostomy is to be permanent. The patient with this type of colostomy usually returns from surgery without a stoma. Instead, a loop of bowel is brought out of the body using a separate wound site and a special rod to keep the bowel from slipping back into the abdominal cavity. Several days after surgery, the surgeon opens the bowel, usually using an electrocautery. This leaves the

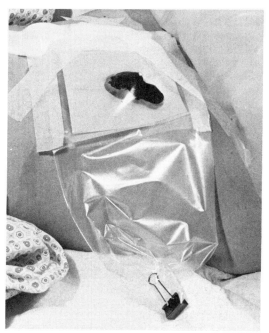

FIGURE 15.16   The bottom of the pouch is folded over twice and then closed securely with a rubber band or clamp. If the appliance is sealed watertight to the ring, it will stay in place at least 24 hours. (From Lamanske, Jacqueline: "Helping the Ileostomy Patient to Help Himself." *Nursing 77,* 7:38 [Jan.], 1977).

patient with the two loops of bowel as described above. It is important to know which stoma or opening is the proximal loop and which is the distal loop in order to report unusual findings and irrigate correctly. For example, the nurse would not expect to observe feces draining from the stoma of the distal loop. Usually, only the proximal loop of the double barrel is irrigated daily. Since it is not always possible to tell the proximal from the distal loop simply by observing, the nurse asks the surgeon and records the information obtained on the Kardex and the patient's chart.

Although the patient with a colostomy does not have voluntary control of the abdominal muscles around the stoma, the passage of fecal drainage can be regulated with irrigations and diet. The first irrigation of the colon following surgery will be prescribed by the surgeon. Enema equipment, a cone-tipped irrigator, or a bulb syringe with an attached catheter may be used to introduce the solution. The tube attached to a disposable enema set generally is not pliable enough to use for a colostomy irrigation.

The purpose of the colostomy irrigation is to empty the remaining portion of the colon of as much fecal material as possible to prevent drainage. Either the catheter or the bulb syringe is inserted approximately 8 to 12 cm (2 to 3 in.) at first. The tip may be inserted further into the colon if no discomfort is experienced by the patient. The tip can be inserted from 15 to 20 cm (6 to 8 in.). The irrigating container should be held no higher than 60.9 cm (24 in.) above the abdomen.

When possible, the patient should be helped to sit on the toilet in the bathroom or on a chair facing the toilet. A plastic drainage sheath is placed over the stoma. The sheath can be held in place with a belt. The distal end of the sheath is placed in the toilet or bedpan if the patient is in bed. As with other irrigations, the pressure of fluid is controlled by the size of the irrigating catheter and height of fluid above the outlet. Remembering these two important factors will help the nurse to know how to adjust the flow of solution for the patient's comfort and safety and to obtain the best results. After all of the solution has returned from the

colon, the nurse and/or the patient should clean the area gently around the stoma with mild soap and comfortably warm water. The stoma should then be covered with gauze or a small temporary stoma pouch. The patient may use an elastic belt, girdle, or shorts containing elastic to hold the gauze in place. A piece of plastic may be placed over the gauze to protect clothing from occasional drainage.

The proximal loop of a double-barrel colostomy leads from the functioning part of the intestine and should be irrigated as described earlier. The nurse also may be advised to irrigate the distal loop to keep it clean. The solution may pass through the patient's rectum when there is no obstruction or it may have to be siphoned through the distal loop. Specific instructions for each patient should be obtained from the surgeon.

The patient with a *wet colostomy* has an artificial opening through which both urine and feces drain. Usually, the patient's bladder has been removed and the ureters have been transplanted into the colon. This patient can be expected to need a bag continuously, and the colostomy is not irrigated.

The physician generally orders a liquid diet for the colostomy patient in the early postoperative period.

As time progresses, the dietitian consults frequently with the patient, family, and nursing staff in helping to adjust the diet to the individual patient. In time, the patient with a colostomy may return to a more normal family diet. However, foods that cause gas and diarrhea generally are avoided. In resuming a relatively normal diet, the patient may need some guidance concerning the foods essential for good nutrition.

Stomatitis

A patient with stomatitis has an inflammation of the mouth. It may occur from many causes. The severity of stomatitis varies widely. A simple inflammation can be associated with digestive disturbance and excessive smoking. Ulcerative stomatitis may occur in a person living in unsanitary conditions. Infections, such as thrush and Vincent's angina, caused by disease-producing microorganisms, result in an inflamed mouth. Stomatitis also may be associated with a nutritional deficiency and may develop following chemotherapy for cancer.

Treatment is directed toward relieving the underlying cause of stomatitis. For example, the patient with Vincent's angina is often given penicillin to combat the infection. The patient with a nutritional deficiency is treated by diet. The physician frequently prescribes a mouthwash for this patient. Good oral hygiene is of utmost importance.

Stricture of the Esophagus

A stricture or narrowing of the esophagus may be present at birth. It can be caused by swallowing a substance, such as lye, that burns the tissues of the esophagus. The scar tissue that forms causes the esophagus to contract. This occurs most often in children. A mass near the esophagus, such as a tumor, may cause a stricture by pressure. A tumor growing within the esophagus will result in narrowing. Such a tumor is usually malignant.

The patient with an esophageal stricture may be treated by dilatation. The physician inserts an instrument into the esophagus in an attempt to stretch the affected area. In some cases the surgeon can remove the narrowed portion. When the obstruction is complete and the aforementioned methods of treatment are not effective, a *gastrostomy* may be done. This is a surgical procedure in which a permanent, artificial opening is made into the stomach through the abdominal wall. A rubber tube is inserted into the opening. This makes it possible for nutrient liquids to be placed directly into the patient's stomach. Additional information about gastrostomy feedings was discussed earlier in this chapter on page 468.

The patient who is unable to tolerate a sufficient amount of gastrointestinal tube feedings or oral feedings may receive *intravenous hyperalimentation* (total parenteral nutrition, or TPN). Nursing observations and interventions appropriate when caring for the patient receiving this form of nutri-

tional therapy were discussed earlier in the chapter on page 469.

Peptic Ulcer

The patient with a peptic ulcer has an eroded area in the mucous membrane, submucosa, and muscular layer of the gastrointestinal tract that is exposed to the acid gastric juice. The areas most likely to be involved by this loss of tissue are the lower part of the esophagus, the stomach, and the first part of the small intestine. A peptic ulcer can develop also in the small intestine adjoining a gastroenterostomy. An ulcer that develops in the duodenum is known as a *duodenal ulcer*, while one that develops in the stomach is called a *gastric ulcer*.

The exact cause is not known. However, a chronic peptic ulcer develops only in portions of the gastrointestinal tract that come in contact with the acid gastric juice. A peptic ulcer develops when a localized portion of the mucous membrane cannot withstand the digestive action of the acid-pepsin gastric juice.

Individuals of all ages are prone to develop peptic ulcers. Newborn infants, children, adults, and aged persons may have ulcers. However, the highest incidence of peptic ulcers occurs in persons between 45 and 55 years of age. Men are more likely to have ulcers than women. The incidence of peptic ulcer in women increases after menopause. Persons in blood group O are more likely to develop an ulcer than those in other blood groups.

Smoking, alcohol, spicy foods, as well as psychologic and physical stress, may cause an increase in the production of gastric secretions and motility that can irritate and weaken the mucosa of the upper gastrointestinal tract. Continued irritation may contribute to the development of an ulcer. Certain personality characteristics seem to be apparent in those who develop peptic ulcers. However, these personality characteristics may be associated with the peptic ulcer rather than the cause. An inherited predisposition for a peptic ulcer is a possibility.

Some drugs used to treat patients can cause peptic ulcers to develop. Drugs such as acetylsalicylic acid, phenylbutazone (BU-TAZOLIDIN), cinchophen, colchicine, indomethacin (INDOCIN), tolbutamide, corticotropin, and adrenal corticosteroids can cause peptic ulcers.

ASSISTING WITH DIAGNOSTIC STUDIES

Members of the nursing staff assist the physician to make a diagnosis. The character of the patient's pain should be observed, reported, and recorded. The nurse should report any apparent relationship of pain to either vomiting or eating. Symptoms of blood in either vomitus or feces should be noted. Specimens of vomitus and feces for examination may be ordered by the doctor.

Such diagnostic measures as gastric analysis, gastrointestinal x-ray, and gastroscopy may be ordered. These tests were discussed earlier in this chapter.

NURSING OBSERVATIONS

The patient with a peptic ulcer generally has a sensation in the epigastric region described as aching, burning, cramplike, or gnawing. The patient may also have a feeling of fullness in the upper portion of the abdomen. The patient's pain generally has a relationship to the ingestion of food.

The pain is caused by the hydrochloric acid in the gastric juice as it contacts the irritated mucosa. Frequently the pain occurs from one to three hours after meals. Relief from the pain associated with a duodenal ulcer results from neutralization of the acid by food or an antacid. Vomiting, which rids the stomach of irritating gastric juice with hydrochloric acid, also may relieve the pain associated with a gastric ulcer.

The patient with peptic ulcer also may experience symptoms related to a complication of the disease such as perforation, hemorrhage, or stenosis. Perforation occurs when the ulcer becomes so deep that it goes through the entire wall of the diseased area. Perforation is especially common in older patients. The sudden escape of the irritating gastric contents into the peritoneal cavity causes chemical peritonitis. The patient with a perforation has a sudden onset of overwhelming, agonizing pain in the abdomen.

Nausea and vomiting may occur. The patient appears pale and anxious, and breathing is short and panting. The patient generally flexes the knees and places the hands over the abdomen. These observations should be reported to the appropriate nurse or physician at once. Emergency surgery usually is needed.

Hemorrhage occurs when the ulcer erodes the wall of a blood vessel. The amount of bleeding is determined by the size of the blood vessel involved. The patient may develop *hematemesis*, vomiting of blood. The vomitus usually resembles coffee grounds. This change is due to the action of gastric juice on the blood. The patient may have *melena*, blood in the stools. Severe hemorrhage causes the patient to develop symptoms of shock as described in Chapter 6. Hematemesis and melena are reported at once to the appropriate nurse or physician so that treatment for hemorrhage can begin early before shock develops. The patient may be treated with gastric decompression and suction, fluids and electrolytes administered intravenously, blood or blood products, and drug therapy. Gastric irrigation via the nasogastric tube with cool normal saline is frequently ordered. In some cases, surgery is indicated. Several procedures are available.

The patient with *stenosis* has a narrowing of the passageway. Scar formation in and around the ulcerated area can result in stenosis. Since scar tissue shrinks and is not elastic, it causes a narrowing of the passageway. An obstruction occurs when this narrowing interferes with the normal flow of food into the duodenum. If the pylorus is obstructed, it is known as *pyloric stenosis*. This patient vomits large amounts of food and often vomits undigested food eaten the preceding day.

Continuous gastric suction in connection with intravenous fluids and electrolytes may be the first method of treatment. Surgery to relieve the stenosis may be performed.

NURSING INTERVENTIONS

ASSISTING WITH DRUG THERAPY. At present, antacids are the drugs most often prescribed for the patient with a peptic ulcer. A typical combination of drug therapy which the physician may prescribe includes cimetidine (TAGAMET) and another antacid from Table 15.9 such as aluminum hydroxide gel, calcium carbonate, magnesium trisilicate, and magnesium oxide.

Occasionally, an antispasmodic drug such as tincture of belladonna and methantheline (BANTHINE) may be prescribed to relax the stomach muscle and reduce pain associated with spasm. However, these drugs are used much less often than they once were. Drugs such as alcohol generally are avoided because they may damage the gastric mucosa. Certain drugs known to irritate the gastric mucosa and stimulate the secretion of acid, *ulcerogenic* drugs, should be avoided. For example, the physician will prescribe salicylates, steroids, indomethacin (INDOCIN), and phenylbutazone for the ulcer-prone patient with great caution.

DIET THERAPY. Most physicians prescribe a regular diet in which the patient selects foods preferred and avoids those foods that cause unpleasant or distressing symptoms. Some patients prefer a bland diet during acute flare-ups, although this diet has not been shown to reduce symptoms. Frequent feedings and bedtime snacks usually are avoided since these eating practices stimulate greater gastric acid secretion. Hourly intake of milk or cream used to be considered an important part of diet therapy. This practice has been discarded in most cases because milk is now known to increase gastric acid secretion. Caffeine-containing beverages such as coffee and cola generally are restricted because they stimulate an increased secretion of gastric acid.

The patient with a peptic ulcer is usually advised to avoid emotionally upsetting conversations and situations just before and after meals. The patient's environment during the mealtime should be attractive, pleasant, and relaxing. The patient usually is instructed to eat slowly in small bites and enjoy the meal.

ASSISTING THE SURGICAL PATIENT. Surgical treatment may be indicated when any one of the three complications (perforation, obstruction, or hemorrhage) occurs. It also may be necessary when the patient's pain is not relieved by medical treatment and when the ulcer does not heal properly. Several procedures are available. For example, a *pyloroplasty* is an operative repair of the pylorus. In some cases, the vagus nerve, which carries impulses to the stomach, is cut. This procedure is called *vagotomy* and its purpose is to disrupt the impulses going to the stomach. This reduces the secretion of gastric juices. Another surgical procedure frequently performed is a *partial* or *subtotal gastrectomy*. In this operation, the lower two thirds to three fourths of the stomach is removed, and the small intestine is attached to the remaining part of the stomach. This procedure also may be referred to as a gastroenterostomy. When the patient has part of the stomach removed and the remaining portion of the stomach attached to the duodenum, the operation is referred to as a Billroth I resection. This type of surgery is used for treatment of an ulcer located in the stomach. The patient with an ulcer in the duodenum may be treated by surgical removal of the diseased portion of the stomach and duodenum. The remaining portion of the stomach is attached to the jejunum. This surgical procedure is called gastrojejunostomy, or a Billroth II resection.

When the patient has gastrointestinal suction, care described earlier in this chapter is indicated. The preoperative and postoperative care of the patient, as discussed in Chapter 6, is applicable to this patient.

Since this patient's incision is high in the abdomen, there is a tendency to take shallow breaths to reduce pain. For this reason, it is extremely important to encourage deep breathing, coughing, and frequent changing of position, as indicated in the postoperative orders.

After having the nasogastric tube removed, the patient should be observed for vomiting or a feeling of epigastric fullness. The ability to tolerate the diet ordered should be reported also.

The "dumping syndrome" is a complication of surgery on the stomach. In this case, the patient has a feeling of weakness, faintness, profuse perspiration, and palpitations. Such symptoms are thought to be associated with the rapid passage of large amounts of food and fluid from the stomach to the jejunum. The patient who has this syndrome is advised to eat frequent, small meals; to drink no fluid with the meal; and to eat a diet high in protein, low in carbohydrate, and moderate in fat. The patient also is advised to lie down for about 30 minutes after eating.

Gastritis

The patient with gastritis has an inflammation of the stomach lining which may either involve all parts of the stomach or may be localized to the fundus and body or antrum portions.

An acute case may be associated with an infectious disease, such as typhoid fever, measles, or influenza. An irritation of the mucous membrane caused by eating highly spiced foods, overeating, drinking too much alcohol, and taking too many aspirin results in gastritis. If a person continues to consume these irritating substances, chronic gastritis may develop. A chronic case also may be associated with an ulcer, cancer, or liver disease.

Generally, the patient with gastritis complains of abdominal discomfort, nausea, and eructation (burping). Hemorrhage may occur. Vomiting and abdominal distention are usually present. The symptoms are more severe in an extremely acute case. The physician usually diagnoses the illness from the patient's report of symptoms and from endoscopy.

Most patients with gastritis do not require treatment. In some cases, a bland diet is advised until symptoms disappear. Antacids may be prescribed. The person with an extremely severe case of gastritis is generally given fluids intravenously. As this condition improves, the patient first takes liquids by mouth and then a bland diet; later, a regular diet is gradually resumed. Irritating substances such as alcohol, aspirin, and cigarette smoke generally are avoided.

The nursing care of the patient with gastritis is similar to that for the one with a peptic ulcer. However, gastritis usually bothers the patient for a shorter period of time.

Hiatal Hernia (Diaphragmatic Hernia)

The patient with a hiatal hernia has an abnormal gap in the diaphragm that permits the stomach and other abdominal organs to slip into the chest cavity. In other words, there is a hernia of the muscle separating the chest and abdominal cavities, the diaphragm—thus, the term *diaphragmatic hernia*.

The hiatal hernia can be a result of congenital defects in the diaphragm, relaxation of tissues supporting the diaphragm, or injury. This condition seems to be more common in older women.

NURSING OBSERVATIONS

The patient with a hiatal hernia may have no symptoms. However, there may be heartburn, which is worse after eating a heavy meal, when lying down, and when bending forward to do something simple such as tying the shoes. The heartburn can progress to painful and difficult swallowing.

The patient may describe the pain as a dull ache behind the sternum, or substernal. Usually there is a feeling of fullness that may be associated with belching. The pain is increased when the patient lies down or moves about after eating. The pain may radiate to the back, jaws, shoulders, and down the inner parts of the arms. Dyspnea, coughing, and palpitations may be present.

The physician makes the diagnosis of hiatal hernia by studying the patient's symptoms, x-raying the upper gastrointestinal tract, and, in some cases, doing an esophagoscopy.

TREATMENT AND NURSING INTERVENTIONS

The patient with a diaphragmatic hernia will probably be treated for relief of symptoms. The doctor advises the patient to avoid overdistention of the stomach with food, lose weight if indicated, avoid lying down after eating, and take a prescribed antacid. Tight clothing around the patient's waist should be avoided. The patient's bed should be elevated about 25 cm (10 in.) at the head. Blocks of wood can be used for this.

Surgical repair may be necessary to correct the abnormality. After moving the stomach back into the abdomen, the surgeon repairs the enlarged opening in the diaphragm. The operation may be performed through the patient's abdomen or through the thoracic cavity. The postoperative care of a patient following surgery for a hiatal hernia is the same as that used for the surgical patient described in Chapter 6. The patient having a thoracotomy generally will have a chest tube in place to provide suction. This tube will be removed in a day or two following surgery. It is left in place until the lung has expanded. Additional information related to nursing observations and interventions for the patient following chest surgery can be located in Chapter 14.

Appendicitis

The patient with appendicitis has an inflammation of the vermiform appendix, which is attached to the cecum. Since the appendix has only one opening, it is easily infected. Contents of the intestinal tract enter and leave the appendix through its one opening into the cecum. If the passageway is blocked by kinking or by fecal material, the appendix becomes infected by bacteria, which are always present.

NURSING OBSERVATIONS

Quite commonly, a person who is developing appendicitis has generalized abdominal pain. It gradually becomes localized in the right lower portion of the abdomen. Fever, nausea, and vomiting frequently occur. The patient may be constipated, but this symptom is not always present. The physician notices that the muscles in the right lower part of the abdomen are rigid and tender. *Leukocytosis* (elevation of the white blood cell count) is found upon examination of the blood.

A hole may develop in an inflamed appendix. In this case it is known as a *ruptured appendix* or a *perforated appendix*. The infected material seeps through the opening into the peritoneal cavity. This may cause either a localized or a generalized infection. When the patient has a localized infection, an abscess develops. In this case, the inflam-matory process is walled off by the body's defenses so that the infection is localized in that area. The patient with a generalized infection has peritonitis. This condition is discussed in more detail later in the chapter.

When the appendix ruptures, the patient's acute pain may suddenly and temporarily stop. After a few hours of relative comfort, the patient generally develops symptoms of more widespread infection and often of shock.

NURSING INTERVENTIONS

The treatment of a patient with appendicitis is removal of the appendix, *appendectomy*.

Since an appendectomy is frequently an emergency operation, the general preoperative care discussed in Chapter 6 is carried out within a shorter period of time. Two specific variations in the care of this patient are the use of an ice bag and the omission of an enema. Frequently, the physician asks the nurse to place an ice bag on the right lower part of the patient's abdomen. In some cases, a preoperative enema is not prescribed in order to prevent stimulation of peristalsis and rupture of the appendix. The care of this patient after surgery is the same as that discussed in Chapter 6.

If the physician thinks the appendix has ruptured and peritonitis has developed, the patient may be treated medically with antibiotics, rest, and intravenous fluids. This is continued until the surgeon is confident that the infection has become localized. Then the patient has surgery to remove the appendix. If an abscess has formed, it may be drained before the appendix is removed.

Because the nurse has knowledge and skills related to health and illness, friends, family members, and neighbors often seek information about abdominal pain and appendicitis. The person with symptoms of appendicitis is advised to consult a physician at once. In addition, the nurse tells the person not to take a laxative or an enema. These self-prescribed remedies can cause the appendix to rupture. This information is so important for the general public to know that it is written on many labels of laxatives sold over the counter. Heat should not be applied to the abdomen of a person with these symptoms unless prescribed by the doctor because heat can hasten the formation of pus.

Irritable Bowel Syndrome

The patient with irritable bowel syndrome has abdominal discomfort and alterations in bowel habits associated with emotional tension and a lack of measurable changes in the bowel tissue. Other terms for this condition are mucous colitis, spastic colitis, and adaptive colitis.

The exact cause of this very common illness is not known. However, it is known that persons with this syndrome have colons that respond abnormally to usual stimuli. For example, meals, emotional stress, drugs, and similar stimuli cause the patient with this syndrome to experience more numerous and more powerful peristaltic contractions. Women in the middle years are affected more often than other groups, and symptoms usually worsen with psychologic and social stress.

NURSING OBSERVATIONS

The patient with an irritable colon generally has pain in the lower part of the abdomen. The discomfort may be relieved by the passage of gas or feces. Other symptoms may include anorexia, nausea, occasionally vomiting, and belching. The patient also may experience sweating, flushing, faintness, and a headache.

There may be alternating diarrhea and constipation. The patient may describe the stools as marbles, or pellets. Mucus and undigested food may be present in the stools, but blood is not. Weight loss and dehydration usually do not occur. Remembering that a change in bowel habits is one of the danger signals of cancer enables the nurse to report these changes in bowel patterns to the appropriate nurse or physician so that early diagnosis can be done.

ASSISTING WITH DIAGNOSTIC STUDIES

The physician will make a diagnosis on the basis of the characteristic symptoms, their proven relationship to emotional tension and the stresses of life, and the ruling out of other disease processes. A barium enema, proctoscopic examination, rectal examination, and the study of stool specimens are some of the measures used to rule out other causes.

When making a diagnosis of irritable bowel syndrome the physician will have to differentiate this condition from other causes of diarrhea, constipation, and abdominal pain. For example, amebiasis, shigellosis, carcinoma, allergy to ingested foods, ulcerative colitis, possible abuse of laxatives, and other conditions will probably be considered.

NURSING INTERVENTIONS

The treatment is directed toward the patient as a person rather than to the colon. The physician will attempt to lead the patient into understanding the relationship of emotional tension to the condition. The patient will need reassurance regarding the benign nature of this illness and an understanding listener. In some cases, psychotherapy is indicated.

The nurse may teach the patient a relaxation exercise such as the one described on page 64 as one measure to reduce the stress associated with symptoms. Drug therapy usually is avoided if possible. Foods that consistently worsen symptoms also may be avoided.

Ulcerative Colitis

The patient with *ulcerative colitis* has an inflammatory condition of the colon characterized by eroded areas. These ulcerative areas involve the mucous membrane as well as the tissue beneath.

The exact cause of ulcerative colitis is not known. The possibilities that it is caused by an infection, psychogenic disturbance, or an allergic or autoimmune response are being explored.

NURSING OBSERVATIONS

The patient with ulcerative colitis may develop symptoms gradually over a period of months or even years, or suddenly and unexpectedly. In some cases, the person cannot remember when symptoms first developed. In other cases, the onset of symptoms is associated with an upper respiratory infection, emotional upset, or antibiotic therapy. Mild symptoms may remain present for years or may become progressively worse.

ABDOMINAL PAIN. In mild cases, the patient may experience vague lower abdominal discomfort. In more severe cases, the patient has severe abdominal cramps which cause disruption of sleep and other activities. Occasionally, pain may become so severe that the patient becomes prostrate and shows symptoms of shock.

DIARRHEA. Frequent, loose stools containing pus, mucus, and blood are characteristic when the patient has ulcerative colitis.

Tenesmus, which is painful straining without having a bowel movement, may be present. Nausea, vomiting, a feeling of weakness, and fever are commonly associated with diarrhea.

The patient is frequently placed on a stool count. This means that the time, approximate amount, and description of each bowel movement is recorded, either on the intake-and-output record or other designated space on the patient's chart.

RECTAL BLEEDING. As previously mentioned, blood in the stools is a common feature of ulcerative colitis. The patient whose illness becomes chronic and/or very severe may develop anemia or other signs of blood loss such as tachycardia, increased respiratory rate, and restlessness. Frequent laboratory tests may be ordered to evaluate the patient's blood loss. Hemorrhage is a possible complication in the patient with this illness. The nurse observes, reports, and records all blood loss so that appropriate action can be taken early, if necessary.

WEIGHT LOSS. Most patients with this illness lose weight associated both with anorexia and reduced intake as well as increased loss of fluids and nutrients via diarrhea. The hospitalized patient usually is weighed daily, and the intake and output are measured carefully and recorded.

FEVER, MALAISE, FATIGUE. These symptoms usually are present in the person with ulcerative colitis. Oral temperatures usually are taken every four hours during the acute phase. Rectal temperatures are avoided because the mucous membrane lining of the rectum is damaged easily during this illness.

OBSERVING FOR COMPLICATIONS. The patient with ulcerative colitis is more likely to develop cancer of the colon than is the person not so affected. For this reason, the person with ulcerative colitis will be examined frequently by proctoscopy and x-ray of the colon for signs of malignancy.

An abrupt onset of abdominal distention in a patient with ulcerative colitis could indicate a bowel obstruction or possible perforation. This, of course, should be reported immediately. The nurse may be asked to measure the patient's abdominal girth during each shift to determine if distention is occurring. The measurement should be taken with the patient lying down and the tape going across the umbilicus.

BEHAVIORAL CHANGES. The patient with ulcerative colitis usually experiences significant changes in behavior associated either with symptoms, and/or therapy. For example, the patient with frequent bloody diarrhea has to change the life-style so that the bathroom is always close and available. Such a situation causes some persons to develop elaborate routines associated with hygiene and elimination. Fatigue, malaise, fever, and pain may cause some persons to feel isolated, depressed, and withdrawn. Imbalances in nutrition, fluids, and electrolytes may be associated with wide mood swings and changes in ability to remember, think, and learn. Such changes in behavior should be reported to the appropriate nurse or physician since they are often the first sign of a change in the patient's condition.

ASSISTING WITH DIAGNOSTIC STUDIES

In addition to a history and physical examination, the physician may order an abdominal x-ray and blood work to evaluate blood loss, and fluid and electrolyte balance. The two studies most often done include sigmoidoscopy and barium enema. Laxatives and enemas normally administered as preparation for these tests usually are avoided when the patient is acutely ill. These preparations may worsen the patient's condition or cause complications such as hemorrhage or obstruction. For these reasons, the nurse asks the physician what special preparation is needed for the patient.

NURSING INTERVENTIONS

PROVIDING A THERAPEUTIC ENVIRONMENT. During an acute flare-up, the patient usually is admitted to the hospital and placed in a room as close to the bathroom as possible. The person who is too ill to walk to the bathroom may be able to use a bedside commode if permitted by the physician. The nurse's assistance may be needed if the patient is too weak to manage alone. The patient who can walk to the bathroom unassisted may need help to return to bed. Remembering that the patient loses blood in the diarrhea and may have severe abdominal cramps enables the nurse to understand the fatigue and weakness which often worsen after an episode of diarrhea.

Deodorizers may be placed in the patient's room to reduce or eliminate unpleasant odors associated with blood and diarrhea. The nurse also can anticipate that the patient will need additional supplies of toilet tissues, towels, and washcloths. The patient who is too ill to use either the bathroom or the bedside commode may need an extra bedpan so that a clean one is always available.

It is important to avoid delays when the patient requests assistance to use the toilet, commode, or bedpan. Delays may cause the patient to have increased worry, abdominal cramping, or an involuntary stool. The patient may have an accident while trying to get to the bathroom or commode alone. After each stool, the nurse empties the commode or bedpan immediately and cleanses it carefully in order to minimize unpleasant odors.

DIET AND FLUIDS. During periods of diarrhea, the physician may prescribe a low-fiber diet. This change requires some restriction of fruits, vegetables, and grains in the diet. Since restriction of these foods results in an inadequate supply of calcium, iron, and vitamins, the low-fiber diet is temporary. A very important nursing action is

the gentle encouragement that helps the patient to increase food and fluid intake. Keeping the patient company during the meal may provide one form of encouragement. Reporting the patient's preferences to the dietitian is another form of encouragement. Praising the patient's efforts to increase intake is still another form of encouragement.

In severe cases, the physician may order nothing by mouth (NPO) in order to rest the bowel. Nasogastric suction as described earlier in the chapter may also be prescribed. Intravenous fluid and electrolyte therapy may be prescribed during this or other times to prevent or correct imbalances caused by excessive losses of electrolytes in the stool. Hyperalimentation, as described earlier in this chapter, may be prescribed to reverse weight loss and/or put the patient in optimal condition for surgery. Blood transfusions may be needed to correct anemia caused by the loss of blood in the stool. Table 15.11 contains a summary of nursing actions related to diet and fluid therapy for the patient with ulcerative colitis.

ASSISTING WITH DRUG THERAPY. A variety of drugs may be prescribed for the patient with ulcerative colitis. *Corticosteroids* may be given orally, intravenously, or rectally to reduce inflammation. *Antibiotics* such as cephalosporins and/or sulfasalazine

TABLE 15.11
SUMMARY OF NURSING INTERVENTIONS IN DIET AND FLUID THERAPY FOR THE PATIENT WITH ULCERATIVE COLITIS

1. Encourage the patient to increase oral intake of food and fluids.
2. Observe the tray after each meal and record how much the patient ate.
3. Monitor the flow rate of all parenteral fluids such as electrolyte solutions, hyperalimentation preparations, blood.
4. Change tubings, dressings, related equipment according to hospital policy.
5. Observe, record, and report abnormal responses to therapy such as fluid overload, transfusion reaction, increased diarrhea.
6. Measure and record food and fluid intake accurately.
7. Observe and report edema, erythema, pain, heat at the intravenous site.

may be prescribed. In some cases, sulfa drugs are prescribed for continuous treatment to lessen the frequency of attacks. *Antidiarrheal agents* such as codeine, paregoric, loperamide (IMODIUM), or diphenoxylate and atropine sulfate (LOMOTIL) may be prescribed very cautiously because they may cause an intestinal obstruction in the patient who is severely ill. Vitamin and mineral supplements may be prescribed to prevent or correct nutritional deficiencies which may develop either from blood loss, diet restrictions, or drug therapy with sulfasalazine.

ASSISTING THE SURGICAL PATIENT. Surgical treatment may be necessary. In this case, the surgeon does a colectomy and an ileostomy. A *colectomy* is removal of the colon and an *ileostomy* is making an opening through the abdominal wall into the small intestine (ileum). Fecal material no longer passes through the rectum but is discharged from the body through the artificial opening in the wall of the abdomen. The care of a patient with an ileostomy is discussed earlier in this chapter.

DEVELOPING A THERAPEUTIC RELATIONSHIP. An important part of the therapeutic relationship involves the nurse's view of the patient with ulcerative colitis as a whole person. The patient's experience with this illness may result in a kind of lopsided self concept in which the bowels are the most important feature. Early in the relationship, the nurse tries to convey friendliness, warmth, understanding, and acceptance of the patient. As the relationship develops, the nurse tries also to convey the message that other aspects of the person are important. For example, the nurse may point out positive aspects of the person's personal, family, or work life that are unrelated to illness.

To understand the patient with ulcerative colitis, the student nurse may imagine what it might be like to plan every day so that a toilet is close and available at all times. Imagine what it would be like to know that any activity, no matter how important or intimate, may be interrupted by abdominal cramps, sudden diarrhea, and blood loss. Every day, time must be planned for medications, medicated enemas, rest, special

meals, and similar treatments. At the same time, the possibility of cancer, complications, an acute flare-up requiring hospitalization, or radical surgery is always present. It is easy to understand why some patients feel like slaves to their own bowels. Such persons can be expected to experience anger, depression, a loss of personal autonomy, changes in body image and disturbances in sexuality.

The first step in developing a helping relationship is establishing trust. The nurse who helps the patient to the commode or bathroom without delay is also promoting trust. Placing extra toilet tissue, towels, and washcloths at the bedside of the patient with ulcerative colitis conveys the nurse's understanding, acceptance, and concern about the patient's illness experience.

Another step in the helping relationship involves the patient's use of the nurse's knowledge and skills as tools for coping with illness. Before this phase can take place, however, the patient must trust the nurse's caring and scientific knowledge. Explaining each procedure and test in advance provides important information to the patient about the nurse's knowledge and caring. The nurse who develops a plan *with* the patient rather than *for* the patient encourages participation and personal autonomy. For example, whenever possible, the patient's usual routines for eating, resting, hygiene, and elimination are followed in the hospital. When adjustments to the usual routine are needed, the patient is asked for suggestions about how to modify the schedule. The nurse uses every opportunity to increase the patient's personal autonomy and participation in care.

Active listening to the patient's concerns is important to the helping relationship. Sometimes, just talking about worries, fears, and problems can help a person feel better. At other times, the nurse may request that selected members of the health team help the patient to solve special problems. For example, the dietitian may be asked to develop a diet that includes the patient's preferences, avoids foods the patient reports as aggravating diarrhea, and provides nutritional value according to the physician's order. The medical social worker may assist the patient with financial difficulties related to illness. An enterostomal therapist may be asked to help the surgical patient with a new or planned ileostomy. A sexual therapist or other qualified person may help the patient to solve problems related to sexuality. Psychologic or other professional counseling may be needed to help the patient identify and cope with emotional conflicts associated with ulcerative colitis. Thus, the patient benefits from the special knowledge and skills of each member of the health team.

Intestinal Obstruction

The patient with an intestinal obstruction has a hindrance to the normal flow of the contents within the intestines. The obstruction may be either partial or complete, and it is a symptom and not a disease. Since the treatment of a patient with an intestinal obstruction is directed toward relieving this symptom first, the care of this patient is given special consideration.

An intestinal obstruction can be caused by paralysis of the intestines, which is known as *paralytic ileus.* In this condition the patient's intestinal muscles become paralyzed or lose their ability to contract. Frequently, paralytic ileus is associated with peritonitis.

A growth, such as a tumor, pressing on the outside of the intestinal wall may obstruct the bowel. Also, obstruction can be caused by growths within the intestine, such as a malignancy or a polyp. An abnormal growth of tissue that appears to be growing on a stalk is known as a *polyp.* It can be thought of as tissue resembling a mushroom.

Swallowing an object large enough to obstruct the passageway can cause this condition; for example, a child may swallow a toy. *Intussusception,* which is the term used when one portion of the intestine slips into another part, results in an obstruction. This may be thought of as a telescoping of the intestine. Intussusception occurs more often in children than in adults. Bands of adhesions, which are masses of scar tissue resulting from an infection, may constrict the intestines. Also, an intestinal obstruction may

be caused by *volvulus,* in which the intestine becomes twisted upon itself. *Diverticulitis* may cause an obstruction.

If the intestinal obstruction is not relieved by medical or surgical therapy, the obstructed portion of the intestine may become strangulated. This life-threatening complication means that the blood supply to the affected tissue is so poor that the tissue may become gangrenous. Emergency surgery is needed in this case.

NURSING OBSERVATIONS

NAUSEA AND VOMITING. The patient with an intestinal obstruction usually has nausea and vomiting. The vomitus may be violent and projectile and may have a fecal odor.

ABDOMINAL DISTENTION. Abdominal distention develops and worsens as the patient's obstruction becomes more complete. Distention is caused both by the collection of fluids and gases in the intestine and a shift in fluids within the abdomen. Bowel sounds are diminished or absent.

ABDOMINAL PAIN. The patient usually reports cramping abdominal pain which comes and goes. The pain is spasmodic in nature, caused by the peristaltic waves hitting the obstruction. Pain is more severe as the obstruction worsens.

CONSTIPATION. At first, the patient with an intestinal obstruction may have a few small, loose stools. As the condition progresses, there are no stools, and the patient passes neither gas nor feces because the passageway is blocked.

VITAL SIGNS. Frequently, the patient has a fever, increased pulse rate, and an increased respiratory rate. If the obstruction is not relieved, serious changes in heart rhythm and other vital signs may develop, caused by an imbalance in fluids and electrolytes.

NURSING INTERVENTIONS

GASTRIC DECOMPRESSION. The patient with an intestinal obstruction may be treated with a nasogastric tube or an intestinal tube as described earlier in this chapter.

As mentioned earlier, it is very important to observe, measure, and record all output from the suction bottle. Gastric decompression and suction may continue for several days. In some cases, this therapy is enough to relieve the patient's obstruction. In other cases, gastric decompression is part of preoperative care.

INTRAVENOUS FLUIDS. The physician prescribes continuous intravenous fluids to prevent the patient from becoming dehydrated and to correct imbalances in electrolytes which develop. Nursing observations and interventions related to intravenous therapy were discussed earlier on pages 78–79.

SURGICAL PROCEDURES. As stated previously, surgery may be done to remove the cause of an obstruction. For example, tumors, polyps, bands of adhesions, and diverticula are removed by the surgeon in cases where this is possible. When the surgeon operates on a patient with an intussusception, the telescoped portion of the intestine may be withdrawn. If the intestine is affected by an inadequate blood supply, it is resected or removed. This type of operation is known as an *intestinal resection*. The patient with volvulus has the affected portion of the intestine untwisted; an intestinal resection is performed if the bowel has become gangrenous.

When the surgeon does an *enterostomy*, an artificial opening in the intestine is created through the abdominal wall. This opening is made above the obstruction so that the intestinal contents can flow through it. Thus, the condition is relieved. The surgeon may perform another operation to remove the cause, to make a permanent opening into the intestine, or to suture the intestine and close the abdomen.

The term *enterostomy* is a general term used in referring to the formation of an artificial opening in the intestine. Frequently, the nurse hears other terms used that tell the site of this operation. The term *ileostomy* means the artificial opening was made in the ileum, *cecostomy* in the cecum, and *colostomy* in the colon.

The surgical patient needs care as described in Chapter 6, as well as nursing observations and interventions related to gastric decompression and abdominal surgery described earlier in this chapter.

Diverticulum

The patient with a *diverticulum* has a sac or a pouch in the intestinal wall. It can be thought of as resembling the appendix. Although diverticula (plural for diverticulum) may occur in parts of the body other than the intestines (for example, diverticula may be found in the esophagus, stomach, and urinary bladder), this discussion deals with those in the lower gastrointestinal tract.

A person may be born with a diverticulum or may develop it later in life. More than one diverticulum may be present. Frequently, it occurs in a middle-aged person who is bothered with constipation. Diverticula occur most often in the colon. The patient with more than one diverticulum is said to have multiple diverticula.

NURSING OBSERVATIONS

Usually the patient has no symptoms unless the diverticulum becomes infected. This is known as *diverticulitis*. Inflammation is encouraged by the collection of feces in the sac. In this case, the patient develops symptoms of an inflammation that resemble those of appendicitis. The patient may experience cramping abdominal pain, diarrhea or constipation, and blood in the stool. Diverticulitis may be complicated by an abscess.

NURSING INTERVENTIONS

The patient with a diverticulum who has no symptoms requires no special treatment ordinarily. A diverticulectomy (removal of a diverticulum) is performed if an inflammation occurs. The patient with multiple diverticula frequently is treated medically if diverticulitis develops. Measures such as low-residue diet, rest, antibiotics, and warm applications to the abdomen may be ordered. Antispasmodics and stool softeners also may be ordered.

Peritonitis

The patient with peritonitis has an inflammation of the peritoneum. It may be localized, such as the inflammatory process around a perforated ulcer, or it may be generalized. In this case, the entire cavity is inflamed. Generalized peritonitis is a serious condition.

Infection is the most common cause of peritonitis. Bacteria spread through a perforation in an abdominal organ. The infected contents of that organ pour into the peritoneal cavity. For example, peritonitis can be caused by a ruptured appendix or a perforated ulcer. Occasionally, peritonitis occurs in the absence of infection. Foreign substances such as urine, bile, and digestive juices in the peritoneal cavity have an irritating effect. These substances may escape from their normal places during surgery; or the cavities in which they are contained may be ruptured in an accident. The following discussion deals with peritonitis resulting from infection.

COMPLICATIONS

As stated earlier in this chapter, peritonitis may be complicated by an intestinal obstruction such as paralytic ileus (absence of peristalsis). Another complication of an inflammation in the abdominal cavity is *adhesions*. These are abnormal unions of surfaces that are normally separate. In other words, the surfaces of structures in the abdominal cavity stick together. This is a result of fibrous bands that form following the inflammatory process. Adhesions can prevent smooth functioning of the organs. After the patient has recovered from the peritonitis, symptoms of adhesions, such as constipation, distention, abdominal pain, and vomiting may develop. The adhesions sometimes cause an intestinal obstruction. The surgeon usually treats a patient with adhesions by cutting them so that the affected organs can once again function properly.

NURSING OBSERVATIONS

The symptoms of a patient with peritonitis vary with the amount of infection present. Frequently, the nurse observes the patient in the supine position (lying on the back) with the knees drawn up toward the abdomen in an effort to relieve severe abdominal pain. The abdomen may be distended and taut. Nausea, vomiting, and constipation are present. Fever and an increased pulse rate develop, and later the pulse becomes weak as the infection progresses. Respiration becomes shallow and rapid because of abdominal distention and pain. The patient also becomes thirsty. The patient's white blood cell count is elevated, and many immature cells are present.

NURSING INTERVENTIONS

Treatment of the patient with peritonitis is directed toward relieving the underlying cause, if possible; it may be surgical, medical, or a combination of both. For example, surgery for a ruptured appendix or gallbladder may be performed. If the physician is not sure of the cause and thinks an operation is necessary, an *exploratory laparotomy* may be done. This is a surgical procedure in which the abdomen is opened so that the doctor can search for the diseased area.

Rest, fluids, antibiotics to combat infection, and either gastric or gastrointestinal suction are important measures in the medical treatment of this patient. These factors may also be used in connection with surgery. It is the responsibility of the nursing staff to make the patient as comfortable as possible. The physician prescribes a drug, such as morphine, when this is necessary to relieve the patient's pain. Fluids are given by infusion until the patient improves and nourishment can be given by mouth. Use of either gastric or gastrointestinal suction is continued as long as the patient's vomiting and distention are marked.

Following surgery, the physician may request that the patient be placed in Fowler's position. To carry out this order, the nurse should raise the head of the bed 45 to 50 cm (18 to 20 in.). It is believed that this position prevents the infection from spreading to the upper part of the abdomen, especially when the infection is in the lower abdomen. Frequently the surgeon leaves a drain in the incision. In this case, the dressing needs to be changed frequently using careful technique to avoid disturbing the drain. The nature of the drainage should be observed and recorded.

The patient's symptoms, such as distention, pain, and fever, begin to decrease as the infection subsides. There is less drainage through the suction tube. The patient begins to pass flatus and feces as peristalsis and the muscle tone of the intestines return to normal. Drainage tubes are often inserted into the peritoneal cavity to remove necrotic or infectious products. These drains may be connected to suction, or they may be placed in a position for irrigation to ensure drainage.

Abdominal Hernia

An individual with an abdominal hernia has a protrusion of a part of the contents of the abdomen through the abdominal wall. It may be congenital (present at birth) or it may be acquired later in life. Additional terms are used to indicate the location of the hernia. For example, an *inguinal hernia* is located in the inguinal canal in the groin. An *umbilical hernia* is in the umbilicus or navel. An *incisional* or *ventral* hernia is located in an operative scar. A hernia is *reducible* when the abdominal contents can be forced back into the cavity by gentle pressure. An *irreducible* hernia is one in which this is not possible.

Two complications of a hernia that may occur are strangulation and an intestinal obstruction. The hernia becomes strangulated when the abdominal contents that protrude through the opening receive an inadequate blood supply. An intestinal obstruction occurs when the intestinal contents cannot pass through the bowel affected by the hernia. Emergency surgery usually is needed for both complications.

NURSING INTERVENTIONS

The patient with an abdominal hernia is usually treated by surgery. A *herniorrhaphy* is done. This is an operation to repair the defect in the wall. The patient needs the usual pre- and postoperative care as discussed in Chapter 6. In addition, the nurse observes carefully for urinary retention and scrotal edema. Prior to discharge from the hospital, the patient needs teaching related to the resumption of usual activities. The surgeon usually advises a temporary restriction on lifting heavy objects. The very active patient may need to change the exercise pattern temporarily or permanently in order to avoid another hernia. For example, certain kinds of weight-lifting and body-building exercises are not recommended for the patient with a hernia. In some few cases, the physician may recommend a *truss* for the patient who does not have surgery. This device is worn over the reduced hernia to keep it from slipping out again.

Hemorrhoids

The patient with hemorrhoids has dilated or varicose veins of the anal canal and the lower part of the rectum. Those that develop around the anal orifice are called *external hemorrhoids*. Dilated veins located in the area of the junction of the anal canal and the rectum are known as *internal hemorrhoids*.

Conditions that interfere with the flow of blood through the veins can cause a person to develop hemorrhoids. For example, chronic constipation and pressure by a tumor may result in this condition. Hemorrhoids may occur during pregnancy as a result of pressure on the veins from the enlarging uterus. The vein walls are weaker in some individuals than in others, and this predisposes to the development of hemorrhoids.

NURSING OBSERVATIONS

Frequently the person with hemorrhoids passes bright-red blood in the stools. Varying degrees of discomfort are present during a bowel movement. The pain is increased if the hemorrhoid becomes thrombosed. In this case, the blood within the dilated vein clots. Another symptom of hemorrhoids is itching around the anus. During perineal care, the nurse may observe swollen, reddened pouches outside the anal opening.

NURSING INTERVENTIONS

HYGIENE. When assisting with perineal care, the nurse is careful to wipe and cleanse gently in order not to cause increased pain. Sitz baths may be prescribed to relieve discomfort. These baths are especially helpful following a bowel movement.

ASSISTING WITH DRUG THERAPY. Local application of an ointment or suppository may be prescribed to relieve the discomfort of hemorrhoids. A mild laxative such as mineral oil may be prescribed to soften the feces. The physician sometimes injects sclerosing medication into the vein. This substance blocks the blood vessel so that blood has to leave the area through another vein.

ASSISTING THE SURGICAL PATIENT. A *hemorrhoidectomy* is a surgical procedure in which the patient's hemorrhoids are removed. In addition to usual preoperative orders, the physician leaves specific instructions regarding the cleansing of the patient's rectum. Usually one or more enemas are ordered. Sometimes the nurse is instructed to give enemas until the solution returns clear. A thorough cleansing of the bowel is important so that the operative field is not contaminated by feces during surgery. The nurse should be sure that all of the enema solution is expelled.

In caring for the postoperative patient, the nurse should check the dressing frequently for blood. This should be reported promptly to the team leader or head nurse. It may be necessary to change the dressing frequently.

Many patients return from surgery with rectal packing in place and a dry sterile dressing over the packing. Within 24 hours, the patient begins sitz baths three or four times a day. During the sitz bath, the packing usually comes out gradually several inches per bath. After each bath, the nurse carefully snips off the packing which has come out of the rectum. Within a day or two, the packing is completely and painlessly out of the surgical area. It is very important to tell the patient with packing what to expect. The patient who finds several inches of packing unexpectedly protruding from the rectum may become very frightened.

Some surgeons want to prevent the patient from having a bowel movement during the first few days after surgery. In this case, the patient's diet consists of liquids. Generally the doctor orders a mild laxative and an oil retention enema several days after surgery. Following this, the patient is permitted to have either a soft or a regular diet.

Other surgeons do not want to prevent the patient from having a bowel movement during the early postoperative days. The patient is given a regular diet soon after surgery. A laxative, such as mineral oil and psyllium hydrophilic muciloid (METAMUCIL), is given as ordered so that the feces are soft.

Many patients have severe pain after rectal surgery. The doctor prescribes narcotics, such as morphine and meperidine (DEMEROL), for its relief. Throbbing pain of increasing intensity should be reported since this may indicate internal enclosed hemorrhage. The patient's first bowel movement following surgery is usually quite painful. In some cases the patient is fearful enough of the anticipated pain to ignore the early sensations of defecation. It is important to tell the patient in advance to request pain medication when the urge to defecate is first noticed. The medication is usually given by injection so that faster onset of action is possible. Ignoring the early urge to defecate may cause a more painful bowel movement later as stools become larger and dryer. Following the bowel movement, the patient receives careful, gentle perineal care. A sitz bath, moist compresses, and/or irrigations may be ordered to relieve swelling and discomfort following the first few bowel movements.

Retention of urine is a frequent discomfort following rectal surgery. The patient should be checked for signs of retention. Nursing measures to stimulate voiding are discussed in Chapter 19. If unable to void, the patient is catheterized.

Before the patient is discharged from the hospital, a specific teaching is needed related to establishing regular bowel patterns, as described earlier in this chapter. Constipation is avoided since straining to have a bowel movement may cause more hemorrhoids to develop.

Anal Fissure

The patient with an anal fissure has an ulcerating crack or crevice in the mucous membrane of the anal wall. The main symptom is pain during and after a bowel movement. An anal fissure has a tendency to become chronic.

The patient with a small fissure may be treated by a diet to correct constipation and by a laxative to soften the feces. Surgery is used in more extensive cases. The ulcer is removed, and the wound is allowed to heal from the inside outward. A drain may be placed in the wound to ensure healing from the inside to the outside. The nursing care of this patient is the same as that discussed for the patient who has had a hemorrhoidectomy.

Ischiorectal Abscess

The patient with an ischiorectal abscess has an abscess in the tissue near the anus. It results from an infection that started in the rectum and spread into the nearby soft tissue. The patient has throbbing pain around the rectum. General symptoms of an infection, such as fever and malaise, may develop.

This condition is treated surgically. The surgeon makes an opening into the abscess to allow the pus to drain. This is known as incision and drainage. The patient has no further difficulty if the infected area heals completely. The nursing care of the patient who has had a hemorrhoidectomy also applies to this patient.

Anal Fistula

The patient with an anal fistula has an abnormal canal leading from either the anus or rectum. It may lead to the outside skin, another cavity such as the vagina, or the tissue of the buttocks. A person develops this condition following an ischiorectal abscess. The infected area heals incompletely, and a small draining canal or fistula develops and leads from the cavity left by the abscess to the rectum. Small particles of feces may enter the canal from the rectum and cause another infection. Another abscess is likely to form unless the opening into the rectum becomes closed.

The patient with an anal fistula is treated with surgery. The tract or canal is opened and excised completely so that healing can take place from the inside outward.

Malabsorption Syndrome

The patient with a *malabsorption syndrome* has one of a family of conditions in which there is an abnormal excretion of fat in bowel movements. This abnormal fecal excretion of fat known as *steatorrhea* eventually results in varying degrees of malabsorption of carbohydrates, proteins, minerals, water, and fat-soluble vitamins; thus, the term *malabsorption syndrome*.

Many conditions cause the malabsorption syndrome. In general, the condition interferes with the digestion of fat in the digestive system. Nontropical sprue involves an intolerance to gluten, a protein found in wheat and rye flour. Eating foods containing gluten stimulates intestinal irritation and decreased absorption. A gluten-free diet is used for the patient with nontropical sprue. Cornmeal and rice are substituted for wheat and rye in the diet. Other conditions causing malabsorption syndrome are stomach resection, pancreatic disease, massive bowel resection, radiation injury to mucosa, parasitic infections, an overgrowth of bacteria, and enteritis.

The patient with malabsorption will experience weight loss, anorexia, abdominal distention, and the passage of stools abnormal in color. The feces frequently are light yellow to gray, appear greasy, and are soft. The patient may develop edema and ascites. Failure to absorb vitamins results in vitamin deficiencies. For example, the patient who absorbs little or no vitamin K bleeds easily. If little or no vitamin D is absorbed, the patient may have bone pain and fractures, weakness, muscle cramps, nocturia, and neuritis, and loss of weight. A list of normal values of laboratory tests frequently used to study absorption is provided for future reference in Table 15.12.

Treatment of the patient with malabsorption is influenced to a large extent by the symptoms and the cause of the condition. When possible, the condition is corrected. Supplementary therapy with appropriate vitamins is an important part of the therapy. When malabsorption is severe, hyperalimentation may be prescribed (p. 469).

Salmonellosis

The patient with salmonellosis, or *Salmonella*, has an infection of the gastrointestinal tract, caused by the ingestion of food or wa-

TABLE 15.12
NORMAL VALUES OF LABORATORY TESTS
FREQUENTLY USED TO STUDY ABSORPTION

TEST	NORMAL VALUE
Blood serum	
Albumin	4.0–5.2 gm/100 ml
Calcium	9.0–10.5 mg/100 ml
Carotene	0.06–0.4 mg/100 ml
Cholesterol	150–250 mg/100 ml
Magnesium	1.7–2.0 mEq/L
Potassium	3.5–5.1 mEq/L
Prothrombin time	12–14 seconds
Stool fat	Less than 6.0 gm in 24 hr
Tolerance tests	
d-xylose	Excretion of more than 4.5 gm in 5 hr
Glucose	35 mg rise
Lactose	Rise
Sucrose	Rise

ter contaminated by one of the many species of *Salmonella* bacilli. The infection is transmitted by the ingestion of the microorganism in food previously contaminated by infected feces of animal or man. Raw eggs, dairy products, poultry, and meat are often the sources of transmittal. Thorough cooking of eggs and other food, proper preservation of the food, adequate refrigeration, and proper handling of the food can prevent the infection.

The patient with salmonellosis has anorexia, nausea, vomiting, fever, and diarrhea. A positive diagnosis is made by isolation of the *Salmonella* microorganism in either stool or blood culture. Dehydration and electrolyte imbalance are frequent complications, especially in children and older adults. The infection may be complicated by the development of abscesses, pyelonephritis meningitis, endocarditis, pneumonia, and arthritis.

Salmonella typhi causes typhoid fever, which is a serious enteric infection. The patient has symptoms of sallmonellosis. However, an infected person may not have clinical symptoms yet may be a carrier of the microorganism. Good handwashing practices are necessary following defecation and before handling foods to prevent the spread of disease.

The patient with salmonellosis generally is allowed no food or fluids until the diarrhea

has subsided. Fluids are administered intravenously until the patient is able to tolerate oral nutrition. Antibiotics are used to combat the infection. An immunization is available to protect those traveling in areas in which typhoid fever is prevalent.

Shigellosis

The patient with shigellosis, or bacillary dysentery, has an infection caused by bacilli of the genus *Shigella*. These microorganisms are transmitted by the fecal-oral route. Water, food, or meat is contaminated primarily by the individual who does not wash the hands after defecating. Asymptomatic carriers may spread the disease. The symptoms, treatment, and prevention are similar to those for *Salmonella* infection.

Staphylococcal Food Poisoning

Staphylococcal food poisoning occurs frequently in the United States. Food contaminated by enterotoxin-producing staphylococci of human origin causes abrupt and often violent gastrointestinal irritation following ingestion. Purulent drainage from an infected finger, eye, or nose may be the source of the microorganisms. The staphylococci produce enterotoxins, several of which are stable at boiling temperature. The staphylococci multiply in unrefrigerated contaminated foods, producing the toxin that causes the poisoning. Within one to six hours of the ingestion of contaminated food, the individual has an onset of severe nausea, cramping, vomiting, and diarrhea.

Positive diagnosis is made by isolation of the organism in the stool or vomitus. Supportive treatment is given until symptoms have subsided, which usually occurs within 24 to 48 hours after the onset. This condition can be prevented by knowledgeable food handlers who store food in a safe manner, handle food in a clean and safe manner, and protect food from contamination.

Neoplastic Diseases

Cancer is the second main cause of death in the United States, and one third of these malignancies occur in the gastrointestinal system. Although a neoplasm may develop in any part of the digestive system, it is most common in the large intestine. Gastrointestinal bleeding, pain, and obstruction are the three most common symptoms experienced by the patient with gastrointestinal cancer. These symptoms occur regardless of the site. Remembering these three common symptoms should reinforce the importance of reporting promptly any evidence of bleeding or change in body function discussed in Chapter 9. The nursing care included in that chapter is applicable to the patient with cancer of the digestive system. Special needs will be discussed in this chapter.

MOUTH

Cancer of the mouth occurs most often in men over 50 years of age. Cancer of the mouth has been linked with tobacco smoking, excessive consumption of alcohol, poor oral hygiene, and improperly fitted dentures that cause irritation. The patient with mouth cancer usually has small painless persistent ulcers. The prognosis for a patient with cancer of the mouth is good because the lesion frequently is observed early enough to enable the physician to remove it. Small, localized lesions may be treated with surgery,

radiation therapy, or a combination of the two. If the tumor is large and/or has spread to the lymph nodes, radical neck surgery may be needed (Figure 15.17). This procedure usually involves a permanent tracheostomy and deformity of the shoulder and neck. At a later time, the patient may undergo plastic surgery to have this remedied. The prosthodontist plays an important role in oral surgery. If the patient has had portions of the maxilla, mandible, or the hard or soft palate removed, a prosthesis may be needed. Frequently, the patient will go to the dentist prior to surgery, and the prosthesis or obturator will be made before the operation is done.

Following surgery, the patient should be observed for signs of bleeding. The patient with radical neck surgery may be placed on carotid precautions postoperatively. As a result of this surgery, the carotid artery may not have as much protection as it did previously. Removal of the muscle tissue and nerves in the area of the carotid artery may cause it to be more susceptible to injury. In this case, the nurse must be aware of the fact that the patient could experience a "carotid blowout." Quick action must be instituted if the carotid artery does rupture.

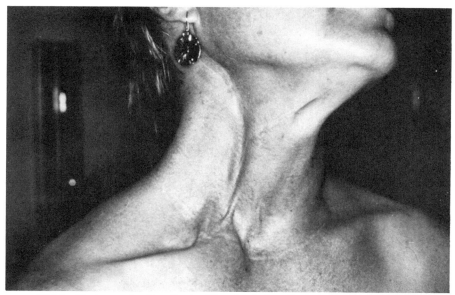

FIGURE 15.17   Photograph of patient with a healed radical neck operation. (Courtesy of Edward F. Scanlon, M.D., Evanston, Illinois.)

A KERLIX roll or a clenched fist should be placed over the area to stop the blood from flowing. The surgeon must be called immediately.

A HEMOVAC suction apparatus may be placed in or near the surgical site to drain blood and fluid. The nurse observes, measures, and records the drainage accurately. The patient can be expected to have a cuffed tracheostomy tube in place. A cuffed tracheostomy prevents the patient from aspirating any secretions and allows a respirator to be used when necessary. Frequent intratracheal suctioning is needed, as described in Chapter 14.

If the patient is receiving radiation therapy and requires a tracheostomy tube, a nonmetal one is inserted. The reason for this is that a metal tracheostomy tube interferes with the rays from the source of radioactivity.

Specific instructions for irrigation of the patient's mouth should be obtained from the surgeon. Oral care is important. The surgeon may prescribe an irrigation of sodium bicarbonate, salt, and water. In some cases, a special spray may be prescribed for use by individuals with special training for this. Special information about mouth care should also be obtained. Mouth care will depend on the extent and site of surgery and may vary from patient to patient.

The type of surgery will dictate the method to be used to feed the patient. The surgeon will leave specific orders about the method of feeding and type of food. For example, the patient may be fed liquid food through a nasogastric tube at first. Later, a shorter nasogastric tube may be used for feeding the patient and, in this case, the end of the tube will be in the esophagus. Another form of nutrition which may be prescribed is hyperalimentation. These methods were described earlier in the chapter on page 468-69.

The patient with a radical neck resection can be expected to have a shoulder deformity. In order to prevent total immobility of the shoulder, the patient should start on exercises as soon as possible. The exercises will be designed to strengthen the remaining muscle tissue, to prevent marked deformity of the shoulder, or to increase use of the remaining muscles.

ESOPHAGUS

Neoplastic disease of the esophagus accounts for nearly 2 percent of all cancer deaths in the United States and the United Kingdom. Carcinoma of the esophagus is more common in men than women and in persons over 45 years of age.

Dysphagia (difficult swallowing) may be present, especially with solid foods. The patient may have a dull or burning sensation in the epigastric region. An accumulation of secretions in the throat following a night's rest, a bad taste in the mouth, and constant thirst may also be symptoms. The obstruction may cause the patient to regurgitate food or get choked while eating, or may result in coughing. The diagnosis may be made by use of a barium swallow, esophagoscopy (which is discussed on pages 458–59), biopsy, and cytologic examination.

Because of the average age of the patient with cancer of the esophagus and because the hope for complete cure is not high, the surgeon may direct treatment toward relieving the symptom of dysphagia. In some cases, radical surgery to remove the tumor and surrounding tissue is done.

Palliative measures to enable the patient to eat and to have less pain frequently are done. A special type of tube can be passed surgically through the tumor to permit the patient to swallow easier.

The surgeon may do a *gastrostomy*, which is the formation of an artificial opening into the stomach. A gastrostomy tube can then be inserted into the stoma. In this way, the patient receives food and fluids that bypass the obstruction. The nursing care of the patient with a gastrostomy is discussed on pages 468.

STOMACH

Carcinoma of the stomach is more common in men than in women. Although cancer of the stomach affects all age groups, it is more common in persons over 50 years of age. Unfortunately, the patient generally does not experience symptoms until obstruction, ulceration, or other complications occur. Weight loss, indigestion or pain, weakness, anorexia, and vomiting may be symptoms experienced by the patient.

X-ray examination of the upper gastrointestinal tract and examination of the patient's stool for blood, gastroscopy, and cytology are diagnostic measures used by the physician when a patient has such symptoms.

The patient with a gastric ulcer must be monitored carefully, as this type of ulcer may become malignant at a later date. The patient with a neoplasm of the stomach usually is treated surgically. All or part of the stomach may be removed, and in some cases adjacent tissue such as lymph nodes, spleen, and part of the pancreas may be removed. In some cases the jejunum is attached to the esophagus, and in others it may be joined to the remaining portion of the stomach.

If the patient has a total gastrectomy, the care needed is similar to that required for a patient following thoracic surgery. When the patient's thoracic cavity is entered, surgical care discussed in Chapter 14 pertaining to thoracic surgery is appropriate. In addition to the chest tubes, a nasogastric tube, discussed earlier in this chapter, usually is present also.

When the patient is allowed to take nourishment by mouth, small amounts at frequent intervals are prescribed because there is no stomach. Injections of vitamin B_{12} usually are prescribed since the patient is no longer able to absorb this vitamin from food.

COLON

Neoplasms of the large intestine are more common in persons over 50 years of age. Cancer of the colon ranks second to carcinoma of the lung as the leading cause of death from cancer in the United States. The most common sites of cancer of the colon are the rectum, sigmoid, and cecum. The patient with a history of polyposis in the family and/ or ulcerative colitis over a long period of time seems to have an increased tendency toward developing cancer of the colon.

The patient with cancer of the colon frequently experiences a change in bowel habits, as mentioned in Chapter 9. Blood and mucus may be lost in the stool and the patient may lose weight. Abdominal pain, weakness, and tenesmus may occur.

A careful history of the patient's symptoms leads the doctor to suspect cancer.

Barium enema with air contrast study will be ordered. Rectal and sigmoidoscopic examinations will be done.

The patient generally is treated by surgery. All or part of the colon may be removed. Regional perfusion with a chemotherapeutic agent may be used also.

There are a variety of surgical procedures for treating the patient with cancer of the large bowel. The malignancy and the surrounding tissue may be removed if the tumor is in the cecum or in the ascending, transverse, or descending colon. Cancer of the lower part of the sigmoid colon generally requires an *abdominoperineal operation*. In this procedure, usually the entire rectum, anus, and part of the colon are removed. Part of the operation is done through an abdominal incision and part through a perineal incision. Thus, the term "abdominoperineal operation" (AP resection) is used. A permanent colostomy is done. In this case the colon is brought through the abdominal wall, and an artificial anus is made. An anterior resection of the colon is an operation in which the tumor of the sigmoid or upper rectum is removed. A temporary colostomy generally is done in this case. A temporary colostomy allows the area to rest and heal.

Preparation of the patient for surgery of the large intestine may take from several days to a week. This time is necessary in order to clean the intestinal tract and to improve the patient's general state of health. In addition to knowing the general nursing care of a prepoerative patient discussed in Chapter 6, the nurse needs an understanding of the special care required by this patient. The physician usually orders a low-residue, but nourishing, diet, enemas, and drugs to combat or to prevent infection. The purpose of the low-residue diet is to avoid the presence of waste material after the operation. Enemas are given to clean the colon. Drugs, such as a sulfonamide or an antibiotic, are used to reduce the number of bacteria in the intestines before surgery. Thus, the possibility of postoperative infection is lessened.

The discussion that follows deals with the special needs of the patient following abdominoperineal surgery. This is in addition to the general postoperative care discussed in Chapter 6. The physician usually does not allow the patient to have fluids or food by mouth for the first day or two after surgery. Intravenous fluids and, at times, blood transfusions may be given. A central venous catheter may be inserted into the patient while in the operating room. This enables the surgeon to monitor changes in the fluid balance before the patient is transferred to the recovery room. The urine output is monitored every hour. Packing is placed in the perineal incision and removed gradually by the surgeon postoperatively. After the packing has been removed, the perineal wound may be irrigated with dilute hydrogen peroxide, which helps to remove necrotic tissue. A sitz bath may be ordered. The patient may wear a perineal pad or a perineal dressing until the wound has healed. Perineal hygiene is of the greatest importance in preventing infection following an abdominoperineal resection. Irrigation and care of the colostomy are discussed earlier in this chapter.

Obesity

The individual with obesity has an excess of body fat as determined by a body weight that is 20 percent or more than that described as ideal for the height, age, and gender. Women in lower economic levels of society develop obesity more often than others. Obesity is associated with other serious illnesses such as cardiovascular disease, diabetes, hypertension, and low pack pain, but the exact relationship is not known. Obesity may precede one of these diseases and/or worsen the patient's condition.

The exact cause of obesity is not known. Causes that have been suggested include heredity factors such as body type, environmental factors such as learned eating patterns, psychologic factors such as depression or disturbances in childhood development, and social factors such as a decrease in the need for physical activity caused by technologic development.

Various medical and nonmedical treatments are currently available for the person who is obese. *Diet therapy* with a restriction of caloric intake is probably the most common method of weight loss. A number of fad diets may be undertaken by the obese per-

son who wants to lose weight quickly. Some of these diets are dangerous to a person's health and should be avoided. In most cases, the person who loses weight on a fad diet quickly regains it when usual eating habits are resumed. *Behavior modification programs* are available to assist obese persons to change eating patterns that contribute to obesity. For example, the individual who eats constantly while watching television is helped to find some other satisfying activity as a substitute for eating. *Exercise programs* may be used to increase the rate of calorie consumption. Before beginning an exercise program, the obese person should consult a physician. *Community resources* for persons with obesity include self-help support groups such as TOPS (Take Off Pounds Sensibly), and Weight Watchers, Inc. These groups usually combine nutrition education, a specific planned diet, an exercise program, behavioral techniques, and group support to achieve and maintain weight loss. *Drug therapy* for obesity may include prescribed or nonprescribed medication to depress the appetite. Dextroamphetamine sulfate (DEXEDRINE) is a drug sometimes used for this purpose. Most experts do not recommend drug therapy for weight loss because drug tolerance and dependency may develop even after short-term use of an appetite depressant. A variety of *surgical procedures* is available for the patient whose life is endangered by obesity. For example, a *jejunoileal* bypass is an operation in which the majority of the small intestine is bypassed and a connection (anastomosis) is made between the two remaining ends of the bowel. Weight loss results from a decrease in the amount of surface area and time available for food absorption. Serious complications that can result from this surgery include uncontrolled diarrhea, fluid and electrolyte imbalance, and liver failure. *Gastric stapling* is a more recent development in surgery for obesity. The surgeon creates a small pouch at the top of the stomach by placing a surgical staple around the top of the stomach. Weight loss results from the patient's inability to consume large amounts of food in the small stomach pouch.

Americans spend over 100 million dollars per year on medical and nonmedical treatment for obesity. Many persons spend dollars needlessly, ineffectively, or dangerously because of incomplete or inaccurate information. As an informed member of the community, the nurse has a vital role to play in assisting persons who are obese. For example, the nurse may provide correct information about obesity, the need for a balanced diet, and weight loss. In addition, the nurse can encourage and assist persons with obesity to develop or continue a planned program for weight loss. The nurse may refer persons with obesity to support groups in the community who share experiences related to obesity and weight loss. Finally, the nurse may set a good example for others by eating a balanced diet, exercising regularly, and maintaining a weight that is consistent with age, height, and gender.

Anorexia Nervosa

The person with anorexia nervosa has an illness associated with self-induced weight loss, amenorrhea, and a disturbance in body image. The cause of this condition is unknown. Girls between the ages of 14 and 17 years are affected more often than others. If the illness is not treated successfully, the patient may develop a chronic condition called *bulimia nervosa*. This illness is characterized by self-induced vomiting, alternating with gorging oneself with food. Death from malnutrition, potassium depletion, or hypothermia also may occur.

NURSING OBSERVATIONS

The person with anorexia nervosa usually has gaunt, hollow facial features. Bony prominences in the face, trunk, and extremities are easily visible. The breasts in the female are shrunken. The extremities look thin and wasted. The hands and feet may feel cold to touch and look blue. The abdomen and buttocks look flat. The patient's skin may be dry with abnormal growth of fine hair on the cheeks, nape of the neck, forearms, and legs. Purpura may also develop on the hands, forearms, and legs. Menstruation stops, and the patient may report constipation when asked. Behavioral changes the nurse, physician, family, and friends may observe include self-induced

vomiting, frequent use of laxatives and/or enemas, excessive solitary exercising, and withdrawal from family and social relationships, especially those with the opposite sex. Changes in eating behavior include elaborate feeding rituals, telling untruths about the amount and kind of food eaten, avoidance of carbohydrates and proteins, and increased consumption of coffee or tea. When asked to describe the body proportion and estimate the body weight, the patient with anorexia nervosa frequently overestimates both the body measurements and body weight. In other words, although the patient looks overly thin to others, the patient sees herself or himself as fat.

NURSING INTERVENTIONS

The patient usually is admitted to the hospital in the initial stage to reverse weight loss and correct nutritional imbalances. Nursing interventions are a vital part of therapy for the patient with anorexia nervosa.

Assisting with Dietary Intake. Initially, the goal of food intake is usually about 1500 calories per day. The patient frequently is permitted to select preferred foods as long as each meal contains foods from the basic four food groups. After a week or so, the physician may increase the patient's calories to 3000 to 5000 per day. The nurse sits with the patient during each meal in order to praise and encourage eating all the food. The patient may require continued close observation after the meal to prevent self-induced vomiting afterward. The daily weight and intake and output are measured carefully and accurately and recorded as indicators of the effectiveness of the patient care plan.

Developing a Therapeutic Relationship. A specific kind of therapeutic relationship usually is planned for the patient with anorexia nervosa. The plan developed and implemented by all members of the nursing staff who interact with the patient includes communication designed to provide positive reinforcement for weight gain. The relationship is usually initiated by a specific nurse who expresses sympathy and concern for the patient's overly thin condition. The nurse works hard to establish a trusting relationship with the patient so that a more realistic picture of body image and appropriate weight can develop. If possible, the patient, physician, and nurse work together to develop specific daily goals related to weight gain and intake of food and fluids. When the goal is reached, the patient may receive praise, encouragement, an increase in independent living privileges, and/or material rewards. The patient who does not gain or loses weight may need closer observation for self-induced vomiting, hiding of food which is later discarded, or the use of laxatives. In addition, the patient may have a restriction of privileges such as watching television.

When assisting with this type of therapeutic relationship, it is especially important to have a specific written plan which is understood by the patient and all members of the nursing staff. The plan must be followed carefully and consistently in order to be effective. For example, the patient with anorexia nervosa may request an individual nurse to modify the plan "just this one time." However, this practice is avoided unless planned in advance with the nurse responsible for the patient's care.

TABLE 15.13
OTHER DISORDERS OF THE GASTROINTESTINAL SYSTEM

DISORDER	DESCRIPTION
Acute gastric dilatation and volvulus	A marked overdistention associated with knotting and twisting of the stomach
Aerophagia	Swallowing of air usually associated with emotional tension
Aperistalsis (cardiospasm, achalasia of the esophagus, megaesophagus)	An obstruction where the esophagus joins the stomach; cardiac sphincter does not relax normally after patient swallows; results in painful swallowing
Congenital megacolon (Hirschsprung's disease, idiopathic megacolon)	A congenital disorder of the colon usually seen first in infancy; characterized by constipation; motility of the intestine is decreased to the extent that the infant may go weeks or months without a bowel movement; toilet training, certain laxatives, and surgery may be used; intestinal obstruction may occur
Diabetic diarrhea	Diarrhea associated with diabetes
Diffuse esophageal spasm (corkscrew esophagus)	A condition of elderly persons in which swallowing is followed by excessive contractions of the esophagus; may or may not be painful
Esophageal diverticula	A pouch or sac caused by herniation of the mucous membrane lining the esophagus through a defect in the muscular wall
Familial polyposis coli	An hereditary condition in which members of a family develop polyps in the colon; incidence of cancer in such patients is high; diarrhea and rectal bleeding are associated with the polyps; treatment is polypectomy or colectomy
Gastrointestinal allergy and food intolerance (food idiosyncrasy)	An antigen-antibody reaction resulting from ingestion of certain foods
Hypertensive esophagogastric sphincter	Spasm of esophagogastric sphincter often associated with emotional stress
Mallory-Weiss syndrome	Vomiting of blood following hours or days of vomiting; blood comes from tear near site where esophagus joins stomach
Malnutrition	A condition resulting when the intake of nutrients is not sufficient to supply metabolic needs. Often found in overpopulated, underdeveloped areas as well as in older age groups
Meckel's diverticulum	A congenital condition in which a blind tube opens into the ileum; it is usually lined with tissue common in another part of the digestive tract, such as the stomach or pancreas; thus, the diverticulum is likely to ulcerate and cause hemorrhage
Megaduodenum	Marked dilatation of the duodenum

TABLE 15.13 (*Continued*)
OTHER DISORDERS OF THE GASTROINTESTINAL SYSTEM

DISORDER	DESCRIPTION
Morbid obesity	A condition in which the client is 20 percent or more above recommended weight. The overweight is caused by an imbalance between the intake of calories and expenditure of energy. Being overweight is considered a hazard to health
Pyloric stenosis	An obstruction of pyloric end of the stomach; may be congenital in infants or associated with peptic ulcer in an adult
Regional enteritis (Crohn's disease)	An inflammatory condition of the intestines usually in the ileum that causes stenosis and fistula formation; acute pain in right iliac region, low-grade fever, and vomiting usually occur; steroids, transfusions, and surgical removal of affected part of intestine
Sideropenic dysphagia (Plummer-Vinson syndrome, Paterson-Brown-Kelly syndrome)	Difficult swallowing involving mouth and throat; occurs mainly in females with low intake of iron and vitamins
Zollinger-Ellison syndrome	A condition in which the patient has a tumor of the pancreas; tumor causes the stomach to secrete large quantities of pepsin and hydrochloric acid; patient develops one or more peptic ulcers that are resistant to treatment

Case Study Involving Peptic Ulcer

Mr. Aaron Johnson, a 35-year-old-man, was admitted to the hospital with a tentative diagnosis of peptic ulcer. The nursing history revealed that Mr. Johnson was married and a tax accountant for a large national company. He had been in good health except for complaints of abdominal pain, usually relieved by TUMS, which he carried at all times. The pain usually occurred late at night or early in the morning. It was described as a burning, gnawing sensation just under his breast bone. The pain has increased in frequency and intensity in the past two weeks.

Routine admission laboratory test results were within normal limits with the exception of hemoglobin. His hemoglobin was 10.5 gm and hematocrit 36 percent. Mr. Johnson smoked three packages of cigarettes a day. He appeared anxious on admission and asked many questions about hospital routine, and his length of stay. The physician's orders were:

• Gastric analysis on Saturday
• Gastrointestinal x-ray series in A.M.
• Gastroscopy on Friday
• HEMATEST all stools and emesis
• Bed rest with bathroom privileges
• MAALOX, 15 ml, at bedside q2h prn
• Diet as tolerated with between-meal snacks

The nurse who entered Mr. Johnson's room found him discussing the latest happenings on the telephone and smoking a cigarette. Mr. Johnson asked for a drink of water.

QUESTIONS

1. What information should the nurse give Mr. Johnson about the diagnostic tests? Where and why should this information be recorded?
2. What nursing observations should the nurse report promptly to the head nurse or physician? (*Hint:* Review the physician's orders.)
3. What information should the nurse give Mr. Johnson before leaving MAALOX at the bedside?
4. What is the relationship between the diet prescribed for Mr. Johnson and his ulcer?
5. What actions should the nurse take to reduce some of Mr. Johnson's anxiety about hospitalization? How is this related to peptic ulcer disease?

Case Study Involving Ulcerative Colitis

Mrs. Frances Kearney, a 46-year-old married female with two college-age children, was admitted to the surgical ward with a diagnosis of recurrent ulcerative colitis. The nurse who admitted Mrs. Kearney noticed she was extremely thin, of medium build, attractive, well dressed, and obviously careful about her appearance. Mrs. Kearney, nervously playing with her wedding ring, told the nurse that this was her seventh hospital admission in the past five years. She also said that she had lost 26.4 kg (12 lb) in the last 12 weeks.

The next day, Mrs. Kearney had 18 loose, watery stools with copious blood and mucus. She reported increasing pain and abdominal distress before each stool. On admission, her hemoglobin was 9.9 gm and hematocrit 36 percent. Mrs. Kearney was prepared for a colectomy with ileostomy. The physician's orders included:

- Daily hematocrit and hemoglobin
- Electrolytes today and qod
- Bathroom privileges—record amount, color, and consistency of each stool
- Type and crossmatch for 4 units whole blood
- Give 1 unit whole blood today

QUESTIONS

1. What is the relationship between the physician's orders for daily hematocrit and hemoglobin and the nurse's observation of the amount, color, and consistency of Mrs. Kearney's stools?
2. What assistance should the nurse anticipate that Mrs. Kearney will need in hygiene? (*Hint:* Consider her frequent trips to the bathroom as well as the effect of frequent stools on the skin.)
3. What nursing observations will be indicated when Mrs. Kearney receives a transfusion? (*Hint:* If necessary, refer to transfusion therapy in Chapter 10.)
4. How do the nurse's personal feelings about ostomy care influence Mrs. Kearney? How can the nurse handle her own unpleasant feelings regarding ostomy care?
5. What information should Mrs. Kearney have about ostomies prior to her surgery? Who should provide the information?
6. What information should Mrs. Kearney's family have about ostomies prior to surgery? Who should provide the information?
7. What persons and organizations are available in the hospital and community to help the patient, family, and nurse with ostomy care?
8. Postoperatively, should the nurse change Mrs. Kearney's ileostomy appliance? What is the effect of ileostomy drainage on the skin? How can the nurse prevent ileostomy drainage from coming in contact with the skin?
9. What changes in behavior should the nurse anticipate in Mrs. Kearney postoperatively? When should the nurse be especially alert for behavioral clues?
10. What patient teaching should the nurse anticipate that Mrs. Kearney will need prior to discharge?
11. What effect could Mrs. Kearney's surgery have on her relationship with her husband and children? What factors in family relationships can influence Mrs. Kearney's response to surgery? What actions should the nurse

take to encourage strong family support for Mrs. Kearney?

Suggestions for Further Study

1. According to the Nurse Practice Act of your state, is it legal for the LPN/LVN to insert a nasogastric tube?
2. Does your community have a local unit of the United Ostomy Association? If so, ask your instructor if one or more of your class may arrange for a visit and report your findings to the class.
3. Review the foods that you have eaten in the past 24 hours. If you were on a low residue diet, which of these foods would have to be eliminated from your diet? Which foods could be added to the diet? Describe to one or more classmates, the impact these dietary changes would have on your life.
4. Mason, Mildred A.; Bates, Grace F.; and Smola, Bonnie K.: *Workbook in Basic Medical-Surgical Nursing*, 3rd ed Macmillan Publishing Company, New York, 1984, Exercise 15.

Additional Readings

Anderson, Marjorie; Aker, Saundra N.; and Hickman, Robert O.: "The Double-Lumen Hickman Catheter." *American Journal of Nursing*, 82:272–74 (Feb.), 1982.

Beck, Marjorie L.: "Preparing Your Patient for an Esophagogastroduodenoscopy." *Nursing 81*, 11:88–96 (Feb.), 1981.

Bromley, Barbara: "Applying Orem's Self-Care Theory in Enterostomal Therapy." *American Journal of Nursing*, 80:245–49 (Feb.), 1980.

Burkhart, Carol: "Upper GI Hemorrhage: The Clinical Picture." *American Journal of Nursing*, 81:1817–20 (Oct.), 1981.

Burkle, Wayne S.: "Tagamet." *Nursing 80*, 10:86–87 (Apr.), 1980.

Ciseaux, Annie: "Anorexia Nervosa: A View from the Mirror." *American Journal of Nursing*, 80:1468–70 (Aug.), 1980.

Claggett, Marilyn Smith: "Anorexia Nervosa: A Behavioral Approach." *American Journal of Nursing*, 80:1471–72 (Aug.), 1980.

Fowler, Evonne; Jeter, Katherine F.; and Schwartz, Arthur A.: "How to Cope when Your Patient Has an Enterostomal Fistula." *American Journal of Nursing*, 80:426–29 (Mar.), 1980.

Hutchison, Margaret McGahan: "Administration of Fat Emulsions." *American Journal of Nursing*, 82:275–77 (Feb.), 1982.

Kroner, Kristine: "Are You Prepared for Your Ulcerative Colitis Patient?" *Nursing 80,* 10:43-50 (Apr.), 1980.

Lamphier, Timothy A., and Lamphier, Robin Ann: "Upper GI Hemorrhage: Emergency Evaluation and Management." *American Journal of Nursing,* 81:1814-17 (Oct.), 1981.

Miller, Barbara K.: "Jejunoileal Bypass: A Drastic Weight Control Measure." *American Journal of Nursing,* 81:564-68 (Mar.), 1981.

Miskovitz, Paul: "Peptic Ulcers: On the Front Lines of Research and Treatment." *Journal of Practical Nursing,* 31:22-23 (Mar.), 1981.

Rambo, Beverly J., and Wood, Lucile A. (eds.): *Nursing Skills for Clinical Practice,* 3rd ed. W.B. Saunders Co., Philadelphia, 1982, pp. 514-50 and 680-707.

Richardson, Thomas F.: "Anorexia Nervosa: An Overview." *American Journal of Nursing,* 80:1470-71 (Aug.), 1980.

Robinson, Corinne H.: *Basic Nutrition and Diet Therapy,* 4th ed. Macmillan Publishing Co., Inc., New York, 1980, pp. 276-91.

Ropka, Mary E.: "Hiatal Hernia." *Nursing 82,* 12:126-31 (Apr.), 1982.

Schlossberg, Nancy: "Easing the Pain of Peptic Ulcers." *Journal of Practical Nursing,* 31:21-24 (Mar.), 1981.

Schumann, Delores: "How to Help Wound Healing in Your Abdominal Surgery Patient." *Nursing 80,* 10:34-40 (Apr.), 1980.

Wilpizeski, Marcia Dunn: "Helping the Ostomate Return to Normal Life." *Nursing 81,* 11:62-66 (Mar.), 1981.

Chapter 16

The Patient with a
Disease of the Liver,
Biliary Tract, or Pancreas

Expected Behavioral Outcomes

Minimum objectives referred to as expected behavioral outcomes have been designed for the practical/vocational nursing student to use as guides in studying this chapter. The student should read these expected outcomes before studying the chapter. The objectives can be used as guides for study.

Using the content of this chapter, the student should return to the objectives and evaluate the ability to:

1. *Prepare a table that shows the manufacturing, storage, metabolic, and detoxifying functions of the liver, gallbladder, and pancreas.*
2. *Describe each of the diagnostic studies in layman's terms.*
3. *Compare nursing observations and related care needed for a person with hepatitis with those needed for a person with pancreatitis.*
4. *Relate the nursing observations and measures needed for a person with cirrhosis to each of the functions of the liver.*
5. *Relate the preoperative and postoperative care described in Chapter 6 to the nursing observations and interventions for a patient having surgery on the gallbladder or biliary tract.*

Vocabulary Development

The following prefixes, suffixes, and combining forms pertain to this chapter. By learning and/or reviewing their meanings, the practical/vocational nursing student will have the keys needed to unlock many exciting new medical terms.

Discover the meaning of these keys in a medical dictionary or in the content of this chapter. How does each key pertain to this chapter? In your notebook write the correct meaning of each prefix, suffix, or combining form listed below. Illustrate each key with an example.

amyl—starch. Ex. *amyl*ase—an enzyme that acts on starch.

anti-	chol-
bil-	cyst-
calc-	glyc(y)-
calor-	hema(at)-

| hepat- | nod- | pan- | rub(r)- |
| lith- | ne- | ret- | zym- |

Structure and Function

LIVER

The liver is a gland located in the right upper portion of the abdomen below the diaphragm. Most of the liver is protected by the rib cage. The lower portion of the gland is adjacent to the right kidney, a portion of the ascending colon, and the stomach at the pylorus. The liver is covered by a capsule and encased in most areas by the peritoneum. There are four lobes in the liver separated by fissures containing blood vessels, nerves, lymph vessels, and bile ducts.

The *lobule* is the working unit of the liver. Each lobule contains hepatic cells, connective tissue, and a complex network of passageways that transport blood and bile. *Sinusoids* are capillary-like networks that contain large amounts of blood and highly specialized *Kupffer* cells important in the filtering activities of the liver. *Canaliculi* are networks of minute channels that transport bile after it is made by the cells. Bile is carried by successively larger channels to the right and left hepatic ducts, which join the cystic duct from the gallbladder to form the common bile duct.

Arterial blood is brought to the liver by the hepatic artery. The portal vein transports blood from the stomach, spleen, pancreas, and intestine to the liver for filtration. Products of digestion are processed in the liver. The hepatic vein transports blood leaving the liver to the inferior vena cava.

As mentioned earlier, the liver is a gland. A gland may be thought of as a manufacturing plant. It takes material from the body and forms a new substance. Most of the material taken from the body arrives in blood via the portal vein. The liver filters out the needed material and returns the filtered blood to the body via the hepatic vein.

Bile is one important substance manufactured by the liver. Approximately 800 to 1200 ml of bile is produced and secreted by the liver each day. Bile is composed of bilirubin, bile salts, and cholesterol. Bilirubin results from pigment (hemoglobin) released by red blood cells at the end of their life cycle. Bile salts aid in the digestion of food in the intestines. Normally, bile is greenish yellow, brownish yellow, or olive green.

In addition to producing and secreting bile, the liver performs many other functions essential to life. Fibrinogen and prothrombin are substances made by the liver that are important in the clotting of blood. Heparin, an anticoagulant substance, is also made by the liver as well as other organs. Aging red blood cells are destroyed by the liver and spleen.

The liver forms vitamin A and stores vitamins A, D, and B_{12}, as well as iron and copper. Vitamin K is needed by the liver to form prothrombin.

The liver is also essential to the metabolism of carbohydrates, fats, and proteins. Glycogen is a form of sugar made and stored by the liver. The liver converts glycogen to glucose to help the body maintain a constant blood sugar. The liver serves as a center for the metabolism of fats and the formation of cholesterol. Amino acids are chemical compounds obtained from the breakdown of protein in the small intestine. The liver breaks down or converts amino acids and makes urea from the ammonia and other chemicals released. Albumin, fibrinogen, and certain globulins, such as immunoglobulins, are important plasma proteins formed in the liver.

The liver plays a vital role in detoxifying substances such as drugs, alcohol, heavy metals, and hormones. In addition, the liver helps to regulate blood volume by storing up to 400 ml of blood in the sinusoids.

The many chemical reactions that take place in the liver produce heat for the body. Laboratory investigation continues into other possible functions of this remarkable organ. However, when the liver ceases to function, so does life.

BILIARY TRACT

As mentioned earlier, bile is delivered from the liver cells through a network of tiny ducts (tubes) which unite to form the hepatic duct. This is a large duct through which bile leaves the liver. The hepatic duct joins a tube from the gallbladder called the cystic duct. These two unite to form the common bile duct, which joins the ampulla of Vater, a short duct leading to the duodenum. Normally, bile takes one of two routes from the hepatic duct; it flows from the common bile duct into the duodenum when food is present in the intestine, or it flows through the cystic duct into the gallbladder when there is no food in the duodenum.

Bile is stored in the gallbladder (see Figure 16.1). This organ is a sac similar to a pear in shape when full and is located under the liver. The gallbladder is approximately 7.5 to 10 cm (3 to 4 in.) long and 2.5 cm (1 in.) wide. The storage of bile by the gallbladder is made possible by the closure of a sphincter muscle called the sphincter of Oddi, located at the end of the common bile duct in the ampulla of Vater. This circular muscle closes when the duodenum is empty. Thus, bile flows through the cystic duct into the gallbladder. The sphincter muscle opens and the gallbladder contracts, forcing bile through the cystic and common bile ducts into the duodenum during digestion. Cholycystokinin is a hormone secreted by cells in the small intestine in response to the presence of fat. It is this hormone that stimulates the gallbladder to contract and to force bile into the duodenum for fat digestion.

PANCREAS

The pancreas is a hammer-shaped gland located behind the stomach and in front of the vertebrae (see Figure 16.2). The pancreas contains lobes, lobules, and ducts. Pancreatic secretions eventually reach the pancreatic duct, which runs from the tail to the head of the gland. The pancreatic and common bile ducts unite to form a short, dilated pouch called the ampulla of Vater, which leads directly to the duodenum.

The pancreas manufactures pancreatic fluid to aid in digestion. About 2500 ml of pancreatic juice is secreted by the pancreas each day. Pancreatic juice is a clear, colorless liquid composed mainly of water, electrolytes, and enzymes. The three important classes of enzymes in pancreatic juice include *amalyse*, which helps to break down carbohydrates; *lipase*, which aids in fat digestion; and *trypsin*, which helps to break down proteins. The pancreas is stimulated to secrete pancreatic juice by hormones (se-

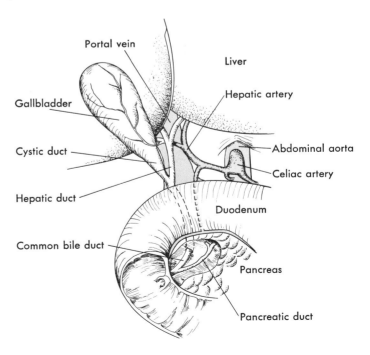

FIGURE 16.1 Diagram of gallbladder, pancreas, and duodenum showing relationships of bile and pancreatic ducts. (From Miller, Marjorie A.; Drakontides, Anna B.; and Leavell, Lutie, C.: *Kimber-Gray-Stackpole's Anatomy and Physiology*, 17th ed. Macmillan Publishing Co., Inc., New York, 1977.)

Portal vein

Liver

Gallbladder

Hepatic artery

Cystic duct

Abdominal aorta

Celiac artery

Hepatic duct

Duodenum

Common bile duct

Pancreas

Pancreatic duct

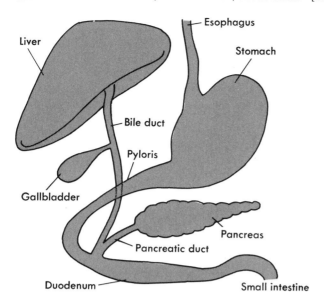

FIGURE 16.2 Diagram illustrating relationship of liver, gallbladder, and pancreas to the small intestine. (From Arlin, Marian: *The Science of Nutrition*, 2nd ed. Macmillan Publishing Co., Inc., New York, 1977.)

cretin and cholecystokinin-pancreozymin, secreted by the small intestine) and by neurogenic and vascular influences.

The islands of Langerhans are highly specialized groups of cells in the pancreas that produce insulin and glucagon. Insulin is needed by body cells in order to use glucose for fuel. Glucagon is needed by the liver to convert glycogen to glucose. These pancreatic secretions are not carried by ducts but are picked up by the bloodstream and transported to the appropriate area.

Assisting with Diagnostic Studies

PHYSICAL EXAMINATION OF THE ABDOMEN

The physician may detect some abnormalities of the liver or the biliary tract by palpating these organs. Since many organs in the abdomen touch each other or lie close to one another, abnormal enlargement of one organ such as the liver may cause the spleen to enlarge also. In addition to enlargment, tenderness, scarring, and masses may be palpated by the physician during the physical examination of the abdomen.

LABORATORY STUDIES

A variety of laboratory studies may be ordered by the physician in order to detect abnormal function of the liver, pancreas, or biliary tract. Table 16.1 contains a list of laboratory tests frequently done.

X-RAY STUDIES

ABDOMINAL X-RAY. The physician usually orders an abdominal x-ray to determine if the disease process has caused enlargement or displacement of organs in the abdomen.

CHOLECYSTOGRAM (GALLBLADDER SERIES). A cholecystogram is an x-ray that permits the physician to visualize the gallbladder. Special preparation is needed before the patient has a gallbladder x-ray.

Generally, the patient is given a fat-free supper on the evening prior to the x-ray in order to avoid contraction of the gallbladder. A special dye, frequently in tablet form, is administered to the patient on the evening prior to x-ray. The dye is picked up from the digestive system by the bloodstream and carried to the liver. The liver then puts the dye into bile, and the gallbladder stores the bile containing the dye. Usually, the patient is not allowed to eat or drink after the dye has been given until the x-ray is completed the next day. Remembering that the presence of fat in the small intestine causes the gallbladder to empty enables the nurse to

TABLE 16.1
NORMAL VALUES OF LABORATORY TESTS FREQUENTLY DONE IN LIVER, BILIARY TRACT, AND PANCREATIC DISEASE

TEST	NORMAL VALUE
Ammonia (plasma)	23–79 mcg/100 ml
Amylase (serum)	40–200 units/100 ml
Amylase (urine)	Below 300 units/hour
Bilirubin (serum)	
Direct	0–0.4 mg/100 ml
Total	Up to 1 mg/100 ml
Bilirubin (urine)	Negative
BSP (serum)	Less than 5 % after 45 minutes
Calcium (serum)	8.5–10.5 mg/100 ml
	4.5–5.5 mEq/l
Cephalin-cholesterol flocculation (serum)	0–2 + in 24 hours
Gamma-glutamyl transpeptidase (serum)	1–20 IU
Lactic dehydrogenase (serum)	90–200 IU
Lipase (serum)	0–1.5 units
Lipids, total (serum)	450–1000 mg/100 ml
Cholesterol, total	150–300 mg/100 ml
Triglycerides	45–170 mg/100 ml
Phospholipids	150–380 mg/100 ml
Fatty acids	9.0–15.0 mM/1
Neutral fat	0–200 mg/100 ml
Phospholipid-P	8.0–11.0 mg/100 ml
Phosphatase, alkaline (serum)	30–85 IU/1
	X2, X3 elevation for children
Protein, total (serum)	6.1–8.6 gm/100 ml
Albumin	3.5–5.5 gm/100 ml
Globulin	2.0–3.5 gm/100 ml
Prothrombin time (plasma)	12–14 seconds
Thymol turbidity	0–4 Maclagan units
Transaminase (serum)	
SGOT	10–50 IU/1 at 37°C
SGPT	5–30 IU/1 at 37°C
Trypsin (stool)	4 + @ 1:10 dilution
Urobilinogen (stool)	
Qualitative, random specimen	Positive
Quantitative, 24-hour specimen	40–200 mg/24 hours
Urobilinogen (urine)	
Male, random specimen	0.3–2.0 Ehrlich units
Female, random specimen	0.1–1.0 Ehrlich units

understand the importance of checking the patient's evening meal to be certain that it is fat free. In addition, the patient should understand that vomiting, eating, or drinking after the dye has been ingested may cause the dye to be lost. The physician should be notified if any of these events occurs.

After the initial films are taken, the patient generally is given a highly fatted substance to drink. This causes the gallbladder to contract and empty the dye-laden bile into the duodenum. Further pictures are then taken to measure the emptying time of the gallbladder.

The nurse should be sure to ask the patient about allergies to iodine and seafood before giving the dye, since iodine may be a component of the dye. The dye should not be given until the physician has been notified if the patient reports an iodine or seafood allergy.

CHOLANGIOGRAM. This is an x-ray procedure that permits the physician to visualize the bile ducts. The dye is usually injected intravenously but may be injected directly into the bile ducts during surgery or into a special drain postoperatively. Generally, the patient experiences burning while the dye is injected. Since the dye used contains iodine, the nurse should notify the physician if the patient indicates an iodine or seafood allergy.

LIVER SCAN. Radioisotopes of certain elements may be injected intravenously. After the isotopes have reached the liver via the bloodstream, a scanning device is passed over the abdomen that records the distribution of the injected isotopes within the liver. By studying the map of the liver made by the scanner, the physician may detect certain abnormalities in the liver, such as cysts or masses.

ULTRASOUND. High-frequency sound waves can be directed toward abdominal organs. The waves are reflected back into a machine which forms them into a picture. Ultrasound may be used to identify tumors, cysts, stones, or an abscess in the liver, pancreas, or gallbladder.

COMPUTERIZED AXIAL TOMOGRAPHY (CT SCAN, CAT SCAN). This relatively new form of x-ray was described on page 71. A CAT scan of the abdomen may provide detailed cross-sectional views of the liver, pancreas, and other intra-abdominal organs.

ENDOSCOPIC RETROGRADE CHOLANGIOPANCREATOGRAPHY (ERCP). During this form of endoscopy, the physician inserts a fiberoptic endoscope through the mouth into the esophagus to the duodenum. The common bile duct and pancreatic ducts may be cannulated. Contrast material is injected into the ducts and x-ray films are taken. In some cases, material from the ducts may be extracted for cytology. An experimental therapeutic use of ERCP is extraction of stones from cannulated ducts.

PERITEONOSCOPY (LAPAROSCOPY). This study permits direct visualization of the peritoneum and the liver via a peritoneoscope which is inserted through a small incision made in the abdominal wall. The patient signs a written consent, and food and fluids are withheld for several hours prior to the procedure. Clotting studies usually are ordered in advance since a clotting defect must be corrected before a periteonoscopy can be done. Bowel, bladder, and skin preparations are also ordered before this test.

ANGIOGRAPHY. Contrast dye may be injected into selected blood vessels, thereby enabling the physician to examine the blood vessels of the liver or pancreas. The dye used frequently contains iodine, which may stimulate an allergic reaction in a person who is allergic to iodine.

LIVER BIOPSY

The physician may wish to obtain a specimen of liver tissue to help establish a diagnosis or determine the progression of diseases such as hepatitis or cirrhosis.

Usually, a liver biopsy is performed at the bedside after the patient has given written consent. Prior to the biopsy, the physician usually orders clotting studies in order to determine if the patient has abnormal bleeding tendencies. In some cases, the physician may prescribe vitamin K intramuscularly to diminish the likelihood of hemorrhage. Usually, the patient fasts for several hours and is given a sedative before the biopsy. Patient teaching and cooperation are essential in order to obtain an adequate tissue sample and avoid complications. The patient must hold the breath for 10 to 15 seconds during the biopsy procedure in order to prevent tearing the liver. This is so important that the physician usually will not do a liver biopsy if the patient is too breathless or disoriented to hold the breath. the nurse may help by timing the patient's ability to hold the breath prior to the biopsy. The nurse also should record the patient's vital signs before the biopsy begins.

During the biopsy, the patient lies on the back. After cleansing the skin and injecting a local anesthetic, the physician aseptically inserts a needle into the liver and obtains the needed specimen while the patient holds the breath after exhaling. After the needle is withdrawn, the patient is instructed to breathe normally. Following the biopsy, the patient usually is instructed to lie on the right side for several hours. This position uses the mattress to apply external pressure on the liver to minimize bleeding. The physician may also instruct the patient to remain in bed for 12 to 24 hours. Vital signs are usually ordered frequently (as often as every 15 minutes) immediately after the biopsy in order to detect the complication of hemorrhage.

Some patients report pain in the right shoulder following liver biopsy. This is not unusual and is believed to be referred pain from the biopsy site. Severe abdominal pain should be reported immediately to the physician since it may indicate accidental puncture of a bile duct during the biopsy. This is a rare but serious complication of liver biopsy that allows bile to escape from the liver, causing peritonitis.

PARACENTESIS

Paracentesis is a procedure in which the physician uses a hollow needle to withdraw abnormal fluid that has accumulated in the peritoneal cavity (ascites). Ascites may be a symptom of liver or other diseases and may cause pressure on abdominal or respiratory organs. Thus, paracentesis may be diagnostic to analyze the components of the ascites fluid and occasionally therapeutic to relieve pressure on compressed organs. Written permission from the patient is generally needed prior to this procedure. The nurse should be certain that the patient has emptied the bladder before the paracentesis begins in order to avoid accidental puncture of the bladder with the needle.

Generally, the patient is positioned in a sitting or a semi-Fowler's position. After the skin has been cleansed, the physician injects a local anesthetic and aseptically inserts the hollow needle into the peritoneum. Tubing may be attached to the needle to allow fluid to drain into a collection bottle, which is placed below the level of the abdomen. The nurse should observe the patient carefully and frequently during and after paracentesis. Circulatory shifts and collapse may occur, causing symptoms of shock. Infection and abnormal bleeding are also infrequent, but serious, complications. Vital signs are generally checked frequently, and fever and/or abdominal pain should be reported to the physician.

Paracentesis is performed rarely as a therapeutic measure. However, if other measures to reduce ascites fail, some persons may be helped temporarily by this procedure.

Nursing Observations

JAUNDICE (ICTERUS)

The patient with jaundice (icterus) has a yellowish color of skin, mucous membranes, and sclerae (white portion of eyes) caused by bilirubin. *Bilirubin* is a yellow pigment made by the reticuloendothelial system from the hemoglobin of aging red blood cells. The *reticuloendothelial system* is a network of specialized cells located mainly in the spleen, liver, bone marrow, lymph nodes, and thymus gland. These very important cells have a variety of functions essential to life, which include:

- Digesting microorganisms or foreign bodies
- Forming antibodies and immune bodies
- Breaking down aged red blood cells
- Storing iron
- Forming certain blood cells such as red cells

Newly formed bilirubin is carried by circulating plasma to the liver, where it is incorporated into bile.

Jaundice may occur in a variety of conditions. *Obstructive jaundice* occurs when the hepatic duct or common bile duct is blocked by a stone or tumor. Bile is prevented from flowing into the small intestine and backs up into the liver. In the liver, the bile pigments are absorbed in the blood.

PRURITUS

The patient with a disturbance of the liver, biliary tract, or pancreas frequently has itching believed to be caused by deposits of chemicals such as bile salts in the tissue. Occasionally, the physician may prescribe a carefully selected drug to reduce itching. Remembering the liver's important function as a detoxifier of many drugs enables the nurse to understand the physician's caution in prescribing medication when liver disease is present.

OTHER SKIN CHANGES

In addition to jaundice and pruritus, a variety of other skin changes may be observed in the patient with a disorder of the liver, biliary tract, or pancreas. The skin may become thickened, scaly, and/or dry. Signs of bleeding may be visible under the skin as petechiae, purpura, and/or ecchymoses. Veins may become visible over the epigastrium or umbilicus. When ascites is present, blood vessels may become visible in the taut skin over the abdomen.

Spider telangiectasia is a small vascular network of dilated capillaries which usually develops on the face, neck, shoulders, forearms, and hands. This skin change may be observed in patients with certain liver diseases such as cirrhosis.

An *xanthoma* is a yellowish papule, nodule, or plaque caused by the deposit of lipids. This skin growth may develop anywhere but is most often seen on the eyelid of a patient with liver disease.

Palmar erythema is a red appearance of the palms of the hands which often develops in patients with liver disease.

The nurse also may observe changes in hair growth caused by hormonal changes associated with cirrhosis. Gynecomastia (breast enlargement) in the male patient may develop from a similar hormone imbalance.

Edema may develop as a result of liver disease. The nurse looks for edema at the sacrum, tibiae, or in the feet.

OBSERVING THE CHEST

The patient's respirations may be affected by swelling in the abdomen, pain in the abdomen, a high abdominal incision, or chemical imbalances. Therefore, an important observation is related to observing the rate and pattern of respirations, as described in Chapter 14.

ASCITES

As mentioned earlier, ascites is an abnormal accumulation of fluid in the peritoneal cavity that can be caused by a variety of conditions. The exact mechanism of ascites is not known, but several events are known to influence the development of ascites. These include:

- Backup of blood in the congested, diseased liver causes increased pressure in the vessels in the peritoneum.
- Decreased production of plasma albumin by the damaged liver changes the pressure relationships between fluid inside and outside the vessels and allows fluid to seep through the vessels into the peritoneum.
- Aldosterone cannot be metabolized by the damaged liver and accumulates in the blood, causing the body to retain more sodium and water.
- As fluid accumulates, the patient's abdomen becomes more taut and swollen.

When the patient has ascites, the physician usually orders daily weights to determine the amount of fluid gained or lost. The nurse may also be asked to measure the person's abdominal girth by placing a tape measure around the abdomen at the level of the umbilicus. Measurements of weight and abdominal girth must be taken meticulously in order to obtain accurate information. For example, the patient should be weighed on the same scale, at the same time every day, wearing the same amount of clothing. Similarly, the patient's abdominal girth should be measured daily at the same time, and the tape measure should be placed next to the skin and not around clothing. Also, the tape measure should be carefully placed at the level of the umbilicus each time the abdominal girth is measured. The nurse can also expect that the physician will order frequent laboratory determination of serum sodium and albumin levels (see Table 16.1). Paracentesis may be done for analysis of fluid and occasionally for relief of uncomfortable symptoms such as difficult breathing.

GASTROINTESTINAL SYMPTOMS

The individual with liver, biliary tract, or pancreatic disease may experience several gastrointestinal symptoms, which vary according to the disease and its severity. Nausea and vomiting frequently occur. Anorexia, indigestion, flatulence, diarrhea, and constipation are common symptoms.

PAIN AND DISCOMFORT

The nurse may often observe that the patient with liver, biliary, or pancreatic disease has pain, which may range from uncomfortable to excruciating in nature.

The individual with liver disease may experience abdominal pain in the right upper quadrant. This is believed to result from stretching of the capsule surrounding the liver as it becomes swollen.

The person with biliary tract disease generally complains of severe, colicky pain in the right upper quadrant or epigastric region. Pain may radiate to the back. Usually, the physician prescribes meperidine (DEMEROL) to relax smooth muscle and control pain.

The individual with pancreatitis frequently has excruciating epigastric pain, which may extend to the back or flank. Meperidine (DEMEROL) usually is prescribed to control this type of pain.

STOOLS AND URINE

The nurse may observe that the appearance of stools and urine may be altered by disease in the liver, biliary tract, or pancreas.

For example, the patient with jaundice may have clay-colored stools since bile cannot reach the intestinal tract to give normal color to feces. The urine may become darker in color and thicker as the kidney removes excess bile pigment from the blood.

The individual with a chronic inflammation of the pancreas may experience frequent foul, fatty stools (steatorrhea). This may be caused by diminished pancreatic fluid containing enzymes that help to break down fats.

Increased bleeding tendency may become visible through blood that appears in the stools. Frequently, the physician requests that all stools be saved and sent to the laboratory to be tested for occult blood.

The nurse should observe and record the frequency, color, amount, and consistency of urine and stools.

BLEEDING

The patient with a disorder of the liver, biliary tract, or pancreas generally has an increased bleeding tendency. This can be caused by a variety of factors, which include:

- Damaged liver cells cannot form prothrombin and other factors needed for clotting.
- Absence of bile in the small intestine reduces absorption of fats containing vitamin K, which the liver needs in order to form prothrombin.
- Pancreatic disease may affect the production of pancreatic juices containing enzymes that affect the walls of blood vessels. This can result in massive hemorrhage.
- Increased pressure in the diseased liver causes enlargement of veins in the esophagus and anus.
- Anemia may occur in the final stages of liver disease and is caused by increased red cell breakdown and dietary deficiencies.

Bleeding may be visible in the skin as ecchymoses or purpura. Another possible source of bleeding is the mucous membranes of the mouth, especially following oral hygiene. Following venipuncture, the site may bleed longer than usual. Any evidence of blood in the patient's urine, stools, vomitus, or other body excretions should be reported to the physician at once.

OBSERVING FOR SIGNS OF INFECTION

The patient with a disturbance in the liver, biliary tract, or pancreas usually has an increased risk of infection. Signs of infection such as chills, fever, and malaise, as well as local signs including erythema, warmth, tenderness, and swelling of a body part should be reported at once.

ASTERIXIS

Asterixis (liver flap) is a flapping tremor of the hands that can be observed when the patient is asked to bend the hands back at the wrist while resting the arms on a flat surface. Asterixis is believed to be caused by the effect of elevated blood ammonia levels on the brain and nervous system. Blood ammonia level rises when damaged liver cells are unable to convert ammonia to urea. A more complete discussion of this process is presented later in this chapter.

BEHAVIORAL CHANGES

As mentioned above, elevated blood ammonia levels have a toxic effect on the brain and nervous system. Memory, attention, concentration, handwriting, speech, and alertness are a few functions that may be impaired by the toxic effect of excessive blood ammonia. The nurse may observe that the patient has wide mood swings. The patient's speed in responding may be slower. In severe illness, the patient may become comatose. Behavior changes also may develop from complications of illness such as bleeding or infection.

The nurse can render valuable assistance by listening to and watching carefully what the patient says and does. Meticulous recording of what the patient actually said or did is more helpful than vague statements such as "seems more confused."

The patient may have a disturbance of the liver or pancreas which is associated with drug or alcohol abuse. When hospitalized, such a patient may develop behavioral changes associated with withdrawal. Such changes should be reported at once in order to prevent life-threatening complications. For example, early behavioral changes associated with alcohol withdrawal include anxiety, jerky, uncoordinated movements, increased irritability, and diaphoresis. These changes are associated with an unexplained rise in blood pressure and pulse. Early behavioral changes associated with withdrawal from drugs include anxiety, sleep disturbances, nausea and vomiting, diaphoresis, muscle spasms, and tremors. An observation guide for the patient with a distur-

bance of liver, biliary tract, or pancreas can be located in Table 16.2.

Nursing Interventions

ASSISTING WITH HYGIENE

During the bath, the jaundiced patient or the nurse may notice that the washcloth, towel or bath water has a slightly yellow color. This may add to the patient's concern and embarrassment. The nurse may help to allay the patient's anxiety by explaining that the coloring is caused by the jaundiced skin cells that are washed off or dried off during bathing.

The physician may prescribe special baths or afterbath lotions for the patient with pruritus. In some cases, the patient may find that scratching the sheets or covers helps to satisfy an overwhelming desire to scratch. In other cases, the patient may need to wear protective mittens or gloves to prevent damage to the skin from scratching.

The patient with an increased bleeding tendency is instructed to brush the teeth gently, using a soft-bristled toothbrush to prevent bleeding from the gums. Also, the patient should blow the nose gently to avoid epistaxis. When moving or turning the patient, the nurse's touch shold be gentle to avoid bruising.

ALTERATIONS OF FLUID AND DIET

Specific alterations of fluid and/or diet depend upon the patient's disease. Some patients may need assistance to eat. Small meals served in an attractive manner by a caring person may help the anorexic patient to eat. Dietary modification is an important aspect of many treatment plans, and the nurse should have a basic understanding of the patient's dietary prescription. Professional assistance from the dietitian should be requested before giving any foods and fluids that are not on the patient's tray or when the patient is not eating.

Usually the physician restricts the dietary intake of sodium for the patient with ascites. In severe cases, the physician may also restrict the patient's fluid intake to 1000 to 2000 ml per day. In some cases, the patient's

TABLE 16.2
OBSERVATION GUIDE FOR THE PATIENT WITH
A DISTURBANCE OF THE LIVER, BILIARY
TRACT, OR PANCREAS

AREA TO BE OBSERVED	OBSERVATIONS
Head and neck	Abnormal distribution of hair in men
	Spider telangiectasia, petechiae
Eyes	Observe for jaundice in sclera
	Observe for xanthomas in eyelids
Nose	Epistaxis may occur from clotting defects
Mouth	Odor of ammonia to breath
	Bleeding from mucous membranes
	Vomiting, hemetemesis
	Eructation, hiccough
Face	Observe for spider telangiectasia
Chest	Observe pattern and rate of respirations which may change from chemical imbalance, ascites, or high abdominal incisions
	Spider telangiectasia, petechiae
	Gynecomastia in males
Abdomen	Abdominal distention from gas or fluid (ascites)
	Prominent veins may be visible through taut skin when ascites present
	Nausea, anorexia
	Pain
Extremities	Palmar erythema
	Spider telangiectasia in forearms
	Tibial and pedal edema
	Asterixis (flapping hand tremor)
	Venipuncture sites may ooze
Back	Sacral edema
Urine	May be darker when jaundice present
	Blood in urine
Stools	Diarrhea or constipation
	Light-colored stools associated with jaundice
	Blood in stools
	Foul-smelling fatty stools (steatorrhea)
Skin changes	Thickened, scaly, or dry
	Pruritus
	Petechiae, purpura, ecchymoses
	Spider telangiectasia
	Jaundice
Behavioral changes	Impairment of memory, concentration, handwriting, speech, alertness
	Restlessness
	Disorientation

Speed in responding may be slower
Lethargy, drowsiness
Coma
Changes associated with withdrawal from alcohol or drugs

disease becomes chronic, requiring a drastic change of life-style. Dietary restrictions that can be lifelong may contribute to feelings of anger and depression. The patient is more likely to follow a special diet that contains foods consistent with cultural values.

POSITIONING

Generally, the patient with ascites is more comfortable in a semi-Fowler's position, which reduces the pressure of excess fluid on the respiratory tract. The patient should be turned and repositioned frequently to prevent skin breakdown caused by increased pressure on vessels that nourish the skin. Other positions may be indicated when the patient has a nasogastric tube. For example, the patient may lie on the right side to improve drainage from a nasogastric tube.

ASSISTING WITH DRUG THERAPY

A variety of drugs may be prescribed for the patient with liver, biliary, or pancreatic disease. Since many drugs are detoxified by the liver, the nurse can understand easily that the patient with liver disease should be observed closely for signs of drug toxicity and interactions. For reasons that are not entirely understood, opiates, sedatives, and tranquilizers appear especially toxic for the individual with liver damage. Therefore, the physician rarely prescribes them. Thus, the nurse must select nursing measures such as backrubs and changes of position and listening to promote rest and reduce anxiety.

Occasionally, the physician may prescribe a carefully selected drug to reduce itching. Remembering the liver's important function as a detoxifier of many drugs enables the nurse to understand the physician's caution in prescribing medication when liver cells are damaged.

In some cases, the physician may prescribe intramuscular injections of vitamin K or other substances to improve the patient's clotting mechanisms. Following an injection or venipuncture, the nurse should apply gentle pressure over the puncture site to prevent oozing of blood.

Diuretics may be prescribed to promote excretion of excess fluid. Table 11.7 (page 300) contains a list of diuretics the physician may prescribe. A careful record of intake and output is maintained by the nurse.

Occasionally, intravenous albumin that is low in salt (salt-poor albumin) is given to reduce ascites and promote excretion of retained fluids. The nurse should observe the patient carefully for signs of circulatory overload.

Narcotics frequently are prescribed to control the severe pain associated with biliary and pancreatic disease. The nurse should watch for signs of respiratory depression when narcotics are needed.

The use of nonprescribed drugs, including alcohol, is especially hazardous for the patient with a disturbance of the liver, biliary tract, or pancreas. This is an important part of patient teaching.

MAINTAINING A SAFE ENVIRONMENT

The patient who is sedated, disoriented, or who has an impairment of memory or attention may need protection from accidents. For example, the nurse may keep the siderails up or apply a restraining vest to prevent the patient from falling out of bed. Safety also is enhanced by placing needed objects within easy reach of the patient so that long stretches for a urinal or tissues are avoided. Short, frequent visits to the patient may enhance safety by reducing confusion associated with lack of contact with others.

PREVENTING THE SPREAD OF INFECTION

As mentioned earlier, the patient with a disorder of the liver, biliary tract, or pancreas often has an increased susceptibility to infection. In some cases, infection may develop as a result of damage to body defenses caused by liver or pancreatic disease. In other cases, the liver, biliary tract, or pancreas becomes infected.

Certain infections may be spread through body substances such as saliva, urine, stool, and blood. Some patients with infections of the liver or pancreas may need to be isolated from others in order to prevent the spread of infection. Special handling of infected substances may be indicated. Good handwashing on the nurse's part both reduces the spread of infection from the patient and the likelihood of introducing infection to the patient from others.

DEVELOPING THE THERAPEUTIC RELATIONSHIP

The patient with jaundice usually experiences embarrassment and concern related to an altered appearance. Such a patient may want to explore these concerns with the nurse. In addition to listening, the nurse may talk with family or friends to explain jaundice and prevent unintentional comments that might be upsetting to the patient. Furniture and mirrors may be moved to avoid constant visual reminders of jaundice to the patient.

In some conditions, the jaundiced patient may have to be isolated from others in order to prevent infection. The nurse should carefully explain that it is not the patient's appearance that requires isolation but the underlying disease. Repeated explanations may be needed to reassure the patient that the illness rather than a change in appearance requires isolation.

The patient who is withdrawing from drugs and/or alcohol needs a restful, quiet environment in which sudden, rapid, unplanned stimuli are avoided. When communicating with such a patient, the nurse uses short, simple sentences and speaks in low tones while facing the patient. The nurse avoids communicating personal moral judgments related to the patient's alcohol or drug dependency. The patient may be referred to other resources in the community for assistance with drug and/or alcohol abuse.

PATIENT AND FAMILY TEACHING

A variety of teaching may be needed. In some cases, a permanent alteration in diet is needed. The nurse may assist with this form of patient teaching by requesting the dietitian to provide information related to shopping, meal planning, and cooking.

Some families and visitors may need information about isolation practices while the patient is hospitalized. Families and visitors are taught to avoid borrowing the patient's personal articles such as combs and brushes. The sharing of food with a patient who is isolated is also avoided. Visitors should be shown the nearest visitor's bathroom and advised not to use the patient's bathroom.

Other opportunities for patient and family teaching relate to the use of nonprescribed drugs and alcohol. One way to present this information is by describing the functions of the liver and pancreas. Next, the effect of drugs and alcohol on these organs may be described in a matter-of-fact way. Most persons respond more favorably to simple explanations of *how* a substance damages the body instead of why such substances should not be used.

Acute Viral Hepatitis

The patient with acute viral hepatitis has an acute inflammation of the liver caused by a virus. The three types of acute viral hepatitis that have been identified are (1) infectious hepatitis, hepatitis A, caused by virus A; (2) serum hepatitis, hepatitis B, caused by virus B; and (3) post transfusion hepatitis associated with a virus currently under investigation which is called non-A and non-B virus.

TRANSMISSION

The virus of hepatitis A most often is transmitted by the fecal-oral route, although other routes are possible. There is a high incidence of hepatitis A in partners, such as coworkers and sexual partners. Poor sanitation, overcrowding, and fecal contamination of water and milk supplies can result in hepatitis A. A concentration of the viruses in shellfish has led to epidemics. Infectious hepatitis can be caused by an infusion of blood infected with the virus; however, this is rare. The incubation period for infectious hepatitis is approximately two to six weeks. After having hepatitis A, the patient is immune against that type of hepatitis but is not protected against other viruses causing hepatitis. The injection of gamma globulin within a few days after having been exposed to infectious hepatitis will help to prevent that person from developing the disease.

Serum hepatitis (B) is thought to be transmitted by the parenteral route as well as by direct contact. For this reason, persons in close contact with patients with serum hepatitis such as physicians, nurses, and sexual partners are more likely to develop it. Heroin addicts who use inadequately sterilized needles are especially prone to hepatitis B, as are persons on hemodialysis and infants born to mothers with hepatitis B.

Other hazards are the use of inadequately sterilized instruments, tattoo needles, and razors. Persons working around whole blood such as laboratory and dialysis unit workers are subject to this occupational hazard. The incubation period for serum hepatitis may range from four weeks to six months.

Persons with this form of hepatitis may develop chronic hepatitis or may become carriers of the hepatitis B virus. Passive immunization from this virus may be acquired by receiving serum immune globulin that has been enriched with hepatitis B immune globulin. Since this treatment is expensive, only persons at high risk receive it. A vaccine currently is being developed to provide active immunity; however, it is not yet available for the general public.

Hepatitis caused by the non-A non-B agent typically develops within two to twenty weeks after a transfusion. Persons with this virus may become carriers or may develop chronic hepatitis.

ASSISTING WITH DIAGNOSTIC STUDIES

The physician confirms the diagnosis by liver function tests. Such studies as urinary urobilinogen, urinary bilirubin, BSP, serum transaminase, dehydrogenase, serum alkaline phosphatase, and 5-nucleotidase may be ordered. Normal values for these and other laboratory tests are included for reference in Table 16.1. Other diagnostic tests are done on the patient's blood to identify specific antigens and antibodies associated with the A and B viruses. For example, persons with the A virus usually have antibodies to that virus (anti-HAV) present in the serum. Persons with the B virus may have an antigen (HBs Ag) or an antibody (anti-HBc) present in the serum. Tests are not yet available to identify the non-A and non-B agent which commonly causes posttransfusion hepatitis.

NURSING OBSERVATIONS

The patient with acute viral hepatitis experiences symptoms similar to those of other viral infections of the respiratory or gastrointestinal tract. Fever, anorexia, weakness, headache, aching muscles, nausea, and vomiting frequently occur. The patient's urine may be discolored with bilirubin and stools clay colored. Abdominal discomfort may be experienced. The patient may or may not become jaundiced.

NURSING INTERVENTIONS

REST. The physician usually advises the patient to avoid fatigue during the acute phase of illness. Bed rest may be prescribed occasionally for the patient whose illness is severe enough to require hospitalization.

DIET AND FLUIDS. The patient with hepatitis usually needs a nutritious diet that favors the regeneration of liver cells. A diet high in calories and protein generally is prescribed. Fat may or may not be restricted. The patient may develop temporary food intolerances during acute illness. Any food intolerances reported by the patient should be communicated to the dietitian so that nutritious substitutes can be provided. An increase of fluid intake is also recommended.

The patient with anorexia may be encouraged to eat small portions with nutritious between-meal snacks. Some patients may need help in feeding themselves, and others may need to have more time to permit them to eat at a comfortable pace. In some cases, it is possible to increase the patient's caloric intake at breakfast. Some physicians request that patients be given the major portion of food early in the day because of nausea in the afternoon.

PREVENTING THE SPREAD OF INFECTION. The hospitalized patient may be placed in some form of isolation in order to prevent the transmission of the virus to other patients or personnel. The specific form of isolation depends upon the virus causing hepatitis and hospital policy.

Remembering that the patient's stools contain the infecting viruses, the nurse can readily anticipate the need for handling fecal waste with care. The feces may have to be disinfected in some cities, depending on the requirements of the local health department. The nurse should avoid contaminating the hands when performing procedures involving the patient's anal area, such as an enema or rectal temperature. Disposable rubber or plastic gloves are suggested for such procedures. Careful handwashing with running water and soap is important.

Needles and syringes used on the patient with acute viral hepatitis should be handled cautiously, as the infection can be transmitted through the patient's serum. A minute particle of contaminated serum from the patient can remain in the needle and syringe.

A careless prick of the skin with the contaminated needle by the nurse can permit the virus to enter the body. Inadequate sterilization can permit the infection to be transmitted to another person if either the same needle or syringe is used. Therefore, the use of disposable syringes and needles has become quite popular. If the nurse does accidently prick the skin with a contaminated needle, the accident should be reported immediately according to the policy of the agency. Gloves should be worn when giving an injection.

Since the hepatitis virus is often found in feces, a disposable bedpan should be used. When a disposable bedpan is not available, the regular bedpan should be sterilized by autoclaving after the patient is removed from isolation or discharged.

Disposable dishware and plastic utensils are also used to prevent the spread of infection.

DRUG THERAPY. Drug therapy generally is avoided when the patient has hepatitis. Occasionally, the physician may prescribe small dosages of an antiemetic or antipruritic drug for the patient with severe symptoms. The patient is cautioned to avoid alcoholic beverages.

Cirrhosis of the Liver

The patient with cirrhosis of the liver has a chronic disease in which liver tissue is gradually replaced by scar tissue. Usually, cirrhosis develops over a period of years. As the normal tissue is replaced by scar tissue, liver function is impaired and finally ceases. Because of the variety of functions performed by the liver, other body organs become involved in the late stages of cirrhosis.

Cirrhosis is the end result of many types of liver injury. At times, the cause of cirrhosis cannot be found. However, cirrhosis is classified by many authorities on the basis of causes that are known, such as:

- Cirrhosis caused by alcoholism (most common cause)
- Cirrhosis caused by hepatitis
- Biliary cirrhosis
- Schistosomal cirrhosis (parasitic)
- Cardiac cirrhosis (associated with chronic congestive heart failure)

Alcoholic cirrhosis frequently develops from two other conditions: fatty liver and alcoholic hepatitis. The patient with fatty liver has large droplets of fat which occupy most of the liver cell. The patient who abstains permanently from alcohol at this point usually experiences a complete resolution of fatty liver. Within weeks or several months, fat droplets disappear from the liver cell. The patient with alcoholic hepatitis has a more serious condition involving inflammation of the liver and sclerosis of central veins in the area. This condition may progress to cirrhosis even if the patient abstains from alcohol. At the present time, the most important factor beside alcohol intake known to influence the development of cirrhosis is poor dietary intake.

Complications of cirrhosis include ascites, bleeding esophageal and gastric varices, disturbances in the spleen, liver failure, and renal failure.

ASSISTING WITH DIAGNOSTIC STUDIES

The physician may order a battery of laboratory tests to assess liver function (see Table 16.1). In addition, liver biopsy may be performed to secure a diagnosis. When ascites or varices are present or suspected, additional studies such as paracentesis, angiography, or esophagograms may be ordered.

NURSING OBSERVATIONS

The patient with cirrhosis develops symptoms associated with a disturbance of blood flowing through the liver and inadequate functioning of the liver. Most of the blood from the digestive organs is carried through the liver. When this flow of blood through the liver is hindered, it collects in the gastrointestinal system. This causes the patient to develop symptoms of abdominal congestion. At first there are digestive disturbances such as indigestion, flatulence (gas), loss of appetite, nausea, and vomiting. Because of this change in the circulation within the liver, the patient may later develop varicose veins in the esophagus known as esophageal varices. One of these may rupture, causing hematemesis, hemorrhage, and death. Increased pressure also causes varicose veins in the rectum and hemorrhoids that may bleed. Bleeding tendency is greatly increased in cirrhosis, for reasons described earlier on page 519.

Because the metabolic functions of the liver are disturbed, the patient may show signs of malnutrition such as thin, wasted arms and legs.

Spider angiomas (vascular lesions) may be visible and especially prominent on the face, probably caused by altered hormone activity in the liver.

Ascites, described earlier as an abnormal collection of fluid in the peritoneal cavity, may develop. Resulting pressure may cause lower-leg edema or disturbances in the functions of the spleen, kidneys, or respiratory system.

Inability of damaged liver cells to use bilirubin usually causes jaundice and related pruritus, clay-colored stools, and darkened urine.

The patient is more likely to develop infections such as pneumonia or tuberculosis. As the disease progresses to its final stages, hepatic failure, renal failure (hepatorenal failure), and death can occur.

In order to monitor the development of these symptoms, the nurse can expect to weigh the patient daily, measure the abdominal girth daily, observe, measure, and record all intake and output, and send all stools to the laboratory to determine if blood is present. Because changes in behavior may indicate undetected bleeding or the development of hepatic coma, the nurse should report them at once to the appropriate nurse or physician.

NURSING INTERVENTIONS

HYGIENE. The patient with cirrhosis usually develops jaundice and needs hygiene related to that condition. Gentle oral hygiene with special sponges or a soft-bristle brush is indicated to prevent trauma and bleeding of mucous membranes. When cleansing or wiping the perineum after a bowel movement, the nurse's touch should be gentle to avoid trauma to hemorrhoids which could initiate bleeding.

DIET AND FLUIDS. In early stages, a high-protein, high-carbohydrate diet usually is prescribed. In more advanced stages, protein, fat, and sodium may be restricted. When esophageal varices are present as a complication, a reduction in fiber is often prescribed to avoid inducing hemorrhage caused by roughage. As previously mentioned, sodium may be restricted severely when ascites is present. When dietary sodium is restricted, fluid intake is also restricted to 1000 to 1500 ml per day.

The patient who is anorexic may benefit from small meals with nutritious between-meal snacks. The patient's participation and cooperation are essential to successful restriction of fluids. For example, the patient may help to determine how much fluid is allotted for meals, medications, and between meals. The patient who is alert may participate in keeping the intake-and-output record.

DRUG THERAPY. Because of disturbances in absorption and metabolism of vita-mins and minerals, supplemental vitamins and minerals usually are prescribed such as B-complex vitamins, ferrous sulfate, folic acid, and vitamins A, D, and K. Potassium also may be prescribed at times to correct losses caused by vomiting, diarrhea, or diuretics.

Diuretics are usually prescribed for the patient with ascites. In some cases, a combination of diuretics is prescribed to decrease ascites. Common drugs used include spironolactone (ALDACTONE), triamterene (DYRENIUM), furosemide (LASIX), and ethacrynic acid (EDECRIN).

REST. Rest is generally indicated. When ascites is present, the patient may be more comfortable in a low or semi-Fowler's position. These positions permit fluid to migrate toward the lower abdomen and reduce the restriction of breathing.

PATIENT AND FAMILY TEACHING. Patient and family teaching is an essential part of the patient's care. Various types of help may be needed. For example, the patient and/or family may be helped by community programs such as Alcoholics Anonymous, ALANON, or ALATEEN when alcoholism is related to cirrhosis, as is frequently the case.

Professional assistance from the dietitian may be needed by the patient and the family in order to understand and prepare the diet at home.

The patient should be cautioned not to take any nonprescription drugs. Aspirin and antihistamines, which are taken frequently, may further damage the liver or increase the bleeding tendency.

ASSISTING WITH COMPLICATIONS

BLEEDING. As previously mentioned, bleeding is a dreaded complication of cirrhosis. Nursing observations and interventions for the patient with gastrointestinal bleeding, described in Chapter 15, apply to this patient.

The patient who is bleeding from esophageal varices requires prompt treatment in order to save life. One or more of the following treatments may be indicated. Vasopressin (PITRESSIN) is a posterior pituitary hormone that may be infused to produce vasoconstriction in the area of the liver and a reduction in blood flow to the liver via the portal vein. A second form of therapy is to insert a gastric tube with balloons, which are then inflated to apply pressure to the bleeding varices. The Sengstaken-Blakemore tube is one type of tube the physician may select. This tube has several balloons. After inserting the tube into the esophagus and stomach, the physician inflates the balloons to apply pressure to the bleeding vessels in the esophagus. The tube has several openings similar to the Foley catheter. One opening allows the inflation of the balloon. Another opening may be connected to suction to empty the stomach of blood that has drained from bleeding varices.

Several operations may be done to stop bleeding by diverting blood from the liver, thus relieving pressure within the liver. A *portacaval shunt* may be done to divert blood flow from the liver by connecting the portal vein to the inferior vena cava. In a *splenorenal shunt,* the splenic vein, which carries blood from the spleen to the portal vein, is connected instead to the renal vein. The spleen is removed. Although these operations are extremely complicated and dangerous, they may save the life of a patient with bleeding esophageal varices.

A third relatively new form of therapy involves injecting the involved vessels with a sclerosing drug while the patient is having endoscopy.

The patient with bleeding esophageal varices is desperately ill. Such a person usually is cared for by specially trained physicians and nurses in the intensive care unit.

HEPATIC COMA. Hepatic coma is another dreaded complication of cirrhosis. It occurs when the liver is unable to remove ammonia from the blood and use it to make urea. Ammonia results from the action of bacteria that break down proteins in the intestine and also may occur as a result of other diseases.

As blood ammonia levels rise, the functions of brain, nervous system, acid-base balance, and kidneys are disturbed. The patient develops mental confusion, asterixis, abnormal breathing patterns, and a characteristic foul odor of the breath. These symptoms

should be reported to the physician at once so that prompt treatment can be started.

Generally, the physician orders a severe dietary protein restriction. Remembering that blood contains a large protein component enables the nurse to understand that bleeding from esophageal varices or other sites in the gastrointestinal tract may cause or worsen hepatic coma.

Cathartics and enemas may be prescribed to remove protein material from the intestine. Neomycin by mouth or rectum also may be prescribed to kill normal bacteria in the intestine so that they cannot act on protein and form ammonia.

Nursing measures that are appropriate to the care of the patient with cirrhosis also apply to this patient. In addition, the patient may be unconscious. Nursing care for the unconscious patient is described in Chapter 21.

Cancer of the Liver

Primary carcinoma of the liver, *hepatoma,* generally complicates cirrhosis of the liver. This form of cancer, which is quite uncommon, also may develop in plastic workers exposed to vinyl chloride. Carcinoma of the lung, breast, and gastrointestinal tract is likely to metastasize to the liver. In such a case, the patient has a secondary carcinoma of the liver. Cancer of the liver is usually fatal. Very few patients live for five years following diagnosis.

ASSISTING WITH DIAGNOSTIC STUDIES

In addition to liver function studies listed in Table 16.1, the physician usually orders a liver scan and a liver biopsy. Ultrasound and CAT scan may help to identify the location of the tumor and differentiate it from a cyst. A rising blood level of alpha-fetoprotein (AFP) also helps the physician to diagnose cancer of the liver.

NURSING OBSERVATIONS

The patient with cancer of the liver frequently has no early signs. Symptoms, which may develop gradually, include weakness, vague upper abdominal pain, and anorexia. Progressive anemia, jaundice, and respiratory distress may occur.

NURSING INTERVENTIONS

The nurse may assist the patient having surgery, radiation therapy, and/or chemotherapy for cancer of the liver. A discussion of these therapies can be located in Chapter 9.

LIVER TRANSPLANTATION

A relatively new experimental surgery involves transplantation of the liver. This surgery may become available for a few patients with chronic hepatic failure or malignancy which is localized. Currently, one of two techniques may be used. In one technique, the patient's liver is removed and the donor organ is substituted. In the other method, the patient's liver is left in place, and the donor organ is placed in a special space next to the vertebral column. The donor liver becomes an auxilliary (helper) liver. Following the transplant, the patient receives immunosuppressive therapy to prevent rejection of the donor tissue. Some patients have survived two or more years following a liver transplant. The interested nursing student may watch for continued developments in this field.

Cholelithiasis

The patient with cholelithiasis has gallstones. These are abnormal formations, calculi, that may develop anywhere in the biliary tract. However, they seem to form most often in the gallbladder. Gallstones are more common in women, especially after 40 years of age.

Factors that seem to favor the development of gallstones include obesity, diabetes, multiple pregnancies, use of oral contraceptives, and bowel resection for persons with Crohn's disease.

Whether gallstones can be visualized by x-ray examination depends upon their content. Some patients with gallstones may have no symptoms, and others develop acute cholecystitis with pain.

Acute Cholecystitis

The patient with acute cholecystitis has an inflammation of the gallbladder which frequently is associated with gallstones. Cholecystitis may be complicated by the formation of pus in the gallbladder, if the wall becomes gangrenous. Contents of the gallbladder escape through the hole into the peritoneal cavity, causing peritonitis. Another complication of cholecystitis may be *cholangitis*. This is an inflammation of the bile ducts. Both those within the liver and those leading from the liver may be inflamed. The patient develops jaundice if the inflammation and/or the stone obstructs the flow of bile from the liver to the intestine.

ASSISTING WITH DIAGNOSTIC STUDIES

The physician usually orders laboratory tests to help diagnose gallbladder disease. Bilirubin may be elevated in the blood and present in the urine. Alkaline phosphatase in the blood usually is elevated, also. Studies may include an abdominal x-ray, gallbladder series, and ultrasound. ERCP (refer to page 516) may be done to visualize the bile duct.

NURSING OBSERVATIONS

Pain is the most frequent symptom experienced by the patient with cholecystitis. Usually the pain is located either in the epigastrium or the right upper quadrant of the abdomen. Pain may radiate either to the right shoulder blade or around the abdomen to the back.

The patient may experience digestive disturbances such as indigestion, nausea, or flatulence, especially after eating fatty foods. Symptoms of inflammation which also may be present include malaise, fever, diaphoresis, and tachycardia. Jaundice does not occur if the infection affects only the gallbladder. As stated earlier, the patient develops jaundice when the flow of bile from the liver to the small intestine is obstructed.

NURSING INTERVENTIONS

SURGERY.   The usual treatment for the patient with cholecystitis is surgery. The surgeon may perform a *cholecystectomy,* which is removal of the gallbladder. In some cases, the surgeon explores the common bile duct at the time of surgery (*choledochostomy*) to locate stones. Following this type of surgery, a special drain, called a T tube, is inserted into the common bile duct. A *cholecystostomy* (incision into the gallbladder) may be done to provide temporary drainage when the patient's condition does not permit lengthier surgery. A larger drainage tubing is sutured into the gallbladder during this surgery. The patient requires postoperative care similar to that described in Chapter 6 with several variations.

Following surgery the patient is usually placed in Fowler's position. If a drainage tube is present, it should be attached to drainage. The amount of drainage should be measured and recorded. The tube is usually checked frequently for excessive drainage and bleeding. The nurse should report the presence of either to the appropriate nurse or surgeon.

In addition, special efforts are made to prevent the patient from developing pulmonary complications. The patient's incision usually is located in the upper right quadrant of the abdomen. Remembering the closeness of the operative site to the diaphragm, the nurse can understand easily why the patient avoids breathing deeply. The patient requires sufficient analgesia to participate actively and frequently in deep breathing, coughing, and turning. Usually, the patient ambulates within 24 hours postoperatively in order to prevent pulmonary complications.

The nurse should observe and report the color of the patient's stools. Knowing the color of the feces aids the doctor in determining when bile is reaching the intestines.

Occasionally, the patient continues to experience symptoms after surgery or experiences recurrent symptoms. This condition is called postcholecystectomy syndrome. The most common causes of the patient's symptoms are residual stones, recurring stones, or stricture of the duct. Additional surgery may be needed.

DIET. The patient with mild disease may be treated with a low-fat diet. In addition, the surgeon may advise a temporary dietary fat restriction for several weeks following surgery. Table 16.3 contains examples of foods permitted on low-fat diets.

Cancer of the Gallbladder

The gallbladder is rarely the site of neoplasm. The person with gallstones is more likely to develop carcinoma of the gallbladder than is the one without stones. Also, women seem to be affected more often than men. The early symptoms are similar to those of cholecystitis and cholelithiasis. The current treatment is surgical removal.

Pancreatitis

The patient with pancreatitis has an inflammation of the pancreas. Oddly enough, the pancreatic juice secreted by this gland begins to digest the cells of its producer. A disturbance to the ducts draining the cells of the pancreas of its fluid allows the juice to come in contact with pancreatic tissue. Pancreatic juice is so strong that it digests the patient's own tissues when it comes into direct contact with them.

Normally the pancreatic duct joins the common bile duct to form a short tube called the ampulla of Vater, which leads to the duodenum. Pancreatic juice and bile enter the small intestine through this tube during digestion. Realizing the close association between the pancreas and the biliary tract helps the nurse to understand that pancreatitis frequently occurs in connection with a disease of the biliary tract. Another cause of pancreatitis is alcoholism. Pancreatitis also may develop as a complication of abdominal surgery.

An acute case of pancreatitis may cause pus to form in this organ or the cells to die (which is referred to as gangrene). Another complication is hemorrhage. Bleeding occurs if a blood vessel is eroded by the pancreatic juice.

Patients having either a mild or a moderate case of pancreatitis have a better chance of recovery than do those with a severe case. Pancreatitis may become a chronic progressive disease.

TABLE 16.3
FOOD ALLOWANCES FOR TWO LEVELS OF FAT RESTRICTION (APPROXIMATELY 1500 KCAL)*

	20 GM FAT	50 GM FAT
Milk, skim	2 cups	2 cups
Meat, fish, poultry (lean)	6 ounces†	6 ounces†
Eggs (3 per week)	½	½
Vegetables		
Dark green leafy or deep yellow	1 serving	1 serving
Potato	1 serving	1 serving
Other	1 or more servings	1 or more servings
Fruits		
Citrus	1 serving	1 serving
Other	3 servings	3 servings
Breads and cereals		
Cereals	1 serving	1 serving
Breads	6 slices	3 slices
Fats, vegetable	none	6 teaspoons
Sweets	3 tablespoons	2 tablespoons
Total fat, gm	20	50
Cholesterol, mg	270‡	270‡
Protein, gm	85	80
Kcal (approximate)	1500	1500

* From Robinson, Corinne H., and Lawler, Marilyn R.: *Normal and Therapeutic Nutrition*, 16th ed., Macmillan Publishing Co., Inc., New York, 1982.
† Only lean cuts of meat, fish, poultry may be used. Each ounce is equivalent to 8 gm protein and 3 gm fat.
‡ Cholesterol level would be reduced to about half this level if eggs were not used. If butter is used instead of vegetable fat, the cholesterol level would be increased.

ASSISTING WITH DIAGNOSTIC STUDIES

The most important diagnostic test is the serum amylase which becomes markedly elevated during pancreatitis. Other tests that may be ordered include abdominal x-ray, ultrasound, and/or CAT scan. Endoscopic retrograde cholangiopancreatography (ERCP) may be done if chronic pancreatitis or neoplasm is suspected.

NURSING OBSERVATIONS

The patient usually seeks help for abdominal pain which tends to be steady and gradually becomes agonizing. At first, the pain may be located in the epigastrium or left upper quadrant of the abdomen. Later, the pain may radiate to the back. Other symptoms such as vomiting, fever, tachycardia, and hypotension also may be present. However, the patient with a more severe attack may have a subnormal temperature, cyanosis, cold and clammy skin, and a rapid, feeble pulse. Some patients have an impaired glucose tolerance, sugar in the urine, and a high blood sugar.

The patient with chronic pancreatitis usually has chronic pain which is less intense. In addition, the patient sometimes develops symptoms of diabetes caused by the gradual failure of pancreatic function. Other symptoms such as fatty diarrhea (steatorrhea) and weight loss are associated with malabsorption of nutrients.

NURSING INTERVENTIONS

DRUG THERAPY. Meperidine (DEMEROL) is the drug most often prescribed to relieve the severe pain associated with pancreatitis. Antibiotics and anticholinergic drugs such as atropine, which were once a common part of drug therapy, are prescribed rarely now. Antacids may be prescribed in some cases. The patient with chronic pancreatitis may need insulin and pancreatic extracts.

NASOGASTRIC SUCTION. A nasogastric tube is frequently inserted and attached to continuous suction when the patient is acutely ill. This therapy is believed to benefit the patient by reducing all stimuli to the flow of pancreatic secretions. Nursing observations and interventions for the patient with nasogastric suction can be located in Chapter 15.

FLUID REPLACEMENT. In severe cases, the inflammatory process may cause an internal loss of six or more liters of body fluids which collects in the patient's peritoneal spaces. Fluid replacement may include blood or blood products as well as electrolyte solutions. An important nursing responsibility is to monitor the patient's response to fluid therapy. The nurse calculates and maintains the correct flow rate, and observes the intravenous site for infiltration or phlebitis.

DIET. The patient with nasogastric suction receives nothing by mouth. As the patient's condition improves, the diet gradually progresses from liquids to a soft or bland diet. The patient with chronic pancreatitis usually requires an alteration in diet which includes a reduction in fat. The patient with associated hyperglycemia usually needs dietary modification for that condition.

Cancer of the Pancreas

The patient with cancer of the pancreas has a malignancy which is usually fatal within one year after diagnosis. The incidence of this form of cancer is rising for unknown reasons. Men are affected more often than women. The incidence of this cancer is also higher in heavy smokers and persons with diabetes mellitus.

ASSISTING WITH DIAGNOSTIC STUDIES

The physician who suspects cancer of the pancreas usually orders a CAT scan and/or ultrasound. Endoscopic retrograde cholangiopancreatography (ERCP) also may be done. A blood test for carcinoembryonic antigen (CEA) is usually elevated; however, this factor may be elevated in other circumstances, also.

NURSING OBSERVATIONS

Nursing observations vary with the location of the tumor. The patient with a neoplasm of the head of the pancreas usually develops jaundice. The patient with a neoplasm elsewhere in the pancreas may develop a dull epigastric pain which sometimes radiates to the back. There may be weight loss, anorexia, a metallic taste in the mouth, an aversion to meat, or diarrhea.

NURSING INTERVENTIONS

The patient with a localized malignancy in the pancreas may have surgery to resect the pancreas (pancreatoduodenectomy) or remove the pancreas (pancreatectomy). These procedures are associated with a high incidence of complications and death. The postoperative patient requires specially trained nurses and physicians and usually is placed in the intensive care unit. Radiation therapy and chemotherapy may be indicated for palliation. Nursing care for patients receiving these therapies can be located in Chapter 9. Examples of other disorders of the liver, biliary tract, or pancreas can be located in Table 16.4.

TABLE 16.4
OTHER DISORDERS OF THE LIVER, BILIARY TRACT, OR PANCREAS

COMMON DISORDER	DESCRIPTION
Choledocholithiasis	Stones in the common bile duct usually in association with cholelithiasis; biliary colic usually occurs; recommended treatment is surgical removal
Chronic persisting hepatitis (prolonged hepatitis) and recurrent hepatitis	A complication of acute viral hepatitis in which the patient has symptoms for several months; these symptoms may continue or they may improve only to be followed by a recurrence

TABLE 16.4 (*Continued*)
OTHER DISORDERS OF THE LIVER, BILIARY TRACT, OR PANCREAS

COMMON DISORDER	DESCRIPTION
Cystic fibrosis of the pancreas (mucoviscidosis)	An inheritable disease causing dysfunction of all exocrine glands as well as the mucus glands; usually seen in childhood but medical control is now enabling some persons with this disease to live to adulthood; pancreatic enzymes are usually lacking and chronic pulmonary disease generally develops
Fatty liver	A condition in which an abnormal amount of fat accumulates in the liver; may be associated with such conditions as carbon tetrachloride poisoning, protein malnutrition, and alcoholism
Fulminant hepatitis (massive hepatic necrosis)	An intense or severe case of hepatitis in which cells of the liver die; patient may die if the condition cannot be reversed
Hepatic coma (hepatic encephalopathy, portal-systemic encephalopathy)	A disturbance of consciousness associated with liver disease; patient may have personality changes, memory loss, or difficulty in concentrating; may go into a deep coma
Hepatic schistosomiasis	An infection of the liver by the ova of the flukes of the Schistosoma genus; in other words, ova of this parasite lodge in the liver and cause an infection
Portal hypertension	Increased pressure of blood in the portal vein of the liver can occur in heart failure, an obstruction of the main veins of the liver, and increased flow of blood; esophageal varices and ascites may occur
Subacute hepatic necrosis (submassive hepatic necrosis)	A complication of acute viral hepatitis in which cells of the liver die; death may be the result

Case Study Involving Cirrhosis

Mr. Daniels, a 50-year-old man, was admitted to the medical unit of the hospital with a diagnosis of cirrhosis with ascites caused by alcoholism. The nurse observed that Mr. Daniels was jaundiced and his abdomen appeared distended and taut. Mr. Daniels told the nurse that he is married and has two teen-aged children. He asked the nurse for some aspirin to relieve his headache.

The physician's orders included:

• Bed rest with bathroom privileges
• Daily weights
• Measure abdominal girth daily
• No sedatives, opiates, or tranquilizers
• High-protein, high-carbohydrate, low-sodium diet
• Spironolactone, 50 mg PO daily
• Strict intake and output
• All stools to lab for occult blood

QUESTIONS

1. What steps should the nurse take to obtain accurate measurements of weight and abdominal girth?
2. What nursing measures are indicated for Mr. Daniels in relation to jaundice?
3. What nursing measures are indicated for Mr. Daniels in relation to ascites?
4. What equipment and explanation should the nurse give to Mr. Daniels in order to maintain an accurate record of intake and output?
5. What is the reason for the physician's order "no sedatives, opiates, or tranquilizers"? What are the implications for the nurse?
6. How should the nurse respond to Mr. Daniels' request for aspirin? (*Hint:*What is the effect of aspirin on bleeding tendency?)
7. What nursing observations and measures are indicated for Mr. Daniels related to bleeding?
8. What effect will Mr. Daniels' jaundice have on the appearance of the stool and urine?
9. What nursing measures will help Mr. Daniels to have an adequate dietary intake?
10. What should the nurse know about spironolactone?
11. What patient and family teaching is indicated?
12. What community programs are available to help Mr. Daniels and the family?
13. How do the nurse's feelings and beliefs about alcoholism affect the care of Mr. Daniels?
14. What behavioral changes in Mr. Daniels should the nurse report at once?

15. What behavioral changes could be anticipated by the nurse in relationship to life-style changes that may be advised?

Case Study Involving Cholelithiasis

Mrs. Gale, a 45-year-old woman, was admitted to the hospital with a diagnosis of cholelithiasis. She told the nurse that she was probably going to have her gallbladder out later in the week. The physician's orders included:

- Cholecystogram in A.M.
- Ambulatory
- Diet as tolerated
- Prepare for cholecystectomy on Thursday

QUESTIONS

1. How should the nurse explain the cholecystogram to Mrs. Gale?
2. What dietary modification is needed prior to the cholecystogram?
3. What information should the nurse have before administering cholecystogram dye tablets to Mrs. Gale?
4. What information should the nurse give to Mrs. Gale about cholecystectomy?
5. What nursing observations and measures should the nurse anticipate for Mrs. Gale following cholecystectomy on Thursday?

Suggestions for Further Study

1. Find out what resources are available in your community to help the patient and his family when alcoholism is the cause of cirrhosis.
2. Visit the dietitian to find out how diets are prepared for the patient who requires a high-protein, high-carbohydrate diet.
3. Prepare a skit in which one person plays an individual displaying obvious behavioral changes and another plays the nurse. Compare feelings, thoughts, and actions.
4. Mason, Mildred A.; Bates, Grace F.; and Smola, Bonnie K.: *Workbook in Basic Medical-Surgical Nursing,* 3rd ed. Macmillan Publishing Company, New York, 1984, Exercise 16.

Additional Readings

Griffiths, Mary: *Human Physiology,* 2nd ed. Macmillan Publishing Co., Inc., New York, 1981, pp. 229–30.

Kosel, Kathy, *et al.:* "Total Pancreatectomy and Islet Cell Autotransplantation." *American Journal of Nursing,* 82:568–71 (Apr.), 1982.

Mar, Dexter D.: "New Hepatitis B Vaccine: A Breakthrough in Hepatitis Prevention." *American Journal of Nursing,* 82:306–307 (Feb.), 1982.

Robinson, Corinne H.: *Basic Nutrition and Diet Therapy,* 4th ed. Macmillan Publishing Co., Inc., New York, 1980, pp. 292–97.

Robinson, Corinne H., and Lawler, Marilyn R.: *Normal and Therapeutic Nutrition,* 16th ed. Macmillan Publishing Co., Inc., New York, 1982, pp. 563–77.

"Test Yourself: Acute Pancreatitis." *American Journal of Nursing,* 82:64, 186 (Jan.), 1982.

Thompson, Donald A.: "Teaching the Client about Anticoagulants." *American Journal of Nursing,* 82:278–81 (Feb.), 1982.

Thorpe, Constance J., and Caprini, Joseph A.: "Gallbladder Disease: Current Trends and Treatments." *American Journal of Nursing,* 80:2181–85 (Dec.), 1980.

Chapter 17

The Patient with a Disease of the Musculoskeletal System*

Expected Behavioral Outcomes

Minimum objectives referred to as expected behavioral outcomes have been designed for the practical/vocational nursing student to use as guides in studying this chapter. The student should read these expected outcomes before studying the chapter. The objectives can be used as guides for study.

Using the content of this chapter, the student should return to the objectives and evaluate the ability to:

1. *Formulate two new terms for each prefix, suffix, or combining form.*
2. *Differentiate between osteoporosis and osteomyelitis in regard to definition, symptoms, and nursing care.*

3. *Discuss the nursing care needed by the patient with arthritis.*
4. *Compare the drugs for arthritis used to treat three patients in your hospital as indicated by their charts with those discussed in this text.*
5. *Compare the similarities and differences indicated for the nursing care of a patient in a cast and of a patient in traction.*
6. *Demonstrate the four-point gait and swing-through gait on crutches.*
7. *Relate the five stages of the grieving process to the feelings likely to be experienced by the patient having an amputation. Outline the preoperative and postoperative measures indicated for the patient having an amputation.*
8. *Differentiate between gout and arthritis in regard to cause, symptoms, and treatment.*
9. *List the five Ps of neurovascular impairment.*
10. *Describe the nursing interventions*

---

*Revised by the authors and Lydia Amores Villanueva, R.N., B.S., who is a Practical Nursing Instructor at the Central School of Practical Nursing in Norfolk, Virginia *that prevent complications associated with immobility.*

Vocabulary Development

The following prefixes, suffixes, and combining forms pertain to this chapter. By learning and/or reviewing their meanings, the practical/vocational nursing student will have the keys needed to unlock many exciting new medical terms.

Discover the meaning of these keys in a medical dictionary or in the content of this chapter. How does each key pertain to this chapter? In your notebook write the correct meaning of each prefix, suffix, or combining form listed below. Illustrate each key with an example.

Ankyl—crooked, looped. Ex. *ankylo*mele—a curved probe.

arthr-	ost(e)-
articul-	ped-
chondr-	peri-
dis-	plas-
dur-	-plasty
fract-	poly-
malac-	scler-
my-	spas-
myel-	tens-
orth-	tract-
oss-	troph-

Structure and Function

The muscular and skeletal systems provide structure, support, and movement for the body. Since both systems work cooperatively, a term often used is *musculoskeletal system.* Another term, *locomotor system,* refers to the function of movement made possible by muscles and bones. This includes movement of internal organs such as the heart and intestines as well as visible movement of arms, legs, and other body parts.

The skeletal system is composed of the bones, joints, and connective tissues, such as ligaments and tendons (see Figure 17.1). These tissues bind the bones and muscles together. The skeletal system helps to support the body, to move the body, to support and protect certain organs, and to maintain such mineral reserves as calcium in the body. Another function of the skeletal system is to manufacture blood cells, which are produced by red marrow of the bones (see Table 17.1 for a listing of laboratory tests performed on blood cells).

Bone is a highly specialized form of connective tissue which contains hard, compact tissue as well as a soft, spongy network of marrow. Compact bone, the exterior part, contains a canal system with blood vessels to nourish bone tissue, bone-forming cells, and special cellular processes which continuously form and resorb bone. Marrow, the inner part, contains specialized cells and processes related to the manufacture of blood cells, as described in Chapter 13.

Bones are covered by a dense connective tissue called periosteum. The inner aspect contains osteoblasts, bone cells that have the ability to produce more bones. The periosteum carries the blood and nerve supplies making this structure essential for bone nutrition, growth, and repair.

A long bone consists of a shaft or diaphysis and expanded ends called epiphyses. During the growing years, a plate of cartilage remains in the area between the diaphysis and the epiphyses. This is called the metaphysis or epiphyseal line which allows for longitudinal growth. The metaphyses calcify into bone tissue by age 17 years. Both epiphyses are capped with an articular cartilage where a joint is formed with another bone.

Joints are places of union of two more bones. The area of a bone that comes into close contact with another bone is known as the *articular surface.* These surfaces are separated by a softer substance, such as cartilage, which helps to absorb the jars of body movement. Most of the joints are freely movable. In this case, the articular end of the bones is protected by a capsule in addition to the cartilage. This capsule is lined with *synovial membrane,* which gives protection by secreting *synovia,* which acts as a lubricant. It is a clear fluid similar in appearance to egg white. Some joints are protected by *bursae.* These are small sacs made of syn-

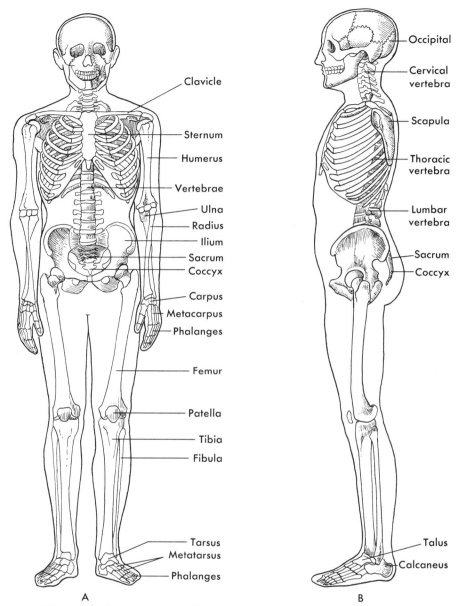

FIGURE 17.1 *A*. The human skeleton, front view. *B*. The human skeleton, side view. (From Miller, Marjorie A.; Drakontides, Anna B.; and Leavell, Lutie C.: *Kimber-Gray-Stackpole's Anatomy and Physiology*, 17th ed. Macmillan Publishing Co., Inc., New York, 1977.)

ovial membrane and filled with fluid. Bursae help to protect joints, bony prominences, tendons, and ligaments from the effects of friction produced by movement.

Muscles are specialized forms of tissue that help to move and support. Skeletal mus-

cle, also called striated muscle, is attached to the skeleton and is capable of rapid, powerful contraction. Contraction and relaxation of skeletal muscles enable the person to move about. Smooth muscle is located on the outer walls of the gastrointestinal tract and

TABLE 17.1
LABORATORY TESTS FREQUENTLY PERFORMED IN CONNECTION WITH THE
MUSCULOSKELETAL SYSTEM

NAME OF TEST	NORMAL VALUE	INDICATION OF ABNORMALITY
Aldolase	3–8 S-L units/ml	Elevation indicates the presence of musculoskeletal diseases, cancer, hepatitis, anemia, or leukemia
Bence Jones protein (urine)	Negative	Positive result indicates presence of bone tumor
Complete blood count	See Table 5.4 (page 93–4)	
Electrophoresis, protein	Albumin: 3.2–5.6 gm/100 ml Alpha-1 globulin: 0.1–0.4 gm/100 ml Alpha-2 globulin: 0.4–1.2 gm/100 ml Beta globulin: 0.5–1.1 gm/100 ml Gamma globulin: 0.5–1.6 gm/100 ml	Decrease may indicate some infection or neoplasm
Erythrocyte sedimentation rate	Men under 50 years <15 mm/hr Men over 50 years <20 mm/hr Women under 50 years <20 mm/hr Women over 50 years <30 mm/hr	Increase may indicate an infection and conditions of cell destruction
Hematocrit	Male: 40–54 volumes % Female: 37–47 volumes %	Decrease may indicate blood loss and increase may indicate dehydration
LE cell preparation	Negative	Positive result indicates lupus erythematosus
Phosphatase alkaline	King-Armstrong units: 4–13 Bodansky units: 1.5–4.5 Bessy-Lowry units: 0.8–2.3	Increase may indicate bone tumors, leukemia, or excessive amounts of vitamin D
Rheumatic factor	Negative	Positive result confirms the diagnosis of rheumatoid arthritis
Serum enzyme tests Serum alpha-hydroxybutyrate dehydrogenase (SHBD)	15–150 units	Increase in these enzymes may indicate cell destructions in the heart, liver, muscles, kidneys, or pancreas
Serum creatine phosphokinase (SCPK)	0–4 units	
Serum glutamic oxaloacetic transaminase (SGOT)	8–40 units	
Serum glutamic pyruvic transaminase (SGPT)	5–35 units	

Table 17.1 (*Continued*)
LABORATORY TESTS FREQUENTLY PERFORMED IN CONNECTION WITH THE
MUSCULOSKELETAL SYSTEM

NAME OF TEST	NORMAL VALUE	INDICATION OF ABNORMALITY
Uric acid	Male: 2.1–7.8 mg/100 ml Female: 2.0–6.4 mg/100 ml	Increase confirms the diagnosis of gout

the walls of blood vessels. Contraction and relaxation of smooth muscle cause the diameters of the intestines and blood vessels to become widened or narrowed. Cardiac muscle is the tissue that forms the heart. The contraction and relaxation of cardiac muscle cause blood to move through the circulatory system.

Ligaments are special forms of tissue that support, strengthen, and connect bones or cartilages. Tendons are special forms of tissue that attach a muscle to bone or other structure. In addition to healthy structures in the musculoskeletal system, an energy supply, intact circulation, and stimulation by the nervous system are needed for movement.

Orthopedics is the branch of surgery that specializes in the treatment of a patient with a disease of the locomotor system. The physician in this specialty is called an orthopedist.

Assisting with Diagnostic Studies

Table 17.2 contains a list of diagnostic tests that may be done when the patient has

TABLE 17.2
COMMON DIAGNOSTIC PROCEDURES

I. Physical Examination

Inspection—The orthopedist may be able to note a deformity, unusual appearance, contour, and color of a part in comparison with the rest of the body as a whole

Palpation—The examiner may detect tenderness, muscle spasm, and temperature changes by palpation

Range of motion—Range of motion can be measured passively or actively. Passive joint motion is carried out by the examiner and active joint motion is carried out by the patient. Motion is limited by pain, muscle spasm, in-

flammation, scarring in the joints, and deformity of the bone

Joint position—The examiner may be able to determine whether a patient is favoring a position of comfort rather than a position of function. A patient with a joint condition naturally assumes a position of comfort that is usually the reverse of the position of function. The physician's responsibility is to support the joint in its position of function in order to minimize disability

II. X-Ray Examination

In order to evaluate the extent or characteristic of the bone lesion or deformity, x-ray pictures are taken at different angles

Arthrogram—A radiopaque dye or air is injected into a joint cavity and visualized by x-ray. This is useful in determining possible tears and other trauma of the soft tissue of the joint not normally seen by ordinary x-ray

Bone scan—A radioactive material is injected intravenously. After a determined time, usually an hour, the patient is taken to the "scan room," where special equipment (scanner) will scan the whole body, in sections, to locate any bone damages resulting from inflammations, degenerations, abnormal growths, and malignancies

Computerized axial tomography (CAT scan, CT scan)—Multiple x-ray beams are passed through the body at various angles and levels and a computerized scanning system recores the image

Laminogram (tomogram)—Visualizes specific layers of tissue or bone. This provides more details of an area than that obtained by a plain or flat film

III. Laboratory Studies

See Table 17.1

IV. Special Tests

Arthroscopy—A telescopic instrument is inserted into the joint to visualize the internal joint structure. Surgery on the meniscus can be done through an arthroscope

Bone marrow aspiration—This is a microscopic examination of bone marrow obtained by needle aspiration. Sites of aspiration are the iliac crest, sternum, or posterior ileum

Electromyography—This is used to test the nerve conduction to the skeletal muscle. Special needles are inserted directly into the muscle for the purpose of recording electrical activities of the muscle

Joint aspiration—This procedure is performed by inserting a long needle into the joint to obtain fluid to be examined for blood, pus, and microorganisms. This is done under aseptic technique with a local anesthetic

Muscle biopsy—The tissue may be obtained through a surgical incision or by a special type of needle or bore introduced through the skin

a disturbance in the musculoskeletal system. When assisting the patient during a diagnostic study, the nurse should remember that such a patient generally has impaired movement. Thus, the patient often needs help to put an x-ray gown on, get into a wheelchair, or change positions when indicated.

Nursing Observations

Many patients have disturbances in the musculoskeletal system that result from ac-

cident and/or injury. When observing such a patient, the nurse is especially alert to undetected conditions that may either cause or result from an accident or injury. For example, one person may fall as a result of dizziness caused by a drug interaction. Another person may trip as a result of rushing to the bathroom because of diarrhea or a urinary tract infection. When musculoskeletal injury has occurred from an accident, other undetected damage also may be present such as head or spleen injury, or fractures. The nurse caring for the patient is often the first one to uncover undetected problems. Therefore, the nurse does not confine observations only to those listed in Table 17.3 but uses the table as a guide to observing the whole person.

OBSERVING THE PATIENT'S AFFECTED PART

When observing the injured body part, the nurse usually finds it helpful to compare it to the uninjured body part on the patient's opposite side. A very important part of this observation is looking for evidence of *neurovascular impairment* (damage to blood and nerve supply). The process of checking for this impairment is sometimes called a *circulation and sensation check*. To do a circulation and sensation check, the nurse looks for the five Ps that indicate damage to the blood

TABLE 17.3
GUIDE TO OBSERVING THE PATIENT WITH A MUSCULOSKELETAL DISORDER

WHAT TO LOOK AT	WHAT TO LOOK FOR
Head and neck	Restriction of movement
	Presence of eyeglasses or hearing aids important to safe ambulation
Chest	Presence of petechiae which may indicate fat emboli
	Adequate respiratory excursion, especially if ribs are injured
Abdomen and back	Presence of petechiae which may indicate fat emboli
Extremities	Obvious deformities
	Restriction of motion or increased pain with motion
	Neurovascular impairment—5 Ps
	Edema, erythema, ecchymoses
Ambulation	Postural deformities
	Gait abnormalities
	Use of aids to ambulation
Behavioral changes	Disorientation may indicate undetected head injury or sensory disturbances from immobility
	Feelings of apathy, anger, helplessness, resentment, withdrawal are common when mobility curtailed
	Restlessness, frequent changes of position may indicate pain

and nerve supply—pallor, pulse changes, paresthesia (abnormal sensations), pain, and paralysis. Remembering the five Ps of neurovascular impairment enables the nurse to report them promptly when observed. As mentioned in Chapter 12, coolness of the patient's skin when compared to the similar area on the uninjured side also may indicate neurovascular impairment.

Other components of the nurse's observation of an injured body part include looking for obvious anatomic deformities, edema, erythema, or ecchymoses. When edema and ecchymoses are observed, the nurse usually measures the circumference of the affected part, if possible. This provides a basis for evaluating an increase or decrease of bleeding. A restriction of movement or an increase of pain during movement is observed and reported. When reporting this observation, the nurse usually describes the type of movement involved (flexion or extension, internal or external rotation).

OBSERVING THE PATIENT'S AMBULATION

The patient with a musculoskeletal disorder often shows a disturbance in ambulation. Observing the patient's ambulation enables the nurse to report abnormalities as well as select nursing interventions that prevent accidents.

One aspect of ambulation the nurse observes is posture, the relative position of the body. A person's posture develops from an interaction of hereditary factors, the condition of the musculoskeletal system, and habit. Posture also reflects the person's self concept. Normal posture is one that maintains physiologic curves in the body and does not place abnormal stresses on the musculoskeletal system. Abnormalities in posture may either cause or result in weak muscles, fatigue, pain, and dysfunction of internal body organs. Postural features the nurse should observe include level shoulders and hips as well as whether vertebrae are straight. Examples of postural deformities the nurse should observe and report include:

- Kyphosis—exaggeration of normal S curve in the thoracic spine.
- Lordosis—exaggeration of normal S curve in the lumbar spine
- Scoliosis—abnormal lateral curve of spine
- Genu varus—bow leg
- Genu valgus—knock-knees

Gait is the patient's pattern of walking which involves a complex interaction of the musculoskeletal and nervous systems. Normal gait is a smooth, even, heel-and-toe walk, accompanied by a coordinated swing of the arms. The patient with a disturbance in the musculoskeletal system may show a disturbance in gait. For example, the patient with *antalgic gait* has a limp adopted to avoid pain on weight-bearing structures. The patient with an *ataxic gait* has an unsteady, uncoordinated walk using a wide base of support. The nurse describes and reports a gait abnormality.

A change in gait may be indicated when the patient uses an aid to ambulation such as crutches, a cane, or a walker. These special gaits are described later in the chapter. In addition, the nurse observes the patient who is admitted to the hospital with an ambulation aid to be sure that it is used safely and correctly.

OBSERVING FOR PAIN

The patient with a musculoskeletal disorder often has pain. Pain may result from the patient's disease or methods used to treat it. In some cases, pain may signal invisible damage occurring under a cast, for example. As previously mentioned, pain is one of the five Ps of of neurovascular impairment. Therefore, the nurse carefully reports the patient's pain with reference to location, intensity, and description. The patient in pain may seem restless and may change positions frequently. When moving, the patient frequently attempts to immobilize the painful area by holding it or keeping it stiff. A common type of pain experienced by the patient with a disturbance in the musculoskeletal system is muscle spasm or cramping, powerful involuntary muscle contractions affecting flexor muscles. Muscle spasms may be caused by ischemia and hypoxia of muscle tissue. Nursing interventions related to relieving the patient's pain are described later in this chapter. A practice the nurse avoids is automatically administering an analgesic without carefully investigating the cause of pain.

OBSERVING BEHAVIORAL CHANGES

The patient with a musculoskeletal disorder may show behavioral changes as a result of pain, undetected head injury, immobility, or complications related to the underlying condition. Since behavior changes often appear before other symptoms develop, the nurse carefully observes and reports unexpected changes. For example, the patient who has been alert and participating in conversation in the morning is expected to be able to continue that activity. Withdrawal from conversation, increasing drowsiness, or agitation and irritability are examples of changes in behavior that should be reported.

A musculoskeletal disorder may cause the patient to become immobilized for a time. When immobilization is extensive or prolonged, the patient may be either deprived of usual environmental stimulation or respond to it differently. A patient lying in a bed actually sees the world differently with respect to depth, length, width, time, and other factors. These distortions, although common, may cause considerable anxiety to the uninformed patient who may be afraid to mention them for fear of seeming "crazy." Other effects of perceptual distortions include dropping things on the floor, over- or underestimating the amount of effort needed to lift, turn, or move, and miscalculating the distance from bed to wheelchair. Occasionally, the patient who is immobilized develops auditory or visual hallucinations (hearing or seeing things not actually present in the environment). These behavioral changes are not expected and should be reported at once.

Behavioral changes also are influenced by a disturbance in body image associated with alterations, immobility, and appearance. The extent of the disturbance is related to the part of the body affected and the meaning to the patient. For example, the patient with a fracture of the nondominant arm may experience less of a disturbance than the person with a fracture of the dominant arm who requires assistance to eat, bathe, and dress.

Nursing Interventions

Nursing interventions for the patient with a musculoskeletal disorder are influenced by the individual patient, the extent of immobility, and the type of medical therapy. Generally, the patient is encouraged to be as active as possible. In addition, the nurse creates opportunities whenever possible for the patient to make decisions and direct aspects of care.

A major goal of nursing interventions when the nurse cares for the patient with a musculoskeletal disorder is preventing complications associated with immobility. For example, *pressure sores* may result from prolonged and continuous pressure from body weight or from appliances. Areas vulnerable to pressure necrosis are the sacrum, heels, ankles, shoulder blades, and the hips where the bony prominences are located. If the redness of these areas does not disappear following release from the pressure, tissue damage most likely has occurred. The nurse may prevent tissue necrosis by relieving the pressure and providing good skin care. *Hypostatic pneumonia* is caused by a pooling of respiratory secretions in the lungs. The recumbent position, inadequate lung expansion, respiratory depression from sedatives, and inadequate fluid intake contribute to stasis of bronchial secretions. Measures to prevent this pooling of secretions include turning, changing positions, alternating the height of the elevation of the head from high to low Fowler's position, deep breathing followed by coughing, and increasing fluid intake. *Thrombophlebitis* is the most common circulatory complication of immobility. Venous stasis usually occurs in the lower trunk and lower extremities. If surgery or trauma is added to the circulatory stasis, blood clots are more likely to develop. Increased viscosity of the blood caused by dehydration or insufficient fluid intake also predisposes to thrombophlebitis. Exercises, especially of the lower extremities, are particularly important in the prevention of venous stasis. Dorsiflexion and plantar flexion of the feet speed up blood flow in the extremities. Elastic support stockings often are ordered for patients on bed rest to prevent thrombophlebitis. The pressure exerted by the stockings on the peripheral blood vessels diverts the sluggish peripheral circulation to the deeper and larger blood vessels which have a more forceful circulation. *Contracture* may result from constant flexion or extension of a muscle group. Flexion contracture is more common because flexor muscles are generally stronger than extensor muscles. *Disuse atrophy* may occur in both muscles and bones. During inactivity, the muscle loses size and strength. An individual placed in prolonged leg traction develops decreasing calf circumference and weakness in the affected leg. *Disuse osteoporosis* (loss of calcium or demineralization) may occur as a result of immobility. Although the mechanisms are not understood completely, a decrease in the rate of normal bone-forming processes is associated with continued normal bone destruction. Complications of osteoporosis are pathologic fractures and urinary tract calculi. Range-of-motion exercises, isometric exercises, early ambulation, weight-bearing, and correct positioning are measures that prevent contractures, disuse atrophy, and disuse osteoporosis. *Renal calculi* are brought about by the increased amount of calcium salts filtering through the kidneys. Disuse osteoporosis, stasis of urine, and alkalinity of urine, which result from decreased activity, favor the precipitation of calcium leading to stone formation. Preventive measures are increased fluid intake, regularly scheduled position change, and bed exercises.

ASSISTING WITH HYGIENE

The client with a musculoskeletal problem may be too uncomfortable or too discouraged to remain well groomed. However, attention to personal hygiene contributes much to lifting the patient's morale. The patient usually is encouraged to perform as many activities of personal care as possible because active movement is beneficial. The

nurse may administer analgesia if pain interferes with the patient's participation. The immobilized patient usually needs assistance with back, perineal, and foot care. The patient on bed rest may require perineal care after each elimination in order to cleanse urine and feces from the skin. It is especially important that the woman patient receive help because she is unable to cleanse and wipe from front to back while in bed. Perineal wiping and cleansing from front to back prevent the introduction of normal flora from the intestine to the urethra or vagina where they may cause infection.

Skin breakdown is a primary concern of the nurse caring for a patient confined to bed or otherwise immobilized. Constant pressure to the superficial capillaries leads to ischemia of the skin and eventual tissue breakdown. Nursing care should be directed at relieving pressure and giving good skin care. Pressure can be relieved by following a schedule of turning and using devices that distribute body weight over a large area. Cleanliness, gentle massage, and maintaining the normal skin oils greatly influence the patient's skin condition.

Lacerations and abrasions may be present as a result of an accident that has caused the patient's injury. Since these breaks in the skin barrier may become sources of infection, they are cleansed regularly. The patient's hair, eyes, ears, nose, fingernails, and toenails may require repeated cleaning in order to remove dirt, gravel, or glass after an accident.

ALTERATIONS IN DIET AND FLUIDS

Good nutrition is essential in order to enhance tissue repair in the musculoskeletal system. A diet high in protein, calcium, and vitamins C and D may be prescribed. Vitamin C aids in wound healing, and vitamin D is needed in bone repair and aids the transport of calcium from the intestinal tract to the bloodstream. Calcium and protein are essential components in bone and tissue repair.

Minor alteration in the diet of patients confined to bed reduces the use of laxatives and enemas for bowel elimination. Increased roughage and increased fluid intake may prevent constipation.

The patient's caloric needs are calculated on the basis of existing weight and activity levels. The patient who is overweight may have difficulty using crutches or regaining muscle strength. The patient who is underweight also may be undernourished. Small, frequent feedings may be indicated for the patient who is anorexic or extensively immobilized.

The patient with a musculoskeletal disorder usually needs an increased fluid intake because of reduced mobility. Prolonged immobility brings about urinary stasis, urine alkalinity, and increased excretion of calcium salt. These events favor the formation of stones in the urinary tract, as described in Chapter 19. Increasing the fluid intake is one intervention that helps to prevent such complications. The patient may drink cranberry juice to make the urine more acid.

ASSISTING WITH ELIMINATION

The patient with a musculoskeletal disorder often experiences difficulties in urinating and defecating as a result of changes in activity, fluids and diet, reduction of privacy, analgesia, and the need to use bedpans and urinals when confined to bed. A complicating factor is the need to wait for help in order to use the bedpan. The combination of these events often results in urinary retention and/or constipation.

A key to preventing elimination problems is early recognition. The informed patient may participate by reporting difficulties to the nurse so that action may be taken early. For example, the immobilized patient who has not had a bowel movement for several days may be given prune juice or some other food or liquid to stimulate defecation. The patient often has a preferred program which has been helpful in the past. When possible, this program should be used in the hospital.

The nurse may help to prevent or correct these problems by assisting the patient to increase fluids and dietary roughage, develop and sustain an exercise program, and by providing as much privacy as possible during elimination. Fracture pans, small flat bedpans, are available for the patient in a cast or in traction. Most patients may be helped by following a pattern of elimination which resembles that of the usual life-style. For example, the patient who usually has a bowel movement daily after breakfast is less likely to become constipated if that pattern continues during hospitalization. Another nursing action that prevents elimination problems is responding promptly to the patient's request for assistance. Stool softeners may be prescribed for the patient who is immobilized. In some cases, laxatives, suppositories, and/or enemas may be needed; however, these often can be avoided by preventive nursing measures.

MAINTAINING A SAFE ENVIRONMENT

In creating a safe environment for the hospitalized patient, the nurse should consider known dangers such as weak and sometimes disabled people, a high concentration of pathogens, oxygen, radiations, waxed floors, and people hurrying. As long as the hospital staff is constantly aware of these hazards, accidents may be prevented. The patient with a musculoskeletal disorder often has additional risks related to changes in usual mobility caused by the injury or the therapy. For example, the patient who is learning to use crutches, a walker, or a leg prosthesis is at risk of falling or tripping. The patient confined to bed may misjudge the distance when reaching for a needed object and fall out of bed. The patient may injure fingers or toes in a wheelchair. Understanding the nature of the increased risk for accidents enables the nurse to maintain a high level of safety awareness when caring for a patient with a musculoskeletal disorder. Table 17.4 contains a summary of nursing actions related to maintaining a safe environment. A good safety practice is to develop a systematic method of observing the environment to identify and correct hazards. An example of one method is to start with the ceiling and work systematically down the wall to and including the floor.

TABLE 17.4
SUMMARY OF NURSING INTERVENTIONS THAT MAINTAIN A SAFE ENVIRONMENT

1. Obtain the patient's cooperation, when possible, by describing facts related to safety and the specific condition.
2. Develop a systematic method of observing the patient's environment to identify, remove, or modify hazards.
3. Place the patient's bed in as low a position as possible.
4. Place objects frequently used within easy reach of the patient, including the call bell.
5. Develop a practice of answering call lights as soon as possible to prevent hazardous activities such as long stretches to reach a bedpan or urinal.
6. Supervise patients who are learning new forms of ambulation such as crutch walking.
7. Discuss the relationship of perceptual distortions and safety with the patient who is immobilized.
8. Remove spills and objects from the floor around the patient's bed, in the bathroom, or in hallways.
9. Ensure that every patient wears appropriate footwear when ambulating.
10. Obtain the number of persons needed for safely lifting and moving the patient with a musculoskeletal disorder.

An additional area of safety relates to the need for frequent lifting, turning, and otherwise moving a patient with altered mobility. The nurse's safety is enhanced by using good body mechanics, appropriate lift techniques, and an adequate number of people.

REPOSITIONING

Appropriate positioning of the patient is a nursing intervention that alternates pressure areas on the skin, prevents contractures and deformities, and provides comfort and additional stimulation. Usually, the nurse is guided in selecting specific positions by normal body alignment as well as the patient's comfort. However, the patient with a musculoskeletal disorder may be positioned in specific ways, either to promote healing of a body part or to prevent complications related to the injury or therapy. For example, the patient whose condition involves the lower extremities usually has the legs positioned in abduction (away from the body) to prevent subluxation (partial dislocation). When specific alignment of a body part is indicated, artificial devices usually are needed. For example, an abduction splint or device may be applied between the patient's legs to keep them apart (abducted). Sandbags may be used to maintain a body part in the prescribed position.

Prolonged positioning of any joint in either continous flexion or extension gener-
ally is avoided to prevent complications such as contractures and footdrop. For example, the patient confined to bed may prefer a sitting position both during the day and for sleeping. During the sitting position, the hip joint is flexed. Prolonged hip flexion may result in a complication known as hip-flexion contracture. This complication, in turn, interferes with a person's ability to walk. Thus, the patient's position is changed frequently so that continuous flexion or extension of the joints is avoided. The informed patient may participate in maintaining positions that prevent complications. For example, the nurse and the patient may develop a schedule for certain position changes which the patient implements using electric bed controls to raise and lower the head and foot.

Before moving the patient to a new position, it may be necessary to administer analgesia to prevent pain. The area on which the patient will be turned may be massaged beforehand with lotion to improve circulation. After turning the patient, the area on which the patient has been lying is inspected for signs of pressure and massaged. Remembering the perceptual distortions described earlier in the chapter enables the nurse to explain the turning procedure in advance. Obtaining the number of persons needed and appropriate positioning devices are nursing measures that help to provide a smooth, safe turn, both for the patient and the nurse (Figures 17.2 and 17.3).

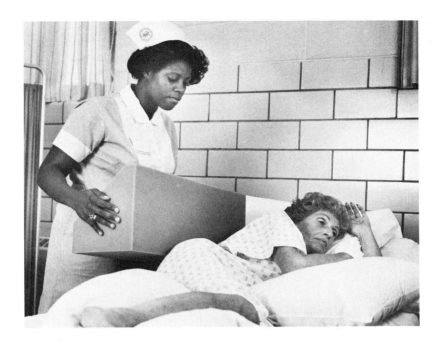

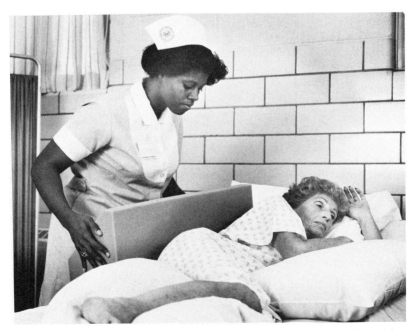

FIGURES 17.2 and 17.3   Using a positioning device to change the patient's position. (Courtesy of Shapero School of Nursing, Sinai Hospital of Detroit, Detroit, Michigan.)

PREVENTING INFECTION

The nurse who is caring for the patient with a musculoskeletal disorder has special concerns about infection. Since many conditions occur as a result of accidents, one common concern of the nurse is the increased hazard of infection caused by abrasions, lacerations, and other breaks in the skin barrier. A second area of concern relates to infection in the pulmonary or urinary systems which may result from prolonged immobility, inadequate fluid intake, and alterations of normal breathing patterns. A third area of concern relates to the patient with surgical intervention into the bone either for traction or repair. This provides a direct entry into bone for pathogens. The patient with a compound fracture also has an increased risk of infection. Last, early signs of infection may be hidden under a cast or dressing. Infection from any of these sites eventually may cause the patient to develop osteomyelitis (infection of the bone). This infection, described later in the chapter, is difficult to treat successfully and may cause permanent disability and chronic pain to the patient. Therefore, nursing measures, such as those listed in Table 17.5 related to the prevention of infection, are a vital component of the nursing care plan. Signs of infection such as fever, malaise, unpleasant odors, unexpected drainage, or a change in usual drainage are reported at once so that the source of infection can be located and appropriate treatment initiated.

MANAGING PAIN AND DISCOMFORT

Clients with musculoskeletal diseases and trauma experience several kinds of pain because of the multiple involvement of bones, muscles, nerves, and other connective tissues. Pain from a bone injury is described as aching or boring, whereas pain from a muscle is sore or aching. Other kinds of pain result from prolonged pressure over bony prominences, described as burning. Swelling under bandages or casts interferes with blood supply and causes excruciating pain. Muscle spasms may occur from disuse and mechanical pressure from the bed or chair on the blood vessels in the muscle.

When responding to the patient's report of pain, the nurse listens carefully to the patient's description before selecting a pain-relieving measure. Practices the nurse avoids include automatically responding to the patient's report of pain by administering an analgesic or permitting a lengthy period to elapse before responding to the patient's report of pain. Such practices may introduce special hazards to the patient with a musculoskeletal disease. Remembering that pain is one of the five Ps of neurovascular impairment enables the nurse to understand that relieving the patient's pain with analgesia will not restore impaired circulation. Thus, the patient who reports pain is observed carefully for the other four Ps of neurovascular impairment in the painful area (pallor, pulselessness, paresthesia, paralysis) before a pain-relieving measure is selected. When

TABLE 17.5
PREVENTING INFECTION IN THE PATIENT WITH A MUSCULOSKELETAL CONDITION

1. Cleanse all abrasions, lacerations, and other breaks in the skin barrier using an antibacterial substance if prescribed.
2. Cleanse the patient's perineum from front to back after each elimination.
3. Encourage and supervise deep-breathing and coughing exercises on a scheduled basis.
4. Help the patient on bed rest to increase fluid intake to at least 1.5 L per day, unless the physician's orders prescribe reduced or increased amounts.
5. Follow the physician's orders or hospital policy related to pin care for the patient with skeletal traction or dressing changes for the surgical patient.
6. Report any indication of infection, including symptoms relating to other body systems such as cough, dysuria, erythema, and warmth around an intravenous site.
7. Take all measures necessary to prevent skin breakdown.
8. Practice frequent handwashing.

evidence of neurovascular impairment is present, the physician is notified at once.

Although careful observation of pain is important, the client should not be allowed to suffer needlessly. In selecting pain-relieving measures, the nurse may refer to Table 7.1 for guidance. As mentioned in Chapter 7, pain is relieved more readily if analgesic is given before the pain becomes too severe. Sometimes pain can be made tolerable by the nurse's comfort measures such as backrubs, tightening linen, fluffing pillows, or saying words of encouragement. Pain or discomfort may be reduced by proper alignment, releasing pressure over bony prominences, supporting painful extremities on pillows, avoiding sharp, sudden movements, or using turning sheets to prevent uneven pulling. Other measures the nurse may select to relieve pain include distraction, repositioning, application of heat or cold, and relaxation. Discussion of these and other interventions related to relieving pain can be located in Chapter 7.

Muscle spasms in the calf may be relieved by flexing the foot forcefully back toward the body. This causes contraction of the opposing muscle group. Other measures helpful in preventing and relieving muscle spasm include a regular exercise program (described later in the chapter), a footboard which permits exercises and also keeps sheets and covers off the feet and legs, and frequent repositioning.

Some patients with musculoskeletal disorders experience a combination of acute and chronic pain. For example, the patient with rheumatoid arthritis who has surgery on a painful joint may have postoperative acute pain related to the surgery as well as the usual chronic pain associated with rheumatoid arthritis. Analgesia is generally more effective for acute than chronic pain. Thus, the nurse is challenged to select a variety of pain-relieving measures, as suggested in Chapter 7.

The patient with a musculoskeletal disorder may be a candidate for the development of chronic pain, as described in Chapter 7. Such a patient may spend many years in and out of the hospitals and doctors' offices in an effort to improve conditions such as low back pain and neck pain. The patient with chronic pain in the musculoskeletal system may benefit from specialized interventions discussed in Chapter 7, such as TENS (transcutaneous electric nerve stimulation), hypnosis, behavior modification, and enrollment in a pain clinic.

ASSISTING WITH AMBULATION AND EXERCISE

Exercise in some form is usually beneficial to the patient with a musculoskeletal disorder. A carefully planned exercise program helps to prevent deformities and other complications related to immobility, to build strength and endurance needed for ambulation, and to improve flexibility in joints. In addition, exercise has a positive effect on the patient's self concept and sense of personal autonomy. An exercise program may provide an opportunity for the discouraged patient to see progress and improvement. The nurse may use the exercise program to focus on positive aspects of the patient's condition, even if the disease is not reversible. For example, the nurse may point out remaining function or strengths. When exercises cannot be done on the affected part, the patient may experience a reduction of frustration and helplessness by exercising unaffected body areas.

When the patient is immobilized in a cast or confined to bed, deep-breathing and coughing exercises are essential to prevent retained secretions in the tracheobronchial tree. Specific instructions for teaching these exercises can be located on page 415–17.

Other common exercises for the patient with a musculoskeletal disorder include range of motion to each joint. Range of motion may be active (done by the patient), passive (done by someone else), or assisted (done by the patient with help from another as needed).

Muscle-setting exercises may be prescribed by the physician to strengthen muscles involved in ambulation. The patient does a muscle-setting exercise by slowly contracting and relaxing a muscle group to a count of three or more without moving the involved joint. Common muscles the patient exercises using this method include the quadriceps (often called quad setting), gluteal muscles, and abdominal muscles.

Pulleys and ropes may be used by the patient in bed to exercise lower extremities by pulling them up gently. This provides stretch to tissues that have become shortened from disuse.

When an ambulatory aid such as crutches is planned, the patient usually needs to increase the strength of the upper extremities beforehand by lifting weights or sandbags. The patient in a wheelchair may strengthen upper extremities and relieve pressure on the buttocks at the same time by pushing the arms down on the wheelchair arms to lift the buttocks several inches off the seat of the chair.

Ambulatory aids include crutches, canes, walkers, and braces. The patient using an aid to ambulation needs properly fitting equipment, appropriate clothing, and instruction and supervision (Figures 17.4 and 17.5). In some cases, these may be provided by the nurse. In other cases, equipment and instruction are provided by the physical therapist and patient practice is supervised by the nurse. Appropriate apparel for the patient using an ambulatory aid includes comfortable clothing which is not likely to get entangled in the aid being used. For this reason, the wearing of long bathrobes is discouraged. Appropriate footwear such as shoes or sneakers with a low, broad heel is needed. Loose-fitting bedroom slippers, high-heeled shoes, and shower slippers are avoided because they may cause trips and falls.

The nurse may be responsible for obtaining crutches and teaching the patient how to use them safely. Unless crutch size is specified in advance by the physician, the patient must be measured. This may be done while the patient lies flat in bed, arms at the side, wearing appropriate shoes as described earlier. The measurement should be taken from the axilla to a point approximately 15 cm (6 in.) to the side of the patient's heel. The hand bar should be adjusted to a level that permits the patient to hold the arm almost straight when leaning on the palms. This can be done when the patient is standing if an adjustable crutch is used. The top of the crutch should be padded with foam rubber to

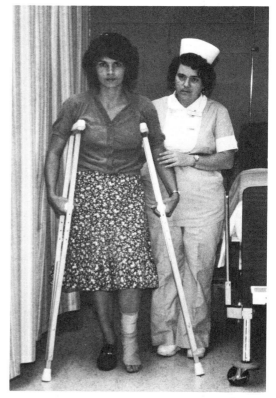

FIGURE 17.4 Using an aid to ambulation. (Courtesy of Loudoun County School of Practical Nursing, Leesburg, Virginia.)

protect the patient's axilla. The crutch should have a firm rubber tip that fits snugly to prevent slipping.

After crutches have been obtained and properly adjusted, the patient is first helped to learn balancing in an upright position. It is important to learn balancing before attempting to walk with crutches. When demonstrating the balanced position, the nurse places the crutches in front near the toe of each foot and leans forward, slightly resting body weight on the palms and wrists rather than the axillae. There should be no pressure on the axillae, as it may injure the nerves there and result in paralysis of muscles in the arm and hand. Crutch tips should be far enough from each other to provide support without allowing the crutches to slip.

Various gaits may be taught to the patient, depending on the amount of weight

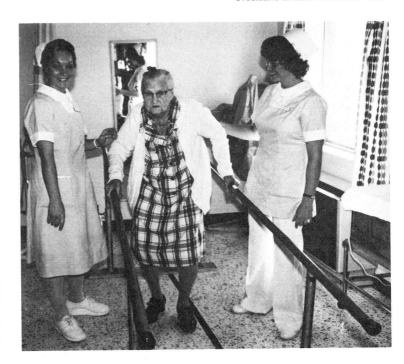

FIGURE 17.5 Learning to walk again. (Courtesy of Northeast Technical Community College Practical Nursing Program, Norfolk, Nebraska.)

bearing permitted by the physician. The *four-point gait* may be used when the patient can bear some weight on each leg. In this gait, the person advances one crutch, the opposite foot; then the other crutch, and the opposite foot. For example, the patient may bring the left crutch forward, then the right foot; the right crutch forward, and then the left foot.

The *two-point gait* is used also when the patient can bear some weight on each limb. The patient learns to use the crutches by putting the weight on one crutch and the opposite leg at the same time. Next, the patient brings the opposite limb and the crutch forward at the same time. The right foot and the left crutch are advanced at the same time. After shifting the weight to them, the patient should advance the left foot and the right crutch.

The *three-point gait* may be used when the patient can bear little or no weight on one leg. The patient advances the weak limb and both crutches at the same time. After shifting the weight to them, the good limb is advanced. The patient may be able to use only one crutch or a cane later. The crutch or the cane is placed on the unaffected side. The weak limb and the crutch are advanced at the same time in order to give support to the affected limb.

The *swing-through* or *tripod gait* is used when the patient's lower extremities are paralyzed. The patient advances the crutches and then swings both legs forward.

Frequently, the patient slouches when learning to use crutches. Good posture is encouraged with shoulders back, chin up, and eyes looking forward. The patient may need to be reminded not to bear weight on the affected foot.

A cane length is selected so that weight bearing occurs with the elbow extended on the hand holding the cane. The cane should have a rubber tip similar to that for crutches. The patient is instructed to hold the cane in the hand on the unaffected side. The patient advances the cane at the same time as the affected leg is brought forward, bearing weight on the cane instead of the affected leg. The patient using a walker without wheels is instructed to advance the walker first. After the walker is securely planted slightly in front of the body, the patient walks toward it leaning on the walker for support.

The physician may prescribe a brace to aid ambulation for the patient with a musculoskeletal condition. Orthopedic braces generally require special fitting by a specially trained person, the *orthotist*. When such an apparatus has been prescribed by the physician and fitted by the orthotist, the nurse inspects all skin areas in contact with the brace to detect irritation and other skin damage which may be caused by a poorly fitted brace. The five Ps are used to look for neurovascular impairment in skin areas in contact with the brace. The nurse may teach the patient how to do this at home, using a mirror if necessary to inspect all skin areas daily. The patient also may need instructions about how to clean and oil some braces. While soft material may be used to protect the skin, padding is not a substitute for a brace adjustment if needed.

An important part of patient teaching related to ambulation aids is the need for unhurried walking to prevent accidents. For example, the patient can anticipate that additional time will be needed for hygiene, elimination, dressing, and similar activities of daily living. A hurried trip to the bathroom may result in a fall. The patient in the hospital may be helped with discharge planning by timing usual activities so that extra time can be allowed at home.

ASSISTING WITH DRUG THERAPY

A variety of drugs may be prescribed for the patient with a musculoskeletal disorder. Drug therapy is complicated by the fact that many clients also have other medical problems requiring different categories of medication that are in no way related to the drugs most commonly prescribed for musculoskeletal conditions. This increases the danger of drug interactions and the need for careful observation. When caring for the patient with a musculoskeletal disorder, the nurse can expect the orthopedist to prescribe analgesia and muscle relaxants. In addition, antibiotics may be prescribed to prevent infection in the surgical patient or treat existing infection. Anticoagulants may be prescribed to prevent or treat thrombophlebitis in the immobilized patient. Sedatives

and hypnotics may be prescribed to help the patient sleep. Other drugs that may be prescribed for the patient with a musculoskeletal disorder can be located in Table 17.6.

PATIENT AND FAMILY TEACHING

Patient and family teaching is an integral part of health care and should be started as soon as the client is admitted to the health care system. All health care team members are teachers to the client because each bit of information or explanation is a form of teaching.

In teaching the patient and family, the nurse must decide what is to be accomplished (objective), what is to be taught (content), how it is taught (technique), and finally determines what the client has learned (evaluation). Every health team member who has anything to do with the client should be aware of the teaching plan because each person is responsible for reinforcing, observing, and reporting the progress of the patient's learning.

Topics generally included in patient teaching are related to the patient's hospitalization as well as how to cope at home. These may include exercise, fluid and dietary intake, correct positioning, reporting pain and discomfort, cast care, elimination, and skin care.

ASSISTING WITH OTHER REHABILITATION

An individual who is temporarily or permanently handicapped from a musculoskeletal trauma may need to go through a rehabilitation program whose objectives include restoration of maximal function, prevention of further impairment, and maintaining existing abilities. Rehabilitation is a very broad field that includes the total effort of a team of health workers. As a member of that team, the nurse is in a position to encourage follow-through of the therapeutic techniques prescribed for the client. The nurse supervises the practice of exercises, works with the social worker to plan the home activities, and works with the family to participate in the rehabilitation program planned for the client.

[Text continued on page 553.]

TABLE 17.6
DRUGS USED IN INFLAMMATORY CONDITIONS OF THE MUSCULOSKELETAL SYSTEM

NONPROPRIETARY NAME	TRADE NAME	AVERAGE DOSE	NURSING IMPLICATIONS
I. Salicylates, Salicylate-like Anti-inflammatory Agents, and Drugs Used for Gout			
Acetylsalicylic acid		600 mg	Because of the gastric irritation, give this with meals. Ringing of the ear is an early sign of toxicity
Allopurinol	ZYLOPRIM	200–300 mg daily	Encourage fluids to assure at least 2 liters of urinary output and alkalinity of the urine
Colchicine		0.5–2.0 mg	Considered very toxic—large dosages are usually prescribed to relieve within a few hours an acute attack of gout. This large dosage is maintained until the patient shows gastrointestinal side effects; then the dose is reduced
Fenoprofen	NALFON	600 mg four times daily	Gastrointestinal side effects such as dyspepsia and abdominal discomfort are common Should be taken on an empty stomach with an antacid
Ibuprofen	MOTRIN	1000–2400 mg daily	Give with meals or with milk to prevent gastric irritation and encourage fluids because the drug increases the acidity of urine
Indomethacin	INDOCIN	50–200 mg daily	Individuals are advised not to drive due to side effects of headache, sensation of drunkenness or unreality
Naproxen	NAPROSYN	250 mg twice daily	May be given with meals to prevent gastrointestinal symptoms
Phenylbutazone	BUTAZOLIDIN	400–600 mg daily	This should be given with meals or with milk due to gastric irritation
Sodium salicylate		0.3–1.0 gm	Give with meals or with milk to reduce gastric irritation
Sulindac	CLINORIL	150–200 mg twice daily	Gastrointestinal side effects are common, including abdominal pain, nausea, constipation May be given with food if gastrointestinal symptoms are present
Tolmetin	TOLECTIN	400 mg three times daily	Give with milk, meals, or antacids to lessen common abdominal discomfort One dose recommended on awakening and one at bedtime

TABLE 17.6 (*Continued*)
DRUGS USED IN INFLAMMATORY CONDITIONS OF THE MUSCULOSKELETAL SYSTEM

NONPROPRIETARY NAME	TRADE NAME	AVERAGE DOSE	NURSING IMPLICATIONS
II. ACTH, Adrenocortical Steroids, and Synthetic Analogs Used for Anti-inflammatory Action			
Betamethasone	CELESTONE	0.6 mg	Corticosteroids are being used with great discretion due to their toxicity. It is often difficult to distinguish between side effects and toxic effects of these drugs. Some of the more common side effects are weight gain, abnormal growth of hair on the face, easy fatigability, and menstrual irregularities.
Corticotropin injection	ACTHAR	20 U.S.P. unit IV in 8 hr	
Cortisone acetate	CORTONE NEOSONE	5–25 mg	
Dexamethasone	DECADRON GAMMACORTEN HEXADROL	0.5–0.75 mg	
Hydrocortisone (cortisol)	CORTEF CORTIFAN CORTRIL HYDROCORTONE	5–20 mg	
Methylprednisolone	MEDROL	2–16 mg	
Paramethasone acetate	HALDRONE	1–2 mg	
Prednisolone	DELTA-CORTEF HYDELTRA METICORTELONE METI-DERM PARACORTOL STERANE STEROLONE	5 mg	
Prednisolone acetate	NEO-DELTA-CORTEF STERANE	25 mg/ml (intramuscular and intrasynovial injection)	These drugs promote sodium retention. The nurse should keep a record of intake and output, daily weights, and blood pressure readings. Withdrawal symptoms are common when discontinued
Prednisolone sodium phosphate	HYDELTRASOL	20 mg/ml (for injection)	
Prednisone	DELTASONE METICORTEN PARACORT	1–5 mg	
Repository corticotropin injection	ACTHAR GEL	40 units/daily	
Sterile corticotropin zinc hydroxide suspension		40 units/daily	
Triamcinolone diacetate	ARISTOCORT KENOCORT	1–16 mg 5 mg/5 ml (oral) 25 mg/ml (injection) 40 mg/ml (injection)	They differ from the other corticosteroids by the elimination of certain side effects such as sodium retention, edema, hypertension, euphoria, increased appetite, and weight gain
III. Gold Compounds			
Aurothioglucose injection	SOLGANAL	50–100 mg/ml	Administration is always intramuscular and preferably into the outer, upper gluteal quadrant
Aurothioglycanide injection	LAURON	50–100 mg/ml	
Gold sodium thiomalate injection	MYOCHRYSINE	10–50 mg/ml	Aurothioglucose should be shaken well, and it requires a large-gauge needle (20) for administration because it is in a suspension

TABLE 17.6 (*Continued*)
DRUGS USED IN INFLAMMATORY CONDITIONS OF THE MUSCULOSKELETAL SYSTEM

NONPROPRIETARY NAME	TRADE NAME	AVERAGE DOSE	NURSING IMPLICATIONS
IV. Immunosuppressive Drugs			
Cyclophosphamide	CYTOXAN		Limited use due to their high toxicity. They are used to suppress autoimmune mechanism. The nurse should observe patient for toxic symptoms
Azathioprine	IMURAN		
Chlorambucil	LEUKERAN		
V. Miscellaneous Drugs			
Chloroquine	AVLOCLOR	Varies with patient	Contraindicated during gold therapy or with phenylbutazone
			Regular eye examinations are needed
Penicillamine	CUPRIMINE	1 gm four times daily	Must be given on an empty stomach

USING THE THERAPEUTIC RELATIONSHIP

In caring for the patient with a musculoskeletal disorder, an understanding of the concepts of immobilization, dependence, and body image is helpful. Most persons have a self-concept in which independence, mobility, and strength are important. A change in any one of these components may lead to an unfavorable change in the patient's self-concept. One's self-concept usually is enhanced by "doing" something successfully and often without help. A person who is unable to "do" and needs a lot of help can be expected to show changes in self-concept in the direction of diminished self-worth and self-esteem.

In some cases, the patient may feel and look well except for a limb suspended in traction or enclosed by a cast. Such a patient sometimes feels as though life has come to a halt and waits impatiently for healing to occur.

Another common situation that affects the patient and the nurse is unexpected hospitalization due to accident and injury. The patient may need days, weeks, or longer to cope with the implications of an automobile accident.

Fear, anger, restlessness, frustration, boredom, and depression are examples of emotions often experienced by the patient with a musculoskeletal disorder. If the trend continues, the patient may not have enough energy, motivation, confidence, or self-discipline to participate in activities vital to recovery.

Active listening to the patient's concerns is the first step in building a trusting relationship. The nurse's attention to details such as skin care, range of motion, and fluid balance conveys concern for the patient.

The patient's participation in care generally is expected and encouraged unless otherwise prescribed. An effective way to encourage someone is to look for and praise successes regularly.

Patients who have prolonged immobility associated with hospitalization generally find it helpful to develop a daily schedule that includes periods of work, rest, and recreation. The patient's work may include personal hygiene activities, eating and drinking appropriate fluids, maintaining an exercise program, and participating in physical or occupational therapy. Recreation may include watching television, visiting with friends, or playing cards or other games. This perspective, when explained to the patient permits a self-concept in which the patient actively "does" something to recover rather than one in which the patient just lies in bed "waiting" for a limb to heal.

Even while accepting the patient's expressions of depression, the nurse may gently point out real strength and progress in a matter-of-fact way. The nurse may use humor in some cases to encourage a more balanced perspective. Some patients benefit from reassurance that their feelings and concerns are normal. For example, a patient may be relieved to learn that many patients have muscle spasms or feel frightened the first time on crutches. When using reassurance, the nurse should be careful that it is realistic. False reassurance is not helpful to the patient.

Assisting the Patient in a Cast

The patient in a cast has a stiff orthopedic dressing applied externally to enclose and immobilize one or more joints. A *cast* is usually made of plaster-of-paris bandage. This consists of crinoline impregnated with powdered plaster. A roll of plaster-of-paris bandage is placed in warm water before being applied by the doctor. The area to be enclosed in a cast usually is covered first with glazed cotton and stockinette. The physician applies the wet plaster-of-paris bandages to form the cast. This hardens or sets as it dries. Another material which may be used for a cast is porous fiberglass tape impregnated with a photosensitive resin which hardens completely when exposed to a special lamp for five to ten minutes. The advantages of the fiberglass cast include lighter weight, lack of deterioration when wet, and quick drying time.

Covering an injured area with a cast may cause serious complications. The nurse's careful observations and skillful interventions are important both in prevention and early detection of neurovascular impairment, infection, and deformities.

NURSING OBSERVATIONS

Edema is expected in a patient's extremity in the early period following the application of a cast. Usually, the extremity is elevated above the level of the heart to reduce swelling. Despite elevation, edema may become severe enough to cause neurovascular impairment. Thus, hourly observation using the five Ps is essential in the early period. Later, observations may be made less often

The patient who reports continuous burning or cramping pain that is not localized to the area of injury may have circulatory impairment. This observation should be reported. Fingers and toes usually are left exposed for this purpose when a cast is applied to the extremity. When a long arm or long leg cast is applied, the orthopedist may leave a hole or "window" over the brachial, radial, or pedal pulses so that circulation can be evaluated. Evidence of neurovascular impairment is considered an emergency since permanent damage may result. The orthopedist relieves the pressure by splitting the patient's cast using a cast cutter or heavy scissors. If this does not restore circulation and sensation within several hours, emergency surgery is usually performed.

Other observations that should be reported include musty, unpleasant odors coming from the cast, unexpected drainage coming through or around the cast, hot spots over a cast area, burning over a bony prominence, and fever.

The nurse observes the patient's skin regularly for reddened areas. At the same time, the cast is inspected for indentations, cracks, or unexpected drainage. A small flashlight may be used to visualize skin areas under the cast which may become irritated by rough edges.

NURSING INTERVENTIONS

The nurse usually prepares for the patient's return from the cast room by placing a bedboard and/or firm mattress on the bed, if necessary. An overhead trapeze or crossbar, suspended from a Balkan frame, may be added to the bed to enable the patient to change position. Sandbags, extra pillows, and positioning devices needed to support the patient in a new cast are placed in the room in advance, also.

In handling the patient's wet cast, the nurse uses the palms of the hand rather than the fingers. This distributes pressure more evenly along the cast and prevents indentations and flattened areas which may damage the skin after the cast is dry. Pillows generally are placed in the patient's normal physiologic curves to prevent flattening of the cast. Thus, pillows may be needed to support the cervical, lumbar, and popliteal areas. In moving the patient to the bed, it is essential to have enough persons to lift gently and distribute pressure evenly in order to prevent cast damage.

The patient is turned frequently to promote even drying from the inside to the outside. The cast is left uncovered, if possible, and the patient is protected from chilling. When covers are needed, a bed cradle keeps them off the cast and allows air circulation. When a cast dryer is prescribed, it must be moved frequently so that drying occurs evenly from the inside to the outside, as previously mentioned.

Specific positions may be prescribed by the orthopedist and, in some cases, certain positions are avoided. The patient with a cast usually is turned away from the cast; however, the nurse should check the physician's orders before repositioning the patient. As mentioned earlier, the nurse elevates the patient's casted extremity to reduce edema unless specifically contraindicated by the orthopedist. The nurse should receive specific instructions when helping to turn a patient in a body cast. When a body cast has been applied, a crossbar frequently is placed between the legs and plastered to the cast in order to provide abduction. The nurse should remember that this crossbar is not strong enough to use when turning the patient in a body cast. The patient is practically helpless in such a cast, and adequate support is needed to prevent the weight of the cast from toppling him out of bed. The careful use of pillows and sandbags to support the patient in a cast aids comfort. After the turn, the nurse should check to see that the patient's body is in good alignment.

Parts of the patient's body that are not casted are bathed and dried thoroughly without introducing moisture under the cast. Skin under the cast edges should be brushed to remove crumbs. The patient's bed is kept free of crumbs of plaster and food as well as wrinkles. Exercises such as those described earlier in the chapter usually are encouraged. When the cast is wet, exercise may be limited to deep breathing or coughing. After the cast is dry, a regular program can be started. Exercises may include one or more of those described earlier in the chapter, depending on the patient's condition and the physician's prescription. Measures related to diet, fluids, and elimination, described earlier in the chapter, apply to this patient. As previously mentioned, continuous burning or cramping pain not related to the area of injury may indicate circulatory impairment. In this instance, the nurse should not administer analgesia until the physician examines the patient or prescribes otherwise. If necessary to visualize a particular area, the physician may cut a *window* in the cast.

Cast care includes cleaning, smoothing rough edges, and preventing moisture damage. Soiling may be prevented by using SARAN WRAP around the perineal edges of a cast. A plastic bag may be used to cover an arm or leg cast for protection from wet weather. Since rough cast edges may damage the skin, the nurse may apply short strips of adhesive around cast edges. The patient should be instructed not to insert objects into the cast to scratch itchy skin. These may injure the skin and cause infection.

After healing has occurred, the cast is removed with either an electric cast cutter or a plaster knife and heavy scissors.

The patient should be informed in advance that feelings of weakness and insecurity may occur because of the loss of support. In addition, the patient should be prepared for the drastic change in appearance caused by disuse and lack of exposure to air.

The skin under the cast is dry and scaly and has a foul odor due to the accumulation of waste products excreted through the skin. The casted area usually looks pale, hairless, small, and withered.

After the cast is removed, the nurse may apply a lubricant or baby oil to soften crusts before bathing the skin with mild soap and water. This process may be repeated over several days to remove all scales and substances from the skin. When the patient is moved, the affected area usually requires support above and below the immobilized joint until muscles become strengthened. The patient usually has physical therapy to improve muscle strength, flexibility, and endurance.

Assisting the Patient in Traction

The patient in traction has a pulling force applied to the musculoskeletal system. Traction may be achieved by the use of weights hung from cords that work from pulleys and other special equipment. The patient may be placed in traction for reduction and immobilization of a fracture. It may be used also to immobilize a joint that is infected, such as a joint infected with tuberculosis. Traction may be used to prevent or to correct a deformity caused by diseases, such as arthritis. In some cases, traction may be prescribed to reduce muscle spasm associated with neck or back pain.

The patient with *skin* or *surface traction*, such as Buck's extension (see Figure 17.6), has traction equipment attached to the skin. Commercially prepared traction equipment or strips of adhesive, moleskin tape, are applied to each side of the extremity and wrapped with elastic bandage. This holds special traction devices to which ropes, pulleys, and weights are attached. Russell's traction is a variation of skin traction during which the limb in traction is suspended with a sling. This allows the patient to move more freely in bed and permits the knee to bend.

Encircling traction transmits a pulling force to the skin using special garments that are placed around the body. For example, the patient in cervical traction wears a head halter. The patient in pelvic traction wears a special girdle. The patient with *skeletal traction* has the equipment attached to the bone. A metal pin, tongs, or a wire may be inserted into the bone and then connected with the traction apparatus. A greater amount of pull is possible with this type of traction. Skeletal traction with a suspension system that balances or floats the limb is commonly used for fractures of the extremities. This is called a *balanced suspension traction* (see Figure 17.7).

Traction may be applied intermittently or continuously. Traction used to immobilize and reduce a fracture is continuous. Traction prescribed to reduce pain and muscle spasm may be either continuous or intermittent. Unless otherwise ordered by the physician, traction is considered continuous. The physician's order for traction includes the type of traction to be used, the limb or area to be placed in traction, the amount of weight to be used, and whether the traction is to be continuous or intermittent. In order

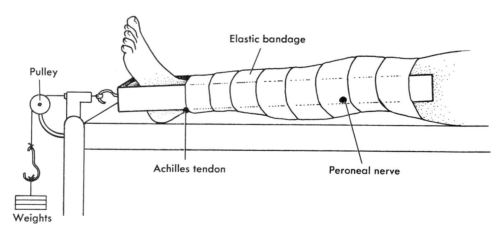

FIGURE 17.6 A patient with skin traction. The part of the patient's body in traction should be kept in the position designated by the physician. The rope should remain on the pulley without touching other objects. The prescribed weights suspended from the rope should not be removed without specific instructions from the physician or the head nurse. The affected part should be observed frequently for symptoms of impaired circulation. Pressure should be avoided on the Achilles tendon and on the area of the peroneal nerve.

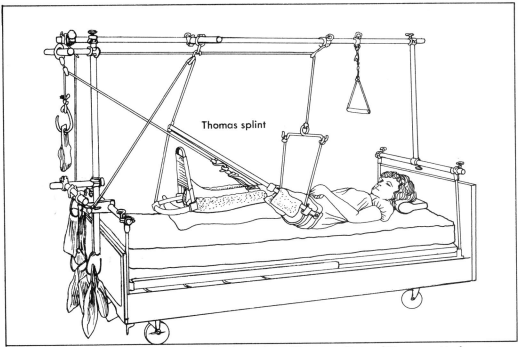

Thomas splint

FIGURE 17.7   Balanced suspension traction using a Thomas splint and Pearson attachment covered with sheep wool. (Adapted from *The Traction Handbook*. Zimmer Co., Warsaw, Indiana, 1975.)

for traction to be effective, the following conditions are necessary:

- Weights, pulleys, and ropes must be free and unobstructed.
- An equal amount of pull (countertraction) is needed to prevent the patient from being pulled against the pulleys.

PREPARING THE PATIENT FOR TRACTION

The nurse may be asked to assist in placing the patient in traction by assembling equipment, preparing the patient's skin, applying manual traction, and providing support for the patient. Equipment needed for traction depends upon the type of traction prescribed and the orthopedist's preference. The nurse can anticipate the need for ropes, pulleys, weights, and spreaders. Generally, a firm mattress and/or bedboard is needed. A traction frame is attached to the bed to which pulleys are attached. When applying a traction frame to the bed, all connections

must be securely fastened in order to prevent accidents (Figure 17.8). Usually, an overhead trapeze is attached to the frame which permits the patient to lift and change position (Figure 17.9).

Skin preparation also varies with the type of traction and the orthopedist's preference. Typical preparation includes washing the affected area with an antibacterial substance and drying it thoroughly. Occasionally, the orthopedist may request that the hair of the affected area be trimmed. Shaving is usually avoided because nicks and scratches increase the hazard of infection and skin breakdown.

The nurse may be asked by the physician to apply manual traction while the patient is being placed in the traction apparatus. The physician positions the limb correctly first. Then the nurse holds the patient's limb in both hands and exerts a constant pull. When providing manual traction, the nurse may prevent self-injury by placing one foot in front of the other, bending the knees

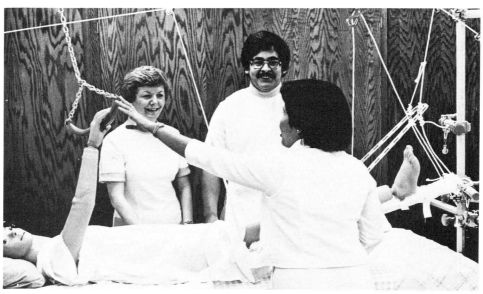

FIGURE 17.8 Learning about traction in the laboratory. (Courtesy of Rochester Area Vocational-Technical Institute Practical Nursing Program, Rochester, Minnesota.)

slightly, and using thigh muscles to pull rather than back and shoulder muscles.

Forms of support when placing the patient in traction may include explaining procedures and equipment and teaching the patient what to expect. For example, the patient may experience temporary muscle spasm when the pulling force is first applied.

NURSING OBSERVATIONS

The patient in traction may be observed systematically in a head-to-toe manner. The patient's head should not be resting against the headboard. The head elevation generally should not exceed 20 to 30 degrees unless otherwise prescribed by the physician.

In observing the patient's traction apparatus, the nurse looks for ropes that are free from blankets, sheets, and other items. Each pulley is inspected to make sure that the rope has not slipped off. The patient's extremities should not be touching the foot of the bed. The weights should be hanging free in the air, not resting on the floor or a footstool.

When observing the body part in traction, the nurse uses the five Ps and observes the skin temperature to check for neurovascular impairment. As previously mentioned, evidence of disturbances in circulation and sensation are reported at once.

The nurse regularly inspects any skin area in contact with a sling, support, or other traction apparatus for evidence of irritation or pressure. The groin, ischial tuberosities, posterior aspects of the knee and leg, Achilles tendon, instep, and heel are areas frequently observed, depending on the type of traction. The patient may be taught to participate in inspecting visible areas. When skeletal traction is used, the nurse inspects both sides of the skin at the pin site regularly for signs of infection such as swelling (edema), erythema (redness), foul odor, and drainage. These are reported at once, if observed.

NURSING INTERVENTIONS

The patient generally is encouraged to participate in personal care activities, as described earlier in the chapter. Because turning usually is restricted, the nurse changes the linens from the head to foot instead of the usual side-to-side method. This enables

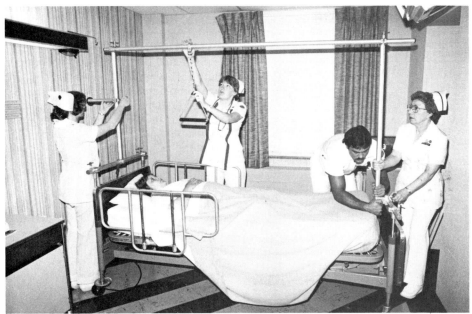

FIGURE 17.9   Applying an overhead trapeze to an orthopedic frame. (Courtesy of North Dakota State School of Science, Practical Nursing Program, Wahpeton, North Dakota.)

the patient to lift up rather than turn. Frequent skin care is a vital part of hygiene for the patient in traction.

Before repositioning the patient in traction, the nurse checks the physician's orders. In some cases, turning is not permitted. In other cases, the patient is permitted to turn slightly toward the traction. Generally, the part of the body placed in traction is elevated. Usually, head elevation is restricted to prevent hip flexion contractures. When pulling a patient up in bed, the nurse instructs the patient to push by placing the unaffected foot flat on the bed and lifting the buttocks slightly to avoid irritating the skin. When the patient is in continuous traction, the nurse may need additional assistance since the weights cannot be removed at any time. Exercises described earlier in the chapter are encouraged for the patient in traction. Dorsiflexion of both feet usually is done more frequently when the patient is in traction because a footboard cannot be used. Thus, the patient is more likely to develop footdrop. Other measures already described

such as alterations in fluids, diet, elimination are used to help the patient in traction, also.

Assisting the Surgical Patient

A variety of surgical procedures may be done when the patient has a disorder involving the musculoskeletal system. Table 17.7 contains examples of common orthopedic surgeries. One important consideration that affects the patient is that surgery on the skeleton causes an intentional fracture. Thus, bone healing occurs in a process similar to fracture healing discussed later in this chapter. A second consideration is the damage to other tissue which occurs in exposing the part of the surgical anatomy. These factors usually influence the patient having orthopedic surgery in the following ways:

- There is an increased hazard of osteomyelitis.
- The surgical procedure usually takes longer.

TABLE 17.7
EXAMPLES OF COMMON ORTHOPEDIC
SURGICAL PROCEDURES

SURGERY	DESCRIPTION
Arthrodesis	Surgical fusion of joint surfaces
Arthroplasty	Plastic surgery on a joint
Arthrotomy	Incision into a joint
Bone graft	Transplantation of bone from one part of the body to another
Open reduction with internal fixation (ORIF)	Alignment of fracture fragments which are held together with metal nails, plates, pins, screws, or wires
Osteotomy	Incision into a bone
Synovectomy	Removal of diseased synovial membrane from the joint
Tendon transplant	Change in the direction or pull of a spastic muscle
Total hip replacement	Replacement of entire hip joint using artificial parts
Total knee replacement	Replacement of entire knee joint using artificial parts

- Recovery from surgery usually takes longer.
- Immobility of some kind is usually present.

Principles of nursing care include those described in Chapter 6. Skin preparation may be done in the operating room in order to reduce the hazard of a break in the skin and infection. A shampoo may be needed preoperatively, especially if surgery will result in prolonged immobility. Meticulous attention is needed for fingernails and toenails, especially if the patient has been in an accident. Elastic stockings may be applied preoperatively to one or both legs to prevent thrombophlebitis.

Postoperatively, the patient may be placed in a cast or traction. When a cast is applied, the orthopedist usually writes on the postoperative orders how much drainage is anticipated. In addition to the usual postoperative observations, the nurse uses the five Ps to look for neurovascular impairment in the surgical area. Skin temperature on the affected limb may be cooler if a tourniquet was used during surgery. This information can be located in the operative note.

Special hazards for the postoperative patient following orthopedic surgery include thrombophlebitis, pulmonary embolism (described in Chapter 12), and fat embolism. The condition is caused by the presence of fat droplets in the bloodstream. These fat droplets have broken away from the injured and exposed bone marrow. Petechiae appearing on the anterior aspect of the chest are frequently an early sign, followed by a steady rise of temperature, pulse, and respiration. As emboli travel to the lungs and brain, the patient becomes restless, apprehensive, dyspneic, and confused and may convulse and lapse into a coma. Observation of the early sign is imperative in order to prevent a fatal consequence. The patient usually is transferred to the intensive care unit, kept absolutely quiet, and is given oxygen, anticoagulants, and other symptomatic therapy.

Sprain

Sprain is an acute injury of a ligament. The injury may include a tearing of the capsule, ligaments, and some muscle fibers after a sudden twisting injury. Sprains are common injuries of the ankle, knees, and the neck (whiplash). The individual has varying degrees of pain, limitation of motion, and edema of the joint.

Immediate intermittent application of ice or cold compress on the area may prevent further capillary bleeding and subsequent hematoma and also prevent further swelling. After 24 hours of intermittent cold application, heat may be applied intermittently to increase the blood supply and hasten the healing process. Elevating the injured joint and applying a compression bandage are effective ways of controlling the edema. Splinting or casting is done to rest and immobilize the joint during the healing period of approximately four to six weeks. Mild analgesics may be needed. X-ray of the injury must be done to rule out an avulsion fracture.

Strain

Strain results from overstretching of a muscle beyond its functional capacity. A strain may occur suddenly after a forced unexpected motion or may occur after repeated overuse of a muscle group.

Management of a strain is the same as that of a sprain, and it also heals within four to six weeks.

Dislocation and Subluxation

The patient with a dislocation has a lack of contact between the articulating surfaces of a joint. This displacement may disrupt the joint capsule and tear the surrounding ligaments and other soft tissues. The patient with a subluxation has an incomplete displacement of joint surfaces. Usually, there is less tissue damage. In adults, dislocation or subluxation usually results from traumatic injury. The patient also may experience these conditions as a complication of certain joint surgeries such as arthroplasty. Pain, abnormal contour, swelling, and loss of motion are the obvious signs and symptoms of dislocation. X-rays are taken that show the abnormal separation.

The most effective treatment is early reduction (realignment) either by manual (closed) or surgical (open) methods. After reduction, the patient may be placed in a cast or traction for several weeks. After healing occurs, the patient gradually increases active motion of the affected part.

Bunion (Hallux Valgus)

The person with a bunion has either a bony overgrowth which is acquired or an abnormal position of the big toe (hallus valgus) which is congenital. The big toe is laterally angulated. As a result of this deformity, increased friction over the head of the metatarsal bone brings about a formation of a bursa which eventually calcifies to a bony overgrowth.

Acquired bunions are caused by wearing shoes that are too narrow or too short. Surgery is aimed at correcting the angulation by removing the proximal portion of the first phalanx (Keller procedure) and removing the bunion or bony overgrowth.

In congenital hallus valgus, the McBride procedure includes osteotomy of the metatarsals and tendon transplant to restore the alignment.

Dupuytren's Contracture

The patient with Dupuytren's contracture has a progressive contracture of the palmar fascia, causing flexion of the little finger, ring finger, and sometimes the middle finger. The cause is unknown, but there is an hereditary tendency. The contracture starts in one hand and eventually involves the identical fingers on the other hand.

Pain is an infrequent complaint, but the main complaint is the interference of the contracture with the use of the hand.

Resection of the palmar fascia gives relief.

Low Back Pain

Pain in the lumbosacral region (low back) is a very common musculoskeletal condition. About 80 percent of all persons are affected by low back pain during their lifetime. Low back pain may occur from strain, osteoarthritis, or herniated intervertebral disk (discussed in Chapter 21). In some cases, no specific cause can be found. Contributing factors include overweight, poor body mechanics, weak muscles, structural abnormalities, and tight muscles.

ASSISTING WITH DIAGNOSTIC STUDIES

The patient usually has x-rays of the lumbosacral spine in addition to an orthopedic examination. Other studies may be indicated to identify or rule out known causes such as osteoarthritis, herniated disk, or bone tumor.

NURSING OBSERVATIONS

The patient's report of pain may vary with respect to intensity, duration, location, and aggravating or relieving factors. The patient's weight and height are measured. The patient may have postural deformities such as increased lumbar lordosis and protruding abdominal muscles.

NURSING INTERVENTIONS

Components of therapy include rest, posture training, mild analgesics, muscle relaxants, low heat, systematic exercises, and pelvic traction. When pelvic traction is prescribed, it may be continuous or intermittent. Correct positioning is important in order to provide traction to back muscles. The hip and knee joints are flexed at 90-degree angles, and the patient's head is placed in a flat or slightly elevated position. After acute pain subsides, the physician usually prescribes a series of back exercises known as *William's exercises* to improve strength and flexibility. These exercises are usually taught by the physical therapist and supervised by the nurse. An important topic in patient teaching is using good body mechanics when lifting, pulling, pushing, and turning objects. Some patients may need help to plan weight loss.

Fracture

The patient with a fracture has a broken bone, which is caused usually by an accident. However, a fracture can result from a disease of the bone. For example, a malignant tumor can weaken the bone to such an extent that it may break during a normal activity such as turning in bed. This type of fracture is referred to as a pathologic or spontaneous fracture. As mentioned earlier, an intentional fracture may result from surgery on the skeleton.

TYPES

A *simple fracture* is one in which the bone is broken, but the skin over the area is intact. When there is a wound leading to the broken bone, the patient has a *compound fracture*. Infection is more likely to develop because the opening allows bacteria to enter. Terms that may be used to describe the direction of the fracture are oblique and transverse. An *oblique fracture* is slanted, and a *transverse* one goes across the bone. Overlapping of the broken bone is present in an *overriding fracture*. In an *incomplete fracture*, the break extends part of the way through the bone. A *greenstick fracture* is an incomplete fracture that usually occurs in children because their bones are still somewhat flexible. It is known as a greenstick fracture because its break resembles the breaking of a young and green branch of a tree. When the bone is broken into at least three pieces, it is called a *comminuted fracture*. In an *impacted fracture*, the bone fragments are driven together. (See Figure 17.10.)

BONE HEALING

When bone tissue is injured or broken, bleeding occurs and a *hemotoma* forms around the broken ends, usually within 24 hours. Gradually, cells and new capillaries invade the hematoma (*cell proliferation*), changing the hematoma into granulation tissue. Within a week to ten days, the granulation tissue changes into a callus (*callus formation*) which now contains cartilages, minerals, and osteoblasts from the adjacent periosteum. Firm union of the fragments occurs when the new bone starts to grow from beneath the periosteum of each fragment and fuses across the fracture site (*callus ossification*). After the osseous callus is formed, *consolidation* and *remodeling* take place. During this stage, necrotic cells are resorbed and new bone is gradually changed to a normal shape, contour, density, and strength. The healing process may require a year to complete.

COMPLICATIONS IN BONE HEALING

Certain factors can disturb the healing process of traumatized bone. In open fractures or open reduction of a fracture, *infection* is often a possibility that can complicate the healing process. When reduction is incomplete or temporary, *malunion* of the bone fragments may cause a deformity of the fracture site. This may be corrected by realignment, continued immobilization, or by surgical intervention. *Delayed union* or *nonunion* of the bone fragments of a fracture also may occur. If the bone fragments are pulled too far apart by traction, the callus cannot fill the gap. Healing also is de-

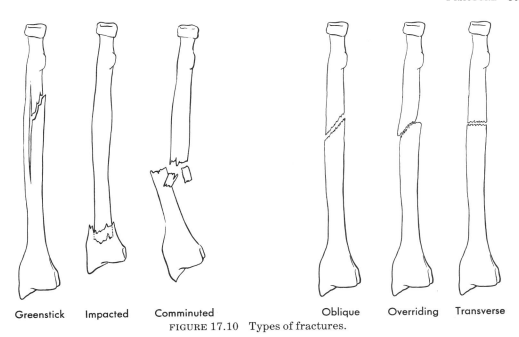

Greenstick   Impacted   Comminuted   Oblique   Overriding   Transverse

FIGURE 17.10   Types of fractures.

layed if there is inadequate blood supply to the affected part or if soft tissue gets caught between the fragments or the callus is broken or torn by too much activity. Nonunion may be corrected by placing a bone graft across the gap (onlay graft). Bones have a highly developed vascular system and will die without adequate blood supply. Some injuries cause irreversible damage to the blood supply of a bone, resulting in death of bone tissue. This complication is called *avascular necrosis*. The patient with a fracture involving the femoral head is particularly susceptible to this late complication because the femoral head has little collateral circulation. The individual with avascular necrosis experiences an increasing pain and increasing deformity. The patient usually needs a joint replacement.

FACTORS THAT INFLUENCE BONE HEALING

The length of each stage in bone healing can be predicted. However, there are factors that influence the length of time required for healing. The healing process is enhanced by good circulation to the part, adequate approximation of bone ends, optimum nutritional status, and good general health. Age also affects the healing process. For example, fractures in children heal more quickly than those in older people.

NURSING OBSERVATIONS

The patient complains of pain after a bone has been fractured. Usually, there is also a loss of normal function. The fracture may cause unnatural movement and a grating sensation known as *crepitus*. The area also may appear deformed. The area soon becomes swollen. The patient may develop symptoms of shock.

An individual with a broken bone usually has an injury of other tissues in the area. The body responds by sending an increased amount of blood to the part. The process of inflammation causes white blood cells and plasma to go from the blood vessels into the tissues. Swelling and pain are caused by increased fluid and damage to soft tissue surrounding the bone and its periosteum, which contains a rich supply of blood vessels and nerves.

Other nursing observations related to neurovascular impairment, shock, and fat embolism, described earlier in the chapter, apply to the patient with a fracture. Specific additional observations depend on the method of treatment such as surgical, non-surgical, traction, or cast.

ASSISTING WITH DIAGNOSTIC STUDIES

When the physician suspects that the patient has a fracture, x-rays are taken. In addition to confirming the diagnosis, the x-rays guide the orthopedist in reducing (setting) the fracture. Another x-ray may be required after the fracture has been reduced so that the doctor can determine whether or not the bone fragments are in the correct alignment. The nurse may be asked to assist by holding an injured part so that the x-ray can be taken.

NURSING INTERVENTIONS

EMERGENCY CARE. Remembering that one of the aims in the care of the patient with a fracture is to prevent further injury to the area, the nurse can realize the importance of gentle handling. This should be a guiding principle in the emergency care of a person suspected of having a fracture. The fracture must be splinted before the patient is moved in order to prevent additional tissue damage.

The patient with a possible fracture of the leg or thigh can have the part splinted with a long board (see Figure 17.11). Rolled newspapers can be used to immobilize the forearm. The upper arm may be bandaged to the chest with a blouse or a coat.

Movement of the patient with a suspected fracture of the spine should be done with utmost caution. If a vertebra is broken, the fragments may damage the spinal cord permanently when the patient is moved. The patient should be moved smoothly along the surface to a rigid surface. The patient can be rolled like a log onto the abdomen on a blan-

ket when a rigid surface is not available. This type of movement should be carried out with at least four persons to facilitate ease of transportation.

The person with a compound fracture should have a sterile dressing or a clean cloth placed over the wound. An open wound leading to the fracture increases the seriousness of the injury. Because of blood loss, the patient should be observed for symptoms of shock. The big danger of secondary infection because of the open wound should serve as a basis for emergency care. In addition to covering the open wound, the person giving emergency care should splint the area to prevent movement of the fractured site. No attempt to replace the bone should be made. This is the physician's responsibility.

ADMITTING THE PATIENT. When helping to admit the patient with a possible fracture, the nurse should handle the patient gently. Clothing should be removed in such a manner that the fractured part is not moved. If movement is necessary, the injured area should be moved as little as possible and supported above and below the fracture, without removing the temporary splint. The patient is kept comfortably warm and closely observed. A narcotic analgesic usually is given to reduce pain.

THE PATIENT WITH A CLOSED REDUCTION. During a closed reduction, the physician realigns the fracture fragments by external manipulation. In other words, no incision is made. When an external manipulation is done, the patient may need a general anesthetic or an analgesic before the orthopedist manually manipulates the extremity. Nursing observations may include those needed for a patient receiving anesthesia as well as those related to neurovascular impairment. After the fracture has been reduced, it may be immobilized in a cast or traction. The care of the patient under these circumstances was described earlier in the chapter.

THE PATIENT WITH AN OPEN REDUCTION. During an open reduction, the orthopedist makes an incision and directly manipulates the fracture fragments to obtain normal alignment. In some cases, the doctor

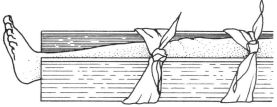

FIGURE 17.11 The fracture should be splinted before the patient is moved.

may have to secure the fragments with a special type of wire, screws, nails, or metal plates. This procedure is called open reduction with internal fixation. A special type of fixation device which may be used in severe fractures is called a Hoffman fixator. This device stabilizes compound fractures which are often difficult to immobilize. A rigid scaffolding holds the fragments in alignment by exerting pressure on pins inserted into the bone fragments above and below the breaks. The perpendicular rods of the scaffold are telescopic and can be lengthened or shortened by turning the compression nuts.

In addition to usual care of the surgical patient, as discussed in Chapter 6, the patient's care is affected by the principles described earlier in this chapter on page 559.

The patient with a fracture involving the head of the femur or the acetabulum usually has an open reduction and internal fixation. The patient with this kind of fracture is frequently an elderly person with osteoporosis who has sustained the injury during a fall. Preoperative preparation frequently includes studies to identify or correct problems in the cardiovascular and respiratory systems. During this time (usually less than 24 hours), the patient may be placed in Buck's traction to reduce tissue damage and pain from muscle spasm.

Postoperatively, the nurse is especially alert for signs of respiratory depression caused by anesthesia and/or narcotics.

A vigorous program of deep breathing and active exercises of the unaffected extremities is started as soon as the patient returns from surgery to prevent pulmonary and circulatory complications. Circulation and sensation checks for neurovascular impairment are hourly at first and every four hours after the first postoperative day.

An abduction splint or abduction pillows are placed between the legs to separate them. After the legs have been placed in abduction, the patient usually can be turned as one unit (log roll), if permitted by the physician.

Exercises are also prescribed as early as the first postoperative day. The patient is helped out of bed to start nonweight-bearing ambulation using a walker or a pair of crutches within a few days after surgery.

The patient is instructed not to bear weight on the affected leg until x-rays confirm the healing of the fracture.

A third method of reduction which may be used is skeletal traction, which was described earlier in the chapter. This method is generally used when powerful muscle contractions cause the fracture fragments to become displaced. Table 17.8 contains a summary of factors that influence the care of a patient with a fracture.

Arthritis

Arthritis literally means an inflammation of a joint. The term *arthritis* is used to describe other aches and pains in joints and connective tissues throughout the body. The word *rheumatism* is used frequently for unexplained aches and pains in joints and muscles. According to the Arthritis Foundation, arthritis is the number one crippler in the United States, claims 600,000 new victims annually, affects one in seven people, is the

TABLE 17.8
SUMMARY OF FACTORS THAT INFLUENCE THE CARE OF A PATIENT WITH A FRACTURE

Factors that Determine the Plan of Treatment and Nursing Care

- Age of the individual
- Health of the individual
- Place of break
- Extent of break

Objectives of Treatment

- Reduce or put fragments together and in alignment
- Immobilize or hold the fragments in position until healing occurs
- Rehabilitate and regain normal function

Methods Used to Reduce a Fracture

- Closed reduction
- Open reduction
- Traction

Methods Used to Immobilize a Fracture

- Splints and elastic bandages
- Casts
- Consistent traction (pull from a significant weight)
- Internal fixation devices
- External fixation device

leading cause of industrial absenteeism, and is second only to heart disease as a cause of disability payments.

There are many types of arthritis. The two main types are rheumatoid arthritis and osteoarthritis. A comparison of these two common types of arthritis can be located in Table 17.9. Less common types of arthritis are caused by an infection of the joint, such as gonorrhea, tuberculosis, syphilis, typhoid fever, streptococcal infection, and staphylococcal infection. An injury and a metabolic disturbance such as gout may result in arthritis.

RHEUMATOID ARTHRITIS

Rheumatoid arthritis is a systemic, chronic, and inflammatory disease of unknown cause. It tends to subside and flare up unpredictably. These periods of intermittent remissions and exacerbations result in damage to the involved tissues.

Any connective tissue may become involved, but the primary sites affected are the joints and the synovial membrane that lines and lubricates the joints. This membrane reacts to the inflammation by secreting more fluid and by becoming swollen and tender. Because of the pain, the individual limits joint movement and assumes a position of comfort which is a joint flexion. Because of the limitation of motion, the muscles surrounding the joints atrophy and flexion contractures develop. As the disease progresses, excess synovial fluid precipitates into a fibrous layer that spreads over the joint surfaces and erodes the underlying cartilage and bone. This fibrous ankylosis eventually leads to permanent bony ankylosis as bone overgrowth develops in the fibrous layers. Loss of motion is accompanied by muscle atrophy and disuse osteoporosis of the affected bone.

Although joint inflammation is characteristic in persons with rheumatoid arthritis, it is not known what initiates the inflammatory process. A current theory is that some type of virus infection results in an abnormal autoimmune response.

Females are affected more frequently with rheumatoid arthritis than are males. Young adults are affected more than older ones. However, individuals of any age may have rheumatoid arthritis.

ASSISTING WITH DIAGNOSTIC STUDIES

In addition to a history and physical examination, the physician usually orders blood tests and x-rays. The erythrocyte sedimentation rate (ESR) usually is elevated. Mild anemia may be evident in hematology studies. A special blood test may be done to detect the presence of rheumatoid factors, special autoantibodies that react with IgG. X-rays, which may be negative in early stages, later show progressive joint damage. Fluid withdrawn from an affected joint (joint aspiration) usually is thick, looks cloudy, and contains increased protein.

NURSING OBSERVATIONS

The patient with rheumatoid arthritis usually experiences a gradual onset of generalized weakness and stiffness. In some cases, the patient has a sudden onset of severe illness. The patient may have anorexia, increased fatigue, and fever. The involved joints become painful, swollen, and stiff, especially after periods of inactivity. Some persons report coldness and abnormal sensations in the hands and feet. As the disease progresses, nodules can be seen over pressure points in the posterior part of the head, trunk, and spine. Visible joint deformities result from destruction of joint structures and muscle imbalances. This causes a loss of function of the part involved.

As the patient loses mobility and function, the nurse may notice a change in appearance related to hygiene, grooming, and dressing. This is especially obvious if the patient lives alone or does not ask for or receive help from family members.

NURSING INTERVENTIONS

Although the cause and cure for rheumatoid arthritis are not yet known, effective measures to control the disease and prevent crippling deformities are known. The Arthritis Foundation recommends the following program of treatment, which should be adapted to the needs of the individual. Variations of the program will depend on the severity of the condition, the joints affected, the client's age, occupation, and life-style.

- Medication
- Rest
- Exercise
- Posture rules
- Splints and walking aids
- Heat
- Surgery
- Rehabilitation

The program of treatment is aimed toward relieving pain, reducing inflammation, preventing joint damage, preventing and/or correcting deformities, and maintaining and/or restoring function of the affected part.

ASSISTING WITH DRUG THERAPY. Drug therapy may be prescribed to reduce pain and inflammation and/or produce a remission of the disease process. The drug of choice for the patient with rheumatoid arthritis is acetylsalicylic acid (aspirin). When this drug is not effective, other drugs the physician may prescribe include nonsteroidal anti-inflammatory drugs or adrenocorticosteroids. Drugs prescribed to produce remission include gold therapy, penicillamine, and antimalarial drugs. Immunosuppresive therapy may produce remission in some patients. Table 17.6 contains a list of drugs commonly prescribed for the patient with an inflammatory condition of the musculoskeletal system.

ASSISTING WITH HYGIENE. The patient with rheumatoid arthritis often requires assistance with daily hygiene. Special areas for which help may be needed include a shampoo, brushing the teeth, washing the back, perineum, and lower extremities. If possible, the patient should receive a tub bath or shower when hospitalized since many patients are unable to do this at home.

REPOSITIONING THE PATIENT. When moving and/or helping the patient to move, the nurse frequently can be guided by the directions of the patient (Figures 17.12 and 17.13). The individual is a better judge of the assistance needed to move from one position to another. In other words, when helping the patient to turn in bed and to perform other similar activities, the nurse should ask the patient for directions about the most comfortable way to move.

When handling the individual's affected joint, the nurse should provide support of the inflamed joint in its most functional position (see Figure 17.14).

Muscles that flex (bend) a part of the body are stronger than those that extend it. Because of this, the patient is likely to develop flexor deformities. The patient should be encouraged to keep the affected joint straight to help prevent a flexor deformity. In general, the patient should not remain for a long period of time in a position with the affected joint bent. For example, the patient with rheumatoid arthritis of the elbows should not remain in a position in which the elbow is bent. The patient with affected knees should not use pillows under the knees, as this encourages flexor deformity of these joints. The nurse may find that sandbags are helpful in keeping the extremities in good position. A footboard can be used to prevent footdrop. A cradle may be used over the patient's feet to keep bedclothing from pressing his toes. A bedboard may be used under the mattress to prevent sagging.

ASSISTING WITH REST AND EXERCISE. Proper rest balanced with proper exercise can help to prevent or correct deformities. Too much rest can result in uncomfortable stiffening of joints, and too much exercise can further damage the joints. Exercise involves putting joints gently through their full range of motion to keep them flexible. Resting the entire body in good alignment helps to take the weight off the affected joint and helps to reduce inflammation.

The physician may immobilize the affected joint by the use of a cast or a splint. The use of these aids increases the amount of rest for the joint in an extended position so that flexor deformities do not develop. Frequently, these orthopedic devices are applied so that they can be removed at specified times. The nurse should receive definite instructions regarding when and how to remove and to replace them. Traction is an-

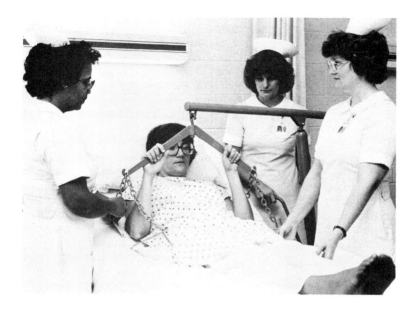

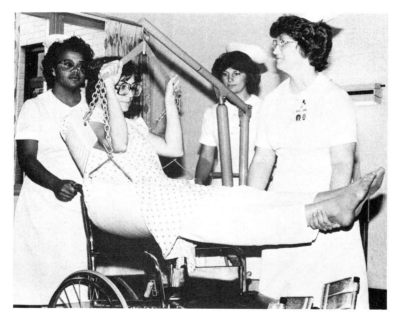

FIGURES 17.12 and 17.13 The patient's wishes are considered when lifting, moving, and turning. (Courtesy of Newport News Public Schools and Riverside Hospital School of Practical Nursing, Newport News, Virginia.)

other type of treatment that may be used to prevent and/or correct arthritic deformities.

The patient should be encouraged to perform the prescribed exercises in an effort to prevent deformity, preserve joint motion, and increase muscular strength. The exercises should be performed slowly and may be less painful after a warm bath or shower. Knowing the purpose of each exercise motivates the client to follow the prescribed routine, which at times is painful and discouraging. The periods of exercise can be increased gradually as the individual's condition improves. If the client notices increased pain

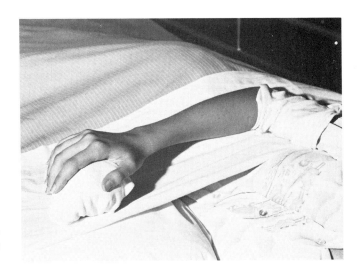

FIGURE 17.14 The patient with arthritis has the hand placed in its most functional position.

that lasts for more than two hours following exercise, the length of the exercise period may be shortened. A swimming pool, if available for exercise periods, provides relaxation and decreases discomfort.

APPLICATION OF HEAT. The physician frequently prescribes the local application of heat. Heat applied to the joints increases the blood supply, which aids in healing. It also relieves pain by relaxing the muscles around the involved joint. Some methods of using heat may be applied by the nurse such as a heating pad or aquapad. A bath or shower provides heat and hygiene at the same time. When using heat, the patient needs protection from burning. In addition, safety measures are needed to prevent falls in the tub or shower.

The physical therapist may be requested to give heat treatments. For example, *diathermy* is the use of a machine that sends an electric current into the tissues underneath the skin. This current produces heat in the arthritic joint. *Ultrasound* uses a machine to send high-frequency sound waves into the affected tissue. The sound waves produce heat in a manner similar to electric current. *Paraffin-dip treatment* is the use of melted paraffin for the application of heat. It is used mainly for an affected hand, arm, or foot. The patient's extremity is dipped a number of times into the warm paraffin until it is covered with a thick coat. The heat is trapped under this coat. The paraffin usually is removed by having the patient dip the part into the warm paraffin after approximately one hour.

ASSISTING WITH POSTURE, SPLINTS, AND WALKING AIDS. Incorrect posture places a strain on inflamed joints. The client should make a conscious effort to maintain proper posture not only when moving about but also when resting. The client should be advised to avoid sudden, jerky motions. Prolonged periods of standing and walking, especially when tired, should be avoided by the client. In addition, the client should be encouraged to sit in chairs having high seats to avoid the tendency toward slouching in a chair, which increases the possibility of injury to the knee and hip joints. Increased weight increases the strain on weight-bearing joints. In other words, obesity increases the strain on an individual's weight-bearing joints. The client should be encouraged to lose excess weight and to avoid obesity.

The individual should select properly fitting shoes for walking and should avoid slippers. Supports such as crutches, braces, and a cane are recommended for use when the individual has an acute flare up of rheumatoid arthritis involving the weight-bearing joints. As mentioned earlier, splints may be used to prevent deformities. In addition to preventing deformities, splints help to relieve pain and muscle spasm. Frequently, the client will be instructed to wear the splints while sleeping. Splints may need to be adjusted for comfort and proper support every several weeks.

ASSISTING WITH REHABILITATION. Rehabilitation usually involves many members of the health care team. For example, the occupational therapist is particularly important to the patient during rehabilitation. The occupational therapist works with the doctor, the physical therapist, and other members of the health team to help the patient regain joint function and spend time in a satisfying, useful way. For instance, the patient with arthritis of the hands may be learning to type not as a means of livelihood but as a means of keeping the mind and body active during convalescence. Another aim of the occupational therapist is to help the patient become adjusted to a disability. Emphasis is focused on the patient's abilities rather than disabilities. Genuine complimentary remarks by members of the nursing staff help to encourage the patient's efforts.

The occupational therapist also may provide a kind of "tool kit" containing special utensils that help the patient continue normal activities. Examples of items in the "tool kit" include zipper pulls for dressing, special handles for turning faucets, and special eating utensils. When occupational therapy is not available, the nurse may provide valuable assistance by suggesting activities and projects that use affected joints and are consistent with the patient's interests.

Most patients with rheumatoid arthritis are able to remain active and mobile. A full rehabilitation for the working client may include vocational counseling and retraining and/or placement.

ASSISTING THE SURGICAL PATIENT. Most of the procedures listed in Table 17.7 may be used either to prevent the spread of inflammation or correct deformities. Total joint replacements are becoming much more common to reduce pain and restore a functional joint. Almost any joint can now be replaced using a prosthesis. For example, arthroplasty of the hip involves two implanted components. In total arthroplasty, the surgeon utilizes a high-density polyethylene cup that allows friction-free motion to replace

the acetabulum. A stainless steel ball and stem replace the head of the femur which is surgically removed. The stem is driven into the femoral canal. A surgical bone cement that hardens rapidly and is resilient to the stress of walking anchors the cup and the stem (Figure 17.15).

Total knee arthroplasty utilizes the same materials. The metal is used for the distal femoral joint surface, and the plastic is used for the tibial joint surface. Elbow and shoulder joints have been surgically reconstructed in a similar manner.

Fingers can be made movable by replacing the ends of bones with silicone plastic spaces that are again cemented to the bones.

Before arthroplasty was developed, arthrodesis, or fusing the joints to make them immobile, was utilized to provide relief from pain to many patients. This type of operation continues to be done for some individuals. The fusion is accomplished by removing the articular cartilages so that the raw bone ends can grow or fuse together.

The most dreaded complication of any orthopedic surgery is infection. If this tragic circumstance occurs, the prosthetic devices must be surgically removed in order to effectively clear the infection and prevent its spread. During this process, the joints may in some instances fuse together, resulting in a nonfunctioning joint.

In addition to the usual complications of orthopedic surgery such as thrombophlebitis, pulmonary embolism, fat embolism, and subluxation, the artificial joint may become unstable after a few years, requiring another surgery.

THE PATIENT WITH A TOTAL HIP ARTHROPLASTY. The patient admitted for a hip arthroplasty usually receives extensive preoperative teaching. The physical therapist teaches exercises described earlier in the chapter including abdominal, gluteal and quadriceps setting as well as plantar flexion and dorsiflexion. These exercises are started preoperatively and continued postoperatively in preparation for ambulation. The patient is also instructed in using a trapeze, a fracture bed pan, crutches, and/or a walker. Practice sessions are a part of the preoperative teaching.

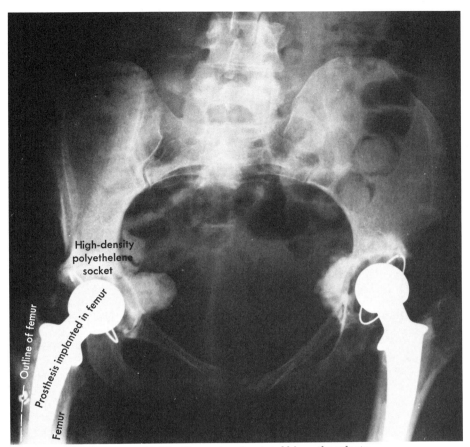

High-density
polyethelene
socket

Prosthesis implanted in femur

Outline of femur

Femur

FIGURE 17.15   X-ray showing total hip arthroplasty.

Postoperatively, the patient's legs usually are wrapped with elastic bandages or stockings to prevent thrombophlebitis. An abduction splint or abduction pillows may be placed between the legs to keep them separated. In some cases, the surgeon may prefer to place the patient in traction to maintain abduction and prevent muscle spasm. Nursing observations and interventions related to the patient in traction apply to postoperative care even if the patient is not placed in traction. The patient usually begins non-weight-bearing ambulation with a walker or crutches within the first postoperative week. Many patients are able to walk without these aids within six months.

The patient usually is discharged within two weeks with instructions to maintain abduction by placing a pillow between the knees when lying on the back or side. Additional instructions include frequent short walks and using a raised toilet seat. Practices that are avoided include sitting in low chairs, crossing the legs, and sitting for prolonged periods. These activities increase the likelihood of hip-flexion contracture and joint dislocation.

THE PATIENT WITH A TOTAL KNEE REPLACEMENT.   Nursing observations and interventions for the patient having a total knee replacement are similar to those for a patient in a cast.

Immediately following a total knee joint arthroplasty, the affected knee is immobilized with splints. Surgical stockings or elastic bandages also are applied to both legs to prevent thrombophlebitis, as mentioned earlier. Because a tourniquet is placed on the leg during surgery to decrease bleeding, a crucial postoperative nursing observation is frequent checks of circulation, motion, sensation. The patient usually is confined to bed for a few days postoperatively. During this time, the patient maintains an exercise program which emphasizes quadriceps strengthening. Range-of-motion exercises usually are started by a physical therapist on the third postoperative day. The patient gradually ambulates with a walker or crutches and is instructed to progressively bear weight on the affected leg or legs.

ASSISTING WITH PSYCHOSOCIAL ASPECTS. The patient with rheumatoid arthritis may become irritable, impatient, and discouraged. Frequent bouts with pain and concern over the crippling effect of the disease are two common causes of worry. Other sources of concern include the cost of care, and possible loss of income and occupation. Sexual relationships may be altered by pain, deformity, and disability. A combination of these events may create or intensify problems in the family or household.

The nurse is in a key position to help the patient in adjusting to illness because of their close daily contact. The nurse's realistic understanding and thoughtful attitude may be uplifting to the patient during trying times.

The nurse should help the individual to avoid premature withdrawal from opportunities and enjoyable activities. In some cases, the nurse may suggest variations of a favorite activity so that it can be continued. In other cases, substitute activities may be recommended.

The nurse's encouragement may be especially helpful when the patient feels too discouraged to continue prescribed treatment such as exercises. In some cases, the nurse may enlist a family member to exercise with the patient.

After spending hours with the patient and family, the nurse may become aware of special problems. Such problems should be reported to the appropriate nurse or physician so that help can be obtained for the patient.

DEGENERATIVE JOINT DISEASE (OSTEOARTHRITIS)

An individual with degenerative joint disease has a chronic disease of the joints. The nurse may hear degenerative joint disease referred to as *osteoarthritis* or *hypertrophic arthritis*. This is a wear-and-tear condition that destroys the cartilage on weight-bearing joints of persons in the older age group. Women are affected more often than men. Additional joints that may become involved include the distal finger joints. These bony enlargements of the finger joints have been referred to as *Heberden's nodes*. The tissue affected by osteoarthritis is the joint cartilage that loses its elasticity, making it more readily damaged because of the stress placed on that particular joint. As the cartilage disintegrates, the joint loses its shape and the bone ends thicken. Bony spurs or cysts may form, causing pain and limited motion. Osteoarthritis does not completely immobilize (ankylose) the joint.

The cause of osteoarthritis is not known. Some experts have suggested a biochemical abnormality of cartilage metabolism as a cause. Familial patterns may occur. Factors that favor the development of osteoarthritis include obesity, trauma, hypermobility of joints, and hyperparathyroidism.

NURSING OBSERVATIONS. An individual with degenerative joint disease complains of pain in the affected joints. Discomfort may be aggravated by changes in the weather. Rising humidity with falling barometric pressure seems to affect this individual more than others. The affected joints become enlarged and stiff. Symptoms may increase following periods of inactivity.

NURSING INTERVENTIONS. Drug therapy may include salicylates or nonsteroidal anti-inflammatory drugs from Table 17.6 to reduce pain and stiffness. Physical therapy, such as heat, may be used to relieve the patient's discomfort. The patient should avoid becoming damp and cold.

When obesity is present, the patient may need a weight-reduction diet and additional help to achieve weight loss.

Activities such as stair climbing and walking are avoided when possible. Non-

TABLE 17.9
A COMPARISON BETWEEN RHEUMATOID AND
OSTEOARTHRITIS

RHEUMATOID ARTHRITIS	OSTEOARTHRITIS
Tissue affected: synovial membrane	Tissue affected: cartilage
An inflammatory condition	A wear-and-tear condition
A systemic disease	General health is not affected
Characterized by remission and exacerbation	There is no remission
Results in ankylosis and deformity	Limitation of motion only
Affects any joint	Affects weight-bearing joints (except Heberden's which affects the finger joints)
Affects all ages, especially the young	Affects the older age group

weightbearing exercises are substituted to improve mobility. Posture training may be needed.

The physician may recommend retirement or a change of work when the patient's occupation places a constant strain on involved joints. Surgical procedures described for the patient with rheumatoid arthritis also may be indicated for the patient with osteoarthritis. Nursing interventions used in caring for the patient with rheumatoid arthritis may be used for the patient with osteoarthritis as well.

Gout

The individual with gout has a disturbance of purine metabolism. Purines are by-products of the digestion of certain proteins. The individual has an excess amount of uric acid in the blood, which tends to precipitate into urate crystals, *tophi*. These crystals settle at various areas where blood flow is sluggish. Most common areas involved are around the joint of the big toe, the knuckles, ankles, knees, and instep. These crystals also settle in the kidneys and in the ear cartilage.

Heredity seems to play a role in the development of gout. Gout affects more men than women. It is classified as a form of arthritis because of the resulting joint involvement from the crystal deposits.

Gout cannot be cured, but the attack can be controlled. Individuals with gout are seldom hospitalized.

NURSING OBSERVATIONS

The patient usually experiences acute pain in the involved joint. The area becomes red, swollen, and extremely tender to the touch. For example, the patient may not tolerate bedclothes touching the affected joint. An acute attack of gouty arthritis generally disappears in about ten weeks.

NURSING INTERVENTIONS

Strict dietary restriction is no longer prescribed because the diet seems to have little effect on urate levels. Avoiding foods high in purine and increasing fluid intake usually are suggested. An increase of fluid intake is especially important to prevent urinary stasis which may promote the crystallization of the uric acids into kidney stones. A low-purine diet frequently is ordered for the patient during an acute attack of gout. Sweetbreads, anchovies, asparagus, brains, kidney, liver, mushrooms, and sardines are high in purine. Foods that may be limited because they result in a moderate amount of purine are poultry, fish, seafood, dry beans, lentils, and spinach.

Reduction of sodium urate in the patient's body will help to prevent recurrent attacks, prevent further formation of tophi, and allow the tophi already formed to dissolve (see Table 17.1). In order to accomplish this the physician may prescribe a *uricosuric drug,* which facilitates the excretion of uric acid in the urine. Colchicine, phenylbutazone (BUTAZOLIDIN), probenecid (BENEMID), sulfinpyrazone (ANTURANE), and allopurinol (ZYLOPRIM) are examples of drugs that may be prescribed (see Table 17.6).

Osteoporosis

The patient with osteoporosis has a decrease in the normal quantity of bony substance. In other words, the bone is more porous than usual. *Disuse osteoporosis* may occur in bones that are immobilized or deprived of normal pull from muscles. For example, the paralyzed person may develop osteoporosis in the bones of the paralyzed extremity. *Postmenopausal* and *senile osteoporosis* occurs in women and in elderly men. *Nutritional osteoporosis* may develop in persons who have a deficient diet or in those who suffer from malabsorption. Endocrine osteoporosis occurs with abnormal functioning of certain endocrine glands. Prolonged steroid therapy also may cause osteoporosis.

NURSING OBSERVATIONS

Osteoporosis is a normal process during the late adult and elderly years and is of no significance until it produces a pattern of symptoms that includes pain induced by activities such as bending or lifting.

Osteoporosis associated with aging frequently results in broken bones, especially a compression of the vertebrae. Vertebral compression may cause back pain and a decrease in height. Bones such as the upper femur may fracture easily. For this reason a fractured hip is seen frequently in the older person.

TREATMENT AND NURSING INTERVENTIONS

Treatment of the patient with osteoporosis is directed toward relieving the symptoms, such as pain, and helping to check the underlying condition. Mineral supplements, physical therapy, and hormones may be prescribed. A diet high in calcium, vitamin D, and protein may be ordered. If the patient cannot drink at least 1 quart of milk daily, calcium may be given as a supplement. An exercise program usually is developed for the patient with osteoporosis.

Osteomyelitis

The patient with osteomyelitis has a localized infection of the bone. The pathogen may enter the area as a result of a penetrating wound, an ulcer, open surgery of the area, or a compound fracture. The pathogen also may enter through the pin sites of skeletal tractions or be brought to the bone by the bloodstream from an infection elsewhere in the body. An abscess and infected tonsils are examples of infections elsewhere in the body that may be the source of pathogens. The most common offending microorganisms are staphylococci and streptococci.

NURSING OBSERVATIONS

An individual developing acute osteomyelitis generally has symptoms of an acute toxic illness with fever. Severe pain in the affected area or referred pain to another portion of the body is the most common symptom. X-ray of the affected area taken several weeks after the onset of infection generally reveals destructive changes.

Chronic osteomyelitis occurs when a person has built up resistance to the infecting organism. There is an intermittent exacerbation of pain and inflammation that may exist for years.

TREATMENT AND NURSING INTERVENTIONS

Early diagnosis of osteomyelitis and prompt treatment with antibiotics will prevent the progression of the disease from acute to chronic. Surgical treatment is reserved mainly for drainage of an abscess in the bone, or *sequestrectomy*. Sequestrectomy is the surgical removal of dead bone that has become separated from the main part of a bone during a disease process.

Chronic osteomyelitis is extremely difficult to erradicate. Treatment includes long-term antibiotic therapy, immobilization, and continued x-ray monitoring. Extensive tissue damage may necessitate multiple surgeries to debride necrotic bone tissue and surrounding tissues that have become involved in the infection. A closed system of irrigation and drainage generally is utilized.

This patient needs nursing care similar to the care needed by other patients with an infection. Measures of particular importance to this individual are rest, adequate fluids, and a nourishing diet. The diet should be high in proteins, vitamins, and minerals to aid in the healing process. Good skin care to prevent a breakdown of tissue and promote comfort is important. When caring for this patient, the nurse should handle the diseased part gently because of the possibility of a fracture. A half cast may be utilized for the purpose of immobilizing the diseased part. A splint may be used for this purpose also. Immobilization decreases the individual's pain and helps to alleviate muscle spasm.

When caring for the patient with osteomyelitis, the nurse should help the patient maintain good body alignment. Comfort measures such as pillows to support other portions of the body may be helpful also in maintaining good alignment. The nurse should wash the hands before and after giving care to the patient with osteomyelitis to prevent cross-infection. The patient may be placed in isolation. The patient should be observed carefully for a sudden rise in temperature, the development of pain or discomfort in other parts of the body, and other symptoms that may indicate the development of a secondary infection in another part of the body.

The drainage has a characteristic odor, and this odor presents a nursing problem. A deodorizer may be utilized in the patient's unit. Discarded dressings should be removed from the patient's unit promptly. The patient should have an explanation regarding the use of a deodorizer and careful removal of any discarded dressings or other contaminated material. Explaining that a bone infection frequently is accompanied by a characteristic odor will help the patient cope with isolation, odor, and the possible reaction of individuals entering the room.

Bursitis

A person with bursitis has an inflammation of a bursa, which was described earlier in this chapter as a sac containing synovial fluid. These sacs are located around joints, beneath tendons, beneath the skin, over bony prominences. Bursae may develop in other areas which are subject to persistent irritation and friction because bursae serve as lubricating devices which diminish the friction of movement. A bursa may become inflamed because of injury or infection. As a response to the infection or injury, the bursa secretes more fluid, causing the sac to be distended and press on surrounding tissues. Bursitis frequently occurs in the subdeltoid bursa, which is located in the shoulder. The

patient with bursitis complains of pain in the region of the inflamed bursa. Movement increases the pain.

The physician frequently prescribes rest of the inflamed part and local application of heat. The inflamed area may be aspirated and injected with procaine and cortisone to relieve the pain (see Table 17.6). Deep x-ray therapy may be needed. In some cases, calcium deposits appear in tendons that lie underneath the bursa. When these get inflamed, the bursa and the calcium deposits are removed surgically.

Bone Tumors

A patient may develop a benign or malignant bone tumor. Pain and swelling are the principal symptoms of bone tumors. Diagnostic studies generally include x-rays, bone scans, skeletal surveys, and a biopsy.

The patient with a benign tumor may have a surgical excision. This patient requires surgical care related to orthopedic procedures, as described earlier in the chapter. The patient may have either a cast or soft bulky dressings.

Primary malignant bone tumor is rare and, if it is diagnosed before it spreads, treatment consists of a combination of amputation, radiation, and chemotherapy. This treatment is not often successful.

The patient with a metastatic tumor of the bone has treatment aimed at the primary lesion in addition to supportive measures. Cancers of the breasts, lungs, kidneys, prostate, and thyroid seem to be prone to spread to the bones.

The nursing care of the patient with a neoplastic disease (see Chapter 9) is applicable to this patient.

Amputation

An amputation is a radical form of treatment for a diseased limb. The extremity may be affected by such factors as severe injury, marked circulatory disturbance, malignancy, and in some cases a chronic infection that promises no hope for the return of function. A deformed, nonfunctioning limb that bothers the patient may be removed in some instances.

Attempts will be made to save as much of the limb as possible. For example, the surgeon would not perform an above-knee (AK) amputation if a below-knee (BK) amputation is feasible. A surgical technique that the surgeon may use is a *disarticulation,* whereby a limb is amputated at the joint. Often the surgeon leaves skin flaps to cover the end of the stump. This is referred to as *skin flap amputation.* Occasionally, it is necessary to sever skin, muscles, and bones at the same level because of uncontrolled infection. In this case, the surgery is called *guillotine amputation.* The wound is left open as the skin is pulled with skin traction until there is enough skin to cover the stump.

PREOPERATIVE CARE

When possible, the surgeon discusses the amputation with the patient and family prior to surgery. The amount of physical disability and the practical possibility of a functioning prosthesis are considered. Psychologic, esthetic, social, and vocational implications should be considered.

When caring for this patient before surgery, the nurse can help by accepting fully the patient's reaction and that of the family to the loss. The nurse should let them discuss their feelings as they need to. A visit from an amputee who has coped with the loss successfully may be of marked benefit to the patient when this is possible.

Some patients will want to know what disposition will be made of the removed limb. In some cases, the patient and the family may want to have it buried.

Tests to determine the status of circulation in the affected limb are often done before surgery. The surface temperature,

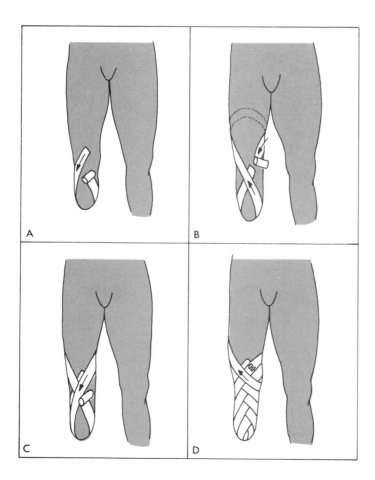

FIGURE 17.16 Bandaging the patient with an amputation of the midcalf.

color changes associated with lowering and elevating the extremity, peripheral vascular studies, and arteriography may be determined.

The limb may be elevated prior to amputation to permit the venous blood to drain from the part. A tourniquet may be applied to compress the blood vessels to decrease the amount of blood going into the extremity.

POSTOPERATIVE CARE

After having an amputation, the patient can be expected to experience the grieving process discussed in Chapter 1. The patient may go through some or all of the stages of denial, anger, bargaining, depression, and acceptance. For example, the patient who first learns of the need for an amputation or the actual loss itself, may refuse to accept it.

An amputation caused by trauma may give the patient and family no time to prepare for the loss.

Although bleeding from loosened ligatures is a rare occurrence, many surgeons order a tourniquet kept at the bedside.

Early ambulation improves circulation in the stump and reduces the need to condition the stump. Some surgeons apply a thin cast over a sterile stump which makes it possible for the patient with a leg amputation to ambulate after 24 hours, with a prosthetic unit consisting of a prosthetic extension and a foot or peg leg.

When the rigid dressing is not used, the patient's stump will need to be conditioned for the prosthesis by bandaging with elastic bandages, using elastic stump-shrinking socks, or a combination of the two (see Figures 17.16 and 17.17). All measures should be

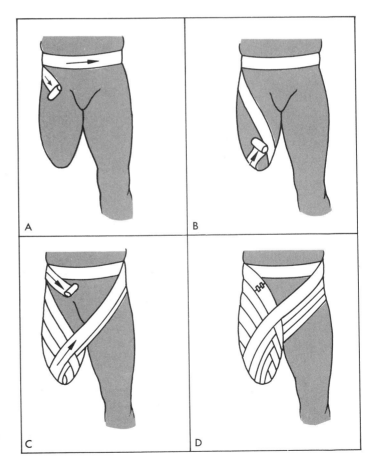

FIGURE 17.17   Bandaging the patient with a midthigh amputation.

taken to place the patient in positions of extension to prevent contractures. After the first day following surgery, the patient should keep the amputated limb extended. Only short periods of flexed position should be allowed. If a leg stump has to be elevated, the foot end of the bed should be raised on blocks. The patient may roll from side to side, but must be encouraged to assume a face-lying position in order to extend the stump.

Bed exercises usually are started on the first postoperative day to prevent contractures and to maintain muscle tone in preparation for ambulation. While on the abdomen, the patient hyperextends the thigh and leg and does push-ups to strengthen the arms and shoulders for crutch walking. While on the back, the patient practices lifting the stump and buttocks off the bed and also does gluteal-setting and quadriceps-setting exercises.

Members of the nursing staff will need to work closely with the physiotherapist in an effort to coordinate activities.

The patient may have a phantom sensation that the amputated limb is still there. In some rare cases, the patient also may experience phantom pain. It is not fully understood whether this phenomenon is a grief reaction or is associated with severed nerve endings. The patient may be reassured to learn that phantom sensation is not uncommon. Disturbing thoughts and feelings often diminish when they can be shared with another person.

After the sutures are removed, the patient may be fitted with a temporary prosthesis until the stump has reached a point at which it can tolerate a permanent one. The specially trained person who makes the prosthesis is called a prosthetist. After learning to use a prosthesis, the patient can expect to experience a marked decrease in awareness of the stump and/or amputated limb. Other disorders of the musculoskeletal system are described in Table 17.10.

TABLE 17.10
OTHER DISORDERS OF THE MUSCULOSKELETAL SYSTEM

DISORDER	DESCRIPTION
Ankylosing spondylitis (Marie-Strümpell disease)	Inflammatory disease of the spine resulting in complete rigidity, either ramrod straight or hunchback; when hip and shoulder joints are involved, an awkward squat gait results
Erythema nodosa	A collagen disease characterized by appearance of red tender nodules under the skin of the legs and arms; it is believed to be an allergic reaction to a viral or bacterial infection or to drugs
Ganglion	A type of cystic tumor that develops on a tendon or aponeurosis; frequently occurs in the wrist
Gonococcal arthritis	A rare disease in which the joints are infected with *Neisseria gonorrhea*
Muscular dystrophies	Progressive atrophy of muscles with no apparent lesion in the nervous system; these conditions are believed to be inherited; main symptom of muscle weakness may appear in childhood
Osteomalacia	A condition characterized by softening of the bones caused by a deficiency of vitamin D or of calcium; pain, tenderness, muscular weakness, anorexia, and loss of weight occur
Paget's disease of bone (osteitis deformans)	A chronic, progressive disease of the bone resulting in deformity; cause is not known; normal bone tissue is replaced by abnormal tissue in the involved areas
Scoliosis	Lateral curvature of the spine beyond normal expectations; frequently occurs during active years of growth; a brace and sometimes spinal fusion may be necessary
Tenosynovitis	An infection of a sheath covering a tendon
Tuberculosis of the spine (Pott's disease)	An infection of the vertebra caused by tuberculosis; chemotherapy and spinal fusion may be used together

Case Study Involving a Fracture

Mr. Reese, a 20-year-old building construction worker, was brought to the emergency room of the local hospital by ambulance stretcher for possible fracture of his right femur. The injury was sustained when a piece of lumber fell on his lap while he was putting up a roof frame.

After being admitted to the emergency room, Mr. Reese received morphine sulfate, 10 mg subcutaneously stat, and had his right leg x-rayed. The x-ray showed a right midfemur transverse fracture. Mr. Reese was admitted to the orthopedic unit with these additional orders:

- Skeletal traction with a 22-kg (10-lb) weight
- Check circulation every hour for 24 hours
- Overhead trapeze
- Meperidine hydrochloride, 50 mg IM every three hours prn, for pain
- Portable chest x-ray
- Complete blood count
- Regular diet

QUESTIONS

1. What is the purpose of the trapeze?
2. Why was a portable chest x-ray preferred to a regular chest x-ray?
3. Plan the nursing care for Mr. Reese, including his activity, eating, personal hygiene, bed making, and recreation.
4. What methods should the nurse use to check Mr. Reese's circulation?
5. What special nursing observations are indicated for a person in skeletal traction and why?
6. What nursing measures will Mr. Reese need to prevent respiratory, circulatory, urinary, and gastrointestinal complications associated with immobility?
7. What life-threatening complications can occur when a long bone is fractured and what observations would indicate this condition?
8. What areas should be examined especially for signs of pressure while Mr. Reese is in traction?
9. What usual site of intramuscular injection should be avoided in the case of Mr. Reese? Why?

Case Study Involving Rheumatoid Arthritis

Mrs. Lori Scott, a 40-year-old homemaker, was admitted to the medical unit of the local hospital because of "an acute flare-up of arthritis."

The nurse who admitted Mrs. Scott noticed that she was overweight, had swollen knees, and appeared to be uncomfortable. The nurse recorded Mrs. Scott's temperature of 38.2°C (100.8°F). Mrs. Scott told the nurse that she had rheumatoid arthritis and had been feeling poorly for about one week. Mrs. Scott requested additional pillows to be placed under her knees. The physician left the following orders:

- Complete bed rest
- 1200-calorie reducing diet—bland
- X-ray both knees tomorrow
- Acetylsalicylic acid, 600 mg po q4h prn, while awake
- Indomethacin, 25 mg po qid, with meals or snack
- Propoxyphene hydrochloride, 65 mg po q3—4h prn, for pain
- Routine admission laboratory studies

QUESTIONS

1. Explain the therapeutic and untoward effects of each drug.
2. If Mrs. Scott takes acetylsalicylic acid, 600 mg every four hours, how many grams will she take in 24 hours?
3. Why is Mrs. Scott receiving a 1200-calorie bland diet?
4. Should fluids be encouraged for Mrs. Scott? Why? Why not?
5. What is the best way for the nurse to respond to Mrs. Scott's request for additional pillows?
6. What can the nurse do to help relieve some of the discomfort of Mrs. Scott's swollen knees?
7. How should the nurse handle Mrs. Scott's affected extremities when movement is indicated?
8. Should Mrs. Scott change position while on bed rest?
9. What assistance should the nurse anticipate giving Mrs. Scott during morning and evening care?
10. How should the nurse respond to Mrs. Scott's statement that she has already been to the bathroom and washed herself?
11. What should the nurse do it is obvious that Mrs. Scott is visibly upset?
12. Plan the nursing care for Mrs. Scott.

Suggestions for Further Study

1. Is there a local unit of the Arthritis Foundation in your community? If so, find out what services are offered.
2. Break a stick, twig, or chicken bone to illustrate as many types of fracture as possible.
3. Is there an emergency rescue squad in your locality? If so, what measures do they take in the emergency care of a person with a fracture?

4. Mason, Mildred A.; Bates, Grace F.; and Smola, Bonnie K.: *Workbook in Basic Medical-Surgical Nursing,* 3rd ed. Macmillan Publishing Company, New York, 1984, Exercise 17.

Additional Readings

Black, Joyce M., and Arnold P. G.: "Facial Fractures." *American Journal of Nursing,* 82:1086–88 (July), 1982.

Buckwalter, Kathleen Coen, and Buckwalter, Joseph A.: "Pain Assessment and Management in the Patient with a Fracture." *Journal of Nursing Care,* 14:17–20 (July), 1981.

Gillette, Ethel: "A Common Sense Approach to Arthritis." *Journal of Nursing Care,* 13:10–12 (Mar.), 1980.

Kryschyshen, Patt L., and Fischer, David A.: "External Fixation for Complicated Fractures." *American Journal of Nursing,* 80:256–59 (Feb.), 1980.

MacLaren, Janet, and Lorig, Kate: "Osteoarthritis." *Journal of Practical Nursing,* 31:17–21 (July-Aug.), 1981.

Meyer, Theresa M.: "TENS: Relieving Pain Through Electricity." *Nursing 82,* 12:57–59 (Sept.), 1982.

Milazzo, Vickie: "An Exercise Class for Patients in Traction." *American Journal of Nursing,* 81:1842–44 (Oct.), 1981.

Nowotny, Mary Lou: "If Your Patient's Joints Hurt, the Reason May Be Osteoarthritis." *Nursing 80,* 10:39–41 (Sept.), 1980.

Porter, Sharon Ferrance; Rovel, Irving; and Dapper, Marcia Johnson: "The Foot and Rheumatoid Arthritis." *Journal of Nursing Care,* 14:18–21 (Apr.), 1981.

Rambo, Beverly J., and Wood, Lucile A. (eds.): *Nursing Skills for Clinical Practice,* 3rd ed. W. B. Saunders Co., Philadelphia, 1982, pp. 260–307 and 734–49.

Robinson, Corinne H.: *Basic Nutrition and Diet Therapy,* 4th ed. Macmillan Publishing Co., Inc., New York, 1980, pp. 240–41.

Walters, Jean: "Coping with a Leg Amputation." *American Journal of Nursing,* 81:1349–52 (July), 1981.

Chapter *18*

The Patient with an Endocrine Disorder

Expected Behavioral Outcomes
Vocabulary Development
Structure and Function
Assisting with Diagnostic Studies
Nursing Observations
Nursing Interventions
The Patient with a Thyroid Disorder
The Patient with a Parathyroid Disorder

The Patient with a Pituitary Disorder
The Patient with an Adrenal Disorder
The Patient with a Pancreatic Disorder
Case Study Involving Graves' Disease
Case Study Involving Diabetes Mellitus
Suggestions for Further Study
Additional Readings

Expected Behavioral Outcomes

Minimum objectives referred to as expected behavioral outcomes have been designed for the practical/vocational nursing student to use as guides in studying this chapter. The student should read these expected outcomes before studying the chapter. The objectives can be used as guides for study.

Using the content of this chapter, the student should return to the objectives and evaluate the ability to:

1. *Prepare a table that describes the effects of each of the main hormones on regulation of body processes.*
2. *Describe each of the diagnostic studies in the chapter using language appropriate for the patient and family.*
3. *Compare the nursing care of the surgical patient as discussed in Chapter 6 to that needed for a patient having surgery on the thyroid gland.*
4. *Compare hypoglycemia and hyperglycemia with respect to immediate causes, underlying causes, nursing observations, nursing interventions, and prevention.*
5. *List the essential parts of a teaching-learning program for the patient with diabetes mellitus.*
6. *Using a head-to-toe format, list nursing observations that could indicate undesirable side effects of the adrenocorticotropic hormone.*

Vocabulary Development

The following prefixes, suffixes, and combining forms pertain to this chapter. By learning and/or reviewing their meanings, the practical/vocational nursing student will have the keys needed to unlock many exciting new medical terms.

Discover the meaning of these keys in a medical dictionary or in the content of this chapter. How does each key pertain to this chapter? In your notebook write the correct meaning of each prefix, suffix, or combining form listed below. Illustrate each key with an example.

acr—extremity. Ex. *acromegaly*—a disease characterized by an enlargement of the extremities.

ad-	horm-
aden-	hyper-
cortic-	hypo-
ede-	insul-
endo-	megal-
exo-	myx-
-gen	ne-
gland-	nod-
glyc(y)-	thyr-

Structure and Function

The endocrine system is composed of *ductless glands* and hormones that help to regulate and control all body systems and processes (see Figure 18.1). Glands of the endocrine system in cooperation with the nervous system take certain chemical substances from the blood and manufacture new chemical messengers called *hormones*. These hormones are then secreted directly into the bloodstream where they are transported to a *target organ* such as the blood vessels, bones, uterus, or another gland. Currently, over 50 different hormones are known to be produced by the body.

Endocrine glands that secrete hormones are (1) the hypothalamus, located next to the pituitary gland; (2) the pituitary, located at the base of the skull; (3) the thyroid, located in the neck; (4) the parathyroids, located on either side of the posterior aspect of the thyroid gland; (5) the adrenals, located above the kidneys; (6) the pineal gland, situated in the skull; (7) the gonads (sex glands); (8) the thymus, situated in the chest; and (9) the pancreas, located behind the stomach in the abdominal cavity. In this chapter, special consideration is given to the patient with disturbances in hormone activity of the thyroid, adrenals, and pancreas.

Hormone production and secretion are affected by a number of factors. In some cases, there is a regular pattern of hormone production and release. Typical rhythmic patterns include *circadian* (over a 24-hour period) and monthly. In other cases, small amounts of a hormone are secreted continuously. Physiologic factors such as activity, body temperature, or illness may affect hor-

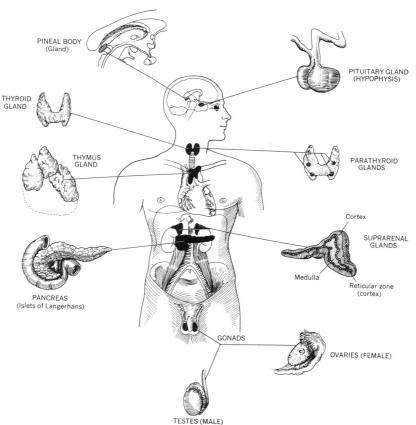

FIGURE 18.1   The endocrine glands. (From Pansky, Ben: *Dynamic Anatomy and Physiology*. Macmillan Publishing Co, Inc., New York, 1975.)

mone production and release. The central nervous system and other hormones are important influences on production and secretion also.

According to recent research, regulation of most hormone activity is accomplished by a mechanism called *negative feedback loops.* The negative feedback loop contains a complex series of interrelated steps to regulate hormone production and release. A rising concentration of hormone in the circulation acts as an inhibitor to further release of that hormone. Similarly, a falling concentration in the circulation of a hormone acts as a stimulator for additional production and release of that hormone. A disturbance in any of the relationships in the feedback loop may cause a person to develop symptoms of an endocrine disorder.

HYPOTHALAMUS AND PITUITARY GLANDS

The hypothalamus and pituitary glands are located in the middle of the head in a portion of the sphenoid bone called the *sella tursica.* The pituitary gland is attached to the hypothalamus by a stalk. Until recently, the pituitary gland was known as the master gland because it was believed to control all other endocrine secretions. It is now known that the hormones secreted by the hypothalamus have an important influence on pituitary activity. Hypothalamic hormones that have been identified include thyrotropin-releasing hormone, gonadotropin-releasing hormone, corticotropin-releasing hormone, prolactin-inhibiting hormone, and somatostatin (growth hormone release-inhibiting hormone).

The pituitary gland is divided into anterior, posterior, and middle lobes. Each lobe secretes different hormones. Table 18.1 contains a summary of information about hormones produced and released by the pituitary gland. Over- or undersecretion of hormones may cause profound physical changes. For example, oversecretion of growth hormone in a child results in giantism, and in the adult causes acromegaly (see Figure 18.2). The client with acromegaly has an overgrowth of the jaw (protrusion) and wide hands and broad fingers. The individual with acromegaly may also develop local manifestations caused by a compression of brain tissues from the existing tumor. The treatment for both giantism and acromegaly

TABLE 18.1
PITUITARY HORMONES

HORMONE	SITE OF ORIGIN	TARGET AREA	ACTION
Adrenocorticotropic hormone (ACTH)	Anterior lobe	Adrenal glands	Increases production and secretion of cortisol
Antidiuretic hormone (ADH); vasopressin	Posterior lobe	Kidneys	Conserves water
Follicle-stimilating hormone (FSH)	Anterior lobe	Ovaries, testes	Stimulates production of ovarian follicles, estrogen, and sperm
Growth hormone (STH)	Anterior lobe	Bones	Stimulates growth of bones, muscles
Luteinizing hormone (LH)	Anterior lobe	Ovaries, testes	Stimulates maturation of ovarian follicle, ovulation, testosterone secretion
Melanocyte-stimulating hormone (MSH)	Middle lobe	Skin cells	Affects skin pigmentation
Oxytocin	Posterior lobe	Uterus, breasts	Stimulates uterine contraction and secretion of breast milk
Prolactin	Anterior lobe	Ovaries, breasts	Stimulates secretion of breast milk and progesterone; affects corpus luteum
Thyroid-stimulating hormone (TSH)	Anterior lobe	Thyroid gland	Regulates manufacture and release of thyroid hormones

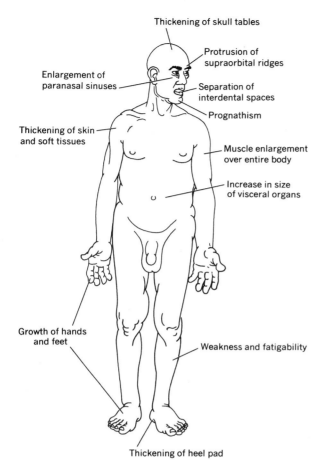

Thickening of skull tables

Protrusion of supraorbital ridges

Enlargement of paranasal sinuses

Separation of interdental spaces

Prognathism

Thickening of skin and soft tissues

Muscle enlargement over entire body

Increase in size of visceral organs

Growth of hands and feet

Weakness and fatigability

Thickening of heel pad

FIGURE 18.2   Physical changes associated with acromegaly. (From Pansky, Ben: *Dynamic Anatomy and Physiology*. Macmillan Publishing Co., Inc., New York, 1975.)

is either surgical hypophysectomy, removal or destruction of the pituitary gland, or irradiation of the pituitary. Dwarfism results when the child produces too little of the growth hormone, STH.

THYROID GLAND

The thyroid gland is located in the neck in front of the trachea. This gland consists of two lobes, which are located on each side of the trachea. The two lobes are connected by a strip of thyroid tissue called the isthmus. The thyroid gland is stimulated by the thyroid-stimulating hormone (TSH), produced by the anterior pituitary gland. TSH regulates the rate at which the thyroid gland clears iodine, which is necessary for hormone production. The thyroid gland produces thyroxine, triiodothyronine, and thyrocalcitonin. The main functions of thyroxine are to regulate the metabolic and oxidation rates of the cells throughout the body and to influence the conversion of glycogen to glucose. Thyroxine also has an influence on the conversion of noncarbohydrates to glycogen. Thyroxine has an effect on the body's quantity of enzymes and stimulates growth and development in children. An absence of thyroxine causes cretinism in the infant. A deficient amount of thyroxine may result in myxedema in the adult. Hypothyroidism can occur as a result of a deficient amount of thyroxine, and hyperthyroidism may result from an excessive amount of thyroxine. The function of triiodothyronine is to stimulate metabolism, especially the catabolic phase.

The hormone thyrocalcitonin lowers the level of calcium and phosphates in the blood plasma.

ADRENAL GLANDS

The adrenal (suprarenal) glands are located above each kidney. Each adrenal gland is divided into two parts: the cortex and the medulla. The adrenal cortex is essential for life. If this structure is destroyed, death occurs in a few days. After being stimulated by the anterior pituitary gland, the adrenal cortex produces steroid hormones called corticoids. Three types of corticoids essential for life are *mineralocorticoids,* which regulate extracellular fluid volume, *glucocorticoids* which regulate metabolism and the stress response, and *adrenal sex hormones* which regulate secondary sex characteristics. The adrenal medulla secretes *norepinephrine* and *epinephrine* which regulate the sympathetic nervous sys-

tem activities. Table 18.2 contains a summary of information about essential adrenal hormones.

Over- or undersecretion of adrenal hormones may cause life-threatening illness. For example, a deficiency of mineralocorticoids may cause hypotension, decreased cardiac output, and severe shock. An excessive amount of mineralocorticoids may result in hypertension. A deficiency of glucocorticoids may cause Addison's disease. Excessive glucocorticoid secretions may produce Cushing's syndrome, diabetes mellitus, tissue wasting, hypertension, impaired healing, and decreased antibody formation. Also, an excessive amount of glucocorticoid secretions may lower the body's resistance to infection. Usually, adrenal secretion of the sex hormones is considered insignificant

TABLE 18.2
ADRENAL HORMONES

HORMONE	SITE OF ORIGIN	TARGET AREA	ACTION
Aldosterone (mineralocorticoid)	Cortex	Renal distal tubules	Regulates extracellular fluid volume by affecting sodium reabsorption
Androgens and estrogens (adrenal sex hormones)	Cortex	Skin, genitalia	Regulates secondary sex characteristics
Cortisol (glucocorticoid)	Cortex	Widely distributed Target area is entire body	Regulates protein, carbohydrate, lipid metabolism Affects physiologic response to stress. Regulates anti-inflammatory activities Affects emotional well-being Necessary for other essential life processes to occur
Epinephrine (catecholamine)	Medulla	Nerve endings in heart, skeletal muscles, sympathetic nervous system	Selective vasodilatation in target areas Stimulates conversion of glycogen to glucose
Norepinephrine (catecholamine)	Medulla	Nerve endings in blood vessels, heart, skeletal muscle, sympathetic nervous system	Increases rate and force of myocardial contraction Peripheral vasoconstriction Dilatation of blood vessels in skeletal muscle and myocardium Stimulates conversion of glycogen to glucose

because androgens and estrogens are se-creted in large amounts by the gonads. When, however, there is excessive produc-tion of sex hormones by the adrenal glands, symptoms may result. One of these is viril-ism, the development of masculine physical and mental traits in the female. Another symptom that may result from excessive es-trogen is retention of sodium and water. All corticoids are important in the body's de-fense against injury and against stress.

An oversecretion of the adrenal medulla usually is caused by a vascular tumor of the adrenal medulla and is called pheochromocy-toma, which produces hypertension and hy-perglycemia (high blood sugar). Removal of the tumor is generally done for correction. A decreased secretion or loss of the adrenal medulla usually does not cause problems be-cause of compensation by the sympathetic nervous system.

Assisting with Diagnostic Studies

A variety of diagnostic studies may be or-dered for the patient with an endocrine dis-order. Most studies involve laboratory anal-ysis of blood and/or urine. Table 18.3

contains a list of common laboratory studies used to evaluate endocrine function. A very important nursing responsibility is correct patient preparation and accurate collection and labeling of urine specimens. In addition, the nurse explains the test using language the patient can understand. Research in en-docrinology is resulting in a wealth of new information about diagnosis and treatment of the patient with an endocrine disorder. The interested nurse may consult nursing journals and other references for new data on diagnosis as it becomes available. Addi-tional information about specific endocrine studies can be located on pages 605–606.

Laboratory Studies

Plasma levels of a particular hormone may be measured using a variety of labora-tory methods. Table 18.3 contains informa-tion about common blood tests ordered to evaluate an endocrine disorder.

Urine collections may be ordered by the physician to measure the amount of a hor-mone or related metabolic substance ex-creted in the urine. In many cases, a 24-hour urine collection is needed to evaluate hormo-

TABLE 18.3
NORMAL VALUES OF LABORATORY TESTS FREQUENTLY USED TO STUDY
ENDOCRINE FUNCTION*

TEST	NORMAL VALUE
Bilirubin (serum)	
Direct	0–0.4 mg/100 ml
Total	0–1.0 ml/100 ml
Calcitonin	0–0.1 ng/ml (basal)
Calcium, total (serum)	8.5–10.5 mg/100 ml
Catecholamines (urine)	Less than 110 mcg/dl in 24-hour urine
Total	
Cortisol (plasma)	
8 A.M. specimen	7–25 mcg/dl
8 P.M. specimen	2–9 mcg/dl
Post-ACTH infusion	30–60 mcg/dl
Dexamethasone suppression (8 A.M. specimen)	
Estriol (serum)	
1st trimester	Up to 1.0 ng/ml
2nd trimester	0.8–7.0 ng/ml
3rd trimester	5.0–35 ng/ml
Estrogens (serum)	
Male	4–14 ng/100 ml
Female, premenopausal	4–60 ng/100 ml
Postmenopausal	3–14 ng/100 ml
Children	Less than 3 ng/100 ml

TABLE 18.3 (*Continued*)
NORMAL VALUES OF LABORATORY TESTS FREQUENTLY USED TO STUDY
ENDOCRINE FUNCTION*

TEST	NORMAL VALUE
FSH, pituitary gonadotropin (urine)	
Male	5–25 IU/24 hours
Female, menopausal	50–100 IU/24 hours
Follicular phase	5–20 IU/24 hours
Midcycle	15–60 IU/24 hours
Luteal phase	5–15 IU/24 hours
Gastrin, fasting (serum)	Less than 300 pg/ml
Glucose, fasting (serum)	70–110 mg/100 ml
Glucose tolerance, IV (serum)	Fasting: 70–110 mg/100 ml
	1 hour: 120–170 mg/ml
	2 hours: below 120 mg/100 ml
	3 hours: fasting level
Glucose tolerance, oral (serum)	Fasting: 70–110 mg/100 ml followed by an elevation to 160 mg/100 ml within 30–60 minutes after ingestion and a return to normal within 2 hours
Insulin (serum)	3–20 microunits/ml
Ketosteroids, 17 (urine)	
Male	6–21 mg/24 hour
Female	4–17 mg/24 hour
Children	2–7 mg/24 hour
Parathyroid hormone (PTH)	Less than 2 ng/ml
Protein-bound iodine (PBI)	3.0–8.0 mcg/100 ml
T-4 (thyroxine), total (serum)	5.0–13.5 mcg/dl
T-3 uptake, *in vitro* (serum)	25–35%
T-3 RIA (serum)	110–200 ng/ml
T-7 male (serum)	2.0–3.8 mcg/dl
Thyroid-stimulating hormone (serum) (TSH)	2–10 micro IU/ml
Testosterone (serum)	
Male	300–1200 ng/100 ml
Female	20–80 ng/100 ml
Vanillylmandelic acid (VMA) (urine)	2–7 mg/dl in 24-hour urine

* See narrative of this chapter for indications and nursing implications.

nal activity. A complete 24-hour collection is essential for accurate diagnostic information. This is accomplished by explaining the collection method to the patient and other members of the nursing staff so that urine is not accidentally discarded. The collection begins immediately *after* the patient empties the bladder. All urine is saved for 24 hours. Each urine specimen is placed in the appropriate container. In some collections, special preservatives are present in the container to prevent chemical breakdown of substances to be analyzed in the laboratory. About ten minutes before the end of the 24-hour period, the patient is asked to urinate so that the bladder is empty at the end of the collection period. If a specimen is accidentally discarded during the collection period, the nurse reports that fact to the physician and the laboratory. In some cases, the collection can be continued with a special notation on the laboratory requisition about the missing specimen. In other cases, the collection must be restarted. When restarting a 24-hour urine, the collection period can begin at the time the discarded urine specimen was voided. For example, if the patient voided 250 ml of urine at 9:30 A.M. and the specimen was accidentally discarded at 9:45 A.M., the new collection period can begin at 9:30 A.M. Table 18.3 includes laboratory tests on urine speciments.

Dynamic tests are available that evaluate the ability of a gland to respond when stimulated. For most tests, a hormone or other substance is administered first to stimulate the gland. Next, blood and/or urine specimens are collected and sent to the laboratory. Remembering that a hormone may have another gland as the target area enables the nurse to understand that the hormone or substance used to stimulate a gland may be different from the hormone or substance measured in the blood or urine. ACTH infusion, dexamethasone suppression, and glucose tolerance (see Table 18.3) are examples of dynamic tests of endocrine function.

Nursing Observations

The widespread distribution of hormone activities throughout the body leads to a variety of possible observations in the patient with an endocrine disorder. Some changes in appearance and behavior are striking and easily noticed. Other changes are more subtle. A family member or close friends of the patient may be helpful in providing information about gradual changes in behavior. Table 18.4 contains a guide to nursing observations when the patient has an endocrine disorder.

TABLE 18.4

GUIDE TO NURSING OBSERVATIONS FOR THE PATIENT WITH AN ENDOCRINE DISORDER

AREA TO BE OBSERVED	OBSERVATIONS
Hair	Changes in distribution, texture, abnormal hairiness (hirsutism)
Eyes	Protuberant eyeballs (exophthalmos), puffiness around eyes
	Vision impairment
Face	Moon-shaped, flushed, downy coat of hair
Ears	Deafness
Mouth	Husky voice, nausea and vomiting, enlargement of tongue
Neck	Enlargement, dysphagia, visible growths
Chest	Apical heart rate may be abnormally fast or slow
	Respirations may be abnormally fast or slow
Abdomen	Protuberant, distended
	May have pink striae (streaks)
Extremities	Abnormal enlargement in proportion to body
	Edema
	Muscle spasms, twitches, weakness (tetany)
	Paresthesias
	Fractures without comparable trauma
	Blood pressure abnormally high or low
Skin	Hirsutism (excessive hair)
	Abnormal changes in skin pigmentation, texture
	Excessive bruising without comparable trauma
Gastrointestinal symptoms	Constipation, flatulence
	Nausea and vomiting
Urine output	Excessive urination (polyuria)
Height	Unusually and abnormally tall or short
Weight	Abnormal gains or losses
	Changes in normal distribution of body fat
Behavioral changes	Appetite changes such as hunger (polyphagia), thirst (polydipsia), anorexia
	Weakness, fatigue, exhaustion
	Wide mood swings
	Feelings of depression, apathy
	Feelings of nervousness, irritability
	Disturbances in all phases of sexuality including menstruation, fertility, sexual interest, performance
	Personality changes such as mental confusion and symptoms of mental illness
	Reports of intolerance to heat and cold
	Memory impairment, disturbances in concentration

Nursing Interventions

Nursing interventions are developed according to the patient's specific endocrine dysfunction. For example, diet therapy is essential for the patient with diabetes mellitus. Hormone replacement is a mainstay of drug therapy for most patients with an endocrine disorder. Table 18.5 contains a list of common drugs prescribed for the patient with an endocrine problem. Patient and family teaching is important for all patients with an endocrine disorder. These interventions are described in greater detail in appropriate sections later in the chapter.

A therapeutic relationship is an important part of nursing care for the patient with an endocrine disorder. The patient often feels and looks different, both to him- or herself and to others. The person who feels and looks different may withdraw from social interaction. This situation may be made worse because people often shy away from contact with those who look or act differently.

The nurse's warmth and friendliness in

[Text continued on page 594.]

TABLE 18.5
SUMMARY OF HORMONES AND HORMONE ANTAGONISTS*

DRUG	USUAL DOSE	METHOD(S) OF ADMINISTRATION	THERAPEUTIC ACTION OR EFFECT	POSSIBLE SIDE EFFECTS AND/OR PRECAUTIONS
Antithyroid Drugs (for hyperthyroidism)				
Methimazole	Dose of these is dependent upon the needs of the patient	Oral	Used in the treatment of hyperthyroidism	May cause agranulocytosis, drowsiness, gastrointestinal disturbances, headache, hepatic damage, and vertigo
Methylthiouracil	As above	Oral	As above	As above
Propylthiouracil	As above	Oral	As above	As above
Sodium iodide	As above	Oral	As above	May cause conjunctivitis, rhinitis, gastrointestinal disturbances, and headache
Sodium iodide (^{131}I) (isotope)	As above	Oral	As above	May induce hypothyroidism
Strong iodine solution (Lugol's solution)	As above	Oral	As above	Contraindicated in tuberculosis—may cause breakdown of lesion
Hypothyroidism Drugs				
Sodium levothyroxine (SYNTHROID)	Dose of these drugs is dependent upon the needs of the patient	Oral	Used in the treatment of hypothyroidism	In general, these preparations may cause such symptoms as angina, diarrhea, dyspnea, headache, nervousness, palpitation, excessive warmth, vomiting, weight loss
Sodium liothyronine (CYTOMEL)	As above	Oral	As above	As above

TABLE 18.5 (*Continued*)
SUMMARY OF HORMONES AND HORMONE ANTAGONISTS*

DRUG	USUAL DOSE	METHOD(S) OF ADMINISTRATION	THERAPEUTIC ACTION OR EFFECT	POSSIBLE SIDE EFFECTS AND/OR PRECAUTIONS
Thyroglobulin	As above	Oral	As above	As above
Thyroid (desiccated thyroid)	As above	Oral	As above	As above
Adrenocorticotropic Hormone				
Corticotropin (ACTH)	As ordered	Intramuscular Intravenous	Diagnostic agent in adrenal insufficiency; may be used in treatment of adrenocortical insufficiency, rheumatoid arthritis, asthma, gouty arthritis, rheumatic fever, contact dermatitis, drug sensitivity, ulcerative colitis	Note: Adrenocorticotropic hormone is produced by the anterior lobe of the pituitary gland and stimulates the cortex of the adrenal gland to produce hormones
Corticosteroids				
Betamethasone (CELESTONE)	The dose of all of these drugs is dependent upon their use	Oral Intramuscular Intrasynovial Intra-articular	Uses of these drugs are similar; they may be used to treat rheumatoid arthritis, scleroderma, lupus erythematosus, dermatomyositis, acute rheumatic fever, as substitution therapy (Addison's disease), certain allergic conditions, as well as various conditions of the eyes, ears, and skin	May cause acne, gastric distress, headache, insomnia, hypertension, muscular weakness, abnormal growth of hair, rounding of the face, vertigo, weight gain, manic-depressive state
Cortisone acetate (CORTONE ACETATE)	As above	Oral Intramuscular		As above
Desoxycorticosterone (DOCA ACETATE)	As above	Subcutaneous Intramuscular Buccal Sublingual		May also cause pulmonary congestion
Fludrocortisone (FLORINEF)	100–300 mcg daily	Oral	As above	Same as betamethasone
Fluprednisolone (ALPHADROL)	Dependent on use	Oral	As above	As above
Hydrocortisone (CORTEF, CORTRIL, HYDROCORTONE)	As above	Oral Intravenous Intra-articular	As above	As above

TABLE 18.5 (*Continued*)
SUMMARY OF HORMONES AND HORMONE ANTAGONISTS*

DRUG	USUAL DOSE	METHOD(S) OF ADMINISTRATION	THERAPEUTIC ACTION OR EFFECT	POSSIBLE SIDE EFFECTS AND/OR PRECAUTIONS
Meprednisone (BETAPAR)	As above	Oral	As above	As above
Methylprednisolone (MEDROL)	Dependent on use	Intramuscular Intrasynovial Oral	Same as betamethasone	Same as betamethasone
Paramethasone HALDRONE	As above	Oral	As above	As above
Prednisolone (DELTA-COR-TEF, PARACOR-TOL, STERANE)	As above	Oral Intravenous Intramuscular Intrabursal Intra-articular	As above	As above
Prednisone (DELTASONE, DELTRASONE, METICORTEN, PARACORT)	As above	Oral	As above	As above Note: 3–5 times more potent therapeutically than cortisone, or hydrocortisone
Triamcinolone (ARISTOCORT, KENACORT)	As above	Oral Intra-articular Intrasynovial	As above	Same as betamethasone
Progestins				
Dydrogesterone	10–20 mg or as ordered	Oral	May be used for functional uterine bleeding, amenorrhea, dysmenorrhea, premenstrual tension, and habitual abortion	May cause nausea and some irregular bleeding
Ethisterone (LUTOCYLOL, PRANONE)	Dependent on use	Oral Sublingual		
Hydroxyprogesterone (DELALUTIN)	125–250 mg as ordered	Intramuscular		
Medroxyprogesterone (PROVERA)	Dependent on use	Oral Intramuscular		
Norethindrone (NORLUTIN)	Dependent on use	Oral		
Progesterone	10–20 mg or as ordered	Intramuscular Subcutaneous		
Androgens				
Dromostanolone propionate (DROLBAN)	100 mg 3 times weekly	Intramuscular	May be used in treatment of hypogonadism, menstrual disorders, and certain cases of breast cancer	May cause abnormal hair growth, and deepening of the voice
Fluoxymesterone	As needed	Oral	May be used in treatment of hypogonadism, testicular hypofunction, and male climacteric	Contraindicated in prostatic carcinoma

TABLE 18.5 (*Continued*)
SUMMARY OF HORMONES AND HORMONE ANTAGONISTS*

DRUG	USUAL DOSE	METHOD(S) OF ADMINISTRATION	THERAPEUTIC ACTION OR EFFECT	POSSIBLE SIDE EFFECTS AND/OR PRECAUTIONS
Methyl- testosterone (METANDREN)	10 mg 3 times daily	Oral Buccal Sublingual	May be used to re- place male hor- mone deficiency, in some cases of breast cancer, to relieve menopau- sal symptoms, to relieve uterine bleeding	May cause abnor- mal growth of hair, deepening of voice, edema, and jaundice
Oxandrolone (ANAVAR)	5–10 mg daily	Oral	May be used in cases of retarded growth and de- velopment in chil- dren	May cause hoarse- ness and abnor- mal growth of hair
Oxymetholone (ANDROYD, ANADROL)	5–15 mg daily	Oral	As above	As above
Testosterone	50 mg 3 times wkly	Intramuscular	As above	As above
Testosterone cypionate	100 to 400 mg 2–4 wk	Intramuscular	As above	As above
Testosterone propionate	10–20 mg daily 25 mg 2–4 times wkly or as or- dered	Buccal Intramuscular	As above	As above
Stanozolol	6 mg daily	Oral	May be useful in treatment of os- teoporosis, burns, decubitus ulcers, and in postoperative treatment of cancer	
Estrogens				
Chlorotrianisene	12–25 mg daily	Oral	In general, all es- trogens may be given to relieve estrogen hor- mone deficiencies during and after menopause, in cases of female hypogonadism, to relieve the symptoms of atrophic vaginitis and pruritus vul- vae, in treatment of functional uterine bleeding, in cases of habit- ual abortion, and	These estrogens may cause ano- rexia, breast en- gorgement, gas- trointestinal disturbances, headache, insom- nia, and vertigo; should be used with caution in cases of history of familial can- cer; contraindi- cated in thyroid dysfunction and liver diseases
Dienestrol	100–500 mg daily or as ordered	Oral Intramuscular Intravenous Subcutaneous Vaginal		
Diethylstilbestrol (STILBETIN)	As ordered	Oral Intramuscular Subcutaneous Vaginal Topical Urethral		
Estradiol (and derivatives) benzoate cypionate dipropionate valerate	Dependent on use and preparation	Intramuscular Subcutaneous Intramuscular Intramuscular Intramuscular		

TABLE 18.5 (*Continued*)
SUMMARY OF HORMONES AND HORMONE ANTAGONISTS*

DRUG	USUAL DOSE	METHOD(S) OF ADMINISTRATION	THERAPEUTIC ACTION OR EFFECT	POSSIBLE SIDE EFFECTS AND/OR PRECAUTIONS
Ethinyl Estradiol		Oral	in treatment of carcinoma of the breast and prostate gland; may also be used to suppress lactation	
Estrogenic substance conjugated (PREMARIN)	Varies—dosage adjusted to control symptoms.	Oral Intravenous Intramuscular Topical	As above	
Estrone	Dependent on use	Oral Intramuscular Intravaginal Topical	As above	
Methallenestril	3 mg daily or as ordered	Oral	As above	

Oral Hypoglycemic Drugs

Acetohexamide (DYMELOR) Chlorpropamide (DIABINESE) Tolazamide (TOLINASE) Tolbutamide (ORINASE)	Dose of these drugs is dependent on needs of individual patient; may be given in one daily dose or in divided doses	Oral	May be given in the treatment of non-insulin-dependent diabetes mellitus	Side effects of the drugs are similar, namely gastrointestinal disturbances, anorexia, headache, dizziness, insomnia, skin rash

Insulin Preparations

PREPARATIONS	APPROXIMATE ACTION ONSET	APPROXIMATE TIME OF DURATION	THERAPEUTIC USE	POSSIBLE SIDE EFFECTS AND/OR PRECAUTIONS
Fast Acting				
Regular insulin	½–1 hour	6–8 hours	Used as replacement therapy in the treatment of diabetes mellitus; indicated in the treatment of insulin-dependent diabetes; it may or may not be considered in the treatment of diabetes mellitus developed in later life	Symptoms of insulin shock include pallor, hunger, weakness, nervousness, sweating, and irritability
Semilente insulin	½–1 hour	14 hours		

TABLE 18.5 *(Continued)*
SUMMARY OF HORMONES AND HORMONE ANTAGONISTS*

PREPARATIONS	APPROXIMATE ACTION ONSET	APPROXIMATE TIME OF DURATION	THERAPEUTIC USE	POSSIBLE SIDE EFFECTS AND/OR PRECAUTIONS
Intermediate Acting				
Globin zinc insulin	1–2 hours	18 hours		
Isophane insulin (NPH)	1–2 hours	24 hours		
Lente insulin	1–2 hours	24 hours		
Long Acting				
Protamine zinc insulin	4–7 hours	36 hours		Peak action and length of action may vary with the dosage, site of injection, and individual response.
Ultralente insulin	4–7 hours	36 hours		

DRUG	USUAL DOSE	METHOD(S) OF ADMINISTRATION	THERAPEUTIC ACTION OR EFFECT	POSSIBLE SIDE EFFECTS AND/OR PRECAUTIONS
Pituitary Hormone, Posterior				
Oxytocin injection (PITOCIN)	2–10 units as ordered	Intramuscular	Given to induce or stimulate labor or treat postpartum hemorrhage	May cause hypotension, nausea, and vomiting
Posterior pituitary injection (PITUITRIN)	5–10 units as ordered	Intramuscular	As above	
Vasopressin (PITRESSIN)	As ordered	Intramuscular	Used to control volume of urine in diabetes insipidus	May cause cutaneous vasoconstriction, and gastrointestinal discomfort

* From Gilman, Alfred Goodman; Goodman, Louis S.; and Gilman, Alfred: *Goodman and Gilman's The Pharmacological Basis of Therapeutics*, 6th ed. Macmillan Publishing Co., Inc., New York, 1980, pp. 1367–1550.

caring for the patient help to reduce feelings of isolation and loneliness. In addition, the nurse sets an example to others about the value and importance of human contact to the person who looks and feels different from others.

The Patient with a Thyroid Disorder

The three basic types of abnormalities of the thyroid gland are (1) enlargement, goiter; (2) hypersecretion, hyperthyroidism; and (3) hyposecretion, hypothyroidism.

In addition to the laboratory studies described earlier in the chapter in Table 18.3, the nurse may wish further information about common diagnostic tests in order to explain and prepare the patient as well as collect the appropriate specimens.

BASAL METABOLIC RATE (BMR)

The basal metabolic rate (BMR) is a measure of the amount of oxygen consumed by the body when the client is in a state of complete physical and mental rest. Preparation of the individual is the responsibility of the nurse. The client has nothing by mouth for

12 hours prior to the test. This includes the ingestion of most drugs. Individuals responsible for caring for the client prior to this examination should explain that the test is painless. Adequate rest, both physical and mental, prior to the examination is necessary. Morning care is generally omitted on the test day in order to avoid disturbing the individual. The normal range of rate is +10 to −10. A rate higher than +10 may indicate an overactive thyroid, and a rate below −10 may indicate an underactive thyroid. This test is rarely used now because newer blood tests provide more precise information.

PROTEIN-BOUND IODINE (PBI)

Protein-bound iodine (PBI) is a test performed on blood serum to measure iodine in the thyroxine released from the thyroid gland, which becomes bound to protein molecules. Table 18.3 includes normal values. Values higher than normal may indicate an overactive thyroid, and values lower than normal may indicate an underactive thyroid. The T-4 (thyroxine test) is currently replacing the PBI in many agencies.

The nursing responsibilities in the PBI are to restrict iodine in any form, such as iodized salt, foods high in iodine such as salt-water fish and shellfish, and iodine-containing drugs. The client and/or the family should be asked if the individual to be tested has recently taken any of the following agents or drugs:

ACTH
Androgens
Barbiturates
Barium sulfate (used in gastrointestinal series and barium enema)
Cortisone
Estrogens
Gargles
Gold salts
Iodine-containing drugs
Isoniazid
Lithium carbonate
Mercurial diuretics
Metrecal
Oral contraceptives
Perphenazine
Reserpine

Salicylates
Sulfonamides
Thiazides

The client also should be asked if any radioiodine substance has been injected or ingested in the last six months, such as that used for a gallbladder x-ray. The client does not have to be without food or fluid prior to this test, which is an advantage.

THYROXINE TEST (T-4)

Thyroxine (T-4) is a test of thyroid function. A high thyroxine level may indicate hyperthyroidism and a low level may mean hypothyroidism. No restriction of food or liquid is necessary prior to the test. Phenytoin sodium (DILANTIN) and related drugs, oral contraceptives, and certain serious illnesses can influence the test results. A normal range is given in Table 18.3, however, the normal range will vary with the laboratory procedure.

RADIOIODINE UPTAKE TEST (^{131}I UPTAKE)

Another procedure that may be used to test the functioning of a patient's thyroid gland is the radioactive iodine uptake study (see Table 18.3). The thyroid gland normally stores some of the iodine that is taken into the body in foods. The remaining portion of the iodine is excreted in the urine. The amount of iodine taken up by the thyroid gland is affected by disease. This amount can be determined by giving the patient radioactive iodine, which gives off rays. A small amount of radioactive iodine is usually given in a glass of water by a specialist trained in this field. The amount of this substance taken up by the thyroid gland is measured 24 hours later by a scintillation scanner. The amount of radioactive iodine passed in the urine may be measured also. The physician assumes that the patient has a toxic goiter when the report shows an increased uptake of radioactive iodine by the thyroid gland. This patient usually excretes less iodine in the urine. If the doctor finds that the patient's thyroid took up only a small amount of radioactive iodine and excreted more in the urine, an underactive thyroid gland is suspected.

Knowing that the dosage of radioiodine is small enables the nurse to allay the individual's fear regarding this substance. The radioiodine will cause no harm. As stated earlier regarding the client scheduled for a PBI, this client also should be questioned regarding a history of drug ingestion and iodine contrast-media diagnostic tests. Information regarding seafood ingestion also should be obtained. Another nursing responsibility is to collect, preserve, and label the 24-hour urine specimen. It is not necessary for the client to be NPO prior to this test.

TRIIODOTHYRONINE (T-3) RESIN UPTAKE TEST

In this test blood is drawn from the client and the serum is incubated with radioactive triiodothyronine (similar to thyroxine) and resin. The amount of triiodothyronine that binds with the protein molecules is measured. Lab values higher than normal may indicate hyperthyroidism, and values lower than normal may indicate hypothyroidism. No special preparation of the patient or restriction of intake is needed prior to this test.

THYROTROPIN TEST (TSH)

The physician may order this test after ordering the ^{131}I uptake and PBI tests to help differentiate between hypothyroidism caused by a malfunctioning thyroid gland and secondary hypothyroidism caused by malfunctioning of the pituitary gland. Thyrotropin is administered by injection. The protein-bound iodine test and ^{131}I uptake test are done 24 hours after the injection. If the client has primary hypothyroidism, the TSH will have no effect on the ^{131}I uptake and PBI tests. However, if the PBI and ^{131}I uptake tests are elevated, it may be an indication of secondary hypothyroidism. The nursing responsibilities are to prepare the client appropriately for the PBI and ^{131}I uptake tests.

THYROID SCAN

The physician may order a thyroid scan to determine the cause of hyperthyroidism in the patient. The patient ingests radioactive iodide first. Next a scanner is moved across the neck in order to record a map of the radioactivity in the thyroid gland. By studying the map and other thyroid tests, the physician is helped to distinguish benign growths from malignant ones. The test is not painful and no special preparation is needed.

ENLARGEMENT OF THE THYROID GLAND

An individual may have an enlargement of the thyroid gland as a result of (1) simple goiter, (2) thyroiditis, or (3) tumors.

SIMPLE GOITER (NONTOXIC). A simple goiter can occur as a result of the thyroid gland compensating for a lack of iodine. Iodine is needed for the manufacture and secretion of hormones by the thyroid gland. A lack of iodine may be caused by an inadequate intake of iodine or a suppression of the production of thyroid hormones caused by other reasons.

Simple goiter tends to be prevalent in regions where there is a deficiency of iodine in the soil and water. However, table salt generally has iodine added. Females tend to have a simple goiter more often than males. Nontoxic goiter seems to be more common during adolescence, pregnancy, and lactation.

Symptoms. The individual with a goiter may experience anxiety, respiratory distress, difficulty in swallowing, and an enlargement of the thyroid gland. The physician will make a diagnosis based on the patient's history, symptoms, and diagnostic studies such as serum T-3, T-4, and ^{131}I uptake.

Treatment and Nursing Care. The client with a simple goiter generally is treated with iodine preparations, such as Lugol's solution or saturated solution of potassium iodide (see Table 18.5). Removal of part of the thyroid gland, subtotal thyroidectomy, may be necessary. The surgery may be done to remove the unsightly enlargement, to relieve respiratory difficulty, and in some cases, if a malignancy is suspected. Care of the patient having thyroid surgery is described later in the chapter.

The patient receiving iodine therapy should be observed for adverse reactions to the drug such as tremors, sweating, increased agitation, palpitations, tachycardia, hypertension, diarrhea, headache, insomnia, nausea, and vomiting. The client also should be aware of the untoward effects of iodine, as the drug usually is administered on an outpatient basis. The patient should be observed for an increase in the enlargement of the thyroid gland. Nodules in or near the thyroid gland should be observed and reported. Nursing care of the patient having surgery, which is discussed in Chapter 6, is applicable to this patient when an operation is necessary.

THYROIDITIS. The patient with thyroiditis has an inflammation of the thyroid gland. Thyroiditis may be caused by an acute bacterial invasion or by a subacute viral invasion of the thyroid gland. A long-term inflammatory process of the thyroid gland may lead to chronic thyroiditis.

The patient with acute bacterial thyroiditis may be treated by having an incision and drainage of the gland. An appropriate antibiotic generally is prescribed. The patient with subacute viral inflammation of the thyroid gland following a streptococcal infection and mumps generally is treated with corticosteroids. Propylthiouracil and desiccated thyroid may be prescribed. The individual with chronic thyroiditis may be treated with desiccated thyroid, x-ray therapy, and/or corticosteroids.

TUMORS. Tumors of the thyroid gland may be either benign or malignant. Benign tumors are more prevalent in young adults than in older persons. Diagnosis of benign tumors usually is done with a tracer dose of ^{131}I because the tumors usually are well encapsulated. Surgical removal of a benign tumor is the treatment of choice.

Malignant tumors of the thyroid gland are rare. The outstanding symptom of a malignant tumor of the thyroid is a hard, painless nodule in the enlarged gland. The malignancy does not take up [131]I. The treatment is generally surgical removal of the thyroid gland and involved lymph nodes. Care of the patient having thyroid surgery is described later in the chapter.

HYPERTHYROIDISM AND GRAVES' DISEASE

The patient with hyperthyroidism has an increased activity of the thyroid gland with excess amounts of thyroid hormone being produced. Hyperthyroidism frequently is part of a syndrome that can include goiter, pretibial myxedema, and exophthalmos. When these occur together, the patient is said to have Graves' disease. *Goiter* refers to an enlarged thyroid gland. *Pretibial myxedema* means that the patient has a dry, waxy type of swelling or edema on the anterior surface of his legs. *Exophthalmos* indicates that the patient's eyeballs protrude abnormally.

NURSING OBSERVATIONS. The individual with Graves' disease generally has symptoms of hyperthyroidism, an enlargement of the thyroid gland, and an abnormal protrusion of the eyes known as exophthalmos. The patient frequently experiences loss of weight in conjunction with an increased appetite, intolerance of heat, profuse perspiration (diaphoresis), tremors, rapid heart rate, nervousness, irritability, agitation, diarrhea, smooth skin, soft hair, fatigue, and mood swings. An abnormal increase in the number of cells in the thyroid gland and increased activity of the thyroid gland result in an enlargement. This enlargement can be three to four times the normal size.

Exophthalmos is a condition in which the patient has protruding eyeballs and a fixed stare. An accumulation of fluid in the fat pads behind the eyeballs causes this appearance. Exophthalmos may become so severe that the patient's eyelids will not close over the globe of the eye. Nonclosure of the eyelids could result in damage to the cornea. If this occurs, the patient's eyelids may be taped over the eye to protect the cornea.

The physician makes the diagnosis of Graves' disease by physical appearance of the enlarged thyroid gland, the protruding eyeballs and fixed stare, personal history of weight loss, evidence of nervousness, and other symptoms of hyperthyroidism. Laboratory values such as PBI, ^{131}I uptake, and T-3 resin uptake are elevated (see Table 18.3).

NURSING INTERVENTIONS. *Creating the Environment.* The patient with hyperthyroidism needs a quiet, calm, and restful environment. This includes the nursing staff responsible for care. The nurse accepts the patient's behavior as an expression of illness. The patient and family also need to understand this. The conversations between the family and patient should be nondisturbing. Radio and/or television programs that are perceived to be disturbing elements to the patient usually are avoided. The patient is encouraged to do activities within the framework of the medical regime and within the framework of personal interests. Becoming involved in some form of diversional therapy frequently helps the patient to divert attention from self.

The physical environment should be maintained at a comfortably cool temperature because of the patient's intolerance to heat. When making the bed, the nurse should use minimum top covering and be prepared to change the linen and clothing as often as necessary.

Alterations in Hygiene. When nursing the patient with exophthalmos, the nurse should observe the eyes closely. If the patient's eyelids are not closing over the globe of the eye, this observation should be reported and recorded immediately. As mentioned earlier, this condition could result in damage to the cornea and eventually lead to blindness. The corneas of the eye need to be moist at all times.

Frequent changes of clothing and/or linen may be necessary because of the profuse perspiration. Alcohol backrubs often have a cooling and relaxing effect on the patient.

Alterations in Diet. The patient's diet should be well balanced and nutritious. Generally, the diet is low in bulk because of the tendency of bulk to increase peristalsis, which may lead to diarrhea. In some cases, the diet will be high in calories and calcium also. An observant nurse will feed the patient or help the patient to eat when hand tremors interfere with eating.

The patient should be weighed regularly and should feel encouraged by a weight gain.

Assisting with Drug Therapy. The patient with Graves' disease may be given antithyroid drugs for two or three months prior to thyroid surgery. Drugs to decrease the size of the gland such as propylthiouracil, saturated solution of potassium iodine, and Lugol's solution may be prescribed, especially for a pregnant woman and for a patient under 18 years of age.

When administering iodine solution, the nurse should dilute the medication in milk or some preferred liquid to reduce gastric irritation. The patient receiving antithyroid drugs should be asked to report a rash, a sore mouth, or a sore throat. A brassy taste in the mouth, headache, and an excessive secretion of the lacrimal and nasal glands also should be noted.

Radioiodine therapy (^{131}I) may be used for a middle-aged person or an elderly individual (see Table 18.5). Surgery generally is performed on the young patient who is relatively free from other organic conditions.

Assisting the Patient with Thyroid Surgery. Surgical removal of the entire thyroid gland is total *thyroidectomy.* Total thyroidectomy usually is performed on the patient with cancer of the thyroid gland. After a total thyroidectomy, the patient is placed on thyroid extract. The patient having a subtotal thyroidectomy has approximately five sixths of the thyroid gland removed. This type of operation generally is done to correct hyperthyroidism.

The patient scheduled for a thyroidectomy because of hyperthyroidism will need the same type of care as the individual with hyperthyroidism and the surgical care discussed in Chapter 6.

Preoperative Care. The purpose of preoperative care generally is directed toward relieving the symptoms of hyperthyroidism. A combination of antithyroid drugs, bed rest, an adequate and nutritious diet, supplemental vitamins, and an environment conducive to rest is used to accomplish this goal.

Postoperative Care. Postoperative care is centered around four goals. These are (1) positioning the patient to relieve strain on the suture line, (2) promoting rest and relieving discomfort of the sore throat, (3) preventing respiratory obstruction, and (4) observing for surgical complications. Examples of surgical complications are hemorrhage, tetany, nerve paralysis, and thyroid storm.

The postoperative nursing responsibilities for the patient having a thyroidectomy include support of the patient's head, neck, and shoulders to prevent strain on the suture line. The nurse should help the patient support the head and neck when changing position and teach the patient how to do this. Usually, the patient is more comfortable in a semi-Fowler's position with pillows supporting the head and shoulders. The dressing over the incision should be checked frequently during the first 24 hours for bleeding. The area around the incision, back of the patient's neck, and back of the shoulders should be checked also for signs of bleeding. Medication prescribed by the physician should be given when the patient becomes restless and experiences pain. An increase in the patient's pulse rate may indicate the need for postoperative medication, also.

The patient should be encouraged to cough and breathe deeply at least every 30 minutes to prevent the collection of secretions in the trachea, bronchi, and lungs. Special attention should be paid to the quality of the patient's voice. Hoarseness, weakness, and inability to speak should be reported as these may be symptoms of injury to the laryngeal nerve. The patient should not be encouraged to talk excessively but is instructed to speak every one to two hours to provide the opportunity for the nurse to notice changes in the voice. Hoarseness generally occurs and is temporary.

The patient should be observed for symptoms of an obstruction to the trachea. An obstruction can be caused by edema of the glottis, hemorrhage, nerve damage, or tetany. Symptoms of an obstruction to the trachea are cyanosis, increased restlessness and apprehension, croupy or crowing-sounding respirations, and retraction of the neck tissue. A suction machine, tracheostomy set, and oxygen should be available in the patient's room. Any symptoms of an obstruction to the airway constitute an emergency and should be reported immediately.

Tetany is a possible complication of a thyroidectomy. This may occur when part of the parathyroid glands is accidently removed during surgery. The patient should be observed for tetany, which may occur from one to seven days following surgery. Twitching of the muscles and muscle spasms are symptoms of tetany and should be reported at once. Intravenous calcium generally is administered by the physician to correct tetany. The patient should be observed for symptoms of a rare complication called thyroid storm (crisis). This condition usually develops from a sudden increase in metabolism, due to excessive amounts of thyroid hormones being released in the blood. The nurse should observe the patient for an elevated temperature, an increased heart rate, extreme restlessness, and unconsciousness. The appearance of any of these symptoms should be reported promptly. The patient may be treated with oxygen therapy, hypothermia blanket, sedatives, and the administration of intravenous fluids.

HYPOTHYROIDISM

The individual with hypothyroidism has an underactive thyroid gland. The condition is known as myxedema in adults and cretinism in infants.

Myxedema seems to be more common in females over the age of 60 years. The symptoms range from mild to severe. The patient with mild myxedema may have only vague symptoms, such as mild sensitivity to cold, slight weight gain, dry skin and hair, some forgetfulness, and fatigue. The client with severe myxedema has more pronounced symptoms. For example, the individual generally has a marked sensitivity to cold temperatures, a weight gain, dry skin and hair, edema, constipation, and marked fatigue. Such complications as arteriosclerosis, angina pectoris, coronary heart disease, mental changes such as delusions and paranoia, and coma may occur.

The infant with cretinism, if not treated, will have stunted growth. The child may be mentally deficient. Such symptoms as dry skin, expressionless face, open mouth with thick protruding tongue, and short neck may be present also.

The physician diagnoses myxedema on the basis of personal history, physical examination, and laboratory tests such as T-3, T-4. Thyroid extract or synthetic hormones may be utilized individually or in combination for the treatment of the client with myxedema (see Table 18.5). The prognosis for myxedema is excellent with treatment.

When caring for the client with myxedema, the nurse should provide a comfortably warm physical environment. This includes adequate clothing and covering for the bed. A diet low in calories generally is prescribed. Foods high in roughage such as lettuce, carrots, raw cabbage, celery, and apples frequently are included. Changes in the patient's physical and mental activities should be observed and recorded. The individual with dry skin will need special care to prevent tissue breakdown. This is especially true when edema is present. When administering narcotics or barbiturates to the individual with myxedema, the nurse should observe for signs of sensitivity to the drugs.

When assisting with thyroid hormone replacement therapy, the nurse is especially alert for tachycardia, palpitations, sleep disturbances, and nervousness since these observations indicate possible overdosage. At the beginning of therapy, the nurse usually counts the pulse before each dose of thyroid hormone. A pulse greater than 100 beats per minute is reported to the physician before giving the drug so that a dosage adjustment can be prescribed if necessary.

The Patient with a Parathyroid Disorder

The parathyroid glands, located on either side of the posterior aspect of the thyroid gland, secrete the hormone parathormone (PTH). The functions of PTH are to control calcium and phosphate metabolism and to maintain serum calcium levels in the blood.

An individual suspected of having a disorder of the parathyroid glands may have various diagnostic tests performed on the blood and urine. A 24-hour urine specimen for the study of calcium generally is obtained. A single urine specimen may be obtained for calcium (the Sulkowitch test). The main specific preparation for these diagnostic studies is that the patient may have a low-calcium diet prescribed for three to six days prior to certain tests. In addition, parathormone level can be measured in the serum using radio immunoassay.

The two basic disorders of the parathyroid glands are hyperparathyroidism and hypoparathyroidism.

HYPERPARATHYROIDISM

The individual with hyperparathyroidism has an excessive amount of parathormone secreted by the parathyroid gland. This condition was once thought to be rare. However, an increased number of persons with hyperparathyroidism has been discovered in recent years, probably due to better diagnostic techniques. In most cases, the exact cause of this condition is unknown. In some cases, tumors have been located in the parathyroid gland. Women are affected more often than men, and the incidence of this condition increases after age 50 in both women and men.

In addition to the measurement of hormone levels in blood and urine, other diagnostic tests such as ultrasound and computerized axial tomograms (CT scans) may be done to identify abnormal lesions.

Hyperparathyroidism causes the individual to have bone damage, characterized by bones becoming fragile and painful. This results in pathologic fractures. Kidney stones, gastrointestinal problems such as poor appetite, loss of weight, thirst, nausea, abdominal pain, and constipation may occur. The individual may also experience impairment of vision, listlessness, depression, and paranoia.

Nursing care of the individual with hyperparathyroidism includes protection of the patient from injury such as pathologic fractures. The patient's urine should be strained for possible kidney stones because of the disturbed calcium level in the blood (see Table 18.3). The intake of fluids should be increased, and, in some cases, the physician leaves an order for a minimum of 3000 ml during a 24-hour period.

Drug therapy is usually prescribed to reduce the elevated serum calcium associated with this condition. Drugs prescribed may include phosphates, prednisone, mithramycin (MITHRACIN), or calcitonin CALCIMAR).

Surgery may be indicated when a parathyroid tumor is found or when the patient's bones, kidneys, and/or pancreas is affected by illness. *Subtotal parathyroidectomy* is the surgical procedure most often done. This procedure includes removal of most, but not all, parathyroid tissue. A small amount of tissue is left so that normal levels of parathormone can be restored and hypoparathyroidism is prevented. Surgical care of the patient is similar to that indicated for a person having a thyroidectomy. The patient usually is placed in Fowler's position postoperatively to improve breathing, promote drainage, and reduce pressure on the neck suture line. The patient is observed carefully for respiratory distress. A wound drain may be present to prevent respiratory distress caused by the accumulation of blood and fluids around air passages. In addition, the patient is observed carefully for signs of calcium deficiency such as nervousness and irritability, muscle spasms, cramps, paresthesias, and laryngeal stridor. These observations are reported to the surgeon at once so that calcium supplements can be prescribed to correct this life-threatening imbalance.

HYPOPARATHYROIDISM

The client with hypoparathyroidism has a deficient amount of secretions from the parathyroid glands, which may be caused by injury to the glands or accidental removal during surgery. The patient with hypoparathyroidism experiences the symptoms of tetany. These symptoms are tingling in the fingers, muscle spasms, tremors, and laryngospasm. The patient may have convulsions if treatment is not started early. Calcium is administered intravenously as an emergency measure and is administered slowly when given by this route. Oral calcium may be prescribed after the patient's condition has stabilized.

The individual should be in a quiet environment that is free of sudden movements, loud noises, and disturbing sounds and that has subdued lights. Symptoms of tetany should be reported immediately. The patient may be urged to select foods that are high in calcium.

The Patient with a Pituitary Disorder

Disorders of the pituitary gland may develop from genetic abnormalities, disorders of the hypothalamus, tumors in the pituitary gland, or disturbances in the target organ. Disorders are more likely to occur in the anterior lobe of the pituitary gland and include hyperpituitarism and hypopituitarism.

A diagnosis may be established by measuring blood levels of circulating hormones and urine specimens for hormone-related substances as described earlier in the chapter. In addition, diagnostic studies of the central nervous system may be done (see Chapter 21) if a pituitary tumor is suspected.

Some or all of the observations described in Table 18.4 may be present when the patient has a pituitary disorder. In addition, the patient may have symptoms of a brain tumor as described in Chapter 21, pages 747–48. The individual with hyperpituitarism has an increased secretion of hormones produced by the anterior lobe of the pituitary gland, usually caused by a benign tumor. Gigantism (giantism), acromegaly, Cushing's disease, and sexual disturbances are some of the disorders that result from hyperpituitarism. The patient is treated by surgical removal of the tumor or radiotherapy of the pituitary. A patient with hypopituitarism has a deficiency of the hormones secreted by the anterior lobe of the pituitary gland. Such factors as a tumor, congenital deficiency of the growth hormone, and destruction or removal of the pituitary gland may cause this disorder. Dwarfism, myxedema, reproductive disorders, and insufficient adrenocortical hormones are the major disorders that may result from hyyopituitarism. The patient with hypopituitarism generally is treated by surgical removal of the causative tumor and hormonal replacement.

A deficient amount of ADH (antidiuretic hormone) produced by the posterior lobe of the pituitary gland is one of the main disorders of that lobe. The patient with this deficiency has diabetes insipidus. Water is not reabsorbed by the kidney tubules, and the individual passes excessive amounts of dilute urine. Such a person may drink as much as 40,000 ml of fluid in a 24-hour period. An excessive intake of fluid results in a low specific gravity of urine. It is necessary for the individual with diabetes insipidus to drink fluids continuously to prevent severe dehydration.

Drug therapy for the patient with diabetes insipidus is the injection of vasopressin tannate (PITRESSIN TANNATE) (see Table 18.5) or the inhalation of posterior pituitary hormones in a "snuff" preparation.

The nursing care of an individual with a pituitary gland disorder varies with the disorder and treatment. For example, surgical removal (hypophysectomy) involves manipulation of the brain. In this case, the patient will need the preoperative and postoperative care discussed in Chapter 6, in addition to the nursing care of the patient having surgery of the brain, discussed in Chapter 21.

The Patient with an Adrenal Disorder

The major disorders of the adrenal cortex are hypocorticism (hypofunction of the adrenal cortex) and hypercorticism (hyperfunction of the adrenal cortex). Hypocorticism causes the individual to have a deficiency of mineralocorticoids, glucocorticoids, and the androgens and estrogens. The individual with adrenocortical deficiency, hypocorticism, generally has developed this condition because of a lack of pituitary gland stimulation to the adrenal cortex, destruction of the adrenal cortex such as by surgical removal, destruction of the cortex from such lesions as tuberculosis, cancer, or fungi, and abrupt discontinuance of steroid therapy. The patient with hypocorticism generally has Addison's disease. The physician makes the diagnosis of Addison's disease on the basis of laboratory tests such as the ACTH stimulation test, the plasma cortisol re-

sponse to ACTH, and 24 hour urine collections for 17-hydroxycorticoids. The client with Addison's disease generally has a gradual onset. There may be early symptoms of weight loss, nausea, vomiting, diarrhea, mild fatigue, irritability, mental changes, postural hypotension, dizziness, an increase in pigment cells of the skin, and the appearance of bluish-black patches on the mucous membrane. As the disease progresses, the patient's symptoms increase. Without treatment the patient will go into an addisonian crisis in which the symptoms of Addison's disease are acute and may result in death.

Steroid drug therapy is the main treatment for the patient with Addison's disease. Cortisone acetate, hydrocortisone, deoxycorticosterone, and fludrocortisone are examples of steroids that may be prescribed.

Nursing responsibilities for the patient with Addison's disease include collecting and maintaining urine for diagnostic tests, preparing the patient for diagnostic tests, recording accurate intake and output, weighing the patient as requested by the physician, encouraging the patient to eat a high-carbohydrate, high-protein diet, checking vital signs, and observing the patient for symptoms of infection. Adverse reactions to steroid therapy should be reported. It is especially important for the nurse and the patient to remember that steroid drugs may irritate the gastric mucosa and should be given with milk or food.

The patient will need emotional support from members of the health team. As stated earlier, the patient generally is irritable and may not understand mental changes common to this illness. Such changes also affect the family. Continuous therapy with steroids for the remainder of one's life may alter the individual's life-style slightly. In some cases, the patient may experience depression, denial, or other coping mechanisms discussed in Chapter 1. The patient will need patience, understanding, tolerance, kindness, and a willingness on the part of the nurse to be an active listener. This is especially important since the patient with Addison's disease may not be able to cope effectively with physical or mental stress until treatment has improved the condition. The patient with an adrenal gland disorder should be advised to have on the person at all times: identification as to name, the name and telephone number of the physician, the name and telephone number of closest relative, and the type of disorder.

The individual with an overactive adrenal cortex has hypercorticism. This condition may be caused by a tumor of the adrenal cortex, pituitary gland, or other organs of the body. Hyperplasia of the adrenal cortex may also cause hypercorticism. The condition also may result from prolonged steroid therapy.

The patient with hypercorticism usually has Cushing's syndrome. The physician generally makes the diagnosis of Cushing's syndrome on the basis of personal history, appearance of the patient, blood studies, and hormonal tests. Examples of the tests that may be used are the ACTH stimulation test, plasma cortisol test, and cortisone suppression test.

Some of the main symptoms experienced by the individual with Cushing's syndrome are edema, marked irregularity in the distribution of fat in the face, moonface, maldistribution of fat in the neck referred to as "buffalo hump," and irregular distribution of fatty tissue in the trunk, especially in the abdomen. Muscular weakness, tissue wasting, hyperglycemia (high blood sugar), renal disorders, mental changes ranging from euphoria to depression, lowered resistance to infection, and development of secondary male characteristics in the female also may occur.

When possible, the cause of Cushing's syndrome is surgically removed, especially if a tumor is present. Radiation and chemotherapy may be used also.

The nursing responsibilities for the patient scheduled for adrenocortical surgery are of great importance. Preoperatively, the patient receives detailed information about the nature of surgery and results that can be expected. The expected changes in life-style are discussed at length with both the patient and family, including the need for lifelong hormone replacement with cortisol preparations (if both adrenal glands are removed). In addition to the usual preoperative prepa-

ration described in Chapter 6, the nurse pays special attention to protecting the patient from exposure to infection and injury, careful measurement of the daily weight and vital signs, and the promotion of physical and mental rest. Postoperatively, the patient usually is placed in the intensive care unit for close observation until stable. In addition to the usual postoperative care described in Chapter 6, the nurse pays special attention to the prevention of respiratory and wound infection, careful administration of cortisone preparations, and meticulous monitoring of the urine output. Patient and family teaching before discharge includes topics such as the prevention of infection, stress-management techniques, rest and relaxation, drug therapy, and the use of a medical bracelet that contains information about the patient's diagnosis and therapy in the event of an emergency.

Major disorders of the adrenal medulla are neuroblastoma, a malignant tumor seen in children, and pheochromocytoma, a tumor that is usually benign and is frequently found in children and women during the middle years. This small tumor causes overactivity of the adrenal medulla, resulting in excessive secretion of epinephrine and norepinephrine. Due to this excessive secretion, the patient will have symptoms of marked hypertension with apprehension, excessive perspiration, rapid pulse rate, nausea, and vomiting. The patient also may have hyperglycemia, nervousness, and emotional instability. The patient with pheochromocytoma generally has the tumor removed surgically. The first 48 hours after surgery is a critical period for the patient because of the possibility of excessive amounts of pressor hormones being introduced into the body during anesthesia or tumor manipulation during surgery. This sudden release causes the blood pressure to rise markedly and may cause cardiac arrhythmia. After surgery, the patient's blood pressure may also drop to an acutely low level. Constant monitoring of the blood pressure is essential during this immediate postoperative period. The surgical dressing should be checked at least every 30 minutes for bleeding, and other signs of hemorrhage should be noted. Vomiting, nausea, distention, and abdominal pain that may indicate internal bleeding should be noted by the nurse. Narcotics generally are given somewhat cautiously because of the possibility of a drop in blood pressure.

The Patient with a Pancreatic Disorder

The pancreas is a large, elongated gland located behind the stomach. The pancreas secretes enzymes that facilitate digestion, as discussed in Chapter 16. It also secretes two protein hormones, insulin and glucagon. These hormones are formed by the islet cells of Langerhans and regulate carbohydrate metabolism. The level of glucose in the blood influences the secretion of insulin. If the individual's blood sugar is above normal, insulin is released into the blood stream; if the blood sugar is normal, insulin secretion slows down. When there is a deficiency of insulin, the blood sugar remains above normal; the sugar spills into the urine and usually the disorder, diabetes mellitus, develops.

The hormone glucagon is secreted to elevate the blood sugar when it is abnormally low. Therefore, if the pancreas is healthy, a blood sugar balance is maintained by insulin and glucagon.

Carbohydrate metabolism is a series of chemical processes involving the hormones insulin, glucagon, epinephrine, ACTH, and thyroxine. The chemical processes that take place are: glucose is converted to energy, and excess glucose is stored as glycogen and fat; glycogen is converted to glucose when needed for energy; fats and proteins are converted to glucose or glycogen when energy is required and there is no glucose or glycogen available. Carbohydrates usually are used by the body for energy. However, if there is an insufficient amount of hormones discussed above to convert glucose to energy and store glycogen, the body converts fats and proteins to glucose and uses these for energy. Carbohydrates must be present in usable form in order for fats to be metabolized completely. Therefore, fat metabolism is faulty and ketone bodies and acetone bodies are in the blood. This condition may result in diabetic ketoacidosis or coma. The

major disorders of the islets of Langerhans are hyposecretion and hypersecretion.

HYPOSECRETION OF ISLETS: DIABETES MELLITUS

Diabetes mellitus results from faulty carbohydrate metabolism associated with the hormone insulin. Diabetes mellitus is the most common disorder of the endocrine system. Complications of diabetes are one of the major causes of death in the United States.

Several types of diabetes have been identified. *Type I insulin-dependent* diabetes most often develops in children, adolescents, and young adults, although it may occur at any age. This form of diabetes is associated with a deficiency or lack of insulin. *Type II non-insulin-dependent diabetes* develops more often in persons over 40 years of age who are overweight. This type of diabetes is associated with ineffectiveness of circulating insulin. *Gestational diabetes* occurs during pregnancy; however, women with this condition are more likely to develop diabetes within five to ten years. Some persons have a condition known as *impaired glucose tolerance*. This means that the glucose level in the blood is abnormal but not diagnostic for diabetes. Finally, a person may develop *secondary diabetes* after taking certain drugs or as a result of another endocrine disorder.

The exact cause of diabetes mellitus is not known. Factors believed to contribute to the onset of diabetes include heredity, obesity, viral infections, severe stress, and pregnancy.

At present, the disease cannot be cured but may be controlled by a planned program of exercise, diet, and medication. Good control is achieved when the patient's blood glucose level is maintained as near to normal as possible. It is important to control diabetes because studies show that persistently elevated blood sugar is more likely to cause complications of diabetes such as cardiovascular disease, peripheral vascular disease, vision problems including blindness, kidney disease, and disturbances in the nervous system.

DIAGNOSTIC TESTS. The diagnostic tests used to determine diabetes mellitus are performed mainly on the blood and urine of the individual. The laboratory tests frequently used and the normal values of each are found in Table 18.3. The nursing responsibilities are to prepare the patient appropriately, collect specimens at the correct time in conjunction with medical laboratory personnel, and provide support and explanations to the patient.

In addition, the nursing staff is usually responsible for teaching the patient how to do diagnostic testing at home. The main diagnostic tests, a brief explanation, and the nursing responsibilities are considered below.

- Fasting blood sugar (FBS)—The patient is NPO for 12 hours before the test. Blood is drawn by venipuncture and taken to the laboratory.
- Postprandial blood sugar—No preparation necessary. Blood is drawn by venipuncture two hours after meal or as ordered by the physician.
- Oral glucose tolerance test (GTT)—The patient is NPO except for water for 12 hours before the test and during the test. Activity should be kept at a minimum, as walking and other activity will affect carbohydrate metabolism. Stress also should be kept at a minimum as epinephrine and cortisone may elevate the blood sugar. Specimens of the blood and urine are obtained. 100 gm of glucose are given orally. Blood and urine specimens are obtained in one and two hours. Occasionally, specimens are obtained for up to 5 hours after the ingestion of glucose. All specimens must be labeled correctly with name, room number, special code number, and time of specimen collection. A diagram of glucose tolerance curves is shown in Figure 18.3.
- Intravenous glucose tolerance test— Glucose is given intravenously rather than orally when the patient is unable to ingest the oral glucose or is unable to tolerate oral glucose. The preparation of the patient is the same as for the individual having an oral glucose tolerance test. 50 ml of 50 percent glucose is given intravenously very slowly. Blood and urine specimens are collected every 30 minutes for two hours or more.

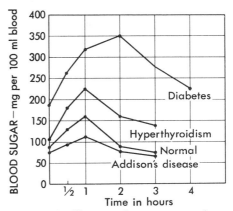

FIGURE 18.3   Glucose tolerance curves in various metabolic disorders. (From Robinson, Corinne H., and Lawler, Marilyn R.: *Normal and Therapeutic Nutrition*, 16th ed. Macmillan Publishing Co., Inc., New York, 1982.)

- Glycosylated hemoglobin A_1C is a relatively new blood test which enables the physician to evaluate the pattern of glucose control over the preceding three to four months. The test is possible because elevated blood glucose forms a permanent attachment to the hemoglobin portion of the red blood cell. Since the life of the cell is approximately 120 days, measuring the amount of glucose-bound hemoglobin provides a kind of backward glance which is helpful to the physician making adjustments in the treatment plan.
- Home blood glucose monitoring is now available for diabetics. This method eventually may replace urine testing because the tests show the exact amount of glucose in the blood at the time of testing. The patient takes a single drop of blood from either the ear lobe or the fingertip and places it on a special strip such as CHEMSTRIP or DEXTROSTRIP. The specific method varies according to the manufacturer. After waiting the prescribed amount of time, the strip color is compared to a color chart. An electronic device is also available that gives the exact amount of glucose present when the chemical strip is inserted into the meter.
- CLINITEST chemical reduction urine test— This test is used to identify glucose, lactose, galactose, fructose, maltose, and salicylates. CLINITEST tablets are used. Five

drops of a second voided urine specimen are put in a test tube with ten drops of water and one CLINITEST tablet (Figure 18.4). When boiling stops, the specimen is read in 10 to 15 seconds (according to the manufacturer) by comparing the color of the urine with the CLINITEST color chart. The nurse must be sure that the CLINITEST bottle cap is on tightly because the tablets deteriorate with air.

A variation of this method is recommended by the American Diabetes Association for type I diabetics. The variation is to use two drops of urine rather than five drops, as described above. This variation is suggested because the two-drop method gives a more accurate reading when the glucose is high. Some types of antibiotics as well as aspirin and vitamin C may cause false readings.

• Enzyme urine test—These tests are used to identify glucose and acetone in the urine. A test tape, or CLINISTIX, is dipped

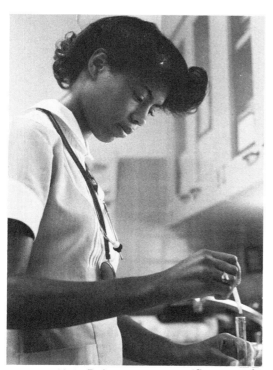

FIGURE 18.4   Doing a CLINITEST. (Courtesy of Henrico County–St. Mary's Hospital School of Practical Nursing, Richmond, Virginia.)

in the urine and compared with a color chart (Figure 18.5). When the ACETEST tablet is used, the nurse should place a drop of urine on the tablet, wait the length of time indicated on the instructions, and compare the moistened tablet with a color chart. A KETOSTIX can be dipped in urine and compared with a color chart also. Both the tape and STIX deteriorate in a few months. The American Diabetes Association does not recommend sticks and tape for regular use by type I diabetics because they do not indicate when large amounts of glucose are present.

When collecting a urine for sugar and acetone, the nurse should be certain that the specimen is fresh. In general, it is preferable to collect a second voided specimen when the information desired is the current status of glucose control. Usually, the client is asked to urinate about 30 minutes prior to the test. This specimen may be saved until a second specimen is obtained. The client may be asked to drink a glass of water so that the second specimen can be obtained. If a second specimen cannot be obtained, the first specimen is tested. However, when recording the results, the nurse labels the results as a *first-voided specimen* on the patient's record.

The times during which a urine specimen is collected and tested vary with the type of diabetes, the physician's orders, the patient's condition, and the type of medication prescribed. For example, type I diabetics may be asked to test the urine before each meal and at bedtime. Type II diabetics may be asked to test before one or more meals. The patient testing the urine at home is instructed to keep a record of the results of each test so that information is available for the physician or clinical nurse specialist if problems arise.

• 24-Hour urine test—This urine test is done to measure the amount of sugar in the urine for a 24-hour period. The patient voids at the start of the test, and this urine is discarded. All urine is saved for 24 hours and sent to the laboratory.

Urinary tract illnesses most likely to develop as a complication of diabetes include

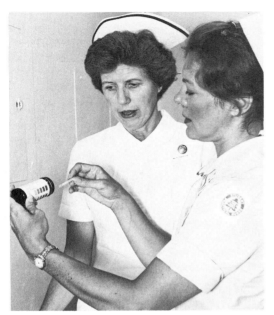

FIGURE 18.5   Using a test tape to identify glucose in the urine. (Courtesy of Bergen Pines County Hospital School of Practical Nursing, Paramus, New Jersey.)

bladder and kidney infections, nephrosis, and renal failure.

The diabetic is highly susceptible to all types of infection. Infections that do develop are more difficult to treat and slower to heal. Carbuncles, furuncles, ulcers, cuts, blisters, burns, and insect bites present special problems for the diabetic. The physician should be notified at once if these lesions are observed.

In pregnancy, the secretions of the hormones estrogen, progesterone, and glucocorticoids increase and antagonize the effects of insulin. The complications of pregnancy, such as miscarriage, preeclampsia, toxemia, and hemorrhage, may occur. Diabetic women usually have large babies, and congenital abnormalities are not rare.

Table 18.6 contains a summary of observations that may develop in the patient with diabetes.

NURSING OBSERVATIONS.   The nurse has several vital responsibilities in observing the patient with diabetes. For example, the nurse may assist the undiagnosed person to recognize symptoms of diabetes and seek

medical attention. The individual with diabetes mellitus has symptoms of excessive thirst (polydipsia), excessive hunger (polyphagia), excessive urination (polyuria), and weight loss. The patient also may experience fatigue, pruritus, skin infections, decreased resistance to infection, blurred vision, lightheadedness, nervousness, anxiety, and depression. The patient will also have an elevated blood sugar (hyperglycemia) and may have sugar and acetone in the urine.

A second important form of observation involves early detection of complications. Two acute complications of diabetes mellitus are *diabetic ketoacidosis* and *hypoglycemia* (described on page 611). Diabetic ketoacidosis develops from the patient's inability to use the glucose in the body. A need for energy causes the body to convert fats and proteins into glucose to meet energy requirements. Factors associated with diabetic ketoacidosis include infection or illness in the diabetic patient, taking too little insulin or omitting insulin entirely, overeating, and/or undiagnosed diabetes. The patient with diabetic ketoacidosis may have one or more of the following symptoms which gradually develop over a period of hours or days:

- Flushed dry skin
- Lethargic, drowsy behavior which can lead to coma
- Fruity odor to the breath
- Deep, labored breathing (Kussmaul respirations)
- Nausea, vomiting, diarrhea
- Dry tongue and thirst
- Abdominal pain
- Large amounts of sugar in the urine
- Hyperglycemia

The patient with diabetic ketoacidosis is treated with insulin and intravenous fluids. The underlying condition (such as infection) also is treated. Hypoglycemia is discussed later in the chapter.

The main chronic complications of diabetes mellitus usually are found in blood vessel and nerve degeneration. The areas most affected are the heart, feet and lower legs, eyes, and kidneys.

Atherosclerosis, hardening of the arteries, may strike diabetics at an early age. This disease leads to coronary artery disease

TABLE 18.6
GUIDE TO OBSERVING THE PATIENT WITH DIABETES

WHAT TO OBSERVE	OBSERVATIONS
Head	Headache may occur
Eyes	Visual disturbances such as blurred vision and double vision may develop
	Redness of conjunctiva
Mouth	Fruity odor to breath
	Lips and tongue may be dry, moist, tingling, or numb
	Vomiting, thirst, hunger
	Dental disease
Chest	Respirations may be deep and labored (Kussmaul) or rapid and shallow
Abdomen	Abdominal pain
Extremities	Trophic skin changes such as hairlessness, color changes, waxy skin may be observed in legs and feet
	Toenails may be brittle and thick
	Leg cramps, weakness, and pain may occur
Genitalia	Vaginitis may occur
	Impotence may develop
Bowel movements	Diarrhea or constipation may occur
Urine	Polyuria may occur
	Urine may show ketones and elevated glucose
Skin	May be moist or dry
	May be flushed in color
	Skin lesions may be present such as carbuncles, cuts, blisters, ulcers
	Rashes may be present on any part of the body
Behavioral changes	Fatigue, lethargy, drowsiness may occur
	Nervousness, irritability
	Coma
	Feelings of anger, fear, and guilt may be verbalized
	Medication, diet, and exercise program may not be followed if emotional conflict and tension persist

and a reduced blood supply to the extremities (mainly feet and lower legs), resulting in inadequate healing of foot infections, lesions, and gangrene.

Peripheral nerve (neurologic) problems may develop in a diabetic patient. The causes usually are vascular insufficiency, high blood sugar levels, and a vitamin B deficiency. The symptoms of peripheral neurologic problems are pain and tingling of the lower extremities, especially at night, which may later change to an inability to feel pain in the lower extremities. This inability to feel pain could be of great importance as the client may be unaware of trauma or injury to the lower extremities, thus a severe infection could develop with inadequate healing.

Ocular changes may occur in the diabetic causing double vision, hemorrhage, cataracts, and diabetic retinopathy. Retinopathy is a condition which, if untreated, may result in blindness.

The diabetic patient can be expected to experience a variety of feelings associated with chronic illness, acute and chronic complications, and changes of life-style. Feelings of fear, anxiety, and guilt are not uncommon. Persistent, unrelieved emotional tension and conflict may affect control of blood glucose by influencing the release of stress hormones. Seven possible crisis periods have been identified in the life of a diabetic including:

- The time of diagnosis
- The start of school
- Adolescence
- College and/or the first job
- Marriage
- Pregnancy
- The onset of complications

When observing the patient with diabetes, the nurse can be alert for behavioral changes associated with crisis. The patient may need additional support and/or professional help at this time.

NURSING INTERVENTIONS. The nurse has a vital part to play in helping the patient with each of the cornerstones of therapy: diet, exercise, and medication. In addition, the nurse teaches the patient how to prevent, identify, and report complications of diabetes.

Diet and Fluids. As previously mentioned, diet is one of the essential components of controlling the disease process in diabetes. The diet is planned on the basis of the patient's weight, age, size, occupation, hobbies, habits, religion, ethnic background, financial situation, and social activities. Personal likes and dislikes play an important part in the dietary regime.

In general, the diet for the diabetic is well balanced with foods from each of the four basic food groups and a total calorie intake consistent with ideal body weight. Type I diabetics need to pay special attention to the time of meals and snacks as they relate to the amount and type of exercise and insulin. In addition, consistency is important related to the daily consumption of proteins, carbohydrates, and fats in the diet. Type II diabetics must pay special attention to the total calories consumed each day in order to achieve and maintain ideal weight.

A diabetic diet is planned using a system of food exchanges. Each food is assigned to one of six exchange lists: (1) milk, (2) vegetables, (3) fruits, (4) breads, cereals, and starchy vegetables, (5) meat, fish, and some cheeses, and (6) fats. Any food on one list may be traded or exchanged for food on the same list in specified amounts. Each prescribed diet contains a certain number of exchanges from each list each day.

In learning to develop a new eating plan, the diabetic patient learns to recognize the names of common sugars that may appear on the labels of foods in the grocery store. These include corn sugar and syrup, fructose, honey, lactose, mannitol, sorbitol, xylitol. Artificial sweeteners may be used in limited amounts, if permitted by the physician. The American Diabetes Association recommends limited use of artificial sweeteners in children, adolescents, and pregnant women.

New research indicates that a high-complex-carbohydrate, high-fiber diet may be helpful to some persons with diabetes. Present evidence indicates the persons most likely to be helped by this diet are type II diabetics who are overweight. The nurse may watch with interest for new developments in diet for the patient with diabetes mellitus.

Exercise. The patient with diabetes mellitus derives many benefits from regular physical exercise. For example, exercise helps to lower blood glucose by increasing the rate of absorption of glucose in the cells. In addition, regular physical exercise helps circulation, eases stress, and helps the overweight person to lose weight. Exercise is a second cornerstone of therapy for the diabetic.

The best exercises for diabetics are continuous and rhythmic such as walking, jogging, running, bicycling, swimming, rowing, skating, and cross-country skiing. Type I diabetics may need a protein snack before exercising in order to prevent symptoms of hypoglycemia. If symptoms do develop, the patient is taught to stop the exercise and take some form of carbohydrate such as orange juice, a soft drink, or hard candies. Type II diabetics should consult a physician before starting an exercise program. Because these patients are usually over 40 years of age, the physician may order a stress (treadmill) test to check for possible coronary artery disease (see Chapter 11). Other variations of exercise indicated for diabetics include exercising on a daily basis, wearing properly fitted shoes, and exercising after a meal as blood sugar is rising, if possible.

Assisting with Drug Therapy. Several medications may be prescribed for the patient with diabetes mellitus. As previously mentioned, type I diabetics are insulin dependent and must inject insulin regularly in addition to adjusting the diet and exercise in order to control blood glucose. For type I diabetics, insulin is the third cornerstone of therapy.

As stated earlier in this chapter, insulin is necessary for carbohydrate metabolism. In the patient with diabetes mellitus, there is a deficiency or lack of functioning insulin.

This may necessitate the administration of insulin.

Insulin is made from the pancreas of pork or beef and must be administered by injection. Recently, scientists have been able to grow and produce insulin by genetic engineering. This insulin, called Humulin, is now on the market. The nurse can expect to care for an increasing number of type I insulin-dependent diabetics who are using this new insulin. The nurse may watch with interest new developments in this field. Since the enzymes of the gastrointestinal system render insulin useless, it must be injected. Insulin is classified according to the time span of action. The three major types of insulin currently being used are:

- Fast-acting insulin, which includes crystalline zinc (regular) insulin and semilente insulin
- Intermediate-acting insulin, which includes globin zinc, NPH (neutral protamine Hagedorn), and lente insulin
- Slow-acting or long-acting insulin, which includes protamine zinc (PZI) and ultralente insulin (see Table 18.5).

Insulin is measured in units, and the vial labels are color coded according to the unit concentration. Insulin comes in 10-ml vials, and 1 ml equals the unit concentration. For example, if the vial label reads U-100, the vial contains 100 units of insulin per milliliter.

Insulin is administered with an insulin syringe, which is calibrated in units to correspond with the insulin. For example, if the patient is to receive 30 units of regular insulin and the vial contains 100 units per milliliter, a U-100 insulin syringe should be used. The syringe should be filled to the mark indicating 30 units. The scale on the syringe should correspond with the strength of insulin. A small-gauge, 25-g or 26-g needle should be used to inject insulin into subcutaneous tissue.

Insulin is very stable and does not have to be refrigerated, although it should be protected from strong light and extremes in temperature. Injecting refrigerated insulin may cause the patient to develop a complication known as lipodystrophy (abnormal fatty deposits) at the injection site. When using insulin, the nurse should check the expiration date and observe the contents for clumping. Evidence of clumping or exceeding the expiration date should prompt the nurse to obtain a fresh vial. When giving semilente, NPH, lente, protamine zinc, and ultralente, the nurse should rotate the vial to mix the insulin. The vial should be rotated between the palms of the hands.

In some cases, the physician orders two different types of insulins for the patient. Typically, regular insulin (short acting) is mixed with a longer acting insulin in the same syringe. Table 18.7 consists of directions that guide the nurse and the patient in mixing two different types of insulin in the same syringe.

When giving insulin, the nurse should have another nurse check the prescribed dosage with that prepared as a safety measure. Insulin generally is not administered when the patient is NPO unless the physician leaves specific orders. The nurse should administer the solution at room temperature into the subcutaneous tissue of the outer aspect of the upper arm, anterior and lateral portions of the thigh, or lateral and anterior portions of the abdomen. The injection site should be systematically rotated to prevent

TABLE 18.7
GUIDELINES FOR MIXING INSULINS

1. Check the physician's orders for the types of insulins to be mixed.
2. Compare the units on the syringe to be used with each insulin vial to be certain that the unit concentration numbers are the same.
3. Rotate the vial of cloudy insulin gently to mix well.
4. Cleanse the stopper on each insulin vial in the usual manner.
5. Into the cloudy insulin vial inject an amount of air equal to the dosage to be withdrawn from that bottle. Do not withdraw this insulin at this time.
6. Into the clear insulin vial inject the amount of air equal to the dosage to be withdrawn and draw this amount into the syringe.
7. Return to the cloudy insulin vial and draw the prescribed dosage into the syringe.
8. Inject the insulin.
9. Follow the same directions if two cloudy insulins are to be mixed in the same syringe.

atrophy or hypertrophy of the tissues. The injection site should be located at least one inch from the previous site. The nurse should select an injection area that appears normal to touch and sight (Figures 18.6, 18.7, 18.8, 18.9, 18.10, and 18.11).

An acute complication that may develop in the patient who takes insulin is *insulin reaction* (hypoglycemia). This condition may develop if too much insulin is administered, if the patient does not eat or eats less than the specified amount, or if vomiting develops. Another factor that can result in an insulin reaction is an unplanned increase in physical exercise. The symptoms of insulin reaction are:

- Hypoglycemia
- Weakness
- Apprehension
- Irritability
- Profuse perspiration
- Pallor
- Hunger

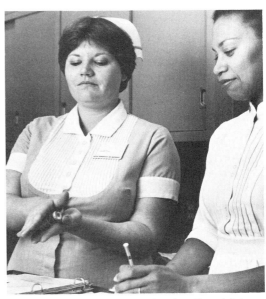

FIGURE 18.7   Rotating the insulin vial between the palms of the hands. (Courtesy of Shapero School of Nursing, Sinai Hospital of Detroit, Detroit, Michigan.)

- Visual disturbances
- Tremors
- Unconsciousness
- Convulsions

Treatment for insulin reaction is determined by the severity of the symptoms. If the insulin reaction is mild, usually a glass of orange juice is given. A second glass of orange juice is followed by a protein snack if symptoms persist. When the insulin reaction is severe, 50 ml of 50 percent glucose is given intravenously or glucagon, 1 to 2 mg, is given subcutaneously.

Another insulin-related complication is called the *Somogyi effect* after the physician who first described it. The patient experiencing this complication has a prolonged insulin reaction without the usual symptoms. The Somogyi effect occurs when a very low blood sugar, which often develops at night, causes the body to compensate by releasing hormones such as adrenalin, glucagon, and cortisol to raise the blood sugar. This, in turn, causes the morning urine test to be high in sugar. A cycle develops in which increased insulin, administered on the basis of elevated blood and urine sugar, causes more

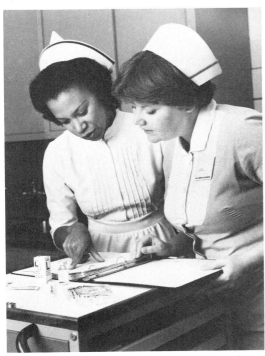

FIGURE 18.6   Checking the physician's order, insulin, and syringe. (Courtesy of Shapero School of Nursing, Sinai Hospital of Detroit, Detroit, Michigan.)

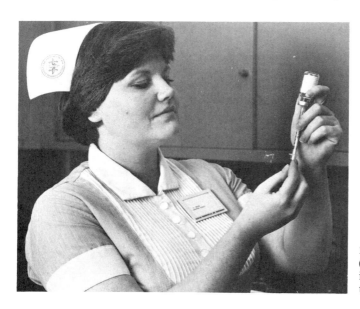

FIGURE 18.8 Filling the syringe. (Courtesy of Shapero School of Nursing, Sinai Hospital of Detroit, Detroit, Michigan.)

hormone to be released. Wide swings of overly high and overly low blood sugars occur. Such a patient may have morning headache, low morning temperature, and morning urine tests high in sugar and acetone. The physician usually treats the patient with this condition by adjusting the insulin dosage and/or redistributing food and exercise times.

A new development for insulin-dependent diabetics is an *insulin pump* which is worn around the waist. A small needle, inserted into the abdomen and connected to the pump, permits the continuous infusion of small amounts of insulin. Additional insulin can be infused at mealtimes or as needed by flicking the switch on the pump. The needle site is changed every few days to prevent irritation. This device is especially useful during pregnancy and for persons whose diabetes is hard to control. The patient receives considerable instruction and assistance in learning how to use the pump successfully.

A *closed loop pump* is currently available for some hospitalized diabetics during surgery and childbirth. This pump, when attached to the patient, monitors blood glucose levels and releases appropriate amounts of insulin on that basis.

It is hoped that future research will result in a similar pump for home use. Re-

cently, a pump was implanted under the collarbone of a diabetic man. The ideal pump could be implanted in a manner similar to a pacemaker (see Chapter 11), could monitor

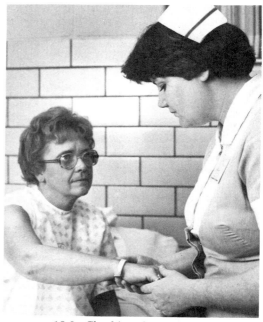

FIGURE 18.9 Checking the patient's identification bracelet. (Courtesy of Shapero School of Nursing, Sinai Hospital of Detroit, Detroit, Michigan.)

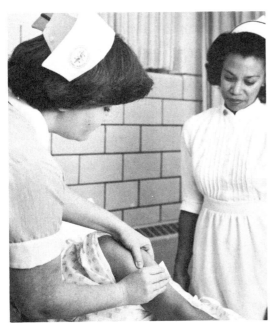

FIGURE 18.10 Cleansing the site. (Courtesy of Shapero School of Nursing, Sinai Hospital of Detroit, Detroit, Michigan.)

An *oral hypoglycemic* agent is a drug taken by mouth that stimulates the release of insulin in the body. This drug is not an oral form of insulin as is sometimes thought. In order for this drug to be effective, the patient must be able to produce some insulin and must achieve and maintain appropriate weight levels using the prescribed diet. Oral hypoglycemics are most likely to be prescribed for the type II non-insulin-dependent diabetic. Several drugs are available including sulfonylureas such as tolbutamide (ORINASE), chlorpropamide (DIABINESE), tolazamide (TOLINASE), and acetohexamide (DYMELOR). The sulfonylureas stimulate the beta cells of the pancreas to release insulin.

The patient taking an oral hypoglycemic agent may also experience hypoglycemia, although this is less common. Reactions are more likely to occur in persons over 50 years old with impaired liver or kidney function. Persons taking oral hypoglycemic agents may experience a drug interaction if other drugs are taken simultaneously. Alcohol, salicylates, dicumarol, and phenylbutazone are examples of drugs that may be involved in an interaction with hypoglycemic agents.

The diabetic patient is taught to avoid using nonprescribed medication without first checking with the physician. Liquid cold medicines and nonprescribed medication for allergies and asthma may contain alcohol,

blood glucose levels, and release appropriate amounts of insulin automatically. As previously mentioned, continuous control of blood glucose levels in the normal range is believed to result in the prevention or delay of complications associated with diabetes.

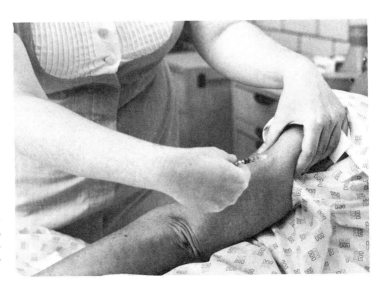

FIGURE 18.11 Injecting the insulin. (Courtesy of Shapero School of Nursing, Sinai Hospital of Detroit, Detroit, Michigan.)

sugar, and/or antihistamines that may interfere with treatment or upset the balance of blood glucose.

Assisting with Skin Care. As previously mentioned, the person with diabetes is more likely to develop arteriosclerosis. As blood vessels become narrow from the disease process, blood supply to the legs and feet is reduced. Tables 18.8 and 18.9 contain a summary of information related to skin care for the person with diabetes.

Assisting the Surgical Patient. In addition to the usual care needed before, during, and after surgery (see Chapter 6), the patient with diabetes needs special attention. Surgery disrupts the usual patient's regime of insulin/hypoglycemic agents, diet, and exercise. The patient should be observed for hyperglycemia and hypoglycemia. The nurse should report any unusual observation immediately. Also, since the diabetic patient is highly susceptible to infection and heals slowly, scrupulous sterile technique is necessary during dressing changes in order to prevent infection.

TABLE 18.8
GUIDELINES FOR CARE OF THE SKIN IN
DIABETIC PATIENTS

- Keep skin clean.
- Inspect the skin daily for any irritation, especially scratches, cuts, splinters, festered eruptions, etc.
- Clean irritated areas carefully with a mild soap and water. Do not use antibacterial soaps or strong skin antiseptics such as iodine and phenol as these may burn the skin. After cleaning the area, apply a sterile gauze bandage and avoid using adhesive tape. If the irritation increases, contact the physician at once.
- When using household cleaning products, use protective gloves.
- Avoid using a sun lamp, heat lamp, hot water bottles, heating pads, ice caps, etc., because they may burn the skin.
- Notify the physician if skin injuries and infections occur, such as ulcers, blisters, abscesses, burns, cuts, boils, carbuncles, and insect, animal, human, and fish bites.
- Avoid overexposure to the sun.
- Avoid using strong deodorants.

TABLE 18.9
GUIDELINES FOR FOOT CARE IN THE
DIABETIC PATIENT

- Wash feet daily with a mild soap (see Figure 18.12). Dry thoroughly.
- Apply mild lotion or oil to prevent dryness.
- When cutting toenails, cut straight across. If toenails are brittle, soak in water before cutting. Do not cut toenails too short.
- Wear clean cotton socks (white socks are preferred). Change daily.
- Wear properly fitted, low-heel shoes of soft leather.
- Do not pick, tear, or cut corns, calluses, or in-growing toenails. Do not use plasters or chemicals to remove corns or calluses. Soak corn or callus in mild soap and water and then gently rub off corn or callus tissue with a towel or file. Do not irritate the skin. If more treatment is needed, see a podiatrist (foot specialist), being sure to mention the diabetic condition.
- Avoid being barefoot.
- Inspect the feet daily for any irritation, scratch, cut, blister, etc. If these occur, wash gently with mild soap, apply sterile gauze, and notify physician. Any break in the skin may lead to gangrene. Do not apply any medication to the feet without being ordered by the physician.
- Never wear garters, as they restrict the circulation.
- Keep feet warm, as cold reduces circulation.
- Do not cross legs when sitting, as this restricts circulation.
- Avoid the use of tobacco, as nicotine constricts blood vessels.
- Consult physician as to proper exercise to increase circulation.

Assisting with Common Concerns. As previously mentioned, the diabetic patient can be expected to have a number of serious concerns related to illness, complications, and therapy. The nurse having daily contact with the patient and family is often the person best able to help. Several forms of help may be given. For example, active listening and careful observation are tools that enable the nurse to help identify specific concerns. Sometimes the patient has feelings of anger or anxiety but has difficulty in recognizing the specific source of those feelings. Common concerns that affect diabetics include the impact of diabetes on career and employ-

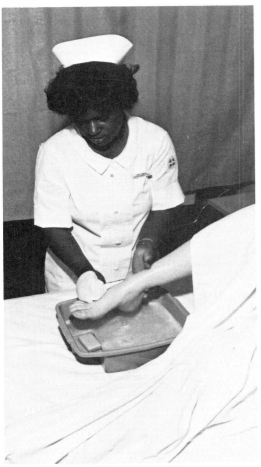

FIGURE 18.12   The patient with diabetes mellitus should keep the feet clean by using water and mild soap daily. When bathing the patient in the hospital, the nurse can explain the important aspects of foot care.

ment plans, sexuality, marriage, pregnancy, and family life, travel, obtaining insurance, eating out, and similar aspects of life.

Once specific concerns have been identified, the nurse may provide accurate and complete information or may refer the patient to others who can help. Since a wealth of new information rapidly is becoming available, the nurse needs to be certain to obtain up-do-date information before counseling the patient.

The local affiliate of the American Diabetes Association is a valuable community re-source for the diabetic patient and family as well as the public and health professionals. This organization provides direct services to diabetics as well as education materials and programs for diabetics and health professionals. Interested persons may contact the national organization to obtain the address of the nearest local affiliate.

The American Diabetes Association, Inc.
2 Park Avenue
New York, New York 10016

Patient and Family Teaching.   Patient and family teaching is one of the most important nursing interventions. The patient's life depends on developing strong skills in controlling the disease process. The information already discussed in this section is typical of the topics included in a comprehensive learning program for the diabetic. A summary of information is presented in Table 18.10. This information is then individualized for the patient on the basis of the specific treatment plan, the patient's learning style, attention span, and attitude.

An environment for learning is of utmost importance. A student learns more readily when the environment is quiet, relaxed, and friendly and a trusting nurse-patient relationship has been established (Figure 18.13). The nurse must constantly keep in mind that the patient may not find it easy to accept and cope with the illness; so an extreme amount of patience, tolerance, and understanding must be displayed by the nurse. A good learning program includes time for presenting information as well as for supervising the patient's newly learned skills. In general, most persons learn by doing.

It is important for the diabetic patient to wear some form of identification at all times. Complete identification includes the type of diabetes mellitus (type I insulin-dependent or type II non-insulin-dependent), as well as the name and telephone numbers of the physician and closest relative.

HYPERSECRETION OF ISLETS: HYPERINSULINISM

The second major disorder of the islets of Langerhans is hypersecretion of the islets,

TABLE 18.10
SUMMARY OF INFORMATION FOR DIABETIC TEACHING-LEARNING PROGRAM

TOPIC	INFORMATION
Diabetes	Description of disease, symptoms, effect of disease process
Monitoring blood and/or urine glucose	How, when, and where to test blood or urine
	How to store supplies
	Interpreting results
	Recording results
Diet	Understanding food exchanges, reading labels, shopping, food preparation, establishing mealtimes
Insulin and/or oral hypoglycemic agents	How to store medication, prepare the dosage, administer medication, rotate injection sites
	How to recognize and manage hypoglycemia
Exercise	Establishing an exercise program
	Prevention of hypoglycemia
Skin care	Regular inspection of the skin for lesions, care of feet
Complications	Preventing, reporting, and managing complications such as eye changes, circulatory changes, infection, diabetic ketoacidosis
Community resources	Kinds of services provided and how to obtain help

which results in an excessive amount of the hormone insulin (hyperinsulinism). This condition may be organic (pertaining to an organ) or functional (affecting the functions, but not the structure).

Organic hyperinsulinism is mainly caused by overgrowth (hyperplasia) of the islets or by a tumor, which is usually benign.

Functional hyperinsulinism usually occurs in anxious and nervous people, and the cause is unknown. Studies have shown that many people with functional hyperinsulinism later develop diabetes mellitus. One explanation of this is that the beta cells over- work and give out, resulting in insulin deficiency. Functional hyperinsulinism may follow a gastrectomy because carbohydrates pass directly into the small intestine, where they are absorbed.

Symptoms of hyperinsulinism are the same as those of hypoglycemia: hunger, weakness, apprehension, irritability, tremors, and profuse perspiration. When hypoglycemia is allowed to persist, complications may result. The complications usually seen are functional disturbances and pathologic changes in the peripheral nervous system, retinal hemorrhages, permanent behavioral

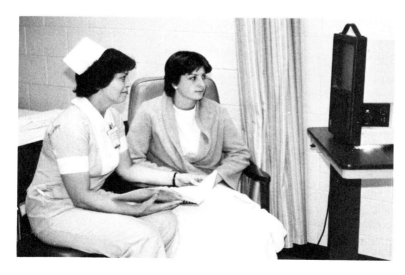

FIGURE 18.13 Teaching the diabetic patient. (Courtesy of Loudoun County School of Practical Nursing, Leesburg, Virginia.)

changes, cerebrovascular accidents, and permanent intellectual damage.

Immediate treatment of acute hyperinsulinism is orange juice with sugar or a solution of granulated sugar. Long-term treatment of organic hyperinsulinism requires surgery, removal of the tumor, or resection of the hyperplasia tissue. In functional hyperinsulinism, the long-term treatment is to relieve tension and anxiety. The patient may need professional counseling by a psychologist or a psychiatrist; a high-protein, low-carbohydrate diet; sedatives and anticholinergic drugs; and regular medical examinations to check for possible diabetes mellitus.

Case Study Involving Graves' Disease

Mrs. Sue Vaughn, a 38-year-old homemaker and mother, was admitted to the medical unit of the hospital with a possible diagnosis of Graves' disease.

The past history of Mrs. Vaughn indicated that at the time her illness began, her children were 17, 7, and 2 years of age. Her husband indicated that she was normally a calm, understanding person who enjoyed keeping house and participating in the children's activities. She had a tendency to gain weight easily and was 4.5 kg (10 lb) overweight. Recently, Mrs. Vaughn had a particularly busy week with overnight guests. She had a ravenous appetite, yet she noticed that she had lost weight during the week. Within a short period of time she lost 11.4 (25 lb). Instead of feeling more energetic, she found herself feeling extremely tired at the end of the day. This tendency toward fatigue progressed quickly to the extent that she no longer wanted to do her housework and engage in the children's activities. She decided to have a physical examination.

During the physical examination, she told the nurse that she had been extremely nervous, irritable, depressed, and then happy at times. She also indicated that she had loose bowel movements, could not tolerate heat, had profuse perspiration, felt that her heart was beating rapidly, noticed tremors of her hands, and noticed that her skin and hair were changing.

After having arranged for the care of her children, Ms. Vaughn was hospitalized for diagnostic studies. She was admitted with a tentative diagnosis of Graves' disease. The doctor's orders were:

- Bed rest with bathroom privileges

- 2200-calorie diet, low in roughage and spices
- DALMANE 15 mg at hs, may repeat × one
- T-3, T-4, ^{131}I tests Monday, Tuesday, and Wednesday
- SMA-20 and routine urinalysis
- Routine serology
- Chest x-ray
- ECG
- Weigh daily and record

QUESTIONS

1. What behavioral changes can be anticipated by the nurse in caring for Mrs. Vaughn?
2. How should Mrs. Vaughn be weighed?
3. Relate the order for a high-calorie diet, low in roughage and spices, to the symptoms of Mrs. Vaughn.
4. What nursing measures are indicated because of Mrs. Vaughn's intolerance to heat?
5. What steps should the nurse take to provide the proper physical environment for Mrs. Vaughn? What attitude must the nurse have to provide good nursing care for Mrs. Vaughn?
6. In what ways can the nurse provide an emotional environment conducive to rest for Mrs. Vaughn?
7. What are the nursing responsibilities in the diagnostic tests: T-3, T-4?
8. What nursing measures will help Mrs. Vaughn understand her behavior as it is represented in her present illness?
9. In what way could the nurse help to allay the family's concern over the behavior of Mrs. Vaughn?

Case Study Involving Diabetes Mellitus

Mary Allen, a 16-year-old high school student, was admitted to the medical unit of a local hospital with a diagnosis of diabetes mellitus, which already had been established by her family physician. She was admitted to the hospital for regulation of diabetes. The physician's orders are:

- 1800-calorie, ADA diabetic diet
- Up ad lib
- Test urine for sugar and acetone tid ac and hs
- Notify Dr. Zumbol if results are positive
- Fasting blood sugar every two days
- 35 units of NPH insulin q A.M.
- Teach patient to give insulin to self
- Have dietitian explain diet to patient
- NEMBUTAL, 75 mg at bedtime—may repeat × one
- Weigh two times a week

QUESTIONS

1. What nursing measures are indicated for Mary Allen in relation to skin care?
2. What equipment and explanation should the nurse give to Mary Allen to obtain the urine for sugar and acetone?
3. What nursing measures are indicated in relation to foot care?
4. What behavioral changes can be anticipated in relationship to a change of life-style? What should the nurse's reaction be?
5. What is the appropriate approach for the nurse to use to encourage Mary Allen to verbalize her feelings concerning diabetes mellitus?
6. What nursing measures would be helpful in providing a learning environment?
7. What information would the nurse give Mary Allen concerning the storage, rotation of vial, dosage, and proper equipment to use, and method of administration of insulin?
8. What information will the patient need in order to administer insulin to herself in regard to route of administration, site of injection, and rotation of sites?
9. What nursing observations and measures are indicated in diabetic acidosis?
10. What nursing observations and measures are indicated for insulin reaction?
11. What nursing measures will help Mary Allen have adequate exercise?

Suggestions for Further Study

1. Review the medication orders for several diabetic patients. What drugs, if any, have been ordered?
2. Is the new insulin pump being used in your locality yet? What are the advantages? Disadvantages?
3. Mason, Mildred A.; Bates, Grace F.; and Smola, Bonnie K.: *Workbook in Basic Medical-Surgical Nursing,* 3rd ed. Macmillan Publishing Company, New York, 1984, Exercise 18.
4. Visit the local affiliate of the American Diabetes Association to learn more about materials and programs available for diabetics and health professionals.
5. Prepare a file of newspaper clippings that describe new developments in diabetes.

Additional Readings

Comunas, Caroline: "Transphenoidal Hypophysectomy." *American Journal of Nursing,* 80:1820–23 (Oct.), 1980.

Fredholm, Nancy Zilinsky: "The Insulin Pump: New Method of Insulin Delivery." *American Journal of Nursing,* 81:2024–26 (Nov.), 1981.

Garofano, Catherine: "Helping Diabetics Live with Their Neuropathies." *Nursing 80,* 10:42–44 (June), 1980.

Guthrie, Diana: "Helping the Diabetic Manage His Self-Care." *Nursing 80,* 10:57–64 (Feb.), 1980.

Jackson, Carol: "Diabetes: How Your Patient Looks at It." *Nursing 81,* 11:82–83 (May), 1981.

Jenkins, Elda: "Living with Thyrotoxicosis." *American Journal of Nursing,* 80:956–58 (May), 1980.

Kiser, Debra: "The Somogyi Effect." *American Journal of Nursing,* 80:236–38 (Feb.), 1980.

McCarthy, Joyce A.: "Diabetic Nephropathy." *American Journal of Nursing,* 81:2030–34 (Nov.), 1981.

McConnell, Edwina A.: "Be Prepared for Double Trouble If Your Surgical Patient's a Diabetic." *Nursing 81,* 11:118–23 (Nov.), 1981.

Miller, Barbara K., and White, Nancy E.: "Diabetes Assessment Guide." *American Journal of Nursing,* 80:1314–16 (July), 1980.

Pelczynski, Linda, and Reilly, Ann: "Helping Your Diabetic Patients Help Themselves." *Nursing 81,* 11:76–81 (May), 1981.

Richardson, Betty: "A Tool for Assessing the Real World of Diabetic Noncompliance." *Nursing 82,* 12:68–73 (Jan.), 1982.

Robinson, Corinne H.: *Basic Nutrition and Diet Therapy,* 4th ed. Macmillan Publishing Co., Inc., New York, 1980, pp. 226–37.

Sackheim, George I., and Lehman, Dennis D.: *Chemistry for the Health Sciences,* 4th ed. Macmillan Publishing Co., Inc., New York, 1981, pp. 457–79.

Stevens, A. Denise: "Monitoring Blood Glucose at Home—Who Should Do It." *American Journal of Nursing,* 81:2026–27 (Nov.), 1981.

Chapter 19

The Patient with a Disease
of the Urinary System*

Expected Behavioral
Outcomes

Minimum objectives referred to as expected behavioral outcomes have been designed for the practical/vocational nursing student to use as guides in studying this chapter. The student should read these expected outcomes before studying the chapter. The objectives can be used as guides for study.

Using the content of this chapter, the student should return to the objectives and evaluate the ability to:

1. *List in sequence the route taken by the normal flow of urine on a diagram of the urinary system.*
2. *Draw a diagram illustrating a nephron.*
3. *Compute the approximate amount of blood that flows through the kidneys in 24 hours and discuss its implications to the nursing staff in caring for a patient with a disease of the kidney.*

4. *Compare the nursing actions indicated for a person with a urethral retention catheter with those indicated for a person with a suprapubic catheter, relating each nursing action to structure and function of the urinary system.*
5. *Demonstrate the behavior to be expected from the patient suffering from kidney colic.*
6. *Compare the nursing observations and interventions indicated for a person with urinary retention with those required for a person with urinary suppression.*
7. *Compare the nursing interventions needed by the patient with an inflammation with those indicated for patients with pyelonephritis and glomerulonephritis, by listing the factors they have in common.*
8. *Relate the symptoms of cancer of the urinary system to the seven danger signals.*
9. *Describe the behavioral changes that are associated with the patient requiring regular hemodialysis to sustain life.*

*Revised by the authors and Lydia Amores Villanueva, R.N., B.S., who is a Practical Nursing Instructor at the Central School of Practical Nursing in Norfolk, Virginia.

10. *Describe the nursing observations and interventions related to each of the diagnostic tests described in this chapter.*

11. *Describe the nursing care of an incontinent patient who also has a urinary tract disease.*

Vocabulary Development

The following prefixes, suffixes, and combining forms pertain to this chapter. By learning and/or reviewing their meanings, the practical/vocational nursing student will have the keys needed to unlock many exciting new medical terms.

Discover the meaning of these keys in a medical dictionary or in the content of this chapter. How does each key pertain to this chapter? In your notebook write the correct meaning of each prefix, suffix, or combining form listed below. Illustrate each key with an example.

calc—stone. Ex. renal *calculus*—a kidney stone.

cortic-	nephr-
cyst-	olig-
electr-	poly-
grad-	pto-
-gram	pyel-
hem(at)-	ren-
hydr-	retro-
lith-	scop-
micr-	ur-

Structure and Function

In addition to carrying food and oxygen to the body cells, blood removes waste products from them. These waste products are carried to appropriate places for disposal. The respiratory system, the intestinal tract, the skin, and the urinary system remove waste material from the body.

One function of the urinary system is (1) to excrete waste products from the body, especially those resulting from protein metabolism, such as uric acid, urea, ammonia, and creatinine. Another function of the urinary system is (2) to help control the fluid and the electrolyte balance in the body. *Electrolytes* are electrically charged particles of acids, bases, and salts. These particles are known as electrolytes because they conduct electricity when in water. Electrolytes, such as chloride, potassium, sodium, and bicarbonate, help to hold fluid within compartments of the body. The urinary system helps (3) to maintain an acid-base balance in plasma necessary for enzyme activities. (4) Certain cells in the kidneys secrete *renin,* an enzyme that leads to an increase in blood pressure. (5) An oxygen deficiency in the bloodstream stimulates the kidneys to secrete a renal factor that changes plasma protein to *erythropoietin.* This protein stimulates the bone marrow to produce more red blood cells.

The normal urinary system is composed of two kidneys, two ureters, a bladder, and a urethra (see Figure 19.1). The kidneys form urine from waste materials taken from the blood. Urine is carried from the kidneys to the bladder by the ureters. The urethra carries urine from the bladder to the outside of the body.

KIDNEYS

The kidneys are shaped like beans (see Figure 19.2). They are approximately 11.25 cm (5 in.) long, 5.0 to 7.5 cm (2 to 3 in.) wide, and 2.5 cm (1 in.) thick. The kidneys are located near the junction of the thoracic and lumbar vertebrae. One is on each side of the vertebral column. The kidneys are behind the abdominal organs and are held in place by cushions of fat and fibrous tissue. The anterior side is in back of the peritoneum. The posterior portion is protected by the muscular wall of the back. The kidneys are continuously purifying the blood in the body. Approximately 1 liter (1 qt) of blood passes through the kidneys every minute. The water and the waste products taken from the blood in the kidneys are known as urine.

The *hilus,* which is the depressed area on the inner side of the kidney, is the location of the entrance and exit of the ureter, blood and lymph vessels, and nerves. Each kidney has a *pelvis,* which is a funnel-shaped hollow

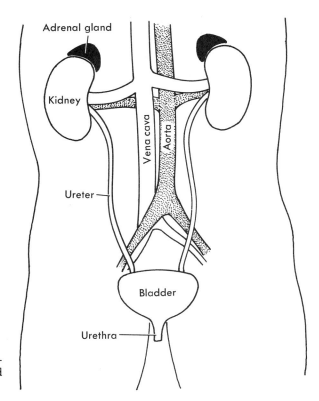

FIGURE 19.1 Diagram showing kidneys, ureters, urinary bladder, adrenal glands, and large blood vessels.

structure. This cavity of the pelvis becomes smaller as it leads outward from the kidney in the hilus. The narrow portion of the pelvis forms the ureter. The larger part of the pelvis is surrounded by tissue known as the *medullary substance* or *medulla*. This substance has cone-shaped projections called *pyramids*, which project into cuplike divisions of the pelvis of the kidney known as *calyces*. The outer portion of the kidney is known as the *cortical substance* or *cortex*.

The cortex and medulla contain many tiny units called *nephrons*. These unique microscopic structures are the functioning units in which waste is filtered from the blood. Each nephron has three main parts: the glomerulus, Bowman's capsule, and a convoluted tubule (see Figure 19.3). The glomerulus is a network of tiny blood vessels branching from the renal artery and pushing into the top part of a hollow ball called *Bowman's capsule*. Water and dissolved substances are filtered out of the blood into the capsule, and the fluid flows down into the

convoluted tubule. Products that the body can use again are reabsorbed along the various parts of the tubules. The capillaries surrounding the tubule carry the blood containing the reabsorbed water, as well as certain reusable dissolved substances, back to the body by way of the renal vein. The fluid remaining in the collecting tubules is known as *urine* and is emptied into the pelvis of the kidney.

URETERS

Two long, small tubes about 25 to 30 cm (10 to 12 in.) long and about 4 to 5 mm (1/5 in.) in diameter, called ureters, connect the pelvis of each kidney to the bladder. The ureters are composed of smooth muscle tissue and are lined with mucous membrane. Urine is carried down the ureters by peristalsis to the bladder.

BLADDER

The bladder is a hollow organ located in the pelvic cavity. The bladder is a muscular

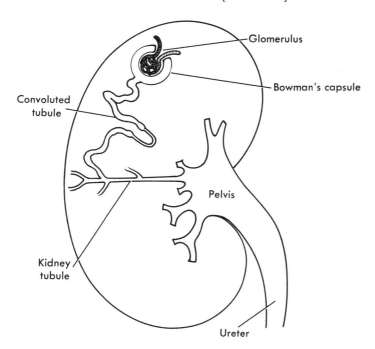

FIGURE 19.2 Illustration showing gross structure of kidney.

elastic sac lined with mucous membrane similar to that which lines the ureters. The bladder serves as a reservoir for urine. After the bladder has collected a sufficient amount of urine, about 250 ml (½ pt), the urge to void is felt, and the smooth muscle tissue in the walls contracts, the sphincter muscles relax, and urine is forced out of the bladder. This process of voiding is called *micturition* or *urination*.

URETHRA

The urethra is a small tube, lined with mucous membrane, that leads outward from the bladder. The urethra of the female is short, about 3.8 cm (1½ in.), and serves only

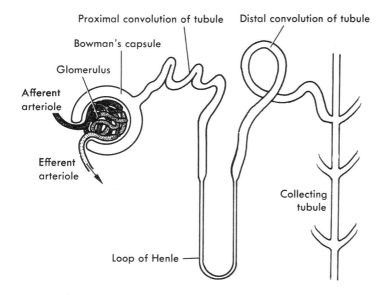

FIGURE 19.3 Schematic drawing of nephron.

as a passageway for urine. The male urethra is longer, about 20 cm (8 in.), and carries urine as well as secretions from the reproductive glands. The urethra has two sphincter muscles surrounding it that prevent the continuous flow of urine from the bladder. These sphincter muscles relax when the bladder contracts and voiding takes place. The opening of the urethra is called the *urethral meatus*.

URINE

Urine is composed primarily of water; electrolytes, including sodium, potassium, chlorides, and bicarbonates; and the waste products of protein metabolism, mainly urea, creatinine, and ammonia. The amount of solid waste products in the urine in relation to the amount of water determines the *specific gravity*. This is the comparison between the weight of urine and the weight of an equal amount of water. Normally the specific gravity of urine may range from 1.010 to 1.030, as compared with water, which has a specific gravity of 1.000. Thus, urine is heavier than water because of the solid waste products. The specific gravity of urine is regulated by the kidneys acting under the influence of the *antidiuretic hormone* (ADH) secreted by the pituitary gland. An unusually high specific gravity or an unusually low one can indicate disease of the kidney or some other organ. A dificiency of the antidiuretic hormone causes large volumes of urine of low specific gravity to be excreted. This occurs in a rare condition known as *diabetes insipidus*.

Normally, the average amount of urine voided by an adult in 24 hours may range from approximately 1200 to 1500 ml (40 to 50 oz). Various factors, such as a change in the amount of perspiration, a change in the fluid intake, and a change in the environmental temperature, can affect the daily output of urine. A variation in the urinary output can also be caused by disease. For example, diarrhea, vomiting, and hemorrhage, as well as a disease of the kidneys, heart, or blood vessels, may cause variations. The patient with *polyuria* passes large amounts of urine. Voiding small amounts is known as *oliguria*. The patient whose kidneys fail to excrete urine has *anuria*. This is known as *suppression* of urine production. The patient with urinary *retention* has urine in the bladder but is unable to void successfully.

Urine generally has a slightly acid reaction, has a faint aromatic odor, and is clear yellow in appearance. The proportion of water and waste products in solution affects the color. For example, if the patient drinks an inadequate amount of fluids, the urine is likely to be concentrated and deep yellow in color. When the patient drinks a large amount of fluid, the urine is likely to be less concentrated and lighter in color.

Common abnormal substances in the urine that may indicate disease of the urinary system are albumin, glucose, acetone or ketone bodies, casts, calculi, red blood cells, bacteria, and white blood cells.

Albumin, a simple protein, may indicate a disease of the tiny blood vessels in the glomeruli. Disease in this part of the kidney allows albumin to seep from the blood into the urine. The patient with albumin in the urine has *albuminuria*.

Glucose may indicate that the patient has eaten more sugar than the body can promptly use or store. This extra amount excreted in the urine exceeds the kidney's ability to reabsorb sugar and it therefore "spills over" into the urine. This is called *temporary glycosuria*. However, glucose in the urine also may indicate a high blood sugar as a result of insulin deficiency or the body's inability to utilize insulin. This condition is known as *diabetes mellitus*.

Acetone or *ketone bodies* indicate that the body is using stored body fat for energy instead of the carbohydrates that are being eaten. The kidneys excrete these end products of the breakdown of the fat as ketone bodies or acetone. They may be excreted in the urine in diabetes mellitus or acute starvation, and the presence in the urine is called *ketonuria*.

Casts may indicate a disease of the tubules. The casts are microscopic bodies that are formed when substances harden in the tubules. These casts are then washed out of the tubules by the flow of urine. There are various types of casts: pus, red cells, granular, waxy, epithelial, hyaline, and fatty.

Their names come either from the substances composing them or from the way they look under the microscope.

Calculi, or stones, are made of crystals of salts and organic material. The reason a person develops them is not fully understood. More discussion will follow in this chapter in the section on nephrolithiasis.

The presence of blood in the urine is known as *hematuria*. It may be seen when it changes the color of urine to cloudy, smoky, or reddish-brown or various shades in between and is then called *gross hematuria*. However, when blood in the urine can be detected only under a microscope as isolated blood cells, it is called *microscopic hematuria*. Hematuria may occur in the patient because of an injury, an inflammation, or a tumor of the urinary tract.

Bacteriuria is a term indicating the presence of bacteria in the urine. This is an abnormal condition, because urine should not contain any microorganisms.

Pus in the urine is the result of an infection or inflammation usually caused by bacteria and is known as *pyuria*. The science of diagnosing and treating disorders of the urinary system is called *urology*. The physician who specializes in this science is a urologist.

Assisting with Diagnostic Studies

The nurse is frequently responsible for the collection of urine specimens to aid in diagnosing a urinary tract disorder. The nurse may also be asked to prepare the patient for a particular procedure or assist the physician in examining the patient. A discussion of various diagnostic studies done to aid the physician in establishing a diagnosis follows.

URINALYSIS

One of the most common initial methods used by the doctor to aid in determining whether or not the patient has a urinary system disease is urinalysis (see Table 19.1). This is a laboratory analysis of the urine. Urinalysis includes a description of the color; determination of the pH (acidity or alkalinity); specific gravity; the amount of protein, glucose, and ketones; and the sediment which may contain red blood cells, white blood cells, and casts.

TABLE 19.1
CHARACTERISTICS OF NORMAL URINE

Amount in 24 hr	1200 to 1500 ml
Color	Clear yellow to deep yellow
Specific gravity	1.010 to 1.030
Acidity	Slightly acid (reported as pH 4.8 to 7.5)
Albumin	0
Glucose	0
Acetone	0
Red blood cells	0
White blood cells	0
Casts	0

The first-voided specimen is preferable because it is concentrated and the abnormal components are more likely to be present. A clean and dry container is provided to catch the urine after cleansing the meatus with a cleansing solution or mild soap and water. At least 30 ml is collected. If the specimen cannot be analyzed immediately, it must be refrigerated.

URINE CULTURE

Another type of examination the doctor may request is the urine culture. This is a laboratory procedure used to determine the possible growth of microorganisms that might cause an infection of the urinary system. Using this information, the doctor can plan a more specific course of treatment. It is important to obtain an absolutely clean specimen. A contaminated specimen may contain organisms from a source other than the patient's urine. This could lead to incorrect interpretation of the culture and inappropriate therapy for the patient.

A specific order may be given by the doctor to obtain a catheterized specimen for culture. The practice of catheterizing the patient to obtain urine for culture is decreasing because of the danger of introducing an infection into the urinary system. A clean voided, or "clean catch," specimen collected midway in the voiding process frequently is requested. When asked to collect a clean specimen for culture, the nurse should refer to the specific procedure approved for the institution.

In general, the area around the urethral meatus is cleansed scrupulously, similar to the preparation for a catheterization. Instruct the client to start voiding, stop the stream of flow after a few seconds, void into the sterile container, and place the cap on the container. The cap is placed on the container to prevent contamination from the air. The specimen is then sent immediately to the laboratory. In the female, the labia are kept separated throughout the procedure. In the male, the foreskin is retracted throughout the procedure. The importance of proper specimen collection cannot be overemphasized which makes the nurse indirectly responsible for the diagnosis and appropriate drug therapy.

SENSITIVITY TEST

A laboratory procedure the doctor often may request in conjunction with the urine culture is the *sensitivity test* (see Figure 5.7). Most clinical laboratories provide a sensitivity test automatically whenever a culture shows pathogens. The sensitivity test is done to determine which antibiotics will eradicate the bacteria. The medical technologist places tiny pieces of paper, each containing different antibiotics, on the culture. Bacteria sensitive to a particular drug do not grow around the piece of paper containing that drug. The doctor uses this information in determining which drug to use in combating the infection.

EVALUATING BLADDER FUNCTION

Residual urine is that amount which remains in the bladder after the patient voids. Normally, a bladder is empty or contains a small amount of urine after voiding. Some conditions in which there is an incomplete emptying of the bladder are prostatic hypertrophy, urethral stricture, or interruption of nerves supplying the bladder.

There are two methods by which residual urine is determined. The procedure most commonly used is catheterizing the client immediately after voiding. A volume of 50 ml or less is considered normal. The other method is an x-ray view of the retained urine. The client is not catheterized; instead a radiopaque substance is injected intraven-ously and allowed to accumulate in the bladder. When there is a sufficient amount of urine, the client is instructed to void. Immediately after voiding, an x-ray is taken of the residual urine containing the radiopaque substance.

CYSTOMETRIC EXAMINATION. Cystometric examination is performed to evaluate bladder tone in individuals who have urinary incontinence or evidence of neurologic dysfunction. A Foley catheter is inserted into the urinary bladder and pressure is exerted by the instillation of normal saline. The amount of pressure being exerted is measured by the cystometer. The client is told to report any feeling of fullness, urgency to void, and discomfort. Select medications may be given to determine their effects on the tone and relaxation of the bladder.

OTHER URINE TESTS FOR RENAL FUNCTION

CLEARANCE TESTS. Another way to identify renal (kidney) function is the clearance test which measures the amount of blood that the kidneys can clear of a substance in a given time. The creatinine clearance test is the most widely used of all the clearance tests. Creatinine is the end product of the breakdown of muscle tissues. It is relatively fixed and it is not influenced by dietary intake.

A precisely timed collection of urine is made for either 12 or 24 hours beginning in the morning, and the total quantity of urine is sent to the laboratory for study. It is usually the nurse's responsibility to make certain all of the urine is collected in the special container and none is discarded. The nurse should keep an accurate record of the collection period and record this information on the patient's chart. Immediately after the last urine is collected, a blood specimen is drawn to determine the serum creatinine level.

The *urea clearance test* is less accurate than the creatinine clearance test and is seldom used.

The *sodium excretion test* measures tubular function. It determines the ability of the kidneys to excrete or conserve the electrolyte sodium. A 24-hour urine collection is analyzed for its sodium content.

Concentration and dilution tests are done to determine whether or not the kidneys are concentrating and diluting the urine properly. One of the first functions lost by a diseased kidney is its ability to dilute or concentrate urine. Thus, the patient with kidney damage may be unable to produce urine with a normal specific gravity. The patient is first dehydrated by restricting fluids to determine the kidney's capacity to concentrate. One or more specimens of urine are collected. The client is then hydrated by drinking a large amount of fluid in a short period of time to test the capacity to dilute. Urine specimens are collected at periodic intervals. The specific gravity is measured in each specimen. The patient's inability to concentrate or to dilute urine may indicate dysfunction of the kidney tubules.

When caring for a patient who is having these tests, the nurse should seek specific instructions from the team leader, or head nurse, as to whether or not the patient may have fluids. The nurse should know also when the urine specimens are to be collected.

Another example of a kidney function test that may be ordered is the *phenolsulfonphthalein, or PSP, test*. A harmless red dye is injected intravenously. This dye is removed from the bloodstream by the kidneys and colors the urine. The nurse may be asked to collect urine specimens at specific times during the test and should collect these specimens promptly. If the patient is unable to void at a designated time, this should be reported to the nurse in charge. The amount of dye in each urine specimen is then estimated in the laboratory and an estimate of kidney tubule function can be made from the results.

X-RAYS

X-ray is one of the visualization tests of the urinary tract. Since the kidneys lie at the back of the peritoneal cavity, feces and flatus in the intestines could obstruct the view of the kidneys. To assure a clear picture, the bowel is emptied prior to x-rays of the kidneys.

KUB (kidneys, ureters, and bladder) is a flat plate x-ray of the abdomen to determine the size and position of the kidneys and to reveal radiopaque stones along the urinary tract.

PYELOGRAM

The patient may have either an intravenous pyelogram or a retrograde pyelogram (see Figure 19.4). When doing an intravenous pyelogram, the doctor or the technician injects the special dye into the patient's vein. The kidneys remove the dye from the blood. This dye causes the kidneys to be visible by x-ray. Both kidneys are x-rayed at intervals after the dye is given. This type of examination helps the doctor determine whether or not both kidneys are picking up and excreting the dye normally. A pyelogram may identify sources of difficulty such as an obstruction in renal blood flow, renal calculi, tumor, and obstruction in urinary flow. In addition to the bowel cleansing, the client usually is not permitted food or fluids for approximately 12 hours before the x-ray, so that the dye will be concentrated and permit a better x-ray. The dye injected during an IVP may cause a severe allergic reaction. An important nursing responsibility is to question the patient about allergy to iodine and seafood. Any allergy should be reported before the x-ray.

In doing a retrograde pyelogram, the physician inserts a cystoscope into the bladder and then passes small catheters through this instrument through the ureters into the kidneys. A special dye is injected through the catheters into the pelvis of each kidney. This dye causes the outline of the kidney, pelvis, and ureters to be visible on the x-ray. The nurse should be familiar with the procedure used in the particular agency for preparing the patient for pyelograms and cystoscopy. Generally an operative permit is required.

CYSTOGRAM

A catheter is inserted into the bladder and a radiopaque solution is instilled to outline the wall and also to evaluate vesicoureteral reflux which is a backing up of urine into one or both ureters.

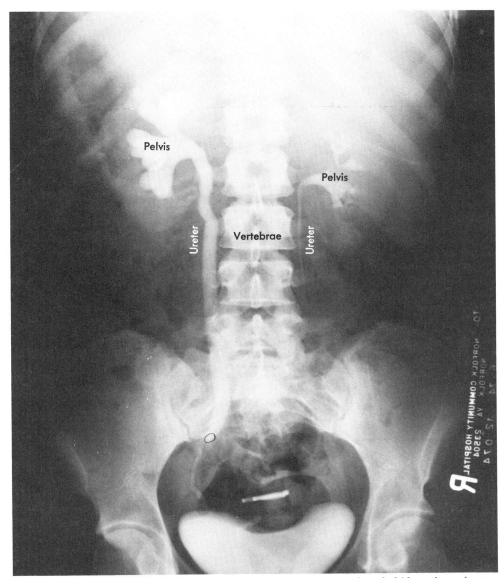

FIGURE 19.4 Retrograde pyleogram. The pelvis and ureter of each kidney have been labeled.

ULTRASOUND

In ultrasonography, high-frequency sound vibrations are sent into the kidneys. The resulting sound echo patterns are recorded as they return. Ultrasonography is useful in evaluating the size of a mass in the kidney and helps in determining whether the mass is solid or cystic.

There are usually no preparations before this test. However, ultrasound of the bladder requires the client to have a full bladder. The patient may have questions concerning the procedure. The nurse can allay anxiety by telling the client that the procedure is done in the x-ray department, is much like other x-ray examinations, and no pain is involved.

RENAL SCAN

A renal scan is still another diagnostic radioactive test to determine an outline of functioning kidney tissue. A tracer dose of radioactive mercury or iodine is given intravenously, after which a probe is passed back and forth over the kidneys, and either a record is made or a special electronic photograph is taken. Nonfunctioning areas of the kidney will show no record of radioactivity since that kidney tissue is not filtering wastes containing the radioactive material from the blood. An explanation of the procedure with the information that is is not associated with pain should be provided for this patient.

COMPUTERIZED AXIAL TOMOGRAPHY (CAT SCAN, CT SCAN)

This noninvasive technique may be used to obtain a cross-sectional view of kidney anatomy in order to locate tumors and cysts. Additional information about this test method can be located in Chapter 4, page 71.

CYSTOSCOPIC EXAMINATION

The cystoscopic examination is a special procedure performed by the doctor, who generally is a *urologist*, a specialist concerned with the diagnosis and treatment of diseases of the urinary system in the female and the genitourinary tract in the male. In this procedure, the urologist inserts an instrument called a cystoscope into the urinary bladder. The doctor looks through the cystoscope to examine the walls of the bladder and the urethra. Urine specimens can be taken from the ureters and kidneys. The doctor also can perform certain treatments of the bladder through the cystoscope. For example, one can remove small stones, obtain a specimen from a tumor, or remove small growths.

This examination may be done with or without anesthesia. A sedative such as diazepam (VALIUM) or meperidine hydrochloride (DEMEROL) is given one hour before the procedure. A local anesthetic may be instilled into the urethra prior to the insertion of the cystoscope. General anesthesia is used if the person is apprehensive or when other procedures are done such as litholapaxy (crushing a stone) or prostate resection. During the cystoscopic examination, a sterile irrigating solution is run in and out of the bladder to distend it for better visualization and to wash out blood clots, tissues, or stone fragments.

The nurse can give a great deal of support to the patient undergoing a cystoscopy and should be available to answer the patient's questions or refer them to the appropriate person. Preparation for a cystoscopy may include giving enemas to cleanse the bowel.

After the cystoscopy, the patient should be encouraged to drink large amounts of fluid to lessen the amount of irritation to the urethra when voiding. Painful micturition and a small amount of hematuria may be expected for about 24 hours after the procedure. If large amounts of blood are seen in the urine and the pain continues longer than usual or is intense, the doctor should be notified.

RENAL ANGIOGRAPHY

Renal angiography visualizes the renal arteries to determine the possibility of stenosis as a cause of hypertension or to reveal a tumor or abnormal renal vessels.

Preparation for this test usually includes special written consent as well as a laxative, enemas, and restriction of food and fluids. The client may receive a sedative prior to the procedure. A special needle is used to puncture the skin and permit insertion of a catheter into an artery. When the femoral artery is used, a catheter is threaded into a puncture made on the groin to the femoral artery upward to the level of the renal artery. At this point, the dye is injected through the catheter. The patient may experience a temporary sensation of heat when the dye is first injected.

After x-rays have been taken, the catheter is removed and a pressure dressing is applied to the puncture site.

The puncture site should be observed for bleeding, swelling, and tenderness; distal pulses should be checked; and vital signs monitored frequently during the first four hours. The client is put on bed rest for at least eight hours, and the pressure dressing is left in place, usually for 24 hours.

Translumbar aortogram is done less frequently than femoral aortogram. The dye is injected with a long needle inserted through the client's back into the aorta. The injection is made while the client is in a position for immediate x-rays. The nursing care is the same as that for the client with femoral aortogram.

KIDNEY BIOPSY

Kidney biopsy is a diagnostic test to determine the type or stage or prognostic outcome of a renal disease, particularly glomerular disease. Kidney biopsy may be done either through a needle puncture or through an incision. The biopsy may be performed in the patient's room, in the x-ray department, or in the operating room.

Preparation for the procedure includes an explanation, written consent, and blood studies to identify potential bleeding problems that could cause hemorrhage after the biopsy. Sedation usually is not required. The individual is placed prone over a sandbag or a firm pillow. The skin is prepared and a lo-

cal anesthetic is injected over the puncture area. The patient is instructed not to breathe during certain parts of the procedure. After the needle is withdrawn, pressure to the site is applied for 20 minutes, and a pressure bandage is secured in place. The client is positioned according to the physician's instructions. The client is instructed to avoid any strain such as coughing or turning. Vital signs are monitored frequently, and all urine is observed for hematuria which may appear with the first voiding. The client is cautioned to remain in bed for 24 hours.

COMMON BLOOD TESTS

BLOOD CHEMISTRY STUDIES. Urine normally contains nitrogenous waste products called urea, creatinine, uric acid, ammonium, and amino acids. When the kidneys are not functioning normally, nitrogenous wastes are not filtered completely from the blood. Blood urea nitrogen (BUN) and serum creatinine level are two commonly ordered tests of renal function. (See Table 19.2 for other blood tests.)

[Text continued on page 633.]

TABLE 19.2
EVALUATION OF KIDNEY FUNCTION*

NORMAL VALUES OF URINE		INDICATIONS OF ABNORMALITIES
Acetone	0	Indicates a metabolic disorder and patient may have symptoms of central nervous system depression
Addis count		
Erythrocytes	0–130,000/24 hr	A comparison of the amount of each suggests the type of kidney disease
Leukocytes	0–650,000/24 hr	
Casts (hyaline)	0–2000/24 hr	
Aldosterone	3–20 mcg/24 hr	An increase may indicate nephrosis, cardiac failure, cirrhosis of the liver
Amino acid nitrogen	64–199 mg/24 hr	An increase may indicate a defect in the renal tubules
Ammonia nitrogen	20–70 mEq/24 hr	
Amylase	35–260 Somogyi units/hr	An increase may indicate pancreatic diseases
Bilirubin (bile)	Negative	Bile pigments are found if there is biliary obstruction. Bilirubin alone is found if there is excessive hemolysis of RBC
Calcium		
Regular diet	Less than 250 mg/24 hr	An increase indicates hyperparathyroidism and osteoporosis. A decrease may indicate hypoparathyroidism
Low-calcium diet	Less than 150 mg/24 hr	
Catecholamines		
Epinephrine	Less than 10 mcg/24 hr	An increase of 3 to 100 times greater than the

TABLE 19.2 (*Continued*)
EVALUATION OF KIDNEY FUNCTION*

NORMAL VALUES OF URINE		INDICATIONS OF ABNORMALITIES
Norepinephrine	Less than 100 mcg/24 hr	normal indicates the prescence of a rare tumor of the adrenal medulla. This tumor produces severe hypertension. Severe anxiety or anger (also in some psychiatric patients) produces slight elevation of catecholamines
Chloride	110–250 mEq/24 hr	Used to evaluate cardiac patients' response to low-sodium diets, to adjust fluid-electrolyte balance
Copper	0–30 mcg/24 hr	An increase may indicate acute or chronic infections, certain malignancies, rheumatoid arthritis, biliary cirrhosis, and thyrotoxicosis. A decrease may be seen in nephrotic syndrome, malabsorption, and malnutrition
Creatine		
Female	0–100 mg/24 hr	Creatinuria occurs in severe muscle disease such
Male	0–40 mg/24 hr	as muscular dystrophy, atrophy, and myositis
Creatinine		
Female	800–1700 mg/24 hr	Abnormal results may indicate glomerular dis-
Male	1000–1900 mg/24 hr	ease
Estrogens		
Female	4–60 mcg/24 hr	Low estrogen levels may indicate pituitary fail-
Male	4–25 mcg/24 hr	ure. An increase may indicate fetal distress in pregnancy
Gonadotropins, pituitary	10–50 mouse uterine units/24 hr	An increase may indicate ovarian failure and testicular insufficiency. A decrease may be seen with anorexia nervosa
Hemoglobin	Negative	The presence of hemoglobin may indicate toxic drug ingestion, viral pneumonia, excessive exercise with low renal threshold
17–Hydroxycortico-steroids (17 OHCS)		
Female	4–10 mg/24 hr	This is primarily a test of adrenal function. An
Male	5–15 mg/24 hr	increase may indicate hyperadrenalism (Cushing's syndrome)
5-Hydroxyindole-acetic acid (5-HIAA)		
Qualitative	Negative	An elevation may indicate carcinoid tumors
Quantitative	Less than 16 mg/24 hr	found in the appendix or in the intestines. Carcinoid tumors have a low degree of malignancy
17-Ketosteroids		
Female	4-13 mg/24 hr	High levels may indicate adrenal dysfunction or
Male	6-18 mg/24 hr	testicular hyperfunction
Osmolality	38–1400 mOsm/kg water	An increase may indicate severe dehydration and a decrease may indicate diuresis. This tests the concentrating and diluting ability of the kidneys
pH	4.6–8.0	The degree of acidity or alkalinity of the urine varies, but changes do not indicate abnormality. However, an acid or alkaline urine is advisable in certain situations
Phenylpyruvic acid, qualitative	Negative	A positive result indicates phenylketonuria in infants—which may lead to permanent mental deficiency if not treated

TABLE 19.2 (*Continued*)
EVALUATION OF KIDNEY FUNCTION*

NORMAL VALUES OF URINE		INDICATIONS OF ABNORMALITIES
Phosphorus	0.9–1.3 gm/24 hr	An increase may indicate hypoparathyroidism and a decrease may indicate hyperparathyroidism
Porphobilinogen, qualitative	Negative	An increase may indicate red blood cell hemolysis as in hemolytic anemia and liver disease. A decrease may indicate obstruction of the bile duct or carcinoma of the head of the pancreas
Porphyrins		
Coproporphyrin	50–250 mcg/24 hr	Elevation may indicate toxic liver damage, lead poisoning, pellagra, and some blood disorders
Uroporphyrin	10–30 mcg/24 hr	
Potassium	25–100 mEq/24 hr	The ratio of sodium to potassium is increased in Addison's disease. Normally the ratio is 2 parts sodium to 1 part potassium
Pregnanetriol	Less than 2.5mg/24 hr	An elevation is seen in Cushing's syndrome and in adrenogenital syndrome
Protein		
Qualitative	0	An increase may indicate glomerular damage
Quantitative	10–150 mg/24 hr	
PSP excretion		
(6 mg dye IV)	20–50% dye excreted in 15 min	A decrease may indicate chronic nephritis and urinary tract obstructions. An increase may indicate certain liver diseases
	16–24% dye excreted in 30 min	
	9–17% dye excreted in 60 min	
	3–10% dye excreted in 120 min	
(6 mg dye IM)	40–60% dye excreted in 60 min	
	20–25% dye excreted in 2 hr, 10 min	
Sodium	130–260 mEq/24 hr	An increase is seen in adrenal insufficiency and a decrease is seen when there is an increase in adrenal aldosterone production as in shock, heart failure, or cirrhosis
Specific gravity	1.003–1.030	This indicates the concentration of dissolved material in the urine, which is descriptive of the condition of the tubules
Titratable acidity	20–40 mEq/24 hr	An increase indicates chronic acidosis
Urea nitrogen	6–17 gm/24 hr	A decrease may indicate filtration insufficiency
Uric acid	250–750 mg/24 hr	A decrease may indicate filtration, reabsorption, and secretory insufficiency of the kidneys
Vanillylmandelic acid (VMA)	1–8 mg/24 hr	A high level may indicate pheochromocytoma, a rare tumor of the adrenal medulla and other parts of the sympathetic nervous system
Zinc	0.15–1.2 mg/24 hr	

NORMAL BLOOD, SERUM, AND PLASMA VALUES		INDICATIONS OF ABNORMALITIES
Calcium	8.5–10.5 mg/100 ml	A decrease may indicate celiac disease, sprue, hypoparathyroidism, multiple myeloma, and respiratory diseases
Carbon dioxide content (CO_2)	24–30 mM/liter	A high CO_2 concentration may indicate inadequate gas exchange in respiratory insufficiency

Table 19.2 (*Continued*)
Evaluation of Kidney Function*

Normal Blood, Serum, and Plasma Values		Indications of Abnormalities
Chlorides	96–106 mEq/L	An elevation occurs in various kidney disorders, Cushing's syndrome, and hyperventilation. A decrease occurs in excessive vomiting, diarrhea, diabetic acidosis, Addison's disease, heat exhaustion, and certain postoperative conditions
Creatinine	0.7–1.5 mg/100 ml	An elevation may indicate a disorder of kidney function
Fibrinogen (plasma)	200–400 mg/100 ml	A decrease will determine that the clotting deficiency is due to the inadequate fibrinogen
Magnesium (serum)	1.5-2.5 mEq/liter	A deficiency may indicate the occurrence of tetany
Nonprotein nitrogen (NPN)	15–35 mg/100 ml	A rise may indicate kidney dysfunction
Phosphatase, acid (serum)	<3 ng/ml RIA 0.4–0.6 U/L Roy, Brower, Hayden	An increase in men may indicate metastatic carcinoma of the prostate. Other conditions that produce elevated serum acid phosphatase include hyperparathyroidism, metastatic mammary carcinoma, multiple myeloma, Paget's disease, some liver diseases, renal insufficiency, arterial and pulmonary embolism, myocardial infarction, sickle cell crisis, thrombocytosis, and osteogenesis imperfecta
Phosphatase, alkaline (serum)	20–70 or 90 U/L depending on method used	An increase may indicate bone diseases, liver diseases, hyperparathyroidism, hyperthyroidism, leukemia, and pregnancy
Phosphate, inorganic (serum)	3.0–4.5 mg/100 ml	An increase may be noted in severe kidney disease, hypoparathyroidism, acromegaly, or excessive vitamin D intake. A decrease may show in certain disease of the kidney tubules, hyperparathyroidism, and rickets
Potassium	3.6–5.0 mEq/L	A decrease may cause cardiac arrhythmias and muscle weakness; an increase produces a series of electrocardiographic changes and arrhythmias. Also, a decrease may be found in severe diarrhea and chronic kidney disease

Proteins (serum)
  Total
  Electrophoresis
    Albumin
    Globulin
      Alpha$_1$
      Alpha$_2$
      Beta
      Gamma
	6.0–8.0 gm/100 ml
	
	3.5–5.5 gm/100 ml
	
	0.2–0.4 gm/100 ml
	0.5–0.9 gm/100 ml
	0.6–1.1 gm/100 ml
	0.7–1.7 gm/100 ml
		The ratio of albumin to globulin is normally high; that is, there is more albumin than globulin. When the ratio is lowered, the condition may indicate chronic nephritis, lipoid nephrosis, liver disease, amyloid nephrosis, and malnutrition

Renin (plasma)	1.6–4.5 ng/ml/hr	Elevated levels are usually present in hypertension and Addison's disease
Sodium	136–145 mEq/L	Increased sodium levels may indicate inadequate water intake and excessive sodium intake. Decreased levels may occur in heat exhaustion, diarrhea, Addison's disease, and certain kidney disorders
Urea nitrogen, blood (BUN) plasma or	10–20 mg/100 ml	Elevation may indicate deficiency in renal ability

TABLE 19.2 (*Continued*)
EVALUATION OF KIDNEY FUNCTION*

NORMAL BLOOD, SERUM, AND PLASMA VALUES		INDICATIONS OF ABNORMALITIES
serum	11–23 mg/100 ml	to concentrate nitrogen wastes, excess in thyroxin, deficiency in insulin, dehydration, and gastrointestinal obstruction
Uric acid		
Female	1.5–6.0 mg/100 ml	An increase may indicate renal failure, violent
Male	2.5–8.0 mg/ml	muscular exertion, coronary artery disease, or gout

* A routine urinalysis usually is the first test done to aid the physician in evaluating the patient's renal function. In summary, the specific gravity indicates how well the tubules are concentrating the urine, an analysis of the protein indicates the effectivness of the tubules, and the microscopic examination aids in identifying disease of the upper and lower part of the urinary tract.

Kidney function tests are performed when the physician suspects renal disease. The ineffective functioning of various parts of the urinary system can be localized by specific kidney function tests that measure that particular function. For example, functioning of the glomeruli in the kidney can be evaluated by the routine urinalysis, creatinine clearance of the blood, urea clearance of the blood, and an Addis count of the urine.

Abnormal elevations of nitrogenous waste products in the blood can be associated with other disease conditions, such as intestinal obstruction, gastrointestinal hemorrhage, dehydration, and shock. When caring for a patient with elevated blood levels, such as urea and creatinine, the nurse should observe especially for disorientation and possible convulsions. Measures to protect the patient from injury should be taken. Siderails and a padded tongue blade may be indicated.

Since the kidneys also regulate the concentration of electrolytes, analysis of the levels of electrolytes also tests renal function. Potassium, sodium, calcium, chlorides, and phosphorus are the electrolytes most frequently evaluated. No special preparation for these blood tests is necessary.

Nursing Observations

Three factors affect the nurse's observation of the patient with a disturbance of the urinary system. First, a functioning urinary system is vital to life. Second, the activities of the urinary system can be observed indirectly in a variety of ways. Third, in Western culture, urine function is usually a private matter and frequently associated with matters of sexuality. Thus, nursing observations should be accurate, complete, and obtained in a tactful, gentle manner which respects the patient's privacy.

WEIGHT CHANGE

Because the function of the urinary system is elimination of the products of metabolism and electrolytes, and because water is used to move these substances, the nurse should be alert to observe the symptoms of electrolyte and water imbalance. An indication of fluid retention in the tissues is weight gain which may be associated with edema. To maintain an accurate record, the client is weighed each day at the same time with the same amount of clothing and on the same scale.

EDEMA

Edema (collection of fluid in the tissue) is first noted in dependent areas such as the feet (swollen ankles), presacral area (buttocks), and periorbital areas (puffiness around the eyes). Edema usually indicates that the circulatory system is overloaded. Pulmonary edema and congestive heart failure are complications of the circulatory overload.

INTAKE AND OUTPUT

Intake and output is a record of the volume of fluids consumed and excreted by the patient within a certain time. This observation helps the physician to evaluate fluid and electrolyte balance which is regulated in part by the urinary system. The nurse is the person responsible for maintaining a complete and accurate intake and output record.

Beside the dietary intake, fluids consumed by the patient and included in the record are liquid medications, water ingested when swallowing pills, tube feedings, and all parenteral fluids. Parenteral fluids may include hyperalimentation solutions, intravenous fluids, blood, blood products, and hypodermoclysis fluids. If the patient has output from sources other than the urinary tract, such as vomitus or drainage from tubes or wounds, the nurse should observe and record these accurately.

The oriented patient and family may be taught to participate in maintaining this important record. In some cases, participation may be limited to saving all fluids excreted so that they can be measured by the nurse. In other cases, the patient and family may be taught to measure and record intake and output fluids.

In order to keep an accurate intake and output record, the patient needs to know why a record is important, which intake fluids to record such as Jell-O and ice cream, which output fluids to record, how to use the measuring devices, and how to record.

GASTROINTESTINAL SYMPTOMS

Gastrointestinal and renal symptoms may occur simultaneously due to the reflex actions between the urinary and gastrointestinal systems and the proximity of the kidneys with the gastrointestinal tract. This explains the nausea, vomiting, anorexia, diarrhea, abdominal distention, and peritoneal irritability which the patient may experience along with renal symptoms. Other gastrointestinal symptoms the patient may report include a bitter, metallic taste and a fetid, fishy, or ammoniacal breath caused by the formation of ammonia from the salivary urea.

OBSERVING THE BLADDER

In conditions such as urinary retention or urinary nerve dysfunction, an individual may or may not be able to feel the pressure of a full bladder. A tense area can be felt above the symphysis pubis or may rise up to the level of the umbilicus. The patient who has received an adequate intake and who has not voided in six to eight hours can be expected to have a full bladder. Inability to void when the bladder is full should be reported to the appropriate nurse.

OBSERVING THE CHARACTERISTICS OF VOIDING (URINATION, MICTURITION)

Normal micturition is painless and occurs five to six times a day and occasionally once at night. The average amount of 1200 to 1500 ml of urine voided in 24 hours is modified in amount by fluid intake, perspiration, outside temperature, vomiting, or diarrhea. The patient with a disturbance in the urinary system frequently reports a change in the usual voiding habits.

Frequency, a relative term which implies urinating more often than usual for that person, may be a symptom of cystitis. *Urgency* is a sudden desire to urinate which may be due to the irritation of the trigone and posterior urethra. *Polyuria*, frequent urination of larger than normal volumes at each voiding, may be due to excessive fluid intake, diuretics, diabetes mellitus, or diabetes insipidus.

Oliguria refers to a small total output, between 100 and 500 ml in 24 hours, and *anuria* is absence of urine in the bladder or an output of less than 50 ml in 24 hours. These conditions occur in shock, drug poisoning, or incompatible blood transfusion and require immediate attention.

Dysuria, painful urination as described by clients, may be actually urethral pain which is felt along the course of the urethra or at the meatus. Dysuria at the beginning of urination is indicative of urethritis, and pain during and after voiding may be caused by bladder infection.

One of the most distressing symptoms is *incontinence* or loss of voluntary urinary control. This may be a result of an injury of the external urinary sphincter or damage to the nerves supplying the lower urinary tract. *Stress incontinence*, an intermittent leakage of urine from sudden strain such as sneezing, coughing, or lifting, may be due to weakness or damage of the sphincter.

Nocturia is excessive urination at night suggesting diminished ability of renal concentration or heart failure. *Enuresis*, an involuntary voiding during sleep, is physiologic to the age of three years, but may be also functional or a symptom of a lower urinary tract condition.

Hesitancy or difficulty in starting to urinate may be caused by a compression on the urethra. *Pneumaturia* is passage of gas in the urine. This may raise a suspicion of a fistula between the bladder and the bowel.

OBSERVATION OF THE URINE

The urine should be observed for amount, odor, degree of cloudiness, sediments, mucus, clots, shreds of materials, or other abnormalities. Normal urine varies in color from pale yellow to dark amber (see Table 19.3).

Hematuria means blood in the urine. The nurse should determine when bleeding first occurred, how long it lasted, and if it was associated with pain. Clots also should be described. A shoestring clot suggests ureteral bleeding. Even though hematuria may not be accompanied by any other symptom, the condition needs a thorough evaluation.

Accurate observation of abnormal color of urine may lead the physician to an early diagnosis. The female patient rarely observes the color of her urine because of her anatomy. The male patient may observe that his urine has an abnormal color, but his description of the color change may not be exactly specific. Therefore, the nurse has the major responsibility when handling urine of observing and recording abnormal color. Some of the abnormal colors of urine with examples of their implication are provided in Table 19.3.

Unless the urine comes from a necrotic urinary tract as in cancer, or from an infected urinary tract, urine is almost odorless as it leaves the body. The characteristic odor is caused by ammonia formed from the urea acted upon by bacteria from the external environment. The longer urine is left standing, the more the odor increases. Thus, the quality of nursing care may be judged by sniffing the air in the patient's room.

FEVER

Fever is a common indicator of urinary tract infection which may be caused by structural and functional abnormalities, obstruction of the flow of urine, and impaired bladder nerve supply. Urinary tract infection is discussed in this chapter.

PAIN

Careful description of pain may help pinpoint the source of the problem of a client with a urologic condition. Kidney pain is a dull, constant ache in the costovertebral angle (below the twelfth rib at the lumbar vertebral area) which radiates to the umbilical region. This pain is caused by distention of the renal capsule.

Ureteral pain is described as colicky pain starting from the costovertebral angle and radiating across the abdomen to the genital area. The pain is produced by the spasm of the renal pelvis and ureteral muscles.

TABLE 19.3
ABNORMAL COLORS OF URINE

COLOR	EXAMPLES OF IMPLICATIONS
Blue-green	Methylene blue, phenol, indigo blue, and acriflavine
Brown-black	Bilirubin, phenol, porphyrin, creasol, and highly concentrated urine
Cloudy white	Epithelial cells from the lower genitourinary tract, pus, bacteria, chyle (lymph)
Colorless	Low concentration associated with excessive fluid intake, chronic kidney disease, diabetes mellitus, diabetes insipidus
Orange	Urobilinogen and such drugs as phenindione (anticoagulant) and santonin (anthelminic)
Orange-red	Varies with pH of urine. Bleeding and such foods as beets, blackberries and rhubarb. Drugs such as aloes (cathartic), senna (cathartic), aminopyrine, phenolphthalein, sulfonal, cascara, picric acid, and pyridium

Bladder discomfort is felt over the suprapubic area. This may be due to overdistention. Burning pain along the urethra is suggestive of bladder infection.

SKIN CHANGES

Skin changes may show the obvious signs of kidney dysfunction. The skin is dry and scaly because of a decrease in the oil gland secretions. Pruritus or a creepy, crawling sensation makes the individual scratch, causing abrasions. The color of the skin is also indicative of renal dysfunction. The skin is pale due to anemia, or it may have a yellow-gray cast because of the inability of the kidneys to excrete carotenelike substances or because of retained urochrome pigments. Uremia crystals may form in areas of concentrated perspiration. The presence of edema increases susceptibility to skin breakdown. Petechiae or large bruises may appear on the skin as a result of capillary fragility.

BLEEDING

Bleeding tendency is a significant characteristic of kidney dysfunction associated with a platelet defect. The bleeding time is prolonged. Increased capillary permeability may cause bleeding from any orifice or bleeding under the skin, mucous membrane, or internal organs.

BEHAVIORAL CHANGES

A person who is usually pleasant may become irritable and disagreeable and report headaches, physical and mental fatigue, malaise, and anorexia. A more detailed description of these changes is discussed in this chapter with renal failure.

The level of awareness and personality of the client with renal failure is often affected. There may be a faltering memory or inability to think clearly. A docile person may become belligerent and vocal. Most of these individuals are able to perceive their own behavioral changes.

The patient with a disturbance in the urinary system may experience embarrassment associated with the symptoms and/or diagnostic studies and treatment that cause a loss of privacy.

Nursing Interventions

HYGIENE AND PERINEAL CARE

Many diseases of the urinary system are associated with the development of infection. In some cases, infection leads to other diseases in the urinary system. In other cases, infection results from underlying abnormalities in the urinary system.

Personal hygiene, adequate cleansing of the perineum, and healthy voiding practices are measures that prevent infection in the urinary tract. Personal hygiene includes wiping the perineal area from front to back after defecation, good handwashing, and regular bathing. Cleaning the perineum includes retraction of the penile foreskin by the male and cleaning from front to back by the female. Healthy voiding practices include urinating as soon as possible after the voiding sensation is felt. Many individuals ignore the first voiding sensation as a regular practice. This habit may lead to irritation of tissue by more concentrated urine and urinary stasis which are factors associated with infection.

Perineal care customarily done by a healthy individual may become inadequate during illness and bed confinement. Efficient hygiene and perineal care under these conditions are relatively difficult, especially for the female patient. If there is a reason to doubt the capacity of a patient to complete this care, the nurse must undertake the cleaning. The perineal region should be cleansed with soap and water, from front to back, after each defecation. Whenever activity permits, showering instead of tub bath is advised. The patient with an indwelling catheter generally needs perineal cleansing more frequently. The nurse should follow agency or hospital guidelines concerning the method and cleaning substances to be used.

ALTERATIONS IN FLUIDS AND DIET

Diet and fluid intake are very important parts of therapy for the client with a disturbance in the urinary system. Many clients with renal disease require some type of sodium restriction. As the patient's edema increases, the sodium restriction prescribed by the physician usually becomes more severe also. Potassium and protein are other parts of the diet that may be restricted. Carbohydrates may be increased in some cases to provide more calories and/or to minimize protein breakdown. The client with kidney disease generally is advised not to use salt substitutes unless the physician has been consulted. Reading labels is important when a dietary restriction is needed.

Changing dietary patterns developed over a lifetime often is frustrating and difficult for the patient and family. The nurse may anticipate behavioral changes associated with grieving when dietary changes are needed. The dietitian's help usually is needed to learn how to make necessary changes.

Unless the doctor orders fluids to be restricted, the patient with a disease of the urinary system needs to drink more fluids than the normal amount, which is 1500 to 2000 ml (1½ to 2 qt) a day. The amount of fluid ordered may be almost double the normal amount, or 3000 ml or more. Within the limits of diet the patient may have beverages such as tea, coffee, soups, gelatin, carbonated beverages, milk, eggnog, and water. The common expression "force fluids" is often just that. The patient may not be accustomed to drinking much fluid, may be nauseated, anorexic, or disoriented, or may not realize the importance of the increased fluid intake. Some patients find it easier to force fluids if they know how much to drink. For example, the nurse may ask the patient to drink "a glassful of fluid every hour while awake." This type of statement may be much more helpful to the patient than to be told to force fluids. The patient should be offered fluids frequently between meals and within the limits of diet. If possible, give a choice of fluids. The patient's preference for liquids iced, at room temperature, or refrigerated should be respected. The nurse should relay success or failure to other members of the nursing team to help determine how the objective of increased fluids can be met more effectively and efficiently. A step-by-step method for increasing fluid intake can be located in Chapter 14, page 410.

Fluids are limited especially when the patient has edema and when kidney failure develops. When fluids are restricted, the patient needs to have the reason explained. Thirst becomes a real problem when fluid intake is limited. Nursing measures to reduce discomfort include special mouth care with a solution that has a taste pleasant to the patient. Sucking on hard candy, a lemon, or ice may be helpful when allowed by the patient's medical routine. Intake of fluid from the ice or lemon must be included in the client's total fluid intake. Application of a lubricant, such as glycerin with lemon juice or mineral oil with lemon juice, can be used to relieve dry lips.

ASSISTING WITH DRUG THERAPY

Drug toxicity is a special danger to patients with renal insufficiency. Clients with decreased renal capacity have a high incidence of adverse drug side effects. Decreased renal function results in abnormal sensitivity and excretion of certain drugs. For example, sensitivity to barbiturates is increased so that a smaller dose usually is prescribed. Sensitivity to insulin or diuretics is decreased, and a larger dose is prescribed by the physician. Delayed elimination of certain drugs such as digoxin can cause toxic blood levels. Drugs that contain sodium and potassium usually are not prescribed.

A variety of drugs may be prescribed for the patient with a disturbance in the urinary system. These may include urinary antiseptics, antibiotics, analgesics, diuretics, and others.

Observation of the adverse side effects of medication prescribed for patients with renal diseases challenges a nurse's knowledge of drug therapy. The nurse should make a special effort to identify each drug's toxic signs in the patient and report them promptly to the doctor.

ASSISTING THE INDIVIDUAL WITH URINARY RETENTION

Some of the causes of urinary retention are damage to nerves in spinal cord injuries and interference of bladder sensation after surgery. Although urinary retention due to spinal injury often may be permanent, retention during the immediate postoperative period is temporary. Prolonged retention and distention of the bladder may result in urinary tract infection or bladder atony.

Inability to void after surgery may be due to sedation brought about by anesthesia and later by narcotic analgesics which suppress bladder sensation. Urinary retention is more common following low abdominal surgery and pelvic surgery involving the rectum or reproductive organs. During these procedures, the nerve supply is disturbed both by the surgery and by pressure caused from local edema in the tissues. Some individuals may not be able to void in a recumbent position or on a bedpan, or may be unable to void due to nervous tension brought about by the surgery or lack of sufficient privacy.

Many men can void if allowed to stand at the bedside, and many women can void if allowed to sit on the commode. If the client is not allowed this activity, many nursing measures can be used to assist a client to void normally. Encouraging more fluids, pouring warm water over the perineum, running water in the sink, and providing privacy are some of the common nursing measures.

The patient who reports inability to push the urine out may be helped to void by instructions to relax and let the urine flow out naturally. The patient who is so relaxed that there is no sensation to void may be helped by a sitting position and bending forward slightly, instructions to push the urine out, and gentle pressure on the bladder. If these measures are not effective, catheterization is ordered by the physician, and if repeated catheterizations are needed, a Foley catheter usually is inserted (Figure 19.5). Since catheterization involves the risk of bladder infection, it should be avoided when simple nursing procedures can result in voiding.

Some individuals who have had long-term problems of urinary retention due to bladder nerve dysfunction may be taught to catheterize themselves, usually every four hours while awake. A clean technique rather than sterile is used in the home for its convenience and the fact that the home environment does not have the pathogenic microor-

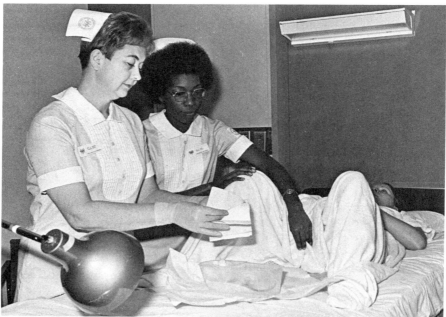

FIGURE 19.5 Sterile technique is essential when catheterizing a patient to avoid introducing pathogens into the bladder. (Courtesy of Shapero School of Nursing, a Program in Practical Nursing of Sinai Hospital, Detroit, Michigan.)

ganisms normally found in a hospital environment.

ASSISTING THE INDIVIDUAL WITH AN INDWELLING CATHETER

When a retention or indwelling catheter is connected to a collecting device and allowed to drain by gravity, the procedure is called a straight drainage system. Closed drainage refers to the setup where the drainage system is sealed from outside air.

The collecting receptacle has a valve opening to enable the staff to empty the bag without contamination. A recent finding indicates that contamination of the tube used to empty the bag is associated with a high incidence of urinary tract infection in the catheterized patient. The bag or receptacle should be emptied every eight hours, and its contents should be measured and recorded accurately. The drainage should be kept at a level below the patient's bladder to prevent the return of urine from the bag to the bladder (see Figure 19.6).

This closed drainage system should not be interrupted unless an irrigation of the

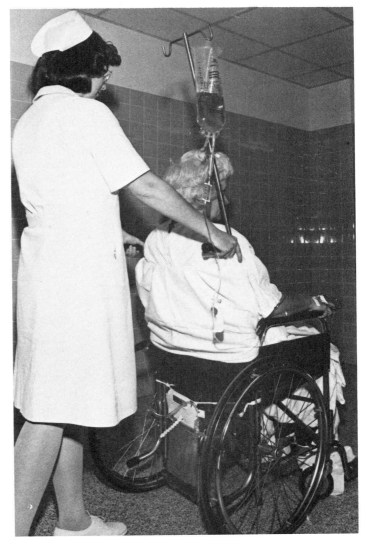

FIGURE 19.6 The patient has an indwelling catheter. Notice that the level of the drainage bag is below that of the patient's bladder. The drainage bag is attached to the back of the wheelchair between the two wheels.

catheter or bladder is ordered. A backflow of urine into the bladder causes pressure on the bladder wall and its blood vessels. This can cause ischemia of the bladder, which increases the likelihood of infection. When a specimen of fresh urine is to be obtained, the nurse can accomplish this without interrupting the closed system of drainage. A portion of the tubing distal to the catheter can be clamped for a few minutes to aid in accumulating urine in the tubing. An alcohol sponge should be used to clean the distal end of the catheter or a built-in insertion site on the catheter or on the drainage tube. The specimen is aspirated with a sterile syringe and a small-gauge needle.

The tissue surrounding the urethral catheter should be cleansed with soap and water twice daily. A prescribed antibacterial agent or an antibacterial ointment may be placed around the junction of the catheter and urethral orifice if permitted by hospital policy. Alert patients can be taught to perform this procedure for themselves, and most patients want to do so.

After a catheter has been removed, it is normal to have some dribbling of urine for a few hours, because of the dilated bladder sphincter. However, if dribbling continues, damage of the sphincter may be suspected and must be reported to the physician. On the other hand, a client may not be able to void after a catheter has been removed. This may be due to edema of the sphincter or neck of the bladder and may necessitate reinsertion of the catheter.

ASSISTING THE INDIVIDUAL WITH CATHETER OR BLADDER IRRIGATION

Irrigating a retention catheter should be done only on specific order of the physician. Sterile technique is used when irrigating a retention catheter. It must be reemphasized here that the safest and most effective way of keeping a catheter open and functioning will be by forcing fluids by oral or intravenous means. The nurse should again refer to a basic book of procedures or to the hospital procedure manual for the steps to be followed in the irrigation of a retention catheter.

Continuous irrigation of the bladder may be ordered for the patient with a closed drainage system. In this case, a catheter with three openings, or triple lumen, is used. One channel of the catheter is used to inflate the catheter bag in the bladder with sterile water, one channel permits urine to drain from the bladder, and one channel is designed for the irrigating solution to flow into the bladder. The three-way catheter is attached to the sterile closed drainage system and to the irrigating system. The irrigating system should have a drip chamber, which enables the nurse to count the drops of irrigation solution used per minute. The prescribed solution rinses the bladder and aids in reducing bleeding following surgery. The flow generally is regulated from 30 to 60 drops per minute or as fast as needed to keep the urine color pink. To measure the urine output of a patient with irrigation, the nurse must subtract the amount of irrigating fluid from the total amount in the drainage bag.

Intermittent irrigation is alternately instilling an irrigating solution into the bladder by way of a catheter and allowing the solution to drain by gravity into the drainage bag. The container of the irrigating solution is hung on a pole above the patient.

ASSISTING THE PATIENT WITH POSTOPERATIVE CARE

In addition to the usual postoperative care described in Chapter 6, the patient having surgery involving the urinary system requires additional measures. For example, many patients returning from surgery have one or more drainage tubes, each connected to a separate drainage system. The nurse should know the location of the drainage tube, the purpose of the drainage tube, and the type of drainage expected. This information usually is available on the operative note in the patient's chart. If it is not available, the nurse should seek this information from the appropriate nurse or surgeon. Drainage from each system is measured and described separately.

In addition to a Foley catheter which was described earlier in this chapter, the patient may have a suprapubic catheter, ureteral catheters, and/or drains as described in Chapter 6. A suprapubic catheter is located in the bladder and exits the body through a small incision above the pubis. The catheter may be sutured in place or secured using special seals or cements. A ureteral catheter is located in a ureter and exits the body through an incision in the skin. This catheter usually is sutured in place. A nephrostomy catheter is located in the kidney pelvis and exits the body through a surgical incision in the flank on the side of the affected kidney. This catheter also is sutured in place. When caring for the patient with a drain, the nurse's primary responsibilities include maintaining the free flow of drainage and observing, measuring, and recording the output of each drain. The nurse should check the drains frequently to prevent blocking, kinking, twisting, or disconnection of tubing. Apparent blockage of drainage should be reported promptly to the surgeon. Another common feature of postoperative care is the use of bulky dressings to collect drainage. The surgeon usually orders dressing changes as needed. Since saturated dressings permit the entry of bacteria to the wound, and urine on the skin causes irritations and odors, frequent dressing changes using sterile technique are needed. Montgomery straps are used for convenience and to prevent bruising the skin from frequent peeling of adhesive tapes. Each dressing change should be recorded as to time, color, and quantity of drainage.

Remembering that a large volume of blood normally passes through the kidney, the nurse observes the postoperative patient frequently and carefully for signs of excess bleeding. Signs of hemorrhage such as pallor, cool, clammy skin, apprehension, drop in blood pressure, rapid pulse, and an increase in respiratory rate should be reported. Bleeding can be observed along drainage tubes and on dressings. The drainages are usually dark red or pink, but should not be bright red or viscous and should not contain blood clots. It takes only a small amount of blood to make urinary drainage red. If there is much bleeding, the urine will be viscous and contain clots.

Atelectasis and other respiratory complications are common in postoperative patients with flank incisions. The proximity of the incision to the diaphragm makes deep breathing painful so that the individual takes shallow breaths or is reluctant to move about. Narcotic analgesia usually is administered every three to four hours. At this time, the client should be encouraged to take deep breaths, to cough, and to turn from side to side. The incision may be splinted while the individual is doing these activities. Early ambulation is strongly encouraged. Additional information about these interventions can be located in Chapter 6.

ASSISTING THE PATIENT WITH URINARY INCONTINENCE

Bladder training is a program that includes increasing the fluid intake, voiding on a regular schedule, and exercises to help a patient regain urinary continence. Patients who benefit from bladder training include the elderly, the acutely ill, and the comatose. The patient whose urinary incontinence is caused by a disturbance of the urethrobladder reflex, a disturbance of nerve pathways, or cerebral clouding also may be helped by a program of bladder retraining. The patient with incontinence caused by a urinary tract infection should wait until the infection is cleared before beginning such a program.

The success of urinary control is maintenance of a sufficient fluid intake of 2500 ml daily and establishment of a voiding schedule that should be followed until the client learns to react to the feeling of having to urinate. An adequate intake is necessary to ensure that there is enough urine to stimulate the voiding reflex at the scheduled time. Most experts suggest that reducing fluid intake at night is acceptable only if the fluid-intake goals can be reached earlier in the day. The interval between voidings and drinking is fairly short during the early part of bladder training and is gradually lengthened as the client gains more control over voiding.

An example of a beginning schedule is to give a measured amount of fluid every two hours, wait 30 minutes, and then let the client void. If capable, the client should assume the normal voiding position. Massaging over the bladder or leaning forward while sitting will help initiate micturition.

Some individuals are able to regain continence by strengthening perineal muscles. The Kegel exercise directs the client to sit in a chair with the feet on the floor, knees spread, and contract the perineal muscles as though stopping a urination. This exercise is done ten times, four times a day.

Another method used to control incontinence is electrical inhibition of the voiding reflex. An electrode is surgically implanted in a pelvic muscle or may be inserted vaginally or anally. The latter appliance can be removed and reinserted as needed. The electrodes are connected to a control box which is activated by the patient.

A variety of surgical procedures has been developed to control urinary incontinence that occurs as a result of urinary diversion (surgical procedures that change the normal route of urine excretion through the bladder and urethra). For example, a recent advance in surgery is called continent vesicostomy. During this procedure, the patient's bladder is sutured to the abdominal wall and the urethral neck is sutured closed. A new exit for urine is made on the abdomen using tissue from the bladder wall to form a nipple valve. As the bladder fills, the pressure causes the nipple to be pulled in and prevents urine outflow. The urine is drained by the client with a catheter using clean technique.

When these methods are unsuccessful or impossible, collecting devices may be used to prevent urine from coming in contact with the skin. An external drainage apparatus may be devised for a man. For example, a rubber sheath may be rolled over the penis. The rubber sheath has a drainage attachment at the tip. Collecting devices for women such as female urinals tend to be unsuccessful, and usually perineal pads or waterproof panty protection is necessary. The woman who uses a perineal pad or waterproof panty to cope with urinary incontinence needs more frequent perineal care in order to prevent skin irritation and urine odors.

The two main objectives of giving nursing care to a patient with incontinence are (1) to keep urine from contacting the skin

and (2) to remove it as soon as possible if and when it does. Urea is a normal constituent of urine. When it is allowed to come in contact with bacteria in the air, ammonia is formed that is very irritating to the skin and offensive to smell. Therefore, if the patient is incontinent, changing the patient's clothes and bed linen is not sufficient inasmuch as urine remains on the skin to cause irritation. A daily tub bath is the most cleansing and effective method of removing urine. Cleansing of the skin after each voiding with soap and water is necessary to prevent skin irritation, breakdown, and the characteristic odor from forming. One can almost predict the condition of an incontinent patient's skin by the odor or absence of it in the room. If the skin does become excoriated, exposure to air and heat is helpful. Ointments may be ordered by the physician to prevent urine from irritating the skin and/or aid in healing. An antiseptic, methylbenzethonium chloride (DIAPARENE), helps inhibit the growth of the bacteria that cause ammonia to form. It is available in powder and ointment form.

USING THE THERAPEUTIC RELATIONSHIP

The anatomic relationship of the reproductive organs and the urinary organs, coupled with social restrictions regarding open discussion of the personal and private act of voiding, may cause the client with a urinary tract condition to feel embarrassed and avoid discussing anxieties and fears. The patient, especially the male, may fear loss of sexual functions because of a urinary tract condition. These individuals generally are concerned about the outcome of a urologic disorder. They may be afraid of incontinence or permanent damage of the urinary system.

The male patient may feel embarrassed and anxious when a female nurse has to catheterize him. However, if the nurse feels confident and does not feel embarrassed, the procedure can be explained to the patient and the feeling of embarrassment reduced. The nurse should explain exactly what is going to be done and the observations that must be made. The nurse should maintain the patient's privacy with adequate draping.

The patient's fears and anxieties must be openly and honestly discussed so that one's own resources can be used to cope with the problems while allaying false fears. If the patient appears to be hesitant to verbalize, the nurse may ask, in a matter-of-fact manner, about possible concerns. The nurse may ask an open-ended question that does not suggest the answer. This communicates the nurse's attitude that urination is a normal and vital function.

When a surgical patient recovers from the postoperative period and begins to realize what has happened, the patient may experience irritation, depression, and anxiety. Urinary incontinence, the odor of drainage, the catheter, and other urinary appliances may add to the fears, apprehension, and feeling of rejection. By keeping the patient clean, dry, and free of odor, and demonstrating acceptance as well as understanding with sincerity in the spoken word, and skill and confidence in the performance of nursing care, the nurse will add to the patient's emotional support.

PATIENT AND FAMILY TEACHING

An important part of patient teaching for the person with a disorder of the urinary system includes hygiene measures. The woman patient is taught to cleanse and wipe from front to back after urinating or defecating. The man patient is taught to cleanse the glans penis daily.

Patients who are continent and have a voiding sensation are encouraged to void when they first become aware of that sensation. A practice that is discouraged is waiting until it is more convenient to urinate. Unless specifically contraindicated by the physician, the patient usually is instructed to increase the fluid intake.

The success of the treatment of any disease condition depends on the client's understanding of that disease, the plan of treatment, and the motivation to get well. The nurse and/or doctor must make a sincere effort to include the client's family or a significant other in the discussion about the condition, because family understanding and cooperation contribute to the client's ability to participate in the treatment.

The client with renal disease and the family need to understand the concept of fluid and dietary restraint and should be taught how to monitor the progress of the illness by observing for edema, decreased output, weight fluctuations, and signs of a downward progression of the disease.

REFERRAL TO COMMUNITY RESOURCES

In most localities, individuals with kidney conditions organize themselves to share their experiences, their problems, successes, and failures. The National Association of Patients on Hemodialysis and Transplantation (NAPHT) is composed of patients throughout the country and has a magazine *NAPHT News*. The National Kidney Foundation raises funds for research and education. The American Kidney Fund provides direct patient assistance such as transportation and money.

Urinary Tract Infections

Infection occurs in any part of the urinary tract. The condition may be diagnosed as urethritis, cystitis, or pyelonephritis, depending upon the location of the infection. The infecting microorganisms may come by way of the urethra or by way of the kidneys. The presence of bacteria in a clean-voided specimen of urine is a sign of infection since the urine is normally sterile.

The bacteria commonly identified in a urinary tract infection are *E. coli, Pseudomonas,* and other enterococci found normally in the fecal flora. Some of the factors that contribute to urinary tract infection are fecal contamination, instrumentation, urinary stasis, and urinary obstruction.

Women are more likely to develop urinary infection than men because of the shorter urethra and its proximity to the rectum. Also, the woman lacks the prostatic fluid protection of the man. Instrumentation from a cystoscope or a catheter is a common source of urinary contamination. One of the most common hospital infections is nosocomial urinary tract infection in patients with catheters. Urinary stasis provides the medium for bacterial growth. Stasis may be caused by urethral stricture, tumors, or an enlarged prostate. Obstruction of urinary flow due to stones and strictures will also contribute to urinary tract infections.

An infection elsewhere in the body may spread by way of the bloodstream to the kidneys. Certain metabolic diseases such as diabetes mellitus and gout also are predisposing factors.

NURSING OBSERVATIONS

The patient with a lower urinary tract infection (cystitis or urethritis) usually has frequent, urgent, painful, burning urination often accompanied by spasms in the suprapubic area, low back pain, and hematuria.

If pathogens ascend the urinary tract causing an upper urinary tract infection (pyelonephritis), the patient may have the symptoms already mentioned as well as fever, chills, and pain in one or both flanks. In both conditions, the patient may have cloudy, foul-smelling urine in addition to hematuria. Diagnosis is made from an examination of a clean-catch voided specimen. Bacterial count in excess of 100,000 per ml of urine indicates an infection.

NURSING INTERVENTIONS

Nursing interventions are related to relieving symptoms, carrying out medical therapy, and preventing recurrence. The nurse may participate in drug therapy that is prescribed to kill the pathogens and relieve symptoms. After urine has been collected for culture and sensitivities, the physician may prescribe a sulfonamide, an antibiotic, or a urinary antiseptic. For example, sulfisoxazole (GANTRISIN), nitrofurantoin (FURADANTIN), broad-spectrum antibiotics such as tetracycline, or penicillin preparations (see Tables 5.7 and 5.8, pages 99 and 103) may be prescribed. Methenamine mandelate (MANDELAMINE) is a commonly used urinary antiseptic that acts on the bacteria by releasing formaldehyde in the urine (see Table 19.4). At times, phenazopyridine hydrochloride (PYRIDIUM), a urinary analgesic, is used to help relieve the pain of micturition, but it has no effect on clearing up the infection. The nurse needs to warn the patient that PYRIDIUM will turn the urine a bright reddish-orange color. Nursing measures generally needed by a patient with an infection include rest, an increased intake of fluids, and a nourishing diet. Unless contraindicated, fluid intake of 3 to 4 liters a day is encouraged in order to make the urine more dilute and less irritating during micturition. Additional fluid also helps to prevent urinary stasis, thereby facilitating the eradication of the microorganisms. A specific oral fluid often suggested is cranberry juice. The liquid makes the patient's urine more acid which reduces bacterial growth.

Urine acidifiers such as ammonium chloride may be prescribed for individuals with chronic urinary tract infection because organisms do not survive well in acidic urine. Patient education should emphasize prompt medical attention to symptoms, continued medication even after symptoms are gone, follow-up urine cultures, and sustained fluid intake of 3 to 4 liters a day. In women, the nurse may need to reemphasize the importance of cleansing the perineal area from the front to the back after voiding and defecation to prevent urethral contamination from the rectum. A voiding pattern usually recommended to prevent recurrence includes voiding every two to three hours and voiding after sexual intercourse.

A woman with cystitis related to sexual intercourse generally receives special instructions from the physician to prevent recurrence. These instructions usually include urinating and drinking two glasses of water along with a prescribed antimicrobial drug after intercourse.

Urinary Bladder Tumor

An individual may have either a benign or a malignant tumor of the bladder. Carcinoma of the bladder occurs more frequently in men than in women. In malignant tumors, metastasis does not usually occur as long as the tumor has not penetrated the muscle wall of the bladder. Known predisposing factors to bladder cancer are exposure to certain chemicals and inhaling the excretory products of tobacco tars. Coffee, artificial sweeteners, and food dyes also have been associated with the development of bladder

TABLE 19.4
URINARY DRUGS

DRUG	ACTION	DOSAGE	NURSING IMPLICATIONS
Bethanechol (URECHOLINE)	Urinary cholinergic which stimulates urinary bladder in acute urinary retention	5 mg subcutaneously to stimulate voiding; 10 mg orally 3 times daily until voluntary voiding begins	Side effects may include sweating, epigastric distress, flushing, belching Usually withdrawn gradually
Flavoxate hydrochloride (URISPAS)	Urinary antispasmodic to relieve spasms associated with frequency, urgency, dysuria in lower urinary tract infections	100–200 mg 3 or 4 times daily	Contraindicated in spasm caused by blockage in gastrointestinal or urinary systems Patient should be cautioned about driving or other hazardous tasks because of drowsiness and blurred vision
Methanamine hippurate (HIPREX, UREX)	Urinary antiseptic	1 gm 2 times daily	Report symptoms of gastrointestinal distress Administer after meals Encourage increased fluid intake Drink cranberry juice to help acidify urine
Methanamine mandelate (MANDELAMINE)	Urinary antiseptic	500 mg–2 gm 4 times daily	Administer after meals Encourage increased fluid intake Drink cranberry juice to help acidify urine
Nalidixic acid (NEGGRAM)	Urinary antiseptic	1 gm 4 times daily	May cause nausea, vomiting, abdominal discomfort Caution patient to avoid ultraviolet light and sunlight because of photosensitivity
Nitrofurantoin (FURADANTIN)	Urinary antiseptic	50 mg 4 times daily	Give with milk or other food to reduce nausea, vomiting, diarrhea Report chills, fever, jaundice Explain that drug causes urine to turn brownish red
Sulfisoxazole (GANTRISIN)	Antimicrobial sulfonamide drug	2 gm initial dosage 1 gm 4 times daily	Encourage increased fluid intake Report headache, nausea, vomiting, jaundice, fever May increase effects of oral anticoagulants, thiazide diuretics, and hypoglycemic drugs

cancer. Painless hematuria is the first symptom of bladder tumors. The individual also may have urgency, frequency, and dysuria.

ASSISTING WITH DIAGNOSTIC STUDIES

A variety of studies may be done to determine the size, location, and type of tumor. Cystoscopy usually is done to visualize the tumor and obtain a specimen, if possible. A urine specimen for cytology generally is collected. In addition, a variety of other procedures such as CAT scan, intravenous pyelogram, and renal angiogram may be ordered to determine if a malignant tumor has spread.

NURSING INTERVENTIONS/ ASSISTING THE SURGICAL PATIENT

Tumors that have not spread to other areas are removed surgically. Table 19.5 contains a description of common procedures the surgeon may choose to remove a tumor. Small tumors generally are removed during cystoscopy or transurethral resection. Electrocautery and fulguration are specific procedures which may be done to destroy the tumor before removing it through the cystoscope or resectoscope. Larger tumors usually have to be removed through an incision in the lower abdomen. Part or all of the bladder may be removed along with the tumor. If the tumor is on the dome of the bladder, a segmental resection is done. Over half of the bladder may be removed, leaving only a 50-ml fluid capacity immediately postoperative. As the elastic tissues of the bladder regenerate and compensate, the individual will be able to retain 200 ml or more within several months. A cystectomy, or complete removal of the entire bladder, may be done if the tumor appears localized and there are no signs of metastasis.

If a cystectomy is done, the urine has to be drained from the ureters in some type of urinary diversion. Table 19.6 contains a description of common procedures for urinary diversion. The specific method used is selected by the surgeon on the basis of factors such as the patient's body build, weight, and state of renal function.

In addition to the usual preoperative care, the patient usually receives a bowel cleansing. The nurse also directs attention to the amount of food and fluids consumed by the patient preoperatively. The patient with a suspected bladder tumor often misses meals during diagnostic testing. Dehydration before surgery may cause hypovolemia and inadequate blood flow through the kidneys during or after surgery. Extensive discussions take place between the surgeon, patient, and family members about the tumor, the type of surgery, and expected results. When urinary diversion results in a stoma the location of the site is planned by the surgeon preoperatively. Marks placed on the abdomen to locate the stoma site should not be washed off. In some cases, patient teaching sessions are held preoperatively to demonstrate collecting devices and permit the patient to practice using them.

Following urinary surgery for bladder cancer, the patient can be expected to have one or more catheters and/or drains as described earlier in this chapter. Because of variations in surgical procedures, it is extremely important for the nurse to know the location and purpose of each catheter as well as the type of drainage expected. For example, fecal drainage would be unexpected from a ureteroileostomy stoma. The nurse should report this unexpected drainage to the surgeon or appropriate nurse. It is especially important to know which of the catheters is expected to drain urine so that a decrease in the urine output can be reported immediately. A fall in urinary output after surgery for a bladder tumor may indicate abnormal bleeding, inadequate fluid replacement, or destruction of a suture line resulting in leakage of urine into a body cavity. Remembering that formation and excretion

TABLE 19.5
SURGICAL PROCEDURES TO REMOVE BLADDER TUMORS

SURGICAL PROCEDURE	DESCRIPTION
Electrocautery	Application of electric current to destroy tissue
Fulguration	Destruction of tissue using electric sparks
Segmental resection (partial cystectomy)	Removal of portion of bladder containing tumor
Total cystectomy	Removal of entire bladder and creation of urinary diversion (see Table 19.6)
Transurethral resection	Removal of tumor or tumor fragments using a resectoscope inserted into the urethra

TABLE 19.6
COMMON SURGICAL PROCEDURES FOR URINARY DIVERSION

PROCEDURE	DESCRIPTION
Cutaneous ureterostomy	One or both ureters are brought to the skin of the lower abdomen
	Urine drains from ureters to collecting device applied to skin
Ureteroileostomy (ileal conduit, ileal bladder)	Portion of ileum is used to form a collecting pouch inside abdominal wall
	Ureters implanted into the ileum
	Stoma is created on abdomen for exit of urine
	Urine drains through stoma into a collecting bag applied to skin
	Remaining ileum reconnected for resumption of normal gastro-intestinal function
Ureterosigmoidostomy	Ureters implanted into sigmoid colon
	Urine excreted through rectum
	Up to 200 ml of urine may be retained before urge to evacuate is felt
	Stools evacuated are soft
	Flatus and leakage may occur

of urine are essential life processes enables the nurse to observe and report changes in urine output.

The patient with a stoma created as a result of urinary diversion needs care similar to that required for a patient with a colostomy or fecal ileostomy as described in Chapter 15. Principles of assisting the patient with a urinary stoma are summarized in Table 19.7. Generally, the patient wears a collecting device which has a valve at the bottom to drain urine.

The patient can be expected to demonstrate some or all of the behavioral changes associated with losing a body part, having a life-threatening illness, and disruption of body image. Additional information about these topics can be located in Chapters 6, 9, and earlier in this chapter.

ASSISTING WITH OTHER THERAPIES

If metastasis has occurred, external radiation is usually done before surgery to retard the growth of cancer cells. Supervoltage irradiation may be given if the individual has an inoperable tumor. External radiation is used more commonly than internal radiation, which involves an implantation of radioisotopes in the bladder. Nursing care of the patient receiving radiotherapy, discussed in Chapter 9, is applicable to this patient.

TABLE 19.7
GUIDE TO ASSISTING THE PATIENT WITH A URINARY STOMA

1. The collecting device is usually changed every five to seven days if there is no leakage.
2. The patient and the nurse plan a convenient time for changing the collecting device.
3. The stoma is generally edematous at first and gradually shrinks over a period of several months. Cyanosis of the stoma and skin excoriation are reported if observed.
4. A variety of appliances may be used including disposable or reusable products.
5. The new collecting device is prepared according to manufacturer's instructions before old device is removed.
6. The opening of a collecting device is usually about 1.3 cm (1/8 inch) larger than the widest part of the stoma.
7. The skin must be clean and dry while a new device is applied.
8. An increase in fluid intake is generally recommended.
9. Reusable appliances require regular cleaning and deodorizing.
10. The patient is encouraged to contact a local chapter of the United Ostomy Association for practical information on living with an "ostomy."

Acute Pyelonephritis

The patient with acute pyelonephritis has an infection of kidney tissue. The infection usually begins in the lower urinary tract and travels up to one or both kidneys. Other factors that favor the development of acute pyelonephritis include pregnancy, blockage of urine flow from a stone, stricture, or tumor, trauma, diabetes, hypertension, and abnormalities of normal bladder reflexes. Women are affected more often than men. Complications of acute pyelonephritis include chronic pyelonephritis. In most infections, the causative microorganism is *E. coli*.

NURSING OBSERVATIONS

The patient with acute pyelonephritis usually develops fever, shaking chills, malaise, nausea, vomiting and diarrhea. There may be tenderness in one or both flanks. The patient may or may not have symptoms of lower urinary tract infection such as frequency, urgency, and dysuria. The patient may have hematuria, cloudy urine and/or pus in the urine (pyuria). The physician usually diagnoses the patient's condition on the basis of the patient's symptoms and a urine culture that shows a bacterial count of more than 100,000 per ml of urine.

NURSING INTERVENTIONS

The physician usually prescribes an antibiotic on the basis of the urine culture and sensitivities. When pyelonephritis results from bacterial infection in the urethra or bladder, the drugs commonly prescribed are ampicillin (POLYCILLIN) or cephalexin (KEFLEX) for seven to ten days. The patient is instructed to remain in bed and increase the fluid intake. When pyelonephritis is associated with other conditions such as kidney stones, an indwelling catheter, or diabetes, additional measures are needed to relieve or improve the underlying condition. The hospitalized patient may need a newer antibiotic such as gentamicin (GARAMYCIN) to eradicate resistant organisms.

A very important part of patient teaching is the need for additional urine cultures after the treatment is completed. It is important to eradicate all bacteria from the urine in order to prevent recurrence. Although symptoms may have disappeared, the only way to be certain that all bacteria have been eliminated is a urine culture that is negative. These facts are explained to the patient by the nurse as part of teaching.

Chronic Pyelonephritis

The patient with chronic pyelonephritis has recurrent persistent infection which causes permanent damage to kidney tissue. This condition may develop if all bacteria are not eliminated from the urine during an acute infection or when an underlying disease is not identified and corrected. In some cases, the patient experiences exacerbations and remissions of infection which do not cause enough damage to threaten life. In other cases, chronic infection may result in extensive damage to the kidneys causing the patient to develop renal failure. The patient with renal failure is discussed later in this chapter.

NURSING OBSERVATIONS

The patient with chronic pyelonephritis often does not experience symptoms in the early stages. At this time, the disease may be discovered when the patient has an abnormal urinalysis or elevated blood pressure during a regular physical examination. Later, the patient may have fatigue, low-grade fever, vague gastrointestinal symptoms, and anemia. During laboratory analysis, the patient's urine has abnormal white blood cell casts and protein. The BUN may be elevated. An intravenous pyelogram usually shows abnormalities caused by recurrent infection and scarring.

NURSING INTERVENTIONS

Antibiotic therapy is prescribed according to the culture and sensitivities test. The client is instructed about the importance of continuing antibiotic therapy as directed by the physician even weeks or months after symptoms subside or after the urine culture becomes negative. Other important nursing measures include helping the client find ways to increase fluid intake on a permanent basis and avoiding sedentary activities which cause pooling of urine. Hygiene practices discussed earlier in this chapter apply to the client with chronic pyelonephritis.

The client should continue to be under medical supervision with follow-up urine cultures at periodic intervals.

Renal Calculi

The patient with renal calculi has kidney stones present in the urinary tract. One or more stones may be present anywhere in the urinary tract. The calculi may range from the size of a pinhead to one large enough to fill the entire pelvis of the kidney.

The reason for the formation of these calculi is not fully understood. When crystalline substances such as oxalate, uric acid, and calcium phosphate are not excreted in the urine, they may precipitate and form stones. Other factors that seem to favor the development of renal calculi include:

- Urinary tract infections that change the pH to alkaline
- Urinary stasis caused by inactivity such as bed rest
- Changes in normal calcium balance caused by diseases such as gout, hyperparathyroidism, leukemia, and certain nutritional deficiencies or imbalances

There are several types of stones. Most stones are composed of *calcium*. Another common type is *uric acid stones*. A third common stone is the *struvite* stone. This type may grow very large and assume the appearance of a stag horn.

NURSING OBSERVATIONS

The patient may have no symptoms until the stone prevents urine from flowing normally or until the stone moves causing irritation and a characteristic colicky pain. Sometimes the patient develops an infection as a result of a stone. A dull ache in the kidney region also may be experienced. The characteristic colicky pain is called *kidney colic* or *renal colic* and occurs when the stone becomes lodged in the ureter or kidney calyces and causes a spasm of the smooth muscle tissue of the ureter. Movement of the stone irritates the tissues around it. The pain that the patient suffers is excruciating and wavelike. It may start in the kidney region and radiate to the lower part of the abdomen and

into the groin. The severe pain may continue to the inner part of the thigh. This acute pain can cause the patient to perspire profusely, develop nausea and vomiting, and go into a mild state of shock. Hematuria may occur because of tissue damage caused by movement of the stone. In some cases, the patient passes small stones. If the patient develops an infection, there is pus in the urine (see Table 19.1), and chills and fever may be present.

Urine which the patient excretes is observed carefully and strained through several layers of gauze or a special strainer to determine if gravel or stones have been passed. All gravel and/or stones collected are labeled and sent for laboratory analysis.

ASSISTING WITH DIAGNOSTIC STUDIES

The physician usually makes a diagnosis of renal calculi on the basis of the patient's symptoms as well as stones visualized during an intravenous pyelogram and KUB x-ray. Other diagnostic tests of blood and urine may be ordered to identify or rule out underlying conditions. For example, a 24-hour urine collection for calcium, a urine Sulkowitch, and a serum calcium test may be ordered if the physician suspects hyperparathyroidism.

As previously mentioned, all gravel or stones excreted by the patient are sent to the laboratory for analysis. The physician prescribes certain drug and diet therapy on the basis of the stone composition.

NURSING INTERVENTIONS

Nursing measures for the patient with renal calculi are directed toward making the client comfortable, removing the gravel or stone(s), and preventing the formation of more calculi.

ASSISTING WITH DRUG THERAPY

Drug therapy includes narcotic analgesics such as morphine and meperidine hydrochloride (DEMEROL) (see Table 7.2, page 159 to relieve severe pain. Atropine or dicyclomine hydrochloride (BENTYL) may also be prescribed to relax the smooth muscle of the ureter and therefore help in relieving pain. An antibiotic may be prescribed when infection is present. Allopurinol (ZYLOPRIM) may be prescribed to prevent additional uric acid stones.

ALTERATIONS IN FLUID AND DIET

An increased fluid intake is an important nursing measure both to help eliminate stones and to prevent the formation of new stones. Three liters or more of fluid per day may be encouraged when the patient has existing stones. Six or more liters per day may be recommended for the patient with cystine stones. Encouraging an increased fluid intake in the patient who is immobilized is an important nursing measure that helps to prevent renal calculi.

The physician may prescribe a dietary restriction to prevent new stones from forming. The specific restriction depends on the chemical composition of existing stones. For example, a low-purine diet may be prescribed for the patient with uric acid stones. An adjustment of calcium in the diet may be needed for the patient with calcium stones.

Simple adjustments in diet may be prescribed to adjust the urine pH. For example, to acidify the urine, the patient may be instructed to eliminate citrus fruits, carbonated beverages and substitute apple or cranberry juice. To make the urine more alkaline, the patient may be instructed to drink 1 to 3 liters of orange juice daily.

AMBULATION AND EXERCISE

The patient with renal calculi usually is encouraged to increase ambulation in order to pass existing stones and prevent the formation of new ones. A key factor in encouraging ambulation when the patient has renal calculi is adequate pain relief. As mentioned in Chapter 7, pain relief is more effective when analgesia is administered early, before pain becomes severe.

Nursing interventions that encourage exercise and activity are especially important in preventing renal calculi in the patient who is immobile. Bedridden patients are ambulated or turned at scheduled intervals. Wheelchairs and a tilt table may be used to prevent urinary stasis. Active and passive exercises are done frequently and on a scheduled basis.

ASSISTING THE SURGICAL PATIENT

When the patient experiences obstruction, infection, serious bleeding or intractable pain, the surgeon may decide that it is necessary to remove the stone from the kidney, ureter, or bladder. Removal of the stone through an incision into the kidney is known as a *nephrolithotomy*. The surgeon does a *ureterolithotomy* to remove the stone through an incision into the ureter. Sometimes, the stone can be crushed (litholapaxy) if it is in the bladder by inserting a special instrument through a cystoscope. After the stone is crushed, the fragments are washed out of the bladder. When a stone has passed to the lower portion of the ureter, it may be manipulated by the surgeon through the cystoscope. A special catheter with a corkscrew tip, expanding basket, and a loop is inserted through the cystoscope to retrieve the stone. This procedure is done under anesthesia. The client is informed that if the manipulation is not successful, surgery may be performed at that time.

With few exceptions, the patient having surgery of the urinary tract needs the same type of care discussed in Chapter 6. The nurse should observe the patient carefully for early symptoms of shock and hemorrhage after surgery. Remembering the large amount of blood that flows through the kidney and the close relationship between the circulatory and urinary systems should help the nurse to realize the importance of watching for early signs of these complications. A drain of some type is often left in place in the wound following the operation and a moderate amount of drainage is to be expected on the dressings or through a drainage tube. The drainage may be mainly urine or of a serous nature. Close observation by the nurse is essential with accurate recording and reporting of the amounts, color, and consistency of drainage and urine. An increased urinary output can be expected following elimination of renal calculi. This results from release of a backflow of urine that was present behind the stone.

Hydronephrosis

An individual with hydronephrosis has a kidney that is distended with urine because of an obstruction somewhere below the kidney. Urine that does not flow normally backs up and slowly fills the pelvis of the kidney. This can cause the kidney tissue to be destroyed because of the pressure of the collecting urine. The kidney eventually may become a fibrous sac filled with urine, and the patient may end up in kidney failure.

The normal flow of urine from the kidney through the ureter may be obstructed or blocked by a stone, a tumor, or a stricture. In older men, an enlarged prostate gland is a common cause of the obstruction. This condition is discussed in Chapter 20. An anatomic defect in urinary structures such as the ureters may cause a person to develop hydronephrosis.

NURSING OBSERVATIONS

Pain is often the first symptom that develops when the patient has hydronephrosis. Pain is caused by distention of the kidney. The degree of pain depends upon the degree of kidney tissue stretching. A gradual stretching may result in a dull flank pain, while a sudden obstruction by a stone may result in a severe renal colic. In addition to pain, the patient may have symptoms of infection in the urinary tract. The patient also may have a decreased urinary output. The patient's urine may contain blood (hematuria), bacteria (bacteriuria), or pus (pyuria).

ASSISTING WITH DIAGNOSTIC STUDIES

The patient with suspected hydronephrosis usually has an intravenous pyelogram in order to locate the obstruction. Other studies which also may be ordered for this purpose include ultrasound and a renal scan. Urine specimens are collected and analyzed to evaluate the presence of infection as well as disturbances in forming urine.

NURSING INTERVENTIONS

Specific nursing interventions depend upon the cause of the patient's hydronephrosis. The physician attempts to remove the cause of the hydronephrosis and renew adequate urinary drainage. Surgical procedures are common. For example, a litholapaxy may be done to remove a stone blocking the ureter. In some cases, the physician may drain the urine from the kidney by surgically placing a nephrostomy tube in the pelvis of the kidney. The entire kidney may have to be removed if it has been damaged severely and can no longer function. This operation is known as a nephrectomy. The nursing care needed by the patient following a nephrectomy is similar to that discussed in the previous section on kidney surgery.

Acute Glomerulonephritis

The patient with acute glomerulonephritis has an inflammation of the glomeruli in both kidneys. The inflammatory process may be initiated by infection, a disturbance in the immune mechanisms, systemic disease such as systemic lupus erythematosus, or drug toxicity. Glomerulonephritis may develop as a complication following streptococcal infection such as pharyngitis or scarlet fever. Since the basic filtering unit of the kidney is affected by the disease process, the patient experiences disturbances in the formation of urine, clearance of waste products, salt and water balance, and regulation of blood pressure.

Most individuals with acute glomerulonephritis recover completely. A few develop chronic glomerulonephritis. It takes up to two years for complete recovery and the individual should continue with close medical supervision and avoid any other type of infection.

NURSING OBSERVATIONS

Changes in the volume and characteristics of urinary output are often the first symptoms noticed by the patient. The volume of urine excreted may decrease. The patient may have gross hematuria, smoky, or coffee-colored urine. The patient may experience anorexia, fatigue, weakness, and headache. Since the disease causes retention of salt and water, the patient can be expected to have considerable edema. Edema or puffiness around the eyes is more noticeable in the morning. Edema of the feet and legs may develop later in the day, especially if one has been in an upright position most of the day.

The patient with a severe case of acute glomerulonephritis may develop cerebral edema, a life-threatening complication. Early indications of cerebral edema are changes in the level of consciousness and behavior. The patient may become less alert or may exhibit behavior unusual for that person. These early observations should be reported at once to the appropriate nurse. Other signs of cerebral edema include visual disturbances, such as spots before the eyes, or even blindness, severe headache, convulsions, and coma. This patient would have a marked decrease in the output of urine and an extremely high blood pressure.

The patient's intake and output as well as weight are carefully measured and recorded in order to detect changes in fluid balance that require an adjustment in therapy.

Retention of salt and water and associated changes often cause the patient with glomerulonephritis to develop hypertension. If the patient's blood pressure remains high over a long time, complications such as heart failure and pulmonary edema may result (Figure 19.7).

ASSISTING WITH DIAGNOSTIC STUDIES

The patient's urinalysis may contain protein (albumin), red blood cells, and red blood cell casts. The blood urea nitrogen (BUN) and creatinine usually are elevated (refer to Table 19.2).

NURSING INTERVENTIONS

AMBULATION AND EXERCISE. The patient is usually placed on bed rest for several weeks until edema subsides and the blood pressure decreases. If after starting ambulation, the blood pressure goes up and the urine shows blood and protein, bedrest is again prescribed.

ALTERATIONS IN DIET AND FLUIDS. The physician usually prescribes sodium restriction to reduce water retention. A mild protein-restricted diet also may be prescribed until the BUN and creatinine levels decrease.

DRUG THERAPY. When streptococcal infection is associated with acute glomerulonephritis, the physician may prescribe an antibiotic such as penicillin or erythromycin. Diuretics such as furosemide (LASIX) or ethacrynic acid (EDECRIN) may be prescribed to reduce edema. When the patient has severe hypertension, a vasodilator such as hydralazine (APRESOLINE) may be prescribed.

Chronic Glomerulonephritis

The patient with chronic glomerulonephritis has a progressive impairment of renal function caused by destruction of the glomeruli. This condition may develop slowly for some unknown reason or may occur following acute glomerulonephritis. The patient with chronic glomerulonephritis may have long symptom-free periods. However, the disease usually progresses to end-stage renal failure which is described later in the chapter.

NURSING OBSERVATIONS

The patient with chronic glomerulonephritis usually experiences recurrent onsets of mild headache, dependent edema, exertional dyspnea, difficulty of sleeping in a flat position, blurring of vision, nocturia, and weakness. In some cases, the patient experiences no symptoms and the disease is first detected by an abnormally high blood pressure or an abnormal urinalysis during a physical examination. Other observations common in the patient with acute glomerulonephritis such as hypertension, edema, and behavioral changes associated with cerebral edema apply to the person with chronic disease also. Careful recording of intake and output and daily weights are indicated as well.

ASSISTING WITH DIAGNOSTIC STUDIES

The patient with chronic glomerulonephritis usually has persistent abnormalities in the urinalysis including protein (proteinuria) and blood (hematuria). A variety of blood tests including BUN and creatinine usually are ordered to evaluate renal function. When chronic disease is suspected, the patient usually has a renal biopsy to confirm the diagnosis.

NURSING INTERVENTIONS

Because there is no way to reverse or stop the disease process, interventions are directed toward relieving the patient's symptoms and preventing complications associated with edema and hypertension. Nursing interventions are similar to those indicated for acute glomerulonephritis. However, these also are influenced by the long-term nature of the patient's condition as well as the unfavorable outcome which is expected.

DIET AND FLUIDS

Diet and fluid restrictions may be more difficult for the patient with chronic disease since they are often permanent yet do not cause the disease process to stop or reverse itself. The nurse may help the patient to live with these restrictions by providing opportunities for the patient to participate in care. For example, the physician may prescribe a fluid intake of 1000 ml per day. The patient may participate by determining how and when fluids will be consumed. One patient may require 30 ml of water to swallow with medication. Another patient may require 100 ml of fluid. The patient may be encouraged to follow a dietary restriction when foods recommended are consistent with cultural influences.

HYGIENE

The patient with considerable edema usually needs special attention to the skin in order to prevent decubitus ulcer. Frequent turning and repositioning, meticulous hygiene, loose-fitting clothing, and appropriate footwear are measures that reduce pressure and irritation to edematous skin. Additional information related to the care of a patient with edema can be located in Chapter 11.

DRUG THERAPY

Drug therapy may include drugs similar to those used for the patient with acute glomerulonephritis. Other drugs prescribed may include anti-inflammatory drugs or cytotoxic agents.

THERAPEUTIC RELATIONSHIP

The patient with chronic illness generally can be expected to experience a variety of emotional ups and downs and behavioral changes associated with chemical imbalances, changes in life-style, drug therapy, fatigue, and a poor prognosis. The nurse can be of great help by listening to the patient's concerns and by referring the patient to others when appropriate. For example, the patient with financial concerns may be helped by a social worker. The nurse's concern may be expressed in attention to details such as helping the patient to plan a fluid restriction or eliciting the patient's participation in measuring intake and output.

When caring for the patient with chronic illness including glomerulonephritis, the patient may be helped by the nurse's encouragement to live each day as completely and fully as possible. One way to express this is by helping the patient to air emotions such as fear and anger. Another way to encourage this is to point out aspects of a situation that are enjoyable or humorous. Before using the latter approach, it is very important to be aware of the patient's immediate concerns. For example, the nurse would not select this intervention if a patient is angry, sad, or extremely frustrated about a loss of income or occupation.

PREVENTION

The patient who is symptom-free generally is advised to avoid activities that increase the workload of the kidneys. These activities include overwork, strenuous exercise, exposure to infection, or overeating.

Nephrotic Syndrome

The patient with nephrotic syndrome or nephrosis has a degenerative noninflammatory disease of the glomerular membrane. Damage to this membrane causes proteins to leak out of the plasma into the urine. This leakage sets the stage for a series of disturbances including inadequate production of albumin by the liver, overproduction of lipoprotein and triglycerides, anemia, and edema.

A variety of conditions is associated with the development of nephrotic syndrome. These include glomerulonephritis, infection, drug toxicity, diabetes, neoplasms, and circulatory disorders.

In severe episodes, disrupted renal function may progress to complications such as renal failure, renal hypertension, and thrombosis in the kidneys, lungs, or extremities. In less severe episodes, there may be regeneration and complete recovery.

NURSING OBSERVATIONS

Edema is often the first symptom the patient notices. In addition to observations related to glomerulonephritis, the patient usually experiences weight gain and anorexia. Intake and output as well as daily weights are important nursing measurements.

ASSISTING WITH DIAGNOSTIC STUDIES

The patient's urine generally contains large amounts of albumin. At the same time, blood tests usually show hypoalbuminemia (low level of albumin in the blood), hyperlipidemia (high level of lipids), and elevated cholesterol levels. Hematology tests (refer to Table 19.2) may indicate anemia and increased clotting tendency in the blood. Immunoglobulin levels may be abnormally low.

NURSING INTERVENTIONS

DRUG THERAPY.   Diuretic therapy with one or more of the drugs listed in Table 11.7 is important to relieve the patient's edema. Corticosteroids may be prescribed for selected patients with specific forms of the disease.

DIET AND FLUIDS.   Currently, there is a controversy among scientists concerning the value of a high-protein diet for the patient with nephrotic syndrome. Fluid restriction and sodium restriction also depend upon the cause of the patient's syndrome.

INTRAVENOUS ALBUMIN.   Intravenous salt-poor albumin may be given in some cases for temporary improvement in the patient with hypotension related to low levels of plasma albumin.

Kidney Tumor

Although tumors of the kidney are not common, they are frequently malignant. Men are more likely to develop cancer of the kidney than women. Children are likely to develop malignant tumors in the kidney. Wilms' tumor is a fast-growing malignancy affecting children under the age of five. Abdominal swelling is usually a sign of this kind of tumor.

NURSING OBSERVATIONS

Often the first symptom of a tumor of the kidney in adults is painless intermittent hematuria. Late in the disease, the tumor can be felt, and the patient may complain of a dull, aching pain in the area of the kidney. There may be a loss of weight as the condition progresses. As the malignancy spreads, the patient develops additional symptoms related to the area of metastasis. The most frequent sites of metastases are the lungs, bones, regional lymph nodes, and liver.

ASSISTING WITH DIAGNOSTIC STUDIES

In addition to blood and laboratory tests related to renal function, the patient may have an intravenous pyelogram, renal scan, CAT scan, or renal angiogram to locate the tumor. Urine cytology and a renal biopsy are needed to identify the malignancy.

NURSING INTERVENTIONS

ASSISTING THE SURGICAL PATIENT.   If the tumor of the kidney is benign or there are no signs of metastasis, a nephrectomy may be done. Nephrectomy may be done either through a flank incision, abdominally, through a thoracic approach, or an abdominal-thoracic approach. The nursing care of the patient with nephrectomy is the same as for those patients with other renal surgeries. If a thoracic approach is selected, the patient usually has chest tubes. Nursing interventions related to the care of the patient with chest tubes can be located in Chapter 14.

ASSISTING WITH OTHER THERAPIES. After surgery of a malignant tumor, radiation therapy is initiated. Radiation therapy also is given to inoperable tumors. Chemotherapy is not usually prescribed.

END-STAGE RENAL DISEASE (RENAL FAILURE)

The patient with renal failure is unable to eliminate waste products or maintain fluid and electrolyte balance. When these wastes accumulate in the blood at a level that causes symptoms, the condition is called *uremia,* which literally means urine in the blood. The term *azotemia* has a more specific meaning which is the presence of excessive quantities of urea and other nitrogenous wastes in the blood.

Acute Renal Failure

Acute renal failure is a sudden rapid deterioration of kidney function which causes wastes to accumulate in the body. The patient may develop this condition as a result of sepsis or absorption of substances such as mercury or poisonous mushrooms. Nephrotoxic drugs such as gentamicin (GARAMYCIN) and tobramycin (NEBCIN) may cause acute failure.

An obstruction in the urinary tract that prevents urine from leaving the kidneys may result in kidney failure. Other causes include conditions that interfere with normal blood flow through the kidneys. For example, shock and resulting low blood pressure due to hemorrhage, myocardial infarction, dehydration, burns, and severe tissue injury will cause a decreased blood flow. Blood clots in the renal artery leading to the kidney can be a contributing factor. A severe blood transfusion reaction that causes the blood cells to disintegrate and allows hemoglobin to filter through glomeruli and block the tubules can result in kidney damage. If the cause can be removed, the prognosis for recovery is good with the nephrons returning to normal function.

The patient usually develops acute renal failure in three phases. The initiating phase begins with the specific agent that damages the cells. Cellular damage results in a buildup of toxic waste products in the blood and variations in the quantity and composition of urine output. The maintenance phase begins when changing other factors cannot reverse the buildup of toxic waste products in the patient's bloodstream. For example, discontinuing a nephrotoxic drug or replacing fluid in the patient who is hemorrhaging does not result in a return of normal kidney function. This phase is often associated with oliguria (urine output of less than 400 ml per 24 hours). The third phase, called recovery, begins when the patient's blood studies (BUN, creatinine) no longer show an increase in the accumulation of waste products. If the patient has been oliguric, there may be a marked increase in the urine output. Complications associated with acute renal failure include infection, gastrointestinal hemorrhage, fatal cardiac arrhythmias, and irreversible brain damage.

ASSISTING WITH DIAGNOSITC STUDIES

In addition to frequent blood tests to evaluate renal function, the nurse can anticipate that most urine output will be sent to the laboratory to analyze the composition. Frequent determinations of serum electrolytes (Table 15.4) also will be ordered to monitor the patient's fluid and electrolyte balance. Hematology studies (Table 19.2) usually are ordered to evaluate the extent and type of the patient's anemia as well as disturbances in clotting. In addition to these studies, the physician can be expected to order whatever diagnostic tests are needed to identify the underlying cause of the patient's acute renal failure.

NURSING OBSERVATIONS

The nurse's observations of the patient in acute renal failure are related to a buildup of toxic waste products, reduction in urine formation, and disturbances in fluid and electrolytes. A head-to-toe guide of selected nursing observations, Table 19.8 applies to the patient in acute renal failure.

A crucial observation in the patient with renal failure is a change in the expected urine output. The amount, color, and characteristics of the patient's urine may vary according to the underlying condition. Variations in intake and output as well as daily weights are carefully observed and recorded.

Laboratory studies are helpful additions to the nurse's observations both because they help to explain the existing observations as well as anticipate future ones. The accumulation of waste products causes a rise in blood urea nitrogen (BUN) and serum creatinine. Potassium may also build up to dangerous levels (hyperkalemia).

Infection is a feared and common complication when the patient has acute renal failure. Observation such as fever, cough, redness or warmth at the intravenous site, or purulent drainage from a body orifice should be reported at once.

NURSING INTERVENTIONS

MAINTAINING SAFETY. Safety precautions are essential for the patient with renal failure who may be weak, disoriented, or sleepy. Siderails are raised, the bed is usually placed in the lowest position, and needed objects placed within easy reach. Simply telling the patient not to get out of bed usually is not effective because of memory loss. Appropriate restraints may be needed. Seizure precautions as described in Chapter 21 also may be needed.

HYGIENE. Meticulous hygiene is needed to prevent infection, skin breakdown, and refresh the patient. Generally, soap is avoided if possible. If used, soap should be thoroughly rinsed from the skin to avoid causing further dryness or pruritus. Tepid bath water may be soothing to the patient with pruritus.

Careful oral hygiene is also important to prevent bacterial overgrowth which can cause infection. Oral hygiene should be given gently to prevent trauma and bleeding of mucous membranes.

DIET AND FLUIDS. Generally, the physician prescribes a diet high in carbohydrates and low in sodium and potassium. The diet may be adjusted regularly depending on the patient's blood levels and losses. It is important for the nurse to check the patient's tray to make sure that the correct diet is served. In addition, the nurse should report to the appropriate person when the patient is not eating. In some cases, smaller, more frequent meals may encourage the patient to eat.

Fluid intake generally is adjusted so that it balances fluid losses. The patient's intake and output as well as changes in daily weight are used to make needed adjustments.

REPOSITIONING. The patient with acute renal failure needs frequent changes of position to prevent skin breakdown, relieve muscle twitches and tremors, and loosen pulmonary secretions. When repositioning the patient, the nurse should check the new position to make sure that full lung expansion is maintained. Deep breathing and coughing using methods described in Chapter 14 are encouraged each time the patient is turned and at regular intervals in between.

ASSISTING WITH DRUG THERAPY. A variety of drugs may be prescribed for the patient with acute renal failure. In some patients, mannitol or a powerful diuretic such as furosemide (LASIX) may be prescribed to enhance urine output. Other drugs may be prescribed to correct dangerous electrolyte imbalance. For example, sodium polystyrene sulfonate (KAYEXALATE) may be administered orally or by enema to correct hyperkalemia. Cimetidine (TAGAMET) may be prescribed to prevent gastrointestinal bleeding. A variety of other drugs may be indicated if the patient develops complications.

ASSISTING WITH OTHER THERAPIES. The patient with acute renal failure may be placed on dialysis therapy to remove toxic waste products that accumulate and/or toxic drugs or substances that caused the kidneys to fail. Dialysis is described in greater detail later in the chapter.

PREVENTION. The nurse has three major roles in preventing acute renal failure. Since reduction of blood flow to the kidneys may initiate acute renal failure, careful observation of vital signs in the hospitalized patient may prevent dangerous hypotension which reduces blood flow to the kidneys. This is especially important for the surgical patient as well as the patient with a blood loss from some other cause. Because formation and excretion of urine are essential to life, the nurse may view the patient's urine output as a vital sign. Unexpected changes in urine output should be reported early when first observed.

The nurse is the person who administers most drug therapy, including nephrotoxic drugs. Awareness that a prescribed drug may cause kidney damage enables the nurse to be especially alert for changes in output. Usually, the physician orders regular blood tests to monitor renal function when the patient is receiving a nephrotoxic drug. The nurse may explain the need for such tests to the patient. In some cases, the patient may need to return as an outpatient to the laboratory for follow-up blood tests. Such a patient may be influenced to return for the test by the nurse's clear explanation.

Finally, the nurse may be consulted by relatives, friends, and neighbors on a variety of symptoms and ailments. Early diagnosis and treatment of other diseases such as hypertension, streptococcal infection, and pyelonephritis may prevent some patients from developing acute renal failure. Therefore, the nurse should advise prompt medical attention when appropriate.

Chronic Renal Failure

The patient with chronic renal failure has a progressive irreversible inability to eliminate waste products and regulate fluid and electrolytes caused by the destruction of nephrons. This condition may develop slowly over a period of years or as a result of acute renal failure from which the patient does not recover. The causes of chronic renal failure may include those agents that cause acute renal failure. Diabetes mellitus, hypertension, sickle cell disease, and polyarteritis nodosa are a few examples of systemic diseases that may cause chronic renal failure.

As the destruction of nephrons progresses, the patient is unable to filter waste products from the bloodstream. A large volume of dilute urine may be excreted. The buildup of toxic waste products produces a wide range of life-threatening disturbances in every body system. The patient's condi-

tion is terminal unless an alternate route for filtering and excreting excess fluids, electrolytes, and metabolic waste is established and maintained.

NURSING OBSERVATIONS

Beside the nursing observations already described in Table 19.8, the nurse may see additional symptoms related to the progressive irreversible nature of chronic renal failure and its effects on every body system. For example, the patient may experience polyuria and nocturia in early stages. In later stages, the patient usually has hypertension caused by retention of salt and water. Changes in blood and blood-forming organs produce anemia and increased bleeding tendency. Changes in the reproductive system result in low sperm count and impotence in men, irregularities in the menstrual cycle, and decreased libido in both men and women. Changes in the musculoskeletal system may result in pathologic fractures in addition to abnormal sensations described in Table 19.8. Changes in the gastrointestinal system include hiccough and metallic taste as well as symptoms described in Table 19.8. Additional changes in the respiratory system include urinary odor of the breath and hyperventilation. The patient's cardiovascular system may be affected by heart failure, cardiac arrhythmias, and pericarditis. The patient's skin may develop a yellow-gray color, a typical frosty appearance caused by the excretion of wastes through the skin. Uremic frost, the term used to describe this condition, causes an increase in pruritus. The patient's sensory nerves may be disturbed, causing progressive loss of vision and hearing. Behavioral changes are varied but may include impaired thinking, remembering, and concentration. Profound alterations in personality may include wide, rapid emotional mood changes, depression and self destructive behavior.

NURSING INTERVENTIONS

The basic goals of nursing care for the patient with chronic renal failure are related to slowing the disease process, preventing complications, and teaching the patient how to live with the illness. Specific interven-

Table 19.8
Guide to Nursing Observations for the
Patient in Renal Failure

Area to Observe	Observations
Head and neck	Visual disturbances
	Edema of eyelids—puffiness around eyes
	Thirst
	Anorexia, nausea, vomiting, hematemesis
	Stomatitis
	Bleeding in mucous membranes of mouth
	Cough and/or hemoptysis
	Alterations in taste
Chest	Alterations in usual respiratory rate and pattern caused by electrolyte imbalances
	Dyspnea caused by fluid in lungs
	Alterations in normal heart rate
	Pleuritic chest pain
Abdomen	Epigastric or gastric distress
	Ascites caused by fluid in abdominal cavity
	Vague, diffuse pain
Extremities	Tremors
	Weakness
	Restlessness in extremities
	Footdrop
	Gait changes
	Edema
	Aches and pains in joints
Urine output	Changes in volume and characteristics of urine depending upon underlying condition
Bowels	Diarrhea, constipation
	Blood in stools
Skin changes	Petechiae, purpura, and/or ecchymosis
	Pallor, pruritus
	Dryness
Behavioral changes	Apathy, fatigue
	Memory loss
	Disorientation
	Convulsions
	Coma

tions are described in general terms. The nurse who is interested in assisting the patient with chronic renal failure requires additional specialized knowledges and skills.

Hygiene. The patient's skin should be kept clean and moist in order to make it a more efficient organ of excretion. For this reason, the individual may require more frequent bathing to prevent body odor of urine. Uremic frost may be washed with vinegar solution of two tablespoons to a pint of water. Frequent gentle oral hygiene may temporarily relieve unpleasant odors and tastes and prevent infection.

Alterations in Diet and Fluids. Dietary protein, potassium, sodium, and phosphorus are restricted and individualized for each patient. A therapeutic dietitian usually visits regularly to plan menus consistent with the patient's preferences, explain the diet, and instruct the patient, family, and others about how to plan, shop, and prepare the special diet at home. The nurse may participate by observing and recording the patient's dietary intake, listening and encouraging the person(s) learning the new diet, and referring questions to the dietitian. The nurse avoids making substitutions on the patient's tray once it has arrived. When the patient's tray is not satisfactory for some reason, the appropriate nursing action is to notify the dietitian. Maintaining adequate nutrition is difficult for an individual who has anorexia, nausea, and an ammonia taste in the mouth.

Nursing measures that encourage the anorexic patient to eat include oral hygiene, providing social interaction, and praising every effort of the patient to eat.

A permanent fluid restriction usually is indicated. The amount of oral fluids prescribed generally is determined by fluctuations in the daily weight as well as blood chemistries. As previously mentioned, the patient who understands and participates in developing a plan for fluid restrictions frequently has more success with it.

Assisting with Drug Therapy. Drug therapy for the patient with chronic renal failure is complicated by the need for a variety of drugs, the high risk for drug toxicity, and the patient's fluid restriction. Prescribed drugs may include stool softeners, antacids, vitamins and minerals, antihypertensives, diuretics, antipruritic agents, anticonvulsants, and sedatives. The clinical pharmacist is the nurse's best resource for questions related to drug therapy.

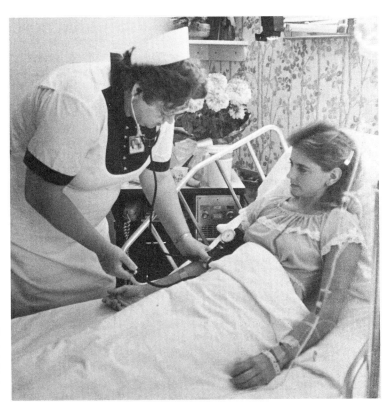

FIGURE 19.7 Checking the patient's blood pressure. (Courtesy of Martinsville-Henry County School of Practical Nursing, Martinsville, Virginia.)

REST. The patient with chronic renal disease usually requires increased rest. The symptoms as well as treatment measures may cause the patient to become exhausted. The patient may benefit from nursing measures that provide uninterrupted rest periods and prevent overexhaustion.

PREVENTION OF INFECTION. The patient requires protection from infection which may be life threatening. In some cases, the hospitalized patient may be placed temporarily in protective isolation. The nurse provides protection by frequent handwashing. The patient receives instructions related to avoiding contact with infected persons and preventing injury.

ASSISTING WITH DIALYSIS. If conservative treatment is not successful in regulating fluid and electrolytes and the accumulation of waste products, the patient may be placed on *dialysis*. Dialysis is a process of removing waste products using a *semipermeable membrane*. A semipermeable membrane is one that allows some but not all particles to move from one side of the membrane to the other. The particles pass from the side of higher concentration to the side of lower concentration of the dissolved particles.

Two methods of dialysis can be used as substitutes for normal kidney function. In peritoneal dialysis, the peritoneal membrane acts as the semipermeable membrane. In hemodialysis, a synthetic material in an artificial kidney machine is the semipermeable membrane.

Peritoneal dialysis can be used in acute or chronic kidney failure. Peritoneal dialysis also might be used to rid the body of an overdose of drugs such as the barbiturates. The peritoneal lining surrounding the abdominal cavity and organs is used as the semipermeable membrane through which the accumulated wastes from the blood will pass. In order to use this method, a catheter must be inserted through a small incision in the skin into the peritoneal cavity. After injecting a local anesthetic, the physician, using sterile technique, makes a small incision in the skin between the symphysis pubis and umbilicus. A catheter is then inserted into the peritoneal cavity, sutured in place to the skin, and covered with a sterile dressing. The TENCK-HOFF catheter is a widely used indwelling catheter for individuals with end-stage renal failure. This silicon catheter is 35 cm long with two attached DACRON cuffs to form a barrier against infection and also to stabilize the catheter in position. It is inserted in the operating room. The catheter is threaded through a subcutaneous tunnel with the first cuff located 10 cm from the external end of the catheter and the second cuff 15 cm from the intraperitoneal end of the catheter. The catheter is attached to tubing, and 2000 ml of dialyzing fluid are allowed to flow into the peritoneal cavity in 10 to 15 minutes. The fluid has a makeup similar to blood. The dialyzing fluid is allowed to remain in the peritoneal cavity as specified by the physician. At the end of that time, the empty bottles are placed on the floor, and the fluids flow out of the peritoneal cavity by siphon drainage and gravity. For the siphon drainage to function, dialyzing fluid must remain in the tubing. The tubing therefore should be clamped before the last few milliliters run out of the bottles and into the peritoneal cavity. The patient also may be rolled from side to side to aid in draining the fluid.

Individuals with end-stage renal failure can be dialyzed either intermittently or continuously. In intermittent peritoneal dialysis (IPD), the individual is dialyzed three or four times a week at a dialyzing center for approximately eight hours. Some individuals are taught how to dialyze themselves at home. An automatic cycling machine has made this procedure simple and convenient for many clients. Most clients dialyze themselves at night while they sleep.

The other method of peritoneal dialysis is called continuous ambulatory peritoneal dialysis (CAPD). Many urologists call this method the closest thing to a portable artificial kidney. The individual on CAPD undergoes a round-the-clock dialysis without machines and without prolonged interruption of activities. The client attaches the tubing

of the plastic bag solution container to the peritoneal catheter and the solution is raised to shoulder level. Once empty, the container is rolled up and tucked under the client's clothing. While the client goes about everyday activities, dialysis takes place. The solution is left four to six hours during the day and eight hours during the night.

When the exchange process is completed, the plastic container is unrolled and lowered below the level of the abdomen and allowed to drain. The drainage and the container are discarded, a new container of dialysate is attached, and the process is repeated. Clients on CAPD do not usually have dietary restrictions.

The length of time required for the dialysis procedure depends on the purpose for the treatment. In acute kidney failure, only one dialyzing treatment may be required to rid the blood of excess waste, with the kidneys regaining normal function. However, more than one treatment is not unusual.

Extremely accurate records must be kept of intake and output. Intake will include not only the dialyzing fluid but also oral and intravenous fluids. The output recorded will be the fluid returning from the peritoneal cavity as well as urinary output, and others such as vomitus and drainage from tubes. Vital signs should be checked frequently as ordered by the physician. The patient will experience a feeling of fullness when the fluid is in the peritoneal cavity. Pain also may be present. Sedatives or analgesics may be given.

The nurse may be asked to assist in initiating the peritoneal dialysis as well as being responsible for caring for the patient undergoing the dialysis. It is the nurse's responsibility to have a clear and complete understanding of the entire procedure, to maintain accurate records, and to observe the patient for complications.

The complications are bleeding, peritonitis, or perforation of the intestine. The bleeding might be around the catheter site or from within the peritoneal cavity. Therefore, the color of the returning dialyzing fluid should be noted carefully. Symptoms of peritonitis might be cloudiness of the returning fluid, temperature elevation, and abdominal pain. The symptoms of a perforation of the intestine probably would be apparent with the fluid returning from the first dialyzing fluid. The returning fluid would be cloudy, brownish, and may even contain bits of fecal material.

Hemodialysis is done with an artificial kidney. Instead of the peritoneal membrane acting as the semipermeable membrane, the patient's blood circulates through a synthetic semipermeable membrane made of cellophane or CUPROPHANE. The semipermeable membrane is immersed in a bath of dialyzing fluid such as that used for peritoneal dialysis. Since the blood of the patient contains more waste products than the dialyzing fluid, the waste passes into the dialyzing fluid and out of the patient's blood. The semipermeable membrane allows only the passage of wastes and not blood cells because the cells are too large for the tiny pores of the cellophane.

A cannula or catheter is placed in an artery of the patient's arm or leg, and this arterial blood flows into the artificial kidney. It flows out of the semipermeable membrane through a tube and back into a vein in the arm or leg that also has been cannulated or contains a intravenous catheter.

There are a few methods by which the client's vein and artery are made accessible for hemodialysis. An external arteriovenous shunt is created by a surgical procedure during which one catheter is placed in an artery and another catheter is placed in a vein. The two catheters are brought out from the skin and connected by a special U-shaped connector (Figure 19.8). The U-shape connector is removed during dialysis.

A method used more often is surgical creation of an internal *arteriovenous fistula*. An adjacent artery and vein are surgically connected causing a fistula. The fistula gradually enlarges to permit entry of one or two needles during dialysis. Variations of this method include special grafts used to connect the artery to the vein. Materials used for the graft include synthetics and bovine animal arteries. The HEMASITE shunt is a recent development of a synthetic fistula. Two buttonlike attachments which protrude from the skin are the external accesses to

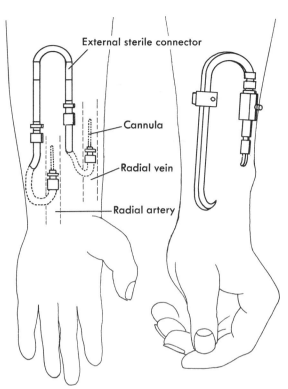

FIGURE 19.8   The cannulation usually is made into an adjacent artery and vein. After the dialysis, the patient has the ends of the cannulas joined by a sterile connector that permits normal circulation of blood between treatments. An external sterile connector between the radial artery and the radial vein is illustrated.

the dialyzing machine. Adaptors are needed to connect them to the machine. These external accesses are covered with sterile plugs when not in use.

Some patients receive hemodialysis by coming to a center at a scheduled time. Other patients and/or family members learn to use hemodialysis at home. This involves an extensive program of teaching, learning, practice, and supervision.

PSYCHOSOCIAL ASPECTS

The patient on maintenance dialysis has many problems. The client is undergoing long-term dialysis and is concerned with very real problems such as restricted meals, unquenched thirst, unpredictable medical status, financial problems, waning sexual desires, impotence, dependency on a machine, and a regimented life-style. Some studies have shown that these individuals go through several phases of adaptation. A "honeymoon" period after the initial depression has been described. At this time the patient feels better due to relief of the symptoms of uremia. But this period usually ends in disenchantment and discouragement. Periods of depression may result in suicidal attempts or just giving up and not following dietary and fluid restrictions. Later, a long-term adaptation may occur when the patient accepts the condition and restrictions. This last phase is not achieved by some patients.

The family also may resent the patient due to necessary changes in their life-style. They may even withdraw from the patient if they view the condition as hopeless.

Members of the health team should be understanding and accepting of the unique needs of the patient and family. They should allow for ventilation of feelings and have an accepting attitude when dealing with the client and family.

ASSISTING THE PATIENT WITH A KIDNEY TRANSPLANT

The most ideal method of treatment for the patient with chronic renal failure is a kidney transplant during which the patient receives another human kidney in a surgical procedure. The donor kidney may come from a sibling, parent, or "brain dead" individuals. Because the patient's immune system is activated by the introduction of foreign material, rejection of the donor kidney may occur. Rejection is less likely when the donor tissue closely resembles that of the patient. For this reason, the best donor is an identical twin, if available. Sibling donors are better than parent donors. Other donors are acceptable if immunologic compatibility is assured. The patient who receives a kidney transplant is freed from the dependency on a machine, but faces lifelong immunosuppressive therapy to prevent rejection which can occur at any time. The survival of the individual depends on the response to the immunosuppressive drugs. Some of the more common drugs are azathioprine (IMURAN), corticosteroids such as prednisone, and anti-

lymphocyte globulin. Side effects of these drugs are numerous. The recipient of kidney transplantation should be reassured that in the event of rejection or failure of the transplant, maintenance hemodialysis can be resumed while waiting for another suitable kidney donor.

A bilateral nephrectomy is often done if both kidneys are equally nonfunctioning. The donor kidney is transplanted into the iliac fossa and the renal artery and vein are sutured to an appropriate and close artery and vein. The ureter is sutured in place into an opening in the bladder wall.

Postoperatively, the patient is placed in a special room in protective isolation to prevent infection. As discussed in Chapter 5, suppression of the patient's immune system causes increased susceptibility to infection. Nursing interventions are related to the care of a patient with kidney, urinary tract, and blood vessel surgery. Other nursing responsibilities are recording and reporting of fluctuations of weight, vital signs, and intake and output. Common laboratory tests to monitor the patient's postoperative course include electrolytes, BUN, creatinine, hematocrit, urine testing for protein, pH, specific gravity, and creatinine clearance.

The patient with a kidney transplant needs lifelong close medical supervision. In addition, the patient becomes an expert in special self-care practices related to testing urine, measuring intake and output, weighing, taking vital signs, and avoiding infections. When these practices are continued regularly, a client with a successful transplantation can resume a normal life including a job, recreation, and sports.

Case Study Involving Glomerulonephritis

Mr. George Henry, a 20-year-old college student, was admitted to the hospital with the following: anorexia, nausea and vomiting, weakness, pallor, blood pressure of 150/90, temperature 38°C (100.4°F), edema of the ankles, and puffy eyelids. He was relatively well until he was sent home from his part-time job two weeks prior to admission with a cold and sore throat. His admitting diagnosis was acute glomerulonephritis.

TABLE 19.9
OTHER DISORDERS OF THE URINARY SYSTEM

DISORDER	DESCRIPTION
Hereditary nephritis (Alport's syndrome)	A form of hereditary renal disease marked by hematuria, proteinuria, and nerve deafness; renal function deteriorates slowly and hypertension develops; patient may need to be treated for urinary infections, hypertension, and renal failure; hemodialysis and kidney transplant may be indicated
Idiopathic membranous glomerular disease (membranous nephrosis)	A disease of the glomeruli in which a portion of the membrane becomes thickened; nephrotic syndrome and hypertension often occur; this condition is usually progressive with no treatment known to change the course
Nephroptosis	An abnormal downward displacement of the kidney associated with excessive movement of the kidney; this condition usually causes no symptoms
Nephrosclerosis	A hardening of the arteries in the kidney usually resulting from renal hypertension
Polycystic disease	An inherited condition in which the kidneys have cysts that may contain water, serum, pus, blood, or urine; hemodialysis may be used when renal failure occurs; some patients may benefit from renal transplant
Renal medullary necrosis	A severe complication of pyelonephritis in which part of the kidney tissue dies; symptoms of pyelonephritis are intensified; treatment is directed toward the control of infection when possible
Renal osteomalacia	A demineralization of bone resulting from inadequate absorption of calcium in uremia
Renal tuberculosis	A secondary tuberculosis infection transmitted by way of the bloodstream from the lungs. Drugs used for pulmonary tuberculosis are used also to treat this condition. The symptoms are similar to those of pyelitis. The urine contains pus, blood, and tubercle bacilli
Renal tubular acidosis	A rare disease in which the tubule is defective in urinary acidification or in reabsorbing bicarbonate; cause of some cases is not known and others can be traced to the intake of such substances as paraldehyde and tetracycline; alkalinizing substances such as sodium citrate or sodium bicarbonate may be prescribed
Renal vein thrombosis	A thrombus can develop in the renal vein in connection with thrombosis of the inferior vena cava, an obstruction of the vein by external pressure such as a neoplasm, and renal disease; anticoagulant therapy and treatment of the complicating neophrotic syndrome may be used; nephrectomy may be done in some cases in which one kidney is affected
Toxic nephropathy	A change in the structure or function of the kidney caused by substances such as bichloride of mercury, the sulfonamides, lead, diuretics, and compounds that cuse an immune reation in the kidney; acute renal failure may occur

Laboratory findings indicated a BUN of 31 mg/100 ml and a serum creatinine of 1.9 mg/100 ml. Urinalysis showed albuminuria, red blood cells, white blood cells, a specific gravity of 1.040, and a pH of 6.5.

The physician's orders were:

- Bed rest
- Measure intake and output
- Weigh daily
- Furosemide (LASIX), 40 mg daily
- Low-sodium (500-mg) and low-protein diet
- Restrict fluids to 1000 ml daily

QUESTIONS

1. What kidney functions of Mr. Henry are altered? What nursing implications do they have?
2. What kind of infection could have happened two weeks prior to Mr. Henry's admission and did it have a relationship to his present illness?
3. Explain each symptom as a forerunner of chronic glomerulonephritis and eventual kidney failure if this present acute condition is not cured. Relate these to nursing actions.
4. What nursing actions are called for in response to the medical orders?

5. What nursing actions should be taken because Mr. Henry is receiving LASIX?
6. Under what conditions should Mr. Henry be weighed?

Case Study Involving Renal Colic

Mr. Gordon, a 20-year-old college student, was admitted to the hospital with a diagnosis of left ureteral caluli. The nurse who admitted Mr. Gordon observed that he was diaphoretic, rolling from side to side in bed, and holding his left side. Mr. Gordon reported nausea and vomited after the nurse left the room. A urine specimen that was grossly bloody was obtained. The nurse recorded the following vital signs on the chart: temperature 38°C (100.4°F), pulse 116, respirations 28, blood pressure 130/68. The physician's orders included:

• Activity as tolerated
• Strain all urine—send any stones to laboratory for analysis
• Force fluids
• DEMEROL, 100 mg IM q3h prn for pain
• TIGAN, 100 mg IM q4h prn for nausea
• KUB and IVP in A.M.
• Cystoscopy on call after x-rays in A.M.
• Uric acid and routine laboratory tests
• Clean-voided urine specimen for culture and sensitivity
• Vital signs q4h while awake

QUESTIONS

1. What actions should the nurse take in caring for Mr. Gordon? List in order of priority and give the reason for each action.
2. What patient teaching and/or equipment is needed for each of the diagnostic studies ordered for Mr. Gordon?
3. What specific actions should the nurse take to encourage increased fluid intake for Mr. Gordon?
4. How should the nurse obtain a clean-voided specimen from Mr. Gordon and why?
5. What is the relationship between the laboratory studies ordered and renal colic?
6. What changes in vital signs should the nurse anticipate and report?
7. What nursing observations and actions will be indicated when Mr. Gordon returns from having the cystoscopy?
8. What are the nursing observations and actions related to each of the procedures used to remove renal caluli?
9. What is the relationship between the physician's order for activity and renal colic?

Suggestions for Further Study

1. How can a specimen for a urine culture be obtained from a female patient without doing a catheterization?
2. What causes the characteristic odor of ammonia around an incontinent patient? How can you alleviate this?
3. Why would the practical nurse be asked to strain the urine of a patient with nephrolithiasis?
4. Why should the nurse caring for a patient who has recently had surgery of the urinary tract observe closely for symptoms of shock and hemorrhage?
5. Mason, Mildred A.; Bates, Grace F.; and Smola, Bonnie K.: *Workbook in Basic Medical-Surgical Nursing,* 3rd ed. Macmillan Publishing Company, New York, 1984, Exercise 19.

Additional Readings

Barrett, Nancy: "Cancer of the Bladder: A Case History." *American Journal of Nursing,* 81:2192–95 (Dec.), 1981.

Boh, Dawn Mare, and VanSon, Allene R.: "The Water-Load Test." *American Journal of Nursing,* 82:112–13 (Jan.), 1982.

Cain, Lyn, and Bigongiari, Lawrence R.: "The Percutaneous Nephrostomy Tube." *American Journal of Nursing,* 82:296–98 (Feb.), 1982.

Chambers, Jeannette: "Assessing the Dialysis Patient at Home." *American Journal of Nursing,* 81:750–54 (Apr.), 1981.

Cianci, Judith, and Lamb, Joann: "Matching Organ Donors and Recipients." *American Journal of Nursing,* 81:544–45 (Mar.), 1981.

Cianci, Judith; Lamb, Joann; and Ryan, Rita K.: "Renal Transplantation." *American Journal of Nursing,* 81:354–55 (Feb.), 1981.

Denniston, Donna, and Burns, Kathryn Taylor: "Home Peritoneal Dialysis." *American Journal of Nursing,* 80:2022–26 (Nov.), 1980.

Hill, Martha N.: "When the Patient Is the Family." *American Journal of Nursing,* 81:536–38 (Mar.), 1981.

Law, Carolyn: "Catheter Care and UTI." *Journal of Practical Nursing,* 31:29–32 (Sept.), 1981.

Luke, Barbara: "Nutrition in Renal Dialysis: The Adult on Dialysis." *American Journal of Nursing,* 79:2155–57 (Dec.), 1979.

Metheny, Norma: "Renal Stones and Urinary pH." *American Journal of Nursing,* 82:1372–75 (Sept.), 1982.

Orr, Martha Lane: "Drugs and Renal Disease." *American Journal of Nursing,* 81:969–71 (May), 1981.

Rambo, Beverly J., and Wood, Lucile A. (eds.): *Nursing Skills for Clinical Practice,* 3rd ed. W. B. Saunders Co., Philadelphia, 1982, pp. 485–513.

Reckling, JoAnn Bell: "Safeguarding the Renal Transplant Patient." *Nursing 82,* 12:47–55 (Feb.), 1982.

Robinson, Corinne H.: *Basic Nutrition and Diet Therapy,* 4th ed. Macmillan Publishing Co., Inc., New York, 1980, pp. 263–75.

Sackheim, George I., and Lehman, Dennis D.: *Chemistry for the Health Sciences,* 4th ed. Macmillan Publishing Co., Inc., New York, 1981, pp. 397–406.

Sheahan, Sharon L., and Seabolt, John Patton: "Understanding Urinary Tract Infection in Women." *Nursing 82,* 12:68–71 (Nov.), 1982.

Stark, June L. "How to Succeed Against Acute Renal Failure." *Nursing 82,* 12:26–33 (July), 1982.

Chapter 20

The Patient with a Disease of the Reproductive System *

Expected Behavioral Outcomes

Minimum objectives referred to as expected behavioral outcomes have been designed for the practical/vocational nursing student to use as guides in studying this chapter. The student should read these expected outcomes before studying the chapter. This will enable the student to use the objectives as guides for study.

Revised by the authors and Lorraine Richardson, R.N., B.S., B.S.N., who is a Practical Nursing Instructor with the Central School of Practical Nursing in Norfolk, Virginia.

After studying the chapter, the student should return to the objective and evaluate the ability to:

1. *Compare the nursing observations and interventions indicated for a patient having an abdominal hysterectomy with those needed for a person having a vaginal hysterectomy.*
2. *List the nursing observations and interventions appropriate when caring for an individual before and after a prostatectomy.*
3. *Compare the nursing observations, treatment, and complications related to an individual with gonorrhea with those related to a person with syphilis.*

4. *Demonstrate the method suggested by the American Cancer Society for monthly breast self-examination.*

5. *Describe the importance of a regular Papanicolaou smear of the cervix as you would to a nonmedical person.*

6. *Describe nursing observations and interventions related to each of the diagnostic studies in this chapter.*

7. *List the nursing observations, interventions, and patient teaching indicated for an individual experiencing a radical mastectomy.*

8. *Describe in a short paragraph or two how the nurse's own values and attitudes about sexuality influence the care of an individual experiencing a disorder of the reproductive system.*

9. *When given an example of venereal disease, describe nursing observations and interventions related to symptoms, drug therapy, preventing the spread of infection, and client education.*

Vocabulary Development

The following prefixes, suffixes, and combining forms pertain to this chapter. By learning and/or reviewing their meanings, the practical/vocational nursing student will have the keys needed to unlock many exciting new medical terms.

Discover the meaning of the keys in a medical dictionary or in the content of this chapter. How does each key pertain to this chapter? In your notebook, write the correct meaning of each prefix, suffix, or combining form listed below. Illustrate each key with an example.

ante—before. Ex. *ante*flexion—forward curvature of the uterus.

aden-	leuk-
andr-	lymph-
ante-	mamm-
-cele	mast-
cervic-	men-
chancr-	metr-
-cid(e)	oo-
colp-	orchi-
fibr-	ov-
-flex	para-
gyn(ec)-	salping-
hydr-	sperm(at)-
hyster-	test-
jact-	vagin-
labi-	vas-
lapar-	vesic-
leuc-	

THE MALE PATIENT

Structure and Function

The male reproductive system consists of the scrotum and its contents, two seminal vesicles, the ducts through which the spermatozoa pass from the scrotum to the exterior, the prostate gland, two bulbourethral glands, and penis (see Figure 20.1).

The *scrotum*, which is a pouch, normally contains two glands known as the testes. The glands produce the male sex hormone by means of the *interstitial cells*, called *isles of Leydig*. The seminiferous tubules, from the age of puberty, continuously form sperm or *spermatozoa* (male germ cells).

The formation of sperm is called *spermatogensis*. The sperm has three main parts: a head, neck, and tail. The head contains the nucleus of the cell, and the tail contains the cytoplasm. Genes are carried by the head of the sperm, while mobility is provided by the tail. Normal sperm move up the female vagina, uterus, and fallopian tube to capture the ovum. Spermatozoa formed in the seminiferous tubules are carried to the epididymis, where they mature. These spermatozoa leave the epididymis by way of the *vas deferens* or *ductus deferens*. The two vas deferens, one for each of the testes, lead from the epididymis to the abdominal cavity and then continue along toward the urinary bladder. There each joins the seminal vesicle to form an ejaculatory duct. The two seminal vesicles are small sacs that store the spermatozoa and add an alkaline fluid that makes them more mobile when ejaculation occurs. The two ejaculatory ducts pass

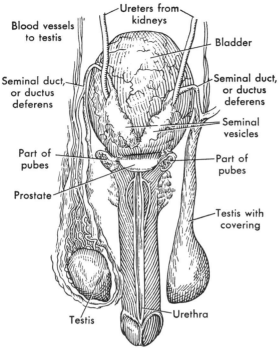

FIGURE 20.1   Diagram of the sagittal section of the male reproductive system. (From Miller, Marjorie A.; Drakontides, Anna B.; and Leavell, Lutie C.: *Kimber-Gray-Stackpole's Anatomy and Physiology*, 17th ed. Macmillan Publishing Co., Inc., New York, 1977, page 575.)

through the prostate gland to the urethra. The *prostate gland* is an organ made of muscular and glandular tissue. This gland surrounds the lower end or neck of the urinary bladder and the beginning of the urethra. The prostate gland secretes an alkaline fluid that is added to the semen during ejaculation. *Semen* is the fluid containing spermatozoa. This fluid is made of substances produced by the two testes, the two seminal vesicles, the prostate gland, and the two bulbourethral glands. The two small glands located below the prostate gland are known as *bulbourethral glands*. These glands produce an alkaline substance that is added to the semen through a small duct, which opens into the urethra. An alkaline fluid is essential to the vitality and length of survival of spermatozoa. The penis is the male organ of copulation or sexual intercourse. The penis is

composed of three separate structures: one *corpus cavernosum urethrae* and two *corpora cavernosa penis*. Blood fills these spaces during sexual stimulation, distending the tissues enough to produce erection of the penis for successful sexual intercourse. The external opening of the urethra is located at the end of the penis, which has a slight enlargement known as the glans penis. The foreskin or prepuce, which covers the glans penis, is frequently removed by circumcision shortly after birth. The urethra serves as a passageway for urine, sperm, and seminal fluid to leave the body.

Assisting with Diagnostic Studies

Men should be encouraged to seek routine examinations as are women. They should be taught the importance of regular self-examination of the prostate gland and testes. Routine health checkups may be embarrassing and uncomfortable for the male, but early prostatic malignancies are often easily detected, diagnosed, and cured. Some sources advocate teaching the male how to go about the examination and what abnormalities to observe for.

RECTAL-PROSTATIC EXAMINATION

A rectal-prostatic examination is essential for every man age 40 or over for early detection of diseases of the rectum and prostate gland. The purpose of the digital examination of the prostate is to determine the size and presence of tumors.

The client should be asked to empty the bladder prior to the examination for easy identification of the prostate, accuracy, and for comfort. The client may be positioned in a knee-chest position on the examining table with the buttocks elevated or be asked to bend from the hips, while placing the elbows either on the examining table or the knees. The client is asked to "bear down" as to help relax the anus, thus making it easier for the physician to insert a well-lubricated, gloved finger.

PROSTATIC MASSAGE

Prostatic massage facilitates the release of small amounts of prostatic fluid. Indications for this procedure are to reduce prostatic edema and perform diagnostic studies.

RENAL AND UROLOGIC STUDIES

Because of the close anatomic relationship between urinary and reproductive structures in the male, a disorder in one system often affects function in the other. Therefore, the nurse can anticipate that one or more of the diagnostic studies described in Chapter 19 may be done when the male client has a disturbance in the reproductive system.

ENDOCRINE STUDIES

As mentioned in Chapter 18, hormones are powerful chemical messengers that regulate body functions, including reproductive functions such as sperm formation and testosterone secretion. Abnormalities in the endocrine system may result in disturbance in reproduction. Examples of hormone levels which may be measured in urine or blood include testosterone, gonadotropins, and 17-ketosteroids. Additional information about these studies can be located in Table 18.3.

SPERM COUNT (SEMEN ANALYSIS)

Semen analysis is done to determine male fertility and to check the effectiveness of a vasectomy. An analysis of semen is done also for medicolegal purposes in such cases as rape and paternity.

In order to obtain an adequate specimen, the client receives written instructions about preparation for the test, collection of semen, and transporting the specimen to the laboratory.

The patient is instructed to refrain from sexual intercourse for two to five days before the test. The most desirable specimen is collected in the doctor's office or laboratory. If this is not possible, the specimen may be collected at home and delivered to the laboratory within two hours without warming or chilling it.

As part of diagnostic studies related to infertility, semen also may be collected from the woman in order to examine sperm movement in the cervix. This examination usually is done during the ovulatory phase of the menstrual cycle and within six to eight hours after sexual intercourse.

CULTURE OF PENILE DRAINAGE

Drainage from lesions on the penis or fluid draining from the penile opening may be examined under the microscope to identify pathogens causing infection or atypical cells that indicate cancer. This diagnostic study usually is done to identify herpes genitalis, *Neisseria gonorrhoeae*, and other similar infections in the male reproductive system.

BIOPSY OF THE PROSTATE

Types of biopsies of the prostate are needle aspiration for cytology, needle punch biopsy for histology, transurethral resection biopsy, and open perineal biopsy. The purpose of the biopsy is to confirm carcinoma or to determine the cause of prostatic hypertrophy. Microscopic tissue examination also can detect benign hyperplasia of the prostate, prostatitis, lymphomas, and urinary or bladder carcinoma. Nursing observations and interventions for the patient having a biopsy of the prostate include those needed for the surgical patient, as described in Chapter 6.

SERUM ACID PHOSPHATASE

Acid phosphatase is an enzyme found mainly in the prostate gland in the adult male's semen, and small amounts are found in the red blood cells, kidneys, spleen, liver, bone marrow, and platelets. An increase in serum acid phosphatase levels almost always indicates prostatic carcinoma with metastasis. This test also may be used to monitor the client's response to prostatic therapy. Serum acid phosphatase levels tend to decrease with successful therapy.

Nursing interventions include telling the client that the reason for the test is to evaluate prostatic function. Food or drink should be restricted prior to the test.

Nursing Observations

OBSERVING FOR GROWTHS AND LESIONS

Because the nurse has close daily contact with the patient, there are opportunities to observe and report abnormalities that may indicate a disturbance in the patient's reproductive system. For example, during the daily bath, the nurse may observe the foreskin in the uncircumcised male. In some cases, the foreskin cannot be retracted for cleaning due to constriction and narrowing. This condition, known as *phimosis*, should be reported. In other cases, the foreskin is completely retracted over the glans penis but cannot be returned to its usual position. This condition, known as *paraphimosis*, may constrict the blood supply causing severe edema, cyanosis, pain, and dysuria. Paraphimosis should be reported at once to the head nurse or physician.

Lesions, ulcerations, growths, rashes, or redness of any part of the external genitalia are described and reported when observed. A description of common lesions can be located in Table 20.1. The characteristics of drainage from either a lesion or the urethral meatus such as color, odor, thickness, clarity, and volume are reported and recorded.

EDEMA

When observing the patient with edema of the scrotum, the nurse should look carefully at the bottom and back of the scrotum for early signs of skin breakdown caused by pressure. In some cases, turning the patient to one side and asking the patient to bend the knee of the top leg enables the nurse to make a more complete inspection.

URINARY FUNCTION

As previously mentioned, the patient with a disturbance in the reproductive system also may experience a disturbance in urinary function. For example, urinary retention usually develops when the patient has an abnormal enlargement of the prostate gland. In thin persons, a distended bladder may be visible above the symphysis pubis. Other disturbances which the patient may report include frequency, dribbling (retention with overflow), dysuria, oliguria, urgency, hesitation, nocturia, hematuria, pyuria, urethral discharge, and incontinence. The nurse also should observe and record the characteristics of the patient's urine. A complete description is located in Chapter 19.

CHILLS AND FEVER

A chill is the body's response to microorganisms. A fever is a sign of infection. Superficial blood vessels constrict, sweating stops, and circulation is diverted to the deepest, more protected blood vessels. A feeling of coldness, and muscle contractions may be followed by shivering and shaking, complaints of extreme heat, sweating, and vasodilation.

TABLE 20.1
COMMON LESIONS OF THE EXTERNAL MALE GENITALIA

LESION	DESCRIPTION
Chancre	Fluid-filled lesion which is hard, oval or round, dark red, nontender, eventually looks like an ulcer
Chancroid	Soft macular lesion with irregular edges
Condyloma accuminatum	Soft, flat top, painless, red or pink warts or papillomas; may have a stem
Erysipelas	Inflammation of the skin and subcutaneous tissue with round or oval patches. These patches readily enlarge and spread
Granuloma inguinale	Small, raised, clear, beefy-red, foul-smelling lesion
Herpes simplex virus, type II	Small, fluid-filled vesicles on an erythematous base which are painless, burning, tingling, and itching. They develop into shallow, painful ulcers which are red, tender
Liposarcoma	The most common soft tissue sarcoma; originating in fatty tissue. Tends to become quite large
Lymphogranuloma venereum	Small, papular, or macular erosive ulcer
Soft tissue sarcoma	Hard or soft mass, superficial tumor causing redness and local heat

Chills and fever may be a direct result of the disease process or complications resulting from an operative or diagnostic procedure, such as prostatectomy, needle punch, or aspiration biopsy. Such disease conditions as balanoposthitis, prostatitis, epididymitis, and orchitis may produce chills and fever.

GYNECOMASTIA

The nurse also may observe and report gynecomastia, breast enlargement in men associated with hyperplasia in the mammary glands. This observation is more likely to be seen in males during puberty and after the age of 40. In some cases, gynecomastia may develop in men who have cancer of the testes (described later in the chapter) or those who are receiving estrogen therapy for cancer of the prostate gland. Occasionally, in older men, gynecomastia may be associated with breast cancer. Biopsy and a mastectomy may be needed in this case.

BEHAVIORAL CHANGES

Many clients put off physical examination of the reproductive system, as this causes intense emotional reactions. Cultural background, fear, and embarrassment play an important role in this type of distress. Persons in today's society are anxious about conditions such as carcinoma, venereal disease, sterility, and sexual problems but may be afraid to discuss or report symptoms with the physician or the nurse. Thus, the nurse's observations are especially important.

Illness, diagnostic studies, and surgery involving the sexual organs can be expected to threaten a person's sexual identity. The threatened male client occasionally may become aggressive, overactive, and immodest toward the female nurse. This behavior is usually an expression of the patient's anxiety and concern over a possible loss of sexual function.

For many persons, successful sexual and reproductive functioning are related to feelings of self-worth and self-esteem. Disturbances in sexual and/or reproductive function may cause such a person to feel weaker, less masculine, or less competent.

Nursing Interventions

Some nursing interventions involving the external genitalia may cause the male client to experience an erection. This situation, although not unusual, may result in considerable embarrassment for the patient. The nurse may be very helpful at this time by explaining in a matter-of-fact way that this is not unusual, and by temporarily discontinuing the particular intervention until the erection is over. In some cases, the nurse may leave the room and return at another time to complete the nursing intervention.

PERINEAL CARE OF THE MALE CLIENT

Perineal care is an important part of hygiene for the client with a disorder of the reproductive system in order to remove secretions, drainage, and/or urine from the skin. Table 20.2 contains a guide to perineal care for the uncircumcised male client. As previously mentioned, the nurse has an opportunity during perineal care to observe the external genitalia for abnormal lesions and drainage.

Perineal care is needed more frequently when the patient has a Foley catheter or following genital or rectal surgery. The exact procedure varies according to hospital procedure and the surgeon's preference. Sterile technique may be used. The perineum is

TABLE 20.2
GUIDE TO PERINEAL CARE IN THE
UNCIRCUMCISED MALE

1. Retract the foreskin of the penis.
2. Holding the penile shaft in one hand and a washcloth in the other, bathe the tip of the penis using a circular motion. Rinse this area.
3. Using a clean section of the washcloth, bathe the penile shaft from top to bottom. Rinse this area.
4. Holding the scrotal sac, bathe all portions of the scrotum and perineum. Rinse this area.
5. Dry the external genitalia thoroughly using a patting motion.
6. Pull the foreskin gently back over the tip of the penis.
7. After turning the client to the side, separate the buttocks and cleanse the rectal area.

washed with soap and warm water. In some cases, an antibacterial soap is used. An antibiotic ointment or disinfectant ointment such as povidone-iodine (BETADINE) may be applied around the urethral meatus, according to local policy, if the patient is not allergic to iodine. The patient's privacy should be carefully protected during perineal care.

SITZ BATHS

Sitz baths may be prescribed to provide moist heat to the perineal and anal regions. The purposes are to cleanse, promote healing and drainage, decrease soreness, relieve vascular congestion, and reduce inflammation. This type of moist heat is used primarily for clients who have had perineal, anal, or rectal surgery. The temperature of the bath may range from 37.8 to 43.3°C (100 to 110°F), depending upon the purpose and condition of the client's skin. The patient's bath usually lasts for 15 to 20 minutes. Plastic disposable sitz baths may be used while the client is hospitalized and sent home with him. Whenever heat is used, the nurse should check the temperature as well as the patient's skin in order to prevent burns.

APPLICATIONS OF HEAT AND COLD

The physician may prescribe applications of heat or cold for a patient with a disturbance in the reproductive system. For example, heat via the sitz bath or lamp may be prescribed following surgery to relieve pain and muscle spasms in the perineum. Cold may be applied via ice bags or chemical cold packs to relieve swelling associated with injury, bleeding, or infection involving the external genitalia. Except for the sitz bath, the hot or cold application is not applied directly to the skin. Instead, the patient's skin may be protected from damage with a towel or other similar covering. Other safety measures include frequent observation of the skin during the application to detect early signs of damage.

ALTERATIONS IN DIET AND FLUIDS

In general, the client with a disorder of the reproductive system should have a nour-ishing diet and an increased fluid intake unless otherwise prescribed.

When an extensive preoperative workup has been done, the nurse may anticipate possible undernutrition and dehydration caused by withholding food and fluids for diagnostic tests. These problems are corrected preoperatively.

Following perineal surgery, a low-residue diet may be prescribed to prevent the client from straining and to reduce risk of postoperative bleeding.

ASSISTING WITH DRUG THERAPY

Drug therapy is often prescribed for the male client with a disturbance in the reproductive system. Often, patient teaching is needed because much of drug therapy occurs at home. Table 20.3 contains a description of observations and interventions commonly used by the nurse when assisting with drug therapy for the patient with a disorder in the reproductive system.

MANAGING PAIN AND DISCOMFORT

Some pain-relieving interventions used to assist the client with a disease in the reproductive system have already been described, including the sitz bath, applications of heat or cold, and drug therapy. Other interventions that may be helpful include backrubs, scrotal support when the scrotum is edematous, repositioning, and rest.

PREVENTION OF INFECTION

All members of the health team are responsible for maintaining high levels of personal practice to prevent the spread of infection. Since nurses are in direct contact with the client, maintenance of asepsis in catheter insertion, instillations and irrigations of catheters, wound cleansing, dressing changes, and perineal care is an important method of preventing the spread of infection.

The reproductive system contains excellent portals for entry and exit of pathogens causing infection. These sites and secretions include mucous membranes of the urethra, vagina, open draining lesions in the genitourinary tract, genital secretions, and urine.

[Text continued on page 675.]

TABLE 20.3
ASSISTING WITH DRUG THERAPY

CLASSIFICATION	DISEASE DISORDER	NURSING IMPLICATIONS
Analgesics	*Most infections*	*Observe for*
Acetaminophen (TYLENOL) Phenacetin (ACETOPHENE-TIDIN)	Prostatitis Epididymitis Urethritis Orchitis	1. Symptoms of methemoglobinemia (bluish color of mucosa and fingernails, dyspnea, vertigo, weakness, headaches—anoxia related) 2. Symptoms of hemolytic anemia (pallor, weakness, palpitations) 3. Symptoms of nephritis (hematuria, albuminuria) 4. Collapse with confusion, dyspnea, weak rapid pulse, cold extremities, clammy hands, diaphoresis, subnormal temperatures 5. Toxicity (CNS stimulation, excitement, delirium)
		Inform client that
		1. Urine may be dark brown or wine color 2. Long-term ingestion of drug may cause toxicity reactions 3. Combinations of salicylates, para-amino derivatives, and caffeine may be more dangerous than aspirin
Antibiotics—Anti-infectives		*General*
Carbenicillin indanyl sodium (GEOCILLIN) Erythromycin (ERYTHROCIN) Kanamycin sulfate (KANTREX) Penicillin Spectinomycin hydrochloride (TROBICIN) Chlortetracycline hydrochloride, tetracycline Minocycline hydrochloride (MINOCIN, VETRIN)	Gonorrhea Syphilis Chancroid Prostatitis Urethritis Granuloma inguinale Abscesses Lymphogranuloma venereum Balanitis Balanoposthitis	1. Check for past hypersensitivity. Hold drug and report if history reveals sensitivity. Mark records appropriately 2. Observe for allergic reaction after administration (anaphylactic shock, skin rash, urticaria). Report and record immediately 3. Have emergency equipment (oxygen, epinephrine) available for allergic reaction 4. If no hypersensitivity exists, observe for therapeutic response (reduction of fever, increased appetite, increased sense of well-being) 5. Observe for fungal infections (black tongue, nausea, diarrhea)
		Inform the client that
		1. The prescribed course of therapy must be continued even after discharge and after symptoms are gone 2. Therapy should only be used under supervision 3. Order must be reviewed ever 5 to 7 days by medical supervision 4. Effectiveness of drug depends upon adequate blood levels. Space administration evenly throughout each 24 hours
Antineoplastics		
Bleomycin sulfate (BLENOXANE) Chlorambucil (LEUKERAN) Dactinomycin, actinomycin O	Carcinoma Penis Testes Prostate Breast	1. Protect client from exposure to communicable disease 2. Use protective isolation and strict medical asepsis, especially when WBC count is below 2000–3000/mm; report any sudden drop in platelets or WBC (indicates a need for drug reduction)

TABLE 20.3 (*continued*)
ASSISTING WITH DRUG THERAPY

CLASSIFICATION	DISEASE DISORDER	NURSING IMPLICATIONS
Mechlorethamine hydrochloride (MUSTARGEN) Methotrexate, amethopterin Mithramycin (MITHRACIN) Cisplatin (PLATINOL)		*Observe for* 1. Symptoms of anemia or bleeding. Report 2. Symptoms of stomatitis (dryness, erythema, white, patchy area on oral mucosa) 3. Symptoms of liver involvement (abdominal pain, increased fever, nausea, diarrhea, jaundice) 4. Edema 5. Nausea, vomiting. Let pass before serving food. Ask doctor to order antiemetic, provide foods liked by the client 6. Symptoms of alopecia and amenorrhea. Advise client these are reversible with termination of therapy 7. Symptoms of bleeding and ulceration of gums. Advise client to rub gums. Provide mouthwashes and a soft, bland diet 8. Symptoms of extravasation of intravenous fluids containing antineoplastic drugs—report at once 9. Enthusiasm of client—share the pleasure of remission
Antispasmodics Papaverine hydrochloride (PAVABID)	Prostatectomy Postoperative urinary distention Neurogenic bladder (bladder spasms)	1. Observe for overdosage (abdominal cramps, fecal incontinance, urinary frequency, asthmatic attacks, substernal pain, decreased blood pressure, atrioventricular block, cardiac arrest)
Sulfonamides Sulfisoxazole (GANTRISIN)	Abcesses Urethritis Lymphogranuloma Venereum Chancroid Herpes	1. Maintain increased fluid intake, even 24–48 hours after discontinuation of drug. Minimum output should be at least 1500 ml daily 2. Drug reactions have been caused by taking another drug at the same time. Question client about drugs being taken 3. Question unusual orders for long-acting drugs 4. Inform client of untoward effects and to report same 5. Observe for side effects a. Blood dyscrasias (sore throat, fever, pallor, jaundice, weakness) b. Serum sickness (eruptions of purpuric spots, limb and joint pains)—starts 7–10 days after beginning of therapy c. Stevens-Johnson syndrome (elevated temperatures, severe headaches, conjunctivitis, urethritis, and balantitis) d. Jaundice (hepatic involvement) e. Renal involvement (renal colic, oliguria, anuria, hematuria, proteinuria) f. Ecchymoses and hemorrhage caused by decreased vitamin K produced by the intestinal flora

Knowing the means of transmission of pathogens enables the nurse to select the methods most effective in preventing the spread of the organisms. For example, pathogens may be spread by *direct contact* when a susceptible person touches an infected person. Pathogens may be spread by *indirect contact* when a susceptible person touches recently used contaminated objects or articles. *Droplet contact* occurs when a susceptible person comes in contact with droplets from an infected person. *Airborne transmission* occurs when droplet nuclei or contaminated dust particles are carried at distances of three feet by air, from the infected person to a susceptible one. Table 20.4 describes nursing interventions that prevent the spread of infection from the reproductive system.

ASSISTING WITH URINARY OUTPUT

As previously mentioned, the close anatomic relationship between the reproductive and urinary systems in the male client is often associated with problems in urinating. Table 20.5 contains a list of interventions that encourage the client to void. Table 20.6

TABLE 20.4
NURSING INTERVENTIONS THAT PREVENT THE SPREAD OF INFECTION FROM THE REPRODUCTIVE SYSTEM

- Use good handwashing before and after each client contact.
- Wear gloves when handling secretions and contaminated articles of persons with active infection.
- Follow hospital policy and procedure related to isolation of persons with known or suspected communicable infection.
- Follow hospital policy and procedure related to the care of bedpans, urinals, sitz baths, dressings, and similar equipment.
- Explain to hospitalized patients the reasons for not loaning or borrowing personal items.
- Explain to hospitalized patients the reasons for not sitting on each other's bed.
- Teach the patient how to avoid the spread of infection.
- Report signs of infection as soon as they are observed.

TABLE 20.5
NURSING INTERVENTIONS THAT ENCOURAGE THE CLIENT TO VOID

1. Increase the fluid intake.
2. Provide adequate privacy.
3. Pour warm water over the perineum.
4. Apply heat, if permitted (hot water bottle, electric pad).
5. Have the client listen to running water, put hands in warm water.
6. Assist the client to a normal voiding position. Stand the male client if possible.
7. Observe the bladder after voiding for distention which may indicate incomplete emptying.
8. Reduce bladder spasms by warm sitz baths, if prescribed.
9. Measure and record each urine output.

contains a list of nursing interventions that favor an adequate urinary output when the client has a catheter postoperatively. Generally, all urine output is carefully measured and recorded.

Some surgical therapies cause the client to experience temporary or intermittent urinary incontinence with frequency and dribbling. Exercises may be done to strengthen perineal muscles and reduce frequency and dribbling. The client is instructed to contract the buttocks and perineal muscles as if attempting to stop the flow of urine; then relax. This exercise, known as Kegel's exer-

TABLE 20.6
NURSING INTERVENTIONS THAT MAINTAIN ADEQUATE URINE DRAINAGE IN THE CATHETERIZED PATIENT

1. Check the tubing frequently for kinks, loops, disconnections.
2. Milk, flush, or irrigate the tube, if obstructed by mucus, small clots, if permitted by physician.
3. Situate catheter over the thigh rather than under the thigh.
4. Administer medications to relieve fear, tension, pain, bladder spasm.
5. Keep the drainage bag below bladder level.
6. Allow client out of bed frequently (as condition permits).
7. Do not clamp the drainage tubing unless ordered by the physician.
8. Measure and record contents in drainage bag.

cise, is repeated ten or more times per hour during the day.

ASSISTING WITH COMMON CONCERNS

As mentioned earlier in the chapter, most patients with a disorder of the reproductive system are intensely concerned about the effect of illness and treatment on sexuality, sexual performance, and reproduction. Impotence, sterility, and urinary incontinence are common concerns at any age for the person with a disease involving the reproductive system. In some cases, the patient is not able to verbalize these concerns but shows behavioral changes, as described earlier in the chapter. When immodest or suggestive behavior is observed, there are several possible responses. One response is to ignore the behavior. Another response is to tell the patient in a matter-of-fact way that the behavior is not appropriate. Another response is to obtain help for the patient from persons specially trained to assist with sexual concerns such as the physician, clinical nurse specialist, chaplain, and sexual therapist. Understanding that the patient's behavior represents serious personal concerns about sexuality enables the nurse to respond in ways that are helpful and effective.

Illness and treatment may temporarily or permanently alter a sexual relationship that is very important to the patient. This circumstance may cause the patient and the partner to experience the grieving process, as described in Chapter 1. The nurse may respond to the grieving patient by active listening and creating privacy for the patient and the partner. In some cases, the patient may be referred to a qualified sexual therapist for assistance in making a successful adjustment in the sexual relationship.

PATIENT AND FAMILY TEACHING

The nurse may include a variety of topics when teaching the client with a disturbance of the reproductive system. For example, many clients do not know the correct names for organs of reproduction and the external genitalia. Lack of knowledge may prevent the client from asking questions or expressing concerns about the illness, symptoms, treatment, and possible outcomes. Thus, early teaching often includes providing the patient with correct names of normal anatomy and physiology.

A second area of possible patient teaching relates to appropriate hygiene. Some patients do not know, for example, how to cleanse the penis and scrotum.

In addition to the usual patient teaching related to planned diagnostic procedures, drug therapy, surgical care, and other aspects of therapy, the nurse may anticipate the patient's need for information about the effect of illness and treatment on sexuality and/or reproduction. Usually, the physician provides this information; however, the nurse may assist by helping the patient develop questions using correct terminology, by asking the physician to talk with the patient, and by translating medical terms used by the physician into language the patient can understand.

Another form of patient teaching can be accomplished by referring the patient to community resources for additional information. For example, Planned Parenthood, Inc., is a community resource which has a wealth of information about contraception. The American Cancer Society may provide information and assistance to the patient and family with cancer. The Public Health Department may provide information and assistance about sexually transmitted infectious disease of the reproductive system.

A very important form of patient teaching is monthly self-examination for testicular cancer, as recommended by the American Cancer Society. Table 20.7 contains instructions on how to do this examination. All men clients should receive these instructions.

Prostatitis

The patient with protatitis has an inflammation of the prostate gland. In some cases, bacteria such as staphylococci, *E. coli*, or *Neisseria gonorrhoeae* may cause prostatitis. In other cases, the cause of inflammation is not known. An acute inflammation of the prostate may become chronic if treatment is unsuccessful.

TABLE 20.7
INSTRUCTIONS FOR SELF-EXAMINATION FOR
TESTICULAR CANCER

Who?	All men
What?	Examination of testicles
When?	Every month after a warm bath or shower
How?	Roll each testicle between the thumb and fingers of both hands to check for hard lumps. Report to physician if lumps are found
Why?	Cancer of the testes may be treated successfully if detected early

ASSISTING WITH DIAGNOSTIC STUDIES

A specimen for urinalysis usually is collected first. Next, the physician may massage the prostate gland to express secretions for microscopic examination. Following prostate massage, urine may be collected in specific quantities for culture. Other studies that may be ordered include urine for cytology and cystoscopy to rule out symptoms caused by cancer.

✳ NURSING OBSERVATIONS

The patient with acute prostatitis caused by bacterial infection usually experiences fever, chills, low back pain, perineal pain, and urinary symptoms including frequency, urgency, nocturia, and burning. The patient with prostatitis from other causes usually experiences voiding symptoms and pain without fever or chills. The nurse should measure the patient's urine output since swelling of the inflamed prostate may obstruct the urethra, causing urinary retention.

NURSING INTERVENTIONS

During the acute stage, the physician usually prescribes rest in bed, an increase in fluid intake, and abstaining from sexual stimulation. Drug therapy may include an antibiotic such as trimethoprim-sulfamethoxazole (BACTRIM, SEPTRA) which the patient is instructed to take for a prolonged period after symptoms subside. The patient with urinary retention may need an indwelling catheter temporarily until swelling sub-

sides. The patient with a chronic condition may be helped by sitz baths and prostatic massage.

Benign Prostatic Hypertrophy

The client with benign prostatic hypertrophy has an enlarged prostate gland. The exact cause is not known. However, it is believed to be caused by an endocrine dysfunction or disorder and occurs in men over 50 years of age.

Enlargement of the prostate gland causes the urethra to become obstructed. Urinary retention, urinary stasis, and residual urine in the bladder lead to infection and back pressure which results in damage to the kidneys such as hydroureter, hydronephrosis, and renal damage, as described in Chapter 19. If the condition continues untreated, the client may develop digestive disturbance, weight loss, and fatal uremia.

ASSISTING WITH DIAGNOSTIC STUDIES

A variety of diagnostic studies may be ordered to rule out malignancy, infection, and urinary tract disorders. Urinalysis, urine culture, cystoscopy, and intravenous urogram are examples of common diagnostic studies. Serum creatinine and acid phosphatase are common blood tests to evaluate renal function and the possibility of malignancy, respectively. *IVP*

In addition, a variety of other studies may be indicated when surgery is planned. Knowing that the average age of the client with benign prostatic hypertrophy is 65 years enables the nurse to understand the need for evaluations of cardiovascular, respiratory, and renal function when surgery is planned. *TURP*

NURSING OBSERVATIONS

The client with an enlarged prostate gland first notices that the urinary stream is smaller and that it is more difficult to start voiding. There also may be a feeling of urgency to void or of hesitancy. There may be difficulty in emptying the bladder because the enlarged prostate gland presses on the urethra. This causes frequent voiding, noc-

30cc balloon

turia, or the inability to void. If the client is not able to empty the bladder completely, the urine left in the bladder is called residual urine. The client may develop pain or symptoms of urinary tract infection, as described in Chapter 19. The nurse observes and measures output carefully to detect and report abnormalities.

In doing a *transurethral prostatectomy,* often abbreviated TUR, the urologist inserts a special instrument called a resectoscope into the bladder (see Figure 20.2). This instrument resembles a cystoscope but has a cutting and cauterizing loop on the end. The cutting is accomplished with a high-frequency electrical current that passes through the loop on the end. The movements of the loop are controlled by the operator while viewing the region through an endoscope. Pieces of the gland are continually chipped away with the instrument while the area is being irrigated. The irrigating solution must be nonelectrolytic because of the electrical current being used. The transurethral procedure has the advantage of not requiring an external incision, and of producing less postoperative discomfort and a more rapid convalescence. However, urethral strictures and incontinence may occur. A Foley catheter is usually inserted postoperatively.

NURSING INTERVENTIONS

Assisting with Catheterization. The client with urinary retention usually is catheterized at once by the urologist in order to prevent damage in the urinary system. Special catheters and/or guides may be needed in order to manipulate the catheter through the obstructed urethra. Occasionally, the urologist is not able to guide the catheter through the obstruction. In this case, a suprapubic catheter may be inserted through the skin above the symphysis pubis into the bladder so that urine can be drained. When urinary retention is severe, the urologist may prescribe alternate clamping and unclamping the catheter to drain specific quantities of urine at a time. This is the only time a catheter may be clamped. Rarely, a client may not be a candidate for surgery to remove the enlarged prostate gland. In this case, the client may have a permanent catheter. Such a client requires considerable teaching related to catheter care, hygiene, and fluids and nutrition.

Assisting the Surgical Patient. Surgical removal of part of the prostate gland is the usual treatment for the client with benign prostatic hypertrophy. The procedure is called a prostatectomy. Although the procedure generally is referred to as a

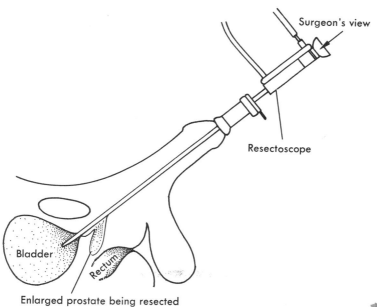

Surgeon's view

Resectoscope

Bladder

Rectum

Enlarged prostate being resected

FIGURE 20.2 Illustration of a transurethral prostatectomy being done with a resectoscope.

prostatectomy, it does not indicate removal of the entire prostate gland as the capsule is not removed. The four main methods of doing a prostatectomy are transurethral, retropubic, suprapubic, and perineal. The selection of a method of operation is specific for each client. Some considerations include the client's physical condition, age, size, and sexual activity. The presence of a urethral stricture also will influence the choice of operation.

When doing a *retropubic prostatectomy,* the urologist removes the prostate gland through an incision made in the lower part of the abdomen. The incision is made into the anterior prostatic capsule. The prostate is incised under direct vision. A Foley catheter generally is inserted. Sometimes a cystostomy catheter is inserted for additional drainage. Tissue drains are brought out through the incision. The retropubic prostatectomy is more time consuming than the transurethral prostatectomy, but the operator can see and control bleeding in the retropubic approach.

When a *suprapubic prostatectomy* is done, the urologist removes the prostate gland through a bladder incision. The incision is made above the pubic region. A urethral catheter is inserted. In addition, a suprapubic catheter usually is inserted through an abdominal incision into the bladder. Controlling the patient's bleeding may be difficult in this procedure. Packing may be used to control bleeding.

A *perineal* prostatectomy is done by removing the prostate gland through an incision made into the perineum behind the scrotum and in front of the anus. After removing the prostate, the surgeon inserts a urethral catheter. A tissue drain or wick generally is brought out through the incision closure. The advantage of this type of procedure is that the surgeon can perform a biopsy on a suspicious lesion and proceed with surgery according to the results of the biopsy. The possibility of urinary incontinence, disturbance of sexual ability, and impairment of rectal tissue may be associated with this type of surgery.

Men who have had suprapubic, retropubic, perineal, or transurethral prostatectomies generally can expect to perform sexual intercourse, maintain an erection, and expe-

rience orgasm. None of the procedures mentioned above involves a total prostatectomy. Crushing a vas deferens, ligation, or prophylactic vasectomy may be done before a prostatectomy to decrease the incidence of postoperative epididymitis and orchitis.

Preoperative Care. The preoperative nursing care discussed in Chapter 6 is appropriate to this client. However, variations in care may be needed because of advanced age. Additional information related to variations in preoperative care associated with aging can be located on page 53–4. Specific attention in the preoperative period is directed toward identifying and correcting fluid and nutritional imbalances, cardiovascular, respiratory, and kidney disorders, and drug interactions.

Preoperative instruction includes a discussion of what to expect after a prostatectomy in addition to the usual instructions related to deep breathing, coughing, turning, exercises, and pain, as described in Chapter 4. For example, the client is told to expect a catheter that drains bloody urine for several days after surgery. The presence of the catheter may cause the patient to experience a strong desire to urinate as well as bladder spasms. The patient also receives an explanation about the need for bladder irrigations postoperatively in order to prevent blood clots from obstructing the catheter.

Preoperatively, the surgeon may prescribe elastic stockings. The bandages or stockings should fit snugly but not obstruct the flow of blood. They should remain on the client postoperatively until the surgeon orders them removed. However, the stockings or bandages should be removed and reapplied every eight hours by the nurse to facilitate observation of the skin, care of the skin, and prevention of possible areas of pressure.

The surgeon describes the operative procedure to the client and family including results expected, possible complications, and the effect of surgery on sexual activity. The nurse sometimes assists by helping the client formulate questions and relating the client's concerns to the surgeon when appropriate.

Postoperative Care. In addition to the nursing care of a postoperative client which was discussed in Chapter 6, this client needs special care from the nursing staff related to the presence of a catheter and/or cystostomy drainage.

The client usually has an indwelling catheter in place when transferred from the operating room. The catheter is attached to the sterile drainage equipment preferred by the urologist, either in the operating room or recovery room immediately after surgery. The catheter must never be clamped. The nurse must remember that the purpose of the catheter is to maintain free urinary drainage. The catheter also makes possible accurate measurement of the urine flow and an estimate of bleeding. The basic nursing interventions for the patient having a retention catheter were discussed in Chapter 19.

The specific character of the urine must be observed and recorded on the client's chart. Thick, bright-red drainage with clots indicates that the client has lost arterial blood. The physician and/or head nurse should be notified. A darker-color drainage resembling red wine may indicate blood lost from the veins. In this case, the nurse may observe dark-colored clots. Irrigation of the bladder may improve this situation.

The client's intake and output must be monitored carefully. The physician should be notified immediately if the urinary output changes significantly and if the Foley catheter is not functioning properly. A sudden cessation of urinary output should be reported promptly. Such a condition could indicate blockage of the catheter with a clot or reduction in output of urine. In general, the urinary output should be at least 30 ml per hour. Less than this for a prolonged period could be associated with renal damage.

Frequent bladder irrigations may be prescribed. The doctor may ask the nurse to carry out this procedure as often as every 10 to 15 minutes. Irrigation of the bladder helps to prevent small blood clots from plugging the catheter or the drainage tube. The procedure varies in different hospitals and with different urologists. However, the procedure should be sterile. The basic equipment necessary is the sterile irrigating solution, bulb syringe, and clean basin for the drainage. The syringe is filled three fourths full with fluid. If the catheter appears to be plugged and the nurse finds a large amount

of resistance when attempts are made to irrigate the catheter, the head nurse or physician should be notified. When doing an irrigation, the nurse should measure the amount of irrigating fluid being used and measure the amount of fluid returning. In the event that an equal amount of fluid does not return, the nurse should discontinue the irrigation and notify the head nurse or physician. If the nurse continues to irrigate the bladder when the return flow is scanty, the bladder may become overdistended, and this may lead to hemorrhage. The bladder should be checked for distention before being irrigated.

In some cases a three-way Foley catheter is inserted into the patient's urinary bladder. "Three way" refers to a catheter with three lumens. One lumen permits urine to drain from the bladder. Another lumen is connected to the balloon in the bladder, which helps to prevent the catheter from being pulled from the bladder. The third lumen is used for the irrigating fluid. This system permits the bladder to be irrigated continuously if necessary. When the continuous drainage is to be stopped, the nurse places a sterile plug in the opening.

The client who has had a retention catheter and who also has had a TUR may have bladder spasms. Since blockage of the catheter frequently causes the client to experience pain, the first thing the nurse should do is to irrigate the Foley catheter when blockage is suspected. However, the client may experience a desire to void even though the catheter is draining well and the bladder is empty. This condition is believed to be caused by the bag on the end of the Foley catheter pressing on the bladder neck or the trigone of the bladder. Suppositories containing medication such as belladonna and opium may be given to relieve discomfort. Narcotics may be required to relieve severe spasms. The client who feels the urge to force the urine through the catheter is advised that this will not relieve the spasms but may even make them worse.

The client with a urethral (Foley) catheter should have the catheter taped to the thigh. Advise the client to avoid pulling on the catheter. The client also should know that the urethral catheter drains because of the force of gravity. Therefore, the drainage bag must be placed below the level of the bladder.

If the client has had a suprapubic prostatectomy, a cystostomy tube or a suprapubic tube usually is present. This tube generally is taped to the client's abdomen and may be sutured in place. In order for the tube to drain properly, the catheter must contain urine because it works as a siphon.

Before the cystostomy or urethral catheter is removed, the surgeon may prescribe an order for the catheter to be clamped on and off. This allows the bladder to regain its tone and resume normal functioning.

The client's dressings are checked frequently for drainage and bleeding. Either of these observations should be reported and recorded. It is important to change soiled dressings frequently, if ordered, to prevent skin irritation and unpleasant odors. Sterile technique is used when changing the client's dressing. When tissue drains are present, care must be taken not to pull them when the dressing is changed. A sterile safety pin may be found on the drain to prevent it from slipping back into the wound. The area around the drain should be kept clean and free from odor. The nurse records the time, color, and quantity of drainage with each dressing change.

An increase of liquids usually is prescribed, often as much as 3000 to 4000 ml per day. When the client is elderly, the nurse carefully observes the patient's respiratory rate and function so that early symptoms of fluid overload can be reported.

Because the rectum is close to the operative area, following a prostatectomy, rectal temperatures and enemas are avoided to prevent bleeding. Mild laxatives or a stool softener such as dioctyl sodium sulfosuccinate (COLACE) may be prescribed to prevent constipation. Other drug therapy may include an antibiotic or one of the sulfonamides, such as sulfisoxazole (GANTRISIN), to prevent infection in the urinary tract.

The retention catheter is removed from four to seven days following a prostatectomy. The client may have some difficulty voiding afterward because of edema of the meatus or urethra. The client also may experience some pain and incontinence. Incontinence, frequency, and dribbling of urine may cause the patient to feel discouraged and frustrated. The nurse may offer encouragement by explaining that these distressing symptoms are not unusual and gradually improve. The client is instructed to continue the increased fluid intake. Each output is measured, observed, and described.

Cancer of the Prostate Gland

Cancer of the prostate gland occurs more frequently in older men. If the malignancy is in an early stage, generally no symptoms occur. In a later stage, the client with a malignancy that presses against the urethra has symptoms similar to those experienced by the client with benign prostatic hypertrophy. In other words, difficulties in emptying the bladder may range from frequent, difficult voiding to inability to void. Cancer of the prostate gland may occur concurrently with benign prostatic hypertrophy. Low back pain or hip pain may be a common complaint if metastasis to the vertebrae, pelvis, and femur is present. The client may complain of pain similar to that associated with sciatica because of involvement of nerve roots. If the pelvic lymph nodes are involved, the client may have edema of the lower extremities.

ASSISTING WITH DIAGNOSTIC STUDIES

Discovery of cancer of the prostate may be made in several ways. The doctor may be able to feel a characteristically hard, nodular gland when a rectal examination is done. For this reason, a rectal examination should be part of an annual physical examination for every man over 50 years of age. An intravenous pyelogram frequently is ordered to determine how much, if any, of the renal system is involved. A cystoscopic examination may be done to visualize the bladder and determine the extent of the tumor. A biopsy of the prostate may be done to confirm the diagnosis. A needle or a punch biopsy obtained through the perineum may be performed for a frozen section to determine if curative surgery is indicated as well as confirm a tentative diagnosis of cancer. A blood test called acid phosphatase level generally is performed. Acid phosphatase is an enzyme that is elevated in 75 percent of the clients with metastatic cancer of the prostate gland. Frequently, the alkaline phosphatase level is elevated when the metastasis is associated with the bone. A Papanicolaou test on the urine may be done. Other tests include a bone scan and bone marrow biopsy to determine if metastasis to the bone has occurred.

TREATMENT AND NURSING INTERVENTIONS

The physician will decide on the treatment of the client with cancer of the prostate on the basis of many factors, such as age, general health, degree of sexual activity, and extent of the tumor. The decision may be to watch carefully the progress of the tumor, use radiotherapy, perform surgery, or use endocrine therapy. Frequently, cancer of the prostate does not progress according to any schedule. Many clients with cancer of the prostate die from other causes. However, this does not mean that individuals do not die from cancer of the prostate. For these reasons, various modes of treatment will be seen.

The physician may decide to remove the prostate gland if the diagnosis is made early enough to offer the client a chance of recovery. A radical prostatectomy generally is done. The prostate gland and its capsule, the seminal vesicles, and the portion of the uretha within the prostate are removed. The surgery may be performed through a retropubic or perineal approach. In doing a radical prostatectomy, the surgeon may make an incision in the perineum or in the lower abdomen and use the retropubic approach. The client will be impotent and sterile after a radical prostatectomy. The client may also have urinary incontinence.

Nursing interventions for the patient following a radical prostatectomy are similar to those needed for other types of prostatectomy already discussed on page 678–87. One variation of this care includes the need for perineal exercises, as described on page 675, to reduce incontinence.

The client may be treated with radiation therapy if the malignancy is in an early stage. Radiation therapy generally will not cause the client to be incontinent or impotent. Nursing interventions for the patient receiving radiation therapy can be located in Chapter 9.

In some cases, the client with an advanced malignancy and metastasis may be treated by having parts of the growth removed, especially if they interfere with voiding. This often is done by a transurethral resection. External radiation therapy may be done in an attempt to reduce the size of the tumor or to relieve some of the bone pain.

Hormones seem to affect certain malignancies. Female hormones may be prescribed to slow the tumor growth. Female hormone therapy may cause the patient to develop engorgement and tenderness of the breasts, nausea, a decrease of facial hair, and voice changes. In some cases, the surgeon may advise additional surgery to remove the sources of hormones. For example, the testes may be removed (bilateral orchiectomy) to remove the source of testosterone. Adrenalectomy (removal of the adrenal glands) and/or hypophysectomy (removal of the pituitary gland) may be done to remove other hormones that contribute to tumor growth. Nursing interventions for the client following endocrine surgery can be located in Chapter 18.

Epididymitis

The client with epididymitis has an inflammation of the epididymis. The original site of infection usually is the prostate gland and seminal vesicles, from which it spreads to the epididymis. It may result from a urinary tract infection, trauma, gonorrhea, syphilis, a chlamydial infection, or as a complication of prostatectomy. The specific organisms causing the condition usually are identified in a urine culture.

NURSING OBSERVATIONS

The client usually experiences pain and swelling in the groin and scrotum. The scrotum may be reddened, tender, and warm. Lymph nodes in the groin may be enlarged and tender. The client may walk with a waddling gait because of the pain and swelling.

Other symptoms of infection the client may experience include fever, malaise, headache, and those related to a urinary tract infection.

NURSING INTERVENTIONS

The client with epididymitis generally is placed on bed rest with the scrotum elevated on a support or on a folded towel. Ice bags may be applied to reduce swelling and discomfort. When applying the ice bag, the nurse should avoid weight that will add discomfort to the patient. When ice bags are applied to the scrotum, they should be removed for 10 to 15 minutes every hour to prevent damage to the tissue of the scrotum.

An appropriate antibiotic is prescribed to combat infection. Aspirin or acetaminophen may be ordered for discomfort and to reduce fever. When pain and swelling subside, an athletic support may be used to prevent pain and promote comfort. Patient teaching includes encouraging the sexual partner to seek medical attention in some cases to prevent reinfection.

Orchitis

The individual with orchitis has an inflammation of one or both testes. This is a serious complication of epididymitis. The condition may be caused by a virus (mumps), bacteria, fungus, testicular torsion, or severe trauma. The primary site of infection generally is elsewhere in the reproductive tract. The male who develops mumps after puberty may have orchitis as a complication. Orchitis may cause atrophy of the testes and, if it is bilateral, sterility.

NURSING OBSERVATIONS

The patient with orchitis usually develops headache, fever, chill, and lower abdominal pain. The involved testis swells and becomes painful and tender.

NURSING INTERVENTIONS

Nursing interventions are similar to those indicated for a patient with epididymitis. A preventive nursing measure is to encourage mumps immunization in persons who have not had that illness.

Cancer of the Testis

The client with cancer of the testis has a malignant tumor in one or both testes. This condition occurs more often in men in their 30s and 40s. The male with undescended testes (cryptorchidism) is more likely to develop cancer of the testes.

ASSISTING WITH DIAGNOSTIC STUDIES

In addition to a complete history and physical, the patient usually has one or more of the tests described in Chapter 19 to evaluate urinary function. Hormone levels in blood and urine also are evaluated. A lymphangiogram may be ordered to detect metastasis or recurrence. The final diagnosis is made when the affected testicle is removed during surgery and examined under the microscope.

NURSING OBSERVATIONS

The patient with testicular cancer usually notices a slight enlargement in the testes which is not painful. The patient also may notice a dull ache in the lower abdomen and groin as well as a heavy, dragging sensation. Often, the patient does not experience early symptoms or ignores them, but seeks medical care for symptoms related to metastases. Common sites of metastases include the lungs, liver, viscera, and bone.

NURSING INTERVENTIONS

ASSISTING THE SURGICAL PATIENT. Surgical removal of the affected testicle (orchiectomy) is both diagnostic and therapeutic. A gel-filled artificial testicle may be implanted during the original surgery or later to preserve a more natural appearance.

Removal of one testicle does not affect sexual potency or fertility. However, if both testes are removed, the patient becomes sterile. The patient who wishes to have children may be referred to a sperm bank preoperatively. Sperm are collected and stored until such time as the client wishes to start a family.

Postoperatively, the patient usually has an inguinal incision, a dressing, and a Foley catheter. Drains may be present if lymph nodes in the area have been removed. Nursing observations and interventions described in Chapters 6 and 9 are appropriate for this patient.

ASSISTING WITH OTHER THERAPIES. Radiation and chemotherapy may be used in some cases. Nursing observations and interventions for the patient receiving either of these therapies can be located in Chapter 9. As previously described on page 677, monthly self-examination of the testicles results in early detection and treatment.

Hydrocele

The client with a hydrocele has a collection of fluid in the membranous sac, tunica vaginalis, surrounding the testes or along the spermatic cord. A hydrocele may occur in connection with an infection of the epididymis and the testes, or it may develop following an injury. However, an individual can develop a hydrocele even though there has been no history of either infection or injury. This condition also may develop as a result of congenital malformation. The client with a hydrocele has an enlargement of the scrotum with or without pain, depending on fluid accumulation.

TREATMENT AND NURSING INTERVENTION

The physician may treat this patient by surgical excision of the sac—hydrocelectomy. The mass then is studied in the laboratory to determine whether it is a neoplasm or a hydrocele. Following the hydrocelectomy, the client has a drain in the operative area. The pressure dressing is applied and the scrotum elevated. A scrotal support may be prescribed during and after the hospital stay. The client should be observed for symptoms of hemorrhage, as bleeding may not be external.

Varicocele

An individual with a varicocele has dilated veins along the course of the spermatic cord. It is more common on the left side. The client may complain of a dragging sensation but frequently has no symptoms.

A scrotal support generally is recommended. If the condition does not disappear, surgical ligation or removal of the veins may be done. The nursing care includes having the client wear the scrotal support and observing the client for bleeding postoperatively.

Circumcision

A circumcision is surgical excision of the prepuce or foreskin. It is still widely recommended for male infants soon after birth and for the patient with phimosis. Some experts believe that circumcision prevents cancer of the penis. The child or adult may be hospitalized for a few hours or days. General anesthesia may be given to the adult. Postoperatively, the incision site is covered with a petrolatum gauze. Bleeding may be controlled by a pressure dressing, which may need to be removed for voiding. The client requires careful observation for bleeding and adequate urine output. The client may need frequent analgesia for several days.

Vasectomy

The client with a vasectomy has a ligation or transection of the vas deferens for the purpose of interrupting the transportation of sperm or preventing recurrent epididymitis. A vasectomy may be performed as a prophylactic measure against orchitis or epididymitis in connection with a prostatectomy. The complication of epididymitis following a prostatectomy can be debilitating, painful, and serious. For this reason, a prophylactic vasectomy may be done in connection with a prostatectomy.

Birth control measures and family-planning methods have influenced the increase of vasectomies during the past few years. The procedure varies according to the surgeon's preference and may be done on an outpatient basis or during hospitalization. The vas deferens may be clamped and cut or ligated laterally with sutures and clamps. Two small incisions are made into the skin of the scrotum below the penis and above the testicles. This procedure does not influence sexual potency, erection, ejaculation, or hormone production. Vasectomy results in sterility which is considered permanent. The sperm cells produced after a vasectomy are short lived, disintegrate, and are reabsorbed by the body. However, sperm remaining at the distal point of interruption need to be evacuated before sterility is assured. A semen analysis is usually done to verify the absence of sperm in the ejaculate.

TREATMENT AND NURSING INTERVENTIONS

PREOPERATIVE CARE. Physical preparation such as cleaning and shaving the operative site should be done. A legal consent must be obtained after an explanation of the possibility of sterility has been made and is understood by the client. A local anesthetic is injected into the scrotal area by the physician.

POSTOPERATIVE CARE. An ice bag may be applied intermittently to the scrotum for several hours to reduce swelling and to relieve discomfort. Scrotal support may be recommended for support as well as comfort. Analgesics may be given to relieve minor aching in the lower abdomen. The client may be advised to avoid strenuous activity for several days.

A period of relaxation and rest may be recommended following the surgery. However, a man generally does not experience any occupational absenteeism. Postoperative complications such as pain, edema, infection, nonbacterial epididymitis, recanalization (spontaneous growing together of the ligated area of the vas deferens), bleeding, and hematoma may occur.

An important patient teaching following vasectomy is the need to continue contraception until the physician reports that sperm-free specimens have been obtained.

Fertility, in some cases, may be restored after a vasectomy by a surgical procedure known as a *vasovasotomy*.

THE FEMALE PATIENT

Structure and Function

The female reproductive system consists of the breasts and the external and internal organs of reproduction, known also as the external and internal genitalia.

The breasts are known as *mammary glands*. Their function is to secrete milk to nourish the newborn. Both sexes have these glands. However, the breasts normally develop and function only in the female. The mammary glands develop at puberty. Some women notice temporary changes associated with the menstrual period. The breasts frequently become smaller after menopause.

Each breast is made of connective tissue, fatty tissue, and 15 to 20 lobes. These lobes contain glandular tissue. A duct leads from each lobe to an opening in the nipple. The nipple is surrounded by dark- or pink-colored skin, which is called the *areola*. The remaining portion of the skin that covers each mammary gland has a color similar to that of the skin which covers most of the body.

Glandular tissue of the breasts becomes active during pregnancy in response to a pituitary hormone, prolactin. This causes the breasts to increase in size and the areola to become larger and darker. A yellowish fluid called *colostrum* is secreted by the glands within the breasts during the latter part of the pregnancy and during the first few days after delivery. This secretion is then replaced by milk.

The external reproductive organs, external genitalia (see Figure 20.3), consist of the anatomic structures viewed when the female patient is in stirrups and prepared for vaginal examination. These are the mons, the labia majora, the labia minora, the clitoris, perineum, urethral meatus, vulvovaginal glands (Bartholin's glands), and openings to Skene's ducts. The internal structures also are identified.

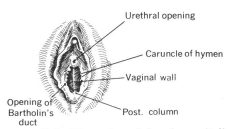

FIGURE 20.3 The external female genitalia. (From Pansky, Ben: *Dynamic Anatomy and Physiology*. Macmillan Publishing Co., Inc., New York, 1975.)

The mons pubis is a pad of fatty tissue covering the symphysis pubis. It is located over the front part of the pubic bone. The mons pubis is covered with hair after puberty. Puberty is the period in which the individual's reproductive organs mature and reproduction becomes possible.

The *labia majora* are two thick folds of tissue that begin at the mons pubis. The outer surface of the labia majora is covered with hair after puberty. The labia minora are two folds of tissue located within the labia majora. The *clitoris* is a small, sensitive organ located at the junction of the labia minora. The *urinary meatus* is located below the clitoris. The opening to the vagina is below the urinary meatus.

The internal organs of reproduction, internal genitalia, consist of the vagina, the uterus, two fallopian tubes, and two ovaries (see Figure 20.4).

The *vagina* is a canal leading from the uterus to the outside of the body. This canal is approximately 7.5 to 10 cm (3 to 4 in.) long and is lined with mucous membrane. The urinary bladder and the urethra are in front of the vagina, and the rectum is behind it. The upper portion of the vagina surrounds the cervix. There is normally a passageway from the vagina through the uterus and fallopian tubes into the abdominal cavity through which ova reach the uterus.

The *uterus* (womb), which is the largest internal organ of reproduction, is a hollow muscular organ that is similar to a pear in shape. The uterus is approximately 7.5 cm (3 in.) long and 5 cm (2 in.) wide. It is located within the pelvis between the urinary bladder and the rectum. Ligaments help to hold the uterus in place. The body of the uterus is known as the *corpus*, and the lower portion is known as the *cervix*. The cervix is smaller than the corpus and projects into the vagina. In other words, the vagina surrounds the lower cervix. The upper part of the cavity within the uterus connects with the hollow fallopian tubes, and the lower part connects with the vagina. Mucous membrane, known as *endometrium*, lines the inside of the uterus. The endometrium is the part of the uterus in which a fertilized egg becomes implanted and begins to grow.

The two *fallopian tubes*, or *oviducts*, are muscular, small, hollow tubes that are approximately 7.5 to 12.5 cm (3 to 5 in.) long. There is an opening from the uterus into each tube. The outer part of each tube opens into the abdominal cavity very near an ovary. The outer end of each fallopian tube is fimbriated, which means that is appears to be fringed. The fallopian tubes are lined with mucous membrane, which is continuous with that of the uterus, vagina, and urinary tract.

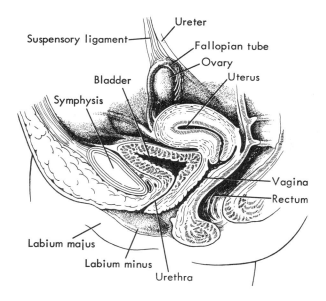

FIGURE 20.4 The female reproductive system and lower urinary tract. (From Keuhnelian, John G., and Sanders, Virginia E.: *Urologic Nursing.* Macmillan Publishing Co., Inc., New York, 1970.)

The *ovaries*, which are known as the female sex glands, are about the size of an almond. One ovary is located on each side of the uterus. The ovaries contain thousands of ova (egg cells). A single ovum matures in the ovary periodically, once a month, and is discharged. The ovaries under the influence of the pituitary gland produce the female hormones, estrogen and progesterone. These hormones not only affect the uterus but also give a woman the secondary sex characteristics of breast development, rounded body contour, and soft skin.

Gynecology is a branch of medical science that deals with diseases involving the reproductive and urinary systems of women. A specialist in this field is known as a gynecologist.

Menstrual Cycle and Menopause

The menstrual cycle is the periodic recurrent changes occurring in the uterus and associated organs. Menstruation is a normal, periodic discharge of endometrium from the uterus. Menstruation usually begins between the twelfth and the fifteenth year of age. However, it may begin at an earlier age or at a later one. The menstrual period usually lasts from four to five days. Menstruation occurs approximately every 28 days, but there is considerable variation in different individuals. In general, each individual tends to have a schedule that is considered to be normal for that individual. The individual schedule may be affected, however, by various emotional stresses and physical illnesses.

One of the many ova begins to mature in the ovary before menstruation. The single ovum is enclosed in a sac known as a *graafian follicle.* Two hormones produced by the anterior pituitary are the *follicle-stimulating hormone* (FSH) and the *luteinizing hormone* (LH). FSH stimulates the graafian follicle in the ovary to grow. It continues to grow until it reaches the surface of the ovary. The ovaries secrete a hormone called estrogen. This hormone stimulates the uterus and causes the endometrium to become more vascular, and this is known as the proliferative phase. The mature graafian follicle ruptures and releases the ovum into

the peritoneal cavity. The ovum is picked up by the fimbriated ends of the fallopian tube. This single cell is carried down the tube by peristalsis and the movement of cilia, which are hairlike projections of the mucous membrane lining the tube. The follicle is called the corpus luteum after it ruptures. The luteinizing hormone released by the anterior lobe of the pituitary gland stimulates the corpus luteum to develop and to secrete a hormone called *progesterone.* Progesterone causes the lining of the uterus to become thicker and more congested with blood in preparation for a fertilized ovum. This is the secretory or progestational phase.

If the ovum, in passing through the fallopian tube, is not fertilized, the body has no further use for the thick, rich lining of the uterus. Menstruation takes place approximately 14 days after the ovum leaves the graffian follicle and enters the oviduct. When menstruation occurs, estrogen and progesterone are at their lowest level. The endometrium, which has become thicker and filled with blood, begins to slough off in the form of a bloody discharge. The menstrual discharge leaves the body by way of the cervix and the vagina. A new cycle begins with the start of the menstrual flow.

Menopause is the period in life when menstruation stops. This period, which is also referred to as the change of life or as the climacteric, usually occurs between the ages of 45 and 50. Some individuals experience the menopause at an earlier age and some at a slightly later age. Artificial menopause occurs after both ovaries have been removed or have been treated by radiation therapy. An individual stops menstruating also after the uterus has been removed—hysterectomy. General changes of menopause are not experienced until later in life when the ovaries stop functioning.

Frequently, the woman notices that the amount of flow with each menstrual period becomes less as she goes through the menopause. However, the periods end quite abruptly in some individuals. In either case, the ovaries stop functioning. The ovaries stop producing ova, and the amount of estrogen is greatly decreased.

Vasomotor instability may occur resulting in hot flashes, periods of increased perspiration, palpitations, severe headaches, and fatigability. Some women may experience a fear of ending a useful life. These fears may be expressed in terms of the loss of the maternal role, marital relationship, attractiveness and femininity, and mental and physical disability. Depression may occur and become incapacitating. This woman needs to be reassured that sexual life need not be influenced, nor is there anything abnormal about menopause. The reproductive organs and the breasts begin to atrophy (become smaller). The vagina loses some of its normal moisture, secretions, and ability to become distended.

The physician may prescribe mild sedatives, tranquilizers, and hormones—estrogen or a combination of estrogen and progesterone. These hormones delay the characteristic sex changes from occurring. There is also the belief that the lack of estrogen in the postmenopausal individual may contribute to the increased incidence of cardiac disease and osteoporosis. Therefore, some physicians believe that these hormones should be given to an individual after the menopause for an indefinite period of time. Some physicians believe use of hormones increases the incidence of uterine cancer.

The incidence of cancer of the reproductive organs seems to increase after the menopause. Therefore, every woman should have at least a yearly pelvic examination, which should include a Papanicolaou smear of the cervix. Breast self-examination should be done monthly to identify any unusual changes.

Assisting with Diagnostic Studies

PELVIC EXAMINATION

The pelvic examination is a fairly simple procedure; however, many individuals tend to be anxious about the procedure for various reasons. Some women might feel embarrassment when the genitalia are examined. Others may have a fear of the results of the examination. Before a pelvic examination is done, the client should void to empty the bladder. The nurse stays with the client during the entire examination and encourages breathing and relaxing exercises. The examination can be more complete and less un-comfortable when the client's muscles are relaxed. The client is most often placed in the lithotomy or dorsal recumbent position. Various types of stirrups are used to support the legs and feet. Adequate draping is imperative with only the vulva exposed.

The pelvic examination includes an inspection of the external genitalia. A clean speculum is then inserted into the vagina to enable the physician to see the walls of the vagina as well as the cervix. The Papanicolaou test is usually done at this time. A digital examination will follow. The physician inserts a gloved, lubricated finger into the vagina and palpates the lower abdomen with the other hand. This examination aids in detecting abnormalities in the pelvic region. A rectal examination usually will be done after completion of the pelvic examination.

CERVICAL CYTOLOGY

A cytologic test is the microscopic examination of any body fluid that contains cells that have been discarded by the tissue through normal scaling. Malignant cells will scale away along with normal cells. The Papanicolaou test is a cytologic test for cancer. Cells in the secretions of the vagina and cervix are studied by a pathologist to detect any abnormalities that may be cancerous. In the past, cells from the cervix and vagina were studied by placing some of the vaginal secretion on a slide. This method has been improved. Now the cervix is cleansed of secretions and some of the cells are scraped from the cervix. The physician uses a tongue-blade-like scraper to remove cells from the cervix and from the posterior portion of the vagina (see Figure 20.5). The cells are immediately spread on a slide. Some physicians insist on holding the slide so that no time is lost. Then a smear is fixed in one of two ways: The slide may be dropped into a solution of alcohol and ether or it may be sprayed with a fixing compound. This preserves the specimen until it can be examined by a pathologist.

ENDOSCOPY

An endoscopy is a visual examination of an interior structure of the body with an endoscope (instrument used for direct visual

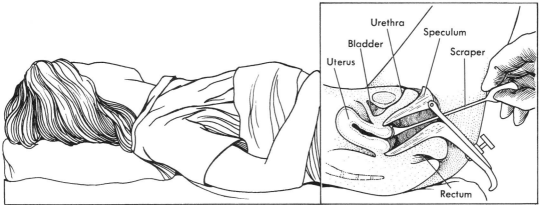

FIGURE 20.5   Pap smear. The physician uses a tongue-blade-like scraper to remove cells from the cervix for later microscopic examination by the pathologist. (Adapted from *Illustrations for Patient Counseling—The Female Reproductive System*. G. D. Searle & Co., Chicago, Ill., 1976.)

inspection of hollow organs or body cavities). An endoscope may vary in design according to the area to be viewed. It has a viewing portion (scope), light, ground cord, and power source. Because endoscopy may be used for diagnostic and therapeutic purposes, the endoscope has a suction tip and pump, forceps for removal of tissue for biopsy, and an electrode tip for cauterization. A variety of endoscopy procedures may be done when the client has a disorder of the reproductive system. Each diagnostic study is named according to the area to be viewed.

Laparoscopy is a type of endoscopy during which the gynecologist visualizes the peritoneal cavity by inserting the laparoscope through a small abdominal incision. The ovaries, oviducts and fallopian tubes can be seen during the examination. This procedure may be indicated for the diagnosis of pelvic pain, infertility, and certain pelvic masses. Laparoscopy may be used therapeutically to ligate the fallopian tubes for permanent sterilization.

Culdoscopy is a type of endoscopy during which the gynecologist visualizes the pelvic organs by inserting the culdoscope through a small incision made in the posterior vaginal fornix. The client usually is placed in the knee-chest position for this examination. Organs that can be seen include the internal organs of reproduction as well as parts of the intestines and rectal wall. The procedure

may be indicated to diagnose pelvic pain, tubal pregnancy, and pelvic masses.

Hysteroscopy is a type of endoscopy during which the gynecologist visualizes the uterus by inserting a hysteroscope through the cervix. This procedure may be indicated to investigate the causes of infertility and bleeding.

Colposcopy is a form of endoscopy during which the gynecologist visualizes the tissues of the vagina and cervix by inserting a colposcope through the vagina. The colposcope magnifies the tissue which permits better visualization than with the naked eye.

Nursing care appropriate for the patient having an endoscopy are similar. The type of anesthesia selected varies according to the procedure. The procedures may be done in the operating room, in the x-ray department, or in an ambulatory surgery center. The nurse observes for abnormal bleeding and adequate urinary output following endoscopy. The gynecologist usually recommends a restriction of sexual intercourse until healing has occurred.

HYSTEROSALPINGOGRAPHY

Hysterosalpingography is an x-ray study of the uterus and fallopian tubes. This study may also be called uterosalpingography. A radiopaque dye is introduced into the uterus, causing the uterus and fallopian tubes to be filled with the dye. The x-ray demonstrates whether or not there is an obstruction in the tubes. This procedure usually is done to aid in determining the cause of sterility. Complications of this procedure include perforation of the uterus, intravascular injection of the contrast medium, and exposure to potentially harmful radiation. Following a hysterosalpingogram, the client may experience temporary cramping, nausea, and dizziness.

ULTRASONOGRAPHY

Ultrasonography is the generation of high-frequency sound waves which are reflected to a transducer. Sound waves are converted into electrical energy, and images of the interior area are formed on an oscilloscope screen. Pelvic ultrasonography is used in the evaluation of symptoms of pelvic disease, to detect foreign bodies, cysts, and tumors, to measure organ size, to detect multiple pregnancy, to confirm maternal and fetal abnormalities, to assist in diagnostic studies (amniocentesis), and to evaluate fetal viability, growth rate, position, and gestational age.

MAMMOGRAPHY

Mammography is an x-ray of the breast when no contrast medium is injected. Mammograms may be ordered to evaluate breast pain, nipple discharge, and/or breast masses. The American Cancer Society recommends that women between the ages of 35 and 40 have a baseline mammogram. After age 50, women are advised to have a yearly mammogram. When the mammogram findings are positive, the patient has additional studies to determine whether or not the breast mass is malignant. The client wears an x-ray gown which opens in the front and removes all jewelry and clothing above the waist for this x-ray.

BIOPSY

A biopsy of any reproductive organ may be obtained for microscopic examination during a pelvic examination, endoscopy, or surgery.

A *cervical biopsy* is the examination of a small piece of tissue from the cervix. This examination may be done if atypical cells are seen when the Papanicolaou smear is examined or if the cervix has an abnormal appearance and the physician suspects cancer. The patient may be placed in the lithotomy position and prepared as for a pelvic examination. The procedure is explained to the patient and she is told there will be no pain involved. A speculum is placed in the vagina and biopsy forceps are used to obtain a sample of the cervical tissue. The sample is either placed in a special solution, usually formalin, or sent to the pathologist. A tampon may be placed in the vagina to control bleeding.

After the procedure, the client should be advised against strenuous exercise for 8 to 24 hours after the biopsy and should rest prior to going home. The tampon should be removed after 8 to 24 hours, as ordered. Any heavy bleeding should be reported to the physician. Sexual intercourse should be avoided up to two weeks. A foul-smelling, gray-green vaginal discharge may exist until the cervix has healed (up to three weeks), at which time normal cervical discharge should return.

Other means of obtaining a tissue specimen for biopsy of the endometrium are the GRAVLEE jet washer and the VABRA aspirator. The physician introduces isotonic solution into the uterus when using the GRAVLEE jet washer and then recovers the solution. The solution with the cells contained in the lining of the uterus is examined. The VABRA aspirator is connected to suction. The aspirator has a plastic chamber in which a specimen from the lining of the uterus is collected. The specimen is then examined in the laboratory.

SCHILLER'S IODINE TEST

The Schiller's iodine test is done on cervical (uterine) tissue to detect normal squamous epithelium. The iodine stains normal squamous epithelium tissue a dark mahogany and fails to color abnormal tissue, which lacks glycogen. An applicator stick is saturated with iodine solution, inserted through the speculum, and stains the cervix. The tissue is removed for histologic studies.

DILATATION AND CURETTAGE

A *dilatation and curettage* of the cervix and uterus is often called a D and C. This is a minor surgical procedure. These procedures are done either to aid in the diagnosis of a disorder of the reproductive organs or to treat certain disorders. The scrapings are sent to the pathologist for microscopic examination. The cervix is first dilated and then the curettage is done. A cervical dilatation may be done to relieve a stenosed cervix, which may be causing dysmenorrhea or sterility.

Since a dilatation and curettage is a surgical procedure, the patient receives surgical care as described in Chapter 6 and on page 696. The patient usually is discharged within 24 hours with instructions to avoid douches, strenuous exercise, and sexual intercourse until the physician prescribes otherwise.

Nursing Observations

CHARACTERISTICS OF THE MENSTRUAL CYCLE

The nurse is often the first person to collect information about the client's menstrual cycle. Data that are important include the date of the last menstrual period (LMP), the length of the menstrual period, the length of the cycle, and unusual characteristics related to flow, pain, and regularity of the cycle.

CHARACTERISTICS OF ELIMINATION

Because the female reproductive organs are close to the organs in the urinary and gastrointestinal systems, a disturbance in one area may affect function in the other. Therefore, the nurse asks, observes, and reports any unusual characteristics related to urination and bowel habits. Additional information on these subjects can be located in Chapters 15 and 19.

OBSERVING VAGINAL DRAINAGE

The nurse is usually the person who assists the patient to change the perineal pad when needed. Careful observation of vaginal drainage is important because the characteristics of vaginal drainage are helpful indicators of health and illness in the reproductive system. *Leukorrhea* is a term that describes whitish vaginal discharge.

Normal vaginal discharge is odorless, nonirritating, thin or mucoid, and clear or cloudy. Some whitish, creamy material is normal. During normal ovulation, the vaginal discharge is a clear, stringy, mucoid discharge. Menstruation produces thin, dark, bloody discharge lasting from two to five days and is 4 to 6 oz. in amount. Following a hysterectomy, the discharge is a bright red or reddish brown which lasts three to six weeks. If a D and C is performed, a reddish-brown discharge may be observed. Following delivery, a red, bloody, mucous discharge is noted for about three days, watery, pink, or slightly brown until about the tenth day, and yellowish-white mucous until about the twenty-first day. It should not be foul smelling or offensive. Table 20.8 contains a description of abnormal vaginal drainage that the nurse should observe and report.

TABLE 20.8 CHARACTERISTICS OF ABNORMAL VAGINAL DRAINAGE	
DESCRIPTION	IMPLICATIONS
Thick, white, cheesy	Characteristic of drainage caused by *Candida albicans*
Dirty, white, malodorous	Characteristic of drainage caused by *Haemophilus vaginalis*
Profuse, watery, frothy, malodorous May be grayish, greenish, or yellow-brown in color	Characteristic of drainage caused by *Trichomonas vaginalis*
Leukorrhea, irregular spotting of blood, malodorous, watery, dark brown	Characteristic of drainages caused by carcinoma
Thick, yellow, purulent	Characteristic of drainage caused by gonococcus

APPEARANCE OF THE EXTERNAL GENITALIA

When bathing a patient, the nurse may observe discolorations, swelling, or lesions of the external genitalia. These observations should be reported to the appropriate nurse or physician so that further action can be taken.

OBSERVATION OF THE BREASTS

The nurse observes and reports abnormalities in skin color, nipple discharge, and appearance. Breast self-examination is described later in this chapter. In some cases, the nurse examines the breasts of a patient who is immobilized or otherwise unable to examine her own breasts.

PAIN

The client with a disturbance in the reproductive system may experience pain either from the disease or treatment. Careful descriptions of the patient's pain lead to more effective measures to relieve it.

Tense pelvic muscles may cause pain during diagnostic studies. Whenever the diagnostic test or treatment involves manipulation of the uterus, a painful uterine contraction may occur. Dyspareunia is pain the patient experiences during sexual intercourse. Postoperative pain occurs when surgery is selected as a treatment method.

BEHAVIORAL CHANGES

Behavioral changes may occur as a result of illness, treatment, or changes in life-style. Changes in reproductive function may cause some women to feel less feminine and less attractive. In other cases, a change in reproductive function may enable the client to meet goals associated with parenthood, career development, or personal relationships. A person who experiences major changes in reproductive function can be expected to show behavior related to anxiety, grieving, and body image. Some clients report a need for increased physical closeness such as touching or hugging at this time. The relationship of self-concept to reproduction, which was described earlier in the chapter, applies to women as well as men.

Nursing Interventions

ASSISTING WITH HYGIENE

Usual perineal care may be altered slightly for the patient with a reproductive disorder. For example, sterile equipment and a disinfectant are often needed for perineal care for the surgical patient. The nurse may wear disposable gloves when giving perineal care to a patient with an infection in the reproductive system.

The physician may prescribe a medicated douche (irrigation of the vagina), to reduce normal flora in the vagina. In some cases, a douche may be prescribed before gynecologic surgery. In other cases, the physician may prescribe a douche to remove unpleasant odors associated with vaginal drainage or destruction of tissue in the reproductive system.

During perineal care, the nurse has the opportunity to provide important patient teaching. For example, the nurse may teach the patient to cleanse the perineum from front to back. The nurse may advise the client to avoid feminine hygiene sprays or douches unless prescribed by the physician.

ALTERATIONS IN FLUIDS AND DIET

In most cases, alterations of fluid and diet are indicated for the patient who has either infection or surgery involving the reproductive system. For example, an increase in fluids is generally needed when the patient has infection. A progressive surgical diet usually is prescribed for the patient after gynecologic surgery.

ASSISTING WITH ELIMINATION

Because the reproductive organs are anatomically close to the urinary and gastrointestinal systems, the female patient may need assistance with elimination. Tables 20.5 and 20.6 describe nursing interventions that encourage the client to void and maintain adequate drainage when an indwelling catheter is present. Special perineal care, according to hospital policy, is indicated when the patient has a catheter.

Congestion in the pelvic area may interfere with bowel elimination. Laxatives, suppositories, and enemas may be prescribed either to relieve constipation or as part of a preoperative bowel preparation for gynecologic surgery. Perineal cleansing is an important part of care after the patient has a bowel movement.

AMBULATION AND EXERCISE

Early ambulation is recommended for most persons with a disorder of the reproductive system. The large volume of circulation normally present in the pelvic area is increased during gynecologic illness and/or surgery. Immobility increases the risk of thrombosis in pelvic veins and veins in the lower extremities.

Intermittent periods of walking and lying down are preferred to sitting positions which increase pelvic congestion. Elastic stockings frequently are prescribed for the hospitalized patient with a gynecologic disorder to prevent venous stasis in the lower extremities. When permitted, leg exercises such as those described on page 120 are also helpful.

Perineal exercises frequently are recommended to strengthen pelvic muscles after surgery. Instructions for these exercises can be located on page 675. Specific exercises to be done after mastectomy are described later in this chapter.

ASSISTING WITH DRUG THERAPY

Drug therapy prescribed for the patient with a disturbance in the reproductive system may include oral contraceptives, other hormones, antibiotics, antiseptics, and antifungal drugs. Many drugs are administered intravaginally.

Often, the nurse provides instruction about how to administer the drugs at home and side effects that should be reported. For example, the client using oral contraceptives is instructed to report severe abdominal pain, chest pain, or shortness of breath, headaches, eye problems (blurred vision, flashing lights, blindness), and severe leg pain in the calf or thighs.

The client on hormonal therapy related to the menopause is instructed to report vaginal spotting, bleeding, and/or postmenstrual bleeding. This client also is instructed

about the need for continuous medical supervision and regular Pap smears while on hormonal therapy.

The patient using intravaginal medication may need instruction about how to measure the prescribed amount and/or how to insert the applicator into the vagina.

MANAGING PAIN AND DISCOMFORTS

The nurse may select a variety of pain-relieving interventions in addition to analgesia. For example, low back massage may be helpful in relieving pain associated with pelvic congestion. Ambulation may be helpful in relieving pelvic pain associated with abdominal distention. Rest and local heat may relieve the discomforts some women experience (Figure 20.6).

PREVENTING THE SPREAD OF INFECTION

Nursing measures that prevent the spread of infection are listed in Table 20.4. These measures apply to women and men clients. The nurse follows hospital policy when disposing of perineal pads and similar equipment. A practice to be avoided is sending a used disposable douche set home with the patient. This practice both encourages the use of nonprescribed douches as a hygiene measure and may introduce pathogens into the patient's vagina.

ASSISTING WITH COMMON CONCERNS

The patient with a disturbance in the reproductive system can be expected to have concerns about alterations in body image, reproductive status, sexual behavior, human relationships, and physical and mental comfort levels. Illness and treatment may either enhance or detract from these areas. For example, removal of the reproductive organs may enhance one patient's life by removing the *fear* of pregnancy. The same operation in another person may result in grieving associated with a lost *opportunity* for pregnancy. Symptoms related to illness or treatment may cause or aggravate problems in the sexual and/or marital relationship.

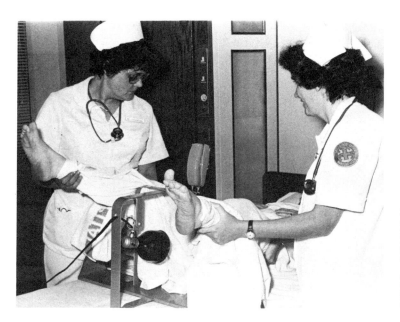

FIGURE 20.6 Perineal lamp provides local heat to relieve pain and promote healing. (Courtesy of Tri-County Area Vocational–Technical School and Jane Phillips Episcopal Memorial Medical Center, Bartlesville, Oklahoma.)

The female client often looks to the nurse to help with concerns related to a disturbance in the reproductive system. The combination of the nurse's knowledge and caring forms the basis for helping the patient address these concerns.

A common form of assistance is active listening. Some patients may be helped to verbalize concerns by the nurse's explanation and description of common concerns shared by others. Another form of assistance is to explain the patient's concerns to others who can help, such as a family member, the physician, or a nurse specialist. For example, a marital partner may be encouraged to meet a patient's need for touching, hugging, and similar physical closeness when sexual relations are not possible. The patient's concerns may be relayed to the physician who often can provide medical help by explanations, special medication, or referral to other specialists. The nurse specialist may provide specific information to the patient and family about how to minimize the effects of illness and treatment on everyday life. A third form of assistance is to provide practical suggestions related to an expressed concern. For example, the patient who feels less feminine as a result of illness or treatment may be helped to comb the hair, apply makeup, or wear a personal item of clothing that enhances feelings of attractiveness. When selecting this intervention, the nurse provides suggestions consistent with the patient's life-style and cultural values. For example, the nurse would not suggest makeup to a woman who does not wear it.

PATIENT AND FAMILY TEACHING

Patient and family teaching includes topics described earlier for the male client such as correct terminology, hygiene, the effects of illness and treatment on sexuality and fertility, and community resources. Every woman should be taught breast self-examination, as described in Figure 20.7.

In addition to these topics, most women benefit from patient teaching related to the use of commercial feminine hygiene products such as sprays, vaginal suppositories, and douches. Secretions normally present in the vagina have a cleansing action. Many women believe that normal vaginal secretions are somehow unclean and should be removed using home-prepared or commercial products. Using these nonprescribed products may change the acid climate in the vagina, remove normal flora, and predispose the patient to infection. Cleansing of the ex-

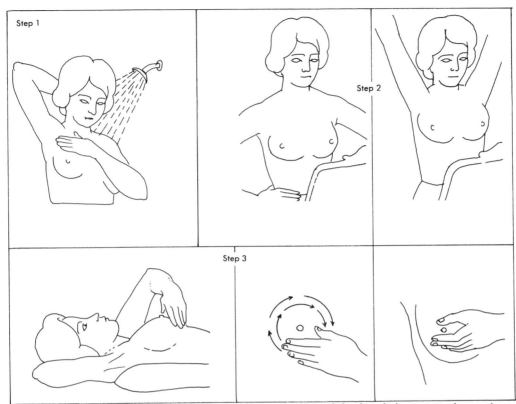

FIGURE 20.7 Breast self-examination. Self-examination of the female breasts each month is recommended by the American Cancer Society as a safeguard against breast cancer. This simple three-step procedure could save your life by finding breast cancer early when it is most curable.

Step 1. Examine your breast during a bath or shower; hands glide easily over wet skin. Fingers flat, move gently over every part of each breast. Use right hand to examine left breast, left hand for right breast. Check for any lump, hard knot, or thickening.

Step 2. Before a mirror: inspect your breasts with arms at your sides. Next, raise your arms high over your head. Look for any changes in contour of each breast, a swelling, dimpling of skin, or changes in the nipple.

Then, rest palms on hips and press down firmly to flex your chest muscles. Left and right breasts will not exactly match—few women's breasts do.

Regular inspection shows what is normal for you and will give you confidence in your examination.

Step 3. Lying down: to examine your right breast, put a pillow or folded towel under your right shoulder. Place right hand behind your head—this distributes breast tissue more evenly on the chest. With left hand, fingers flat, press gently in small circular motions around an imaginary clock face. Begin at the outermost top of your right breast for 12 o'clock, then move to 1 o'clock, and so on around the circle back to 12. A ridge of firm tissue on the lower curve of each breast is normal, toward the nipple. Keep circling to examine every part of your breast, including nipple. This requires at least three more circles. Now slowly repeat procedure on the left breast with a pillow under left shoulder and left hand behind head. Notice how your breast structure feels.

Finally, squeeze the nipple of each breast gently between thumb and index finger. Any discharge, clear or bloody, should be reported to your doctor immediately. (Courtesy of American Cancer Society, Inc. © 1975.)

ternal genitalia with warm, soapy water from front to back is all that is needed, unless otherwise prescribed by the physician.

The woman client also may benefit from instruction related to abnormal vaginal discharge that should be reported to the physician. Any discharge that is a change from that described on page 691 should be reported.

The patient may request information about contraception from the nurse. This very important information is best provided by an expert. Accidental pregnancy may result from incomplete or inaccurate information. Expert resources to whom the patient may be referred include the gynecologist, a nurse specialist, and Planned Parenthood, Inc.

ASSISTING THE SURGICAL PATIENT

Table 20.9 contains descriptions of common gynecologic surgical procedures which may be done when a patient has a disturbance in the reproductive system. Information related to the care of the surgical patient can be located in Chapter 6. This section considers only special features of caring for the patient having gynecologic surgery.

TABLE 20.9
COMMON GYNECOLOGIC SURGICAL
PROCEDURES

PROCEDURE	DESCRIPTION
Abdominal hysterectomy	Removal of the entire uterus through an abdominal incision
Anterior colporrhaphy	Repair of a defect in pelvic muscles causing a cystocele
Dilatation and curettage (D & C)	Widening of cervix and scraping of endometrium for diagnosis and/or treatment
Oophorectomy	Removal of one or both ovaries
Posterior colporrhaphy (perineorrhaphy)	Repair of a defect in pelvic muscles causing a rectocele
Salpingectomy	Removal of one or both fallopian tubes
Vaginal hysterectomy	Removal of the entire uterus through the vagina

PREOPERATIVE CARE. In addition to the usual preoperative care discussed in Chapter 6, psychologic preparation includes one or more discussions among the surgeon, the patient, and the partner about the effects of surgery on reproduction and sexuality. For example, when both ovaries are removed (bilateral oophorectomy), the patient is informed that this procedure results in permanent sterility and artificial induction of the menopause. When a hysterectomy is done, the patient is informed that the menses stops, conception is no longer possible, and the ovaries remain. The nurse may be helpful at this time by assisting the patient to formulate questions for the surgeon and by translating medical words into understandable language. It is extremely important that the patient have complete and accurate information. Therefore, the patient's specific questions about surgery usually are referred to the surgeon.

Additional preoperative teaching includes perineal exercises, leg exercises, and preferred patterns of intermittent walking and lying down already described in this chapter.

Specific physical preparation usually includes a bowel cleansing with enemas and a liquid diet on the day before surgery. Following the enemas, the surgeon often prescribes a disinfectant douche such as povodone-iodine (BETADINE) and/or an antibacterial intravaginal tablet or ointment. Local skin preparation depends on hospital policy and the surgeon's preference. Antiembolism stockings usually are applied as part of immediate preoperative care. A Foley catheter frequently is inserted either in the immediate preoperative period or in the operating room. A nasogastric tube may be inserted preoperatively when an abdominal approach to the reproductive organs is used.

POSTOPERATIVE CARE. Postoperatively, the patient may have an abdominal dressing, perineal dressing, vaginal packing, or some combination of these, depending upon the surgical approach and the specific procedure. A perineal pad may be applied to absorb drainage either from the vagina or indirectly through the vaginal packing. The characteristics and amount of vaginal drainage are observed, recorded, and reported. Expected drainage varies from dark red to pink to serous, depending on the specific surgery. Bright-red blood is not expected and should be reported. In some cases, the number of perineal pads used by the patient during each eight-hour shift are recorded in order to provide a rough estimate of bleeding. Other sites the nurse observes frequently for bleeding after gynecologic surgery are the urinary and gastrointestinal systems. The intestines and ureters are close to the operative site and may be injured inadvertently during surgery. Rectal bleeding and blood in the urine are unexpected observations that should be reported at once.

The patient's elimination is an area of concern to the nurse. During the first several days after surgery, the nurse carefully observes and measures the patient's urinary output. Within 72 hours, the nurse's attention focuses also on whether or not the patient is expelling flatus or has had a bowel movement. Frequent ambulation and sufficient food and fluid intake are positive actions that prevent postoperative abdominal distention and constipation.

Following gynecologic surgery, careful perineal care is needed. The specific substances and technique used depends upon hospital policy and the surgeon's preference. Sterile technique usually is indicated after vaginal and perineal surgery. A heat lamp may be prescribed to aid healing in the perineal area. The lamp should be placed about 16 inches from the patient in order to prevent burning. Other measures already discussed such as ambulation and lying down and leg exercises also are used when caring for the patient following gynecologic surgery.

Discharge instructions should include a list of activities to be temporarily avoided such as driving, lifting, stair climbing, and sexual intercourse.

Menstrual Disorders

PREMENSTRUAL SYNDROME

The woman with premenstrual syndrome experiences characteristic cyclic symptoms such as weight gain, edema, breast engorgement, abdominal bloating, headache, and feelings of irritability, depression, and lethargy. Symptoms generally develop about 7 to 14 days before the onset of menses and disappear with menses. The exact cause of this syndrome is not known. However, cyclic hormone imbalances leading to fluid retention have been associated with this condition. The physician may suggest a mild dietary restriction of sodium and caffeine during the premenstrual period. In some cases, the physician may prescribe hormonal therapy such as dydrogesterone (GYNOREST) to help relieve symptoms.

DYSMENORRHEA

A woman with dysmenorrhea has excessive, incapacitating pain at the time of menstruation. She usually complains of cramplike pains in the lower part of her abdomen. She also may have a headache, backache, nausea, and vomiting. Dysmenorrhea frequently occurs in women with normal reproductive tracts. However, it can result from other factors such as displacement of the uterus, a tumor of the uterus, an endocrine disturbance, allergy, an abnormally small opening in the cervix, and endometriosis. Symptoms of dysmenorrhea may be made more severe by fatigue, cold, and tension.

The woman with dysmenorrhea should consult a gynecologist so that the cause can be identified and corrected, if possible. Treatment of this condition may include measures such as rest, local heat, regular exercise, and reduction of emotional stress. Drug therapy may include a prostaglandin inhibitor such as aspirin and/or hormone therapy with small doses of an oral contraceptive containing estrogen and progestin. Surgery may be indicated to correct a displaced uterus, uterine stricture, or other anatomic abnormalities associated with dysmenorrhea.

AMENORRHEA

A woman who does not menstruate has amenorrhea. It normally occurs during pregnancy, lactation, and the menopause. Amenorrhea can occur as a result of diseases of the endocrine glands, especially those of the thyroid, the pituitary, the ovaries, and the adrenals. Extreme anxiety can cause a woman to stop menstruating. Amenorrhea also may be associated with other diseases, such as tuberculosis, anemia, and anorexia nervosa. A change of climate or activities can cause a woman to miss a number of menstrual periods.

After determining the cause of a patient's amenorrhea, the physician prescribes treatment when it is indicated.

MENORRHAGIA

The woman with menorrhagia has excessive menstruation. She may have a period that lasts too long or she may have a profuse flow. Anemia may result from the loss of blood, which is more than normal.

Menorrhagia may occur from retained products of conception after a pregnancy has ended. Tumors of the uterus, an infection of the uterus, tubes, or ovaries, or a tumor of the ovaries also can cause menorrhagia. A special type of tumor known as a polyp frequently causes this condition. A *uterine polyp* is an abnormal growth of tissue that appears to be growing from a stalk. A disturbance of the endocrine glands, especially in young girls, also may cause excessive menstruation.

TREATMENT AND NURSING INTERVENTIONS

Treatment and nursing interventions are directed toward reducing blood loss and relieving the cause of menorrhagia. The gynecologist may prescribe bed rest to diminish excessive flow. A dilatation and curettage (D and C) may be done to diagnose abnormal conditions in the uterus that may cause excessive flow. This procedure also may relieve menorrhagia caused by bleeding endometrial tissue. Other forms of treatment include hormone therapy (refer to Table 18.5) or surgical removal of the uterus (hysterectomy). Nursing observations and interventions related to caring for a patient having gynecologic surgery can be located on pages 696–97.

METRORRHAGIA

The woman with metrorrhagia has bleeding between menstrual periods. Spotting may occur when the ovum is discharged from the graafian follicle. Metrorrhagia can occur as a symptom of either a benign or malignant tumor of the uterus and should be investigated.

Infections of the Female Reproductive Tract

VAGINITIS

The woman with vaginitis has an inflammation of the vagina, which is frequently caused by microorganisms. *Senile vaginitis* is a special type of vaginitis that occurs in women past the menopause. The woman's resistance to organisms found frequently in the vagina may become decreased after the menopause. These organisms can cause a mild inflammation of the mucous membrane lining the vagina, which is greatly thinned because of a lack of estrogen.

A variety of microorganisms may cause vaginitis. The most common causative organisms include *Candida albicans* (a yeast), *Haemophilus vaginalis* (a bacteria), and *Trichomonas vaginalis* (a fungus). Other organisms such as those causing venereal disease also may cause vaginitis. Additional information about venereal disease is presented later in this chapter. Factors that favor the development of vaginitis include pregnancy, destruction of normal flora from antibiotic therapy, frequent douching or feminine sprays, diabetes mellitus, oral contraception, constant irritation from tight clothing, and nylon underclothes.

ASSISTING WITH DIAGNOSTIC STUDIES

In addition to listening to the client's description of symptoms and vaginal discharge, the gynecologist usually inspects the vagina during a pelvic examination. A smear of vaginal secretions is placed on a slide so that the specific organism can be identified under the microscope.

NURSING OBSERVATIONS

The client with vaginitis usually notices a change in vaginal drainage. The characteristics of the vaginal drainage depend upon the causative organism. Table 20.8 includes descriptions of abnormal drainage. Other symptoms the client may experience include local pruritus, burning, and dyspareunia.

NURSING INTERVENTIONS

Drug therapy prescribed for the client depends upon the cause. For example, metronidazole (FLAGYL) is the oral drug prescribed for vaginitis caused by *Trichomonas*. Both partners may be given this drug since the male may harbor organisms without having symptoms. The patient taking this drug is cautioned not to drink alcohol, since it results in a drug interaction. A vaginitis caused by *Candida albicans* may be treated with nystatin (MYCOSTATIN) vaginal cream or tablets. Ampicillin and/or sulfonamide vaginal creams may be prescribed for the client whose causative organisms *Haemophilus vaginalis*.

During antimicrobial therapy for vaginitis, the male partner is instructed to wear a condom in order to prevent reinfection caused by the transfer of pathogens from one partner to the other.

Medicated creams, douches, or jelly may be prescribed to make the pH in the vagina more acid because this environment discourages the growth of pathogens. The doctor may recommend suppositories containing estrogen for the patient with senile vaginitis.

Patient teaching is an important nursing intervention that encourages successful treatment and helps to prevent recurrence of vaginitis. The following instructions may be given to the client by the nurse:

- Follow the physician's instructions related to the prescribed medication.
- Avoid douches, feminine sprays, and other vaginal products unless prescribed by the physician.
- Avoid wet bathing suits, nylon underclothing, and tight pants that cause friction and increased heat in the vagina.
- See a physician when symptoms appear.

CERVICITIS

The woman with cervicitis has an inflammation of the cervix. Cervicitis may be either acute or chronic. The client with endocervicitis has an inflammation of the mucous membrane lining the cervix.

The infectious microorganism may be staphylococcal, streptococcal, or gonococcal. One of the more common causes of acute cervicitis is the gonococcus. A change in the acid-alkaline reaction of the cervical secretions may promote cervicitis. In chronic cervicitis, various microorganisms may be responsible, such as the gonococcus, *Staphylococcus*, *Streptococcus*, or *herpes simplex II virus*. The patient with cervicitis also may have an erosion of the cervix. In this case, an ulcer of the cervix is present.

ASSISTING WITH DIAGNOSTIC STUDIES

The patient usually has a pelvic examination so that the cervix can be visualized. A smear of cervical secretions is placed on a slide so that the specific pathogen can be identified under the microscope.

Since it is difficult to distinguish between a cervical erosion and malignancy, the physician usually does a Papanicolaou smear and/or biopsy. Colposcopy usually is done so that all parts of the cervix can be visualized.

NURSING OBSERVATIONS

The main symptom experienced by a woman with cervicitis is leukorrhea. The term *leukorrhea* refers to a whitish or yellowish discharge. The amount of leukorrhea varies. Sometimes the woman has a large amount and at other times a small amount. Spotting or abnormal bleeding may be present. In some cases, the woman may have no symptoms of cervicitis. This condition is recognized by the physician when a pelvic examination is done.

TREATMENT AND NURSING CARE

When the patient has acute cervicitis caused by the gonococcus, she will be treated with appropriate antibiotics. The patient with chronic cervicitis may be treated with a procedure known as *cauterization*. This means that tissue is destroyed by applying a chemical or by using electricity passed through a thin blade or a wire loop. In this procedure, the physician aims to destroy the infected areas. The patient should be advised that a grayish-green discharge may occur for approximately two to three weeks after cauterization because of necrotic cervical tissue. The discharge may have an unpleasant odor. Sexual relations should be avoided until the physician indicates that intercourse will not be harmful. Seven to eight weeks generally are required for healing.

Cryosurgery, use of extreme cold to destroy tissue, may be employed. The care of the patient following cryosurgery is similar to that for the individual having a cauterization.

The physician may do a *conization*, which is removal of the eroded area by means of a fine, high-frequency electric current. The patient may or may not be hospitalized for cauterization, cryosurgery, or conization. The nursing care of a patient following a conization is concerned mainly with observing for signs of postoperative bleeding.

PELVIC INFLAMMATORY DISEASE

The patient with a pelvic inflammatory disease has an inflammatory reaction in the pelvis that often affects the organs of the reproductive tract as well as adjacent structures. This disorder is often abbreviated to PID. The inflammation may include the ovaries (oophoritis) and fallopian tubes (salpingitis). There may be pus in the fallopian tubes (pyosalpinx). The peritoneum lining the pelvis, the veins in the pelvis, and the connective tissue in the pelvis may also be affected—pelvic cellulitis.

The cause of PID is usually a bacterial infection. Staphylococci and streptococci can cause an infection after childbirth (puerperal infection) or after a septic abortion. A complication of this may be PID. Gonorrhea can also result in PID. The microorganisms causing the infection pass up the vagina, through the uterus, and cause inflammatory reactions in the sites that have been mentioned. The risk of developing this infection is greater in women wearing an intrauterine device (IUD).

If the infection causing the PID is not eradicated completely, the condition can become chronic. The most serious complication of PID is sterility. Adhesions and strictures can form in the fallopian tubes as a result of this infection. The ovum and spermatozoon therefore cannot unite. An ectopic (tubal)

pregnancy may occur if the sperm, which is smaller, can pass a stricture but the fertilized ovum cannot. Adhesions also can form in the pelvic cavity.

NURSING OBSERVATIONS

The patient with a PID has local symptoms of inflammation that may produce severe lower abdominal and back pain. General symptoms of an infection may be noted, such as fever, nausea, vomiting, and malaise. The patient's heart rate usually is increased. A copious vaginal discharge also may be present. Upon examination, the lower abdomen may be tender, and a pelvic examination is often quite painful for the patient.

NURSING INTERVENTIONS

The patient with PID usually receives an antibiotic or sulfonamide drug such as those listed in Tables 5.7 and 5.8 on pages 91 and 103. The hospitalized patient often receives antibiotics via the intravenous route. Thus, an important nursing intervention is to prevent the intravenous tube from becoming kinked, twisted, or disconnected and to report erythema, edema, and induration at the site.

The patient usually is placed on bed rest in semi-Fowler's position to encourage drainage of infectious material through the vagina. The perineal pad is changed frequently and discarded appropriately to prevent the transmission of infection. Good handwashing, gloves, and disposable equipment are indicated when giving perineal care to the woman with a pelvic infection.

The physician may prescribe local heat to relieve discomfort and improve pelvic circulation. Heating pads, warm moist packs, or sitz baths are the methods most commonly used. Other interventions indicated for a patient with infection, such as an increased fluid intake and a nourishing diet, apply to this patient also.

Surgery is necessary sometimes to free adhesions, drain a pelvic abscess, or remove the damaged organs. Removal of either one or both fallopian tubes is known as a *salpingectomy*. When either one or both tubes and ovaries are removed, it is called a salpingo-oophorectomy. The patient requires care similar to that described in Chapter 6 and pages 696–97 following surgery.

The nurse plays an important part in preventing PID. Careful attention to sterile technique during delivery and gynecologic surgery is one form of prevention. Appropriate clean and/or sterile techniques in the postpartum and postoperative periods is another example of prevention. The nurse contributes to prevention by instructing and encouraging the patient with gonorrhea to complete the prescribed treatment, even when symptoms are not present. In addition, the nurse encourages and explains the need for treatment of the sexual partner to prevent recurrence. Early detection and treatment of other infections such as vaginitis, cervicitis, and urinary tract infection also help to prevent the development of pelvic inflammatory disease. To prevent recurrence, the patient with a pelvic infection usually is advised to avoid tampons and refrain from sexual intercourse until the infection clears.

The patient with PID may experience a temporary or permanent change in reproductive status, significant personal relationships, and life-style. In developing a therapeutic relationship, the nurse uses listening skills to help the patient identify and verbalize concerns. Some nurses erroneously believe that all patients with PID have bad morals. This judgment error may prevent the nurse from developing a helping relationship which the patient badly needs. An accepting, compassionate nurse may reduce typical feelings of uncleanliness and unworthiness in the patient with PID.

Tumors of the Ovaries

OVARIAN CYST

The client with an ovarian cyst has a sac containing fluid or some other material in her ovary. For example, the *dermoid cyst* is a sac containing different kinds of tissue, such as teeth and hair. A cyst can develop in either one or both ovaries. An ovarian cyst

may be benign or malignant. A benign cyst may become malignant. The size of the cyst varies. It may be the size of a small pea or it may reach the size of a grapefruit or even a watermelon.

NURSING OBSERVATIONS

The client with a small ovarian cyst may not experience any symptoms, and the cyst may not be detected by the physician during a pelvic examination. The cyst may interfere with the menstrual cycle, causing the client to experience menstrual irregularity. She may feel a mass in the abdomen or a dull, pressing pain. If the pedicle (stalk) to which the cyst is attached becomes twisted, it causes the person to have a sudden attack of acute pain. Twisting of the pedicle cuts off the blood supply to the tissues below it. This lack of blood to the area (ischemia) results in pain.

The client with a large ovarian cyst may have symptoms caused by pressure on surrounding structures. For example, she may have constipation because of pressure on the rectum and have edema of the legs because of pressure on the blood vessels. The abdomen may become enlarged also. The client also may have a heavy feeling in the pelvis. The abdomen may become rigid, and there may be nausea and vomiting. A cyst may rupture. If the client has a large amount of bleeding, symptoms of shock may be observed.

NURSING INTERVENTIONS

The gynecologist often chooses a surgical procedure such as a *wedge resection* to remove the cyst. In some cases, the entire ovary may be removed (oophorectomy). Whenever possible, a portion of ovary is left in place in order to avoid producing an artificial menopause. However, the woman who has already experienced menopause may have a total hysterectomy. The patient has an abdominal incision and requires care similar to that described for the surgical patient in Chapter 6 and page 696. The patient can be expected to need support for concerns related to an altered reproductive status, possible cancer, or possible recurrence. After surgery, the client usually is advised to avoid tampons, douches, strenuous activity, and sexual intercourse until the surgeon reports that sufficient healing has occurred.

Cancer of the Ovaries

The woman with cancer of the ovaries has a malignant tumor in one or both ovaries. This form of cancer is now the leading cause of death from genital cancer in women over age 50. Women who have breast cancer are more likely to develop ovarian cancer and the reverse is true also. A lack of early symptoms contributes to late diagnosis and a poor survival rate for most patients with ovarian cancer.

NURSING OBSERVATIONS

The woman with ovarian cancer usually experiences no symptoms until the tumor has spread throughout the abdomen. However, the physician may detect a small tumor during a regular pelvic examination before symptoms develop. Symptoms related to advanced disease include abdominal pain, weight loss, abdominal pressure, ascites, intermittent vaginal bleeding, dysuria, frequency, and/or constipation.

NURSING INTERVENTIONS

When the physician detects a tumor during a pelvic examination, the patient usually has exploratory abdominal surgery to identify and biopsy the abnormal tissue. A hysterectomy with removal of the oviducts and ovaries is done when the tumor is malignant and if found early. Chemotherapy and radiation therapy can be used as a palliative measure. ^{32}P can be injected into the peritoneal cavity after the hysterectomy has been done. The nursing care of the patient receiving chemotherapy or radiotherapy, discussed in Chapter 9, applies to this client.

An important nursing measure related to early detection is to encourage all women to have yearly pelvic examinations throughout the life cycle. Even after a partial hysterectomy, the patient who retains the ovaries may develop ovarian cancer.

Tumors of the Uterus
FIBROID TUMOR

The woman with a fibroid tumor of the uterus has an abnormal localized growth arising from muscle cells. Such a tumor is also known as a leiomyoma. One or more of these abnormal growths may occur. A myoma can develop within the muscle wall, on the outer surface of the uterus, or beneath the endometrium. The cause of leiomyoma is not definitely known, but it is thought to be a result of hormonal influence (estrogen and the growth hormone). During pregnancy, the tumor increases in size, and it reduces in size when the pregnancy has terminated. Fibroid tumors are the most common types of uterine tumors. These are benign and occur most frequently between the ages of 30 and 50. These benign tumors rarely become malignant.

NURSING OBSERVATIONS

The most common symptom the patient with a fibroid tumor is likely to experience is abnormal bleeding from the uterus. Menorrhagia is the most common type of abnormal bleeding. Excessive bleeding can result in anemia. The client also may complain of backache and heaviness in the abdomen. Pressure on the secondary organs may produce pain. Intestinal obstruction can occur depending upon the size of the tumor. In some cases, a large tumor may press on structures in the area. This results in symptoms associated with these organs, such as frequent voiding and constipation. A woman may become pregnant if she has these tumors. However, abortion may occur. Birth control pills may cause enlargement of a fibroid tumor.

Diagnosis may be made by palpation, radioimmunoassays of plasma growth hormone and estrogen, D and C (submucous leiomyomas), laparoscopy, and barium enema (to rule out tumors of the large intestines).

NURSING INTERVENTIONS

The gynecologist may not recommend treatment for the patient with small fibroids that cause no symptoms. The surgeon may remove the tumor, *myomectomy*, and leave the uterus in the woman who is young and wants more children. However, the older woman with more severe symptoms usually has a removal of the entire uterus (hysterectomy). The operative procedure is called an *abdominal hysterectomy* when the uterus is removed through an incision in the abdomen. Removal of the uterus through the vagina is known as a *vaginal hysterectomy*. As previously mentioned, removal of the uterus causes permanent sterility and cessation of menses. However, since the ovaries usually are retained when a hysterectomy for fibroids is done, symptoms of the menopause will not occur and hormone therapy is not required.

The client whose condition contraindicates surgery may be treated with radiation therapy to reduce the size of the tumor and slow its growth. A D and C may be done to stop the bleeding and to aid in diagnosing the cause of the menorrhagia. Since radiotherapy stops the functioning of the ovaries as well as that of the uterus, this therapy causes the patient to have an artificial menopause. This type of therapy is used most often for women nearing their menopause who are not good candidates for surgery.

The preoperative nursing care indicated for the surgical patient is applicable to the patient scheduled for removal of the uterus or a part of the uterus. The perineal, abdominal, and anal areas usually are shaved prior to surgery. An indwelling catheter usually is inserted either before surgery or in the operating room. In some cases, a suprapubic catheter is inserted during surgery.

The nursing care of the patient following surgery discussed in Chapter 6 and on pages 696–97 applies to this patient. The patient's output of urine should be observed, measured, and recorded. The appearance of blood in the urine may indicate a complication such as a nicked ureter. Prompt reporting of this observation is necessary. Perineal cleansing using sterile equipment frequently is prescribed. Other nursing interventions related to ambulation, exercise, elastic stockings, and perineal pads, which were described earlier in the chapter, apply to this

patient. Variations in care indicated for the patient following a vaginal hysterectomy may include observing vaginal packing and using a heat lamp and/or sitz baths to promote healing. The patient usually receives specific instructions from the surgeon prior to discharge concerning the gradual resumption of usual activities including sexual intercourse.

Cancer of the Cervix

The patient with cancer of the cervix has a malignancy located at the opening of the uterus. This form of cancer is more likely to develop in women over 35 who began sexual intercourse in the early teens. Other factors linked to cervical carcinoma include recurrent genital infections caused by bacteria or herpes simplex II virus and many sexual partners. Invisible cancerous changes in cervical tissue may be present for five to ten years before invasive carcinoma develops. These changes may be detected by the Papanicolaou smear. If detected in the earliest stage, cancer of the cervix is 100 percent curable. This favorable outlook diminishes considerably after cancer spreads from the primary site in the cervix to the vagina, pelvic wall, bladder, and rectum.

ASSISTING WITH DIAGNOSTIC STUDIES

If cancer is suspected on the evidence of the Papanicolaou smear, the physician usually does a colposcopy which enables the examiner to see the cervix and vagina under magnification. At that time, multiple tissue specimens for biopsy may be obtained. Schiller's test may be done to identify the location of suspicious cells. Conization (excision of a cone-shaped piece of tissue) may be done to examine a suspicious lesion. Other studies may be done as needed to determine the extent and location of invasion in order to determine the appropriate therapy.

NURSING OBSERVATIONS

The patient usually has no early symptoms of cervical carcinoma. Symptoms that may indicate cancer include unusual bleeding or vaginal discharge (leukorrhea) between menstrual periods, following sexual intercourse, or after menopause. In more advanced stages, anorexia, weight loss, anemia, pelvic pain, and fistulas may be present. The nurse who observes these symptoms in a client should report them to the physician. Friends, family, and neighbors who have these symptoms are encouraged to seek medical attention.

NURSING INTERVENTIONS

ASSISTING THE SURGICAL CLIENT. Surgery usually is recommended in early stages. The exact procedure varies according to the stage of cancer, the patient's desire for children, and the surgeon's preference. The patient with carcinoma in situ (confined to the epithelial tissue in the cervix) who does not wish to bear children or who is past menopause usually has a simple hysterectomy. Some gynecologists recommend removing only the area containing cancerous tissue and close follow-up for the patient who wants children. A radical hysterectomy includes removal of all of the reproductive organs as well as pelvic lymph nodes and may be done in more advanced cancer. This patient usually has one or more drains that require additional attention during postoperative care.

The patient with cancer of the cervix that has spread beyond the uterus and the pelvic lymph nodes may have a *pelvic exenteration*. Basically, a pelvic exenteration includes a radical hysterectomy with removal of the lymph nodes from the pelvis. The three types of pelvic exenteration are anterior pelvic, posterior pelvic, and total pelvic exenteration. The decision to do a pelvic exenteration generally is made if radiotherapy has been unsuccessful and if the surgeon believes the patient can benefit from this procedure. An *anterior pelvic exenteration* involves removal of the bladder, a *posterior pelvic exenteration* involves removal of the rectum, and a *total pelvic exenteration* involves removal of both the bladder and the rectum. In an anterior or total exenteration, the ureters from the kidneys are placed in the bowel. If the loop of the intestine is brought out to the surface of the abdomen and a stoma from the ileum is created, the patient will have an ileal conduit. If the loop

is not brought out to the surface of the abdomen, the patient will evacuate urine with stool; or if a colostomy has been performed, as in the case of a total exenteration, she will have a wet colostomy. If a posterior or total exenteration is performed, the patient basically has undergone the removal of all of the contents of the pelvis with the creation of a colostomy. The care of these patients involves the same care given to a patient who has had a radical hysterectomy plus the care given to the patient following an ileal conduit and/or a colostomy.

Radical pelvic surgery does not necessarily end sexual expression. However, both the client and the sexual partner may experience profound changes in interest and frequency levels caused by visible anatomic changes, physical discomfort, and fear of injury. Most clients need closeness and reassurance from the sexual partner. The nurse may provide welcome assistance to the patient and/or partner by listening to expressed concerns and by obtaining expert help for the client and partner.

ASSISTING THE PATIENT RECEIVING RADIOTHERAPY. The patient with invasive carcinoma of the cervix may be treated with radiation therapy. Radiation can be done in two different ways: (1) external or (2) internal. When doing internal radiation, the physician uses radium, radioactive cobalt, or iridium. Sometimes both internal and external radiation will be used. The patient who is treated with internal radiation goes to the operating room, where the cervix is dilated and an applicator with radium tubes is placed into the uterus. The surgeon usually places packing around the applicator to keep it in place.

The patient scheduled for internal radiation therapy usually has a preoperative enema and douche. Postoperatively, the patient usually is restricted to lying on her side or back with the head slightly elevated. A low-residue diet may be ordered because a strain when having a bowel movement could displace the radium implant. The nurse should watch for the signs of radiation sickness discussed in Chapter 9. The position of the applicator should be noted by the nurse. The patient has a urinary catheter in place, and the nurse must check the output frequently. If the patient complains of a full feeling in her bladder, has an unexplained decrease in urinary output, or has a leakage around the catheter, these symptoms should be reported promptly to the nurse in charge and/or the physician. The patient with urinary drainage is at increased risk to sustain overexposure of the bladder to high-dose radiation.

Additional information about nursing interventions appropriate when caring for the patient receiving radiotherapy can be located in Chapter 9. Radiation therapy seems to produce a more negative impact on sexual activity than other forms of treatment. Nursing interventions described for the client with sexual concerns related to surgery apply to the client receiving radiation therapy also.

Cancer of the Endometrium

The woman with cancer of the endometrium has a malignancy of the mucous membrane lining the corpus (body) of the uterus. This type of cancer occurs more often after menopause. Factors linked to endometrial cancer include infertility, late menopause (after age 55), obesity, diabetes, hypertension, and long-term diethylstilbesterol (DES) therapy. The patient often experiences bleeding between menstrual periods or bleeding after menopause initially. Usually, the pathologist diagnoses the client's cancer from tissue samples obtained during a dilatation and curettage. The patient usually has intracavity radiation first, followed by a total hysterectomy and bilateral salpingo-oophorectomy. In later stages, external radiation may be added to the treatment plan. Nursing interventions related to these forms of therapy can be located on pages 233–35 and in Chapter 9.

Cancer of the Vulva

The patient with cancer of the vulva has a malignancy involving the external organs of reproduction. This form of cancer occurs in a small percentage of women between the ages of 50 and 70. Early detection and treatment of localized lesions result in a higher

five-year survival rate. The diagnosis is usually made by the pathologist by examining tissue samples obtained from a punch biopsy with or without colposcopy.

NURSING OBSERVATIONS

A precancerous lesion, known as *leukoplakia*, may be observed on the external genitalia when giving perineal care. Leukoplakia is a white, thickened, plaque type of lesion which may ulcerate. The nurse who observes this or any other lesion on the external genitalia should report it so that further investigation can be started. The patient may also experience vaginal discharge, pruritus, and bleeding.

NURSING INTERVENTIONS

The patient usually has a surgical procedure which is selected according to the size of the lesion and extent of involvement. A simple vulvectomy involves removing leukoplakia and resection of the vulva. When lesions are identified as cancerous by the pathologist, the surgeon usually does a radical vulvectomy. This procedure includes excision of the inguinal lymph nodes as well as a wide margin of tissue around the malignant tumor. Plastic surgery usually is needed following this extensive surgery. Care of the client is influenced by a drastic alteration in the appearance of the perineum, characteristic slow healing, the need for bed rest during healing, and the hazard of infection.

Preoperatively, the patient practices changing positions slightly, range-of-motion exercises, leg exercises, and deep breathing. The patient may have questions about the effects of surgery on sexuality. In most cases, this surgery does not interfere with reproduction, sexual interest, or sexual response once healing is complete. The patient usually receives a preoperative enema and extensive local skin preparation. An indwelling catheter also may be inserted. More often, however, the client has a suprapubic catheter inserted during surgery.

Postoperatively, the patient usually has one or more wound catheters, each connected to HEMOVAC suction. The wound may be either left open or covered by a dressing held in place by a T-binder. Wound care may include meticulous cleansing by the nurse and a heat lamp prescribed by the physician. A new sterile setup is used for each wound site to be cleansed.

The patient usually is placed in a low Fowler's position to avoid discomfort caused by sitting on the operative site. The usual postoperative exercise and turn schedule is maintained.

After recovering from anesthesia, the patient may be placed on a low-residue diet to avoid disturbances in bowel function such as constipation or diarrhea. The patient who is constipated may place undesirable pressure on the sutures. The patient with diarrhea is at risk to develop a wound infection from fecal contamination. Carefully cleansing of the anal area is needed after each bowel movement.

Drug therapy usually includes antibiotics to prevent infection and analgesics for pain. Since pain often lasts longer after this surgical procedure, the nurse is challenged to select a variety of pain-relieving measures in addition to analgesia.

The physician also may treat the patient with radiotherapy or chemotherapy. Although surgery may be the treatment of choice, other treatments may be instituted, especially if the malignancy has spread or if the patient is unable to withstand surgery.

Endometriosis

The client with endometriosis has a progressive condition in which patches of endometrium are distributed outside the uterus. As described earlier, the endometrium is the mucous membrane lining the uterus. The patient with endometriosis may have patches of endometrium in the ovaries, fallopian tubes, uterosacral ligaments, bladder, intestines, rectum, and/or pelvic wall. These displaced patches of endometrium are influenced by hormones as is uterine endometrium and therefore proliferate and bleed. When the ovary contains displaced endometrium, cyclic bleeding causes the formation of masses known as chocolate cysts because of their typical color. Bleeding in areas outside the uterus results in an inflammatory reaction. This, in turn, may cause adhesions

and subsequent sterility. The cause of this condition is unknown. Women in the reproductive years are affected. After menopause, the displaced endometrium usually atrophies because there are no hormones to cause proliferation and bleeding.

NURSING OBSERVATIONS

The client frequently reports progressive dysmenorrhea and pelvic pain. Dyspareunia, abnormal uterine bleeding, lower abdominal and back pain are other common symptoms. There may be bowel and/or bladder symptoms if those organs are affected. Pregnancy, lactation, and menopause usually relieve symptoms since the endometrium does not normally proliferate or bleed during those times.

In some cases, the client may have no painful symptoms, but the condition is discovered during an investigation of infertility. Should a chocolate cyst rupture, the symptoms are quite similar to those of appendicitis or a ruptured ectopic pregnancy.

NURSING INTERVENTIONS

Because a woman is in her reproductive years during the course of endometriosis, the treatment usually is directed toward relieving the symptoms and preserving the reproductive organs. The client who desires children is advised to become pregnant as soon as possible after marriage because endometriosis often results in sterility. There are two methods of treatment: hormonal and surgical.

Hormone therapy is directed toward producing a pseudopregnancy (false pregnancy), the result being a nonbleeding endometrium. Birth control pills such as norethynodrel (ENOVID) and norethindrone (ORTHO-NOVUM) are given to produce the pseudopregnancy. The client may take these drugs for months, and it is hoped that when they are discontinued, the endometrium will function more normally. Because the drugs are given in large doses, symptoms of early pregnancy may occur. These symptoms are nausea and vomiting, tender breasts, and weight gain. Bleeding from the endometrium also may occur. Despite these possible side effects, the client usually feels much better with the symptoms relieved. The client receiving hormone therapy usually is not seen in the hospital but is treated on an outpatient basis.

Surgery may be required in endometriosis to loosen adhesions, to remove cysts, and to remove the patches of bleeding endometrium. However, if the endometriosis and/or adhesions and cysts are severe, removal of the uterus, fallopian tubes, and ovaries may be required. Nursing interventions for the surgical patient, described in Chapter 6, apply to this client.

Vaginal Fistula

The client with a vaginal fistula has an abnormal canal leading from the vagina to the ureter (ureterovaginal fistula), bladder (vesicovaginal fistula), or rectum (rectovaginal fistula). A fistula may form due to tissue damage as a result of cancer or internal radiation therapy to the uterus. A fistula also can occur after injury during childbirth or after surgery of the reproductive organs.

NURSING OBSERVATIONS

Ureterovaginal and vesicovaginal fistulae result in constant leaking of urine from the vagina. As a result of the constant irritation to the vagina by the urine, the tissue often becomes excoriated and an infection can result. A rectovaginal fistula causes flatus and feces to pass through the vagina. This contamination easily causes a bad odor and infection. The nurse who notices these situations should report them at once to the head nurse or physician.

NURSING INTERVENTIONS

Surgery is the treatment for fistulae that do not close of their own accord. However, the inflammation and infection must be treated and should have subsided before surgical repair is possible. A lengthy preoperative period of weeks or months may be needed. The patient may be hospitalized to learn the procedures and then be discharged to carry them out at home.

The preoperative treatment to decrease the infection may include douches (often sterile), perineal care, enemas, sitz baths, and a heat lamp. For a rectovaginal fistula, an antibiotic (see Table 20.3) may be given to rid the bowel of bacteria. The resulting infection of the vagina then will be treated. A deodorizing douche may be required for a rectovaginal fistula. A mild solution of CLOROX may help in eliminating the odor. A nourishing diet and increased fluid intake are usually prescribed.

After surgical repair of a vesicovaginal fistula, the patient usually has a retention catheter. An increased fluid intake is a very important part of postoperative care. Special wound care using sterile technique may be prescribed by the surgeon, including perineal care and/or a heat lamp. All nursing interventions that involve the operative area are performed very gently to avoid undue stress and strain to the repair. The usual postoperative nursing observations and interventions, such as increasing the fluid intake, measuring intake and output, exercise and ambulation, and observing for excess vaginal bleeding, apply to this patient.

A temporary colostomy may be done along with the repair of a rectovaginal fistula. The colostomy prevents contamination of the operative site with feces. The nursing care of the patient with a colostomy is discussed in Chapter 15. If a colostomy is not done, the patient is often on a clear liquid diet for several days postoperatively. The diet progresses slowly to a low-residue diet and eventually to a general diet. The operative site and external genitalia are kept clean with perineal care, and a heat lamp may be ordered to promote healing and relieve discomfort.

The patient with a vaginal fistula has been affected emotionally. The smell of urine and feces may be hard to control, and, as a result, she may withdraw from social as well as family contacts. Friends and family also may withdraw from the client, resulting in feelings of uncleanliness, loneliness, and isolation. The nurse makes every effort to convey acceptance, warmth, and compassion for the client and the family. These attitudes may be conveyed by active listening, gentle touching of the client's body during care, and assistance in hygiene and grooming. Visiting the client at times when physical care is not needed conveys an interest and concern that goes beyond physical aspects of care.

Not all surgical repairs for fistulae are successful, and some fistulae cannot be repaired. If this is the case, frequent deodorizing sitz baths and douches may be done to control infection and reduce odor. A perineal pad and protective pants may have to be worn to protect the clothing. High enemas to rid the bowel of fecal material help to prevent a bad odor and fecal discharge. These patients are often depressed and withdrawn. The nurse can assist the patient with care if necessary and help her to become clean and presentable to others.

Relaxed Pelvic Muscles

The muscles and tissues of the pelvis normally lose their tone as age progresses. The tissue may relax as a result of childbirth without repair of the perineum or as a result of multiple deliveries. Some degree of pelvic muscle relaxation is a common disorder of older women.

PROLAPSE OF THE UTERUS

The client with a prolapse of the uterus has a uterus that has slipped down below its normal level. There are three degrees of prolapse. In a first-degree prolapse, the cervix is low but remains within the vagina. A second-degree prolapse means the cervix is at the vaginal opening. A third-degree prolapse means the cervix hangs outside the body. The patient may also have a cystocele or a rectocele.

NURSING OBSERVATIONS

The client may report a feeling of heaviness in the lower abdomen and a backache which is aggravated by standing. Stress incontinence, dyspareunia, and constipation also may be present. The nurse may observe the displacement of the cervix into the vagina when giving perineal care or inserting a catheter. These observations should be reported.

NURSING INTERVENTIONS

Surgery may be indicated to correct uterine prolapse. The client beyond childbearing years usually has a vaginal hysterectomy and repair of surrounding tissue. Another method of surgical repair is resuspension of the uterus. The patient requires the usual postoperative nursing care with special attention to the prevention of constipation because straining may damage the surgical repair. A mild laxative may be prescribed, along with ambulation, increased fluid intake, and a balanced diet.

A *pessary* may be prescribed for the patient whose condition is not suitable for surgery. A vaginal pessary is a ring-shaped device that is fitted to the cervix and holds the uterus in place. When inserted and correctly fitted, the client does not experience any discomfort. Since this foreign object often causes an inflammatory response, the patient usually receives instructions to douche regularly to remove inflamed material. An important client teaching is the need for regular follow-up examinations to check on the placement of the pessary and for excessive irritation. Difficulty voiding, a return of symptoms, and leukorrhea are problems the patient should report at once to the gynecologist.

CYSTOCELE

The patient with a cystocele has a prolapse of the urinary bladder into the vagina which generally results from injury during childbirth.

NURSING OBSERVATIONS

The client usually reports passing a small amount of urine when coughing, sneezing, or laughing. This condition is called stress incontinence. Other urinary symptoms the patient may experience include frequency, urgency, and incomplete emptying of the bladder. Residual urine in the bladder may cause the client to develop cystitis.

NURSING INTERVENTIONS

Anterior colporrhaphy is a surgical procedure that includes a repair of the defect in pelvic muscles and return of the bladder to a normal position. The client receives the usual postoperative perineal care. A heat lamp may be prescribed. Special attention is directed toward urinary output, maintaining a patent Foley catheter, and increasing the fluid intake. The client is encouraged to perform perineal exercises, as described earlier in the chapter. After the catheter is removed, the client is encouraged to continue the exercises and drink sufficient fluids to urinate frequently. A catheterization for residual urine may be ordered postoperatively to check for incomplete emptying of the bladder. The client is instructed to avoid sexual intercourse, lifting, straining, prolonged periods of standing, sitting, or walking until the surgeon determines that adequate healing has occurred.

RECTOCELE

A woman with a rectocele has a bulging of the rectum into the vagina. This condition generally is caused by injury to the muscles of the perineum during childbirth.

NURSING OBSERVATIONS

The patient with a rectocele may complain of a backache and constipation. She also may have hemorrhoids.

NURSING INTERVENTIONS

Nursing interventions are related to the surgical repair of the client's weakened tissues. This operation is known as a *posterior colporrhaphy*. It also may be called a *perineorrhaphy*. A cystocele and rectocele can occur at the same time. Frequently, a woman with a rectocele has a cystocele or a prolapsed uterus. An anterior and posterior colporrhaphy may be performed at the same time. A vaginal hysterectomy also may be done. If the pelvic floor and perineum are weak, a perineorrhaphy may be done. This procedure is a repair of the old tears in the perineum that occurred during childbirth.

Preoperatively, a patient who is to have a posterior colporrhaphy usually has enemas to empty the bowel.

After the surgical procedure, the nursing care of a patient having posterior colporrhaphy is similar to that after an anterior colporrhaphy. Clear liquids or a low-residue diet may be given for a longer period of time to prevent defecation. Stool softeners (see Table 15.7) such as dioctyl sodium sulfosuccinate (COLACE), mineral oil, and oil-retention enemas may be ordered to prevent constipation. Some doctors advise the patient to exercise the muscles of the perineum by trying to close the gap between the buttocks. Patient teaching is similar to that following anterior colporrhaphy.

Retroversion of the Uterus

A woman with retroversion of the uterus has a backward displacement of it. In other words, the uterus is tilted backward. Another type of uterine displacement is antiflexion (forward displacement of the uterus). This condition may be present at birth or may develop as a result of injury, surgery, childbirth, or endometriosis.

NURSING OBSERVATIONS

The patient with retroversion of the uterus frequently has no symptoms. However, she may have dysmenorrhea, backache, dyspareunia, or infertility.

NURSING INTERVENTIONS

The client who is asymptomatic usually is not treated. The client with symptoms may be treated with a temporary vaginal pessary to hold the uterus in a normal position. Nursing interventions related to this treatment method have already been described on page 708.

In some cases, the physician recommends that the client assume the knee-chest position for portions of each day. Occasionally, the client may have a surgical procedure during which the uterus is resuspended in the pelvic cavity. Nursing observations and interventions are similar to those indicated for a client having abdominal surgery.

Breast Conditions
CANCER

The client with cancer of the breast has a malignancy of one or both breasts. Breast cancer is the most common of all cancers in women between the ages of 25 and 75. Although it is more common in women over 40 years of age, cancer of the breast can develop at any age. It also may occur in men, although this is rare.

removal of the breast and nipple. A *modified radical mastectomy* involves removal of the breast, the pectoral fascia, and lymph nodes of the axilla. A *radical mastectomy* involves the removal of the breast, pectoral muscles, and lymph nodes of the axilla. An *extended radical mastectomy* includes the radical mastectomy with removal of a portion of the sternum, ends of the ribs, and the internal mammary lymph nodes. Experimental surgical procedures currently under investigation include partial mastectomy and lumpectomy. A variety of reconstructive mammoplasty procedures using skin grafts and silicone implants are also available to some women following mastectomy.

Preoperative Care. In addition to the usual preoperative care described in Chapter 6, the client has several discussions with the surgeon about the surgery and expected results. Also, during this time, the client and her husband, partner, or family member often need time and privacy to share thoughts and feelings about impending surgery. The client may experience anticipatory grieving over the loss of an important and valued body part. As mentioned in Chapter 9, the client often begins treatment for neoplasm while still in denial. The client may or may not want to express these fears and concerns to the nurse. The nurse tries to reduce any additional fear and anxiety by explaining all activities and procedures in advance. Repetition of information and instructions may be needed when the client's anxiety level is high. Postmastectomy exercises such as those illustrated in Figure 20.8 are taught in advance so that the client has time to practice.

POSTOPERATIVE CARE

OPERATIVE AREA. In addition to the usual postoperative care described in Chapter 6, the patient's dressing should be checked frequently during the early postoperative period. The color, approximate amount of drainage, consistency, and odor should be observed and recorded. Bloody drainage in the immediate postoperative period gradually becomes serous.

The patient may have a drain inserted in the operative area for drainage of excess fluid. In some cases, the drain is attached to low-pressure suction such as the HEMOVAC. A pressure dressing may be used during the immediate postoperative period. However, the surgeon generally tries to allow for arm movement as soon as possible.

The patient's dressing, in addition to the discomfort from surgery, may cause her to avoid taking deep breaths. The patient must be encouraged to breathe deeply and cough at frequent intervals and to change position to aid in the prevention of pulmonary complications. The dressing helps to support the incision so that coughing is less painful. The patient should be told this also. The patient with an extended radical mastectomy has a chest tube. Care of the patient with a chest tube as discussed in Chapter 14 is applicable in this situation.

After the dressing has been removed, the patient needs to care for the area. Gentle washing with mild soap, warm water, and a soft washcloth is encouraged. Gently rubbing cold cream or petroleum jelly into the healed scar may be beneficial. When possible, the patient is encouraged to see the incision before leaving the hospital while she has the support of the health team to make an initial adjustment to the change. Members of the nursing staff should be receptive listeners when the patient needs to express feelings and/or fears. Visits from a person who has recovered from a radical mastectomy, such as a member of the local Reach to Recovery Society, may be of invaluable assistance to the patient.

POSITION AND CARE OF ARM. During a radical mastectomy, the surgeon, as stated earlier removes the lymph nodes in the axilla. Removal of these may cause the patient to have lymphedema in that arm since the lymph drains through these nodes. In order to reduce this possibility, the patient's arm and hand may be elevated above the heart on one or more pillows after surgery.

In some cases, the surgeon may immobilize the arm during the immediate postoperative period by bandaging it to the body. This may be especially helpful when the pa-

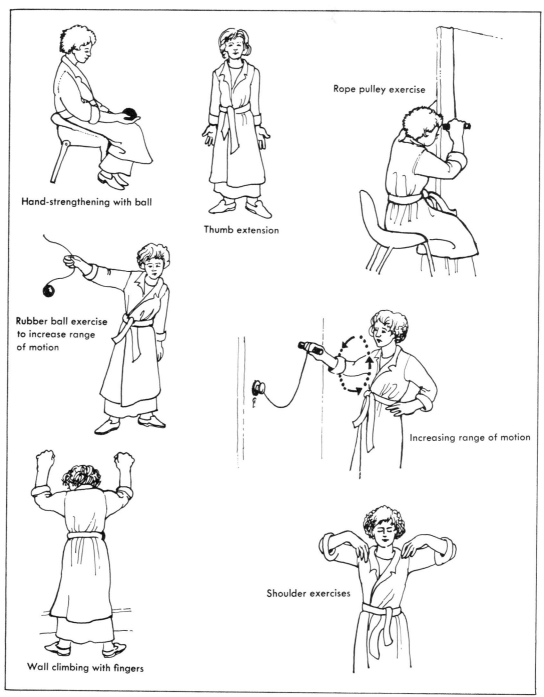

Hand-strengthening with ball

Thumb extension

Rope pulley exercise

Rubber ball exercise to increase range of motion

Increasing range of motion

Wall climbing with fingers

Shoulder exercises

FIGURE 20.8 Exercises following a mastectomy. (Courtesy of American Cancer Society, Inc.)

tient has had a skin graft. When the arm is bandaged to the body, the patient's hands should be checked for symptoms of disturbed circulation, such as paleness, swelling, cyanosis, tingling, and coldness. These symptoms should be reported promptly.

If the lymph nodes of the axilla have been removed, the patient's arm should not be used for venipunctures, injections, intravenous needles, or blood pressures. This is done in an attempt to avoid lymphedema and infections. The patient should know that the axillary lymph nodes have been removed and the implications. In other words, she needs to know that she should not have an injection in that arm and that the blood pressure should not be measured in that arm. The patient also needs to be aware of the importance of avoiding burns and infections on that extremity. For example, a thimble should be used when sewing and a padded glove when removing anything from the oven.

EXERCISES. The surgeon indicates when the patient's arm can be moved and when active exercises should begin. In caring for the patient after a skin graft or an extended radical mastectomy, the nurse should receive specific instructions before beginning exercises of the arm (see Figure 20.8). Perhaps one of the earliest exercises is the opening and closing of the hand on the affected side. A planned program of progressive exercises designed to enable the patient to perform the same functions with the affected arm that she did before surgery should be initiated. In some hospitals, the physical therapist plans the exercises and solicits the cooperative efforts of the patient and the nursing staff to carry them out. In other agencies, the nursing staff may have much of this responsibility.

Exercise to prevent limitation of motion of the shoulder on the affected side is encouraged. At the beginning, the patient may need considerable encouragement and assistance from members of the nursing staff. Using the hand of the affected side to comb her hair is encouraged as an early exercise. The patient should be encouraged to abduct the arm of the affected side and swing it in a circular manner. Another exercise fre-

quently recommended by the doctor or physical therapist is to have the patient walk the fingers up and down the wall. In doing this, the patient stands within reach of a wall and moves the fingers stepwise up the wall as far as possible and then repeats the procedure downward. Information regarding appropriate exercises, which must be approved by the patient's physician, can be obtained from the local cancer society. This information is especially helpful when the services of a physical therapist are not available.

The American Cancer Society conducts a program called Reach for Recovery. This program provides volunteer guidance from individuals who have had mastectomies, suggestions about exercise and prostheses, and other information helpful to the patient and the family. Educational pamphlets are also available for this purpose. The American Cancer Society recommends exercises such as ball throwing, rope pulling, and walking the wall with fingers as in Figure 20-8.

LYMPHEDEMA. After recovering from a mastectomy with an axillary node dissection, the patient should try to avoid injuring or irritating that arm. The reason for this is that an infection may lead to the complication of lymphedema.

The patient with lymphedema has swelling of the subcutaneous tissue of her hand and arm caused by an excessive amount of lymph fluid. An elastic sleeve or bandaging the arm with an ACE bandage may help to reduce lymphedema. In some cases a special air-pressure machine with a sleeve is used. The patient's arm is placed in the sleeve, which is automatically filled with air and exerts alternating pressure on the fingers, wrist, and arm. This pressure forces fluid through the lymphatic system.

PROSTHETIC FORMS. Prosthetic forms can be purchased that match the size and shape of the breast removed. A temporary prosthesis usually is worn until the wound heals and the dressing is removed. Some surgeons prefer to recommend the type of prosthetic appliance to be used.

ASSISTING THE CLIENT RECEIVING RADIATION THERAPY. The client with breast cancer may receive radiation therapy before surgery to shrink the tumor or after surgery to prevent recurrence. This form of treatment also may be indicated for the client with inoperable, recurrent, or metastatic breast cancer. The patient who receives radiation therapy for a malignancy of the breast should be observed for such systemic reactions as nausea, vomiting, fever, loss of appetite, and malaise. The patient's skin over the affected area may be either dry or moist. Erythema, dilation of the capillaries, tanning, and desquamation may occur. Desquamation refers to the shedding of portions of the skin. These reactions generally are temporary and subside when the radiation therapy has been completed.

A new treatment option when the entire tumor has not been excised is an internal implant of radioactive iridium-192. The implant is done in the operating room while the client is under general anesthesia.

Additional information related to the care of a patient receiving external and internal radiation therapy can be located in Chapter 9.

ASSISTING THE PATIENT RECEIVING DRUG THERAPY. The patient with breast cancer may receive chemotherapy if the malignancy is advanced, recurrent, or metastatic. The drugs usually used include alkylating agents, antimetabolites, antibiotics, and mitotic inhibitors (refer to Table 9.3). Chemotherapy also may be used as adjuvant therapy following mastectomy or radiation therapy. Appropriate nursing observations and interventions when caring for the patient receiving chemotherapy can be located on pages 235–37.

ASSISTING WITH OTHER THERAPIES. Hormonal therapy may be indicated for a woman with advanced breast cancer that is hormone dependent. Treatment usually is indicated after surgery and radiation therapy have been unsuccessful in slowing or stopping the disease process. The basis of therapy is that altering the client's hormone balance, especially estrogen, deprives certain tumors of hormones needed for growth and development. To determine hormone dependency, a *hormone receptor assay* is

done in the laboratory on a tissue sample obtained during a biopsy.

One form of therapy is surgical removal of the ovaries, adrenal glands, or pituitary gland. Another form of therapy is administration of large doses of certain hormones such as estrogen, androgen, or progestin.

MASTITIS

The woman with mastitis has an infection of the breast, usually caused by staphylococci or streptococci. Mastitis occurs most often in a woman who has delivered recently. Bacteria usually enter through a crack in the nipple and spread to other parts of the breast.

NURSING OBSERVATIONS

The infected breast is swollen, tender, hard, and painful. The area also appears inflamed. The client usually has general symptoms of an infection, such as fever and malaise. Mastitis can result in a breast abscess. Cracks that appear in the nipple should be reported.

NURSING INTERVENTIONS

The nurse plays an important role in the prevention of mastitis by cleaning the woman's nipples before breast feeding, using good handwashing technique before caring for the mother who is breast feeding, and arranging for cleanliness of the mother. Antibiotics such as penicillin G (CRYSTICILLIN), erythromycin (ERYTHROCIN), and kanamycin (KANTREX) may be prescribed. Antibiotic therapy is continued for about ten days even though the symptoms disappear after two or three days. Analgesics may be given to control pain. Incision and drainage of the abscess, if present, is done. Ice packs, uplift support, increased fluids, and rest usually are indicated.

CYSTIC HYPERPLASIA (FIBROCYSTIC DISEASE)

The woman with cystic hyperplasia has an excessive growth of certain tissues in the breast. Normally, breasts grow in a specific pattern. Probably as a result of a hormonal imbalance, some tissues grow at different rates than others. As a result, cysts or lumps occur. Cysts or lumps usually develop in the upper outer quadrants of the breasts. The cysts may come and go. Usually, changes in the breast tissue stop after menopause.

NURSING OBSERVATIONS

The client may consult the doctor because she notices lumps and feels pain in her breasts. The pain usually is most severe immediately prior to a menstrual period. Sometimes the woman has a discharge from the nipple.

NURSING INTERVENTIONS

Nursing interventions generally are related to diagnostic measures to rule out cancer. Cysts or lumps associated with cystic hyperplasia must be confirmed as such. For this reason, the physician generally orders a Papanicolaou smear of the nipple discharge or a mammogram. A biopsy to rule out the possibility of cancer also may be done. After ruling out cancer, the physician generally treats cysts that recur by needle aspiration. In other words, the fluid contained within the cyst is removed. A Papanicolaou smear is done of the fluid. If the physician cannot obtain fluid from the cyst or if blood is obtained, an incision is made into the breast to remove some of the tissue for a biopsy. Generally, if a cyst recurs within two months after aspiration, the patient has a biopsy.

BENIGN TUMOR

A benign tumor of the breast usually is freely movable and does not spread. However, the physician who finds that a woman has a breast tumor generally removes tissue from it or the entire tumor for examination. A definite diagnosis can be made only after the tumor has been removed by the surgeon and examined microscopically by the pathologist.

VENEREAL DISEASE

An individual with a venereal disease has a communicable disease that is almost always transmitted through sexual contact. There has been a steady increase in the num-ber of cases of venereal disease (VD) in recent years, especially in young people. With the advent of the use of penicillin in the 1940s, it was believed that VD would become extinct, and the number of cases did dramatically decrease. As a result, control measures decreased and the treatment was left to individual efforts. Since some persons, principally women, may have VD without symptoms, they serve as reservoirs for infecting many more persons. Therefore, the contacts of those treated for venereal disease must be persuaded to obtain treatment.

Another reason for the increase in venereal disease is the trend toward more sexual partners. Another factor in the increased rate of VD probably pertains to the methods of birth control used today. Birth control pills and the intrauterine device (IUD) do not prevent transmission of venereal disease, as does the condom.

The control of venereal disease will be brought about mainly by education. The objective of this education will be to teach the facts of VD. Infected persons also must be encouraged to seek early treatment and to cooperate in bringing in for treatment persons with whom they have had sexual contact. Syphilis, gonorrhea, and herpes genitalia, which are three of the main venereal diseases, are included in this discussion.

Syphilis

Although syphilis may attack any part of the body, it frequently starts in the reproductive system. For this reason, it is included in this chapter.

The person with syphilis has an infectious disease that is caused by *Treponema pallidum*. This delicate organism is called a spirochete because it is similar to a corkscrew spiral in shape. These spirochetes may continue to live in the patient's body throughout life. *Treponema pallidum* lives only a short period of time outside the body and is killed in a short time by exposure to cold or heat. Soap and water also destroy this spirochete.

Syphilis is almost always transmitted by sexual contact but also may be transmitted to the fetus by an infected mother. Syphilis is classified as primary, secondary, latent, and late.

PRIMARY SYPHILIS

In primary syphilis the client has a chancre, as mentioned earlier. This is called the *initial lesion* or *primary chancre*, and it usually is found on the penis of the male and on the cervix or external genitalia of the female. The chancre also may be found in the anal canal, on the lips, on the fingers, tonsils, or eyelids. The chancre is usually painless and starts as a papule which becomes indurated and erosive with raised edges and clear bases. It disappears after three to six weeks without treatment.

SECONDARY SYPHILIS

The client with secondary syphilis has a rash which may contain macules, papules, pustules, or nodules. They are uniform in size and generalized. The lymph nodes around the chancre usually are enlarged and may remain so for several months. The diagnosis of syphilis can be made at this time by a dark-field examination of material from the lesion and serology tests such as the Venereal Disease Research Laboratory slide test (VDRL) and the fluorescent treponemal antibody absorption test (FTA-ABS). The rapid plasma reagin test (RPR) is another example of a serology test for syphilis. The VDRL and RPR commonly are used for screening purposes. If the physician believes that the VDRL or RPR results are incorrect, usually the FTA-ABS test is ordered. Cerebrospinal fluid (CSF) examination identifies neurosyphilis when the total protein is above 40 mg/100 ml.

Although the client usually passes through a period during which there are few, if any, symptoms after the chancre heals, the body continues to be invaded by the spirochetes which have already spread by the lymph and blood. The patient develops a *generalized lymphadenopathy*, which means that many lymph nodes are involved. The nodes are enlarged, firm, painless, and freely movable. The patient develops a skin rash. The skin has pale, red,

roundish patches that do not itch. The rash may appear on the trunk, arms, palms, soles, face, scalp, perineum, and vulva. The lesions may enlarge and erode.

Eventually, this rash may change and lesions containing pus may develop. The patient may lose patches of hair. In areas such as the vulva and scrotum, condylomata lata may develop. These are large, pinkish, or grayish-white lesions that are highly contagious.

The client's mucous membrane may be involved. Areas of the mucous membrane become eroded. Fingernails and toenails become brittle and pitted. Other symptoms which may develop include headache, weight loss, anorexia, malaise, fever, nausea, vomiting, and sore throat. The eyes may become inflamed. The client may report severe pain if bones are infected by the spirochetes. The patient's liver and kidneys may be affected by the spirochetes.

LATENT SYPHILIS

The next stage is referred to as *latent syphilis*. After the early symptoms of syphilis have disappeared, the untreated or the inadequately treated patient goes through a period during which he has no symptoms. Latent syphilis is divided into early latent and late latent periods. The early latent period includes the first two years after the patient has been infected with the spirochete. During this time, the lesions of the skin and mucous membranes may reappear. The late latent syphilis period follows, and during this time the lesions usually do not recur.

LATE SYPHILIS

What a person has late syphilis, lesions known as *gummata* may develop. A gumma appears similar to a mole. The center frequently is a mass of dead cells. The surrounding area is made of fibrous tissue. The patient may develop a gumma in the internal organs, on the mucous membrane, or on the skin.

Since any system of the patient's body can be attacked by the spirochetes, a variety of symptoms may occur. The symptoms vary in different individuals. The two systems frequently affected by late syphilis are the nervous and the circulatory systems. A person with syphilis of the nervous system has *neurosyphilis*. The individual with syphilis of the circulatory system has *cardiovascular syphilis*. An example of neurosyphilis is seen in the person with general *paresis*. This patient develops mental changes, abnormal reflexes, and changes in speech. An example of cardiovascular syphilis is seen in the person with an *aneurysm* of the aorta. The aorta, which is the large artery leading from the heart, may be attacked by spirochetes. When this happens, it causes the wall of the aorta to become weak. The diseased part of the aorta, which becomes dilated as a result of this, is known as an aneurysm. The nurse may find it helpful to think of an aneurysm as resembling the bulging of a weak spot in a balloon. The weak part of the aorta, like the weak part of a balloon, is likely to rupture.

NURSING INTERVENTIONS

Nursing interventions for the client with syphilis are related to antibiotic therapy, preventing the spread of infection, and client teaching.

The client with syphilis is usually treated in the doctor's office or special VD clinic. Hospitalization is seldom necessary.

Penicillin generally is prescribed for the patient with syphilis (see Table 5.7). The doctor may use another antibiotic, especially when the client is allergic to penicillin. The client is encouraged to visit the doctor regularly in order to determine whether or not the treatment was effective. In some cases, treatment must be repeated in order to eradicate all spirochetes.

When caring for the patient with syphilis, the nurse should remember that the client with an open lesion or a rash is usually infectious. Gloves should be worn when touching an open lesion. The nurse's hands should be washed thoroughly with soap under running water after caring for the patient.

Before teaching the client, the nursing student must first deal with personal feelings about syphilis. Usually the patient is young and afraid and may have feelings of guilt. The fear that friends and family will learn of the disease may be a strong one.

As stated in Chapter 1, the nurse must accept the client as is, without attempting to criticize or judge. The client must know that the information disclosed will be given only to those responsible for the care and to absolutely no one else. The client must have confidence in those in a caring role if the client is to feel free to discuss the various aspects of the problem.

All persons with whom the client with primary syphilis has had sexual relationships within the past three months may have syphilis, and all persons with whom the client with secondary syphilis has had sexual relationships within the past six months may have syphilis. The client with early latent syphilis may have transmitted the disease to all sexual partners within the past 12 months. These persons are known as contacts and should be examined for syphilis. This information is reported to the client so that diagnosis and treatment of sexual partners can be started. The client is also instructed to refrain from sexual intercourse with previous partners not under treatment in order to prevent reinfection. There is also a need for continued medical supervision and blood tests in order to be sure that all spirochetes have been eradicated.

Gonorrhea

The client with gonorrhea has an infection caused by *Neisseria gonorrhoeae* and transmitted by sexual contact. However, gonorrhea is not always transmitted by sexual intercourse. For example, an infant may develop *ophthalmia neonatorum* after coming in contact with the gonococcus while passing through the genital tract during delivery.

The sites most commonly affected by the organisms are the urethra, anal canal, cervix, pharynx, and conjuctiva. The infectious process may spread to regional organs such as the endometrium, fallopian tubes, peritoneum, or epididymis. Gonococcal infections in the fallopian tube may result in sterility caused by scarring, narrowing, and/or blockage of the tube. In addition, serious systemic disease may develop such as arthritis, meningitis, pericarditis, or hepatitis. Gonorrhea, the most common venereal disease, is considered epidemic.

ASSISTING WITH DIAGNOSTIC STUDIES

The physician can confirm the diagnosis of gonorrhea by having the patient's discharge examined in the laboratory under a microscope. Culture sites in the female consist of the cervix and anal canal, and in the male, the urethra and anal canal. The pharynx also may be a culture site. In men, a gram stain of the urethral discharge is considered accurate. In women, a sample of the cervical discharge is taken and cultured.

NURSING OBSERVATIONS

The individual develops a discharge that contains pus approximately two to six days after contact with an infected person. The man usually notices a urethral discharge that is purulent. Urinary symptoms that usually accompany the discharge include urgency, frequency, and dysuria. The female may not experience early symptoms until infection spreads. The woman may have this purulent discharge from the vagina. She also may have painful and frequent urination, perineal itching, burning, and pain. When gonorrhea spreads through the fallopian tubes, the spread may cause various symptoms in the female. Such symptoms as fever, nausea, vomiting, and abdominal pain may occur.

The client may have symptoms in other areas infected with gonorrhea such as a sore throat, rectal burning and itching, redness, swelling, and discharge from the eyes.

NURSING INTERVENTIONS

Drug therapy with a penicillin, tetracycline, or spectinomycin (refer to Table 5.7) usually is prescribed. Probenecid (BENEMID) may be given by mouth to block the excretion of penicillin and provide a longer lasting effect. The nurse instructs the client to take the medication exactly as prescribed so that effective treatment is received. Inadequate or incomplete drug therapy may relieve

symptoms without eradicating all the organisms. This situation may lead to the spread of infection and permanent damage to affected body organs.

The nurse prevents the spread of infection by good handwashing and appropriate disposal of equipment and supplies contaminated by the client's infected secretions. The patient prevents the spread of infection by refraining from sexual intercourse until the infection is cleared and good handwashing.

The instillation of 1 percent silver nitrate solution or an appropriate antibiotic in the newborn infant's eyes is done to prevent gonococcal ophthalmia neonatorum, as mentioned earlier. Using a condom during sexual intercourse can provide a high degree of protection to the uninfected partner. Treatment of the client's sexual partners is another important preventive measure.

Genital Herpes—Venereal Herpes

The client with genital herpes has an acute infection of the genital area caused by the herpes simplex virus, usually acquired by sexual contact. There are two different herpes viruses: type 1 and type 2. Most genital herpes infections involve the type 2 virus. All the modes of transmission are not yet known. As previously mentioned, sexual contact is the most frequent mode of transmission; however, the client may transmit the virus to the eye if the hands contain infectious material. Contamination from toilet seats, towels, and bathtubs sometimes may occur. It can be transmitted during pregnancy by an infected expectant mother via the placenta. It can cause congenital malformations and lead to abortion or premature labor. Infection of the fetus may occur during passage through the cervix and vagina. A large number of newborns die or have serious eye and central nervous system involvement. Genital herpes in women also has been linked to cervical cancer, although the exact relationship has not yet been proved. The incidence of genital herpes is rising. Currently, it is the second most common venereal disease. The herpes virus is identified in the laboratory from microscopic examination of fluid in the lesion.

NURSING OBSERVATIONS

The client usually notices a cluster of painful vesicles in the genital area. Common sites include the labia, clitoris, vaginal opening, urinary meatus, perianal tissue, glans penis, foreskin, or penile shaft, and on the mouth. The lesions may ulcerate, forming larger round or oval lesions, covered with a grayish-white exudate and surrounded by diffuse erythema and inflammation. The male client may experience burning, urgency, and frequency. The female client may experience paresthesias and burning of the vulva, dyspareunia, and dysuria. Both men and women usually experience generalized symptoms of infection such as fever, headache, malaise, and enlargement of inguinal lymph nodes (lymphadenopathy). Symptoms usually subside gradually over a period of days. However, lesions may recur at intervals of weeks to months. Some persons remain asymptomatic but become carriers of the virus which is then transmitted to others.

NURSING INTERVENTIONS

At present, there is no known cure for a genital herpes infection. Nursing interventions are related to relieving the discomforts of acute illness, preventing the spread of infection, and client support and education.

The lesions are kept clean and dry. Sitz baths may be soothing during acute attacks. The client may be advised to rest in bed, increase the fluid intake, and take a mild antipyretic analgesic such as aspirin. In severe cases, a local anesthetic or stronger analgesia may be indicated. Acylovir (ZOVIRAX Ointment 5%) may be prescribed to shorten acute episodes by promoting faster healing of lesions. This drug is applied with a glove so that all lesions are covered. The drug does not cure the illness or prevent the transmission of infection.

To prevent the spread of infection, hospitalized clients are usually isolated from others. The nonhospitalized client is advised to refrain from sexual intercourse until lesions are healed completely. Good handwashing is important both for the client and the nurse when active lesions are present. Good handwashing on the client's part prevents autoinoculation of other body areas such as the eyes and lips.

As previously mentioned, genital herpes is presently incurable, has a devastating effect on the fetus, and is associated with cervical cancer. Thus, this disease can be expected to have a devastating impact on the client and loved ones. For example, sexual relationships may be altered temporarily or permanently. This, in turn, may affect the ability of the client to give and receive love

TABLE 20.10
OTHER CONDITIONS INVOLVING THE REPRODUCTIVE SYSTEM

CONDITION	DESCRIPTION
Abortion	Interruption of pregnancy before fetus is viable
	Dilatation and curettage may be needed to remove products of conception
Habitual	Unintentional interruption of three or more consecutive pregnancies
Missed	Failure to expel uterine contents after the death of the embryo
Spontaneous	Unintentional interruption of pregnancy from unknown causes
Therapeutic	Intentional interruption of a pregnancy
Bartholin cyst	The abnormal collection of fluid in a Bartholin's gland located at the base of the labia majora
Bartholinitis	An inflammatory condition of the Bartholin's gland located at the base of the labia majora; abscess may have to be incised by the doctor to allow for drainage
Condylomata acuminata (venereal warts)	Warts that develop around genitalia and anus; may or may not be acquired by sexual contact; chemically or surgically removed

in a romantic relationship. The nurse's warmth, compassion, and understanding are especially important when caring for this client.

Research into genital herpes is continuing. An important nursing responsibility is to collect new facts that become available so that complete and accurate information can be provided for the client. A community resource available to clients with herpes is the Herpes Resource Center. Information about local chapters can be located by writing to:

Herpes Resource Center
Box 100
Palo Alto, California   94302

Case Study Involving Uterine Cancer

Mrs. Sally Jones was admitted to the hospital on her thirtieth birthday for a vaginal hysterectomy. Her past history indicated that she consulted the doctor because of a whitish vaginal discharge and a slight bloody vaginal drainage following intercourse. A Papanicolaou smear of the cervix was positive for malignant cells.

Mrs. Jones's mother died three years ago from metastatic breast cancer. Her father is alive and well. Mrs. Jones has no children. She and her husband planned to have a child two years ago. When first married, they could not afford a child.

After having a vaginal hysterectomy, Mrs. Jones was transferred from the postanesthesia recovery room to the surgical unit. She had a perineal pad in place, an urethral (Foley) catheter draining, and an IV of 5 percent dextrose in saline.

The physician's orders were:

- Force fluids
- I and O
- Perineal care
- Heat lamp to perineum for 20 minutes tid
- COLACE, 100 mg (PO) qd

QUESTIONS
1. What are some of the concerns and fears that Mrs. Jones could be experiencing?
2. Mrs. Jones asked the nurse, "Why can't this operation wait until I have a baby?" What would be the nurse's best reply?
3. The nurse noticed that Mrs. Jones was crying when she asked if her operation would cause her to go through the menopause before her time and become an old lady. What would be the nurse's best response?
4. While being given an enema, Mrs. Jones told the LPN/LVN that she had promised God that she would go to church every Sunday if only she could keep her uterus for one year. What stage of the grieving process according to Kübler-Ross is Mrs. Jones probably experiencing? (*Hint:* Refer to Chapter 1 if necessary.)
5. What area of Mrs. Jones's body should be shaved prior to surgery?
6. When should the nurse give perineal care? How often? How should this be done?
7. What distance should separate the heat lamp from the patient?
8. Mrs. Jones asked the nurse if this operation would interfere with her sex life. Describe the best response to be made by the nurse.
9. How often should the nurse check Mrs. Jones's perineal pad during the first 24 hours following surgery?
10. How should the nurse carry out the doctor's order to force fluids?
11. What positions are indicated and contraindicated following pelvic surgery?

Case Study Involving Gonorrhea

Mr. James Colden, a 24-year-old male, visited the doctor because of frequent and painful urination. His history indicated that he had noticed a purulent urethral discharge recently. He was married two weeks ago and had just returned from his honeymoon. The physician did a smear of the discharge and discovered gonococci. The physician ordered Probenecid, 1 gm orally, to be followed by penicillin G procaine suspension, 4.8 million units (2.4 units IM in each buttock).

QUESTIONS
1. Mr. Colden told the nurse in the doctor's office, "Oh! I can't tell my wife. Please don't make me tell my wife." What would be the best response for the nurse to make?
2. Mr. Colden told the nurse that he had "one last fling" before getting married. What is the law in your state regarding a person with gonorrhea and the sexual contacts of that person?
3. What agency is responsible for follow-up regarding venereal disease in your locality?
4. Examine your feelings about Mr. Colden's behavior and consider how they could influence your nursing care.
5. Having had only the contact mentioned of giving Mr. Colden an IM injection and an oral medication in the doctor's office, is the nurse likely to become infected with gonorrhea?
6. What could happen to Mr. Colden if he were not treated?

7. What are some of the reasons for an increase in the incidence of gonorrhea?
8. Mr. Colden asked the nurse why the gonorrhea was not detected when he came to the doctor for a premarital examination. What knowledge would the nurse need in order to answer his question accurately?
9. What nursing measures should the nurse take before and after administrating penicillin to Mr. Colden?
10. What is the desired effect of probenecid?

Suggestions for Further Study

1. What services are offered through your local family planning center?
2. What is the similarity between a varicocele and varicose veins discussed in Chapter 12?
3. What program does the local public health agency in your area have for the prevention and control of venereal disease?
4. What personal feelings about venereal disease will you have to consider in preparing to nurse the patient currently infected?
5. Mason, Mildred A.; Bates, Grace F.; and Smola, Bonnie K.: *Workbook in Basic Medical-Surgical Nursing*, 3rd ed. Macmillan Publishing Company, New York, 1984. Exercise 20.

Additional Readings

Bettoli, Elena J.: "Herpes: Facts and Fallacies." *American Journal of Nursing*, 82:924-34 (June), 1982.

Campbell, Charles E., and Herten, R. Jeffrey: "VD to STD: Redefining Venereal Disease." *American Journal of Nursing*, 81:1629-35 (Sept.), 1981.

Gorline, Lynne L., and Stegbauer, Cheryl C.: "What Every Nurse Should Know About Vaginitis." *American Journal of Nursing*, 82: 1851-55 (Dec.), 1982.

Hoeft, Rhoda Tigert, and Jones, Anne G.: "Treating Metastasis with Estramustine Phosphate." *American Journal of Nursing*, 82: 828-30 (May), 1982.

Jones, Anne G., and Hoeft, Rhoda Tigert: "Cancer of the Prostate." *American Journal of Nursing*, 82:826-28 (May), 1982.

Levinger, Gloria E.: "Working Through Recovery After Mastectomy." *American Journal of Nursing*, 80:1119-20 (June), 1980.

Lynch, Jane M.: "Helping Patients Through the Recurring Nightmare of Herpes." *Nursing 82*, 12:52-57 (Oct.), 1982.

Pearson, Linda: "Climacteric." *American Journal of Nursing*, 82:1098-1102 (July), 1982.

Rambo, Beverly J., and Wood, Lucile A. (eds.): *Nursing Skills for Clinical Practice*, 3rd ed. W. B. Saunders Co., Philadelphia, 1982, pp. 389-97.

Seefeld, Bert: "Breast Cancer Part II: Prostheses and Reconstructive Techniques." *Journal of Practical Nursing*, 30:15-19 (Apr.), 1980.

Stromberg, Marilyn: "Screening for Early Detection." *American Journal of Nursing*, 81: 1652-57 (Sept.), 1981.

"Test Yourself: Stage II Breast Cancer." *American Journal of Nursing*, 82:271, 317 (Feb.), 1982.

Wilcox, Patti M.: "Benign Breast Disorders." *American Journal of Nursing*, 81: 1644-51 (Sept.), 1981.

Wiley, Katherine Rudolph: "Postbiopsy Care." *American Journal of Nursing*, 81:1660-62 (Sept.), 1981.

Chapter 21

The Patient with a Disease
of the Nervous System

Expected Behavioral Outcomes

Minimum objectives referred to as expected behavioral outcomes have been designed for the practical/vocational nursing student to use as guides in study this chapter. The student should read these expected outcomes before studying the chapter. The objectives can be used as guides for study.

Using the content of this chapter, the student should return to the objectives and evaluate the ability to:

1. *Describe the responsibilities of the LPN/LVN in your agency when assisting with diagnostic studies included in this chapter.*
2. *Describe nursing observations that indicate rising intracranial pressure in each part of the neuro check.*
3. *Compare the nursing measures discussed in Chapter 6 for the postoperative patient with those discussed in this chapter for the neurosurgical patient.*
4. *Relate the nursing care of the patient with an inflammation discussed in Chapter 5 to that indicated for the patient with an inflammatory condition of the nervous system.*
5. *Describe nursing observations and interventions appropriate for the patient having a seizure.*
6. *Compare the care needed for the unconscious patient with that indicated for the person with spinal cord injury.*
7. *Contrast the nursing measures needed by the patient with Parkinson's disease with those needed by the patient with multiple sclerosis.*

Vocabulary Development

The following prefixes, suffixes, and combining forms pertain to this chapter. By learning and/or reviewing their meanings, the practical/vocational nursing student will have the keys needed to unlock many exciting new medical terms.

Discover the meaning of these keys in a medical dictionary or in the content of this chapter. How does each key pertain to this chapter? In your notebook write the correct meaning of each prefix, suffix, or combining form listed below. Illustrate each key with an example.

cell—room, cell, Ex. *cella* lateralis ventriculi lateralis—the lateral enclosure of the lateral ventricle of the brain.

centr-	cerebr-	crani-	neur-
cephal-	chord-	disc-	par-
cept-	-cipient	front-	quadr-
		lep-	rachi-
		lumb-	semi-
		mening-	sens-
		ment-	spas-
		mne-	spin-
		myel-	vuls-

[handwritten: Afferent receive / Efferent send out transmit]

Structure and Function

The nervous system is composed of the brain, spinal cord, and nerves (Figure 21.1). Although this system consists of only a few organs, it plays a vital role in the functioning of the body. It helps to regulate and to coordinate the body's activities. In general, the nervous system influences the body processes in the following ways:

- Receives, transmits, and processes information in the external and internal environment
- Generates impulses that regulate and control various voluntary and involuntary motor activities
- Stores information

The functional unit of the nervous system is the nerve cell or *neuron* which receives, processes, and transmits impulses. The neuron consists of a cell body, dendrites, and the axon. The cell body (also known as gray matter) conducts activities necessary to cell life. *Dendrites* are thin, branchlike projections which extend from the cell body and carry impulses toward the cell body. The *axon* is a long projection extending from the cell body that carries impulses away from the cell body. The axon is covered by a special layer of cells called *glia*. A nerve fiber includes both the axon and glia. About one third of all nerve fibers are further covered by a special sheath composed of a substance called *myelin*. Myelinated nerve fibers (also know as white matter) are able to conduct impulses more rapidly than other fibers. *Afferent nerve fibers* carry information about changes in the internal and external environment to the central nervous system. *Efferent nerve fi-* bers transmit information from the central nervous system to skeletal muscle, smooth muscle, and glands.

A *nerve* is a collection of nerve fibers which transmits messages to and from the brain and spinal cord. The number of fibers varies from dozens to thousands, depending upon the size of the nerve. Practically all nerves contain both afferent and efferent fibers bundled together. *Somatic nerves* refer to those located in the skin, skeletal muscles, and joints. *Splanchnic nerves* lead to the viscera (internal body organs).

An impulse conducted by the neuron travels down the axon until it reaches the *synapse* (junction between two neurons). At the synapse, a chemical known as a *neurotransmitter* is released which may either excite the next neuron (cause it to discharge an impulse) or inhibit it (prevent the discharge of an impulse). *Acetylcholine* is an example of an important neurotransmitter that excites the next neuron. Inhibitory neurotransmitters include gamma-aminobutyric acid (GABA) and glycine. Impulses may travel either from one neuron to another or from the neuron to smooth or skeletal muscle. *[handwritten: acetecholine excite / GABA glycine inhibit]*

CENTRAL NERVOUS SYSTEM

[handwritten: ganglia] The central nervous system is made up of the brain and the spinal cord (see Figure 21.2). Both of these are surrounded by membranes and a bony case for protection. The three membranes—dura mater, arachnoid, and pia mater—that cover the brain and the spinal cord are known as *meninges*. The *cranium* or *skull* is the bony case protecting the brain and its meninges. The spinal cord and its meninges are protected by bones known as *vertebrae*.

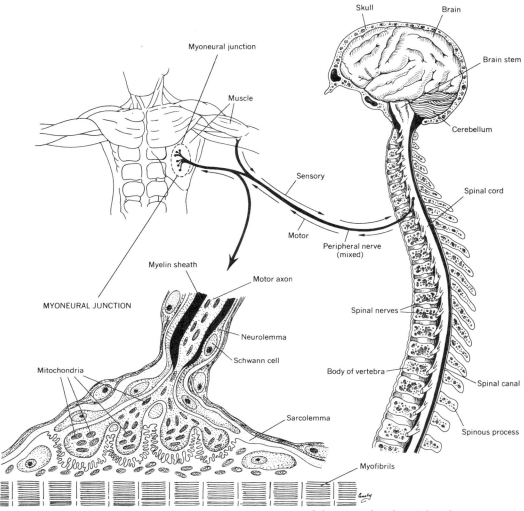

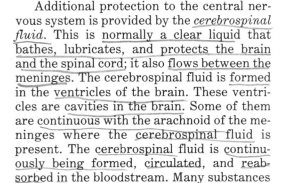

FIGURE 21.1 Illustration of some of the major parts of the central and peripheral nervous systems. A schematic drawing of a myoneural junction is on the lower left. (From Pansky, Ben: *Dynamic Anatomy and Physiology.* Macmillan Publishing Co., Inc., New York, 1975.)

Additional protection to the central nervous system is provided by the *cerebrospinal fluid*. This is normally a clear liquid that bathes, lubricates, and protects the brain and the spinal cord; it also flows between the meninges. The cerebrospinal fluid is formed in the ventricles of the brain. These ventricles are cavities in the brain. Some of them are continuous with the arachnoid of the meninges where the cerebrospinal fluid is present. The cerebrospinal fluid is continuously being formed, circulated, and reabsorbed in the bloodstream. Many substances in the bloodstream, including some drugs, do not enter into the cerebrospinal fluid. This invisible protective mechanism is called the *blood-brain barrier*. Whenever a drug is needed to treat the meninges, the physician will order a drug that is known to cross the blood-brain barrier and enter the cerebrospinal fluid.

BRAIN

The brain is composed of both gray and white matter; that is, it contains nerve cells and nerve fibers. The brain is the largest

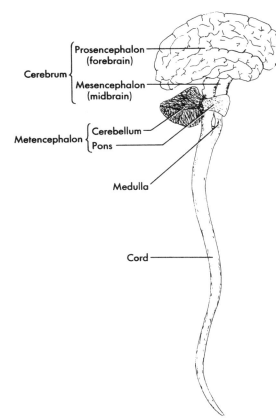

Cerebrum { Prosencephalon (forebrain)
Mesencephalon (midbrain)

Metencephalon { Cerebellum
Pons

Medulla

Cord

Cerebrum—memory, association, personality. Synthesizes sensory impressions into perceptions. Highest level of somatic motor control. Receives impulses from and sends impulses to all lower levels.

Midbrain—contains many nuclei for control of ocular reflexes, eye movement, higher postural reflex actions. Motor nuclei of cranial nerves III and IV. Nuclei for control of many visceral activities.

Cerebellum—vestibular and postural reflexes, equilibrium and orientation in space. Helps to maintain muscle tone and regulate muscle coordination.

Pons—relay station from lower to the higher centers. Contains nuclei for cerebrocerebellar relay of impulses. Nuclei and pathways for regulation of skeletal muscle tones. Contains nuclei for cranial nerves V, VI, VII, and VIII. Connects both halves of the cerebellum.

Medulla—contains nuclei of many cranial nerves. Location of many vital centers. Contains nuclei for relaying sensory impulses to higher centers. Contains fiber tracts for all ascending and descending impulses.

Cord—only means by which impulses from the periphery can reach higher centers and impulses from higher centers can reach the periphery. Contains neurons which form ascending sensory pathways. Receives incoming sensory fibers and their impulses. Centers for intersegmental and segmental reflexes.

FIGURE 21.2 Diagram of the central nervous system—cerebrum, midbrain, and medulla pulled apart to show parts. (From Miller, Marjorie, A.; Drakontides, Anna B.; and Leavell, Lutie C.: *Kimber-Gray-Stockpole's Anatomy and Physiology*, 17th ed. Macmillan Publishing Co., Inc., New York, 1977.)

mass of nervous tissue in the body. The five main parts of the brain are the cerebrum, the midbrain, the cerebellum, the pons varolii, and the medulla oblongata. The cerebrum, which is the largest part of the brain, is located in the upper portion of the cranium. The five lobes of the cerebrum are the frontal, the parietal, the temporal, the occipital, and the insula. Mental activities, such as reason, intelligence, memory, and consciousness, are controlled by the cerebrum. The cerebrum also controls such activities as seeing, smelling, talking, and voluntary movements, such as picking up a pencil.

The cerebellum is behind and below the cerebrum. It helps to control equilibrium and muscular coordination. The cerebellum helps to coordinate nerve data.

The brainstem is composed of the mid-brain, the pons varolii, and the medulla. The midbrain connects the cerebrum and the cerebellum with the pons. The pons varolii is located between the medulla oblongata and the midbrain. The pons connects the midbrain and the medulla. The brain is connected to the spinal cord by the medulla oblongata. Many of the motor nerves (those responsible for motion) cross in the medulla. The vital centers that control automatic activities of the body, such as respiration, heartbeat, and blood pressure, are in the medulla oblongata. Such activities as sneezing and coughing are also controlled by this part of the brain. The 12 pairs of cranial nerves are attached to the base of the brain and control the activities of the head. These nerves serve as pathways for special senses, such as sight, smell, taste, and hearing.

SPINAL CORD

The spinal cord goes from the medulla to the lower part of the back (see Figure 21.2). It contains both gray and white matter. The gray matter is located in the center of the cord. Nerves going to and from the brain pass through the spinal cord. The nerves that branch off from the cord are known as *spinal nerves*. The spinal nerves eventually form the peripheral nerves, which are located near the surface of the body. The spinal cord and the spinal nerves serve as pathways for the impulses between the brain and parts of the body below the head. In the lumbar and sacral regions of the vertebral column, the spinal cord ends, and the spinal nerves are grouped together and look like a horse's tail. They are referred to as the *cauda equina*, meaning horse's tail.

AUTONOMIC NERVOUS SYSTEM *ANS*

The autonomic nervous system is not a separate structure, but a separate function of the nervous system. The autonomic nervous system, in general, regulates activities of structures that are not under voluntary control and that operate below the level of consciousness. Activities of the body such as metabolism, respiration, circulation, sweating, regulation of body temperature, digestion, and secretion of some endocrine glands are controlled, at least in part, by the autonomic nervous system.

The autonomic nervous system (ANS) is divided into two divisions: the *sympathetic* and the *parasympathetic*. These two divisions have contrasting functions but work together to regulate the internal environment of the body.

The sympathetic system helps to prepare the body for "fight or flight." It increases the pulse rate, increases the blood pressure, increases the concentration of blood sugar, helps shift the blood supply to the skeletal muscles, dilates the pupils, and dilates the bronchioles. Drugs that mimic this response are called *sympathomimetics* or *adrenergics*.

The parasympathetic system acts more to conserve and restore energy. It decreases the blood pressure, decreases the pulse rate, stimulates activity of the gastrointestinal system, empties the bladder and rectum, and constricts the pupils (to protect the retina from excessive light). Drugs that mimic the parasympathetic system are called *parasympathomimetics* or *cholinergics*.

CIRCULATION

The circulation to the brain is supplied by the vertebral arteries originating from the subclavian artery and the carotid arteries originating from the aorta. Major branches of these arteries include the anterior, middle, and posterior cerebral arteries and their branches. Circulation to the spinal cord is supplied by the anterior and posterior spinal arteries and their branches.

A short temporary disruption in the blood supply to the nervous system may result in permanent irreversible damage to the nerve cells (neurons). However, nerve fibers may heal or be repaired in some cases.

Venous drainage in the brain is provided primarily by the superior longitudinal sinus and the dural sinuses. These, in turn, empty blood into the jugular veins for return to the heart. In the spinal cord, the venous system includes a network of drainage vessels located in the abdomen, neck, and thorax.

Assisting with Diagnostic Tests

NEUROLOGIC EXAMINATION

The neurologic examination is a highly specialized procedure done by the doctor. A *neurologist*, who is a physician specializing in diagnosing and treating patients with disorders of the nervous system, is the person who may be responsible for this examination. The examiner tests the patient's reflexes and special senses, such as sight, smell, and touch. The patient's ability to coordinate movements, such as those involved in walking, are examined and evaluated. The physician also tests the strength of various parts of the patient's body. The patient may be asked to squeeze the physician's hand. The neurologist also determines whether or not the patient knows the exact location and position of the extremities. For example, the patient may have to look at the feet to know where they are. The neurologic examination will include a very detailed history. A complete neurologic examination may be tiring

Checking patellar reflex

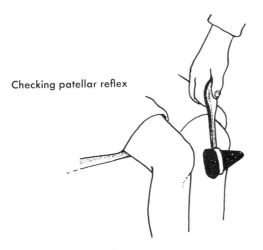

Checking Achilles reflex

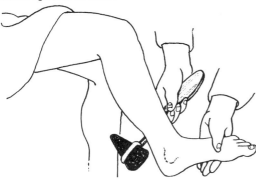

Checking triceps reflex

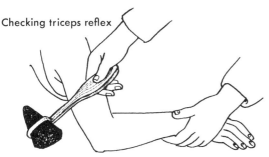

FIGURE 21.3   A percussion hammer is used by the neurologist to check the patient's reflexes. (Adapted from Pansky, Ben, and House, Earl Lawrence: *Review of Gross Anatomy*, 3rd ed. Macmillan Publishing Co., Inc., New York, 1975.)

for some patients and may have to be done in stages. The nurse may be asked to assist the physician during this examination. In ad-

dition to the usual equipment needed for a general physical examination, some added equipment and supplies needed for a general physical examination, some added equipment and supplies will be required. A special tray with the necessary equipment may be available in some hospitals. Some of the more common items required are a percussion hammer (see Figure 21.3); a straight pin (see Figure 21.4); a safety pin; cotton (see Figure 21.5) or a fine brush; tuning forks (see Figure 21.6); substances with distinctive odors such as onions, vanilla, or coffee (see Figure 21.7); substances with distinctive tastes such as sugar, salt, vinegar (sour), and quinine (bitter); hot and cold water (see Figure 21.8); and test tubes. A special blank diagram may be requested by the physician to indicate the results of the tests.

SKULL AND SPINE X-RAYS

Most patients with a disturbance in the nervous system have skull and/or spine x-rays. Skull films provide information about the size and shape of skull bones as well as fractures, calcifications, erosions, and vascular abnormalities. Before the x-

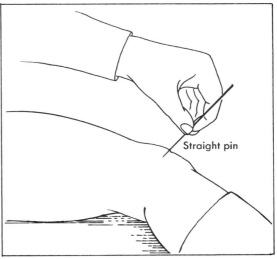

FIGURE 21.4   A straight pin may be used to measure response to superficial pain. (Adapted from Pansky, Ben, and House, Earl Lawrence: *Review of Gross Anatomy*, 3rd ed. Macmillan Publishing Co., Inc., New York, 1975.)

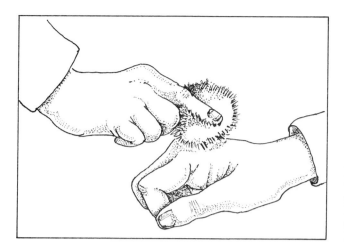

FIGURE 21.5   Cotton may be used to determine superficial tactile sensation. (Adapted from Pansky, Ben, and House, Earl Lawrence: *Review of Gross Anatomy*, 3rd ed. Macmillan Publishing Co., Inc., New York, 1975.)

ray, hairpins and other metal objects should be removed from the patient's hair. Spine films may show fractures, erosions, narrowing of the vertebral canal, or abnormal bony growths such as spurs. Before spinal x-rays, the patient should be helped to remove undergarments containing metal fasteners.

LUMBAR PUNCTURE

The doctor may do a *lumbar puncture*, which is known also as a *spinal tap*, to aid in diagnosis. In this procedure, a needle is inserted between the vertebrae into the spinal canal. This is known as a lumbar puncture since it usually is done in the lumbar region, lower part of the back, between L4 and L5 or L5 and S1. The needle is inserted below the level of the spinal cord into the area of the cauda equina; hence, there is very little danger of damage to the nerves. The physician usually determines the pressure of the cerebrospinal fluid during a lumbar puncture by attaching a manometer to the hub of the spinal needle. The nurse may need to steady the manometer by holding it lightly well above the area where the physician might have contact with the sterile glove. Usually, several specimens of cerebrospinal fluid are sent to the laboratory. These specimens should be labeled accurately. Normal characteristics of cerebrospinal fluid are listed in Table 21.1.

The nurse is often asked to assist the physician during a lumbar puncture (see Figure 21.9) by preparing the necessary equipment. In some agencies, the patient must sign a consent form. The nurse may assist the patient to assume a position suitable for the examination, which is on the side and near the edge of the bed or examining table.

Following a lumbar puncture, the patient may be encouraged to lie flat in bed from 6 to 24 hours, depending on the physician's preference, hospital policy, and the neurologic disturbance. The nurse observes the patient frequently for headache, abnormal neurologic or vital signs, temperature elevation, temporary difficulty in voiding, and backache. Oral fluids are usually encouraged.

Some patients develop a headache following this procedure which is aggravated by the upright position. The cause of a post-lumbar-puncture headache is believed to be leakage of cerebrospinal fluid through the opening made in the dura at the puncture site. The headache usually disappears spontaneously within several days. The patient

TABLE 21.1
NORMAL CHARACTERISTICS OF CEREBROSPINAL FLUID

Appearance	Clear
Glucose	45–75 mg per 100 ml
Total protein	15–45 mg per 100 ml
White cell count	0–5 lymphocytes
	0 neutrophils

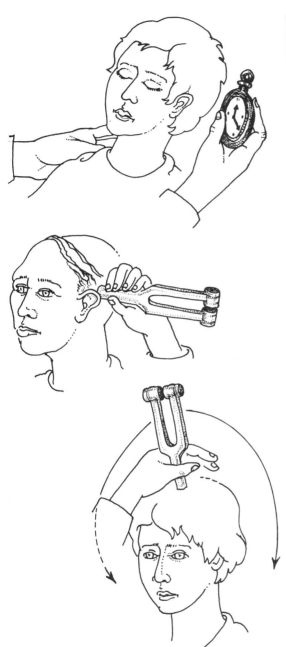

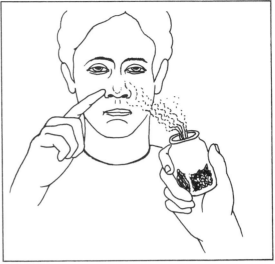

FIGURE 21.7 A substance with a distinctive odor is used to test the sense of olfactory function or smell. (Adapted from Pansky, Ben, and House, Earl Lawrence: *Review of Gross Anatomy*, 3rd ed. Macmillan Publishing Co., Inc., New York, 1975.)

may be helped by lying flat in bed and taking a mild analgesic such as aspirin and/or codeine.

COMPUTERIZED AXIAL TOMOGRAPHY (CT SCAN, CAT SCAN)

Computerized axial tomography uses an x-ray beam and a computer to make a detailed image of thin cross-sections of the brain and skull without physically penetrating the skin or body cavities (Figure 21.10). The wealth of information about the brain and skull helps the physician with early diagnosis of brain tumor, abscess, hematoma, cyst, and blood vessel abnormalities. Because the body barriers are not invaded, the procedure is painless and safe.

The patient lies on a table in front of the scanning device. The head is placed in a chamber which prevents movement while the scanner rotates around at various angles to collect information (see Chapter 4, page 71). In some cases, a radiopaque dye may be injected to provide sharper images.

In preparation for the CT scan, the patient's hair may be shampooed to remove

FIGURE 21.6 A watch and a tuning fork are used to measure air and bone conduction. (Adapted from Pansky, Ben, and House, Earl Lawrence: *Review of Gross Anatomy*, 3rd ed. Macmillan Publishing Co., Inc., New York, 1975.)

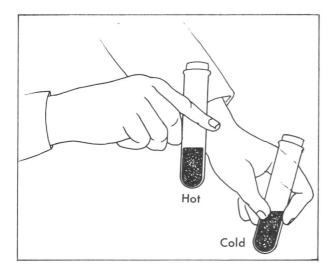

FIGURE 21.8   The patient's response to temperature is determined with hot and cold water. (Adapted from Pansky, Ben, and House, Earl Lawrence: *Review of Gross Anatomy*, 3rd ed. Macmillan Publishing Co., Inc., New York, 1975.)

hair spray. Metal hair clips and bobby pins are also removed. If a radiopaque dye is used, food and fluids may be withheld for four to eight hours prior to the test. Because the CAT scan provides a wealth of detailed information without complications, it gradually has replaced other studies such as pneumoencephalogram, when possible.

CISTERNAL PUNCTURE *BRAIN*

A *cisternal puncture* may be done to obtain spinal fluid for examination by a highly trained specialist. This procedure is done less frequently than a lumbar puncture. A needle is inserted into the cisterna magna at the base of the brain. The back of the neck is

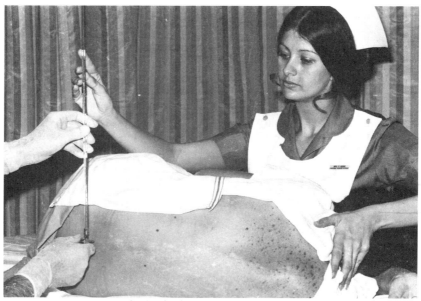

FIGURE 21.9   Assisting with a lumbar puncture.

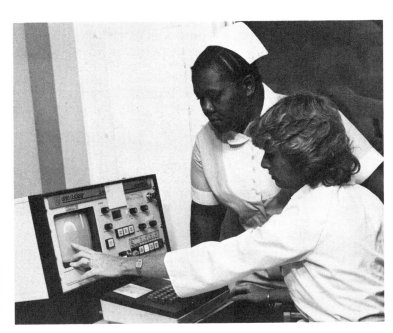

FIGURE 21.10 A CAT scan of the skull. (Courtesy of Shapero School of Nursing, Sinai Hospital of Detroit, Detroit, Michigan.)

shaved and an operative permit may be signed. The patient's head is bent forward and held by the nurse while the doctor obtains the sample of fluid.

Following a cisternal puncture, the patient's neurologic and vital signs are monitored carefully. The patient usually is kept flat in bed for six to eight hours. Oral fluids generally are encouraged. Pain, chills and fever, and nuchal rigidity (stiff neck) should be reported at once since these symptoms indicate complications.

ENCEPHALOGRAPHY

A patient having *encephalography* has x-rays taken of the head after some of the cerebrospinal fluid has been replaced by air or oxygen.

To perform a *pneumoencephalogram* or *air encephalogram* air is injected into the spinal canal. The air then rises to the ventricles in the brain as the patient is assisted to a sitting position. An x-ray is taken and the size and shape of the ventricles can be visualized. For example, the shape of the ventricle may be changed if a brain tumor is taking up space near a ventricle. The patient is prepared for a pneumoencephalogram as for surgery because a general anesthesia may

be given for the procedure. Food and fluids are withheld for a period of time, a sedative may be given, and a permit signed. The procedure usually is done in the x-ray department. After the procedure, the patient usually remains flat in bed for a certain period of time. Vital signs and neurologic checks (see page 734) are taken as ordered, and food and fluids may be taken as tolerated. The nurse should observe the patient for symptoms of increased intracranial pressure, discussed in detail later in this chapter. A headache may occur, for which analgesics and ice caps often are given. The patient usually can be up the day after the procedure.

A ventriculogram usually is done when a pneumoencephalogram is not possible. A patient having *ventriculography* has air placed into the ventricles (small cavities) within the brain. In order to do this examination, the neurosurgeon makes surgical openings in the patient's skull so that air or some other suitable substance can be injected into the ventricles. These openings are called burr holes. After the air is injected, the patient's head is x-rayed. This type of examination, which is done in the operating room, enables the neurosurgeon to visualize the size and shape of the ventricles on x-ray. The patient is prepared for a ventriculogram in much the same way as for a pneumoencephalogram. The hair that covers the area where the burr holes will be made is removed. This may be done in the operating room. After the procedure, the patient needs care similar to that indicated following a pneumoencephalogram. Dressings will cover the areas of the burr holes.

Pneumoencephalograms are done much less frequently now since the development and increasing use of computerized axial tomography (CAT scan) which provides more accurate and complete information at less risk to the patient.

CEREBRAL ARTERIOGRAPHY

The patient having a *cerebral arteriogram* has x-rays taken of the head immediately after the injection of a radiopaque dye into either the carotid or vertebral arteries (Figure 21.11). The dye may be injected directly into the above arteries or indirectly via the brachial, femoral, subclavian, or axillary arteries. This diagnostic test enables the physician to visualize blood vessels inside the brain and the cranium. Abnormalities in blood vessels such as narrowing, thrombosis, and occlusion may be identified. In addition, displacement of blood vessels by tumors, cysts, and swelling may be detected.

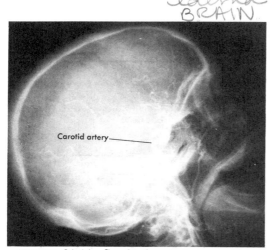

FIGURE 21.11 Cerebral arteriogram. Contrast media injected through carotid artery. Lateral view.

The cerebral arteriogram may be done in the x-ray department or the operating room. After a permit has been signed by the patient, the injection site may be shaved and scrubbed with an antiseptic according to hospital policy and the physician's preference. A sedative usually is prescribed. The patient may be told that a burning sensation in the eyes, tongue, teeth, lips, and jaw is common during the dye injection.

Following the procedure, the patient usually is placed on bed rest for 12 to 24 hours. The head may be elevated and an ice bag usually is placed on the injection site(s) to reduce edema and control bleeding. If an extremity has been used for an indirect injection site, sandbags may be used for immobilization to prevent bleeding. The patient's neurologic and vital signs are carefully monitored in order to detect complications. For example, bleeding and/or excessive swelling at the carotid injection site may cause the patient to have respiratory difficulties. The injection of dye into the brain may cause symptoms of increased intracranial pressure (see pages 746–47). The dye may cause an allergic reaction. If an extremity has been used for arterial injection, the area distal to the injection site is closely observed for disturbances in circulation using the five Ps (pulse, pain, paralysis, pallor, paresthesia). Any unusual observations are reported to the appropriate nurse or physician immediately. Cerebral arteriography is another diagnostic procedure that is done less frequently because of the valuable information provided by computerized axial tomography (CT scan).

BRAIN SCAN

A brain scan is a test in which a radioisotope is used to help localize a brain lesion. A substance such as radioactive albumin or mercury is injected intravenously. A few hours later, a scanner is passed over the head. The lesions will pick up an increased amount of the radioactive substance from the blood. These areas of concentration will be recorded by the scanner. No special preparation is necessary. No special observations are required after the procedure.

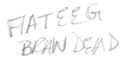

ELECTROENCEPHALOGRAM

An electroencephalogram, which is referred to as an EEG, is a tracing of the electrical waves of the brain. The brain waves of a healthy person have a definite pattern. An individual with certain brain diseases has an abnormal pattern.

During the test, special electrodes are placed on the scalp to record electrical activity in the brain. An alternate method is the insertion of tiny electrode needles just under the scalp. The electrodes then are connected to a machine that records the electrical waves coming from the brain onto special paper so that the pattern can be analyzed.

There is no special preparation for this procedure other than explanation to the patient and reassurance that there is no pain involved. However, if needles are used, they may cause discomfort. After the EEG is completed, a shampoo may be needed to remove electrode paste from the hair. No special observations pertaining to the test need to be made.

ECHOENCEPHALOGRAM

The echoencephalogram uses ultrasound to determine the size, shape, and position of the deep structures within the skull. Vibrating sound waves are aimed at the brain, and the echo that is reflected is recorded. The patient should be informed before the test that it will be painless and noninvasive.

MYELOGRAM

A myelogram is the injection of a gas, air, or a radiopaque dye into the spinal canal. The vertebral column is then x-rayed to determine if there is any deviation from the normal. A spinal cord tumor or ruptured intervertebral disk may be visualized in this manner. If a dye is used, it will be removed through a lumbar puncture. After the procedure, the patient remains flat in bed for a certain period of time. The nursing care given to this patient is similar to that given after a pneumoencephalogram or lumbar puncture.

ELECTROMYOGRAPHY

The patient having electromyography has a recording of electrical activity in the peripheral nerve and a particular muscle. This diagnostic test may be ordered when the physician suspects a neuromuscular disorder such as muscular dystrophy.

During the procedure, small needle electrodes are inserted into the specific muscle being tested. A recording is made of electrical activity in the muscle both at rest and during contraction. The patient is told to expect discomfort as the needles are inserted. In addition, the patient is asked to contract and relax certain muscles during the test.

NERVE CONDUCTION STUDIES

Nerve conduction studies are measurements of the speed at which nerve impulses are conducted along a peripheral nerve fiber. An electrical stimulus is applied to the specific nerve being tested. The stimulus, in turn, initiates a nerve impulse which travels along the nerve and is recorded by an electrode placed a measured distance away from the stimulus. The transmission time and distance from the stimulus to the recorder are used to calculate the conduction velocity.

This diagnostic study may be helpful in identifying injury, compression, or disease affecting peripheral nerves. The patient usually has a mild shock sensation as the electrical stimulus is applied.

Nursing Observations

The nurse's observations are crucial to the patient with a disturbance in the nervous system. As mentioned earlier in the chapter, the nervous system receives, processes, stores, and transmits information. Disruptions of these vital functions cause mental, emotional, and physical changes which range from minor annoyances to life-threatening crises. Most nursing observations are based on the fact that the brain and spinal cord form a closed system protected by the skull which permits little room for expansion. An abnormality that occupies even a small space usually causes symptoms.

Some or all of the observations discussed in this section may be present when the pressure in the brain increases, a life-threatening condition known as rising *intracranial pressure*. Tables 21.2 and 21.3 contain guidelines to assist the nurse when

TABLE 21.2
LEVELS OF CONSCIOUSNESS

STATE OF CONSCIOUSNESS	OBSERVED PATIENT BEHAVIOR
Conscious	Awake and alert; participates appropriately in conversation; oriented to time, place, others, and self
Lethargic	Asleep unless aroused by verbal stimulus. When touched or spoken to, verbal response is slow but appropriate. After stimulus, falls back to sleep
Disoriented	When asked, unable to identify time, place, person, or self. May not remember even after this information is provided
Delirious	Restless, hyperactive, agitated, fearful, suspicious, disoriented. Visual and/or auditory hallucinations may be present
Obtunded	Requires repeated vigorous stimulus such as shaking in order to respond. Painful stimulus may be needed to obtain response. Verbal response may be short and inappropriate. May respond to painful stimulus slowly but appropriately
Stuporous	Makes no verbal response even to painful stimulus. Moves in response to painful stimulus, but movements are not appropriate to stimulus
Comatose	Does not respond to any stimulus

OBSERVING THE LEVEL OF CONSCIOUSNESS

Consciousness can be thought of as complete awareness of the self in the environment. A completely conscious person is awake and able to participate appropriately in conversation. Such a person can correctly identify the time, place, familiar persons, and the self.

Research has demonstrated that changes in the level of consciousness are the earliest indicators of a change in the patient's neurologic condition. Consciousness may change rapidly within moments or slowly over a period of weeks or months, depending upon the patient's underlying condition. For this reason, the nurse regularly observes, reports, and records the level of consciousness in the patient with a disturbance of the nervous system. This observation is so important that it is one of the parts of the neurologic assessment done by the nurse. In clinical practice, this assessment is often called the *neurocheck*.

The patient's level of consciousness is observed by providing a stimulus and observing the response. The two stimuli most often used are verbal and physical. For example, the nurse may ask a question or try to engage the patient in conversation. If there is no response to verbal stimuli, the nurse may

observing the patient with a disturbance in the nervous system.

TABLE 21.3
GUIDE TO THE NEURO CHECK

PROCEDURE	NURSING IMPLICATIONS
Check the level of consciousness (LOC)	Changes in LOC are first sign of changes in patient's condition
Observe pupil size, shape, equality, and reaction to light	Changes may develop in patients with drug overdose, brain hemorrhage, rising intracranial pressure, and metabolic disturbances
Observe posture and movement	Specific postural changes and changes in strength and symmetry of movement help to locate part of the brain affected by disease
Check the vital signs	Bradycardia, rising systolic blood pressure, and widening pulse pressure occur late in the patient with rising intracranial pressure. Irregular pulse may indicate cardiac arrhythmia. Breathing pattern may help to identify anatomic location of disease process in brain

provide a physical stimulus by shaking the patient, applying pressure over the eye or sternum, or pricking the skin with a pin. Uniform descriptions of altered states of consciousness are not yet available. For this reason, the nurse describes both the stimulus applied and patient's response when recording and reporting the level of consciousness. In addition, the nurse should consult hospital or agency policy about stimuli to be used and the next procedure to be followed in observing and reporting the level of consciousness. Table 21.2 contains descriptions of levels of consciousness and related patient behavior that the nurse may use as guidelines.

OBSERVING THE PUPILS

The patient with a disturbance in the nervous system may have a change in normal pupil size, shape, and reaction to light. These changes can be detected by observing the pupils and shining a light into them. Normal pupils are round and of equal size (2 to 6 mm). When light is shone into the pupils, they constrict immediately. When the light is withdrawn, the pupils dilate rapidly.

A number of abnormal findings are possible. For example, the pupils may be abnormally small or large or unequal in size (Figure 21.12). These findings usually are recorded using a diagram to show the abnormal or unequal size. Both pupils may react sluggishly to light or one pupil may react more slowly than the other. The pupil(s) is called *fixed* or *nonreactive* when it dos not react to light. The pupil check is a part of the neurocheck as listed in Table 21.3.

BEHAVIORAL CHANGES

In addition to observing and recording the level of consciousness, the nurse looks for behavioral changes that develop in the patient with a disturbance in the nervous system. In order to detect subtle changes, it is important to know something about how the person usually acts. This information often can be obtained from family members and friends. For example, the person who is usually very energetic and becomes listless may be demonstrating a behavioral change associated with illness. The person who is

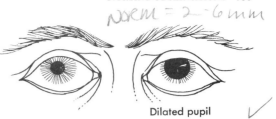

FIGURE 21.12 The pupils of the eye should be checked for position, reaction to light, and whether dilated or constricted.

usually very calm and becomes easily excitable and highly emotional may be having a behavioral change caused by illness. The patient having seizures or other unusual physical activity is demonstrating behavioral changes associated with illness. A detailed description about observing seizures is presented later in this section. When reporting and recording the patient's behavior, it is more helpful to describe what the person actually said or did. Labels such as cooperative, uncooperative, and confused are generally avoided because they do not provide enough detail to be helpful in evaluating the patient's condition.

OBSERVING POSTURE AND MOVEMENT

Abnormalities of posture or movement may occur in some persons with a disorder of the nervous system. Such abnormalities may occur on one side of the body (unilateral) or on both sides of the body (bilateral). *Decorticate posture* is the term used to describe hyperflexion of the upper extremities accompanied by hyperextension of the lower extremities. *Decerebrate posture* is the term used to describe hyperextension of both the upper and lower extremities. These abnormal postures may occur in the patient when stimulated or at other times. The presence of these postures or a change in them indicates that the patient is extremely ill. Postural changes are reported to the appropriate nurse or physician at once.

When observing the patient's movement, the nurse looks to see if it is equal and strong on both sides of the body. For example, when the patient is asked to squeeze the nurse's fingers, the handgrasps should be firm, equal, and strong. Similarly, when the patient is asked to push and pull both feet against the nurse's hands, the observed force should be firm, strong, and equal. The nurse observes and records the strength and symmetry of the patient's movements as part of the neurocheck.

VITAL SIGNS

A number of changes in vital signs may occur in the person with a neurologic disorder. Remembering the function of the autonomic nervous system enables the nurse to understand that temperature, pulse, respirations, and blood pressure may fluctuate considerably when the patient has a neurologic disease. Although changes in vital signs are usually late signs of changes in the patient's condition, they are part of the neurocheck (see Table 21.3).

The patient with rising intracranial pressure develops characteristic changes in vital signs. These include a slow pulse (bradycardia), rising systolic blood pressure, and widening pulse pressure (increased difference between the systolic and diastolic blood pressure). Because these changes occur late in the deterioraton of the patient's condition, it is important to observe and report early signs such as a change in the level of consciousness as described earlier in this chapter.

When the hypothalamus is affected by the patient's condition, the temperature may be either subnormal or greatly elevated. Hyperthermia (elevated temperature) is of special concern because it produces changes in cell metabolism and body chemistry that further affect the brain.

When observing the patient's pulse, the nurse notes and records the rate, rhythm, and quality. In certain neurologic conditions, the patient is more likely to develop a cardiac arrhythmia (see Chapter 11). Therefore, the nurse reports an irregular pulse at once so that an ECG or cardiac monitoring can be initiated if necessary.

The patient's respiratory pattern provides important information about the specific anatomic area of the brain affected by disease. Characteristic patterns of breathing develop according to the specific part of the brain involved. Additional information related to abnormal breathing patterns can be located in Chapter 14.

OBSERVING DRAINAGE

Following injury or surgery to the brain, leakage of cerebrospinal fluid from the nose and/or ears should be reported at once. Cerebrospinal fluid is normally clear in color. The *halo sign* helps the nurse to identify cerebrospinal fluid when it is mixed with blood or other drainage. The halo sign is an area of bloody or dark drainage encircled by a lighter ring (halo) of fluid which is cerebrospinal fluid. This fluid distinguished from mucus by testing the drainage with a DEXTROSTIX to identify the presence of glucose. Glucose is present in cerebrospinal fluid but not in mucus.

OBSERVING SEIZURES

The patient with a seizure has a sudden episode of excessive discharge of impulses from the neurons which causes a change in the level of consciousness, as well as abnormal sensory and motor activity. Several kinds of seizures have been identified. For a detailed description of common seizures, refer to page 761.

A variety of conditions are associated with seizures. These include head injury, brain tumor, brain surgery, increased intracranial pressure, alcoholism, and epilepsy (described later in the chapter). When observing a patient during a seizure, it is important for the nurse to collect the following information:

- Warning signs, if present
- Specific location of the beginning of the seizure (such as hand, foot, face; also, note which side of the body)
- Sequence or progression of seizure activity from one part of the body to another
- Presence of urinary and/or fecal incontinence
- Presence of dilated pupils or deviation to one side of body
- Changes of pulse, respirations, skin color during seizure
- Level of consciousness before, during, and after seizure
- Length of time of seizure

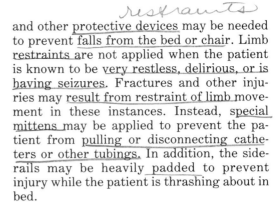

- Patient's condition following the seizure (as determined by the neurocheck)

Table 21.5 (page 762) contains a summary of nursing interventions appropriate when a person is having a seizure.

OTHER OBSERVATIONS

The person with *vertigo* experiences a sensation of whirling or spinning which is often accompanied by nausea, vomiting, pallor, diaphoresis, and tinnitus. Symptoms may be helped by lying down with the eyes closed and worsened by moving, turning the head, and sitting up.

The person with *dizziness* has a feeling of swaying or swimming which is often accompanied by palpitations and trembling. The individual with *syncope* has a fainting spell associated with a temporary loss of consciousness, generalized loss of postural tone, and rapid recovery.

 The patient with *headache* (cephalgia) has pain in the head which may develop from a variety of conditions. The nurse collects and records information related to the location, description, intensity, and duration of the headache, as well as factors that make the pain better or worse.

Nursing Interventions

MAINTAINING SAFETY

The safety of the patient is a primary concern of the nurse. The need for usual safety measures is enhanced when the patient has a disorder of the nervous system because of altered sensation, perception, and judgment, as well as a disturbance in motor function (movement). This combination results in increased risk of accident and injury. Accident and injury often can be prevented by (1) regular systematic inspection of the environment for safety hazards, and (2) immediate correction of hazards when first observed.

The patient in bed may have siderails up at all times to serve as reminders of the location of the edges of the bed. The call bell and other needed objects may be placed within easy reach to avoid long stretches which may result in a fall. Special vests, jackets,

and other protective devices may be needed to prevent falls from the bed or chair. Limb restraints are not applied when the patient is known to be very restless, delirious, or is having seizures. Fractures and other injuries may result from restraint of limb movement in these instances. Instead, special mittens may be applied to prevent the patient from pulling or disconnecting catheters or other tubings. In addition, the siderails may be heavily padded to prevent injury while the patient is thrashing about in bed.

The patient who is ambulating in the hospital corridors needs appropriate nonskid footwear, a shorter length gown, robe, or pajama bottoms to prevent trips and falls. The corridors should be free from dangerous obstacles such as wheelchairs, stretchers, laundry hampers, and spills. The patient who uses a cane or walker for ambulation needs appropriate instruction and supervision on how to use it safely.

ASSISTING WITH HYGIENE

The patient with a disturbance in the nervous system may need more frequent baths and oral hygiene because of changes in the regulation of temperature, perspiration, respiration, and elimination. Good skin care is especially important when the patient's normal protective mechanisms such as sensation and movement are disturbed by illness.

When helping the patient with bathing and oral hygiene, the nurse has an opportunity to observe important changes in the level of consciousness, communication, muscle strength and flexibility, and perception. For example, the nurse may observe that the patient does not wash a body part. The reasons for this might include lack of awareness of the body part; weakness, tremors, or stiffness of the washing hand, arm, or shoulder; or pain.

Range-of-motion exercises normally done during the bath may be altered for some patients to prevent an increase in intracranial pressure. For example, the exercises may be passive (done by the nurse) instead of active (done by the patient). When helping the patient with passive range of motion, the nurse stops the specific exercise when pain, resistance, or fatigue occurs.

ASSISTING WITH POSITIONING AND MOVEMENT

When moving and repositioning the patient with a neurologic disorder, the nurse selects those positions that promote good air exchange, maintain normal alignment of body parts, and prevent pressure areas (Figure 21.13). In addition, specific positions may be either indicated or avoided, depending upon the patient's specific disease.

The patient's position may be changed as often as every two hours around the clock. Positions to be used or avoided are recorded in a place which is seen easily by members of the nursing staff. In some hospitals, diagrams of positions to be used are placed at the bedside of each patient. Practices that help to achieve and maintain good positioning include having enough personnel available as well as pillows and other positioning devices before moving the patient.

LOG ROLLING PT

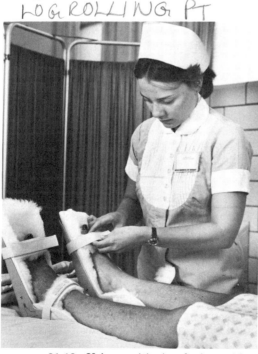

FIGURE 21.13   Using positioning devices with lamb's wool. (Courtesy of Shapero School of Nursing, Sinai Hospital of Detroit, Detroit, Michigan.)

FOOD AND FLUIDS

Alterations in the diet may be needed because of neurologic changes such as alterations in the level of consciousness, difficulty in swallowing, surgery, or motor weakness. Aspiration of food particles is a special hazard for the patient with a neurologic disorder because normal protective mechanisms such as the gag reflex may be changed. The patient with changes in consciousness, sensation, or movement needs careful observation during the mealtime. Good positioning is helpful in preventing aspiration of food particles.

Some patients may need help to eat. Special eating utensils are available for the person with muscle tremors, weakness, or paralysis. The unconscious patient may require gavage feeding in order to remain well nourished.   NG — suprapubic

The physician may prescribe a specific amount of oral or intravenous fluid intake for the patient with a neurologic disorder. Because the patient is less able or slower to adjust to changes in the internal and external environment, it is important to follow the physician's orders carefully. For example, the patient who receives too much fluid may be slow in compensating by making and excreting more urine. This increases the likelihood of fluid overload. Increasing or decreasing the flow rate of intravenous fluids is undertaken cautiously for the same reason. Careful intake and output as well as daily weights help the physician to evaluate the patient's fluid balance.

ASSISTING WITH ELIMINATION

The patient with a disturbance in the nervous system often has associated difficulties with elimination. These difficulties may take the form of urinary retention, infection, or incontinence as well as constipation or stool incontinence. Factors that contribute to problems with elimination include:

- Diminished awareness and impairment of memory
- Disturbances of normal bowel and bladder reflexes
- Changes in usual dietary, fluid intake, and exercise patterns

• Motor weakness or paralysis with difficulty getting to the bathroom

Some elimination problems can be avoided by keeping a careful record of the patient's pattern of urinating and defecating. Stool softeners may be prescribed to help prevent constipation. Intermittent catheterization (page 638) may be needed for some patients to prevent urinary retention.

Urinary and fecal incontinence may cause the patient to feel helpless, guilty, and ashamed. Whenever a pattern of incontinence develops, the nurse may initiate a training program to help the patient regain continence. Additional information about bowel- and bladder-training programs can be located in Chapters 3 (pages 51–52), 15 (pages 470–72), and 19 (pages 641–42).

ASSISTING WITH HYPOTHERMIA

The patient with a disturbance in the nervous system is more likely to develop a fever which results in increased body metabolism and a depletion of oxygen. Brain tissue is so susceptible to oxygen deficiency that permanent irreversible damage to the cells results if body temperature exceeds 41°C (106°F). Hypothermia is a process of reducing the patient's body temperature to normal or below normal levels. A variety of methods is available. Drug therapy with antipyretics to reduce fever and sedatives to prevent shivering may be prescribed. The patient may be bathed or sponged with solutions of alcohol and/or cool water. Ice bags may be placed at the groin, axilla, and neck.

The hypothermic blanket or mattress is another way to reduce body temperature. This device uses a refrigerating machine to circulate a cooled solution of alcohol and water through coils of a rubber or vinyl pad which is placed under and/or over the patient. Before using the hypothermic blanket, the nurse explains why it is necessary and how it works both to the patient and family members. Vital signs and a neurocheck usually are taken and recorded as a baseline from which changes can be evaluated. In some cases, a thin layer of lotion, oil, or cream may be applied to the skin. The specific temperature setting is determined by the physician.

During the time the patient is cooled by the hypothermia blanket, the nurse carefully observes the skin for discolorations, pressure areas, and swelling. The patient is turned frequently and areas of pressure are massaged. When turning or moving the patient, the nurse carefully observes and protects the intravenous site if present. Hypothermia usually causes peripheral veins to collapse, making it much more difficult to insert an intravenous needle or catheter. Vital signs and the neurocheck usually are monitored frequently while the patient is receiving induced hypothermia. Shivering is reported immediately to the appropriate nurse or physician so that the temperature setting can be adjusted if desired. Shivering increases the body heat and raises body temperature.

When the physician decides to terminate hypothermia, the cooling blankets are removed and the patient is covered with regular blankets for rewarming. An alternate method used less often is to raise the temperature setting so that warm liquid circulates through blanket coils. The patient's temperature is observed closely during the rewarming period since wide fluctuations may develop as the body adjusts to the change in environmental temperature.

ASSISTING WITH DRUG THERAPY

A variety of drugs may be prescribed for the patient with a disturbance in the nervous system. Most drugs are prevented from affecting the central nervous system by a network of cells and membranes called the *blood-brain barrier*. When prescribing a drug for a patient with a nervous system disorder, the physician chooses one that can move across the blood-brain barrier. This barrier also affects the dosage of drug needed to produce a therapeutic effect as well as the duration of the drug's action.

Anticonvulsants such as those listed in Table 21.4 are drugs used to prevent or control seizures. Osmotic diuretics such as those listed in Table 11.7 page 301 are prescribed to reduce brain edema. These drugs are administered intravenously to increase osmotic pressure in the bloodstream. This, in turn, causes fluid to leave brain cells and

TABLE 21.4
DRUGS TO CONTROL CONVULSIVE DISORDERS

NONPROPRIETARY NAME	TRADE NAME	AVERAGE DOSE	NURSING IMPLICATIONS
Carbamazepine	TEGRETOL	600–1200 mg/day	Carbamazepine appears effective in generalized and psychomotor seizures. Side effects include drowsiness, irritability, fatigue, hallucinations, and thrombocytopenia
Clonazepam	CLONOPIN	1.5 mg/day in divided doses	Many patients experience drowsiness, somnolence, fatigue, and lethargy
Diazepam	VALIUM	2–10 mg/2–4 times/day	Diazepam has been found effective in status epilepticus, psychomotor seizures, and petit mal seizures. It has a wide margin of safety
Ethosuximide	ZARONTIN	500–1500 mg/day	Ethosuximide is the most effective drug for the treatment of petit mal seizures. Side effects are rare but include nausea, drowsiness, and skin rash
Mephenytoin	MESANTOIN	300–600 mg/day	Mephenytoin has actions similar to those of phenytoin
Mephobarbital	MEBARAL	120–400 mg/day	Mephobarbital and metharbital have actions similar to those of phenobarbital with no apparent advantages
Metharbital	GEMONIL	100 mg 2–3 times/day	
Paramethadione	PARADIONE	900–2100 mg/day in divided doses	Paramethadione is similar to trimethadione, but is less toxic
Phenacemide	PHENURONE	1.5–5 grams/day	Phenacemide is effective in generalized as well as psychomotor seizures. Serious side effects, such as insomnia and personality changes, limit its use
Phenobarbital	LUMINAL	60–200 mg/day	Phenobarbital is one of the oldest and still most effective drugs available for treatment of epilepsy. It is relatively inexpensive for the patient and rarely has toxic effects
Phenytoin	DILANTIN	100 mg/twice daily	Phenytoin is one of the most powerful anticonvulsants available. It is used in control of generalized seizures and has some usefulness in treatment of psychomotor seizures. A common side effect of phenytoin is hypertrophy of the gums. This can be lessened by brushing of the teeth, massaging of the gums, and proper dental care. Other side effects include ataxia, tremors, gastrointestinal disturbances, and occasionally leukopenia
Primidone	MYSOLINE	500–1500 mg/day in divided doses	Primidone is used particularly in the treatment of psychomotor seizures
Trimethadione	TRIDIONE	900–2100 mg/day in divided doses	Trimethadione is effective in the treatment of petit mal seizures. However, side effects of this drug are common and serious. Sedation, visual disturbances, skin rashes, hepatitis, and nephrosis may occur
Valproic acid	DEPAKENE	1000–3000 mg/day in divided doses	Currently used to treat absence (petit mal) seizures. A few persons experience anorexia, nausea, and vomiting

enter the bloodstream so that the kidneys may eliminate it. Corticosteroids such as dexamethasone (DECADRON) may be prescribed to reduce intracranial pressure. When corticosteroids are ordered, the physician frequently prescribes an antacid such as MAALOX and/or cimetidine (TAGAMET) to prevent gastric irritation which can lead to bleeding. Antibiotics are frequently prescribed to prevent or treat infection.

Drugs usually avoided for the patient with a disturbance in the nervous system include narcotic analgesics and alcohol. These drugs can mask important symptoms.

ASSISTING WITH COMMON CONCERNS

To understand fully the concerns of the patient with a disturbance in the nervous system, the nurse can consider some of the basic functions of the system such as receiving and processing information as well as regulating and coordinating motor activity. A disturbance in these functions may cause the patient to experience problems in some or all areas of human living including thinking, feeling, sexuality, movement, working, and judgment. Personality changes may cause the patient to become unrecognizable to him- or herself as well as family and friends.

An early form of assistance is active listening to the fears and concerns expressed by the patient, family, and friends. A second form of assistance is explaining the source of the patient's behavior. For example, Mr. Jones is normally a calm, patient man. Because of his illness, Mr. Jones gradually became more irritable, angry, and frustrated. The nurse was able to help Mrs. Jones by explaining the illness as the source of Mr. Jones's change in behavior. A third form of assistance is to obtain expert help for the patient when indicated. For example, the patient with a disturbance in sexual interest or performance may benefit from help from a qualified sexual therapist.

Denial, anger, and depression are common mental mechanisms used by the patient whose life is disrupted by illness in the nervous system. These mechanisms permit the patient to make a gradual adjustment to the

often drastic changes illness brings. In communicating with the patient, the nurse tries to convey genuine concern, hope, and realistic expectations that do not interfere with the protective mechanisms present.

ASSISTING THE NEUROSURGICAL PATIENT

BRAIN SURGERY. Some neurologic conditions can be corrected surgically. For example, the neurosurgeon may be able to remove tumors, growths, blood clots, or pus from the brain. Certain defects in blood vessels within the brain can be repaired during surgery. The most common neurosurgical procedure on the brain is called a *craniotomy*, a surgical opening into the skull which provides access to the brain. A *supratentorial craniotomy* includes procedures done on the cerebrum. An *infratentorial* or *subtentorial craniotomy* includes procedures involving the cerebellum and/or brainstem. *Burr holes* are small openings drilled into the skull bones that permit the neurosurgeon to obtain tissue for a biopsy, remove accessible blood clots, insert drains, or implant an intracranial monitoring device. *Stereotaxic surgery* involves the introduction of a surgical probe to a target area in the brain. The probe is used to create a tiny lesion that relieves or modifies symptoms such as pain, tremors, or seizures. Local anesthesia is used during stereotaxic surgery so that the patient can provide information and activity needed to pinpoint the target area.

Preoperative Care. In addition to the usual preoperative care described in Chapter 6, special attention is given to the need for informed consent before neurosurgery. A responsible family member usually is asked to be present during the discussions about surgery to prevent misunderstandings that may develop from impairment of the patient's memory, understanding, and judgment. The patient also is told in advance that it is necessary to cut the hair and shave the scalp completely before surgery. This may be done after the shampoo on the nursing unit or after the patient is in the operating room. In some hospitals, an additional permit is signed for removal of the hair.

Hair loss usually causes considerable distress and grieving to the patient and family. The nurse encourages the expression of feelings during the preoperative period and reports evidence of severe persistent emotional conflict to the appropriate nurse or physician.

Vital signs and the neurocheck are recorded regularly during the preoperative period to establish a baseline from which postoperative changes can be evaluated. The anesthesiologist or neurosurgeon may substitute a barbiturate for the usual narcotic in the preoperative medication. Narcotics usually are avoided because they depress respirations and may mask neurologic changes. Barbiturates have been found to reduce metabolism in the brain and therefore reduce the requirement for oxygen. A Foley catheter may be inserted either on the nursing unit or in the operating room to monitor fluid balance during and after surgery.

Postoperative Care. The patient returns from the recovery room often with considerable swelling and discoloration about the eyes and face. This may worsen in the first few postoperative days before gradually decreasing. The family or friends of the patient are told in advance of the patient's drastically changed appearance. A large, bulky turban dressing may be in place also. A drain, if present, may be connected to an external drainage system such as HEMOVAC, Jackson-Pratt drainage, or gravity drainage. If no external drainage system is used, frequent dressing changes or reinforcements usually are needed to prevent saturation of the turban dressing and bacterial contamination from the environment.

Following supratentorial craniotomy, the patient's head usually is elevated 30 to 50 degrees and a large pillow is placed under the head and shoulders. Following infratentorial craniotomy, the patient initially may lie flat with a small pillow under the nape of the neck. The head gradually is elevated over a period of days. The patient usually is turned as one unit (log rolled) every two hours from side to side.

Vital signs and neurocheck are monitored carefully, and even small changes are reported to the neurosurgeon. Sudden ap-nea is a special hazard following infratentorial surgery because of the closeness of the surgical procedure to the respiratory control center in the brain. Increased intracranial pressure is another complication. The patient's urinary output is monitored carefully, and the urine specific gravity may be measured often to help evaluate fluid balance.

The patient may remain NPO for 24 hours or longer following surgery. The diet usually progresses from clear liquids to regular if the patient's swallowing and gag reflexes are normal and if there is no nausea or vomiting. Often, the neurosurgeon prescribes a fluid restriction to prevent or reduce cerebral edema which increases intracranial pressure.

Drug therapy after surgery usually includes osmotic diuretics, antibiotics, anticonvulsants, and corticosteroids. To prevent gastrointestinal irritation and bleeding associated with corticosteroids, an antacid such as MAALOX or cimetidine (TAGAMET) usually is ordered also. Analgesics are prescribed cautiously in the postoperative period. Acetaminophen (TYLENOL) and/or codeine sulfate may be prescribed for headache. However, narcotics such as morphine are not prescribed because they depress respirations and mask important neurologic signs such as pupil changes. A stool softener usually is prescribed as soon as the patient can tolerate oral fluids and medication because constipation and straining to have a bowel movement greatly increase intracranial pressure.

If the patient's postoperative course is uncomplicated, rehabilitation usually begins after about a week or two. The nurse participates in the early phase of rehabilitation by encouraging the patient with self-care activities such as eating, bathing, careful positioning, and range of motion. Later, the patient may receive the services of the physical therapist, occupational therapist, and/or speech therapist.

A variety of complications is possible following cranial surgery. Many can be prevented by meticulous postoperative nursing care as described in Chapter 6. Increased intracranial pressure (see pages 746–47) is a special hazard following cranial surgery.

Certain changes in the usual nursing interventions help to prevent an increase in intracranial pressure. For example, the nurse organizes care to avoid clustering many activities together in a short time. Specific activities known to increase pressure include coughing, sneezing, pushing against a footboard, pulling, and turning. The patient usually is instructed to exhale while moving and turning to prevent the glottis from closing and causing an increase in pressure. Isometric exercises are also omitted following cranial surgery since these increase the patient's intracranial pressure. Other postoperative complications following cranial surgery include hydrocephalus, meningitis, diabetes insipidus, and personality changes which may be temporary or permanent.

SPINAL CORD SURGERY. Surgery on the spinal cord may be done to repair a ruptured disk (cushion between the vertebrae), remove a tumor, drain an abscess, or repair injuries and malformations of blood vessels. In order to reach the diseased areas, the neurosurgeon removes a portion of the vertebra known as the lamina in a procedure called *laminectomy*.

Additional terms may be used to describe which vertebrae are involved. For example, cervical laminectomy denotes procedures on the cervical vertebrae. Thoracic or lumbar laminectomy denotes procedures on those vertebrae. A decompression laminectomy is done to relieve pressure on the spinal cord. If several vertebrae are involved, a spinal fusion may be needed to increase strength and stability in the vertebral column. During a spinal fusion, a wedge-shaped piece of bone is removed from a donor site (usually the iliac crest) and grafted between the vertebrae to prevent motion between them.

Preoperative Care. In addition to the usual preoperative care described in Chapter 6, the patient is taught how to log roll postoperatively (Figure 21.14). Log rolling is the term used to describe a method of turning the patient as one unit. Two or three nurses position themselves on the side to which the patient is to be turned. One nurse supports and turns the patient's upper body, while the second nurse supports and turns

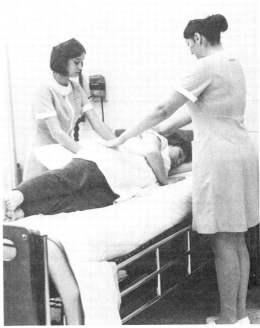

FIGURE 21.14 The neurosurgical patient is being turned in log fashion with the use of a supportive pillow. (Courtesy of Giles County Vocational School, Pearisburg, Virginia.)

the lower body. If the patient has had a cervical fusion, a third nurse supports and turns the head and neck. At a signal from one nurse, all nurses simultaneously roll the patient toward them as one unit. Neurologic and vital signs are taken and recorded as a baseline. Elastic stockings usually are applied preoperatively also.

Another important part of preoperative care is the discussion among the neurosurgeon, patient, and family concerning the possible effects of surgery. The patient's underlying condition has considerable influence on the outcome of surgery. For example, the patient with spinal cord injury may or may not experience a partial return of function after surgery. In some cases, surgery is done to prevent further injury and additional loss of function from edema and/or fractures of the vertebrae. In addition to postoperative complications described in Chapter 6, the patient may develop a cerebrospinal fistula, nerve root injury, arachnoiditis, postural deformity, or severe muscle spasms following a laminectomy. In some cases, the underlying disease process continues and repeated surgery is needed.

Postoperative Care. Before the patient returns from the recovery room, an extra-firm mattress and/or a bedboard is placed on the bed. The patient usually is placed in the side-lying position, either flat or with the head slightly elevated. A pillow may be placed under the patient's head. Following cervical laminectomy, the patient usually wears a cervical collar to support the operative area. A small pillow may be placed at the nape of the neck. The patient is repositioned every two hours using a log roll, as described earlier in this section. After about 48 hours, the patient assists in the log-roll turn, and only one nurse is needed.

Vital signs and the neurocheck are taken and recorded frequently. Following cervical laminectomy, the nurse carefully observes and reports changes in sensation and movement in the shoulders, arms, and hands. Following lumbar laminectomy, the nurse is especially observant for changes in sensation and movement in the legs and feet. Deep-breathing exercises, as described in Chapters 6 and 14, are especially important following laminectomy. The neurosurgeon, however, may avoid the postoperative coughing regimen for some patients to reduce strain on the operative area and aggravation of pain. Following cervical laminectomy, the patient's respirations are observed carefully for impairment caused by swelling around the operative site.

The dressing is observed carefully for the halo effect (see page 736) which indicates leakage of cerebrospinal fluid. Dressing changes or reinforcement, depending on the neurosurgeon's preference, may be needed to prevent contamination of saturated dressings. Following spinal fusion, the dressing on the donor site usually is expected to have more drainage than the dressing over the incision.

In addition to the usual postoperative pain, the patient may have muscle spasms in the upper body following cervical laminectomy or the lower body following lumbar laminectomy. Muscle spasms are believed to result from nerve root irritation during surgery and usually decrease gradually within a few days. Some patients may be helped by a combination of repositioning, relaxation exercises, reassurance, massage, and medication. Following cervical laminectomy, the patient usually has a sore throat which may be relieved by viscous lidocaine (XYLOCAINE), if prescribed.

The patient's intake and output are monitored carefully. Urinary retention is a special hazard following lumbar laminectomy. Every effort is made to help the patient void without catheterization. Typical efforts include standing the male patient to void, running water, placing the patient's hand in warm water, and similar methods as described in Chapter 19, pages 637–38.

The patient usually is helped to ambulate within the first postoperative week, according to the surgical procedure and the neurosurgeon's preference. Following lumbar laminectomy, the flat, standing, or walking positions are preferred to sitting, which increases stress on the operative area. Following cervical laminectomy, pulling of the arms is avoided when helping the patient to move from the erect position since this practice increases the stress on the operative site. The patient continues to wear a cervical collar when ambulating.

Following some types of laminectomies with fusion, the patient may return from the recovery room wearing a cast to immobilize the fused area. Common casts used include the Minerva cast or a body cast. The patient with a cast requires additional nursing observations and interventions, as described in Chapter 17, pages 554–56. After a fusion, the patient experiences a loss of flexibility and permanent stiffness in the fused area. As the patient gradually recovers from surgery, however, increased motion in the joints above the fusion develops to compensate for the loss.

THE UNCONSCIOUS PATIENT

The unconscious person is unable to respond to stimuli in the external environment because of an underlying condition affecting the brain. In addition to brain injury, tumor, thrombosis, or hemorrhage, unconsciousness may develop from respiratory, kidney, or liver failure, drug overdose, diabetic acidosis and other conditions. In other words, unconsciousness is not an illness but the result of other illnesses.

NURSING OBSERVATIONS. The unconscious patient may appear to be asleep but does not awaken or respond to verbal stimuli during a neurocheck. There may be an inappropriate response to painful stimuli or no response. Signs of increased intracranial pressure may or may not be present depending upon the underlying condition. The patient is unable to move or turn when requested. Urinary and/or fecal incontinence may be present. If unconsciousness persists, signs of complications as may be observed. These include problems related to respirations, abdominal distention, kidney stones, urinary tract infection, fecal impaction, decubitus ulcers, and thrombophlebitis.

NURSING INTERVENTIONS. Most nursing interventions for the unconscious patient are based on the need to provide activity essential for survival and prevent complications from immobility. The patient whose unconsciousness is caused by an increase in intracranial pressure needs adjustments in some interventions as discussed on pages 746–47.

Hygiene. The unconscious person needs total assistance with all areas of hygiene. Oral hygiene is especially important to prevent the overgrowth of bacteria in the mouth which later can migrate to the lower respiratory tract to cause life-threatening infection. Careful attention is needed for skin folds and bony prominences in the unconscious person. Changes in normal body functions that occur during this period may cause the skin to break down with the formation of decubitus ulcers. Shaving, combing the hair, and trimming the finger- and toenails may be done by the nurse during the time the patient is unconscious.

Positioning, Turning, and Exercise. The unconscious patient usually is turned at least every two to four hours. After each turn, the exposed bony prominences are massaged generously to prevent pressure areas. For most patients, the positions for turning include side-to-side and the prone position. The supine position usually is avoided because there is danger that the tongue can fall back in the pharynx and obstruct the patient's airway. Special positions indicated for the patient with increased intracranial pressure are described later in this chapter. Mechanical positioning devices such as trochanter rolls, boots, and hand rolls may be used to keep the joints in anatomically correct positions.

Range-of-motion exercises usually are done several times each day to prevent stiffening of the joints and the development of contractures. The family may be taught the exercise program so that they can participate in the care needed to preserve joint function.

The unconscious patient may be lifted to a chair regularly in order to provide an upright position. Special chairs, safety belts, and positioning devices are available that make it possible to place the patient in a safe comfortable position.

In general, the nurse attempts to change the patient's position as often as possible. A practice to be avoided is placing the unconscious patient in a chair for the morning. This practice may result in complications such as pedal edema and decubitus ulcer formation.

Diet and Fluids. The unconscious patient is unable to swallow food and fluids normally. The most common adjustment made is the insertion of a feeding tube and the use of commercial tube feedings to nourish the patient. Special continuous feeding pumps are now available that make possible small or larger amounts of feeding to be instilled, depending upon the patient's needs. The feeding tube should be checked regularly to make sure that it is placed correctly and that residual feeding is not building up in the stomach. The patient should be placed in an upright position, if possible, during and after the feeding.

Elimination. As previously mentioned, the unconscious patient may have fecal and/or urinary incontinence. An external collecting device can be placed on the male patient to prevent urine from saturating the skin and bed linens. Diapers may be needed for the female patient. If the patient's voiding pattern can be identified, a bedpan or urinal may be placed at the anticipated time of voiding. Foley catheters are associated with a high incidence of infection in the urinary tract. Since infection in the unconscious patient may be fatal, catheterization is avoided, if possible.

Stool softeners and suppositories may be needed to encourage elimination of stool in the unconscious patient. In some hospitals, the patient is given a suppository at the same time each day and placed on the bedpan.

The unconscious patient needs meticulous skin care when incontinence is present. In some cases, a protective cream or ointment may be placed on the perineal skin to prevent irritation from urine.

Preventing Complications. Special interventions may be needed to prevent complications. For example, the patient may receive chest physiotherapy and other forms of respiratory therapy, as described in Chapter 14, to prevent complications in the respiratory system such as pneumonia. Elastic stockings may be placed on the patient's legs to prevent thrombophlebitis. Artificial tears may be instilled in the unconscious patient's eyes to prevent drying of the corneas. An older practice which is now avoided is taping the patient's eyes shut. This practice is associated with an increase in eye infection.

Communicating with the Patient and Family. Although the unconscious patient cannot respond, the sense of hearing may remain. For this reason, the nurse continues to explain each procedure in advance. Private conversations in the patient's room are avoided. The family needs this information as well so that disturbing conversations can be avoided.

The patient's family usually is distressed greatly both by the unconscious condition and the underlying disease causing it. The nurse may need to explain more than once the need for certain procedures and/or tests. Specific questions related to the disease process and eventual outcome of unconsciousness may be referred to the physician.

In some cases, the patient's unconsciousness is a prelude to death. In other words,

the unconscious patient is also a dying patient. The family and friends of the patient can be expected to show one or more of the grieving processes described in Chapter 1. The family greatly benefits from the same tender understanding and concern that are given to the patient at this time. The interested family can be encouraged and shown how to participate in care such as range of motion, bathing, massaging body prominences, and similar activities.

THE PATIENT WITH INCREASED INTRACRANIAL PRESSURE

The patient with increased intracranial pressure has a life-threatening elevation of normal pressure in the brain. This condition may develop as a result of edema in cerebral tissue caused by infection, injury, surgery, or tumor in the brain. If the pressure is not relieved successfully, the patient may die from compression and failure of vital brain centers related to temperature, pulse, and respirations as well as blood pressure.

NURSING OBSERVATIONS. Observing and reporting signs of increased intracranial pressure is a major responsibility of the nurse when caring for a patient with a disturbance in the nervous system. The primary purpose of the neurocheck (Table 21.3) is early detection of rising intracranial pressure. The first sign that pressure in the brain is rising is a deterioration in the level of consciousness (LOC). The pupil on the same side as the brain lesion, if present, usually progresses from constriction to dilation, and reaction to light is sluggish. On the side of the body opposite to the lesion, the patient usually experiences progressive loss of sensation and movement. Decorticate or decerebrate posture may be observed in later stages. Characteristic changes in vital signs as described on page 736 develop in later stages also. Another late change is *papilledema* or swelling around the optic nerve which can be seen with an *ophthalmoscope.* Some patients experience headache, nausea, and projectile vomiting.

A recent technologic development for early detection of rising intracranial pressure is the intracranical monitor. A variety of monitors is available. Most systems include a sensor which is implanted into a part of the brain, a transducer which converts impulses to electrical waves, and a recording device. Rising intracranial pressure is detected by analyzing recordings. The patient with this monitoring system usually is placed in an intensive care unit.

NURSING INTERVENTIONS. The patient with increased intracranial pressure needs care similar to that indicated for the unconscious person described earlier in the chapter. Some variations in the usual interventions are needed in order to prevent a rise in pressure associated with the *Valsalva maneuver.* This maneuver is a kind of bearing down with the glottis closed which occurs during many voluntary activities such as turning, exercising, using the bedpan, and pushing up in bed. As the patient bears down, pressures in the abdominal, thoracic, and cranial cavities rise. In order to prevent this rise in pressure, the nurse avoids planning clusters of activities known to increase intracranial pressure. For example, turning, using the bedpan, and suctioning the patient when done in the same 15-minute period may cause an unacceptable rise in the patient's intracranial pressure. Other variations in nursing care are described below.

Positioning and Movement. The patient usually is placed in a semi-Fowler's position with the head elevated about 30 degrees to reduce pressure in the brain. The prone position and exaggerated hip and neck flexions are avoided because they increase intracranial pressure. The patient may be turned every two hours. The conscious patient is instructed to exhale slowly during the turning process to avoid closing of the glottis and the Valsalva maneuver. In addition, the conscious patient is cautioned not to push, pull, or dig in with the heels. Range-of-motion exercise is usually passive (done by the nurse) instead of active. Isometric exercises are avoided.

Diet and Fluids. If the patient is alert enough to swallow safely, a light diet may be prescribed. The patient may be fed the prescribed diet slowly and carefully. Some physicians prescribe a fluid restriction to reduce the volume of fluid in the body. Fluid intake is recorded carefully.

osmolytics

Elimination. A Foley catheter may be inserted to monitor urine output. Urine specific gravity may be measured frequently to evaluate brain function and the effectiveness of drug therapy.

Enemas and straining to have a bowel movement are avoided since these activities cause a rise in intracranial pressure. Instead, stool softeners and mild laxatives may be prescribed to prevent constipation. It is especially important to report constipation early—after 24 hours pass without a bowel movement. Early action is needed to prevent severe constipation.

Drug Therapy. Drug therapy is an important part of treatment for the patient with increased intracranial pressure. Osmotic diuretics, anticonvulsants, corticosteroids, and antacids are prescribed usually. An antipyretic such as acetaminophen (TYLENOL) may be ordered, if the patient is febrile.

Other Therapies. While taking measures to reduce the patient's intracranial pressure, the physician also tries to identify and treat the underlying cause. A brain tumor may have to be removed surgically. An infection usually requires a course of antibiotic therapy. The patient with a brain injury may require time and rest. The specific therapy depends upon the underlying condition.

Tumor of the Brain

The patient with a *brain tumor* or an *intracranial tumor* has an abnormal growth of cells within the skull. The tumor may be *primary* (that is, it started in the brain), or it may be *secondary* or *metastatic* (that is, the tumor started in another part of the body and spread to the brain). An intracranial tumor may be either benign or malignant.

The patient with a malignant tumor that has spread from another part of the body is more likely to have an unfavorable outcome than is the patient with a malignant tumor that started in the brain and is diagnosed early.

NURSING OBSERVATIONS

The patient's symptoms depend a great deal upon the size of the tumor, its rate of growth, its type, and location. This underscores the need for careful observations and accurate, complete recording.

The patient may have headache and/or a loss of sensation of a body part. A tumor in the part of the cerebrum that controls movement may cause the patient to have weakness, convulsions, and paralysis. These symptoms occur in the part of the body that receives its nerve supply from the diseased area of the brain. If the patient's tumor is on the left side, the right side of the body is affected. A tumor in the part of the cerebrum that controls behavior may cause the patient to have personality changes. There may be sudden outbursts of crying and laughing that are unlike the person's usual behavior. Such a person may also become untidy or use vulgar language. Another example of the tumor's location affecting the patient's symptoms is seen in the patient with a tumor in the occipital lobe of the brain. This patient may have visual disturbances, such as difficulty in reading, spots before the eyes, and blindness, since the occipital lobe controls sight.

A brain tumor usually produces symptoms of increased pressure within the cranium, which is known as increased intracranial pressure. Remembering that the brain is soft and is housed in a bony cage helps the nurse to understand the changes that take place. The soft brain yields to pressure and the hard bones of the skull do not. Thus, an abnormality such as a tumor, bleeding, or edema, increases pressure within the cranium.

The neurocheck usually is done frequently when a brain tumor is suspected (see Table 21.3). The nurse reports abnormal findings or changes to the appropriate nurse or physician at once. The patient may be transferred to the intensive care unit for intracranial monitoring and treatment of increased intracranial pressure as described on pages 746–47.

ASSISTING WITH DIAGNOSTIC STUDIES

The patient with a brain tumor is examined carefully by the neurologist or neurosurgeon during a neurologic examination as described earlier in the chapter. The family and/or friends may be asked to provide information related to mental or personality changes, if present.

Skull x-rays usually are done early in the diagnostic process. Other x-rays, such as the chest x-ray, also may be done to identify or rule out brain metastasis from a primary tumor in some other part of the body. A brain scan and CT scan usually are done to help identify the location of the tumor. Other common diagnostic studies when a brain tumor is suspected include lumbar puncture (if increased intracranial pressure is not a problem), arteriograms, and pneumoencephalogram.

NURSING INTERVENTIONS

When possible, the tumor is removed surgically during a craniotomy. The patient requires care as described earlier for the neurosurgical patient. Every effort is made to preserve as much brain tissue as possible. Still, the patient may have permanent mental, emotional, and physical changes as a result of brain surgery. Specific changes depend upon the location of the tumor, size of the tumor, and remaining functional neurons. In some instances, surgery is not indicated, and radiation therapy may be done instead. The patient requires care similar to that described in Chapter 9, pages 233–35.

The patient's convalescence may be longer than that of a patient recovering from other types of surgery. Throughout this period, understanding and encouragement are needed from all members of the health team. Rehabilitation plays an important role in this patient's recovery. For example, it may be necessary for the patient to learn to talk or to walk again. There may be other disability as a result of the tumor. Emphasis should be placed on remaining capabilities rather than disability. The aim of the health team in caring for this patient is to help him or her to live most happily and effectively with disability.

Injury of the Brain

Although a bony cage protects the brain, it may become injured. Damage to the brain can vary from slight bruising to severe destruction of tissue. Brain injury is known also as an *intracranial injury*.

A *concussion* is a minor head injury that usually follows a fall or a blow on the head. Some concussive blows cause only temporary visual disturbances and loss of equilibrium. Severe concussive blows cause loss of consciousness, temporary paralysis, and amnesia for the event that occurred. The patient's skin becomes pale and cold, and the pulse is weak. As consciousness returns, the patient may vomit and complain of a headache.

A severe head injury usually causes brain tissue to be damaged and blood vessels to be torn. Such injuries may be called *cerebral contusions* and lacerations. Blood flowing from the torn blood vessels collects within the cranial cavity and forms a clot. This condition is known as a *hematoma*. The hematoma may form above the dura and is then called an *extradural* or *epidural* hematoma. If the clot forms under the dura, it is called a *subdural* hematoma. An extradural hematoma usually occurs suddenly after the head injury. A subdural hematoma however, can be acute, subacute, or chronic, and symptoms of this condition can occur months after the head injury. A *depressed fracture* of the skull also can cause brain damage. The patient's head should be checked for obvious signs of fracture. In this type of fracture, the bony fragments are driven inward into the brain. Blood flowing from torn blood vessels, fluid escaping from the damaged brain tissue, and a depressed fracture cause the patient to have increased intracranial pressure. The amount of damage to the brain and the location of the injury determine the seriousness of the patient's condition. A *linear skull fracture* is a fracture of the skull resembling a line. The bones are not out of line, and the fracture usually will heal without surgery. A concussion or contusion may occur with a linear fracture.

Meningitis, a brain abscess, encephalitis, epilepsy, and paralysis may result from a brain injury. The individual's mentality is affected sometimes. Another complication is severe headaches. The patient may suffer with headaches long after other sypmtoms have disappeared.

NURSING OBSERVATIONS

The patient with a head injury frequently is admitted to the hospital for observation. The primary concern is the possibility of increased intracranial pressure and/or leakage of cerebrospinal fluid. A special hazard exists for the patient with other injuries who also may have an undetected head injury. For this reason, the nurse may develop a practice of doing the neurocheck on all patients admitted for injuries.

The patient with an intracranial injury may have local symptoms of injury, such as a bleeding wound or a fracture. However, an external wound is not always seen. There is sometimes a period in which the patient appears to have recovered completely and seems to be well oriented. Later, however, the patient may develop the symptoms of increased intracranial pressure. The symptoms are determined by the amount of brain damage. In addition to symptoms of increased intracranial pressure, the patient may have bleeding from the nose, throat, or ears. There also may be clear liquid draining from the ears and nose. This means the meninges have been torn and spinal fluid is escaping. The nurse may look for the halo sign and test the drainage with DEXTROSTIX, as described earlier in the chapter, to identify cerebrospinal fluid. The pupil of the patient's eye on the injured side may be dilated. The patient may have visual disturbances such as blurring or seeing double (diplopia). Weakness or paralysis of an extremity and convulsions can occur also.

A severe head injury usually causes the patient to lose consciousness immediately. A deep state of unconsciousness over a period of time usually indicates an unfavorable outcome. The patient should be observed for symptoms of increased intracranial pressure discussed earlier in this chapter. The doctor may ask the nurse to check the patient's blood pressure, temperature, pulse, respiration, and neurologic signs every hour.

In addition to checking the vital signs, pupillary reaction and the level of consciousness should be checked. The patient who appears to be sleeping should be aroused gently to check the level of consciousness. Even when sleeping, the patient must be awakened for otherwise there is no way of knowing the state of consciousness. The nurse also should observe the patient for signs of deafness, visual disturbances, neck rigidity, convulsions, drainage from the ears and nose, and weakness and/or paralysis of the extremities. A change in any of the above signs, or their appearance, should be reported immediately. The centers that control these vital functions are located in the brain. Thus, injury of one of these centers may cause serious results. For instance, damage to the respiratory center causes the patient's respirations to become slower. A marked decrease in the respiratory rate indicates that the patient needs help in breathing. Such a symptom should be reported immediately.

NURSING INTERVENTIONS

Whenever a head injury is suspected, the patient is placed on bed rest. Nursing interventions described earlier for the unconscious patient and the person with increased intracranial pressure apply to the patient with head injury.

If fluid is draining from the nose, ears, or other body openings, no attempt is made to stop the flow or clean the orifice (Figure 21.15). Free drainage is encouraged. The patient is instructed not to blow the nose.

Generally, the physician performs surgery on the patient with either a depressed fracture or a hematoma. The area around the wound is cleaned and shaved before surgery. The surgeon removes damaged scalp tissue. Bone fragments may be either removed or raised from the brain. It may be necessary for the doctor to place a plate of metal or polyethylene over the opening in the scalp. The surgeon makes an opening through the scalp and skull when it is necessary to remove a hematoma (blood clot). The neurosurgeon will do a craniotomy when a large opening is indicated. Burr holes may be made if the patient's hematoma is located by x-ray examinations and neurologic signs. The patient having brain surgery because of injury needs the same type of care that was discussed in relation to the patient having surgery for a brain tumor.

If surgery is not required, the patient will be treated medically. As previously mentioned, nursing interventions include those needed for the patient with increased intracranial pressure and the unconscious patient. Hypothermia may be needed when temperature elevations cannot be reduced by acetaminophen (TYLENOL).

The patient's family is usually very apprehensive. The nurse can provide emotional support by providing skilled care and genuine interest. Specific questions regarding the patient's condition should be referred to the professional nurse or physician.

Tumor of the Spinal Cord

An individual may have a tumor on the outside of the spinal cord and develop symp-

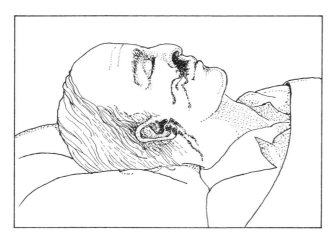

FIGURE 21.15 No attempt should be made to clean fluid from the orifices.

toms when it presses on the cord, or there may be a tumor within the spinal cord. The tumor may be either benign or malignant.

NURSING OBSERVATIONS

Pain is generally an early symptom experienced by the individual with a spinal cord tumor. The pain may be localized in the back over the area of the tumor and may persist over a long period of time. The pain also can occur in the part of the body that receives its nerve supply from the affected area of the spinal cord. For example, a tumor in the upper part of the spine could cause the patient to have chest pain, since the chest receives its nerve supply from that part of the spinal cord. A tumor in the lower region could cause the patient to have pain in the abdomen or legs.

The patient's pain may be associated with numbness and tingling. The affected part of the body may become weak. This usually is caused by an enlargement of the tumor. The patient may lose all sensation in regions of the body that receive their nerve supply from the part of the spinal cord below the tumor. Paralysis also may develop. The patient has *paraplegia* when the lower limbs are paralyzed, and *quadriplegia* when all four of the extremities are paralyzed. The patient may have urinary disturbances, such as incontinence, retention, and urgency to void.

ASSISTING WITH DIAGNOSTIC STUDIES

The diagnosis is made by careful history and neurologic examination. An x-ray of the vertebral column, a lumbar puncture, and a myelogram also may be done to aid in confirming the diagnosis. Specific tests may be done on the blood and spinal fluid. A CAT scan assists the physician to identify the location of a spinal cord tumor as well as malformations of blood vessels, if present. Arteriograms may be done when the tumor is highly vascular (contains many blood vessels).

During the diagnostic period, the nurse can anticipate and appreciate the patient's anxiety and concern. Active listening encourages the patient to verbalize such concerns. Repeated explanations may be needed about the specific tests to be done. In some cases, the patient is helped by the nurse's presence during the physician's visit so that all questions can be asked and answered in understandable language.

NURSING INTERVENTIONS

A tumor of the spinal cord is treated by surgical removal, when possible. The tumor is made accessible when the neurosurgeon does a laminectomy. Nursing care for the patient having a laminectomy was described earlier in the chapter on pages 743–44.

Radiation therapy may be used instead of, or in addition to, surgery. In this case, the patient requires additional nursing observations and interventions as described in Chapter 9, pages 233–35.

Drug therapy may include a corticosteriod such as dexamethasone (DECADRON) to relieve pressure in the spinal cord temporarily. Throughout therapy, the nurse continues to observe and record changes in sensation and motion.

Unsuccessful medical or surgical therapy results in tumor growth, a progressive loss of sensory and motor function, and chronic pain. In this case, the nurse's efforts are directed toward pain relief and prevention of complications. The patient needs care similar to that indicated for a person with spinal cord injury, described later in the chapter. In addition, the person needs tender loving care appropriate for the dying patient. Such a patient can be expected to be alert and oriented and to show behavioral changes associated with grieving, as described in Chapter 1.

Injury of the Spinal Cord

An individual may receive an injury to the spinal cord by an object penetrating the vertebrae, such as a bullet. Also, a fracture or a dislocation may result in spinal cord injury. The cord may be severed completely or it may be destroyed partially. Bleeding and edema following an injury to the spinal cord may cause the patient to have paralysis, which disappears when the blood and edema fluid are absorbed.

Spinal cord injury results in catastrophic changes in a person's life. Such changes include disturbances in human functions such as breathing, eating, dressing, ambulation, sexuality, elimination, and emotions. Recovery from illness and adjustment to disability are measured in years rather than weeks or months.

NURSING OBSERVATIONS

The patient with a spinal cord injury can be expected to show partial or complete loss of sensory and motor function below the level of injury. Specific symptoms depend upon the location and extent of injury to the spinal cord. Injury to the cervical portion of the cord may interfere with normal respirations and other vital signs.

Immediately after the injury, the patient experiences a condition known as *spinal shock,* which usually lasts from one to six weeks. At this time, there is usually flaccid muscle paralysis below the level of injury. Some or all of the spinal reflexes may be absent. There is a partial or complete loss of sensations of pain, temperature, position, touch, and pressure below the level of injury. Instead the patient may report pain above the injured area. The ability to perspire in the involved area may be impaired. There may be partial or complete loss of bowel and bladder function. The male patient may experience *priapism* (abnormal, continuous, painful erection).

As spinal shock subsides, a change in observations may be seen. In some cases, a partial return of function occurs. In other cases, the nature of the patient's paralysis changes.

Paraplegia describes paralysis of the lower half of the body. Quadriplegia refers to paralysis of all four extremities. The patient may or may not have sensation and reflex action in the paralyzed area.

When observing the patient's paralyzed muscles, the nurse may see either spasticity (increased muscle tone with involuntary spasms), flaccidity (weakness and softness or lack of muscle tone), or fasciculations (brief muscle contractions visible through the skin). These observations are recorded with descriptions of the specific areas involved and whether the observations were noted with or without stimulation. Muscles may atrophy (wither away) following some injuries. Trophic skin changes such as dryness, hairlessness, and cyanosis may develop in the involved areas.

When observing a person soon after spinal cord injury, the nurse looks carefully for other undetected injuries such as internal bleeding and head injury. Lack of painful sensations may cause such injuries to remain hidden until a crisis develops.

NURSING INVENTIONS

EMERGENCY CARE.   Emergency care of the patient with suspected spinal injury is directed toward preventing further cord injury. The patient is not moved at all until sufficient trained persons are available. At least three or four persons are needed to transfer the adult patient as one unit or a stiff board onto a stretcher to a neutral supine position. The vertebrae are kept as motionless as possible, and the head and neck are supported so that there is no movement before, during, or after the transfer. Sandbags may be used to prevent rotation or flexion of the head and neck. The conscious patient is instructed not to move at all. The unconscious patient is treated as having possible spinal cord injury until it has been determined by x-rays and the physician that no injury is present.

In the emergency room, careful attention is directed toward maintaining the patient's airway, ensuring adequate oxygenation of vital organs, and establishing the extent of the injury.

DRUG THERAPY.   Corticosteroid therapy with dexamethasone (DECADRON) may be given to control edema of the spinal cord. Antacids usually are given simultaneously to prevent gastric irritation. Other drugs may be prescribed as needed to control pain and muscle spasm, treat infection, and prevent constipation.

IMMOBILIZATION.   The patient is often placed in some form of skeletal traction initially to maintain correct anatomic position. When injury has resulted from fractured vertebrae, cervical traction may be accomplished by inserting special tongs into the skull bones and attaching weights using ropes and pulleys, as described in Chapter 17. Common types of cervical tongs include Vinke, Cone, or Crutchfield tongs. The patient requires care similar to that described in Chapter 17, pages 556–59. As mentioned in Chapter 17, traction is never released or removed until therapy is complete. Removing the weights may result in further injury to the spinal cord. The neurocheck is done frequently and changes are reported immediately to the appropriate nurse or physician.

The patient in cervical tongs is on complete bedrest. A Stryker or Foster frame or CIRC-O-LECTRIC bed may be used for ease of turning. If turning is permitting, a nurse is always present at the head to prevent movement and flexion during the turn.

Halo traction is another type of immobilization used for cervical, thoracic, and some lumbar cord injuries. A metal ring (halo) is attached to the skull bones using four pins. Often, halo traction is used together with a body jacket cast made of fiberglass or plaster. If paralysis is not present, the patient may be encouraged to ambulate. Several variations are used when the thoracic and lumbar spine are involved. Frequent neurochecks and care similar to that indicated for the patient in a cast (Chapter 17, pages 554–56) are needed.

SURGERY. A decompression laminectomy and spinal fusion may be done to stabilize the spinal column and prevent further injury. When surgery is needed, it usually is done within five days after injury. The patient requires care similar to that described earlier in this chapter on pages 743–44. A recent development in surgery is to cool the spinal cord with cold saline irrigation to reduce edema. This method currently is not widely used; however, the interested nurse may look for new developments in the field.

RESPIRATORY CARE. The patient with spinal cord injury is more likely to develop respiratory infection because of restricted mobility. A regular program of turning, coughing, deep breathing, and postural drainage begins during hospitalization and continues during the patient's rehabilitation. Additional information related to these interventions can be located in Chapter 14.

FOOD AND FLUIDS. A nutritious diet which enables the paralyzed patient to maintain a normal weight is indicated. Fresh fruits and vegetables as well as added fiber help to prevent constipation. A greatly increased fluid intake is needed to prevent respiratory and urinary tract infection.

SKIN CARE. Meticulous skin care is needed to prevent decubitus ulcers. Special beds, mattresses, and flotation pads may be used to prevent pressure areas. All areas of the skin are inspected, washed, dried, and massaged daily to prevent decubitus ulcer.

ELIMINATION. A *neurogenic bladder* is a disturbance in urinary function that develops as a result of disease in the nervous system. Urinary retention, incontinence, stones, and infection are more likely to develop following spinal cord injury. These conditions are more serious in the paralyzed patient because permanent damage to the kidneys and urinary tract develops more often. Nursing interventions that encourage normal urinary tract function include:

- An accurate intake-and-output record
- A fluid intake of at least 3000 ml/day unless otherwise ordered
- Observe and report signs of urinary tract infection, if present (see Chapter 19)
- Meticulous perineal hygiene
- Regular catheter care

In some cases, a bladder-training program or intermittent catheterization, as described in Chapter 19, is indicated to prevent urinary incontinence.

A bowel-training program, as described in Chapter 15, is helpful in preventing constipation, impaction, and incontinence. The program is developed according to the individual patient and local custom.

REHABILITATION. After the acute phase of injury, the patient usually is transferred to a rehabilitation unit to learn how to progress to a more independent life-style. *Autonomic dysreflexia* is an emergency situation which can develop in some patients with spinal cord injury during rehabilitation. This life-threatening crisis occurs when an irritating stimulus triggers a mass discharge of sympathetic impulses. This, in turn, causes a sudden elevation of systolic blood pressure to 240–300 mg Hg, pounding headache, seizures, profuse sweating, and gooseflesh above the lesion.

Irritating stimuli most likely to trigger autonomic dysreflexia include distended bladder, plugged catheter, fecal impaction, decubitus ulcer, leg spasms, and overdistention of the stomach by tube feeding.

Emergency drug therapy with intravenous diazoxide (HYPERSTAT) or hydralazine (APRESOLINE) may be needed if the irritating stimulus cannot be identified and removed immediately. Nursing interventions related to the prevention of irritating stimuli are important in preventing the development of autonomic dysreflexia.

A number of factors influence the patient's rehabilitation process. These include:

- Level of cord injured
- Extent of injury
- Readiness to learn
- Skill of teachers
- Community and family support available
- Stage of adjustment to injury

Many paraplegics live alone and support themselves. The patient may wear braces and be able to use crutches for ambulation. Others may use a wheelchair (Figure 21.16). The psychologic problems are great for even the most well-adjusted person. In the initial stages, the patient has to accept being dependent on others for much care. In later stages, the patient has to become as independent as possible while accepting help needed for some aspects of living. During the rehabilitation process, a major task is to redefine body image, sexuality, life goals, career plans, educational objectives in light of the abilities and disabilities that result from the spinal cord injury. At any point in the process, the nurse can provide important help by listening to the patient's concerns, encouraging another try, consoling a temporary failure, and teaching a new way to do something (Figure 21.17).

Ruptured Intervertebral Disk

Vertebrae are separated by a piece of dense tissue containing cartilage. This tissue is known as an *intervertebral disk*. This serves as a cushion between the vertebrae. Each disk is surrounded by a covering. This covering may rupture and allow the inner

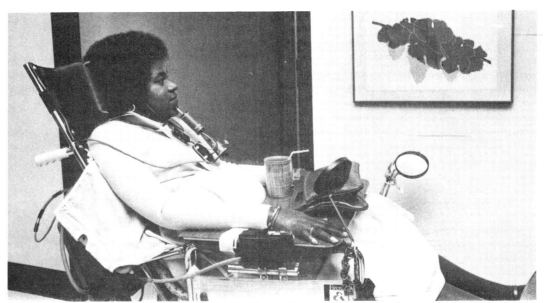

FIGURE 21.16 Using a motorized wheelchair. (Courtesy of Bergen Pines County Hospital School of Practical Nursing, Paramus, New Jersey.)

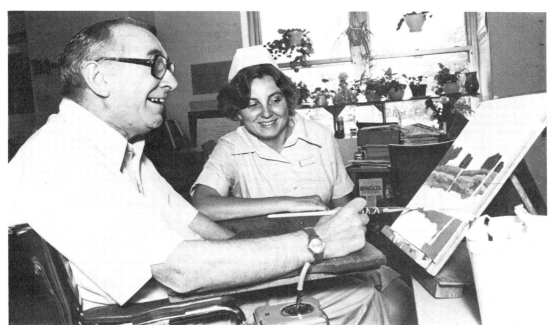

FIGURE 21.17   Providing encouragement and support during rehabilitation. (Courtesy of Bergen Pines County Hospital School of Practical Nursing, Paramus, New Jersey.)

portion of the disk, called the nucleus pulposus, to push outward (see Figure 21.18). The nucleus pulposus is a soft cartilage. The patient has a ruptured intervertebral disk, sometimes called a herniated nucleus pulposus.

NURSING OBSERVATIONS

An individual often develops a ruptured intervertebral disk following an injury of the back, such as a strain. Frequently, the patient gives a history of feeling as though something slipped in the back while bending,

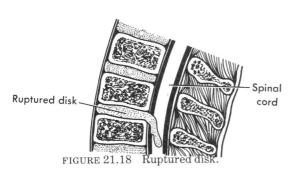

FIGURE 21.18   Ruptured disk.

lifting, or reaching. The misplaced disk may press against nerve roots and cause pain, or it may press against the spinal cord. The patient's pain is usually in the lower part of the back as this is the most common location of ruptured disks. However, the injury may take place in the neck vertebrae. In this case, the patient's pain would be in the neck. The patient with a ruptured disk in the lower vertebral column may have pain that radiates down one leg. Exertion such as coughing, lifting, and bending increases the pain. The patient may have weakness and a loss of feeling in the part of the body supplied by the spinal nerves coming from the injured area.

ASSISTING WITH DIAGNOSTIC STUDIES

The physician usually does a myelogram when a ruptured intervertebral disk is suspected. Spinal x-rays often show a narrowing of the usual space between the vertebrae. Electromyography is another diagnostic test that may be done when a ruptured disk is suspected.

NURSING INTERVENTIONS

The physician may prescribe medical treatment, which consists mainly of rest and traction. The purpose of these two measures is to allow the disk to return to its normal position. The doctor usually recommends bed rest on a firm mattress with a fracture board beneath it. Traction may be used on both legs to obtain extension of the lower vertebrae. Head traction may be used if the ruptured disk is in the neck. These measures help to relieve pain. In addition, local application of heat or ice may be prescribed to relieve the patient's pain. Massage also may be recommended for the same purpose. Analgesics and muscle relaxants may be prescribed.

If the above conservative measures do not relieve the symptoms or if the symptoms recur, it may be necessary for the surgeon to remove the ruptured disk. This is often done by performing a laminectomy, which enables the surgeon to remove the ruptured intervertebral disk. A bone graft (spinal fusion) may be done by the surgeon if the area must be strengthened.

The patient having surgery for a ruptured disk needs, with few variations, the same care as other surgical patients, which was discussed in Chapter 6, and care described earlier in the chapter for a patient having a laminectomy. A back brace may be prescribed by the physician before the patient is allowed out of bed. After the brace has been applied, it should not be removed until permission to do so is given by the doctor. When the patient is out of bed, shoes instead of bedroom slippers may be needed to give more support and lessen the possibility of falling.

The resumption of activity postoperatively depends on the surgical procedure done, the surgeon's preference, and the patient's occupation. Heavy lifting for a certain period of time is avoided, as are twisting, turning, and bending. The patient may have to obtain another job if the previous occupation required heaving lifting. This may cause a problem for the patient and family. The patient's employer and/or vocational counselors may be consulted in an effort to modify the requirements of the patient's occupation.

Inflammatory Conditions of the Nervous System

MENINGITIS

The patient with meningitis has an inflammation of the meninges, the membranes that cover the brain and spinal cord. Meningitis usually is caused by pathogenic microorganisms, such as the meningococcus, the pneumococcus, the streptococcus, and the tubercle bacillus. Viruses also can cause a form of meningitis that may or may not be milder than the type caused by bacteria.

The invading organism frequently enters the body through the nose and throat. It passes from the nose and throat into the bloodstream. The organism is carried by the blood to the meninges. Remembering that the body responds to an invading organism by increasing the blood supply to the area, the nurse easily can understand why the cerebrospinal fluid is increased. White blood cells enter the cerebrospinal fluid in an effort to combat the infection. Pathogens also may invade the meninges and cerebrospinal fluid directly as a result of a head wound, an infectious process in the middle ear, paranasal sinuses or brain abscesses.

NURSING OBSERVATIONS

The patient has symptoms of an infection as well as symptoms of increased intracranial pressure when the inflammation is caused by pathogenic microorganisms. During the early part of this disease, the patient may have symptoms of an upper respiratory infection. Fever, malaise, and vomiting soon follow. The patient is more comfortable when lying on the side with the knees flexed and the head back. There may be headache, and nuchal rigidity (stiff neck), and the fever goes higher as the infection continues. The patient may develop inflamed lips, sensitivity to light (photophobia), irritability, skin eruptions, and convulsions. As intracranial pressures increases, the patient may become delirious or lose consciousness. The neurocheck is done often for this reason (Figure 21.19). Meningitis may be complicated by pneumonia and infections of the ears, sinuses, and eyes.

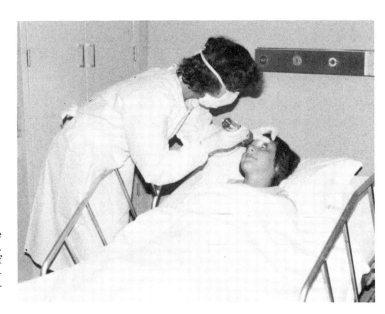

FIGURE 21.19 Checking the pupils of a patient in isolation. (Courtesy of Halifax School of Practical Nursing, Halifax–South Boston Community Hospital, South Boston, Virginia.)

ASSISTING WITH DIAGNOSTIC STUDIES

The physician generally does a lumbar puncture to diagnose meningitis. During the procedure, the doctor will measure the spinal fluid pressure, which is usually higher than normal. The fluid obtained will be examined for the presence of blood cells and the amount of sugar. The cerebrospinal fluid may be cultured and tested for sensitivity to antibiotics. Blood cultures may be obtained, as well as nose and throat cultures, in order to identify the primary site of infection, if possible. Skull and spine x-rays usually are ordered, as well as a chest x-ray to identify undetected injury or sites of infection.

NURSING INTERVENTIONS

The principles of caring for a patient with an infection, such as rest, increased intake of fluid, diet high in calories, and good skin and mouth care, apply to this patient. These are discussed in more detail in Chapter 5.

The patient should have bed rest in a quiet, darkened room. During the acute stage, the patient may convulse when stimulated by loud noises and bright lights. Siderails should be used and the patient observed very carefully and almost constantly. The patient who is unconscious needs the type of nursing care for the unconscious patient as discussed earlier in the chapter (pages 745–46).

The patient may be placed in strict isolation if the infecting organisms are either unknown or believed to be bacterial. When assisting in the care of a person with meningitis, the nurse should follow the isolation procedure used in that particular hospital. The nurse should wash the hands thoroughly before and after caring for the patient. This helps to prevent carrying infection to the patient as well as away from the patient to others.

The physician prescribes one of the antibiotics, such as penicillin, oxytetracycline (TERRAMYCIN), or one of the sulfonamides, such as sulfadiazine, after determining which drug is effective against the specific bacteria. (See Tables 5.7 and 5.8, pages 99 and 103.) Frequently, an antibiotic is given with intravenous fluids in an effort to get the antibiotic into the blood faster than by oral or intramuscular routes. The intravenous fluids also prevent dehydration from the high fever as well as the inability to take fluids orally. A high fever is often treated with aspirin, sponging, and/or hypothermia. Anticonvulsants may be ordered to prevent or treat seizures. Osmotic diuretics may be prescribed to reduce cerebral edema associated with increased intracranial pressure.

Because of antibiotic therapy, most patients recover completely from meningitis. However, the complications that can occur are hearing loss or deafness, visual disturbances, and brain damage that may cause mental deterioration and/or a convulsive disorder.

ENCEPHALITIS

Encephalitis is an inflammation of the brain. It may be caused by a virus or chemicals such as lead and carbon monoxide. Encephalitis may be a complication of another viral disease such as measles or influenza, or a vaccination for smallpox. The virus may be transmitted by the bite of a mosquito or tick. This condition may be called sleeping sickness by the public.

NURSING OBSERVATIONS AND INTERVENTIONS

The patient's symptoms may occur suddenly or slowly. They include headache, fever, drowsiness, restlessness, convulsions, visual difficulties, and signs of increasing intracranial pressure. The diagnosis is made mainly by the symptoms of the patient. The spinal fluid, which is collected by a lumbar puncture, may be normal. If a virus is causing the condition, it can be isolated and identified only by special techniques.

The treatment of encephalitis is symptomatic. Antibiotics are not effective if a virus is causing the inflammation. The patient may not need to be isolated, for the virus cannot be transmitted to another person. The nursing care of this patient is similar to that of a patient with meningitis. The patient may recover completely or there may be neurologic disorders, such as mental changes, convulsive disorders, and Parkinson's disease.

BRAIN ABSCESS

The patient with a brain abscess has a collection of pus inside the skull. The cause may be a systemic infection such as sinusitis or pneumonia. A complication of meningitis may be a brain abscess. A compound depressed skull fracture also may cause a brain abscess. The most common sites for brain abscesses are the frontal and parietal lobes. The most common organisms involved include streptococci, *Staphylococcus aureus,* pneumococci, and meningococci. Diagnostic tests may include x-rays of the skull and other organs to identify sites of infection, CT scan, EEG, and white blood count.

NURSING OBSERVATIONS AND INTERVENTIONS

The patient often has the signs and symptoms of an inflammation, a headache, and signs of increased intracranial pressure. Careful, frequent observations, vital signs, and the neurocheck help to determine the location of the abscess in some cases.

Intravenous antibiotics are given to treat the infection. A craniotomy may be required to drain the pus if the abscess is causing symptoms of increased intracranial pressure. The preoperative and postoperative care for the patient having a craniotomy was described earlier in the chapter on pages 741–43. If the patient is treated medically, the care of the patient with meningitis, which is discussed on pages 756–58, is applicable.

POLIOMYELITIS

The patient with poliomyelitis has an infectious disease caused by a filterable virus. This is a virus so small that it can pass through a fine filter, such as porcelain. After entering the body, the virus can spread to the central nervous system and affect the spinal cord and the brain. The infection frequently involves the anterior portion of the gray matter in the spinal cord. (This gray matter, which is in the center of the cord, is made of nerve cells.) In this case, the patient has *acute anterior poliomyelitis.* The part of the brain most often affected is the medulla. In this case, the patient has *bulbar poliomyelitis.* The respiratory and the circulatory centers in the medulla may be involved. This can result in respiratory and circulatory failure.

The patient regains use of the affected muscles if the nerve cells are not injured too severely. Muscles supplied by nerve cells that die are paralyzed permanently. However, this does not mean that other muscles cannot be trained to take over some of the work previously performed by the paralyzed muscles.

Poliomyelitis may occur in epidemic form, especially during the summer and fall. It can affect older children and adults, but is more common in young children. The exact manner in which poliomyelitis is spread is not understood completely. However, it is thought that the virus may be spread by fecal contamination of food or water supplies and droplet infection.

PREVENTION

Two vaccines are used to prevent paralytic poliomyelitis. Since the 1950s when the vaccines first were used, the incidence of poliomyelitis has decreased dramatically. The first vaccine, developed by Dr. Jonas E. Salk, is prepared from the three types of poliomyelitis viruses. Although the viruses are inactivated, they retain the ability to cause the human body to produce antibodies. Two injections are given at monthly intervals, followed by a booster dose at six months and a supplementary dose at six or seven years of age. A live oral poliovirus vaccine was developed by Dr. Albert Sabin. This is a liquid vaccine containing inactivated strains of the three main types of paralytic poliomyelitis viruses. The person who has received the poliomyelitis vaccine develops antibodies in the blood that combat the poliomyelitis virus if it enters the bloodstream. The oral vaccine is administered by placing two or three drops on a lump of sugar at two-month intervals for three doses. Children receive a booster dose at 18 months of age and when entering school.

However, the fact that vaccines exist does not wipe out the disease. Individuals likely to develop poliomyelitis must receive this preventive medicine if they are to benefit by it. The nurse is often in a position to encourage relatives or friends to consult their doctor about being given the poliomyelitis vaccine. If the level of immunized persons is not kept high, the incidence of poliomyelitis will increase.

NURSING OBSERVATIONS AND INTERVENTIONS

The patient frequently has symptoms of an infection, such as fever, malaise, and headache, during the early stage of poliomyelitis. Symptoms of a gastrointestinal disturbance, such as vomiting and diarrhea, are common. Symptoms of an upper respiratory infection, such as a sore throat, are likely to develop during this stage. The infection may end here. This patient makes a rapid recovery and may not know that he or she has had poliomyelitis.

Infection that spreads to the spinal cord causes the patient to have pain in the muscles supplied by the inflamed area. The neck also may become stiff and sore. The affected muscles may become weak and paralyzed. They soon begin to atrophy or become smaller. Muscles in legs, arms, back, and shoulders frequently are affected. Muscles of the face and chest may be involved also. The patient is likely to have difficulty in talking, in swallowing, and in breathing when the medulla is affected. The location and the amount of paralysis depend upon the area of the central nervous system that is affected, as well as the amount of damage. The acute symptoms of fever, malaise, and pain usually disappear in five to six weeks. The patient may be left with paralyzed muscles, which can result in deformities, or there may be no paralysis.

The patient with poliomyelitis should be placed in isolation during the acute stage, either with a group of patients who have the same disease, or separately. The care of the patient with poliomyelitis is symptomatic and palliative since there is no antibiotic available to act against the virus. Actually, the main efforts of treatment are directed toward prevention. Bed rest is prescribed for the patient during the acute stage of poliomyelitis. If respiration is affected severely, a tracheostomy and the use of a ventilator will be required. Specific care and rehabilitation is similar to that needed for a patient with a spinal cord injury, discussed earlier in the chapter on pages 751–54.

HERPES ZOSTER

The patient with herpes zoster (shingles) has an infection that is thought to be caused by the same virus that causes chickenpox. The patient develops an inflammation of either the skin or mucous membrane along the course of the nerve from the involved area.

The inflammation often occurs along the course of an intercostal nerve (one between the ribs). The pain that results may be called *intercostal neuralgia*. One or both sides of the body may be affected.

Generally, the first symptom experienced by the patient is severe pain along the path of the nerve. This is soon followed by the formation of vesicles, which are tiny sacs containing fluid. The patient may continue to have pain after the vesicles have disappeared. The course of the inflammation takes from one to three weeks. Herpes zoster can be serious in either a debilitated or an elderly patient.

The doctor directs treatment toward making the patient comfortable, since no specific therapy for the virus is available. Calamine lotion may be prescribed as topical therapy for pruritic skin lesions. A solution of 5 percent idoxuridine in 100 percent dimethylsulfoxide may be applied topically to painful lesions. Analgesics such as aspirin, codeine, or propoxyphene (DARVON) may be helpful in relieving pain. In severe cases, corticosteroid therapy with methylprednisolone (PREDNISONE) may produce dramatic pain relief.

NEURITIS

The patient with neuritis has an inflammation of one or more nerves. Neuritis may be caused by injury of a nerve. For example, the nerve in the arm may be injured by pressure from the improper use of crutches. Infections, pressure from a growing tumor, deficiency of vitamins, metabolic disturbances such as diabetes, and poisons, such as arsenic, lead, and mercury, are some additional causes of neuritis.

The nurse may hear of different types of neuritis. It is helpful to know that this condition may be classified in various ways. For instance, neuritis may be classified according to its cause. Alcoholic neuritis is caused by drinking an excessive amount of alcohol and by the nutritional deficiency that usually results from the inadequate intake of vitamins. Neuritis also may be classified according to the number of nerves involved. The term *multiple neuritis* is used to refer to a patient having several nerves inflamed,

whereas the patient with *mononeuritis* has one nerve inflamed. These are only a few of the different types of neuritis.

The patient with neuritis has varying degrees of pain, depending on the location and amount of inflammation. The amount of pain may range from a burning and uncomfortable sensation to severe pain. The patient may develop weakness and paralysis of the part supplied by the affected nerve or nerves.

The physician directs treatment toward removing the underlying cause, if possible. For instance, the patient with a vitamin deficiency is treated with vitamins, the patient with diabetes is treated for this disease, and the patient with an injury is treated for this.

Nursing care will be given to aid the patient in becoming more comfortable. Analgesics often are given to relieve the pain. The underlying disease condition with the applicable nursing care also is to be considered.

Epilepsy

An individual with epilepsy has periodic seizures with recurrent excessive discharge of electricity from cerebral neurons. Symptoms include a loss of consciousness, involuntary movements, abnormal sensations, changes in autonomic activities, and/or psychic disturbances. The exact cause of epilepsy is unknown in most cases, a condition known as *idiopathic epilepsy*. However, epilepsy may occur in an individual following brain damage from a tumor, an infection, or an injury.

An individual can inherit a tendency toward developing epilepsy. A child born of parents either of whom has epilepsy or who has ancestors with this disorder is more likely to develop it than is the child born into a family with no history of epilepsy. The person who has a tendency toward developing epilepsy usually starts having seizures in childhood or during adolescence. Other conditions associated with the development of epilepsy include developmental defects, birth trauma, cerebral anoxia, and drug toxicity. Most patients with epilepsy can be controlled by drug therapy.

NURSING OBSERVATIONS

The single most important nursing observation needed for a person with epilepsy is a complete description of the events before, during, and after the seizure until the patient regains consciousness. The nurse may review the guidelines on pages 736–37 in order to obtain a complete description of the patient's seizure activity.

Many patients experience symptoms before an epileptic seizure. These symptoms are recognized by the patient as a warning that the seizure will occur. There are two types of these warning signals: *premonitory symptoms*, which last for hours or even days before the seizure, and an *aura*, which occurs seconds or minutes before the seizure.

The person with epilepsy commonly will experience either *generalized* or *partial* seizures.

Generalized seizures can be either *convulsive or nonconvulsive*. Frequently seen are generalized convulsive *tonic and clonic seizures*, also called *grand mal* seizures. For the patient with this type of seizure, loss of consciousness occurs and all the muscles contract. Most grand mal seizures last only a few minutes.

A nonconvulsive generalized seizure frequently seen in children is the *petit mal* seizure, also called *typical absence*. This type of seizure is characterized by brief periods of loss of consciousness, lasting 5 to 15 seconds. The child during this time stares with a vacant expression while other activity stops. Occasionally, there may be blinking of the eyelids, swallowing, or movement of an arm.

Partial seizures are also called *focal seizures*. They begin at a specific site and consist of movements of one or more muscles on one side of the body.

Occasionally, a partial seizure will begin in one area, such as the thumb, and spread in an orderly fashion to the fingers, wrist, forearm, and upper arm, and may involve one entire side of the body. This type of "marching" seizure is called *jacksonian epilepsy*.

Partial seizures may spread to become generalized convulsive seizures. This is called *secondary generalization*.

Partial seizures with complex symptomatology are also called *psychomotor seizures*. The patient having a psychomotor seizure has a temporary mental disturbance. Such a person acts in a peculiar manner for a short period of time and does not remember what happened during the episode. Patients may have a variety of symptoms during a psychomotor seizure. One patient may make swallowing noises, one may act dazed and mutter, and another may pull at clothing.

A condition called *status epilepticus* can occur. In this case, one seizure follows another before consciousness is regained. Status epilepticus can be fatal because of the lack of oxygen to the brain for extended periods. It is considered a medical emergency and must be treated immediately. Fortunately, with improved methods of treatment, this condition occurs less frequently than formerly.

ASSISTING WITH DIAGNOSTIC STUDIES

When seizures occur in an undiagnosed person, a complete diagnostic workup is done to try to discover underlying causes, if possible. Skull and spine x-rays may be done to rule out growths and tumors. Similarly, brain and CT scan also may be done. Blood work usually includes fasting blood sugar and serum calcium and phosphorus to rule out chemical imbalances in the bloodstream as a cause of the seizures. An EEG usually is done to identify abnormal wave forms that indicate epilepsy.

NURSING INTERVENTIONS

If the doctor determines that the seizures are being caused by a brain tumor or hematoma, surgery may be performed to remove the cause. However, if there appears to be no organic change in the brain, the condition is called idiopathic epilepsy. There is no cure for this type of epilepsy. Most persons are given anticonvulsant drugs, which are often helpful in eliminating or reducing the number of convulsions.

Table 21.4 contains a list of drugs commonly prescribed to reduce seizure activity in the patient with epilepsy. A very important responsibility of the nurse when assisting the patient on drug therapy is teaching the patient about the importance of continuing the medication as prescribed. The patient who stops taking the medication may experience a resumption of seizure activity.

Some physicians believe that some patients have fewer seizures if they are mildly dehydrated, and a diuretic such as acetazolamide (DIAMOX) may be given. A general diet usually is followed. Alcoholic beverages, fatigue, and emotional stress are avoided.

Special nursing interventions are indicated when a person is actually having a seizure. Table 21.5 contains a guide to nursing interventions at this time. During a tonic and clonic grand mal seizure, additional precautions may be needed to preserve the patient's airway.

The first phase is usually the *tonic* state, in which all the muscles contract. The patient is unconscious and is not breathing. This state lasts few seconds, and the patient may become cyanotic. Secretions may gather in the mouth. Some patients may have an "epileptic cry" that occurs as the air is forced out of the lungs.

The following state of the convulsion is called the *clonic* state. It consists of rhythmic jerking movements and may last moments or minutes. During this phase, the patient breathes and color improves.

If the nurse has enough warning prior to the seizure, a soft rag or padded tongue blade may be inserted into the patient's mouth to prevent the tongue from being bitten. If, however, there was no warning and the teeth already have clamped shut, the nurse should not attempt to wedge anything

between the teeth because it could result in bruised gums or cracked teeth.

The patient's head should be protected from pounding by the use of a pillow, blanket, or even the nurse's lap. The nurse should not try to restrain the extremities during a seizure because this could result in fractures. Furniture should be moved away from the patient and privacy provided if possible.

After the seizure, allow the patient to sleep until he or she wakes. Headache or confusion may be present during the neurocheck after the patient awakens.

The person with epilepsy needs to live as normally as possible with the disease, since no specific cure is known. A regular daily regimen should be established that includes adequate rest, relaxation, work, and exercise. Activities that would involve a risk in the event of a seizure may be avoided or modified. For example, the Epilepsy Foundation of American recommends that only persons who have been without seizures for two years be allowed drivers' licenses in order to prevent accident and injury from a seizure while driving. The patient may swim if accompanied by someone who can help if a seizure occurs.

Because of the public attitudes toward epilepsy, the patient has to cope with numerous social, emotional, and economic factors. If the seizures are not completely controlled, the patient will be very concerned about having a seizure in public. This affects a person's emotional outlook. The intelligence of the person with epilepsy is not affected by the disease. However, these persons often have emotional problems because of society's attitude toward the condition. This may affect the patient's ability to learn, find and keep a job, as well as relationships with coworkers, social acquaintances, and family.

The nurse not only can give good nursing care to the person with epilepsy, but also can help educate the public about the nature of epilepsy. Some communities have local organizations to inform the public about epilepsy, its treatment, and current research. The Epilepsy Foundation of America carries on a program of public education and research. In August, 1975, the Commission for

TABLE 21.5
GUIDE TO NURSING INTERVENTIONS DURING A SEIZURE

1. Stay with the patient.
2. Loosen constricting clothing, if possible.
3. Turn head to one side, if possible.
4. Do not restrain extremities during a seizure.
5. Do not pry a clenched jaw open to insert tongue blade or other device.
6. Carefully oserve the seizure activity.
7. Take vital signs and a neurocheck when the patient awakens.

the Control of Epilepsy and Its Consequences was established. It will study the medical and the social aspects of managing epilepsy in the United States and develop a national plan.

Parkinson's Disease

The patient with Parkinson's disease has a chronic disease of the nervous system. It is a slowly progressive degenerative disease. The nurse may hear Parkinson's disease referred to as *paralysis agitans, parkinsonism,* or *shaking palsy.*

An individual may develop Parkinson's disease at any age following encephalitis. It may also occur in a person with cerebral arteriosclerosis or as a result of certain drugs such as reserpine or phenothiazines. The cause of most cases of parkinsonism is not known although a deficiency of the neurotransmitter dopamine is usually present. Recent studies have shown that the condition may be due to a metabolic disorder. An individual is most likely to develop this disease during late middle life.

NURSING OBSERVATIONS

During the early stages of the disease, the patient may notice weakness, trembling, and rigidity (stiffness) of the muscles in one part of the body. These symptoms gradually spread to other parts of the body. A tremor may develop while the patient is still and lessen when the shaking part is moved.

The patient with a fully developed case of Parkinson's disease has an expressionless face because of the rigid muscles. Weak, rigid muscles cause movements to be slow and stiff. When walking, the patient moves slowly and stiffly, does not swing the arms, and leans forward as if going to fall. This abnormal posture causes the person to take steps that become increasingly shorter and faster. Eventually, a running pace is easier than walking. Rigidity also causes the patient to have difficulty in chewing, swallowing, and talking. Speech may become weak and slurred. The tremor, which developed earlier, usually becomes more noticeable.

The patient also loses the ability to perform fine movements. Drooling may result from a difficulty in swallowing. Constipation and incontinence also can become problems. The patient's ability to perform various activities decreases with emotional and physical fatigue and excitement.

Despite all of the neurologic symptoms, the patient's intelligence generally is not affected. Because of this and a deteriorating physical condition, such a person easily can become discouraged and depressed.

ASSISTING WITH DIAGNOSTIC STUDIES

The patient's characteristic movements can be observed during the neurologic examination by the neurologist. Serial records of the patient's handwriting and drawing of simple figures may be collected to evaluate the progression of illness. CAT scan of the brain may be done to detect underlying disease or atrophy of brain tissue which is characteristic of this disease.

NURSING INTERVENTIONS

Unfortunately, there is no specific cure for a patient with Parkinson's disease. Treatment is directed toward making the patient comfortable and relieving symptoms, such as tremors and rigidity. In general, the three methods of treatment are drugs, surgery, and physiotherapy. A combination of these approaches may be used.

Drug therapy is an important part of the treatment plan for most persons with Parkinson's disease. The drug of choice for the treatment of Parkinson's disease is levodopa, which crosses the blood-brain barrier and is changed into dopamine in the brain. With additional dopamine present, the symptoms of parkinsonism decrease for most patients who take the drug.

Various other drugs which may be given to relieve the symptoms of Parkinson's disease include antispasmodics such as cycrimine (PAGITANE), trihexyphenidyl (ARTANE), and benztropine mesylate (COGENTIN) (see Table 21.6). Amantadine (SYMMETREL) and carbidopa are recently introduced drugs that may help to relieve symptoms (see Table 21.6). Antihistamines, cerebral stimulants, and muscle relaxants also may be used to relieve symptoms.

Table 21.6
Drugs Used for Parkinsonism

Nonproprietary Name	Trade Name	Average Dose	Nursing Implications
Replacement Therapy			
Amantadine	Symmetrel	200 mg/day in divided doses	Believed to encourage release of dopamine in the body. Confusion and nightmares occur occasionally. Insomnia, drowsiness, slurred speech are usually temporary
Carbidopa-levidopa	Sinemet	Varies	Contains combination of levodopa and carbidopa; this combination helps to reduce dose of levodopa needed and reduce side effects
Levodopa	Bendopa Dopar Larodopa	3–4 gm daily	Side effects of levodopa include nausea, vomiting, and mental confusion. Over-dosage may lead to involuntary movements such as grimacing the teeth and sucking movements of the mouth. Phenothiazines, amphetamines, monamine oxidase inhibitors, and vitamin preparations containing pyridoxine interfere with the actions of levodopa and should not be given
Anticholinergics (Antispasmodics)			
Benztropine mesylate	Cogentin	2–6 mg	The anticholinergic drugs are given to control rigidity, tremor, and akinesia. Side effects include dry mouth, blurred vision, constipation, and heart palpitations
Biperiden	Akineton	2–10 mg	
Cycrimine	Pagitane	2.5–10 mg	
Ethopropazine	Parsidol	50–60 mg	
Trihexyphenidyl	Artane	6–15 mg	
Antihistamines			
Chlorphenoxamine hydrochloride	Phenoxene	150–400 mg	The antihistamines are given to control tremor. Side effects include drowsiness, dry mouth, and disturbance of the gastrointestinal tract
Diphenhydramine hydrochloride	Benadryl	50–150 mg	

Surgical treatment may be done in selected cases to relieve rigidity and tremors. Portions of the globus pallidus and thalamus in the brain are destroyed by cautery, injection of alcohol, or surgical removal. The procedures are called *chemopallidectomy* and *chemothalamectomy*, respectively. *Cryogenic* surgery, which is cooling or freezing certain portions of the above structures, has been done. These stereotaxic neurosurgical procedures have been successful in varying degrees. The patient requires care similar to that described for the person having brain surgery (pages 741–43). Fortunately, the use of levodopa has made much of the surgery for parkinsonism unnecessary.

In physical therapy, ambulation and continuation of the activities of daily living are the goals in the early stages of the disease. Regular exercise, continuing to work as much as and for as long as possible, and maintaining social activities have much to do with slowing down the progression of the disease. Occupational therapists may help the patient adapt clothing, home, furniture, and facilities to permit self-care and independence. An unhurried, relaxed atmosphere helps the person to function more normally. The diet often must be modified because of difficulty in chewing and swallowing. The food must be either cut in small pieces or chopped to a consistency that the patient can handle. Constipation is often a problem, which can be avoided by including fruits and vegetables in the diet and establishing a regular time for bowel elimination. When the patient's intelligence is not impaired, psychotherapy may be helpful as well as the avoidance of emotionally upsetting situations. As the disease progresses and the patient becomes more and more incapacitated, physical therapy is aimed at preventing contractures and maintaining muscle function with active and passive range-of-motion exercises. In the late stages, the patient may become irritable, hypersensitive, demanding, and generally hard to care for. The nurse often cares for the patient in the hospital in these late stages of the disease. Pneumonia is often the cause of death.

Multiple Sclerosis

The patient with multiple sclerosis has areas of degeneration of the myelin sheath surrounding the nerve fibers in the brain and spinal cord. Nerve fibers are covered by *myelin*, which is a fatty sheath or covering. It may be helpful for the nurse to compare this sheath with the insulation on an electric wire. Electricity cannot pass through the wire if the insulation is worn away. Neither do the impulses pass through a nerve properly if the myelin sheath is diseased. When the impulses do not pass through the nerve, they do not reach the muscles. This results in either a disturbance of the function of this part of the body or in paralysis. The area has a disturbed function when it receives fewer impulses than usual. The patient is paralyzed if no impulses pass through the nerve because of the diseased myelin sheath. For example, if the patient's larynx and tongue receive fewer nerve impulses than normal, speech difficulties develop.

Areas of the myelin that degenerate are replaced by scar tissue. This is known as *sclerotic tissue* because of its hardness. The patient develops many areas of sclerotic tissue in the brain and spinal cord. Thus, the disease is known as multiple sclerosis.

The life expectancy of a patient with multiple sclerosis usually is decreased. The disease may progress either rapidly or slowly. In some cases the person lives out a normal life-span, and in others the patient may die in five to ten years. The amount of disability from multiple sclerosis varies. Some individuals become confined to bed, whereas others have only a moderate amount of disability. Infections of the lungs and urinary tract, decubitus ulcers, and malnutrition are frequent complications. The patient is more likely to develop one of these complications during the later part of his illness.

The cause of multiple sclerosis is unknown. At the present time, research theories suggest either a slow virus infection, an autoimmune disease, or some combination as possible causes. The National Multiple Sclerosis Society collects funds to finance part of the research. The Society also works in public education.

NURSING OBSERVATIONS

Since demyelination may occur in any part of the nervous system, the patient's symptoms may be extremely varied. When an area of the myelin sheath begins to degenerate, it comes edematous or swollen. The patient has symptoms of disturbed function of the part of the body supplied by that nerve. Disappearance of the edema can result in disappearance of the patient's symptoms unless the area is filled with scar tissue. This accounts for periods of time when the patient may have no symptoms; however, these reappear when the area becomes swollen again and the symptoms recur. When an area becomes sclerotic, the patient's symptoms are permanent.

The patient may go through periods in which symptoms seem to improve (period of remission), only to have the symptoms return in a more exaggerated form. Intervals between the periods when the patient is not bothered with symptoms become shorter as the disease progresses. As additional areas of the central nervous system become sclerosed or hardened, the patient becomes more handicapped. Such a patient may begin to tire more easily and lose the ability to move properly. The patient also may become incontinent and paralyzed. Early initial symptoms frequently include fatigue, lack of energy, motor weakness, and numbness and tingling of a particular area. Early visual symptoms often include blurring, impairment of vision, and diplopia (double vision). The patient's voluntary muscles, those under the control of will, may become spastic. The muscles that receive their nerve supply from the affected part of the central nervous system may tremble. For example, the patient's hand begins to shake when starting to pick up a glass of water. The tremor usually increases as the glass is replaced. The shaking generally disappears when the hand and arm are rested.

The patient may have difficulty in seeing. Common visual disturbances are blurred vision, difficulty in focusing the eyes, inability to control movement of the eyes, and blindness.

In addition to having difficulty with the eyes, the patient with multiple sclerosis is likely to have speech difficulties. Such a person may talk in a hesitant manner with slurred words. As previously mentioned, spinal cord involvement may result in progressive paralysis and disability.

ASSISTING WITH DIAGNOSTIC STUDIES

Some or all of the diagnostic studies described earlier in the chapter may be done to identify the patient's disease. Usually, a combination of positive findings in the neurologic examination, cerebrospinal fluid IgG (immunoglobulin G), CT scan, and nerve conduction studies helps the neurologist to form a diagnosis.

NURSING INTERVENTIONS

Unfortunately, no cure is known at the present time for the patient with multiple sclerosis. However, this does not mean that nothing can be done. A combination of interventions help to slow the progression of the disease process, alleviate symptoms, prevent or treat complications, and adjust to the illness.

REST. The person having an acute attack is placed on bed rest or limited activity until symptoms improve. Throughout the course of illness, the patient is encouraged to plan a life-style that includes frequent rest periods and the prevention of fatigue.

DIET. A high-polyunsaturated-fat diet may be prescribed for the patient with multiple sclerosis. Daily vegetable oil supplement containing linoleic acid such as sunflower oil may be prescribed to replace lineolate which becomes depleted in the brain during the course of illness. Some research indicates that this dietary change results in fewer and less severe relapses.

DRUG THERAPY. Steroid therapy is an important part of treatment for the acutely ill patient. Both cortisone and adrenocorticotropic hormone may be prescribed. As the patient's condition stabilizes, steroid therapy may be discontinued gradually to prevent complications (refer to Chapter 18, pages 590–91). In some cases, immunosuppressive therapy may be prescribed. Diazepam (VALIUM) may be needed for the patient with muscle spasms. Antibiotics are prescribed to treat infection.

PHYSICAL THERAPY. The physician may prescribe physical therapy, such as massage, warm baths, and exercise. These baths, and active and passive exercises, help to strengthen the muscles, to prevent or to correct deformities, to increase muscular coordination, and to prevent atrophy (wasting away) of the muscles from lack of use. Physical therapy may be used also to relieve muscle spasm in an effort to make the patient more comfortable. The nurse may be asked to help the patient with active and passive exercises. Braces, crutches, and other ambulation aids assist the patient to remain ambulatory as long as possible.

Other interventions related to positioning, skin care, adequate fluid intake, and elimination described earlier for the patient with spinal cord injury (pages 752–54) apply also to the person with multiple sclerosis.

Psychotherapy may be needed intermittently or regularly as the patient's disease process continues. Communication problems often develop in the family as the patient's speech and other physical abilities deteriorate. The nurse often may help at this time by listening patiently to the patient's communication. The nurse also may report the patient's emotional difficulties to the appropriate nurse or physician so that additional help can be obtained. Families also need an understanding listener as they struggle to cope with the progressive decline of a loved one who is often a young adult.

Myasthenia Gravis

The patient with myasthenia gravis has a progressive condition in which there is weakness or paralysis of voluntary muscles after activity followed by a recovery of strength after a rest period of several minutes to several hours. It is believed that the nerve impulses do not pass from the brain to the muscles because of a chemical defect at the junction between the nerve and muscle (myoneural junction). The exact cause of the disorder is unknown, but a disturbance in the immune system is linked with this condition.

Myasthenia gravis is rare. Women are affected more often than men and most persons develop this disease in their 20s and 30s.

NURSING OBSERVATIONS AND INTERVENTIONS

The patient usually experiences some kind of weakness which is more severe in the evening. Many patients experience visual disturbances such as diplopia (double vision) and ptosis (dropping eyelid) which appear in the early afternoon, gradually worsen through the evening, and disappear by morning.

Some patients may progress to crisis in which there is generalized weakness including paralysis of respiratory muscles. Such a patient requires emergency care to prevent death.

The diagnosis is confirmed by the muscle response to a test dose of edrophonium (TENSILON). This drug will revive the muscle function within a few minutes.

There is no cure for myasthenia gravis. However, drug therapy can help relieve the muscle weakness and resulting complications, such as pneumonia. The drugs that may be used are neostigmine (PROSTIGMIN)

and pyridostigmine (MESTINON) (see Table 21.7).

The nursing care of this patient is directed toward preventing upper respiratory infections and conserving the patient's energy for the essential activities of life. With rest periods, some patients are able to work during the early stages of the disease. Acute episodes of the condition can occur. In these instance, suctioning is necessary, a tracheostomy may be required, and tube feedings also may be necessary.

Trigeminal Neuralgia # 5

Trigeminal neuralgia may also be called *tic douloureux*. It is a condition resulting in periods of severe, stabbing pain on one side of the face. It occurs mainly in older persons. The pain occurs along the course of the branches of the fifth (trigeminal) cranial nerve, which is the sensory nerve of the face, scalp, and teeth. The nerve also has a function in chewing. The cause of the condition is unknown.

NURSING OBSERVATIONS AND INTERVENTIONS

Stimulation of areas along the course of the nerve branches called "trigger points" may cause an attack. These trigger points may be sensitive to a cool breeze, a slight touch, chewing, or any facial movement. Because of the severity of the pain, these patients are very unhappy and anxious. They are concerned with preventing an attack and try to avoid stimulating the trigger points. As a result, they may be poorly nourished, for chewing may cause pain. Men may be unshaven, their hair may be uncombed, the affected side of the face unwashed, and mouth and dental care may have been avoided because of the resulting pain. During an attack, the patient usually stops talking and flinches the face. Watering of the eye and contraction of facial muscles on the affected side are common.

When caring for the patient during acute episodes, the bed should not be jarred or placed in a draft. The patient should not be approached suddenly. The patient is encouraged in self-care activities such as washing,

Table 21.7
Drugs Used for Myasthenia Gravis

Nonproprietary Name	Trade Name	Average Dose	Nursing Implications
Ambenomium Neostigmine Pyridostigmine	MYTELASE PROSTIGMIN MESTINON	10-mg tablets 15-mg tablets 60-mg tablets	Ambenomium, neostigmine, and pyridostigmine are cholinergic drugs, or drugs that mimic the parasympathetic nervous system. The nurse should be aware that overdosage may aggravate the patient's fatigue, may cause muscle twitching, and may cause nausea, abdominal cramping, vomiting, and diarrhea
Ephedrine		25-mg tablets	Ephedrine is an adrenergic, or sympathomimetic, drug. It is most effective when added to the patient's drugs after optimum dosage of the cholinergics is reached. Ephedrine stimulates the respiratory center in the medulla and helps relax smooth muscle in the gastrointestinal system
Corticosteroid hormones Prednisone Methylprednisalone		Dosage varies	See Table 18.5

oral hygiene, and shaving, if these can be done without causing an attack.

Drug Therapy. A number of drugs may be tried in some cases to treat and prevent attacks. The two drugs most often prescribed are phenytoin (DILANTIN) or carbamazepine (TEGRETOL). Another drug which may be helpful if others are not is clonazepam (CLONOPIN).

Surgery. If medical therapy has not been successful, surgery may be needed. Branches of the nerve may be injected with alcohol, the nerve may be removed, or the ganglion may be destroyed.

A particular disadvantage of most surgical therapies is the total anesthesia that develops in the part of the face supplied by the involved nerve. As a result, the affected part of the face is insensitive to heat, cold, and pain. The patient therefore must take care in shaving and closely observe the temperature of the food. There may be some difficulty in chewing, and mouth care is required after each meal for bits of food may be retained in the affected side. The corneal (blink) reflex also may be lost. An eyeshield is often required, as are ointments and irri-

gations, to prevent ulceration and injury to the cornea.

The surgical patient requires care as described in Chapter 6. If the cranium has been opened during surgery, the patient needs care described earlier in the chapter on pages 741–43. If facial anesthesia has resulted from surgery, the nurse uses the same precautions described earlier for shaving, feeding, and helping the patient with eye care.

Sciatica

An individual with sciatica has pain that radiates down the thigh and the back or side of the leg. This neuralgia pain follows the course of the sciatic nerve, which leaves the lower part of the vertebral column and goes down the back of each leg. Exercise such as walking usually increases the pain. Numbness, tingling, and tenderness along the pathway of the sciatic nerve also may be present.

Sciatica may result from injury, inflammation of the nerve, and unknown causes. A ruptured intervertebral disk, spinal cord tumor, arthritis, and sprain of the lower part of the back are examples of some of the causes of injury to the sciatic nerve. An individual may have an attack of sciatica after becoming chilled.

The person with sciatica is treated for the underlying cause of the pain. The care of the patient with a ruptured intervertebral disk has been discussed in this chapter on pages 754–56 and for a spinal cord tumor on pages 750–51. The care of the patient with arthritis and a sprain is discussed in Chapter 17.

Headache

The person with a headache has head pain that may or may not extend into the back of the head. A headache is an unusually common symptom.

A headache can be associated with tension, fatigue, eyestrain, and acute diseases of the eye, nose, throat, sinuses, or ear. The patient may develop a headache as a symptom of such conditions as an acute generalized infection, head injury, cerebrovascular accident (stroke), brain tumor, meningitis, hypertension, and allergic reactions. For example, monosodium glutamate in certain foods such as soy sauce causes a dilation of blood vessels of the brain in some persons. Dilation of the blood vessels supplying the brain results in a headache that resembles a migraine headache.

The patient with a migraine headache has head pain associated with an episode of vasconstriction followed by dilation of blood vessels supplying the brain. The patient at this time may experience certain symptoms, such as flashes of light, that warn of the onset. The pain begins with the dilation of the blood vessels. The pain frequently is located on one side of the head and is associated with nausea and vomiting. The patient generally is rendered helpless with pain. In addition to the pain, nausea, and vomiting, the patient experiences photophobia (average light in the room cannot be tolerated).

Migraine headache occurs in both men and women. However, it may be associated with the menstrual cycle and stress. An individual with a family history of migraine headaches is more likely to suffer from them

than is the person with none present in the family.

When attempting to determine the cause of the patient's headache, the physician will do a careful medical history, physical examination, and neurologic examination. Other diagnostic studies will be done as indicated.

The physician may prescribe analgesics for the patient's headache (see Table 7.2). Aspirin, 600 mg (10 grains); phenacetin, 300 mg (5 grains); or acetaminophen (TYLENOL), 600 mg (10 grains), may be prescribed. Compound analgesics such as EMPIRIN, APC capsules, and the A.S.A. compound are sometimes ordered. The compounds usually contain a combination of aspirin, phenacetin, and caffeine. Codeine phosphate, a narcotic, may be added to a compound analgesic.

Drugs that have a vasoconstrictive action on the blood vessels of the brain are prescribed. Ergotamine tartrate has been used for years in treating migraines. The patient is advised by the doctor to take the ergotamine tablets when the first signs of headache appear. Frequently ergotamine tartrate, 1 mg, is combined with caffeine, 100 mg, in a preparation called CAFERGOT. The specific amount and time for administration are decided by the physician for each patient.

Methysergide maleate (SANSERT) is effective in preventing the development of migraine headaches in some patients when taken regularly every day.

Reducing the light and noise levels in the patient's room may enhance his comfort. A cool, damp cloth or an ice bag often feels soothing when applied to the patient's forehead.

Brain Death

Brain death is a term generally used to describe a patient with total irreversible brain destruction resulting in an absence of voluntary and reflex response. This condition often develops while the patient is attached to a technical life-support system.

After brain death has been established by the physician using medical, legal, and ethical criteria, the patient is considered dead.

TABLE 21.8
OTHER DISORDERS OF THE NERVOUS SYSTEM

DISORDER	DESCRIPTION
Amyotrophic lateral sclerosis	A progressive condition characterized by degeneration of the motor neurons in the stem of the brain and spinal cord; weakness of muscles supplied by the affected nerve results; more common in later life; no specific treatment is available at this time
Bell's palsy	A facial paralysis of rather rapid onset; patient usually has pain at the angle of his jaw and a retraction of the mouth and difficulty in closing his eye; patient usually begins to recover within a week; however, some patients are left with distressing muscle spasms of the face; steroids may be used in treatment
Guillain-Barré syndrome	An inflammatory response in the nerve roots thought to be due to a hypersensitivity reaction following a viral infection; symptoms include paresthesia and weakness followed rapidly by flaccid paralysis of muscles; most patients make complete recovery unless complications such as respiratory failure develop; good nursing care and physical therapy are essential to treatment
Huntington's disease (postinfectious polyneuritis)	An inherited condition causing atrophy of the cortex of the brain; patient develops continuous, writhing, involuntary movements, especially in the hands; mental deterioration occurs; involuntary movements increase and mental deterioration continues resulting in invalidism; death occurs 10 to 15 years from infection
Nutritional amblyopia (tobacco-alcohol amblyopia, nutritional retrobulbar neuropathy)	A visual disturbance encountered in undernourished persons; may occur in association with those who overindulge in alcohol and tobacco and neglect their dietary requirements; improved dietary intake and B vitamins are used in treatment
Nutritional polyneuropathy (dry beriberi, alcoholic neuropathy	A condition in which the patient has muscular weakness especially of the legs, abnormal sensations, and muscular wasting in the affected extremities; cause is believed to be a nutritional deficiency especially of the B vitamins; B vitamins are used in treatment
Syringomyelia	A condition in which abnormal cavities form in the spinal cord; these cavities are filled with a liquid substance; cause is not known; symptoms vary with the location of the cavities; no specific treatment is known at this time
Tuberous sclerosis (epiloia, Bourneville's disease)	A congenital condition in which the patient has malformations of the brain, skin, and other organs, mental retardation, and epilepsy; condition often is progressive; treatment generally is directed toward control of epilepsy
Vitamin B_{12} deficiency	A deficiency of vitamin B_{12} can result in neurologic symptoms such as numbness and tingling of the feet and hands and generalized weakness; patient may have difficulty in walking; early treatment with B_{12} can reverse the symptoms
Wernicke-Korsakoff syndrome	Nutritional disorder resulting in unsteady gait, visual disturbances, muscular incoordination, and other neurologic symptoms; lack of vitamin B_1, which is usually associated with alcoholism, generally is the cause; vitamin B_1 is used for treatment

Body organs may be donated and/or life support systems may be terminated. Currently, there is no uniform definition of brain death. Criteria for identifying this situation vary according to medical, legal, and ethical concerns.

A major role of the nurse is the tender care given to the grieving family during this difficult period. An important part of grieving for the family of the patient with brain death is the conclusion that everything possible was done. Thus, it is extremely important that questions, concerns, wishes, and feelings conveyed by family members to the nurse are reported fully and accurately to the appropriate nurse and physician. When family members express such concerns to the nurse, they are treated with understanding, respect, and sympathy. Nurses and other members of the staff make every effort possible to provide support and guidance for the family at this time. For example, the nurse may comfort one crying family member, make coffee for another family member, and call the spiritual counselor or hospital chaplain for still another. The nurse's continuous caring efforts help the family to reach the conclusion that everything possible was done.

Case Study Involving A Brain Tumor

Mr. David Hubbard has just returned from the postanesthesia room following a craniotomy for the removal of a brain tumor. You note that his blood pressure is 156/88; his pulse is 68 and strong; there is some drainage on the dressing that appears clear; he is sleeping soundly and responds only to painful stimuli. Both pupils constrict when exposed to light, but the left responds more slowly than the right. Some of the postoperative orders read:

Vital signs every 15 minutes
Notify physician of changes in respiration, blood pressure, pulse, and pupillary reaction
No sedation
Strict record of intake and output

QUESTIONS

1. When Mr. Hubbard begins to awaken, how will you determine his level of consciousness?
2. What specific nursing actions are needed in the immediate postoperative period?
3. Why did the physician order no sedation?
4. Describe nursing observations that might indicate rising intracranial pressure in Mr. Hubbard.
5. Why would you consider this patient a candidate for seizures? What nursing precautions will you take?
6. Describe drainage that might indicate leakage of cerebrospinal fluid.

Case Study Involving Multiple Sclerosis

Mrs. Judy Smith is a 24-year-old mother of two small children. Recently, she has been experiencing periods in which vision is blurred and she is uncoordinated. She now feels that she has postponed seeing a physician too long and consults one. After several days of diagnostic studies and very careful history taking, Mrs. Smith receives a diagnosis of multiple sclerosis. The physician explained to both the patient and her husband that there would probably be periods of remission, in which the symptoms improved considerably and would perhaps even disappear temporarily. A public health nurse was asked to visit the family regularly, assist the patient with physical therapy, and provide information regarding neighborhood services available.

QUESTIONS

1. What, if any, physical changes will need to be made in the home?
2. What neighborhood services might the Smiths need in the future?
3. What would be the interventions related to drug therapy, diet, ambulation, rest, and complications appropriate for a patient with a diagnosis of multiple sclerosis?
4. How might the National Multiple Sclerosis Society help this family?

Suggestions for Further Study

1. Which of the diagnostic studies included in this chapter are performed in your agency? What additional ones are done?
2. Do you know of a person in your community who has epilepsy? If so, what is the attitude of those with whom he or she comes in contact?
3. Is there a local society concerned with epilepsy in your community? Multiple sclerosis? If so, what functions does it have?
4. Does your community or hospital have policies regarding brain death? If so, what are they?
5. Mason, Mildred A.; Bates, Grace F.; and Smola, Bonnie K.: *Workbook in Basic Medical-Surgical Nursing*, 3rd ed. Macmillan Publishing Company, New York, 1984, Exercise 21.

Additional Readings

Barry, Laura: "The Patient with Myasthenia Gravis Really Needs You." *Nursing 82*, 12:50–53 (July), 1982.

Carbary, Lorraine Judson: "Myasthenia Gravis: The Mysterious Masquerader." *Journal of Practical Nursing*, 30:21–36 and 36–37 (Oct.), 1982.

Catonzaro, Marcie: "MS: Nursing Care of the Person with MS." *American Journal of Nursing*, 80:286–91 (Feb.), 1980.

Gresh, Cindy: "Helpful Tips You Can Give Your Patients with Parkinson's Disease." *Nursing 80*, 10:26–33 (Jan.), 1980.

Howard, Marrianne, and Corbo-Pelain, Sally Ann: "Psychological Aftereffects of Halo Traction." *Nursing 82*, 82:1839–43 (Dec.), 1982.

Kinley, Anne E.: "MS: From Shock to Acceptance." *American Journal of Nursing*, 80:274–75 (Feb.), 1980.

McDonnell, Margaret, and Holland, Nancy: "MS: Problem-Oriented Nursing Care Plans." *American Journal of Nursing*, 80:292–97 (Feb.), 1980.

McManus, Joan C., and Hausman, Kathy A.: "Deciphering Diagnostic Studies: Cerebrospinal Fluid Analysis." *Nursing 82*, 12:43–47 (Aug.), 1982.

Plank, Charles: "ALS, MS, MD—What's the Difference?" *American Journal of Nursing*, 80:282–83 (Feb.), 1980.

Price, Gail: "MS: The Challenge to the Family." *American Journal of Nursing*, 80:283–85 (Feb.), 1980.

Rosal-Grief, Victoria L. F.: "Drug-Induced Dyskinesias." *American Journal of Nursing*, 82:66–69 (Jan.), 1982.

Santilli, Nancy, and Tonelson, Stephen: "Screening for Seizures." *Journal of Practical Nursing*, 32:16–20 and 24 (Mar.), 1982.

Sherry, Deborah: "Head Injuries: Your Care Counts." *Journal of Practical Nursing*, 32:31–33 (Apr.), 1982.

Slater, Robert J., and Yearwood, Alma C.: "MS: Facts, Faith, and Hope." *American Journal of Nursing*, 80:276–81 (Feb.), 1980.

Trekas, JoAnne: "Managing Epilepsy: Don't Forget the Patient." *Nursing 82*, 12:62–65 (Oct.), 1982.

Walleck, Constance Anne: "A Neurologic Assessment Procedure That Won't Make You Nervous." *Nursing 82*, 12:50–58 (Dec.), 1982.

Weeks, Carolyn C.: "MS: The Malignant Uncertainty." *American Journal of Nursing*, 80:298–99 (Feb.), 1980.

Wehner, Robert: "Respiratory Care for Patients with Amyotrophic Lateral Sclerosis." *Journal of Practical Nursing*, 31:24–25 and 37 (Apr.), 1981.

Yearwood, Alma C.: "MS: Being Disabled Doesn't Mean Being Handicapped." *American Journal of Nursing*, 80:299–302 (Feb.), 1980.

Chapter *22*

The Patient with a Disease of the Eye

Expected Behavioral Outcomes

Minimum objectives referred to as expected behavioral outcomes have been designed for the practical/vocational nursing student to use as guides in studying this chapter. The student should read these expected outcomes before studying the chapter. The objectives can be used as guides for study.

Using the content of this chapter, the student should return to the objectives and evaluate the ability to:

1. *Relate the structures involved in sight to the physiology of seeing.*
2. *Describe seven eye problems that should serve as a basis for the nurse to recommend that the client consult an ophthalmologist.*
3. *Compare the two main functions of lenses in relation to purpose and characteristics.*
4. *Compare the differences between strabismus, ulceration of the cornea, cataract, glaucoma, and detached retina as a basis for planning nursing care.*
5. *Develop a nursing care plan for an elderly lady being admitted for removal of a cataract.*
6. *Describe the main effect of miotics, anesthetics, cycloplegics, mydriatics, and ophthalmic dyes as a basis for nursing actions.*
7. *Describe the visual impairment, if any, associated with myopia, hyperopia, astigmatism, glaucoma, cataract, and presbyopia.*
8. *Explain the importance of having a patient continue using medication for glaucoma.*
9. *Outline the nursing care of a patient having eye surgery.*
10. *Describe the rehabilitation of a blind person in relation to self-care, communication, and recreation.*

Vocabulary Development

The following prefixes, suffixes, and combining forms pertain to this chapter. By learning and/or reviewing their meanings, the practical/vocational nursing student will have the keys needed to unlock many exciting new medical terms.

Discover the meaning of these keys in a medical dictionary or in the content of this chapter. How does each key pertain to this chapter? In your notebook write the correct meaning of each prefix, suffix, or combining form listed below. Illustrate each key with an example.

blephar—pertaining to eyelid or eyelash. Ex.
   blepharitis—inflammation of the eyelid.
ambly-   cili-
aque-   diplo-
blephar-   emmetro-

fract-   phac-
glauc-   photo-
iso-   presby-
mio-   tropia-
ocul-   vitre-
ophthalm-   xero-
opia-

Structure and Function

Eyes are the organs of vision. Each eye is a firm, rounded organ located in a bony cavity of the skull. This cavity, which is cone shaped, has an opening in the back portion. The *optic nerve,* which is the nerve leading from the eye, and blood vessels pass through this opening into the cranial cavity. The front part of the eye is covered by eyelids and eyelashes that protect it. The eyelids are lined with a mucous membrane known as the *conjunctiva.* A thin layer of this membrane covers the front part of the eyeball. Six muscles are attached to each eye for movement. Eyebrows also help to protect the eye.

The exposed surface of the eyeball is moistened by tears. This fluid is produced by the tear glands, which are called *lacrimal glands.* These glands are located above the eyeballs. After moistening the outer surface of the eye, the tears drain into lacrimal ducts that lead to the nose. This fluid overflows and runs down the cheek when it is not carried away fast enough.

The three coats, or layers of tissue, that make up the eyeball are the fibrous coat, the uvea or uveal tract, and the retina (see Figure 22.1).

The sclera and the cornea form the outer *fibrous coat,* which is strong and flexible. The *sclera* is the white, outer membrane that covers most of the eyeball. It extends from the back of the eyeball to the iris, which is the colored part of the eye. The sclera joins the cornea in the front part of the eye. The *cornea* is the transparent (clear) membrane that covers the iris and the pupil. Light enters the eye through this transparent window, which is approximately 1.2 cm (½ in.) in diameter. The cornea normally has no blood vessels, and it receives nourishment from lymph.

The middle layer of the eyeball, which is known as the *uvea* or *uveal tract,* is made up of the choroid, the ciliary body, and the iris. The *choroid* is the structure that lines the sclera. The choroid has a rich supply of blood vessels. The *ciliary body,* which is attached to the front part of the choroid, contains blood vessels, nerves, and a muscle called the *ciliary muscle.* The third part of the uveal tract is the *iris.* This is the rounded, colored portion of the eye behind the cornea. The black circle in the middle of the iris is an opening known as the *pupil.* Light passes through the center of the eyeball by way of this opening. Muscles in the iris control the size of the pupil.

The *retina* is the inner coat of the eyeball. It is a sensitive membrane containing many nerve cells. Light rays are normally focused on the retina, and an image is formed.

The *crystalline lens* is a transparent body filled with a jellylike substance and is surrounded by an elastic capsule. The lens is located behind the pupil. The ciliary muscle attached to the side of the lens can change the shape of the lens by contracting and relaxing.

The crystalline lens divides the cavity within the eyeball into two parts. The cavity in front of the lens is filled with a clear, watery fluid known as *aqueous humor.* The cavity behind the lens is filled with fluid called the *vitreous humor.* This fluid resembles clear jelly. The vitreous humor plays an important role in helping the eye to maintain its shape.

VISION

Perfect vision depends upon proper accommodation, refraction of the light rays, proper functioning of the pupils, teamwork between the two eyes, and transmission of

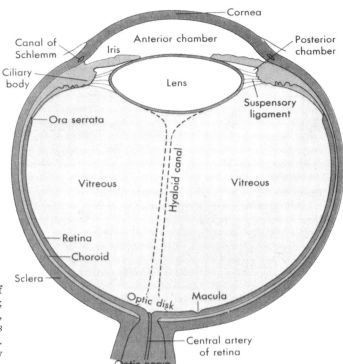

FIGURE 22.1 Horizontal section of the eye. (From Miller, Marjorie A.; Drakontides, Anna B.; and Leavell, Lutie C.: *Kimber-Gray-Stackpole's Anatomy and Physiology*, 17th ed. Macmillan Publishing Co., Inc., New York, 1977, page 285.)

nerve impulses to the brain. The ability of a person to adjust or focus the eyes on objects at varying distances is known as *accommodation*. This is made possible by a change in the shape of the crystalline lens. The ciliary muscle attached to the side of the lens contracts and relaxes. This causes the lens to change its shape so that rays of light from various distances can be focused properly on the retina. An individual loses the ability to focus the eyes properly during the aging process because the tissue involved becomes less elastic.

Refraction is the bending of light rays. These rays must be bent so that they are brought into focus on the retina in order for a person to see properly. The cornea, the aqueous humor, the crystalline lens, and the vitreous humor refract (bend) the light rays so that they are focused properly on the retina. The direction of a light ray is changed when it passes through a transparent substance of different density. For example, the direction of a light ray is changed when it passes at an angle from the air into water. This light ray is refracted, or bent.

The pupils must become larger and smaller in order to control the light rays entering the eye. The size of the pupil is controlled by the circular muscle in the iris. When the muscle contracts, it causes the pupil to become smaller. This reduces the amount of light entering the eye. When the muscle of the iris relaxes, it causes the pupil to become larger. This increases the amount of light entering the eye as in darkness.

An individual normally has two eyes that function as a team so that when both eyes are used, one object is seen instead of two. Teamwork between the two eyes enables a person to determine distance and depth more accurately.

Nerve impulses caused by the light rays that form an image on the retina must be carried to the brain in order for a person to see. These impulses are carried by the optic nerve to the center of sight in the brain. A person is able to see when this area in the brain interprets the impulses as a sensation of color and form. An individual has good vision when (1) there is proper accommodation of the lens, (2) the clear structures within the eyeball refract the light rays so that they are focused on the retina, (3) the pupils react to light properly, (4) the two eyes work together, and (5) the nerve impulses are transmitted to the center of sight in the brain.

The *ophthalmologist,* who is also called an *oculist,* is a physician specializing in the diagnosis and treatment of a person with a disease or a defect of the eye. Such a physician has been prepared to treat a person with an eye defect or disease either medically or surgically. An ophthalmologist frequently can determine whether or not the patient has a condition in the eye caused by a disease elsewhere in the body, such as syphilis, arteriosclerosis, diabetes, certain types of kidney disease, or a brain tumor. The ophthalmologist gives the patient a prescription for glasses when necessary. This prescription can be filled by an *optician,* an individual who grinds the lenses according to the doctor's recommendation. The optician can be compared with the pharmacist who fills the doctor's prescription for medicine. The optician is not licensed to examine a person's eyes or to test vision.

The *optometrist* is an individual who is licensed to measure the visual powers of a person. Glasses or exercises may be prescribed by an optometrist to correct a visual defect. However, the optometrist may not use drugs in either the examination or treatment of the eye. Only a physician may use drugs to examine or treat the eye.

An *orthopist* is an individual who is skilled in the technique of eye exercise used to correct faulty eye coordination.

Assisting with Diagnostic Studies

EXAMINATION OF THE EYES

Visual acuity refers to the person's ability to see. The Snellen eye chart is commonly used to determine an individual's acuity of vision. The chart has rows of letters or a big E, which varies in sizes and positions. Use of the E is necessary when the individual is unable to read letters. The letters and/ or the E are arranged in rows that a person should be able to see at various distances from the chart. The person who can read the letters marked 20 at a distance of 20 feet is

considered to have 20/20 vision, *emmetropia,* or normal vision. The individual who can read only rows of larger letters marked 30, 40, or 200 at 20 feet is said to have 20/30, 20/40, or 20/200 vision. This indicates that the individual has a loss of vision. The eyes are tested separately as well as together. Vision may be perfect in one eye, but there may be a loss of vision in the other eye. Generally, the test is done twice on the individual wearing glasses, once with glasses and again without glasses. A person has defective vision when the light rays entering the eyes are not focused properly on the retina. This type of visual defect is known as an *error of refraction.* An eye examination to determine this type of visual defect is spoken of as *refraction of the eye.* In other words, the doctor measures the ability of a person's eyes to bend light rays.

The *ophthalmoscope* is an instrument used to examine structures inside the eye. The examiner can study the retina, the optic disk, the site of entry of the optic nerve, and the condition of other blood vessels in the patient's body as well as the condition of the patient's eye.

TONOMETRY AND TONOGRAM

The *tonometer* is an instrument used to measure pressure within the eye, *intraocular pressure.* The patient with glaucoma has increased intraocular pressure. Pressure within the eye increases because of improper drainage of the normal fluid (aqueous humor) between the anterior and posterior chambers of the eye.

A *tonogram* is made by placing a tonometer on the eye for about four minutes while a recording device traces intraocular pressure on graph paper. The graph patterns are then measured and analyzed to detect abnormal drainage or an obstruction to normal drainage.

BROMICROSCOPY

Examination of the client with the slit lamp microscope is referred to as bromiscroscopy. The *slit lamp microscope* is an instrument used to study the anterior segment of the eye. The ophthalmologist can visualize the sclera, cornea, iris, anterior chamber, lens, and anterior portion of the vitreous humor with the slit lamp microscope. These structures are illuminated and magnified by this instrument. Early signs of disease may be detected.

FLUORESCEIN ANGIOGRAPHY

Fluorescein angiography is a test useful in diagnosing abnormalities in blood vessels in the retina. A dye known as sodium fluorescein is injected into the patient's antecubital vein and reaches blood vessels in the eye about 12 seconds later. As molecules of dye pass through the blood vessels, a light shone into the eye causes them to become fluorescent. The fluorescence is then recorded by a camera. Normal blood vessels do not permit leakage of dye into surrounding tissue.

A few patients develop temporary nausea and vomiting within seconds after the dye is injected. These symptoms usually disappear within a minute. Following fluorescein angiography, the dye is excreted by the kidneys about one hour after injection. The dye causes the urine to turn green. This color change is explained by the nurse in advance to prevent fear and anxiety in the patient.

ELECTRORETINOGRAM (ERG)

An electroretinogram is a record of electrical changes in the retina following exposure to light. First, the cornea is anesthetized. Next, an electrode is applied to the cornea using a special contact lens. The retina is then exposed to light and subsequent changes are recorded in a manner similar to an electrocardiogram.

ULTRASOUND

An ultrasonogram may be done to examine the retina when hemorrhage, cataract, or neoplasm prevents normal visualization. Sound waves are directed to the retina and reflected back through the different substances present such as blood, tumor, or cataract. By analyzing the sound waves, the expert can detect certain abnormalities in the retina.

Nursing Observations

As a member of the health team, the nurse frequently is asked about health matters by family members, friends, and neighbors. In daily life, the nurse may observe symptoms of eye disease either in persons in the community or in patients hospitalized for another illness. Knowing the symptoms of eye disease enables the nurse to suggest medical attention when indicated. These symptoms are also reported and recorded when observed in the patient. Common symptoms are listed below for easy reference.

- *Persistent redness of the eye,* which may be caused by infection, inflammation, and pressure disorders.
- *Continued pain or eye discomfort,* particularly after an injury to the eye.
- *Disturbances of vision,* such as difficulty in seeing objects that are far or near. Blurred vision is a common symptom of eye conditions.
- *Fogginess of vision and rainbow-colored halves around lights.* These symptoms may occur in acute glaucoma or edema of the cornea.
- *Loss of peripheral vision,* which may indicate detached retina or occluded retinal arteries.
- *Persistent double vision,* which may be due to paralysis of the cranial nerves.
- *Floating spots* that develop suddenly. These may be caused by inflammation or hemorrhage.
- *Crossed eyes.* A child with crossed eyes does not outgrow this defect. Sight cannot be restored if lost because of a lack of early treatment. A child affected with strabismus, or crossed eyes, should be treated before the age of six by an ophthalmologist.
- *Infection,* which usually is the cause of ocular discharge, crusting, and tearing when these symptoms are of a continuing nature.
- *Pupillary irregularities* or changes in the shape and size of the pupils, and unequal pupils. These are indications of a disease of the brain or eye.

- Photophobia (intolerance to light) may signify certain abnormal conditions.
- Nausea and vomiting may occur in acute glaucoma.
- Headache is commonly associated with eye strain and common visual disturbances.

In addition to the symptoms listed above, nursing observations include the presence and use of eyeglasses, magnifying glasses, contact lenses, and sunglasses.

Medications taken by the patient often affect vision. Therefore, it is important to record information about all prescribed and nonprescribed drugs, including commercial eyedrops, the patient uses.

Eye cosmetics worn by the patient are another source that may be associated with eye disease. The nurse may be asked to list the brand of each eye cosmetic used by the patient so that the ingredients may be checked, if necessary.

Nursing Interventions

The ability to see is a priceless gift that is made possible by the proper functioning of our eyes. In many cases these organs of sight are unknowingly subjected to harmful conditions. People are becoming more interested in learning how to avoid these harmful conditions and to conserve sight. The nurse should be familiar with the interventions that are important to eye health. Many interventions appropriate in caring for the patient with a disease of the eye should be taught to the patient, family, and other members of the community.

HYGIENE OF THE EYES

Cleanliness is an important measure in the prevention of eye infection. The skin about the eyes should be kept clean by the use of soap and water. Clean washcloths and towels should be used. Also, they should not be used by another person. When cleaning the eyelids, the nurse moves in a direction from the inner canthus toward the outer canthus. The habit of rubbing the eyes with the fingers is not safe because of the possi-

bility of carrying an infection to them. The use of patent medications to cleanse the eyes should be discouraged as the eye cleanses itself. The use of an eyecup is not recommended because infected material can be carried by the solution to the surface of the eye.

PREVENTION OF EYESTRAIN

Eyestrain frequently results from using the eyes for close work, especially under unfavorable conditions. For example, reading in a moving car can cause eyestrain. The muscles that control the movement of the eyeball as well as those within the eye that control the entrance of light rays attempt to carry out the individual's wishes regarding his or her vision. The muscles become tired because of this abnormal effort to pull the eye into focus. The person's eyes become strained. Remembering that eyestrain frequently follows use of the eyes for close work, the nurse easily can understand the importance of good lighting for such activities. The light should come from above and behind the person engaged in close work. The individual should rest the eyes frequently by gazing into the distance. This allows the eye muscles to relax.

Glare such as that which comes from an unshaded lamp in front of a person's work should be avoided. The muscles of the iris react to glare by contracting in order to reduce the amount of light entering the eye. This can result in eyestrain.

An individual should protect the eyes from direct rays of the sun, as these may destroy parts of the retina. Sunglasses are used commonly for this purpose. Sunglasses that distort vision should not be used. Also, sunglasses should not be worn for night driving.

Many industries have active programs directed toward protecting the workers' eyesight. For example, they provide adequate lighting for their employees; they also provide protection for their workers' eyes from extreme heat and light. Another example of interest in the conservation of sight is seen in the construction of new schools. Adequate lighting is now considered an essential factor.

OBTAINING MEDICAL EYE CHECKUPS

Medical attention is imperative when any of the warning symptoms described earlier in the chapter is observed. As the number of symptoms increases, the severity of the patient's eye disease increases. An individual under 40 years of age generally has warning signals that precede eye disease. After reaching the age of 40, an individual may not have these warning signals. Eye examinations should be done whenever warning signals occur—at birth, between the ages of four and five years, at least every five years after the age of 40, or as often as indicated by the patient's condition and physician. Individuals with hypertension and diabetes mellitus may require more frequent eye examinations. If the client has a family history of glaucoma or intraocular pressure, more frequent visits to the ophthamologist may be needed.

MAINTAINING EYE SAFETY

Legislation was passed in 1972 to require the use of impact-resistant lenses in eyeglasses and sunglasses. Although the lenses are not unbreakable or shatterproof, they are less likely to break and injure the eyes.

Persons who are employed in areas where their eyes are exposed to extreme heat and light or flying objects are required to wear safety goggles to protect the eyes. Medical personnel employed in areas that administer emergency care should be instructed to examine the eye for contact lenses, as described in Chapter 8. Nurses, parents, childcare workers and others who care for children, the elderly, or retarded persons, need to be especially aware of eye safety measures.

Proper training and eye goggles can prevent many eye injuries. For example, injury to the eye may occur when an individual holds the air hose in a service station too close to the face. The compressed air used to inflate tires can cause burns of the eye and conjunctival hemorrhage. The trend in the United States toward self-service necessitates an awareness on the part of the public regarding the proper use of an air hose in service stations.

ASSISTING THE PATIENT WEARING GLASSES OR LENSES

Glasses and lenses are transparent devices worn to correct common eye defects or to protect the eyes from dangers such as flying objects in the air or from extreme heat or light. Corrective lenses may be prescribed in varying degrees of strength. For example, many lenses are prescribed with a single refractory power. *Bifocals* are those lenses in which there are two refractory powers in each lens. The lower portion of the glasses is for viewing objects that are near. The upper portion of the glasses is for seeing objects that are farther away. *Trifocals* are those lenses in which there are three refractory powers in each lens. One lens is for viewing objects that are close, another is for objects that are at a distance, and the third is for objects that are nearer to the individual than either of the two previously mentioned.

Safety lenses or safety glasses are heat treated or heat resistant. The lenses are plastic and will not shatter when broken. Plastic lenses are not as heavy as glass lenses but cost more and are easily damaged by scratching. Hardened lenses have been exposed to high temperatures and are hard. These lenses are resistant to forceful contact. Sunglasses have tinted lenses that decrease the amount of light entering the eye.

Glasses should be kept clean and free from scratches. The glasses should sit straight across the bridge of the nose, and lenses should be the same distance from each eye. Adjustment of glasses should be done by a specialist.

The practice of borrowing glasses from another is discouraged since this can result in damage to vision. Eyeglasses are prescribed on an individual basis as are medications.

Contacts are small plastic lenses designed to float on the liquid surface of the eye over the cornea to correct refractive errors. These lenses are specially suited to individuals in certain occupations and contact sports, and are popular with many for their cosmetic value. However, an ophthalmologist should be consulted by those seeking the use of contacts, as they are not recommended for all medical conditions and all individuals. Another lens that absorbs water is used for those who cannot tolerate a hard lens. This lens is referred to as soft because it is pliant. The soft lens does have disadvantages. It is more costly than a hard lens, it has to be replaced more frequently than a hard lens, and it does not correct vision as well as a hard lens. Extended-wear soft contact lenses are now available. Many patients enjoy these lenses because they can remain in the eye for several weeks, can be worn during sleep, and require less maintenance. Regular medical examination is important to ensure that the cornea is receiving an adequate oxygen supply.

The method of inserting, removing, and caring for contact lenses varies with the type of lens, the physician, and the patient. Specific information and instructions should be obtained before assisting the patient with these activities.

The patient may require encouragement and/or instruction to wear the prescribed glasses or lenses according to the physician's directions. For example, accidents may occur from ambulating without appropriate glasses or lenses. Glasses should be worn while driving, if they are needed.

ASSISTING WITH EMERGENCY EYE CARE

Appropriate emergency care following injury to the eye can prevent a loss of vision. A complete discussion can be located in Chapter 8, pages 195–97.

An individual with a black eye resulting from injury requires medical attention and observation to determine the extent of injury to the tissue around the eye. Many cases of blindness can be eliminated with appropriate first aid measures following an eye injury and regular consultation with an ophthalmologist. Vision can be preserved following an eye burn from toxic chemicals if prompt, adequate first aid measures are taken. As indicated in the chapter pertaining to the emergency patient (Chapter 8), an individual who has suffered a burn of the eye should have the eye washed with copious amounts of plain water immediately. The eye can be opened by the first aider by push-

ing the eyebrow up and the cheek down. Care should be taken not to apply pressure on the eye. In the case of a penetrating wound of the eye, pressure on the eye should be avoided also. The foreign body and eye should be covered with a sterile dressing or a clean cloth while the individual is being transported to a medical facility. No pressure should be placed on the eye. Emergency measures discussed in Chapter 8 are applicable to the person with a foreign body in the eye.

A foreign body in the eye sometimes can be removed with the moistened edge of a clean handkerchief or cotton-tipped applicator. Having the client blink may dislodge the particle and increase tearing. The increased flow of tears may wash the foreign object out of the eye. The person should not rub the eye as this action may cause injury to the cornea.

PREVENTING INFECTION

Infection is a special hazard for the patient with eye disease because of the danger of tissue damage, scarring, and visual impairment or blindness. In some hospitals, each patient receives a special eye kit on admission. The kit contains dressings and supplies to be used only for that patient during hospitalization.

In addition to the usual eye hygiene already discussed on page 778, the nurse takes other actions to prevent the introduction of pathogens into the eye including:

- Careful handwashing before and after each interaction with the patient, when changing the dressing, instilling medication
- Wash the hands before and after touching each eye since pathogens in one eye easily can be transmitted to the other
- Cleanse the eyelid, if necessary, before instilling medications
- Use only those eye medications that belong to the specific patient. Borrowing and/or using stock eye medications are unsafe practices which can lead to eye infection
- Use only sterile supplies for eye dressings

ASSISTING WITH DRUG THERAPY

A unique feature of drug therapy for the patient with a disease of the eye is that most medications are administered locally in the form of drops and ointments. This method is needed because of natural protective mechanisms that prevent the movement of many drugs from the bloodstream to the eye. Table 22.1 contains a list of drugs commonly prescribed for the patient with eye disease.

Since ointments usually provide higher concentrations of the prescribed medication, they cannot be used interchangeably with drops unless there is a physician's order.

Because drug absorption and concentration rise as contact with target tissues increases, the pouch method is recommended when eyedrops are instilled. Table 22.2 contains guidelines for correct instillation of eyedrops.

Dissolvable ocular inserts containing medication may be applied either to the lower or upper cul-de-sacs (spaces under lids). For example, pilocarpine, a pupil constrictor, is available in a sustained-release elliptical unit (OCUSERT) which is placed in a cul-de-sac. This unit is designed to supply a constant release of medication over a seven-day period. The availability and use of sustained delivery systems such as OCUSERT are expected to increase in the future.

CHANGING THE EYE DRESSING

Eye dressings may be applied to one or both eyes to limit eye movement, prevent exposure to light, absorb blood or drainage, prevent injury, and/or apply pressure. Eye dressings are not changed by the nurse unless there is a specific order to do so. When a dressing change is needed, scrupulous handwashing should be done both before and after the procedure.

Eye dressings consist of special oval pads composed of layers of absorbent gauze and cotton. When applying an eye pad, the patient's eyelids should be closed to prevent irritation of the cornea by the gauze. Unless specifically ordered, the dressing should be only tight enough to hold the eyelid closed. Additional pressure is not desirable unless specifically ordered by the physician. The

dressing is held in place by plastic adhesive tapes applied diagonally across the eye pad from the forehead to the cheek.

The eye dressing may be further covered by a plastic or metal patch or shield which serves as protection from rubbing or pressure on the eye. The shield is molded to rest on bony prominences of the eyebrow, cheek, and inside of the bridge of the nose.

ASSISTING THE SURGICAL PATIENT

Some persons with eye disease may be helped by surgery. Advances in technology are resulting in new surgical procedures and some changes in pre- and postoperative care. Table 22.3 contains a description of common surgical procedures on the eye. The interested nurse can consult nursing journals for new information as it becomes available.

PREOPERATIVE CARE. The usual preoperative care, described in Chapter 6, applies to the patient having eye surgery. A shampoo and shower are especially important since these activities may be restricted for some time following surgery. The patient may need help with a shampoo and shower because of visual impairment.

Although preoperative enemas rarely are ordered, the nurse should ask the patient about possible constipation preoperatively. This problem should be resolved before surgery to avoid straining which creates undesirable stress on the suture line and increased pressure in the eye after surgery.

Preoperative teaching includes specific instructions related to the prevention of stress on the suture line, increased intraocular pressure, and postoperative infection. The patient can anticipate the need to lie on the back or unoperated side after most procedures. Activities to be avoided include bending from the waist, lifting, jerky movements, straining to move the bowels, rubbing the eyes, and coughing or sneezing. Thus, it is especially important to assist the visually impaired person to become familiar with the surroundings before surgery. Items

Text continued on page 784.

TABLE 22.1
DRUGS USED IN EYE DISORDERS

NONPROPRIETARY NAME	TRADE NAME	AVERAGE DOSE	NURSING IMPLICATIONS
I. Anesthetics Relieve Pain in the Eye Following Local Application			
Benoxinate	DORSACAINE	0.4%	Prevent healing; anesthetic not used after foreign body removed
Lidocaine	XYLOCAINE	2%	
Procaine		1–2%	
Proparacaine	OPHTHAINE	0.5%	
Tetracaine	PONTOCAINE	0.5%	
II. Antimicrobial Drugs are Used Locally to Combat and/or Prevent Infection			
Bacitracin	CHLOROMYCETIN		Culture done before antibiotic given
Chloramphenicol			
Erythromycin			
Neomycin	MYCIFRADIN		Viruses not susceptible
Neomycin with bacitracin and polymyxin	NEOSPORIN		
Penicillin			
Sodium methicillin	STAPHCILLIN		
Sulfacetamide	SULAMYD		
Sulfisoxazole	GANTRISIN		
III. Carbonic Anhydrase Inhibitors Decrease the Production of Aqueous Humor; These Drugs May be Given Orally for Glaucoma			
Acetazolamide	DIAMOX	250 mg	Observe patient for potassium depletion
Ethoxzolamide	CARDRASE	62.5–125 mg	
Dichlorphenamide	DARARIDE	25–100 mg	Benoxinate
Methazolamide	NEPTAZANE	50–100 mg	
IV. Cycloplegics Produce Paralysis of the Ciliary Muscle which Facilitates an Ophthalmic Examination			
Atropine		1%	See Mydriatics
Cyclopentolate	CYCLOGYL	0.5–1.0%	
Eucatropine		2–5%	
Homatropine		2–5%	
Scopolamine hydro-bromide		0.5%	
Tropicamide	MYDRIACYL	0.5–1.0%	

V. Miotics Cause the Pupils to Contract; They are Applied Locally; They May be Used to Control Glaucoma

Drug	Trade Name	Concentration	Nursing Interventions
Carbachol	CARCHOLIN	0.75–3%	1. Wipe excess solution away. May cause systemic effects: asthma, nausea, or fall in blood pressure
Echothiophate	PHOSPHOLINE	0.06–0.25%	2. Tell patient that visual acuity may be decreased
Demecarium	HUMORSOL	0.25%	
Physostigmine, eserine		0.25–0.5%	
Philocarpine		0.5–2%	

VI. Mydriatics Cause the Pupil to Become Dilated

Drug	Trade Name	Concentration	Nursing Interventions
Atropine		1%	1. Wipe excess solution away. May cause coma, fever, delirium, dryness of mouth, inhibition of sweating, and tachycardia
Cyclopentolate	CYCLOGYL	0.5–1.0%	2. May produce glaucoma in predisposed clients
Epinephrine	EPITRATE	1–2%	3. Wash hands after use to avoid transferring to own eyes
Eucatropine		2–5%	
Homatropine		2–5%	
Scopolamine		0.5%	

VII. Ophthalmic Dyes are Used to Stain the Cornea to Enable the Examiner to see Abrasions

Drug	Trade Name	Concentration	Nursing Interventions
Fluorescein			Fluorescein solution usually has an added antibacterial agent. Strips are available also and are moistened with sterile water
Merbromin	MERCUROCHROME	2%	
Rose Bengal		2%	

VIII. Steroids are Used to Treat Allergic Reactions of the Eye, Inflammation, and Severe Injuries

Drug	Trade Name	Concentration	Nursing Interventions
Cortisone	CORTONE ACETATE	1.5–2.5% suspension	When drug is given for more than two weeks, the patient's intraocular pressure should be checked to detect early signs of glaucoma
Dexamethasone	DECADRON	0.1% solution	
	HEXADROL	0.05% ointment	
Hydrocortisone	CORTEF	2.5% suspension	
	HYDROCORTONE	1.5% ointment	
Prednisolone	METICORTELONE	0.12, 1% suspension	
	HYDELTRASOL	0.125, 0.5, 1% solution	
		0.25% ointment	
Fluoromethalone	OXYLONE	0.1% suspension	
Medrysone	MEDROCORT	1% suspension	

IX. Drug is Used to Inhibit Growth of Herpes Simplex Virus

Drug	Trade Name	Concentration	Nursing Interventions
Idoxuridine	DENDRID	0.1% solution	Boric acid should not be used as combination may cause irritation
	HERPLEX	0.5% ointment	
	STOXIL		

Table 22.2
Guide to Instillation of Eyedrops and Ointments

1. Wash the hands before instilling medication into the eye.
2. Gently grasp the lower lid using the thumb and index finger of one hand to pull out slightly and create a pouch.
3. Apply the prescribed dosage of medication into the pouch.
4. Close the eyelid after instilling eyedrops and apply pressure to bridge of nose to prevent overflow.
5. Because of limited volume in the spaces under the lids, wait 5 minutes before instilling another medication in the same eye.

needed often are placed on the bedside on the unoperated side even before surgery. One common preoperative teaching that is not appropriate for the patient having eye surgery is coughing exercises. Instead, deep-breathing exercises are demonstrated and encouraged.

In some hospitals, preoperative preparation includes clipping the eyelashes. Lubricant may be applied to the scissor blades so that cut lashes stick to the lubricant and do not fall into the patient's eyes. The patient

may be reassured to learn that lashes grow back in six to eight weeks. Eyebrows that are especially long and bushy may be trimmed preoperatively, if desired by the surgeon. A preoperative facial scrub with bacteriostatic soap or solution is ordered by some surgeons.

Preoperative medications include several kinds of eyedrops to prepare the eye for surgery. Specific medications depend upon the procedure to be done but may include one or more of those listed in Table 22.1.

Postoperative Care. The patient often returns from the recovery room fully awake since many procedures are done under local anesthesia. As previously mentioned a general guideline is to position the patient either on the back or unoperated side. The postoperative orders should be checked carefully for special instructions related to positions and activities to be included or avoided.

Deep-breathing and passive range-of-motion exercises are encouraged, and coughing is avoided. In most cases, the patient may be helped to the bathroom to urinate. Bedpans are avoided unless specifically ordered because using the bedpan increases stress on the suture line and raises

Table 22.3
Guide to Selected Surgical Procedures on the Eye

Name	Description
Cryotherapy	Outpatient surgery using a freezing probe applied to the outside of the eye to seal a hole or tear in the retina
Extracapsular extraction of cataract (phacoemulsification)	Removal of lens by breaking it into small pieces which can be irrigated and aspirated out
Intracapsular extraction of cataract	Removal of lens by using cold probe or special forceps
Iridectomy	Excision of part of the iris
Keratoplasty (corneal transplant)	Excision of diseased corneal tissue and replacement with corneal graft from human donor; artificial cornea may be used instead, if previous transplants have not been successful
Photocoagulation	Outpatient surgery using a laser beam to seal holes or tears in retina
Scleral buckling procedure	Incision made into conjunctiva and special instruments used to alter contour of the retina and create a chemical process which causes the layers of retina to adhere to each other.
Trabeculectomy	Removal of trabecular meshwork to create a new channel for drainage of aqueous humor in persons with glaucoma
Vitrectomy	Incision made via the sclera to remove vitreous membrane and repair retinal detachment

intraocular pressure. Early ambulation usually is encouraged.

Drug therapy includes an analgesic for pain. Severe, sharp pain or presssure in the operated eye is reported at once to the appropriate nurse or physician since these findings may signal hemorrhage or infection. The patient who reports nausea is medicated at once with an antiemetic to prevent vomiting and associated increased pressure in the eye. If the patient does vomit postoperatively, the head is turned to the unoperated side. Other drug therapy may include one or more eyedrops from Table 22.1.

The patient usually returns from surgery wearing an eye dressing, as described on page 781. Most procedures are associated with a small amount of serous drainage. Eye dressings are not removed during the immediate postoperative period unless there is a specific order to do so. When dressing changes are permitted, the nurse uses the procedure described earlier on page 781.

Activities associated with hygiene such as washing the face, shaving, and toothbrushing may be modified or avoided postoperatively. The postoperative orders should be checked carefully for restricted activities.

As previously mentioned, items needed frequently should be placed at the unoperated side of the patient's bedside unit. The patient should be reoriented to the location of items and reminded of activities and positions to be used or avoided.

Some behavioral changes postoperatively may either signal or cause complications and should be reported to the appropriate nurse or physician. Examples of changes that should be reported include restlessness, disorientation, coughing and sneezing, pain that is unrelieved by medication, and nausea and vomiting that are unrelieved by medication.

Before discharge, the surgical eye patient needs written instructions related to:

- Bathing at home
- Shampoo of the hair
- Specific activities and positions to be avoided
- Use of eye dressings, shields, glasses
- Medications to be taken
- Correct instillation of eyedrops

CARING FOR THE VISUALLY IMPAIRED PATIENT

Most patients with eye disease have some type of visual impairment. In addition, the nurse cares for patients with other conditions who are also visually impaired. In some cases, eye medication and/or patching may cause a further reduction of vision at a time when the patient's greatest fear is becoming blind. Long hours in the hospital without visual stimulation or diversion activities may result in feelings of anger, boredom, fear, and frustration. In some cases, intense emotional states may further worsen the patient's condition.

The nurse's caring is often the key to a successful recovery. In communicating with the visually impaired person, it is especially important to speak in low, pleasant tones. Each person who enters the patient's room should announce him- or herself even if going to see another patient in the room. A thorough explanation is needed before beginning any procedure. The thoughtful nurse also tells the patient before leaving the room.

In order to compensate for partial or complete loss of visual sensation, the nurse may decide to increase stimulation via other senses. For example, increased conversations, a gentle touch when bathing, or providing a radio helps the patient to maintain contact with others.

When admitting the person with eye disease to the hospital, the nurse collects and records information about visual impairment. This information provides the basis for altering nursing interventions to provide safe, effective nursing.

The newly admitted patient needs a thorough orientation to new surroundings. Usually, the location of objects in the patient's environment is described according to the hands on the clock.

When assisting the visually impaired person to eat, the nurse similarly describes each item on the tray according to the hands on a clock (Figure 22.2). For example, the meat may be placed at six o'clock. The patient's clothing should be protected with a napkin.

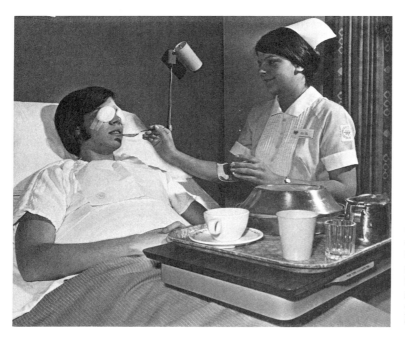

FIGURE 22.2 The practical/vocational nursing student is feeding the patient recovering from eye surgery. (Courtesy of Shapero School of Nursing, a Program in Practical Nursing of Sinai Hospital, Detroit, Michigan.)

If the patient must be fed, the nurse asks what food is to be eaten next.

When assisting the visually impaired person to ambulate, the nurse walks a few steps ahead. The patient takes the nurse's arm for guidance. The patient should be told approximately how far they plan to walk and should be helped to locate both the arms and the back of the chair before sitting down (Figure 22.3).

Safety is important for the visually impaired patient. The combination of unfamiliar surroundings, medication, and anxiety can result in accidents, if special precautions are not taken. Siderails usually are kept up to remind the patient of the location of the edges of the bed. The call bell is placed within easy reach of the patient. Nurses who work with visually impaired persons are especially alert for calls for help to the bathroom, since lengthy waits may tempt the patient to get out of bed unassisted. Rooms, bathrooms, and corridors should be well lighted and free from obstacles such as spills, laundry hampers, and wheelchairs. A particularly important safety intervention is encouraging the patient with glasses to wear them at the appropriate times. The nurse may clean the glasses, if the patient

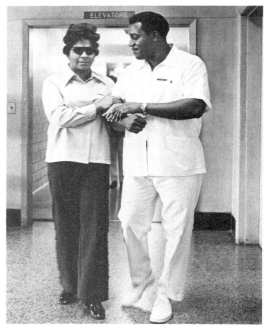

FIGURE 22.3 When walking the patient who has both eyes bandaged or is blind, the practical/vocational nurse should walk slightly ahead of the patient. The patient's hand can be placed on the nurse's arm as shown above. In this manner, the patient is guided by the nurse.

cannot do this alone. Moving familiar objects or rearranging furniture is avoided when possible. When the environment must be changed, an important safety measure is to reorient the visually impaired person to the new surroundings.

Providing diversionary activities is a special challenge for the nurse. Some patients enjoy listening to the radio. Others enjoy being read to. Many patients are particularly interested in listening to local news. The recreational therapist may be asked to suggest additional activities for each level of visual impairment. Volunteers from the family, church, hospital auxilliary, or community may be helpful in providing diversionary activities.

Common Visual Defects

NEARSIGHTEDNESS (MYOPIA)

The person with *myopia* can see better when objects are close. Myopia or nearsightedness occurs when an individual's eyeball is too long or the crystalline lens is too rounded. Light rays entering the eye are focused in front of the retina rather than on it (see Figure 22.4). Nearsightedness can be corrected by lenses that cause the light rays to be focused properly on the retina.

FARSIGHTEDNESS (HYPERMETROPIA, HYPEROPIA)

A person with *farsightedness* can see better when objects are at a distance (see Fig-

ure 22.4). Hypermetropia occurs when an individual's eyeball is too short or when the lens or cornea is too flat. Light rays entering the eye are focused on a theoretic point behind the retina rather than on it. Farsightedness can be corrected by lenses that cause the light rays to be focused properly on the retina.

ASTIGMATISM

An individual with *astigmatism* has an irregular curvature of the cornea or of the crystalline lens. This prevents the light rays from focusing at one point on the retina. As a result, the image formed on the retina is blurred. Thus, the patient with astigmatism has blurred vision and may complain of discomfort when using the eyes. Astigmatism can be corrected by lenses also.

PRESBYOPIA

A person with *presbyopia* may see distant objects distinctly but close objects cannot be seen clearly. This condition occurs with the aging process. The crystalline lenses become less elastic. This decreases the power of accommodation of the lenses. Glasses can be prescribed to improve this type of visual defect. Bifocals, described earlier as lenses with two refractory powers, may be prescribed. The lower portion of the glasses is for reading and viewing objects at close range, and the upper portion of the glasses is for viewing objects at a distance.

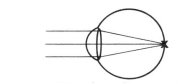
Normal rays focus on retina

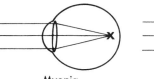
Myopia
Rays focus in front of retina

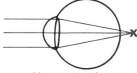
Hypermetropia
Rays focus in back of retina

FIGURE 22.4 Diagram illustrating farsightedness and nearsightedness.

When assisting the patient with a common visual defect, the nurse may teach about the use of glasses or lenses, as described earlier on pages 779–80.

The Patient with an Inflammatory or Infectious Condition of the Eye

STYE

The individual with a stye has a common infection on the edge of the eyelid. The infection generally results in the formation of an abscess. Staphylococci frequently cause a stye. The eyelid becomes red, swollen, and painful. An individual who uses an excessive amount of cosmetics or practices poor hygiene is more likely to develop a stye than one who is more meticulous with hygiene. The staphylococci generally spread from one hair follicle to another, causing infection to occur in clusters.

The physician generally recommends the application of moist, warm compresses to the infected area. Application of heat often causes the stye to drain. The patient's head should be turned to the side so that the solution or drainage will not drain into the unaffected eye. Hands should be washed before and after applying the compresses to prevent the spread of infection. The patient should be instructed not to squeeze or touch the inflamed area with the hands, for the infection can spread and involve a major portion of the eyelid. If the stye does not drain, it may have to be incised to permit drainage. Antibiotic therapy may be used (see Table 5.7).

CONJUNCTIVITIS

An individual with conjunctivitis has an inflammation of the mucous membrane that lines the eyelids and covers the front portion of the eyeball. Conjunctivitis may be caused by an infection, an allergy, or an injury. Such microorganisms as staphylococci, viruses, streptococci, or gonococci may cause conjunctivitis. The Koch-Weeks bacillus is another causative organism commonly found in schoolchildren affected with pinkeye. Pinkeye is transmitted easily from one child to another.

The patient usually has redness and swelling of the conjunctiva. Discomfort may range from a feeling of having grit in the affected eye to acute pain. Usually, the patient has an increased amount of tears. Burning and itching may be present, especially when the inflammation is caused by an allergy. A discharge containing pus generally occurs when the inflammation is caused by the gonococcus. The patient with conjunctivitis may develop an infection of the cornea, if not treated.

The doctor directs treatment toward relieving the underlying cause of the inflammation. For example, suitable drugs are prescribed to combat infection. The doctor may prescribe an antihistamine for the patient with an allergy. In addition, attempts may be made to identify and remove the substance to which the patient is allergic. Irrigation of the affected eye and the instillation of mild antiseptic drops may be ordered. The use of warm compresses also may be prescribed. To prevent the transfer of infection, the person with conjunctivitis should not allow anyone else to use his or her towel. The patient who has only one eye involved should be instructed not to touch the unaffected eye and to wash the hands before and after caring for the affected eye.

UVEITIS

The patient with uveitis has an inflammation of the ciliary body, iris, and choroid, which make up the uveal tract. One, two, or all three of these structures may be involved. The patient with uveitis generally has pain in the affected eye, redness, blurred vision, tearing, edema of the eyelid, uneven pupils, and photophobia. The ophthalmologist determines the form of uveitis and varies treatment accordingly. Uveitis is difficult to cure and may lead to glaucoma, cataract, or retinal detachment. Medication and warm compresses to relieve pain, antibiotics, and steroids may be prescribed. Drugs such as atropine may be instilled in the eye to dilate the pupil and reduce the formation of adhesions (see Table 22.1).

The client may be on bed rest during the acute stage with the eyes covered to increase rest of the affected eye. The environment may be darkened, if necessary. As the patient's condition improves, glasses may be worn to relieve discomfort from bright lights.

KERATITIS

The client with keratitis has an inflammation of the cornea. Keratitis is a serious condition because it may result in blindness. The infectious process may cause perforation and opacity of the cornea. Keratitis may be caused by tuberculosis, syphilis, an allergic reaction, a vitamin deficiency, or a virus infection.

The individual will complain of a feeling similar to having sand in the eye. The eyelid may have spasms, and the patient may experience photophobia. The eye may tear and will appear red.

The individual with keratitis has the treatment designed to combat the cause. After determining the cause of keratitis, the ophthalmologist will direct treatment toward relieving that condition. Bed rest, warm compresses to relieve pain and promote healing, antibiotics, and steroids may be prescribed. The eyes may be covered to promote rest. Drugs such as atropine will dilate the pupil and rest the iris and ciliary body. Idoxuridine (DENDRID, HERPLEX, or STOXIL) may be prescribed as an ophthalmic ointment or eyedrops to treat the patient with keratitis caused by the herpes simplex virus.

BLEPHARITIS

An individual with blepharitis has an inflammation of the edges of the eyelids. The inflammation may be caused by an infection, an allergen, or trauma. Staphylococci, viruses, streptococci, or gonococci may be the causative organisms in blepharitis.

The affected eyelid or eyelids will be irritated and red and have crust formations. Ulcerations of the eyelid may develop. The area is cleansed by the application of warm compresses and a prescribed antibiotic. The nurse should wash the hands thoroughly using meticulous technique before and after touching the inflamed area. The eyes should not be touched before handwashing. The pa-

tient should be instructed not to rub the eyes.

CHALAZION

The client with a chalazion has a cyst of the meibomian gland located within each eyelid. The individual has a hard, shiny lump within the eyelid. If the individual is bothered by the chalazion, it may be removed surgically under local anesthesia in the physician's office. An antibiotic ointment generally is applied and an eye pad left in place for a few days. It is important for members of the health team to remember that handwashing is important to the patient as well as others. The nurse should wash the hands carefully before and after assisting with the procedure. Again, the nurse should remember that the eyes should not be touched before washing the hands thoroughly.

Strabismus

An individual with strabismus cannot direct both eyes toward the same object. Strabismus is known also as cross-eye, wall-eye, and squint. Strabismus is caused by a lack of coordination between the muscles that control the movement of the eyes. The individual with strabismus who looks straight ahead with one eye while the other eye moves toward the nose is said to have *convergent strabismus* or is *cross-eyed*. The individual whose eye moves outward has *divergent strabismus* or is *wall-eyed*. *Esotropia* is convergent strabismus, and *exotropia* is divergent strabismus.

Strabismus may be congenital. This is the case commonly found in children. An individual also may develop strabismus because of paralysis of the nerves that supply the eye muscles.

Early treatment prevents poor vision and helps to prevent the development of emotional problems associated with strabismus. If strabismus is not treated before the child is six years of age, treatment often is not successful and permanent visual impairment may result. The ophthalmologist prescribes glasses and orthoptics (muscle exercise) in some cases. In early childhood, the condition may be treated with occlusion of the unaffected eye or covering the unaffected eye and forcing the child to use the affected eye. Surgery generally is done if the above methods are not successful. During surgery, eye muscles may be lengthened or shortened to straighten the eye. The ophthalmologist may need to do surgery several times to correct the defect. The patient requires care similar to that described earlier in the chapter on pages 781–85. Unlike the patient having eye surgery involving the eye globe, this patient usually is allowed to be out of bed soon after the operation. The reason for this difference is that the surgeon has not performed an operation on the inner structures of the eye but is dealing with muscles around the eyeball.

Ulceration of the Cornea

A person suffering from an ulceration of the cornea has an open lesion on the transparent membrane that covers the front of the eye. The open lesion may be small or it may spread over the entire cornea. The lesion may be deep or shallow. Perforation of the cornea and a loss of vision may occur. Also, loss of the affected eye is a possibility. The ulcer may be the result of trauma, irritation from contact lenses, or infection. A scar may form in the area of the corneal ulcer during the healing process. This is a serious condition because the cornea normally is transparent. Light rays must pass through this clear window into the eye to permit vision. If the scar is located directly over the pupil, light rays are prevented from entering the eye. Thus, the person has diminished vision or no vision in the affected eye.

NURSING OBSERVATIONS

A perforated cornea may cause the patient to have no discomfort, or it may cause marked discomfort. The patient's eyes may be sensitive to light and increased lacrimation may be present. In addition to redness of the eye, pus may form behind the cornea, and a herniation of the iris through the cornea may result. The decreased amount of vision is directly related to the extent of the ulceration of the cornea.

NURSING INTERVENTIONS

Nursing interventions described earlier for the patient with keratitis, such as warm compresses, steroids, antibiotics, and atropine, may be indicated. Idoxuridine may be prescribed for local application.

An operation called keratoplasty (corneal transplant) may be done on a patient who has little or no vision because of a scarred cornea. However, the patient with any infection is not a candidate for a transplant. In doing a corneal transplant, the ophthalmologist removes the damaged cornea and puts in its place another piece of cornea. This tissue, which is transplanted into the patient's eye, was removed earlier from the eye of a deceased person. Ideally, the cornea must be removed within six hours after death and should be used within 24 hours. Eye banks are located in various areas throughout the United States to receive donor eyes and to make corneas available to the ophthalmologist. Some civic organizations aid in obtaining donor eyes by encouraging individuals to donate their eyes to a specific eye bank. These eyes are shipped immediately. Such groups as local police, volunteer motor corps drivers, and airline employees work together closely to speed the delivery of the eye to the eye bank or to the recipient.

Three types of corneal transplants are being used. Lamellar keratoplasty replaces only a thin layer of corneal tissue. The entire thickness of the donated cornea may be used (penetrating keratoplasty). A small part of the total thickness of the cornea, or partial penetrating keratoplasty, may be utilized. A combination of lamellar keratoplasty and penetrating keratoplasty may be utilized. The patient receives pre- and postoperative care similar to that described for the surgical patient earlier in the chapter on pages 781–85. The patient with a penetrating transplant is kept in bed for one or two days with both eyes bandaged to keep the graft in place. The other type of corneal graft allows the patient to be up within 24 hours or be out of bed and able to feed him- or herself the day of surgery. The physician's order regarding activity should be followed meticulously for the patient who has received a corneal transplant. Healing requires from weeks to months because there are no blood vessels in the cornea. Sutures may not be removed for up to a year following surgery. During this time, the cornea is weak and there is increased danger of trauma caused by sudden increases in intraocular pressure.

Prior to discharge from the hospital, the patient should be instructed regarding activities and positions to be aovided at home. Information should be provided regarding the activities allowed as well. Lifting, bending, and sudden rapid movements usually are not permitted.

Complications can occur following keratoplasty. The cornea may become cloudy for no obvious reason, or it may become cloudy because of a growth of blood vessels in the transplanted cornea. The surgical procedure may be required again if the patient's eye is in a condition to receive another donated cornea.

If several transplants are not successful, an artificial cornea may be placed in the affected eye. During this procedure, a cylinder-shaped prosthesis is inserted through the upper eyelid and cornea and sutured in place. The eyelid of the affected eye is permanently closed. A pinhole in the eyelid permits light to enter the eye and pass through the artificial cornea. Nursing care is similar to that needed by other patients having eye surgery. Swelling of the lid and around the eye which is common following this type of surgery may be decreased by placing a small bag of ice chips over the eye dressing. This procedure is also associated with an increased amount of pain.

Cataract

The patient with a *cataract* has a cloudy opacity of the crystalline lens. The capsule surrounding the lens may become cloudy also. Cataracts may develop in one or both eyes. Light rays normally entering the eye through the clear lens cannot enter through a cloudy lens. Thus, the patient will have a decreased amount of absence of vision. Coagulation of protein in the lens and a decrease in vitamin C and vitamin B_{12} because of changes in metabolism may be the cause of opacity.

An infant may be born with cataracts. When this occurs, the condition may be hereditary in nature or it may have been caused by a viral infection in the mother during early pregnancy. An individual may develop a cataract later in life because of injury or a disease affecting another part of the eye, such as an inflammation of the choroid. This condition also may be associated with a disease elsewhere in the body, such as diabetes. A person is more likely to develop a cataract later in life in connection with the aging process. Thus, cataracts are more common in older people.

NURSING OBSERVATIONS

The patient with a cataract has blurred or hazy vision. Reading material or work must be held closer to the eyes. Glare from bright lights may cause some discomfort. These symptoms occur as a result of local areas of cloudiness within the crystalline lens. The patient continues to lose vision as the clouding process continues within the lens. The patient's pupil may appear gray or milky white.

NURSING INTERVENTIONS

Nursing interventions for the patient with a cataract are associated with complete or partial surgical removal of the lens containing the cataract. This offers the patient a good chance for having the sight restored. Surgery for removal of the cataract usually is carried out under local anesthesia in order to prevent strain on the incision of the eye from nausea and vomiting, which sometimes follow a general anesthetic. Frequently, the patient who has cataracts in both eyes has only one cataract removed at a time.

Intracapsular removal of the lens indicates that the capsule containing the lens is removed intact. Cryosurgery, a type of intracapsular extraction, partially freezing the cataract and extracting it with a cold probe, may be used. A decrease in the temperature is produced by use of a probe that contains liquid nitrogen. The subfreezing metal adheres to the cataract, facilitating removal.

In *extracapsular extraction,* the surgeon uses a process known as phacoemulsification. The tip of the instrument introduced into the lens capsule breaks up the lens by high velocity vibrations, after which the minute particles are aspirated. The posterior capsule may be left in place.

Care of the patient having cataract surgery is the same as that described for the surgical patient earlier in the chapter on pages 781–85. The patient requires a thorough orientation to surroundings since visual impairment is present at the time of hospital admission. Preoperative teaching, as described on page 781, is important.

Postoperatively, the patient is positioned carefully either on the back or unoperated side. Drug therapy usually includes a mydriatic (pupil dilator), steroid, and antibiotic in the form of eyedrops (Table 22.1). Activities known to increase intraocular pressure are avoided. Eye dressings are changed using sterile technique, as described on page 781.

Symptoms that may indicate complications such as severe pain, restlessness, and tachycardia should be noted and reported promptly. These symptoms may be indications that the sutures have ruptured, or they may indicate the presence of bleeding. Nausea should be controlled by the administration of antiemetics, as vomiting increases intraocular pressure.

Dark glasses usually are used after the eye dressings have been removed. Taping an eyeshield over the affected eye to prevent accidental injury during the night is a precautionary measure. The patient may be fitted for temporary corrective lenses for the first six weeks. Six to eight weeks after surgery, the ophthalmologist will generally prescribe permanent lenses. Contact lenses now are becoming more popular than regular lenses. Properly fitted lenses should enable the patient to have almost normal vision. The patient's vision does not change to near perfect as soon as the glasses are fitted. The return of improved vision is slow. The patient has to become adjusted to the new lenses before maximum amount of vision can be achieved. It is important for the patient and nurse to remember that the return of normal vision may be gradual following cataract surgery.

A recent development in cataract surgery is the placement of an artificial lens in the eye either at the time of cataract surgery or in a later surgery. A variety of intraocular lenses is available which are named according to the site of placement in the eye. For example, an anterior chamber lens is placed in front of the iris. The selection of a specific lens is based upon which method of surgery is used and the individual patient.

The implanted lens offers advantages of improved depth perception, full visual fields, and binocular vision. The lens is invisible to most persons looking at the patient and is not removed and reinserted as contact lenses are. Some persons have conditions for which implanted intraocular lenses are not suitable. For example, the person with a history of glaucoma, diabetic retinopathy, retinal detachment, or congenital cataracts is not a candidate for an intraocular lens.

A variation in usual postoperative care when an intraocular lens has been implanted is the use of miotic drugs (pupil constricting) instead of mydriatics (pupil dilating). Constriction of the pupil with drugs reduces the likelihood of displacement of the lens. In addition, the nurse may be asked to observe and record the location of the lens at specified times.

Glaucoma

Glaucoma is characterized by increased pressure within the eyeball referred to as increased intraocular pressure. Glaucoma is a serious eye disease that eventually results in blindness if not treated. Glaucoma is one of the leading but preventable causes of blindness in the United States. This condition is more common in persons over 40 years of age—thus, the importance of routine testing for early glaucoma.

Normally, the aqueous humor is produced by the ciliary body and flows in through the pupil and out of the network located at the junction of the iris and the cornea. If the network becomes faulty because of clogging by cells, blood, or fibrin, the outflow of aqueous humor is decreased and pressure builds up in the eye. An abnormality elsewhere in the eyes also may place pressure against the network and cause increased intraocular pressure.

Individuals over 40 years of age should have an eye examination by an ophthalmologist at least once every two years. Diagnostic tests that establish glaucoma include tonometry, tonograms, gonioscopy, and elevation of the visual fields.

NURSING OBSERVATIONS

An individual may have either acute or chronic glaucoma. In an acute case, the patient often complains of pain in the diseased eye and may have nausea and vomiting. The pupil of the affected eye is dilated, and the eye looks red and hazy. The patient reports a decrease of vision and feelings of general malaise.

The person with chronic glaucoma may be only vaguely aware of gradual impairment of vision. Halos may be noticed around lights. There may be episodes of blurred vision and headaches. Frequently, this patient has one eye involved and then the other one. Symptoms develop slowly over a period of time. One of the main symptoms noticed by the patient is that side vision is not as good as it used to be. An instrument used to test the side vision or peripheral vision is a *perimeter*. There also may be difficulty in adjusting the eyes to darkened rooms.

NURSING INTERVENTIONS

The ophthalmologist prescribes drug therapy for the patient with glaucoma to reduce tension within the eyeball. *Miotic* drugs may be prescribed. These drugs, instilled in the eye several times daily, cause the pupil to constrict. This improves aqueous outflow and reduces intraocular pressure. Miotics do not cure glaucoma but will control the pressure and prevent further loss of sight. The patient using miotics for glaucoma will have to remember to use the drugs every day for the rest of his or her life. It is essential that a nurse instilling myotics use the prescribed drug. Use of a pupil-dilating drug (*mydriatic*) could make glaucoma much worse. Other drugs taken orally may be used to reduce the rate of formation of aqueous fluid. These drugs, carbonic anhydrase inhibitors (DIAMOX), also cause diuresis. Other commonly used diuretics do not reduce intraocular pressure.

If the patient has chronic glaucoma and does not respond to medical treatment, surgery may be needed. The individual with acute glaucoma may have surgical treatment also. This type of surgery is performed to improve drainage of aqueous humor. The patient may be treated with a combination of methods.

Surgical procedures that may be done are an *iridectomy*, in which a portion of the iris is excised, an *iridencleisis*, where an opening is made between the anterior chamber and the space behind the conjunctiva to drain the aqueous humor, and a *corneoscleral trephine*, where an opening is made at a point where the cornea and sclera meet. Aqueous humor is absorbed by the conjunctiva. Trabeculectomy involves removal of a portion of trabecular meshwork to create a new channel for drainage of aqueous humor. Nursing care is similar to that described earlier for the surgical patient on pages 781–85. Table 22.4 contains information related to patient teaching for the patient with glaucoma.

TABLE 22.4
GUIDELINES TO TEACHING THE PATIENT
WITH GLAUCOMA

- Avoid activities known to increase intraocular pressure such as lifting, bending at the waist, sudden turning of the head.
- Develop a life-style that avoids intense emotional upsets such as worry and overexcitement.
- Practice good dietary habits that prevent constipation and straining to have a bowel movement.
- Use only prescribed medications and follow the physician's directions carefully.
- Continue regular visits to the eye doctor for examinations.
- Report glaucoma to any other physicians and ask specifically how prescribed drugs for other conditions affect glaucoma.
- Carry glaucoma medication at all times.
- Wear identification that alerts others to the presence of glaucoma.

Detachment of the Retina

Normally the retina fits against the choroid. An individual has a detachment of the retina when this membrane becomes separated from the choroid vessels. The separation may be partial or complete. The nurse may find it helpful to think of a detached retina as being similar to wallpaper that has become loose from the wall. The retina receives the image and transmits the impulses to the optic nerve. An opening in the retina allows the vitreous humor and fluid from the choroid vessels to get behind the retina and separate it from the choroid, its source of nourishment. The part of the retina detached and deprived of nourishment becomes blind.

Detachment of the retina may be caused by such factors as a tumor, an eye injury, or an accident that causes the person to be shaken up, although no direct injury to the eye has occurred. An individual with a severe case of myopia may develop this condition. An older person may have a detached retina because of degenerative changes in the eye associated with the aging process. It also can occur for no apparent reason. Retinal detachment occurs more often in men, Jews, and persons over 40 years old.

NURSING OBSERVATIONS

The patient may experience flashes of light and movement of particles across the line of vision. Later, the patient may report a shadow, spider web, or veil that floats across the visual field. Light rays must be focused properly on the sensitive retina in order for a person to see. With a detached retina, the individual has a loss of vision. This loss of vision may be partial or complete, depending on the location and amount of retinal detachment. The symptoms are frightening, and the patient usually is apprehensive. Because the retina does not perceive pain, a detachment or tear does not hurt.

ASSISTING WITH DIAGNOSTIC STUDIES

The patient who reports symptoms of retinal detachment usually has direct and indirect ophthalmoscopy. A slit lamp examination and ultrasound also may be done.

NURSING INTERVENTIONS

Most patients with retinal detachment are placed on bed rest with both eyes patched. Surgical repair of the retina causes the formation of a scar that seals the hole or tear. Several procedures may be done. Photocoagulation is a process in which an argon laser beam is directed toward the area to be sealed. In about two weeks, scar formation at the site prevents further separation of the retina caused by leakage of retinal fluids. A new form of laser currently under study is the krypton laser beam.

Holes in the peripheral retina caused by degenerative changes may be repaired using *cryotherapy*. During this procedure, a freezing probe is applied to the outside of the eye. The ice ball that forms at the end of the probe travels through eye tissue to seal the damaged area. A scar forms several days later. The patient may experience an achy, cold sensation for a few minutes during the procedure. Another surgical procedure is called *scleral buckling*, in which a portion of the sclera is surgically excised about two thirds of its depth and the two sides sewed back together, sometimes over a plastic tube. This causes the sclera to buckle or bend inward. Before a scleral buckling surgery, the patient is carefully positioned in bed to encourage a settling of the retina against the choroid using gravity. In addition to the usual postoperative care already described on pages 784–85, cool compresses may be applied to reduce swelling and promote comfort. Drug therapy includes mydriatics (pupil dilators) and steroid eyedrops.

When retinal hemorrhage is associated with detachment, the surgeon may do a *vitrectomy*. During this procedure, the vitreous body is removed through an incision in the sclera and replaced with a basic salt solution. A bubble of air or gas may be injected into the vitreous cavity to hold the retina against the choroid. The bubble is absorbed after several days and replaced by aqueous humor.

Nursing care for the patient having this procedure is the same as that needed for the surgical patient. Drug therapy includes mydriatics (pupil dilators), steroid, and antibiotic eyedrops. The patient usually is discharged about a week after surgery with instructions related to the correct use of eyedrops and avoidance of activities that increase intraocular pressure.

Neoplastic Disease

A tumor can develop within the eye as well as in the eyelids and other structures associated with vision. The main symptom experienced by an individual with a tumor of the eyeball may be a bloodshot eye. This symptom should be reported to the physician because early diagnosis and prompt treatment may save the patient's eye and life. Malignant melanomas grow slowly and spread early to the lungs and liver. Enucleation, radiation therapy, chemotherapy, and plastic surgery may be utilized. The patient and family need emotional support, as in other cases of malignancy. They also need to express their feelings and concerns as well as to be accepted. Both the patient and family will need help in adjusting to the illness.

Enucleation, removal of an eye, may be necessary to treat a malignancy. Following enucleation, a firm pressure dressing may be applied for several days. Early ambulation is encouraged, and there usually is no restriction of the activities as there is with other forms of eye surgery. After an enucleation, the patient will have a metal or plastic ball implant placed into the connective tissue from which the eyeball was removed and have the eye muscles attached to the implant. The muscles then will move the implanted ball. When the socket is healed, usually within a month, a prosthesis of glass or plastic will be made to match the patient's other eye. The prosthesis will fit over the buried ball implant and move as the intact eye moves to focus. The prosthesis is a rather fragile shell, and care should be taken to teach the patient to put it in and remove it. Preferably, the patient should learn to lean over a bed while inserting the prosthesis and removing it to avoid breaking it if dropped.

To insert a prosthesis, the individual should place the more pointed end next to the nose. The upper eyelid should be pulled up and out and the prosthesis slipped in place under the upper lid. Holding the prosthesis in this position, the lower lid should be pulled down and the edge of the prosthesis slipped in.

To remove the prosthesis, the individual should pull the lower lid down, and the edge of the prosthesis should be pulled out in front of the lid. Then, while holding a hand to catch the prosthesis, the person should press gently on the upper lid and the prosthesis will slip into the cupped hand.

Careful hygiene of the eye socket and care of the prosthesis will prevent infections and irritations of the socket. The prosthesis generally is removed for sleeping and cleaned. The prosthesis should be stored carefully to prevent scratches. Careful rinsing with saline of the socket and prosthesis will help to prevent irritation of the conjunctiva. The nurse and/or patient should always wash hands thoroughly before touching the prosthesis or eye socket. The individual who has lost one eye should be taught ways of preventing damage to the other. For example, the client should avoid hazardous situations. Safety goggles should be worn if necessary, and unbreakable lenses always should be used. Regular eye examinations by the ophthalmologist should be encouraged.

The nursing of a patient receiving radiation therapy and/or chemotherapy for a malignancy is applicable to this patient also.

Rehabilitation of the Blind Person

Members of the nursing staff share the responsibility of helping the patient who is losing sight, or has lost sight, to live a satisfying life. Such a person needs to learn to be as independent as possible. The individual faced with permanent blindness needs specialized help in adjusting to a loss of sight. Specialists in this field or other individuals who are blind may teach the patient the new skills needed.

TABLE 22.5
OTHER CONDITIONS OF THE EYE

DISORDER	DESCRIPTION
Acid and alkaline burns	Chemical burns of the eye from either an acid or alkaline substance are considered emergencies; lids, conjunctiva, and cornea should be flushed immediately with large amounts of water; this irrigation should last for approximately 15 minutes
Actinic trauma	Injury to the cornea from excessive sunlight, a welder's arc, or a sun lamp; eyedrops to relieve pain and eye patches over both eyes are frequently used by the doctor
Corneal abrasion	Laceration of the cornea which is detected by use of a dye, sodium fluorescein; anesthetic and antibiotic drops may be used; patient's eye may be covered with an eye patch
Pterygium	A winglike fold of membrane that extends toward and onto the cornea from the nasal side of the eye; surgical removal may be necessary
Sympathetic ophthalmia	Following injury of one eye, the patient's uninjured eye develops uveitis; removal of the injured eye (enucleation) may be necessary to avoid loss of sight in the uninjured eye; steroid therapy may be helpful
Trachoma	An infectious disease of the eyes caused by a virus, especially in hot, dry parts of the world; if untreated, blindness may occur; tetracyclines and sulfonamides are used in treatment

After losing vision, the person has the need to accept this fact. Frequently, a period of depression and feelings of isolation develop.

Vocational rehabilitation programs throughout the United States are rendering an invaluable service in the rehabilitation of blind citizens. Many individuals learn to live a satisfying life because of these programs. In many cases, the person is taught a new vocation. The older individual can learn to be independent in the activities of daily living, such as eating, dressing, and walking. Learning to take care of daily needs helps the person to regain and to maintain self respect. Carving, knitting, crocheting, and other diversional activities play an important part in the total rehabilitation program.

The Library of Congress provides a complete library service for persons with visual handicaps through a talking-book program. A wide variety of magazines and books is made available on records, tapes, and phonographs designed for individuals with disabilities in addition to visual handicap. Information about Talking Books generally can be obtained from the local library or directly from the Library of Congress, Washington, D.C. 20542.

Because of successful rehabilitation programs, blind persons can be seen on college campuses, in church, on the job, in the grocery store, or in the dentist's office. Individuals inexperienced in associating with blind persons frequently are overprotective. This attitude does not encourage the person to become as independent as possible. Blind persons prefer to be treated as individuals just as most persons do. Another error of inexperienced people in dealing with a blind person is to talk too loudly. Although the person is blind, he or she is not necessarily deaf.

Case Study Involving Cataract

Mrs. Boggs, an 86-year-old blind widow, was admitted to the surgical unit for cataract removal from the left eye. She told the nurse that she has cataracts in both eyes and will be readmitted at a later date to have the cataract removed from the right eye. Mrs. Boggs is scheduled for surgery tomorrow. She expects to return to the nursing home where she resides.

QUESTIONS
1. What information should accompany Mrs. Boggs from the nursing home?
2. What information about Mrs. Boggs should the nurse communicate to other members of the nursing staff and health team? How can this be communicated?
3. What safety measures are indicated for Mrs. Boggs because of her blindness?

4. What teaching will Mrs. Boggs need prior to surgery?
5. What information should Mrs. Boggs have about postoperative care prior to surgery?
6. How should the nurse adapt the following nursing actions to Mrs. Boggs:
Entering Mrs. Bogg's room?
Serving Mrs. Bogg's tray?
Helping Mrs. Boggs to ambulate?
Talking with Mrs. Boggs?
Orienting Mrs. Boggs to her surroundings?
7. Postoperatively, what observations related to Mrs. Boggs' eye surgery should be reported to the physician promptly?
8. What precautions should the nurse take when instilling eye medication or changing eye dressings?
9. What patient teaching will Mrs. Boggs need prior to discharge?
10. What information should accompany Mrs. Boggs when she returns to the nursing home?
11. As an important member of the health team and the community, what actions of the nurse are related to the prevention of blindness?

Case Study Involving Detached Retina

Mrs. Frederick, a 69-year-old retired teacher, consulted the ophthalmologist for disturbed vision. She told the nurse that she could not understand her trouble as she had not been involved in any activities that would have damaged her eye. She had been planning a program for her senior citizens' meeting and had experienced flashes of light, the feeling that particles were moving in her line of vision, and partial loss of vision in her left eye. Mrs. Frederick appeared quite anxious because of her loss of vision and expressed concern over total loss of vision in the affected eye.

After a thorough examination of both eyes, the ophthalmologist decided that Mrs. Frederick should be hospitalized because of a detached retina.

The doctor's initial orders were:

- Bed rest, allow use of one pillow
- Regular diet
- Eye patches for both eyes
- Schedule for scleral buckling surgery of right eye in two days

QUESTIONS

1. Mrs. Frederick asked the nurse to explain a detached retina to her. What explanation is best?
2. How could the nurse explain the need for bed rest to Mrs. Frederick?
3. How could Mrs. Frederick's daughter be included in the plan of care?
4. In what ways can the nursing staff help to alleviate some of Mrs. Frederick's anxiety about surgery? Loss of vision in the right eye?

Suggestions for Further Study

1. Is there an eye donor bank in your area? If so, who can make arrangements to donate eyes after death? How are these arrangements made?
2. How does the body's reaction to an inflammation of the eye differ from the inflammatory process discussed in Chapter 5.
3. Select a classmate for a partner and arrange to have him or her feed you while you are blindfolded. Change roles and feed your blindfolded classmate. How can this help you when feeding a blind patient?
4. Mason, Mildred A.; Bates, Grace F.; and Smola, Bonnie K.: *Workbook in Basic Medical-Surgical Nursing,* 3rd ed., Macmillan Publishing Company, New York, 1984. Exercise 22.

Additional Readings

Boyd-Monk, Heather: "Conjunctivitis." *Nursing 82,* 12:67 (Nov.), 1982.
Carbary, Lorraine Judson: "The Spirit That Wins." *Journal of Nursing Care,* 13:17 (May), 1980.
Gallagher, Mary Ann: "Corneal Transplantation." *American Journal of Nursing,* 81:1845 (Oct.), 1981.
MacFadyen, Jean S.: "Caring for the Patient with a Primary Retinal Detachment." *American Journal of Nursing,* 80:920–21 (May), 1980.
Norman, Susan: "The Pupil Check." *American Journal of Nursing,* 82:588–91 (Apr.), 1982.
Perrin, Elizabeth D.: "Laser Therapy for Diabetic Retinopathy." *American Journal of Nursing,* 80:664–65 (Apr.), 1980.
Stern, Elizabeth J.: "Helping the Person with Low Vision." *American Journal of Nursing,* 80:1788–90 (Oct.), 1980.

Chapter 23

The Patient with a Disease of the Ear

Expected Behavioral Outcomes

Minimum objectives referred to as expected behavioral outcomes have been designed for the practical/vocational nursing student to use as guides in studying this chapter. The student should read these expected outcomes before studying the chapter. The objectives can be used as guides for study.

Using the content of this chapter, the student should return to the objectives and evaluate the ability to:

1. *Match the following structures of the ear with their specific function associated with hearing: external auditory canal, tympanic membrane, malleus, incus, stapes, inner ear, and auditory nerve.*
2. *Differentiate between conductive and perceptive deafness with a diagram or in writing.*
3. *Describe the nursing responsibilities of the nurse in your agency when helping with an ear examination.*
4. *Outline the nursing interventions when helping the physician remove cerumen.*
5. *Discuss two common dangers of inserting objects into and removing objects from the ear.*
6. *Relate the nursing measures described in Chapter 5 for the patient with an inflammation to those needed by the patient with an ear infection.*
7. *Differentiate between the symptoms of mastoiditis and otosclerosis as a basis for nursing actions.*
8. *Describe the nursing care of a patient being treated surgically for otosclerosis.*
9. *Discuss the rehabilitation of a deaf person in relation to factors influencing rehabilitation, such as communications, attitude, employment, and recreation.*

Vocabulary Development

The following prefixes, suffixes, and combining forms pertain to this chapter. By learning and/or reviewing their meanings, the practical/vocational nursing student will have the keys needed to unlock many exciting new medical terms.

Discover the meaning of these keys in a medical dictionary or in the content of this chapter. How does each key pertain to this chapter? In your notebook write the correct meaning of each prefix, suffix, or combining form listed below. Illustrate each key with an example.

acou—hear. Ex. *acou*metry—testing hearing.

aur-
cer-
dis-
mes-
metr-
oid-
oss-

ost(e)-
ot-
para-
scler-
scop-
vert-

Structure and Function

Hearing is made possible by normal functioning of the two ears and the auditory (acoustic) nerves that lead to the centers of hearing in the brain. Each ear is composed of the external ear, the middle ear, and the internal ear (see Figure 23.1).

The external ear consists of the part that protrudes from the side of the head and the external auditory canal. The part that projects from the side of the head is known as the *pinna*. It is composed mainly of cartilage, fatty tissue, muscles, and skin. The pinna helps to funnel sound waves into the *external auditory canal,* which leads inward. This passage is approximately 2.5 cm (1 in.) in length. The external auditory canal is lined with skin that contains a few hairs near the external opening. The inner part of

the canal has glands that secrete the yellowish, pasty earwax known as *cerumen*. The hair and the cerumen help to prevent foreign substances from entering the ear. The external auditory canal is separated from the middle ear by a membrane known as the *tympanic membrane* or the *eardrum*.

The middle ear is a small bony cavity located in the temporal bone of the skull. This cavity contains three small movable bones that connect the tympanic membrane with the internal ear. These three bones are the *malleus,* which is similar in appearance to a hammer; the *incus,* which resembles an anvil; and the *stapes,* which is similar to a stirrup. The malleus connects the tympanic membrane with the incus, and the incus is connected with the stapes. Part of the stapes fits into the small oval window of the thin bony wall that separates the middle ear

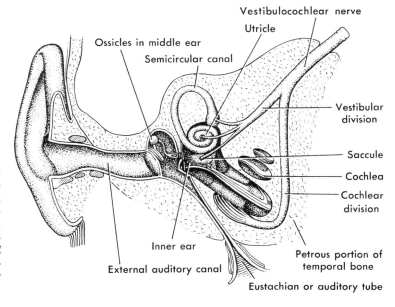

FIGURE 23.1 Section of the ear showing structures of the middle and inner ear. (From Miller, Marjorie A.; Drakontides, Anna B.; and Leavell, Lutie C.: *Kimber-Gray-Stackpole's Anatomy and Physiology,* 17th ed., Macmillan Publishing Co., Inc., New York, 1977, page 274.)

Vestibulocochlear nerve
Utricle
Ossicles in middle ear
Semicircular canal
Vestibular division
Saccule
Cochlea
Cochlear division
Inner ear
External auditory canal
Petrous portion of temporal bone
Eustachian or auditory tube

from the internal ear. The oval window is known also as the *fenestra vestibuli.*

The middle ear has five openings. There is one opening between the external auditory canal and the middle ear. It was stated earlier in this discussion that this opening normally is covered by the tympanic membrane.

Two small openings, the oval window and the round window, are situated in the bony wall that separates the middle ear from the inner ear. The small tube leading from the middle ear to the pharynx (throat) is known as the *eustachian* or *auditory tube.* Normally, air enters the middle ear from the throat through the eustachian tube. This helps to equalize the pressure of air on both sides of the eardrum. Another small opening in the middle ear leads to the mastoid cells. The part of the temporal bone that projects downward behind the ear is known as the mastoid. This contains spaces filled with air, which are known as the mastoid cells.

The inner ear is located beyond the middle ear in the temporal bone. The inner ear is also called the *labyrinth* because it contains an intricate system of connecting canals and cavities. There is a bony labyrinth, which contains a membranous labyrinth. The bony labyrinth is filled with perilymph. The membranous labyrinth consists of a series of fluid-filled sacs and tubes. The fluid that fills these structures is called *endolymph.*

There are three bony parts of the bony labyrinth. They are the cochlea, the semicircular canals, and the vestibule.

The *cochlea,* which is similar in appearance to a snail shell, contains endolymph, perilymph, branches of the auditory nerve, and the organ of hearing known as the organ of Corti. The three small *semicircular canals,* which help to control equilibrium, contain endolymph and perilymph as well as nerve endings.

The *vestibule,* which is the cavity between the cochlea and the semicircular canals, also contains perilymph and endolymph and helps to control equilibrium. The vestibule is connected with the middle ear by the small oval window.

Objects or bodies that produce sound vibrate to cause waves. These waves travel through air, enter the external auditory canal, and cause the stretched tympanic membrane to vibrate. These vibrations rapidly pass through the three small movable bones in the middle ear to the endolymph and perilymph of the inner ear. Movement of this liquid stimulates the endings of the auditory nerve. The impulses are then carried to the centers of hearing in the brain and interpreted as sound.

Assisting with Diagnostic Studies

EAR EXAMINATION

The nurse is often asked to assist the physician to examine the patient's ear. This may be done as part of a general physical examination, or it may be done as a single procedure. In either case, the nurse should provide adequate lighting, a head mirror, ear specula (plural of speculum) of different sizes, an otoscope, and cotton-tipped applicators. A movable lamp placed behind the patient can be adjusted so that its light is reflected from the doctor's head mirror into the ear. The *ear speculum* is a small hollow instrument that is similar to a funnel in shape. The physician inserts it into the external auditory canal to see its walls as well as the tympanic membrane. Several ear specula are needed so that the doctor can select the proper size for a particular patient. The *otoscope* is another instrument used for examination of the external auditory canal and the tympanic membrane. It contains a light that can be directed through an attached speculum. A small magnifying lens in the otoscope enables the doctor to see the tympanic membrane better. The physician may need the cotton-tipped applicators to remove wax and other secretions from the external auditory canal that interfere with examination. A cerumen spoon may be used to remove the wax.

The nurse may be asked to have the patient either lying down or seated in a chair for an ear examination. During the examination, the nurse may hold the patient's head when a special chair with a head support is not used. A special chair such as this usually is found in the clinic and in the doctor's office. The physician is not able to do a complete examination if the patient's head is not still. Sudden movement of the head also may cause injury from the speculum. When the patient is unable to hold the head still or is too young to cooperate, the assistant is responsible for holding the head still.

The physician sometimes has to irrigate the external auditory canal in order to complete the examination. This may be done to remove substances such as a mass of earwax or drainage. Unless otherwise specified by the doctor, the nurse should have the temperature of the solution near body temperature, as the use of warmer or colder solution can cause the patient to have an earache. Nausea and dizziness also may occur. The doctor may order the instillation of a small amount of warmed substance, such as sweet oil or hydrogen peroxide, before doing an irrigation. This is done to soften the plug of earwax.

A variety of tests can be used to determine the person's ability to hear. In general, the ear not being tested is closed. Rough estimates of the patient's hearing can be made by the use of either a ticking watch or a tuning fork. The tuning fork may be used to determine whether the patient has conductive or perceptive deafness, discussed on pages 810–11. The examiner also may whisper to the patient for this purpose.

AUDIOMETRY

An *audiometer* is used for more specific information. This is an instrument used to measure an individual's ability to hear. The *otologist,* a physician who specializes in conditions of the ear, can determine more definitely the exact amount of hearing loss. Audiometry also helps the specialist to determine the amount of sound conducted through the air by way of the external auditory canal as well as the amount conducted through the mastoid. Knowing whether sound is conducted through either the air or the bone and the amount of hearing loss guides the otologist in diagnosis and treatment.

X-RAYS

The patient with symptoms of a disease process in the ear usually has x-rays of the skull, mastoids, and sinuses.

BITHERMAL CALORIC TEST

A bithermal caloric test may be done when the physician suspects a tumor or Ménière's disease (see pages 808–809). In this test, warm as well as cold water is placed into the ear. This test causes dizziness in a normal individual. A bithermal caloric test is done when the patient has no vertigo. The patient with a tumor of the acoustic nerve will have no reaction to this test. The person with Ménière's disease responds with dizziness, tinnitus, reduced hearing, headache, nausea, vomiting, and incoordination.

ELECTRONYSTAGMOGRAPHY (ENG)

Another test, *electronystagmography* (ENG), may be done. In an electronystagmography, the patient has electrodes attached to the face around the eyes. Charges are picked up by the electrodes and recorded on graph paper. Nystagmus, the movement of eyes when closed, is measured. The bithermal caloric test and electronystagmography may be used jointly or individually to diagnose Ménière's disease.

Nursing Observations

The nurse's careful observations and recordings may be helpful in identifying the patient with a disease of the ear and detecting changes in the patient's condition. An early observation includes the appearance of the outer ear for obvious injury, deformity, foreign bodies, or a hearing aid. The characteristics of any drainage present such as color, amount, odor, and viscosity should be observed, reported, and recorded. The presence of the halo sign (refer to page 736) around drainage should be reported at once since this indicates leakage of cerebrospinal fluid from the ear.

The patient may report pain in one or both ears. In this case, the nurse collects pertinent information such as location, intensity, onset, and what makes the pain better or worse.

Some patients with ear disease experience dizziness (a swimming or swaying sensation), vertigo (a sensation of spinning or whirling), or tinnitus (hearing ringing, roaring, or other sounds without an external source). The patient may also report general symptoms such as malaise, nausea or vomiting, and fever.

When conversing with the patient, the nurse looks carefully at the position response. For example, leaning forward, or turning the head to one side may indicate compensation for an undetected hearing loss. The nurse also listens carefully to the patient's speech. Excessively loud speech, mispronounced words, and omission of word endings such as *-ing* or *ed* may indicate undetected hearing loss.

When collecting information from the patient with a disease involving the ear, the nurse asks how the ears usually are cleaned and what drops, if any, are placed in the ear.

Nursing Interventions

CLEANING THE EAR

When cleaning the ear, the washcloth may be placed over a fingertip. Only the outer ear can be cleaned. An alternate procedure for persons who shower is to let warm water from the shower run in and out of the ear (not recommended for persons with a history of ear infections). Cotton-tipped applicators, hairpins, matchsticks, and similar items should never be inserted into the ear for cleaning since they may cause scratching, infection, perforation of the eardrum, or other damage.

PREVENTING INFECTION

Ear infection is a special concern of the nurse when caring for a patient with a disease involving the ear. The location of the ear close to the brain increases the chance of serious secondary infection such as meningitis. Infection in one ear may spread to the other ear or other nearby structures such as the sinuses or pharynx. For these reasons, the nurse pays careful attention to interventions that prevent infection.

Frequent handwashing is the single most effective intervention for preventing infection. The nurse's hands should be washed before and after each contact with the patient, before instilling eardrops, and between caring for each ear.

Medications in the form of eardrops should be ordered for each patient. Borrowing another patient's eardrops is avoided since this practice may lead to contamination between patients. Some experts believe that separate droppers should be used for each ear to avoid introducing pathogens from one ear to the other.

IRRIGATING THE EAR CANAL

An irrigation of the external ear canal may be ordered to remove impacted cerumen, apply heat, cleanse the canal, remove drainage, or apply an antiseptic medication. The physician prescribes the amount and type of solution to be used. Unless otherwise ordered, the solution is warmed to body temperature.

In order to irrigate the external ear canal, the nurse must first straighten the canal. The ear of an adult should be lifted upward and backward in a glentle manner to straighten the canal. The external auditory canal of a child can be straightened by drawing the ear downward and backward gently.

The solution is directed toward the roof of the canal at low force so that the canal is not completely occluded at any time by the irrigating liquid. After the irrigation, the patient is helped to lie on the irrigated side for about 3 to 5 minutes so that remaining fluid can drain out of the ear by gravity.

ASSISTING WITH DRUG THERAPY

A variety of drugs may be instilled into the ear in the form of eardrops. Antibiotics and local anesthetics are the most commonly prescribed eardrops. When ordering the instillation of a drug into the external auditory canal, the doctor usually specifies the number of drops to be used. The prescribed drug should be warmed to body temperature unless otherwise ordered. The patient should be lying down with the ear to receive the drops upward. After straightening the external auditory canal, the nurse drops the prescribed number of drops into the canal. The patient should remain in this position for at least 5 minutes after the drops have been instilled to permit adequate absorption of the drug. The nurse may be requested by the doctor to place a cotton or earwick loosely into the ear opening.

Systemic drugs also may be prescribed for infection or symptoms such as pain, nausea, dizziness, tinnitus, and vertigo.

CHANGING THE EAR DRESSING

Ear dressings may be used to collect drainage and/or protect the ear. One form of dressing frequently used is called an earwick or plug. This small gauze or cotton dressing is inserted gently and loosely into the ear canal which has been straightened. The wick should be easily visible when observing the external ear. As previously mentioned, the wick should be inserted loosely so that the canal is not completely blocked since this may cause harmful pressure on the eardrum.

Following surgery, a bulky turban-style dressing may be present. When this type of dressing is used, the nurse can anticipate an increase in drainage and the need for more frequent reinforcement.

Ear dressings are not changed unless there is a specific order to do so. Specific orders are needed about which parts of the dressing may be changed. Frequently, the surgeon changes the inner ear dressing or packing, and the nurse changes the outer dressing. Unless otherwise ordered, a point to remember when changing the ear dressing is to avoid constricting dressings which may cause a dangerous increase of pressure inside the ear.

COMMUNICATING WITH THE HEARING-IMPAIRED PERSON

Alterations in usual communication methods may be needed when the patient has a hearing impairment. As a first step, the nurse should check to see if the patient has a hearing aid. Next, the hearing aid should be checked to see if it is functioning correctly (see Table 23.1).

People with a hearing impairment have difficulty in communicating which causes them to withdraw from others. The nurse's skill in communicating reduces social isolation and may help others such as family and friends to draw closer to the patient rather

TABLE 23.1
ASSISTING THE PATIENT WITH A HEARING AID

- Wash the ear mold daily according to the manufacturer's directions.
- Turn off hearing aid when it is not being used. Store according to directions.
- Set volume according to information from patient, family, or physician.
- When problems arise, the following areas should be checked first: the on-off switch should be on, the ear mold should be clean, the cord should be undamaged and correctly plugged in, and the battery should be correctly positioned.

than shy away. Table 23.2 contains guidelines in communicating with the hearing-impaired person.

An individual with a hearing impairment may have difficulty with self-expression in addition to hearing. This is especially true when the impaired hearing either prevents or complicates the process of learning to talk. For example, a person who is deaf at birth or becomes so in early childhood needs special instruction in order to speak and to

TABLE 23.2
GUIDELINES TO COMMUNICATING WITH A HEARING-IMPAIRED PATIENT

- Face the patient and have lighting on your face so that lips and facial expressions can be seen by the patient.
- Talk to the patient in a quiet environment, if possible. Turn radio and television volumes down, if necessary.
- Speak slowly and clearly in a slightly louder tone of voice. Avoid dropping the endings of sentences.
- Do not speak with food, gum, cigarettes, cigar, or pipe in the mouth. Keep hands away from the mouth.
- If the patient has trouble understanding, try to rephrase the sentence rather than repeat it. Avoid shouting since this distorts sounds and shapes of the lips.
- When speaking to the patient, state the topic first. Example: "X-ray. The doctor has ordered a chest x-ray for you this morning."
- When speech impairment is present, concentrate on identifying the speaker's topic rather than details.

lip-read. Speech may be difficult to understand because the voices of other people cannot be heard and used for comparison. If the patient is totally deaf and has not learned to talk, communication with others may be done in writing. Then the nurse must write messages to the patient who is unable to understand speech by watching the talker's lips.

To understand the hearing- and speech-impaired person, the nurse should pay close attention by listening and looking at the speaker. Concentration should be directed toward identifying the speaker's main topic rather than details. If the speech cannot be understood, the nurse should not try to give the patient the false impression that it is. Instead, the speaker may be asked to write the message first and then repeat what has been written. This process helps the listener become accustomed to the patient's speech.

ASSISTING THE PATIENT WITH A HEARING AID

The patient with a hearing aid wears a specially made device to improve hearing by amplifying vibrations. One type of hearing aid, worn behind the ear against the skull, uses bone conduction (Figure 23.2). Another type of hearing aid, worn inside the ear, uses air conduction. Most hearing aids have similar parts including a microphone, amplifier, receiver, and a battery.

The hospitalized patient may need help from the nurse with usual maintenance, storage, and trouble-shooting of the hearing aid. A summary of these activities can be located in Table 23.2.

Remembering that a hearing aid is important to the patient as well as expensive, the nurse is careful when handling it. The thoughtful nurse remembers to give the patient the hearing aid. The patient may need help in some cases to put on the hearing aid. The hearing aid should be attached securely. The type that is attached to the clothing can be pinned in the patient's pocket. The hearing aid that is a part of the eyeglasses should be placed comfortably and securely on the patient's face. The nurse usually can find out from the patient or from some member of the family how to turn the hearing aid on

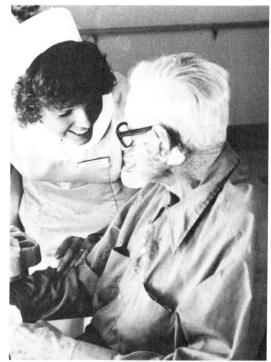

FIGURE 23.2 Communicating with a patient with a bone conduction hearing aid. (Courtesy of Northeast Technical Community College Practical Nursing Program, Norfolk, Nebraska.)

and how to adjust the volume, if necessary. Since water can harm a hearing aid, it should not come in contact with the instrument. The hearing aid should be turned off and put in a safe place at night.

PREVENTION OF HEARING LOSS

Either a partial or complete loss of hearing causes limitations to the individual. Because of this, measures to prevent the loss of hearing are important. The nurse, as a member of the community with special knowledge and skill related to health and illness, has opportunities to share information about the prevention of hearing loss.

For example, the nurse may suggest periodic examinations of children in an effort to discover the conditions that could result in deafness. An individual with the common cold or other upper respiratory infections may develop complications that could result in deafness. The proper care of an individual with such infections helps to prevent complications involving the ears. The person with symptoms associated with an ear infection or with a loss of hearing should be encouraged to consult a physician.

The habit of putting nothing into the external auditory canal is a safe one. Hard objects, such as a hairpin or a matchstick, are likely to scratch the delicate tissue. A tiny splinter from the matchstick may become embedded in the earwax and cause a plug to form. The use of a washcloth, soap, and water should be all that is needed to keep the canal from becoming blocked. If an individual does have a collection of wax in the ear, the doctor may be consulted to remove the plug of earwax by irrigating the canal or removing with a cerumen spoon, as discussed earlier in this chapter.

Many industries have active programs to conserve the hearing of their employees. This is especially important when the workers are exposed to loud noises over a long period of time. Reduction of noise in the vicinity of the employee; the use of material on the walls, ceilings, and floors to absorb sound; the use of ear protectors; and periodic testing of the employees' hearing are examples of noise abatement programs that help to prevent deafness.

In the home, loud volumes from radios, television, and audio systems can cause progressive hearing losses. Parents and children of all ages should know about possible damage from loud volumes so that home noise abatement can be practiced.

Foreign Bodies

The individual with a foreign body in the ear should be advised to see the doctor. Since there is danger of injuring the tympanic membrane and the external auditory canal, an inexperienced person should not attempt to remove the foreign body.

First aid measures to be taken for the individual with a foreign body in the ear are discussed in Chapter 8, in relation to care of the emergency patient. For example, insects may be attracted to light and crawl out of the ear. The application of either alcohol or ether on a cotton ball, which is then placed at the entrance of the ear, may be used to render insects immobile. Water should not be placed in the ear, as this may cause the insect to become more active. If the foreign object is vegetable, such as a bean or pea, the object will swell when water is added.

Otitis Media

The patient with otitis media has an inflammation of the middle ear. Microorganisms that may cause otitis media are streptococci, staphylococci, pneumococci, and *Haemophilus influenzae*. The infection may follow such diseases as the common cold, a sore throat, tonsillitis, scarlet fever, or measles. If the nurse recalls that the middle ear is connected to the throat by the eustachian tube, it is easier to understand that an infection can spread from the nose and throat to the middle ear.

NURSING OBSERVATIONS

The patient may complain that the affected ear feels full and stuffy, and aches. *Tinnitus,* which is a sensation of ringing, may be present in one ear or in both ears. Upon examining the ear, the physician may find a reddened and bulging eardrum. The patient may also have general symptoms of an inflammation, such as malaise and fever.

If the patient is not treated or does not respond to treatment, symptoms can cause fluid to form in the middle ear and result in a temporary loss of hearing. Pressure from the fluid can cause the eardrum to rupture. In this case, the patient has a discharge from the ear. The infection can spread from the middle ear to the mastoid cells by way of the opening between the two structures. A patient sometimes develops chronic otitis media. This may result in a discharge from the involved ear for months. A permanent loss of hearing can result from otitis media. It is important for all parents to learn that a child with an earache should be taken to the doctor.

NURSING INTERVENTIONS

Treatment is directed toward relieving the cause of otitis media as well as relieving the inflammation. For example, the patient with tonsillitis complicated by otitis media is treated for both conditions. A suitable drug to combat the infection, such as an antibiotic or one of the sulfonamides, almost always is prescribed. Dry heat may be used to relieve discomfort, and fluids generally are encouraged.

The physician may, on occasion, do a *myringotomy*. This is a surgical procedure in which an opening is made into the tympanic membrane, fluid is aspirated, and a culture is made. A myringotomy is not done very frequently as many infections of the middle ear respond to drug therapy. A general anesthetic or topical anesthesia is used for a myringotomy since it is quite painful. The nurse should observe, report, and record the type and amount of drainage. A change in the drainage should also be reported. The patient should know that the drainage is infectious. The nurse should wash the hands before changing the cotton plug and cleaning the ear. They should be washed again after the procedure is finished. The external ear may be cleaned with wipes, and petroleum jelly may be applied to the ear to prevent excoriation.

If the patient complains of headache, has an elevated temperature, is drowsy, or appears irritable or disoriented, the physician should be notified. These symptoms may indicate complications, such as brain abscess, meningitis, or mastoid cell involvement, or may indicate that the tympanic membrane needs to be reopened. However, the incision usually heals completely and does not impair hearing.

Other treatments the physician sometimes may order are bed rest, analgesics, nasal constrictors, forcing of oral fluids, irrigation of the ear (see page 802), and instillation of drops of medication into the external auditory canal if the inflammation becomes chronic.

Mastoiditis

Mastoiditis is an inflammatory process generally caused by the spread of an infection from the middle ear to the mastoid, which is located behind the ear.

Although mastoiditis is not commonly seen now, it is a serious disease when it does occur. Remembering that a thin piece of bone separates the tiny air cells of the mastoid from the membranes that cover the brain will help to enforce the realization that mastoiditis can indeed be a serious infection and may spread to the brain.

Staphylococci, streptococci, pneumococci, and *Haemophilus influenzae* microorganisms frequently are the causative pathogens.

NURSING OBSERVATIONS

The patient usually complains of pain around and behind the ear and of headache on the affected side. The tip of the mastoid is tender. An increased amount of drainage from the ear may be present, as well as a loss of hearing. Such general symptoms of infection as malaise and fever are present. Edema, exudate, pus, and necrosis occur as a result of the formation of an abscess and pressure on the blood vessels.

NURSING INTERVENTIONS

The aim of treatment for the patient with mastoiditis is to relieve otitis media as well as mastoiditis. An antibiotic or a sulfonamide generally is prescribed to combat infection. Pain may be relieved by the use of an ice bag or an analgesic. Measures such as bed rest, increased intake of fluids, antipyretics, and a nourishing diet are generally recommended for the patient with an infection. These are important for the patient with mastoiditis also.

Surgery may be indicated when the patient does not respond favorably to the medical treatment. A *simple mastoidectomy*, which is removal of the infected part of the mastoid, is usually done. The incision is made in front of or behind the ear. A small drain is inserted, and the incision is sutured around the drain. The middle ear is not disturbed, and hearing is not impaired. Sometimes a radical mastoidectomy may be necessary. This is especially true in a chronic case that did not respond to other treatment. In a *radical mastoidectomy*, the surgeon removes the tympanic membrane and nearly all of the contents of the middle ear as well as the infected portion of the mastoid. Following a radical mastoidectomy in which the stapes was removed, the patient's hearing is lost. If the stapes or cochlea is not damaged, hearing in the affected ear may improve with a hearing aid. The nursing care of a patient before surgery, discussed in Chapter 6, is applicable to this patient. In general, an area of approximately 5 cm (2 in.) around the affected ear should be shaved in preparation for surgery.

In addition to the nursing care needed by most patients following surgery, discussed in Chapter 6, this patient should be encouraged to move the head frequently. Such movement helps to prevent and to relieve the painful, stiff neck that often follows a fixed position of the head and neck during surgery.

The patient may have a cling-type dressing, which can be reinforced but not changed by the nurse. The surgeon will change the dressing, usually every other day. Small amounts of serosanguineous drainage may be expected, but any bright-red drainage should be reported. The patient should be observed for edema around the face since this may cause the dressing to become too tight. The surgeon should be notified of a tight dressing so that it can be loosened. The patient should be observed for possible paralysis of the face. Of course, this should be reported immediately. Headache, vomiting, stiff neck, dizziness, irritability, and disorientation should be observed, reported, and recorded promptly. These symptoms may be indicative of beginning meningitis or brain abscess. They also may indicate a formation of a blood clot in the brain.

Otosclerosis

An individual with otosclerosis has a growth of new bone that is usually around the oval window. It was stated earlier in this chapter that sound vibrations were carried through the middle ear to the inner ear by the chain of three movable bones in the middle ear. Part of one of these bones, the stapes, fits into the oval window of the thin bony wall that separates the middle ear from the inner ear. Sound vibrations reaching the stapes cause it to move. Movement of the part that fits into the oval window causes the fluid in the inner ear to move. An abnormal growth of bone around the oval window prevents the stapes from moving. Thus, the sound waves do not reach the inner ear. This results in a progressive loss of hearing as the new bone continues to develop. Deafness caused by otosclerosis is known as *conductive deafness* because the sound waves are not transmitted or conducted properly.

The cause of otosclerosis is unknown. More women are affected by otosclerosis than are men. The condition is aggravated by pregnancy.

NURSING OBSERVATIONS

The patient with otosclerosis has a gradual hearing loss that is noticeable by the age of 30 years. However, symptoms of beginning deafness can begin at puberty. Positional changes such as turning the head or leaning forward may be observed. There may be misunderstandings in communications with others or a decline in performance at school. Both ears are affected. However, one may be affected more than the other. The patient generally complains of tinnitus and speaks softly, and, upon examination, bone conduction is better than is air conduction of sound. The eardrum usually is normal.

NURSING INTERVENTIONS

The hearing loss of the patient with otosclerosis may be improved by hearing aid or by surgery. An example of surgery is the *stapedectomy,* which is the preferable treatment. The chance of successful results is 90 percent. A stapedectomy is the surgical excision of the stapes, which is replaced by a piece of wire or a plastic piston that is attached to a fat graft, a vein, or gel foam that covers the oval window. The procedure is done under local anesthesia. An incision is made near the eardrum by the otologist. In doing the operation, the otologist uses an operating microscope with a light. This instrument magnifies the tiny ossicles in the middle ear to the extent that they can be visualized and manipulated by the surgeon. The surgeon frees the footplate of the stapes and removes it, leaving an opening in the oval window. The surgeon must seal the oval window and then connect the oval window with the incus. Wire with gel foam may be used, which turns into a mucous membrane in a few days. Gel foam seals the oval window, seals one end of the wire to the gel foam, and the other end is attached to the incus. Sound travels from the incus to the wire, which vibrates the oval window. Perilymph and endolymph pick up the vibrations, and nerve impulses are started.

Hearing is improved gradually after stapedectomy as swelling and drainage subside. The patient should be told in advance not to expect dramatic hearing improvement. Following surgery, the patient may experience vertigo for a few days. The patient should be advised to move with deliberation and slowness in order to reduce vertigo. Siderails should be raised on the bed as a precautionary measure and to provide a support for the patient to use when turning or moving around in bed. The patient generally is allowed out of bed and walks with assistance. The amount of assistance will be determined by the amount of vertigo. Preoperative teaching should include the postoperative aspect of the plan of care. For example, the patient should know that vertigo and dizziness can be expected, that assistance may be needed to walk, and that dizziness is generally temporary.

The patient generally is advised not to blow the nose for a week, as this forces air through the eustachian tube and dislodges the prosthesis before healing is complete. Postoperative positions differ. Some surgeons request that the head of the patient be turned to the operative side to permit drainage. Others request that the operative ear be uppermost to prevent dislodging the prosthesis. In some cases, patients are allowed to turn their heads to the most comfortable side if dizziness does not occur. For these reasons, members of the nursing staff must determine the exact position preferred and prescribed by the operating physician.

Following surgery, the patient generally is directed to take a tub bath for at least six weeks instead of showers. The hair should not be washed for at least two weeks during the healing period. The patient needs to know that these measures will prevent water from getting into the ear. Realizing this,

the nurse can readily understand that the patient should not go swimming following a stapedectomy.

Antibiotics may be prescribed for infection, and drugs to prevent and/or relieve motion sickness, such as dimenhydrinate (DRAMAMINE), and analgesics to relieve pain may be prescribed. The patient should be instructed to open the mouth as wide as possible in the event that a sneeze is unavoidable. The length of time spent in the hospital may range from two to five days. The packing generally is removed within six days, and cotton is placed in the patient's ear or ears for the first week. The patient may return to work within two weeks. The patient generally is advised to avoid flying for six months and to avoid a common cold. Following a successful stapedectomy that has healed entirely, the patient generally is advised to engage in almost all activities except diving in deep water.

Ménière's Disease

The patient with Ménière's disease has an increase in the pressure of the endolymph in the cochlea due to an increase in the production of endolymph or a decrease in the absorption of the endolymph. A wasting away of the hearing structures eventually occurs. However, the exact cause of Ménière's disease is unknown. The patient has an illusion of body movement that involves her- or himself or the environment. This illusion is known as *vertigo*. Hearing loss and *tinnitus*, an unusual noise in the ears such as ringing, roaring, buzzing, and clicking, occur also.

NURSING OBSERVATIONS

As stated in the preceding paragraph, the patient with Ménière's disease has vertigo, hearing loss, and tinnitus. Personality changes in the form of irritability, depression, withdrawal, and lack of desire to eat also may develop. Attacks of vertigo last a few minutes or hours. The patient may suffer attacks several times a week, or there may be long periods of remission. During an attack, the patient experiences nausea, vomiting, and pallor. A temporary loss of consciousness may occur at times. The loss of hearing may be temporary during an attack, but later, the deafness becomes progressively worse and continues between attacks. As the condition continues, the patient experiences tinnitus between attacks. Symptoms may stop when the auditory nerve dies.

Diagnosis is made on the basis of the patient's history, caloric tests, and electronystagmography (see page 801).

NURSING INTERVENTIONS

An individual with Ménière's disease needs to be protected from falls during an acute attack. Siderails should be used for the patient when in bed. Assistance for ambulation is necessary when vertigo is present. The nurse should explain anticipated movements associated with nursing care to the patient and carry out the movements with deliberation and slowly. Sudden motion should be avoided.

Drugs to counteract vertigo, nausea, and vomiting may be prescribed. Dimenhydrinate (DRAMAMINE), cyclizine (MAREZINE), and meclizine (ANTIVERT) are examples of drugs often prescribed. Fluid intake may be limited; diuretics, a low-sodium diet, vasodilators such as nicotinic acid, sedatives, and tranquilizers may be prescribed. In the event that medical treatment does not relieve the incapacitating vertigo, the patient may have a labyrinthectomy.

Ultrasonic surgery involving use of ultrasonic energy may be done to relieve vertigo and to preserve hearing. An incision is made near the mastoid, and ultrasonic energy is applied to the semicircular canal by way of a probe in the bone in the canal. An endolymphatic shunt may be done. In this case, the endolymphatic sac is decompressed and the vestibular nerve is sectioned.

Postoperatively, the patient may experience vertigo, which can last as long as four to six weeks. Bed rest may be ordered for several days followed by progressive assisted ambulation. All changes in position and movement should be done gently and slowly to avoid vertigo.

The loss of one's ability to hear and to ambulate is indeed threatening and frightening. It may threaten an individual's ability to earn a living, and it will threaten self-image. Reactions associated with loss of a body function discussed in Chapter 1, can be expected in this person. Periods of denial, anger, bargaining, depression, and final acceptance may be expected. These periods are not clearly defined and may occur simultaneously and in various sequences. The patient needs the encouragement, acceptance, and understanding of a caring health team.

Impacted Earwax (Cerumen)

Cerumen is a protective secretion produced by the wax and oil glands of the ear canal. The consistency of earwax varies with the individual and climate. Infection caused by fungus or bacteria increases the production of cerumen. Cerumen can become hard, and removal by an otologist may be necessary.

Cerumen occluding the external auditory canal is a common problem. Individuals should be cautioned against cleaning the ears with sharp objects or cotton-tipped applicators because of the danger of impacting cerumen against the eardrum and the danger of puncturing the eardrum. Earwax may be softened by placing a few drops of mineral oil or olive oil into the auditory canal. The time required for softening is several hours. A mixture of one-half hydrogen peroxide and one-half mineral oil may be used for this purpose. The client should be informed that a bubbling noise may be experienced when hydrogen peroxide is used. Such a noise may be frightening to the patient.

Some authorities have successfully used a WATER PIK with low pressure to remove cerumen (see Figure 23.3). When a WATER PIK is used, the water temperature should be close to that of the body temperature. If the water is too cold or too warm, it could cause nausea and dizziness. When inserting the WATER PIK, the nurse should leave a space around the tip so that water can escape. A towel should be draped around the patient's shoulder, and the patient should hold the emesis basin below the earlobe. A pulsating fine stream of water breaks up cerumen and washes it out into the basin in only a few seconds of irrigation. A piece of cotton on a for-

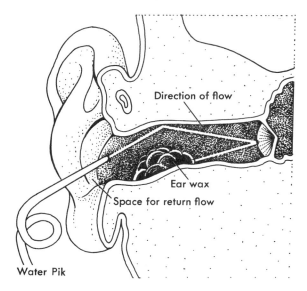

Direction of flow

Ear wax

Space for return flow

Water Pik

FIGURE 23.3   A WATER PIK or an ear syringe may be used to irrigate gently for removal of excess cerumen. The temperature of the water should approximate that of the body. The water stream should be directed toward the anterior wall of the canal.

ceps should be used to dry the external orifice of the auditory canal.

Deafness

The person handicapped by deafness has either a complete loss or a partial loss of hearing. It may be caused by poor conduction of sound waves or by inadequate perception. Two types of deafness are conductive and perceptive.

Conductive deafness occurs when the sound waves do not reach the inner ear properly. Since the waves must pass through the external auditory canal and the middle ear to reach the inner ear, an abnormal condition of these structures can cause a loss of hearing. A plug of earwax or a foreign body in the external auditory canal, perforation of the eardrum, and otitis media can cause conductive deafness. Chronic otitis media may result in either impairment or destruction of the bones in the middle ear. Thus, sound is not conducted properly to the inner ear. Otosclerosis, which was discussed earlier in this chapter, is another cause of conductive deafness. Also, a person may be born with a defect in the part of the ear responsible for the conduction of sound.

Perceptive deafness occurs when the sound waves go through the middle ear but are not received properly by the brain. This is caused by damage to the auditory nerve or to its sensitive branches in the inner ear. An individual may be born with a defect in the part of the ear responsible for the perception of sound. Injury of the auditory nerve may cause perceptive deafness. For example, a brain tumor pressing on this nerve, a skull fracture, and prolonged exposure to loud noises may result in deafness. Toxins associated with certain diseases, such as syphilis, mumps, and measles, can damage the auditory nerve. It also can be injured by an infection of the middle ear.

NURSING INTERVENTIONS

The otologist attempts to relieve the underlying cause of deafness in order to prevent further loss of hearing and to improve the patient's hearing when possible. For example, the patient with chronic otitis media is treated for this condition or the patient with otosclerosis may have a stapedectomy done.

If the physician is unable to improve the patient's hearing, a *hearing aid* may be recommended to amplify vibrations. The patient in this case may need assistance from the nurse as described earlier in the chapter on page 804.

If a hearing aid does not provide sufficient help, the patient may be directed to classes in lipreading and/or sign language. A

TABLE 23.3
OTHER CONDITIONS OF THE EAR

DISORDER	DESCRIPTION
External otitis (infection of ear canal)	A bacterial or a fungal infection may occur in the external ear canal especially after swimming in polluted water; an abrasion of the canal may lead to an infection; analgesics, heat, and antibiotics may be ordered
Furuncle of external canal	An infection of the skin in the external canal can result in the formation of a painful nodule; pain, tinnitus, headache, fever, and enlarged lymph nodes occur; antibiotic therapy is the usual treatment; however, the furuncle may have to be incised and drained in some cases
Malignancy	Basal cell or squamous cell carcinoma may be found in the external ear; this type of malignancy resembles an infection or furuncle of the auricle; surgical excision generally results in success; plastic reconstruction may be indicated for cosmetic purposes

combination of these methods may be used to maximize communication with others. Speech therapy also may be needed to correct speech problems that develop as a result of a hearing loss.

Special efforts are needed to explain diagnostic studies, medications, and similar procedures to the deaf person. Guidelines from Table 23.2 may be helpful in planning communication. In addition, it is especially important to determine whether or not the patient understands what is being described or explained.

A person with defective hearing may respond to what is said by saying "yes" without really understanding, in order to be friendly and pleasant. Knowing this, the nurse can often avoid a misunderstanding by talking further with the patient when a "yes" response is obtained. For example, the nurse was to tell the patient not to eat anything and not to drink any fluids after midnight in preparation for an x-ray the next morning. In order to determine whether the patient understood the procedure to be followed, the nurse asked if the instructions were familiar. After being told "yes" by the patient, the nurse asked when this was done. The patient replied that similar instructions had been given several years ago for a stomach x-ray. By spending a few extra minutes in talking with this patient, the nurse felt assured that the patient understood and was able to follow instructions. A brief description of other conditions of the ear can be located in Table 23.3.

Case Study Involving Otosclerosis

Mrs. Cupola, a 46-year-old woman, was examined by the otologist for a progressive hearing loss in both ears. The nurse observed that Mrs. Cupola was very soft-spoken when she mentioned that her right ear had been buzzing for days. The otologist diagnosed Mrs. Cupola's condition as otosclerosis and asked the nurse to arrange for Mrs. Cupola's admission to the hospital for a stapedectomy of the right ear. A hearing aid was prescribed for the left ear. Later, Mrs. Cupola's husband called the doctor's office requesting information about the operation. The otologist was not available to talk with Mr. Cupola.

QUESTIONS

1. How should the nurse adapt communications skills in talking with Mrs. Cupola?
2. What information will Mrs. Cupola need prior to being hospitalized?
3. How should the nurse respond to Mr. Cupola's request for information?
4. What patient teaching will Mrs. Cupola need about postoperative care prior to having surgery?
5. How could the nurse best describe otosclerosis to a neighbor?
6. What nursing actions are indicated when Mrs. Cupola enters the hospital with a hearing aid?
7. What communication problems should the nurse anticipate when talking with Mrs. Cupola?
8. What patient teaching will Mrs. Cupola need before being discharged from the hospital?
9. As an important member of the health team and community, what is the nurse's responsibility in relation to the prevention of deafness?

Case Study Involving Perceptive Deafness

Roxanne Neal, a 20-year-old woman, was recovering from a fractured skull obtained in a motorcycle accident. She was progressing nicely except for perceptive deafness in both ears. Auditory nerve injury associated with the accident was cited as the cause by the otologist.

QUESTIONS

1. Roxanne is scheduled for lipreading classes before being discharged from the hospital. In talking with Roxanne, what nursing actions can the nurse take to improve communications?
2. Can Roxanne be expected to experience varying phases of the grieving process as described in Chapter 1? Justify your answer.
3. Roxanne is a junior in the local college and plans to become a medical technologist. She is especially interested in hematology. In your opinion, will Roxanne need to make major changes in her career goals? Verify your answer by discussing this case with a local medical technologist.
4. Roxanne asks the nurse why she cannot be fitted with a hearing aid. Describe the best answer that could be given by the nurse. In what way can the nurse communicate an answer to Roxanne?
5. To what extent will Roxanne's loss of hearing influence her ability to resume the following recreational activities?

Swimming?
Motorcycle riding?
Hiking in the mountains?
Having talk sessions with friends?

Suggestions for Further Study

1. What agency in your locality is designed to teach a deaf person to read lips? Or the sign language?
2. How can you determine whether a deaf person understands what you have said?
3. Why is it important to help the patient to walk for the first time following surgery for otosclerosis?
4. Mason, Mildred A.; Bates, Grace F.; and Smola, Bonnie K.: *Workbook in Basic Medical-Surgical Nursing,* 3rd ed. Macmillan Publishing Company, New York, 1984. Exercise 23.

Additional Readings

Carbary, Lorraine Judson: "Tuning Out Tinnitus." *Journal of Nursing Care,* 13:8–11 (Aug.), 1980.

Griffiths, Mary: *Human Physiology,* 2nd ed. Macmillan Publishing Co., Inc., New York, 1981, pp. 392–99.

Miller, Marjorie A.; Drakontides, Anna B.; and Leavell, Lutie C.: *Kimber-Gray-Stackpole's Anatomy and Physiology,* 17th ed. Macmillan Publishing Co., Inc., New York, 1977, pp. 274–81.

Chapter 24

The Patient with a Disease of the Skin*

Expected Behavioral Outcomes

Minimum objectives referred to as expected behavioral outcomes have been designed for the practical/vocational nursing student to use as guides in studying this chapter. The student should read these expected outcomes before studying the chapter. The objectives can be used as guides for study.

Using the content of this chapter, the student should return to the objectives and evaluate the ability to:

1. Relate the observations of a patient with a skin disorder to nursing implications in regard to open lesions and reddened areas.

2. Describe the psychosocial impact that could be associated with a marked facial disfigurement.

3. Describe the adaptations in the daily bath likely to be needed by the patient with a dermatologic condition.

4. Relate the specific danger signals of cancer discussed in Chapter 9 to those likely to be present in the patient with a neoplasm of the skin.

5. Describe the nursing actions indicated for the patient with a decubitus ulcer.

6. Describe the nursing actions of a patient with a serious burn in relation to the prevention of shock, infection, fluid loss, and edema.

Vocabulary Development

The following prefixes, suffixes, and combining forms pertain to this chapter. By learning and/or reviewing their meanings, the practical/vocational nursing student will have the keys needed to unlock many exciting new medical terms.

Discover the meaning of these keys in a medical dictionary or in the content of this chapter. How does each key pertain to this chapter? In your notebook write the correct meaning of each prefix, suffix, or combining form listed below. Illustrate each key with an example.

anti—against. Ex. *antibiotic*—a substance from microorganisms that acts against life of other microorganisms.

*Revised by the authors and Kathy Hancock Grillo, R.N., M.S., who is a Practical Nursing Instructor at the Central School of Practical Nursing in Norfolk, Virginia.

-angenion	derm(at)-	esthe-	re-
bi-	-ektasis	pell-	tela-
cut-	epi-	pil-	therm-
de-	erythr-	py-	top-

Structure and Function

The body is covered by skin, which comprises 15 percent of the total body weight. Some of the many functions of the skin include protection of the body from infection, injury, and loss of fluid. The rich blood supply and the sweat glands of the skin help to regulate body temperature by eliminating water and cerain salts. The sense of touch known as *tactile* is a result of the many nerve endings in the skin. These nerve endings help an individual decide whether an object is hard or soft, hot or cold, rough or smooth, and whether touching the object causes pain. The tactile sense also gives the individual information about his surroundings.

The two main layers of the skin are the epidermis and the dermis. The *epidermis*, the outer layer, is a tough, protective covering composed of four distinct layers of cells. The epidermis provides protection and acts as a barrier to the loss of water and electrolytes. This outer layer also helps to maintain body temperature and thus provides a stable environment for internal homeostasis by releasing water in the form of perspiration. The amount of water lost cannot be measured and is therefore called an insensible loss. The estimated amount of fluid lost in this manner is 500 to 600 ml per day. The epidermis contains numerous nonpathogenic microorganisms including many strains of both staphylococci and streptococci. The epidermis is continuously shedding cells, which are replaced by cells from the dermis. These cells die and are pushed upward by newly formed dermal cells. (See Figure 24.1.)

The second layer of the skin, the *dermis*, lies immediately below the epidermis. The dermis contains many small blood vessels; lymph vessels; nerves; hair follicles; *sebaceous* glands, which are oil glands; *sudoriferous* glands, which are sweat glands; and *collagen*, which is fibrous protein.

Beneath the dermis lies a layer of subcutaneous tissue, which is also known as superficial fascia. The amount of subcutaneous tissue varies in different parts of the body and is composed of loose adipose tissue and dense connective tissue. The dermis is at-

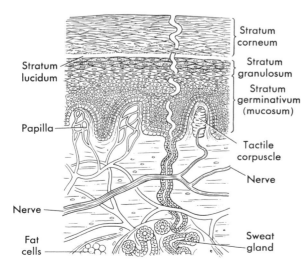

FIGURE 24.1 Diagram of a section of the skin. (From Miller, Marjorie A.; Drakontides, Anna B.; and Leavell, Lutie C.: *Kimber-Gray-Stackpole's Anatomy and Physiology*, 17th ed. Macmillan Publishing Co., Inc., New York, 1977.)

tached to the subcutaneous tissue by collagen fibers which, in turn, connect the dermis to the muscles and bones. The subcutaneous tissue forms a continuous sheet under the dermis, and any breaks in this sheet will provide an entranceway for bacterial invasion. Bacteria that spread in all directions through subcutaneous tissue result in a widespread and diffuse inflammation called *cellulitis*.

The science of diagnosing and treating skin disorders is called *dermatology*. The physician who specializes in this science is called a *dermatologist*.

Assisting with Diagnostic Studies

When assisting with the examination of the individual with a skin disorder, the nurse must provide adequate lighting and have the fully undressed patient correctly draped so that embarrassment is minimized.

In order to determine if a red lesion is the result of a dilated blood vessel or if the blood is outside the vessel, a *diascope* may be used. A diascope is a hand lens, glass slide, or clear plastic instrument used to press gently on the skin to observe the effects. If the lesion is red because of a dilated blood vessel, it will have a decrease in redness or the redness may disappear with pressure. The redness will not disappear when the diascope is pressed against the skin if it is caused by blood outside a vessel.

A Wood's lamp is a high-frequency pressure mercury lamp designed to transmit only long-wave ultraviolet wavelengths. The lamp is used to diagnose fluorescing-type fungus infections and certain bacterial diseases. For example, *Pseudomonas* and certain skin conditions such as *vitiligo*, a complete loss of pigmented cells, may be detected with this lamp.

Scrapings from the skin may be stained and placed under a microscope to be observed for the presence of bacteria and to aid in the identification of microorganisms.

Another type of diagnostic test that may be performed is the dermatologic test medium (DTM) culture. This culture medium inhibits the growth of bacteria and nonpathogenic molds and turns red when a disease-causing fungus is present.

PUNCH BIOPSY

A punch biopsy is a rapid and simple test that gives valuable diagnostic information to the physician. A small punch, which has the appearance of a small drill or cookie cutter, is stamped on the skin. The biopsied skin is fixed and stained for study under a microscope. The biopsy site usually heals with a tiny scar and requires only a small bandage for a day.

CURETTAGE

Curettage is a scraping or scooping away of the skin tissue with a circular cutting edge. This test is useful in diagnosing skin cancer and in the removal of warts, keratoses, and other skin lesions.

When the physician suspects that the patient's skin condition results from a disturbance in another body system, the nurse can anticipate additional diagnostic tests related to that system. For example, the patient may have tests related to the endocrine system if the skin condition is thought to result from an imbalance in hormones.

Nursing Observations

The nurse's observations are very important when the patient has a skin disease. Because of the nurse's knowledge, friends, relatives, and neighbors often seek information and advice about skin lesions. The nurse's close observation of the hospitalized patient during daily activities such as bathing often results in early detection of skin lesions. In addition, the patient with existing skin disease often talks with the nurse and provides information valuable for the physician in treating the condition.

When observing the patient with a skin disease, good lighting should be used. Touching the patient's skin lesions should be done gently in order to prevent further damage. Good handwashing is essential to prevent transferring bacteria to the patient or from the patient to others via the nurse's hands.

Information collected during the nursing observation includes the presence of continuous or intermittent itching, burning, or pain. In addition, characteristics of the patient's life-style, such as eating and sleeping patterns, occupation, and emotional stressors may help to identify factors that cause or worsen symptoms.

When observing the patient's skin, the nurse looks at the hair, nails, skin color, and behavior as well as specific lesions that may be present. Table 24.1 contains a general guide to observing the patient with a skin lesion. When skin lesions are present, the nurse may refer to Tables 24.2 and 24.3 to locate terms related to appearance and shape.

Specific observations of the skin may vary considerably according to the patient's race. For example, gradations of normal skin color in the black patient are determined by the rate of melanin production, a genetic trait. Healthy black skin has a reddish base or undertone to it. The buccal mucosa, tongue, lips, and nails of the healthy black patient are pink.

Erythema usually indicates that an inflammatory process is present and, although not always detected on black skin, may cause the skin to assume a purplish or grayish cast. When erythema is observed or sus-

pected, the nurse also should check for additional warmth, edema, or signs of unusual smoothness which may indicate edema or hardness. Rashes in the black patient can be detected by stretching the skin gently to decrease the reddish skin tone and make the rash stand out. Borders of the rash may be detected by running the tips of the fingers lightly over the rash.

Cyanosis in the black patient causes the skin to assume a grayish cast. The nurse should also check around the mouth, the lips, the skin over the cheekbones and earlobes, and buccal mucosa for signs of cyanosis. Observations relating to special skin conditions that may be present in the black patient are described in Table 24.4.

OBSERVING MOLES, SCARS, BIRTHMARKS

Moles, or nevi, are benign tumors or melanocytes and occur in about 95 percent of the population. The skin color may vary from yellow to black, and elevation of the skin may range from flat macules to elevated nodules. A change of benign moles to malignant growths is rare, but black hair-

TABLE 24.1
GUIDE TO NURSING OBSERVATIONS OF PATIENT WITH SKIN LESIONS

WHERE TO OBSERVE	WHAT TO OBSERVE
Hair	Observe color, texture, distribution
Nails	Observe for soft, hard, discolored, thickened, brittle, broken nails
	Check color of nails for pallor or cyanois
Skin color	Redness (erythema) may indicate vasodilation
	Whiteness may indicate anemia, cold, shock, swelling (edema), or poor circulation
	Yellowness may indicate hepatic disturbances, chemical imbalance, myxedema
	Blueness may indicate poor circulation or inadequate oxygen in tissues
Skin lesions	Look for lesions in scalp, behind ears, in skin folds of eyelids, neck, axilla, breasts, elbows, wrists, groins, gluteus, and popliteal areas. Also, check between fingers and toes
	Observe and record shape, size, location, color, and distribution of lesions
	Report and record itching, burning, pain of lesions
	Report and record drainage from lesions
Moles, scars, birthmarks	Observe and describe location, size, color
Behavioral changes	Patient with visible lesions may isolate self from others
	Disturbances of sleep may occur when lesions itch or burn
	Others may withdraw from patient with visible lesions
	Fatigue associated with sleep disturbances and continuous focus on skin lesions may be present
	Irritability

TABLE 24.2
COMMON SKIN LESIONS

LESION	DESCRIPTION	EXAMPLE
• Bleb	A large bulla	Pemphigus
• Bulla	A large blister or skin vesicle filled with fluid	Large blister
• Callus	A thickening of the outer layer of the skin that occurs as a result of repeated pressure or trauma	Callus
• Crust	A collection of dried-up serum on the surface of the skin caused by damage to the outer skin barrier. The fluid dries and mixes with dirt and skin to form a crust or scab	Eczema
• Cyst	A thick-walled lesion containing fluid or semisolid material. It forms slowly and is covered with a layer of normal-appearing epidermal tissue	Cyst
• Fissure	Ulcer or cracklike sore	"Chapped" skin
• Macule	A flat, nonraised discoloration of the skin or the mucous membrane that cannot be felt. If the lesion is greater than 1 cm, it is called a patch	Freckle
• Nodule	A raised, solid lesion felt deeper in the skin than a papule. If the nodule is greater than 1 cm, it is called a tumor	Mole
• Papule	A raised, solid lesion. Lesions larger than 1 cm are called plaques	
• Pustule	A collection of pus beneath or within the epidermis	Pimple
• Scale	An abnormal thickening of the outer layer of epidermal tissue, which may be dry or greasy. The appearance may also range from thin and silvery to thick, hard, and adherent. The flaking of this skin is known as desquamation	Psoriasis
• Telangiectasia	A fine, often irregular red line, usually permanent, caused by dilation of a normally invisible capillary	Birthmark
• Ulcer	An irregular excavation resulting from necrosis including complete loss of dermis. An ulcer causes a scar after healing	Decubitus
• Vesicle	A fluid-filled, superficial, elevated lesion of the skin or mucous membrane that is less than 1 cm in size. If it is greater than 1 cm, it is called a bulla	Blister
• Wheal	An irregularly shaped, elevated lesion of skin or mucous membrane caused by edema	Hives

less, smooth nevi, especially on the hands, palms, soles of the feet, or genitals, should be observed closely for the development of a malignant melanoma. Other moles that should be observed closely and removed if necessary are those that are frequently or continuously irritated such as a mole on the neck or waist which may be rubbed against clothing.

Birthmarks are superficial or capillary hemangiomas, which are tumors involving the blood vessels. Common birthmarks are "stork bites" or "salmon patches" on the neck or forehead which are usually transient and often disappear in early childhood.

"Strawberry" or cavernous hemangiomas generally grow during the first few months of life, but then regress and may disappear. Those that do not disappear should be treated early in childhood since these angiomas tend to become resistant to treatment with the increasing age of the child. "Port wine" stains are broad, thick, vascular areas which may be either red and superficial or purplish and thick. These birthmarks usually do not disappear and usually are not responsive to surgical treatment. They often may cover one side of the face, and patients who have this type of birthmark will usually resort to make-up to cover up or blend in the hemangioma.

An angioma causing dilated blood vessels is a *telangiectatic angioma,* and an angioma giving the appearance of a spider is a *spider angioma*. The lymph vascular tumors described above usually affect the skin. Such

TABLE 24.3
TERMS THAT DESCRIBE SHAPES OF
SKIN LESIONS

SHAPE	DEFINITION
Annular	Circular, ring shaped
Arcuate (arciform)	Bowed
Borders	Outer part or edge; boundary
Circinate	Circular
Confluent	Running together
Discoid	Like a disk
Discrete	Separate
Eczematoid or eczematous	Dry, pinkish, ill-defined patches with itching and burning, slight swelling with tendency to spread and coalesce; scaling roughness and dryness of skin
Erythema	A form of macule showing diffused redness over the skin
Generalized	To become or render general, to become systemic as a local disease
Groupings	Bunch
Guttate	Resembling a drop
Gyrate	Ring shaped, convulated
Keratosis, keratotic	Condition of the skin characterized by formation of horny growths or excessive development of the horny growth
Linear (striate)	Resembling a line
Moniliform	Resembling a necklace or string of beads
Multiform	Having many forms or shapes
Nummular	Coin shaped; arranged like a stack of coins
Polymorphous	Occurring in more than one form
Punctate	Having pinpoint punctures or depressions on the surface
Reticulated or retiform	Resembling a network
Serpiginous	Creeping from one area to another
Symmetric	Exhibiting correspondence in size and shape of parts
Telangiectasis	Spot formed by a dilated blood vessel, usually on the skin
Zosteriform	Resembling herpes zoster, an acute inflammatory disease with vesicles grouped in the course of cutaneous nerves

tumors also may occur in the internal organs. An example of this is the *arteriovenous angioma of the brain,* a congenital tumor causing convulsive seizures.

Scars are tough fibrous tissues that have been formed at the site of an injury. Scar carcinomas may develop at the site of burns received 20 to 30 years previously, as well as at the sites of chronic osteomyelitis, chronic skin ulcerations (especially of the lower extremities), or from sinuses or fistulas that may have been present for a long time.

The person with a *keloid* has an overgrowth of connective tissue at the site of a scar or an injury. A keloid is most likely to develop on an individual's face, neck, or over the sternum. The practice of piercing ears in today's society seems to have increased the number of keloids. The involved area becomes raised, pink in appearance, and may

increase in size. A keloid often disappears, leaving a scar. The scar, which is enlarged, may have to be removed surgically. However, liquid nitrogen cryosurgery or the injection of corticosteroid into the lesion may be the method of treatment selected by the physician.

When moles, birthmarks, or scars are present, the nurse should record the location, size, and appearance. The appearance and shape may be described using Tables 24.2 and 24.3. The location of these and other skin lesions often may be pinpointed by drawing a simple diagram either on the nursing history or in the nurse's notes.

PRURITUS

The patient with pruritus experiences a sensation of itching of the skin which causes an intense desire to scratch. This desire to

TABLE 24.4
GUIDE TO OBSERVING SELECTED SKIN CONDITIONS IN THE BLACK PATIENT

OBSERVATION	DESCRIPTION	NURSING INTERVENTION
Congenital ichthyosis	Also known as "fish skin" disease. The epidermis becomes thick, hard, and dry and is broken up into scales. Patients with ichthyonic skin are usually unable to tolerate hot water and soap	Use plain warm bath water with teaspoon of bath oil added. Report and record. Cool saline soaks or mineral oil may be soothing after bath. Special creams and emulsions may be prescribed
Dermatosis papulosis nigra	Small wartlike growths which resemble moles	Report and record. Physician may remove using liquid nitrigen, electrodesiccation, cautery, or curettage
Hyperpigmentation	Local areas of darker skin caused by trauma	Report and record
Keloid folliculitis	This condition is characterized by pustules and hardfollicle papules which usually begin at the nape of the neck and extend upward into the occipital region of the scalp forming keloid plaques	Report and record. Physician may treat this condition with steroids and antibiotic drugs
Pseudofolliculitis barbae	Because the hair follicles of the black male are curved, shaving with a straight razor may cause the pointed ends of the hair to reenter the hair follicle and become ingrown	Some patients use electric razors to reduce ingrown hair problems. Some patients grow beards temporarily or permanently
Traction alopecia	Baldness in certain areas on head. May result from trauma, tight pinning, cornrowing, comb picking, hot combing practices	Usually reversible when trauma is discontinued. Inform patient about hair care practices causing condition. Record presence of alopecia
Vitiligo	Slow symmetric progressive loss of pigment which may be preceded by erythema and itching. May be caused by trauma, hyperthyroidism, achlorhydria, Addision's disease, pernicious anemia, diabetes, autoimmune diseases, congenital factors	Report and record. Anticipate disturbances of body image

scratch is caused by internal and external nerve endings in the skin that have been stimulated by chemical, thermal, mechanical, or electrical means. Itching also may be produced as a result of the release of histamine. Heat dilates blood vessels which makes the nerve endings more sensitive and may, therefore, increase the desire to scratch. Itching also may occur as a result of lack of oxygen to tissues or by venous stasis. In observing the patient with a skin disease, the nurse asks if itching is present as well as which factors worsen or relieve it.

BEHAVIORAL CHANGES

Emotions are registered and reflected by our skin in blushing, perspiring, and becoming pale. Skin glows, glistens, and tingles. The cosmetic industry is one of the biggest industries in the world. Skin texture, tone, and color are exaggerated for cosmetic purposes. A healthy, smooth, wrinkle-free skin is considered attractive. Minute changes in an individual can be communicated by touch. A tender touch is known to be necessary not only from an emotional standpoint but a physical one as well. The patient with a skin disease may feel untouchable. Such a person frequently withdraws from others as a result of feeling unattractive, inadequate, worthless, or guilty. People with skin problems experience prejudice. Skin disease may be equated with being unclean. Some persons believe that all skin conditions may be transmitted from one person to another. These prejudices may cause others to withdraw from the patient, increasing isolation.

Many patients have secret fears that their skin lesions are cancerous. Even when cancer is not suspected and lesions are known to be benign, the patient may harbor fears of cancer. Such a patient may show behavioral changes associated with anxiety, fear, or even panic.

Nursing Interventions

APPLICATION OF LOTIONS, CREAMS, OINTMENTS

A number of lotions, creams, and ointments may be applied to the skin to control itching, reduce bacteria or fungi on the skin, or soften and moisturize the skin. A physi-cian's prescription is needed before any substances are applied to the skin of a patient with a skin disease. Specific instructions regarding use of lotions, creams, and/or ointments should be obtained before applying.

SPECIAL BATHS

Balneotherapy, or use of a *bath* for therapy, sometimes is prescribed for its cooling, drying, antipruritic, or emollient effects. The bath also may be used as a means of removing crusts and old medications, and as a means of applying fresh medications. When drying the skin, a patting or blotting motion is used instead of a vigorous rubbing motion. Safety precautions that protect the patient from chilling, burns, falls, and other injuries apply to the person receiving a special bath also.

APPLICATION OF COMPRESSES AND SOAKS

The physician may prescribe compresses or soaks to relieve the patient's itching and reduce inflammation. Compresses and soaks are also helpful in cleaning the skin and removing crusty materials. Compresses are usually normal saline, Burow's solution (aluminum acetate 1:100, 1:20), or an equal mixture of milk of magnesia and water. These compresses are applied with a light covering of gauze (four to eight layers) and may be applied as often as on one-half hour, off one-half hour for the first few days of treatment. Frequency of treatment after this time then will decrease usually to twice or four times a day. Wet soaks are usually mild antiseptic solutions that are used for acute or weeping conditions or infections on the extremities. They are done usually for 15 to 30 minutes several times a day. After a compress or soak is removed, a patting or blotting motion is used to dry the skin instead of a vigorous rubbing motion.

ASSISTING WITH DRUG THERAPY

TOPICAL STEROIDS. When caring for the patient with a skin disorder, topical glucocorticoids (KENALOG, ARISTOCORT) may be prescribed for an anti-inflammatory effect. The effectiveness of steroids is enhanced when a transparent plastic wrap is applied over it, as this increases absorption by the skin. The nurse also should be aware that wrapping plastic over the application will increase the systemic absorption of the steroid. Thus, the nurse should observe the patient for side effects, as described. Prolonged use of topical steroids may produce a rebound reaction of the skin condition if the steroid is withdrawn suddenly. Care should be taken that the drug is not discontinued abruptly. Steroids also are contraindicated in herpes, viral, or fungal infection because they suppress the patient's immune system.

Antibiotics may be prescribed when infection is causing the patient's skin condition or when secondary infection results from open lesions. Table 5.7 contains a list of antibiotics which the physician may prescribe. Antihistamines, such as those listed in Table 10.3, may be prescribed to relieve itching which is present. Chemotherapeutic drugs such as mechlorethamine (MUSTARGEN) or methotrexate have been prescribed for some patients with skin disease. Because these drugs have life-threatening side effects, they are used rarely.

MEASURES TO ASSIST WITH PRURITUS

In addition to topical drug therapy, antihistamines, and special baths, a variety of other measures may be used to help reduce the patient's pruritus. Applications of cold may relieve pruritus caused by dilated blood vessels. Measures used to improve blood flow, such as heat and exercise, may relieve itching caused by venous stasis. Distraction, as described in Chapter 7, may help in some cases. Some patients obtain temporary relief by scratching sheets or blankets instead of the skin. In some cases, the patient who is unable to refrain from scratching the skin may need protective mittens, gloves, or hand restraints to avoid injuring the skin.

ASSISTING WITH HYGIENE

The patient with a skin disease often has the additional problem of dry skin. Fewer baths usually are indicated for such a person. A few drops of oil, if permitted by the physician, may be added to the bath water. Bath water is generally cooler rather than hot. Soap is avoided because it dries the

skin. The patient with skin lesions needs to be protected from chills during normal baths a well as therapeutic baths.

Nail care is an important part of hygiene. The patient with a skin disease should have clean, well-trimmed nails. Injuries to the nail should be reported and recorded. Nails that are not too thick may be softened before manicuring by petroleum jelly, warm olive oil, or bath oil.

DEVELOPING A THERAPEUTIC RELATIONSHIP

Understanding the patient's experience enables the nurse to plan communication which conveys acceptance, warmth, and optimism. Some patients who are silent may be helped to verbalize concerns by the nurse's reassurance that it is common for patients to experience feelings of loneliness, anger, and uncleanliness.

In planning nursing care, the nurse creates opportunities for the patient to participate in care as often as possible. For example, some patients may remoisten compresses, apply topical medications, or decide when to take a special bath. These interventions help to reduce feelings of helplessness and increase the patient's personal autonomy, as described in Chapter 1.

Frequent interactions are indicated when the patient has visible lesions and seems withdrawn. The nurse should not wait for the patient to initiate conversation or activity. When possible, the nurse should initiate conversations that are not related to the patient's disease or therapy. This may help to reassure the patient who feels totally unacceptable because of skin lesions.

In talking with the patient, the nurse has an opportunity to identify and praise other important personal qualities such as kindness, strength, friendliness, and honesty. This helps to restore a balance between a person's appearance and other important personal qualities.

ASSISTING WITH PATIENT AND FAMILY TEACHING

The client with a skin disease usually carries out most of the therapy at home. Thus, patient teaching is important. The nurse's knowledge of the patient's life-style is especially important in planning patient teaching. For example, the patient who lives in an apartment or house without a bathtub will need help to modify a bath routine, if a therapeutic bath is prescribed.

Some clients need help in changing lifestyle practices that influence disease. For example, fatigue and emotional factors may worsen symptoms for some patients. Such persons may need help to prevent fatigue and avoid or modify emotional stress.

Specific written directions are important when teaching the patient how to use topical medications, compresses, and special baths. Side effects of drug therapy are another important topic included in patient teaching.

The patient with pruritus should know about other measures such as heat, cold, and loose clothing, which were described earlier in this chapter. The patient should know about the skin ailment. In some cases, the physician uses terms the patient does not understand. In some cases, the nurse assists with this aspect of family teaching by reporting the patient's confusion to the physician so that misunderstandings can be resolved.

ASSISTING WITH OTHER THERAPIES

ELECTROSURGERY. Many small lesions may be removed by *electrodesiccation,* which is superficial destruction of the skin caused by a burst of electricity aimed at the lesion. Electrocoagulation destroys the tissue at a deeper level and produces more scarring. In electrocoagulation, the patient is grounded for electricity, and the electrical charge that is delivered creates enough heat to coagulate the tissue. Benign superficial lesions such as warts may be coagulated and then removed by curettage.

CRYOSURGERY. Skin lesions may be destroyed also by freezing, *cryosurgery.* Solid carbon dioxide or liquid nitrogen may be used to produce a subfreezing temperature. The procedure is rapid, is done easily, usually requires no anesthesia, and leaves little or no scarring. A mild analgesic or sedative may be used after the surgery. The healing process is usually completed within a month.

ULTRAVIOLET LIGHT THERAPY. Ultraviolet light therapy is used to treat such conditions as acne vulgaris, psoriasis, and chronic eczema. The patient must be instructed to avoid overexposure to this light. Eye goggles, a timer, and the presence of another person should be employed as safety measures against overexposure.

Dermatitis

ACNE VULGARIS

The individual with acne vulgaris has a disorder of sebaceous glands and hair follicles which may or may not be associated with inflammation. A combination of hormonal, genetic, and bacterial factors produce characteristic lesions.

NURSING OBSERVATIONS

Skin lesions include comedomes, papules, pustules, nodules, and cysts which are seen most often on the face and neck. Lesions also may develop on the back and chest. *Comedomes* are dilated follicles that have been plugged by lipids and keratin. Whiteheads are closed comedomes, and blackheads are comedomes that have opened, revealing the impacted keratin inside.

Behavioral changes related to visible skin lesions and disturbances in body image may be present.

NURSING INTERVENTIONS

ASSISTING WITH DRUG THERAPY. Topical preparations, such as vitamin A (RETIN-A) and benzoyl peroxide may be prescribed for acne. Benzoyl peroxide helps peel the tops from the comedomes. Systemic antibiotics such as tetracycline or erythromycin also may be prescribed. Tetracycline should be taken either one or two hours after meals to enhance absorption, and the nurse should observe for such side effects as photosensitivity, nausea, diarrhea, and moniliasis. Clindamycin (CLEOCIN) is sometimes used in resistant cases of acne, but should be monitored carefully because of frequent incidences of colitis. Estrogen therapy is sometimes given to young females whose acne tends to flare up at certain times in the menstrual cycle.

HYGIENE AND SKIN CARE. The client with acne is instructed to wash the face twice a day to remove surface oils and prevent obstruction of oil glands. Frequent scrubbing of the face is avoided because it may damage the skin. All forms of friction and trauma to affected areas are avoided. For example, pimples should not be squeezed because of the possibility of scarring and spreading infection.

OTHER THERAPIES. The physician may use a comedome extractor to remove comedomes. Ultraviolet light may be prescribed in some cases.

The individual with extensive scarring from acne vulgaris may be treated with dermabrasion, a surgical planing of skin layers including the epidermis and dermis to the level of the scar. The patient is hospitalized for the surgical procedure and receives a general anesthetic. Postoperatively, the patient may have a petrolatum gauze or medicated bandage. Edema, which is present after surgery, usually subsides within two or three days. The patient's face usually feels sunburned. Patient teaching after surgery includes avoiding sunlight for four months and avoiding commercial skin products and cosmetics.

ASSISTING WITH PATIENT TEACHING. In addition to teaching the patient about hygiene and drug therapy already discussed, the client is advised to wear a hairstyle which keeps hair away from affected areas on the face and neck. The client also may need help in selecting a balanced diet. Prevention of stress and fatigue is an additional topic that may be included.

HERPES

The individual with herpes has an infection caused by a herpes simplex virus. Two different viruses may cause this infection, herpes simplex virus I and herpes simplex virus II. Viruses may enter the body through the mouth, skin, vagina, cornea, esophagus, or penis. The infection spreads from one person to another by direct contact with infected persons. The virus may be transmitted from the mother to the fetus, causing severe infection in the newborn. Recurrent infections are frequent once a person develops herpes simplex.

Respiratory infections, minor gastrointestinal disturbances, emotional strain, pregnancy, fever, and sunlight may trigger a recurrent infection. This disease has been linked to other conditions such a multiple sclerosis and cervical carcinoma.

The incidence of herpes infection is rising dramatically. Presently, there is no cure for this disease, although there is promising new research related to drug therapy.

NURSING OBSERVATIONS

The person with a herpes simplex I infection usually develops painful vesicles on the lips, face, or tongue. Before oral lesions appear, the client may notice burning, itching, and tingling. Vesicles may rupture, leaving ulcerative lesions which usually crust over in about seven to ten days.

The person with a herpes simplex II infection may develop painful vesicles on the perineum, penis, vagina, cervix, urethra, or buttocks. Vesicles rupture, leaving ulcers covered with a grayish-white exudate. During the acute stage, the patient usually has fever, malaise, and enlarged lymph nodes in the groin which are exquisitely tender. Dysuria may occur when the urethra is involved.

After lesions have healed, some patients remain well and never have recurrences. Other patients may have recurrent symptoms. In addition, some clients become carriers of the virus even when symptoms are not present.

NURSING INTERVENTIONS

ASSISTING WITH DRUG THERAPY. At present, no drugs are available to cure herpes infections that develop around the mouth or genitalia. Special antiviral agents are available for herpes infections which develop in the cornea (keratitis) and those associated with encephalitis. The rapid rise in the number of persons developing herpes infections is causing researchers to work hard to develop new drugs that can cure this disease.

PATIENT TEACHING. The patient with a herpes infection should be instructed to avoid direct contact with others when active lesions are present. Frequent handwashing is important. It is especially important to avoid rubbing the eyes since this may result in serious herpes infections in the cornea.

The patient should be instructed how to avoid other infected persons, prevent fatigue, and reduce emotional stress in order to prevent recurrent infections. When active lesions are present, bed rest, liquids, and similar measures may be used to relieve symptoms such as malaise and fever.

PYODERMA

The individual with pyoderma has a skin infection that generally involves one or more hair follicles and may be caused by *Streptococcus* group A or by *Staphylococcus* microorganisms. When the patient has a primary streptococcal or staphylococcal infection of the skin, the condition is known as *impetigo contagiosa*. Impetigo is easily transmissible and occurs most frequently in early childhood, especially during hot, humid weather. Sources of infection may include dirty fingernails, other children, contaminated swimming pools, secondary infections following bites from insects such as mosquitos, and other individuals.

NURSING OBSERVATIONS

The lesions of the patient with impetigo are thin-walled vesicles that rupture and become covered with a honey-colored crust. The lesions tend to spread in circles or arcs. The exposed parts of the body usually are affected, such as the face, hands, neck, and extremities.

NURSING INTERVENTIONS

PREVENTING THE SPREAD OF INFECTION. The patient with a streptococcal or staphylococcal infection of the skin should be isolated to prevent the spread of infection to others and to avoid carrying additional microorganisms to the patient. When possible, the patient is placed in a private room. A protective isolation gown should be worn when giving direct care to the patient. Gloves are indicated when the nurse is giving care to the infected area such as changing a dressing, and the nurse also should wear a mask.

ASSISTING WITH DRUG THERAPY. After skin lesions have been cultured, the physician usually prescribes an appropriate antibiotic such as penicillin.

OTHER MEASURES. The measures discussed in Chapter 5 such as rest, increased fluid intake, a nourishing diet, and approprite antibiotics are needed by the patient with a streptococcal or staphylococcal skin infection.

ASSISTING WITH HYGIENE. The environment should be cool and dry in order to promote drying. Towels and other personal items used by the infected individual should be separated carefully from the family's personal articles.

PATIENT AND FAMILY TEACHING. The family of the patient with impetigo contagiosa should use a bacteriostatic soap at least once a day. Since impetigo is contagious, family members should be instructed to avoid contact with the member who has the infection. Family members, including the client, should be instructed to practice frequent handwashing. Practices to be avoided include sharing towels and personal articles such as clothing, combs, and cosmetics.

FURUNCLES AND CARBUNCLES

A furuncle is an acute inflammation of a hair follicle caused by *Staphylococcus aureus*. A carbuncle is an abscess involving skin and subcutaneous tissue which develops from a furuncle. These skin conditions occur more frequently in the patient with another underlying disease such as diabetes mellitus.

NURSING OBSERVATIONS

Furuncles resemble pimples and occur most often in the back of the neck, axillae, buttocks, and similar areas subjected to irritation, pressure, friction, and perspiration. When the center becomes yellow or black in color, the boil is said to have "come to a head."

Carbuncles frequently are located on the back of the neck and buttocks. Because infection is more extensive, the patient may experience fever, painful enlargement of lymph nodes, and other signs of infection, as described in Chapter 5.

NURSING INTERVENTIONS

Drug therapy usually includes a systemic antibiotic after a culture and sensitivity have been obtained.

Hot moist compresses may be prescribed to localize the infection. Once localization has occurred, the physician may make a tiny incision to evacuate infected materials. The draining lesion is covered with a dry sterile dressing. The nurse should follow the agency or hospital policy carefully when disposing of soiled dressings. In some hospitals, wound and skin precautions are taken in order to prevent the spread of infection.

Special patient teaching includes a warning never to squeeze boils on the face since this may result in a fatal infection. The area, especially around the mouth and nose, is drained directly into the cranial sinuses. This area is known as the danger triangle. Transmission of pathogenic microorganisms into the brain and other parts of the body could result in a fatal infection.

ATHLETE'S FOOT (TINEA PEDIS)

The individual with athlete's foot has a common superficial fungal infection, which may be either an acute inflammatory process or a chronic condition. In the acute stage, the involved areas have vesicles; in the chronic stage, the involved areas scale and have an erythematous rash. The soles of the feet and the spaces between the toes generally are involved. Toenails may or may not be infected. The itching can range from moderate to severe.

NURSING INTERVENTIONS

During the acute or vesicular stage, soaks of Burow's solution, saline or potassium permananate may be prescribed to remove crusts, scales, and other debris and to decrease inflammation. Drug therapy includes fungistatic creams such as tolnaftate (TINACTIN), haloprogin (HALOTEX), miconazole (MICATIN), or clotrimazole (LOTRIMIN). This therapy often lasts for weeks. If the infection becomes extreme or resistant to topical therapy, an oral antifungal agent such as griseofulvin (FULVICIN) may be prescribed.

Patient teaching includes encouraging the client to keep the feet as clean and dry as possible. Areas between the toes are especially vulnerable because of the moisture naturally present. One suggestion for keeping the area dry is to place cotton between the toes at night to help absorb moisture. Socks should be lightweight and clean. It may be advisable for the individual to wash and boil the socks to prevent reinfection. Medication in the form of an ointment or a powder may be prescribed to combat the infection. The person generally is directed to apply the ointment at night and to remove it in the morning. The powder is then dusted on the feet. The client may be advised to sprinkle powder into the shoes. The individual may be advised to wear shoes alternately. The shoes should be exposed to air and sunlight to facilitate drying before they are worn again. When in public places such as swimming pools, the client should wear shoes.

Dermatoses

PSORIASIS

Psoriasis is a chronic inflammatory disease of the skin in which the epidermal cells are produced at six-to-nine times their normal rate. Psoriasis is one of the most common skin disorders. Although the exact cause of the condition is not known, it is thought that a combination of an individual's specific genetic make-up and environmental stimuli may trigger the onset of the disease. It is also thought that periods of emotional stress and anxiety may aggravate the disease.

Psoriasis usually occurs before the age of twenty, but all age groups may be affected. The patient may go through many cycles of improvement and exacerbation of the condition throughout a lifetime. At present, there is no known cure.

When observing the patient with psoriasis, the nurse sees heavy, dry, silver scales which are in sharp contrast to the normal-appearing skin around them.

Drug therapy for the client with psoriasis may include topical and/or systemic medications. Examples of topical preparations are resorcinol, anthralin, zinc oxide, and preparations of sulfur (sublimed sulfur) and thiosulfate (WHITE LOTION). Coal tar products may be combined with salicylic acid and sulfur and prescribed in the form of ointment, shampoo, bath emulsion, gel, paste, or lotion. Two examples of systemic medications are methoxsalen (OXSORALEN) and methotrexate.

In general, topical preparations should be applied after bathing and after loose scales have been brushed away with a soft brush. A tongue blade or a gloved hand can be used to apply the medication. The area then is covered with a gauze dressing, stockinette, or old pajamas to avoid staining. When topical steroids are prescribed, a plastic dressing is applied, as described earlier in this chapter.

ASSISTING WITH OTHER THERAPIES

Another method of treating the person with a difficult or extensive case of psoriasis is known as photochemotherapy. In this case, the patient is treated with a combination of ultraviolet light and a sunscreening drug such as methoxsalen (OXSORALEN). Because of the possibility of toxic effects, the physician prescribes specific periods of time for the patient to receive ultraviolet light treatments in relation to the time of drug administration. For example, methoxsalen, 20 mg, may be prescribed once a day, to be followed in two hours with an exposure of two minutes to ultraviolet light therapy. Treatments usually are done two or three times a week. Between treatments, the client should be observed for signs of ultraviolet light burns.

While receiving photochemotherapy, the individual should be cautioned to avoid exposure to the sun. Sunglasses should be worn, and frequent eye examinations should be made to make sure no damage to the eyes has occurred. Methoxsalen should be taken with foods to help prevent nausea, which is one of its side effects. Nonmedicated creams and bath oils may be used to remove scales and decrease excess dryness; however, no medicated creams or oils should be used. Again, because of the potential toxic effects of the treatment, the patient should remain under constant and careful medical supervision.

The client with psoriasis needs considerable nursing support, as described earlier in this chapter. Treatment is costly, time consuming, and frequently unappealing.

PEMPHIGUS

The patient with pemphigus develops various-sized blisters on the skin. This condition is believed to be an autoimmune disease. The patient may have periods of exacerbations and remissions, and most who are affected first notice the disease in middle age.

NURSING OBSERVATIONS

Blisters and bullae may develop in a local area or may be widespread, depending on the type of disease. The bullae rupture and leave eroded areas that eventually become encrusted. These areas heal so slowly that new areas may appear before old ones have healed, so that large areas of the body may become involved. When large areas of the body are involved, the patient may lose considerable serum and/or develop secondary infection.

NURSING INTERVENTIONS

ASSISTING WITH DRUG THERAPY. Because the disease is believed to result from a disturbance in the patient's immune system, large doses of corticosteroids may be prescribed to suppress the immune response. Nursing responsibilities related to this form of drug therapy are described in Chapter 18. Systemic antibiotics such as those listed in Table 5.7 may be prescribed to prevent secondary infection.

HYGIENE. Oral hygiene with a nonirritating substance is important in order to prevent secondary infection in mouth lesions. Special skin care may be prescribed to prevent fluid losses from the skin and promote comfort.

DIET AND FLUIDS. Careful intake and output are indicated when the patient sustains fluid losses from widespread lesions. The physician may prescribe a high-protein, high-calorie diet to improve nutrition. An increase in fluid intake usually is recommended. In severe illness, the physician may prescribe intravenous therapy to replace fluids lost from the skin.

Skin Diseases Caused by Insects and Parasites

SCABIES

The patient with scabies has skin lesions caused by a crab-shaped mite which burrows into the skin. The mite is transmitted from one person to another by direct contact as well as from affected clothing and bed linen. Outbreaks of scabies are more common in schools and other institutions where large numbers of persons come in close contact.

NURSING OBSERVATIONS

Usually the person with scabies first notices itching which increases at night and may persist for several days after treatment. Lesions may develop on the skin between the fingers, wrists, axilla, waist, under the breasts, abdomen, buttocks, and genitalia.

Using a magnifying glass and penlight, the physician will search for small raised burrows. The burrows may be multiple, straight or wavy, brown or black lesions. However, burrows are not always seen as the symptoms may also include the presence of only a rash. Secondary lesions from scabies are common and include vesicles, papules, pustules, excoriations, and crusts. Because the integrity of the skin is broken, a bacterial infection may develop.

NURSING INTERVENTIONS

Drug therapy for the patient with scabies includes application of a cream or lotion such as gamma benzene hexachloride (KWELL, GAMENE), or crotamiton (EURAX). These drugs are applied to the skin from the neck down and left on for 8 to 12 hours. In applying these drugs or instructing others, the nurse should wear gloves and avoid the eyes and mucous membranes. The drug is washed off the next day or after the prescribed time. Additional treatments may be prescribed at seven- to ten-day intervals. Antibiotics may be prescribed if secondary infection is present. Antihistamines may be prescribed to relieve severe itching. Family members and others in close contact with the client also are treated at the same time to prevent recurrence.

Prevention of outbreaks includes laundering all bed linen and clothing in very hot water, good handwashing, and reporting of rashes observed in a hospitalized patient.

PEDICULOSIS

The individual with pediculosis has an infestation of body lice. These lice live on blood sucked from the skin and may be on the head, pediculosis capitus; on the body, pediculosis corporis; or on the pubic area, pediculosis pubis. Body lice may be transmitted by direct contact or via discarded clothing in which they can survive for up to a week. The patient develops itching and a characteristic rash in the affected area. In some cases, the body lice or nits (eggs) can be seen.

Nursing interventions include drug therapy using gamma benzene hexachloride (KWELL, GAMENE). For head lice, the hair is first shampooed with ordinary shampoo. Then, the medicated shampoo is applied and left on for four minutes before rinsing. Then, a fine-tooth comb is used to remove nits (eggs) from the hair. This treatment is repeated in seven days. For body lice, the shampoo is used to lather the body for four minutes. After rinsing and drying, KWELL, GAMENE, or other similar lotion is applied to involved skin areas and left for 24 hours. The treatment is repeated in seven days.

When the nurse assists the hospitalized patient who has pediculosis, gloves are worn during the shampoo and body lather in order to prevent the transfer of head or body lice. Bed linens and personal articles, including clothing, hairbrushes, and combs, should be handled according to agency or hospital policies.

Patient and family teaching includes how to separate and clean personal articles belonging to the person with pediculosis. For example, clothing and bed linens should be machine washed. Combs and hairbrushes may be disinfected by soaking them in commercial preparations containing phenol. Another important topic in patient teaching is not to share personal items such as combs, brushes, and hats. Persons are advised to avoid sharing these personal items in order to prevent further outbreaks.

WARTS (VERRUCA)

The individual who has a wart has a common skin tumor caused by a virus. Although the virus is communicable, susceptibility to the virus varies with the individual. Once a wart (verruca) has developed, an individual may spread the virus from one area of the body to another by autoinnoculation (scratching or through another broken area on the skin). A wart also can disappear spontaneously. A verruca generally produces no symptoms unless it is located on an area of the body that bears weight. A wart usually is treated by the application of liquid nitrogen, carbon dioxide, salicylic acid, electrocautery, or curettage.

Decubitus Ulcers

Decubitus ulcers, commonly known as bed sores, are caused by pressure exerted on the skin and subcutaneous tissue by the bony prominences of the patient. These pressure areas come into contact with an object that also exerts pressure. Anoxia, which causes ischemia in the area, occurs. Tissue ischemia soon causes a break in the epidermis and is followed quickly by involvement of the soft tissue below the area. This break in the body's defense system makes invasion by pathogenic microorganisms likely.

Anything that interferes with circulation, such as leaning on an extremity, moisture, heat, wrinkles and crumbs in bed linen, and friction, contributes to the development of decubitus ulcers. Incontinence and poor hygiene may cause skin breakdown. Poor nutrition, with anemia, hypoproteinemia, and vitamin, mineral, or trace element deficiencies rob the cells of needed food sources. Edema interferes with the blood supply to the cells and may cause skin breakdown. Motor paralysis and associated atrophy of the muscles reduce padding between the skin and the bone underneath and may cause a decubitus ulcer to develop.

Sensory loss in the skin causes an absence of awareness of pain or pressure, and the patient loses an important warning sign of circulatory impairment. In the hospital, probably one of the most frequent causes of decubitus ulcer is the shearing force created by having the head of the bed raised. This shearing force is created when the head of the bed is raised 30 degrees or more.

NURSING OBSERVATIONS

Usual observations made by the nurse are heightened when the particular patient has one or more factors associated with the development of decubitus ulcer. For example, the nurse may increase the frequency of observations in an elderly patient who is undernourished and unable to move. The nurse inspects anatomic areas receiving major pressure in a systematic fashion from head to toe. Such areas include the back of the head, shoulders, elbows, sacrum, hips (ischial and trochanter areas), malleoli (ankles), and heels of the foot.

An early sign of skin breakdown and ulcer formation is erythema (redness) of a local skin area which blanches (turns white) when pressure is applied. Next, the involved skin turns purple, then bluish-gray. The first break in the skin may be a blister or a crack. As skin breakdown progresses, the nurse may observe drainage, as well as widening and deepening of the ulcer to involve muscle, connective tissues, and even bone.

NURSING INTERVENTIONS

Prevention of decubitus ulcers is the most effective intervention available. A prevention program begins when the nurse is aware that the patient is at risk to develop decubiti, even before a reddened area appears. An effective program includes good nutrition, adequate hydration, frequent changes of position, massage, and meticulous hygiene.

DIET AND FLUIDS

The patient needs a nourishing diet and a good fluid intake in order to maintain healthy tissue. In some cases, the nurse may need to feed the patient, consult with the dietitian, and instruct the patient in order to prevent or correct undernutrition and dehydration.

REPOSITIONING

Changing the patient's position every one to two hours helps to relieve the pressure, which may deny nutrition to the skin tissue. Shifting weight allows blood to flow to all areas of the skin. Sheepskin or foam rubber, when placed under the sacrum, heels, elbows, hips, and back of the head where decubitus ulcers frequently form, will help reduce the development of ulcers. Keeping the bed clean, dry, smooth, and free of wrinkles will discourage development of decubiti. A footboard used to keep bed linen away from the feet and legs also seems to help. An alternating-pressure mattress, which shifts pressure over several sites, is beneficial in situations in which the patient cannot turn without help. Water beds and flotation therapy also help to distribute the body's weight and pressure more evenly.

MASSAGE

Stimulation of the skin increases circulation and reduces tissue hypoxia. Therefore, frequent skin massages using gentle, circular strokes are useful in the prevention of decubitus ulcers. Care should be taken, however, to remove any excess lotion on the patient's skin since overly moist skin will quickly macerate in addition to being uncomfortable for the patient. Active and passive range-of-motion exercises increase muscle, skin, and vascular tone and improve blood flow.

HYGIENE

The patient's skin should be washed with mild soap and water, or with no soap at all, and blotted rather than rubbed dry with a soft towel. Urine, feces, and other irritating substances should be removed from the skin as often as necessary to keep it clean and dry.

ULCER CARE

The individual with decubitus ulcer requires special care related to the skin breakdown in addition to preventive measures already discussed. A culture of the wound usually is obtained to identify pathogens. The ulcer is cleansed usually daily to remove tissue debris. Special agents that may be prescribed for cleansing the wound include hydrogen peroxide, acetic acid, or normal saline.

After the ulcer is cleansed, topical therapy may be prescribed. A myriad of topical agents has been used to promote healing. These include antibiotic, antiseptic, or enzyme ointments, creams, or sprays, ultraviolet light, sunlight, local application of oxygen, and pressurized air. Recently, a new transparent skin barrier called OP-SITE has been used to cover decubitus ulcers. The nurse should follow directions carefully when using this material. In some cases, surgery may be needed to remove dead tissue, promote drainage, and graft new skin to close large ulcers.

Neoplasms of the Skin

Cancer of the skin occurs more frequently than cancer of any other organ. Basal cell carcinoma, squamous cell carcinoma, and melanoma are three examples of skin cancer. Basal cell carcinoma is the most common of the three types, with exposure to the sun being the most common cause of basal cell carcinoma development. Those people who are at high risk for the development of basal cell carcinoma include people with fair skin, blue eyes, and red hair, those with light or "ruddy" complexions, people who "burn" but do not tan, outdoor workers such as farmers, sailors, and fishermen. Workers who are exposed to certain chemical agents such as arsenic, nitrates, tar, pitch, oils, and paraffins are also at high risk for basal cell cancer development.

The second most common type of skin cancer is squamous cell carcinoma. Squamous cell cancer is true invasive carcinoma, and metastasis of this cancer is related to the level or depth of invasion.

The individual with a malignant melanoma has the most dangerous type of skin cancer. A melanoma has a marked tendency to metastasize and usually is resistant to chemotherapy. Whether the tumor is curable depends on the depth of skin invasion and spread. The malignancy may be curable only if confined to the primary site. Metastasis takes place through both the lymph channels and the bloodstream.

NURSING OBSERVATIONS

Since cancer of the skin is visible, the patient usually seeks medical attention relatively early. Early diagnosis and early treatment result in a high cure rate. The nurse's observations may be very helpful in early detection of skin cancers. As previously mentioned, skin rashes and lesions are recorded and reported.

The appearance of skin lesions in the patient with a skin cancer depends upon the type of malignant cell involved. For example, a smooth, waxy, noninflamed nodule is common in basal cell carcinoma (Figure 24.2). The nodule may contain tiny vessels visible near the surface as well as tiny dots of melanin pigment. A skin lesion typical of squamous cell carcinoma is a firm, red nodule or plaque with vesicle scales on the surface ulceration and crusting may occur on these lesions (Figure 24.3). The back of the hands, ears, or face may be affected. Areas surrounding the mouth, anus, or urethra may develop squamous cell carcinoma also.

The patient with a malignant melanoma may have an early lesion with an irregular border and characteristic colors including shades of red, white, blue, brown, or black. A malignant melanoma freuently starts as a change in a wart or mole. For this reason,

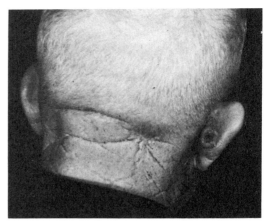

FIGURE 24.3 A squamous cell carcinoma. (From McCredie, John A. [ed.], and Donner, Carol [illustr.]: *Basic Surgery*. Macmillan Publishing Co., Inc., New York, 1977.)

any change in a wart or mole should be reported to one's physician immediately.

NURSING INTERVENTIONS

Nursing interventions are related to a variety of treatments which may include surgical excision, electrodesiccation, cryotherapy, curettage, radiotherapy, and chemotherapy. Additional information about current cancer therapy can be located in Chapter 9.

The nurse's knowledge about factors associated with skin cancer provides a basis for teaching others to avoid prolonged exposure to the sun, use care in handling certain chemicals, and report skin lesions to the physician. The patient with metastatic skin cancer needs emotional support, as described in Chapter 9.

Systemic Diseases with Skin Involvement

The patient with systemic disease may have skin lesions in addition to other local and general symptoms. Often, the appearance of a characteristic rash causes the patient to seek treatment or the physician to diagnose a systemic disease.

Scarlet fever (scarlatina) is caused by a streptococcal infection that results in painful pharyngitis. The pharyngitis is followed

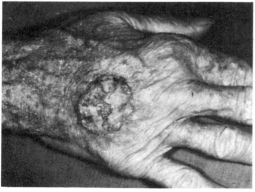

FIGURE 24.2 A basal cell carcinoma of the hand. (From McCredie, John A. [ed.], and Donner, Carol [illustr.]: *Basic Surgery*. Macmillan Publishing Co., Inc., New York, 1977.)

by the appearance of a diffuse erythematous rash. Redness generally appears on the neck first, then rapidly spreads to the trunk and the extremities with total body involvement within 36 hours.

Measles (rubeola) is a contagious systemic virus disease characterized by coryza (coldlike symptoms), conjunctivitis, a barking cough, and blotchy macular erythema on the soft palate. A purplish-red rash appears first on the neck, behind the ears, and over the forehead. The rash slowly spreads over the entire body and gradually takes on a brownish hue. It may last a week or longer.

German measles (rubella), which poses a great threat to the fetus of a pregnant woman, produces a rash that starts near the hairline and on the face. In contrast to rubeola, the rash of rubella often disappears from one site as it spreads to another.

The rash of typhoid fever appears as rose spots seven to ten days after the appearance of high fever. The rash usually appears on the lower anterior chest, the upper abdomen, and the middle portion of the back. The individual lesions last three to four days and become brownish in color before disappearing. Bacteria may be found in these skin lesions.

Smallpox (variola) is a serious virus infection characterized by papules and pustules that become deep and necrotic. These may cause extensive scars.

In Rocky Mountain spotted fever, the rash first appears on the wrists, ankles, and forearms and gradually involves the entire body. Ulcers may occur from this rash, and gangrene may develop in the earlobes and fingertips.

Systemic diseases involving the blood, such as gonococcemia, staphylococcemia, meningococcemia, *Pseudomonas* septicemia, and subacute bacterial endocarditis, are also manifested by skin involvement as are metabolic upsets, malfunction of the pituitary gland and thyroid gland, and diabetes mellitus.

SYSTEMIC LUPUS ERYTHMATOSUS

Systemic lupus erythmatosus (SLE) is a systemic inflammatory disease that pro-

duces inflammation, biochemical and structural changes in connective and vascular tissue, and typical skin lesions. Although the cause of this condition is not known, it is thought to be an autoimmune disease. Other factors associated with the development of SLE include viral infections and genetic abnormalities. Certain drugs such as hydralazine (APRESOLINE) and procainamide (PROCAPAN, PRONESTYL) may produce a syndrome that is similar to SLE. Women are affected more often than men. There is no cure for this disease yet. The physician may prescribe a variety of therapies to suppress flare-ups and prolong life.

ASSISTING WITH DIAGNOSTIC STUDIES

In addition to a history and physical examination, the physician may request a blood test to measure the level of circulating autoantibodies. A high level of antinuclear antibodies (ANA) in the blood indicates the presence of disease. Another blood test may be ordered to try to identify the lupus erythematosus cell (LE cell prep). A variety of other tests may be ordered, depending on the patient's symptoms.

NURSING OBSERVATIONS

Skin lesions the nurse may observe include a characteristic butterfly rash which appears over the bridge of the nose and across the cheeks. Another skin lesion which may develop is called discoid lesion which usually occurs on the forehead, ears, and scalp. Discoid lesions have scales, changes in skin pigment, and scarring. Permanent hair loss may occur. Skin lesions are more likely to occur in areas exposed to the sun. Painless ulcers may also develop in the mucous membranes in the nose and mouth.

The patient may develop a variety of other symptoms, depending on which body systems are involved. For example, the patient may have swelling and pain in the joints when the musculoskeletal system is involved. Hematuria and proteinuria may occur when the patient's renal system is involved. Respiratory symptoms related to pneumonitis and pleural effusion may occur. Convulsions and/or psychosis may occur when the patient's central nervous system is involved.

In addition, the nurse can expect to see general symptoms of inflammation, as described in Chapter 5. The patient usually experiences fever, malaise, fatigue, and weight loss, and tender, enlarged lymph nodes.

NURSING INTERVENTIONS

Nursing interventions include measures to promote comfort, relieve symptoms, improve function in the body system affected, and prevent relapses. During an acute relapse, the patient is generally advised to rest in bed and eat a nourishing diet.

ASSISTING WITH DRUG THERAPY

Drug therapy frequently includes a systemic corticosteroid from Table 17.6. Other drugs that may be prescribed during acute flare-ups include salicylates and/or a nonsteroid anti-inflammatory drug from Table 17.6. Additional drug therapy may be prescribed according to the body system involved. Topical corticosteroid creams may be prescribed for skin lesions.

ASSISTING WITH PATIENT TEACHING

Preventing acute flare-ups is the goal of patient teaching. The patient is taught how to avoid infection, fatigue, sunlight, and emotional stress. Surgery, penicillin, sulfonamides, and blood transfusion are also avoided since these may cause a relapse. The patient is also instructed on correct usage and side effects of drug therapy to be maintained at home.

SCLERODERMA

The individual with scleroderma has a progressive hardening and shrinking of connective tissues of the skin and internal organs such as the lungs, heart, kidney, and gastrointestinal system. The cause of this condition is not known. Present evidence suggests that abnormalities in the vascular system and an overproduction of collagen tissue are important associated factors. Women are affected more often than men. When lesions affect the function of vital organs, the patient is unlikely to recover.

NURSING OBSERVATIONS

The patient with scleroderma may notice sweating of the hands and feet or stiffness in early stages. A characteristic appearance of the skin is its firm, thickened, leathery appearance which usually is first visible in the hands. As the disease progresses, skin ulcers and changes in skin pigmentation are observed. As connective tissue involvement spreads, the patient generally experiences diminished hand and finger mobility, a loss of normal skin wrinkles, a loss of facial expression, and an inability to open the mouth. As other body systems become involved, the patient experiences symptoms related to the dysfunction of that system.

NURSING INTERVENTIONS

Nursing interventions are selected on the basis of relieving symptoms and promoting comfort. Skin care includes meticulous, gentle cleansing and also may include the application of a bland cream. Measures important in preventing complications associated with reduced mobility apply to this patient. These may include frequent repositioning, a nutritious diet, adequate fluid intake, and active or passive exercises. Particular attention is devoted to care of the hands, since loss of function in the hands greatly affects a person's ability to work and care for him- or herself. The person with scleroderma can be expected to require a considerable amount of emotional support. In developing a therapeutic relationship, the nurse's warmth, acceptance, and compassion may help the patient come to some acceptance also. The patient who is encouraged to verbalize feelings of anger, frustration, and despair then may be able to enjoy other aspects of living and focus on remaining function.

POLYARTERITIS NODOSA

Polyarteritis nodosa is a disease of unknown cause characterized by inflammation and necrosis of medium-sized and small arteries resulting in altered functions to the systems the artery supplies. It is thought to be a disease of altered immunity that causes antigen-antibody complexes to locate on blood vessel walls. The onset of the disease also has been known to follow sensitivity reactions to such drugs as sulfonamides, io-dides, and penicillins.

Symptoms of polyarteritis nodosa may vary according to the organ involved and the amount of necrosis produced. Systemically, the disease produces such symptoms as prolonged fever, weakness, myalgia, arthralgia, gastrointestinal symptoms such as abdominal pain, nausea, vomiting, and diarrhea, coronary insufficiency and myocardial infarction, renal problems, pneumonia or bronchitis, and retinal exudates and hemorrhage. In the skin, the patient may develop various-size painful nodules which may ulcerate. Overlying skin in necrotic areas may become reddened or ulcerated and purpuric macules may be present.

Treatment of polyarteritis nodosa is symptomatic and supportive. Steroids such as prednisone may be given, as well as immunosuppresive drugs and antibiotics.

Burns

A *burn* is an injury to the body caused by heat. A major portion of burns each year occurs in homes. An injury resulting in a burn can be caused by thermal, electrical, irradiation, or chemical sources. A thermal burn can be either moist or dry. A hot flame burn and a hot metal burn are examples of dry burn. A moist burn can be caused by boiling water or live steam. An electrical burn results from contact with an electric current. Although the extent of the burn depends on the type, voltage, and amperage, most individuals with electrical burns have an outlet and an inlet burn. Irradiation burns occur from such sources as radium therapy, sunlight, x-ray treatments, and ultraviolet light. Chemicals such as strong acids or alkali products coming in contact with the body may cause a severe burn also. Such factors as duration of heat application, source of heat, and conductivity of involved tissue influence the amount of tissue injury.

Emergency care of the person suffering from a burn was discussed in Chapter 8. This chapter will focus on the care of the patient after first aid has been rendered. Because the management of burns is extremely demanding, many communities have set up units to take care of patients with burns. In this specialized unit, quality care is rendered by personnel who have had additional training in the area of nursing the patient with a burn. All members of the health team in the burn unit are utilized to continuously encourage and maintain social, spiritual, physical, and psychologic well-being of each patient. The continuity of health care is aimed at promoting complete rehabilitation, or as near complete as possible, and in teaching the patient and his family prevention of accidents. Posthospital care utilizing community health agencies is also planned.

NURSING OBSERVATIONS

Meticulous, frequent observations are crucial in order to identify and prevent complications in the burned patient. Because the patient usually receives continuous nursing care, the nurse's observations are especially valuable.

OBSERVING THE BURN. A burn is classified according to the amount and depth of the injury. In a first-degree burn, the tissue is red, discolored, painful, and may have some edema. In a second-degree burn, the skin is red, mottled, blistered, painful, and has a red appearance. In a third-degree burn, the skin is mottled, discolored, white, or charred. In a fourth-degree burn, the tissue resembles that of a third-degree burn, but the damage is more extensive with bone, deep tissue, and internal organs having been destroyed.

Burns also may be referred to as partial thickness, deep partial thickness, and full thickness. A partial-thickness burn involves only the upper layers of the epidermis (for example, sunburn). In a deep partial-thickness burn, the entire epidermis is destroyed, but the dermis remains. In a full-thickness burn, the dermis is destroyed, as may be underlying muscles and bones. Differences in sensation, color, texture, retention of hair, and blisters help to distinguish between full- or partial-thickness burns. Therefore, the nurse observes and describes burns using Tables 24.5 and 24.6 as a guide. A fluorescein dye also may be injected after hydrotherapy. When the patient's burns are exposed to ultraviolet light in a darkened room, partial-thickness burns show the dye because circulation is maintained.

TABLE 24.5
GUIDE TO NURSING OBSERVATIONS OF THE BURNED PATIENT

AREA TO BE OBSERVED	NURSING OBSERVATIONS
Head and neck	Observe and report blurred vision, dizziness
	Report wheezing, stridor, dyspnea, cough, sooty or bloody sputum, hoarseness
Chest	Observe and record pattern of respirations (Chapter 14)
	Report irregularities of heart rhythm, tachycardia (Chapter 11)
Extremities	Report edema, waxy, gray or white skin appearance, coldness, absence of pulse
Abdomen	Report nausea, vomiting, epigastric pain, hematemesis, indigestion, abdominal distention
Bladder	Report bladder distention
	Report urine output below 30 ml/hour or greater than 100 ml/hour
	Report hematuria
	Record characteristics of urine
	Observe Foley catheter for kinked, twisted, disconnected tubing
Bowels	Report diarrhea, constipation, blood in stools
Vital signs	Report changes indicating hypovolemic shock (increased heart rate, falling blood pressure, increased respiratory rate)
	Report fever
Skin	Describe characteristics of burn including color, odor, sensation, appearance (refer to Table 24.6)
	Report diaphoresis, skin temperature, and color in nonburned areas
Behavioral changes	Report changes in level of consciousness, including alertness and orientation to surroundings
	Report restlessness, especially if vital signs are also changing

A full-thickness wound will not be fluorescent because the blood vessels in that area have been destroyed. The nurse can explain to the patient that this procedure is harmless, although a slight feeling of nausea from the dye is not uncommon. The dye is excreted through the kidneys and may cause the urine to be fluorescent. The patient should know this. The procedure and how it was tolerated by the patient should be charted in the nurse's notes.

Burns are also classified as being major or minor, major being those that involve second-degree burns over 30 percent of the body or third-degree burns over 10 percent of the body.

Factors included in this category, besides the size of the burn, are the specific area involved and age. For example, burns involving the head and neck are major because respiratory complications are more likely. Children under the age of two years and adults over the age of 60 years have higher mortality rates from burns than do those individuals who do not fall within these two age groups.

TABLE 24.6
CHARACTERISTICS OF BURNS

	PARTIAL THICKNESS	FULL THICKNESS
Blisters	Thick-walled blisters which may drain and refill with fluid, become larger, or disappear and reappear	Little or no blistering. If present, blisters have thin walls and disappear
Color	Appears red and blanches upon pressure, redness returns with release of pressure	Charred to white, no blanching with pressure
Hair retention	Hair cannot be plucked easily	Hair can be plucked easily
Texture	Feels normal or firm	Feels leathery
Sensation	High sensitivity to pain, heat, and cold	Virtually anesthetized to pain

In determining the percentage area of the body burned, two methods are used commonly. The rule of nines, which computes the percentage of the adult patient, assigns 9 percent of the total body surface to each arm, 9 percent to the head and neck, 18 percent to the anterior torso, 18 percent to the posterior torso, 1 percent to the genital region, and 18 percent to each leg (see Figure 24.4). An alternate method is used in the child whose body proportions change during growth and development.

In addition to observing the burn, the nurse observes the entire patient for early signs and symptoms of complications. Table 24.5 is a guide to nursing observations in the burned patient. The nurse can expect to use a variety of high-technology monitoring systems when the patient has extensive burns. For example, the nurse may determine the patient's pulse with an ultrasonic blood flow detector, Doppler, which magnifies the sound of the pulse in the area of the patient's body touched by the sensitive equipment. The sound of the patient's pulse can be heard by members of the health team as they render care to the patient. Central venous pressures may be monitored using a central venous line, as described in Chapter 11. Arterial blood pressure may be measured directly through an arterial catheter. A Foley catheter is inserted to measure urine output.

OBSERVING FOR COMPLICATIONS. Burns cause dilation of capillaries and small blood vessels. This allows fluid to seep into tissues and escape through the burns. A decrease in circulating fluid volume deprives vital organs of an adequate blood supply and causes the patient to experience symptoms of hypovolemia, as described in Chapter 6.

Infection is another major problem for the burned patient. As the eschar or dead tissue separates from the living tissue beneath it, microorganisms, usually of the gram-negative type, invade the living tissue, which is now open. This invasion of microorganisms may cause a partial-thickness burn to change to a full-thickness burn, as the sepsis penetrates and eventually destroys the dermis. If an infection is present, the pulse rate of the patient usually will increase, while the temperature may increase or decrease, depending on the microorganism involved.

Gastrointestinal bleeding is a frequent complication in the patient with extensive burns. An increase in anorexia, hematemesis, blood in the stool, and a drop in the blood hemoglobin indicate gastrointestinal ulcer.

Grief, terror, pain, sleep disturbances, disfigurement, and isolation may trigger a psychotic episode that includes disorientation, auditory and visual hallucinations, and combative behavior. Thus, the patient should be observed for changes in behavior throughout the recovery period.

NURSING INTERVENTIONS

MAINTAINING ADEQUATE VENTILATION. In caring for a burned patient, maintaining an open airway is the nurse's first priority. The nurse should be especially alert for signs of respiratory distress when the patient has inhaled smoke or when burns are located around the face, neck, or chest. In

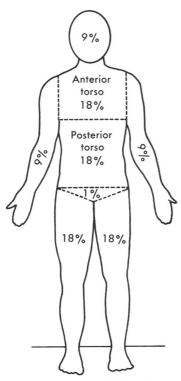

FIGURE 24.4   Rule of nines.

these instances, edema of the patient's air passages can block the airways. Endotracheal intubation, a tracheostomy, and mechanical ventilation may be needed. When repositioning the patient, the nurse should take special care to ensure that the new position does not block the patient's airway or restrict ventilation.

ASSISTING WITH FOOD AND FLUIDS. In the first few hours following an extensive burn, the patient is usually not given fluids by mouth. A nasogastric tube may be inserted to relieve or prevent abdominal distention or paralytic ileus. Later, the nasogastric tube may be used to provide nourishment by tube feedings (Figure 24.5). Hyperalimentation, as described in Chapter 15, also may be used in some cases. When the patient is able to tolerate solid foods, a diet high in protein, calories, and vitamins generally is prescribed. Small, frequent feedings should be given since the patient usually will experience a certain amount of loss of appetite. The patient's nutrition is important to promote healing of burned areas. The patient is usually anorexic and may need encouragement to eat. Food that is consistent with the patient's usual eating practices is more likely to be eaten.

Maintaining fluid balance is another important priority of the nurse. The physician prescribes the fluids to be administered and the rate of flow. The nurse monitors the rate of flow, the patient's response to fluid therapy, and the intravenous site. In the first several days following an extensive burn, the patient can be expected to show evidence of dehydration. After about 72 hours, the patient is monitored for circulatory overload caused by movement of fluid from the tissues back into the circulatory system. As previously mentioned, strict intake-and-output records, as well as daily weights, help the physician to estimate fluid loss. Fluids that may be prescribed include whole blood plasma, plasma expanders, and solutions containing electrolytes.

REPOSITIONING. Frequent repositioning of the burned patient is important to improve blood flow, reduce swelling, prevent contractures, and relieve pressure. Splints, sandbags, rolled towels or blankets, footboards, and other devices may be used to maintain anatomically correct positions. Kinetic beds, which gently rotate the patient from side to side, and CIRC-O-LECTRIC beds, which move the patient from a prone to supine position, are helpful in positioning the

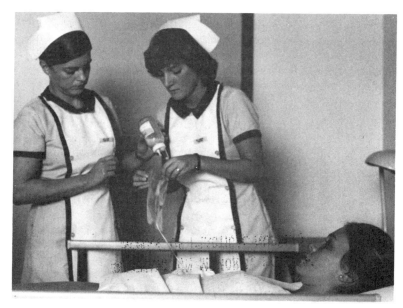

FIGURE 24.5 Preparing a tube feeding. (Courtesy of Southhampton Memorial Hospital School of Practical Nursing, Franklin, Virginia.)

patient who must be turned frequently. Frames such as the Stryker and Foster may be used also.

Elevating a swollen-extremity above the level of the heart helps to reduce edema. Active and passive range-of-motion exercises are especially important. The nurse may consult the physician about exercising a burned extremity.

ASSISTING WITH HYGIENE. The patient with burns needs meticulous hygiene. When hydrotherapy is used, the patient's skin is cleansed in the Hubbard tank. The patient with burns needs protection from chilling since the skin barrier is broken. Oral hygiene is important to promote comfort and prevent overgrowth of bacteria. Nails should be cleansed and trimmed when necessary to prevent the growth of bacteria that could contaminate wounds.

PREVENTION OF INFECTION. The patient with burns may be placed in protective isolation in order to prevent life-threatening infection. Special burn units usually are equipped to control airflow in the room to prevent outside bacteria from entering the patient's room. Antibiotics generally are prescribed to prevent infection.

ASSISTING WITH PAIN AND DISCOMFORT. Pain is a common experience for the patient with burns. Intravenous morphine may be given in early stages because the duration of action is usually short and the patient's response can be monitored closely. Analgesics and other methods of pain control, as discussed in Chapter 7, may be needed for painful procedures such as debridement, hydrotherapy, dressing changes, and physiotherapy.

ASSISTING WITH DRUG THERAPY. The patient with extensive burns can be expected to receive a variety of drugs in addition to analgesics.

A booster dose of tetanus toxoid usually is given to a patient known to have been actively immunized recently. The patient who has not been actively immunized is generally given human immune globulin (HYPER-TET).

An appropriate antibiotic may be prescribed after a culture and sensitivity report has been received.

An antacid from Table 15.11 may be instilled into the patient's nasogastric tube. Another drug frequently prescribed to prevent gastrointestinal bleeding is cimetidine (TAGAMET), which may be given intravenously or orally to help decrease the production of stomach secretions.

A variety of topical agents may be applied to the burned area. The wound may be cleansed with antiseptics or bacteriostatic agents.

Enzymatic ointments also may be applied to help remove necrotic tissue that prevents the formation of granulation (healing) tissue. Such agents as sutilains ointment (TRAVASE) and collagenase (SANTYL OINTMENT) help dissolve necrotic tissue. Before applying an enzymatic agent, the wound must be cleansed of antiseptic or heavy metal antibactericidals (such as hexachlorophene, silver nitrate, BETADINE, and others), which interfere with the enzymatic action.

Silver sulfadiazine (SILVADENE), a cream, is used to prevent wound sepsis. When applying this antibiotic, the nurse should wash the hands and apply sterile gloves. The cream is then applied so that it covers the wound but is not caked. Sterile drapes may be placed under the area to be treated to avoid contact with unsterile surfaces.

Silver nitrate (0.5 to 1 percent) is used as a continuous wet soak. The gauze must be saturated constantly to be effective. This method causes no pain in administration, is easy to apply, is readily available, and is bactericidal. It does have the disadvantage of turning many things black; therefore, great care must be taken by the nursing staff to prevent staining of clothes and skin.

Mafenide acetate (10 percent) (SULFAMYLON CREAM) is an antibiotic cream that may be prescribed for local burn areas. The cream is applied once or twice a day in a thick layer about 1 to 2 mm with a sterile gloved hand. The patient may experience burning pain when the cream is applied.

ASSISTING WITH HYDROTHERAPY. As mentioned earlier in this chapter, upon admission to the hospital, the patient may be placed in a shower, bath, or whirlpool to remove eschar. This therapy is continued on a twice-daily basis using, most often, a Hubbard tank and may be referred to by the staff as tubbing. Tubbing helps to keep the burned area clean and free of excess drainage. It increases the comfort of the patient and is used to facilitate motion of the joint and completion of active and passive exercises to include a full range of motion. This minimizes the formation of contractures. Hydrotherapy also helps with mechanical debridement and with the removal of dressings that may have adhered to the wound. The temperature of the water should be no higher than 37.7°C (100°F). Often an antiseptic solution such as BETADINE or chlorine bleach is added to the water to reduce the number of microorganisms. (See Figures 24.6 and 24.7.) The patient usually remains in the tub from 15 to 30 minutes while the

eschar is debrided. The patient usually is covered with a sterile blanket after having been removed from the tub in order to prevent chilling. Preparation for hydrotherapy may include a nourishing meal, analgesia, weight, and intake and output. Following hydrotherapy, ointments, creams, or dressings may be applied.

The nurses who assist with hydrotherapy wear gloves, gowns, and masks and practice strict aseptic technique throughout the procedure. The hydrotherapy room and the Hubbard tank are scrupulously cleansed with disinfectant between patients.

ASSISTING WITH BURN CARE. The patient may be placed in a shower, tub, or Hubbard tank if possible. The whirlpool action of the Hubbard tank creates a disturbance in the water that helps to debride, cleanse

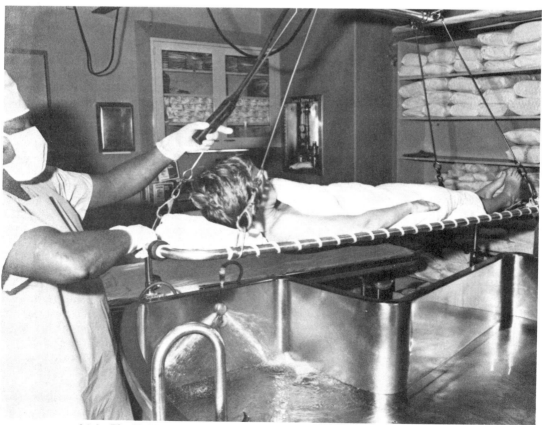

FIGURE 24.6 The Hubbard tank is being filled with water as the patient is lowered into the tank. Notice the jet action of the spray beneath the plinth (carrying litter).

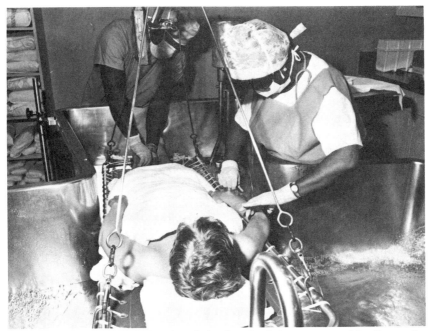

FIGURE 24.7 The newly burned patient is having dead tissue removed by the mechanical action of the water. The nurses are helping to remove some of the eschar also.

away, the *eschar,* which is dead or sloughing tissue. Removal of eschar in this manner is referred to as mechanical debridement and helps in the assessment of the extent of burns and prevention of bacterial growth on the eschar, which could further destroy living tissue.

Surgical debridement may be done instead of mechanical debridement with water (see Figure 24.8). Also, surgical removal of burned tissue may be done in connection with water cleansing.

Once mechanical debridement has taken place, the area of the burn is assessed, and the burned area may be treated in one of several different ways. The area and extent of the burn, as well as the facilities available and the psychologic state of the patient, may help to dictate the method of treatment used.

Dry dressings are used to protect the burn wound from exposure and to protect and secure underlying dressings. When using a dry dressing, the area of the burn is covered by sterile dry sponge and wrapped in sterile KERLEX.

Wet-to-dry dressings are applied wet and allowed to dry. These help to facilitate the removal of eschar in order to prepare the burn area for grafting by removing any overlying film on the wound. When applying wet-to-dry dressings on an extremity, the nurse should begin at the distal end of the extremity and wrap toward the direction of the heart with KERLEX. This enhances circulation and prevents constriction of the extremity. When applying a wet-to-dry dressing of the proximal thigh, a sterile towel folded lengthwise around the upper thigh will help prevent contamination by urine or feces. The dressing should be snug but not tight and have no wrinkles. With burns of the fingers, each finger should be wrapped separately to prevent webbing between the fingers.

Occlusive (Pressure) Dressings. Bulky dressings may be applied for compression, for splinting the affected part, and for support. Usually a topical agent is applied lightly to a cleansed burn area and a bulky material is next applied. Abdominal pads

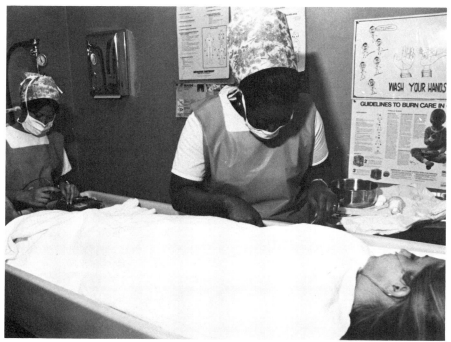

FIGURE 24.8   A newly burned patient is being prepared for surgical débridement by the nurse on the right. The nurse on the left is checking the patient's pulse with an ultrasonic blood flow detector, the Doppler. Notice that oxygen has already been started by means of a nasal cannula.

and elastic bandages or stockinette may also be used. Occlusive dressings tend to impair circulation. Symptoms such as tingling, pain, numbness, coldness, and blanching around the area of the dressing should be reported at once. Functional alignment of each body part must be maintained, such as having thumb and fingers curved over a bandage roll, the foot positioned to prevent pronation and footdrop, and support placed under the knees. The occlusive dressings are changed frequently until skin grafting is done. Because the procedure is very painful, a general anesthetic may be given or the administration of an analgesic may be given before changing the dressing.

In wound dressings, a topical antibiotic may be used.

Semiopen Methods. In the semiopen method, the burn area is covered with a topical ointment. A dressing may or may not be used. When a dressing is used, it consists of a few layers of sterile gauze that has been saturated with a topical agent. The wound is

cleansed once or twice a day. This can be an effective management of contamination by keeping the wound as clean as possible during débridement and requires skilled nursing care from a highly trained, specialized staff.

When changing a patient's dressing, the nurse should tell the patient what is to be done, what to expect, and how long it will take. If an analgesic is required, it should be given 20 to 30 minutes before beginning the dressing change to achieve its maximum effect.

Open Method. In the open method of burn treatment, the burned area is left open to the air. No dressing is applied, but the wound is kept clean, and exudate (drainage) from the wound is removed frequently to prevent the growth of bacteria. This method of treatment is preferred for minor or partial-thickness burns, for newly grafted areas, and for body areas on which dressings are difficult to apply. The open method of treatment allows for frequent inspection of the wound and requires less actual nursing care than other methods. However, the patient is more susceptible to chilling; the wound soils linen, which requires frequent changing; and infection control is difficult because the wound is open to direct and indirect transmission of contamination. The patient must be placed in strict isolation.

GRAFTING. Once the wound has been debrided, grafting is often necessary to aid healing. Skin grafting is a surgical procedure in which the surgeon implants skin from other parts of the body, or from another person, onto the burned area. An *autograft* is removal of full- or partial-thickness skin from the patient (the site of removal is referred to as the donor site), in order to place it on the clean granulation tissue of the burned area. When obtaining an autograft, the surgeon uses an instrument called a *dermatome* to obtain the graft. A new wound, the donor site, is created. The nurse must then employ principles of aseptic technique to prevent contamination of the donor site, and to help dry and heal the donor site to provide for the patient's comfort.

A *homograft* is a temporary dressing. Since the skin tissue is taken from another person (usually a cadaver), the body will, in a few days, reject the skin as being foreign protein. For a short time, however, homografts do provide protection of the wound surface and allow the wound to heal.

Porcine, or pigskin, grafts are another form of temporary biologic dressings used to cover a full- or partial-thickness skin graft. The use of these temporary dressings helps to decrease the pain the patient experiences as well as reducing the loss of body water. The use of temporary skin grafts helps facilitate movement of unused joints and decreases contractures. Temporary biologic dressings also help to prevent protein and electrolyte loss while they increase the vascularity of the new tissue. When the temporary dressings are changed, mechanical debriding takes place. EPIGARD is a new type of synthetic barrier dressing that helps promote granulation of the skin.

Human amniotic membranes are now being used in some areas as a temporary biologic dressing.

DEVELOPING A THERAPEUTIC RELATIONSHIP. The patient with a burn frequently sustains many losses. Home, furnishings, even family members may perish in the tragedy which caused the patient's burns. Lengthy hospitalization and disability may cause further losses such as a job and income. Such a patient can be expected to show one or more signs of grieving, as discussed in Chapter 1, and to use defense mechanisms such as denial.

Feelings of anger, guilt, and depression are not uncommon as the patient tries to cope simultaneously with losses, pain, isolation, disfigurement, and a lengthy, unpleasant recovery period. Nursing actions that favor a successful resolution of these feelings include:

- Active listening to patient's concerns.
- Encourage the patient to describe feelings about the experience. Provide pictures, songs, other objects to represent feelings.
- Provide information and explanation about procedures, medications, and all interventions that involve the patient.
- Create opportunities for the patient to direct and participate in care whenever possible.
- Praise all positive gains in healing, appearance, patient participation.
- Provide environmental stimuli such as clocks, calendars, radios.
- Initiate conversations about subjects unrelated to hospitalization.
- Avoid disrupting normal processes such as grieving, using defense mechanisms.

REHABILITATION. Rehabilitation of the patient with burns usually involves the entire health team. For example, the social worker may be particularly useful in helping the patient's family prepare for discharge, securing financial assistance, and contacting community agencies. Occupational and physical therapists help the patient to reach the maximum amount of mobility possible. Vocational rehabilitation may be indicated to help the patient prepare for the work world. Thus, the burned patient benefits from the special skills of each member of the health team.

Plastic Surgery

Plastic surgery accomplishes one of two basic purposes—reconstruction or cosmetic changes in a patient's appearance. Reconstructive surgery repairs extravisceral deficits and malformations, restores function, or prevents loss of function. Cosmetic surgery may improve the physical appearance of an individual.

Dermabrasion is the scraping, sandpapering, or brushing of the skin to remove the epidermis and some of the superficial dermis, while allowing for new epithelial cells to grow. It usually is done on those patients who have facial disfigurements ranging from scars from acne and trauma to tattoos, nevi, freckles, and chickenpox or smallpox. The procedure may be done in a physician's office or clinic, or in the hospital under general anesthesia.

Preoperative preparation of the patient who is to undergo dermabrasion usually involves an assessment of the patient's nutritional status to determine if additional vitamin and protein intake is needed to assist with postoperative healing. A hemoglobin and clotting time are done, as these levels may affect the healing process. The skin usually is washed with a detergent germicide for three days prior to surgery. Hair may be washed the night before.

Edema occurs during the first postoperative day and usually subsides within 48 hours. Petrolatum gauze dressings which have been applied usually are removed after 48 hours. The patient looks and feels severely sunburned. Lanolin, cocoa butter, or hypoallergenic creams may be used to soften crusts that form and relieve the sensation of tightness. The patient should be cautioned to avoid exposure to the sun.

Rhinoplasty is a type of cosmetic surgery designed to change the shape of the nose. It is a widely performed type of cosmetic surgery. Patients who have noses that have become deformed through a fracture, or who have a congenital malformation such as a large lump, or bulbous or drooping tip may decide to have this type of surgery. If the condition is congenital, the patient usually is advised to wait until the nose is mature, or about 16 to 17 years of age. The surgery is done through an intranasal incision and may

be done under either local or general anesthesia. The hospital stay is brief but postoperative edema and periorbital bruising may last for several days.

Other types of cosmetic surgery are *mentoplasty* (for a receding chin), *rhytidoplasty* (a face lift), *otoplasty* (to change the shape of the ears), and *blepharoplasty* (for the eyelids).

Basic postoperative care for all of these types of surgeries may include maintaining the patency of any suction drains used, administration of antibiotics to combat infection, and tranquilizers to decrease movement that may disturb the grafts.

Cosmetic surgery usually results in a changed body image. In talking with the patient, the nurse selects communication that conveys warmth, interest, and acceptance. In helping the patient explore a changed body image, the nurse may ask an open-ended question such as, "What changes in your life do you expect from surgery?"

Reconstructive surgery usually involves the application of skin grafts. *Free grafts* are separated completely from the donor site and connected to the vascular bed of the recipient site. *Pedicle grafts* are still attached at some point either to their point of origin or to an intermediate transfer site. They carry their own blood supply and, therefore, do not depend on the blood supply of the recipient site for survival. For the graft to take, it must be in complete contact with the recipient site, it must have an adequate blood supply, the area must be free from infection, and immobilization must be assured.

Grafts may be obtained by the use of razor blades, skin graft knives, or dermatomes. The grafts may or may not be sutured or stapled into place and may or may not be covered with dressings. If dressings are used, the base layer is usually a single layer of fine mesh gauze impregnated with an ointment to make it nonadherent. Fluffy gauze dressings are placed on top of this and then secured with a wraparound type of dressing. The donor site usually is covered with a layer of scarlet-red gauze and is left exposed to the air.

Certain alterations in the usual postoperative care occur when the patient has a graft. For example, range-of-motion exer-

TABLE 24.7
OTHER DISORDERS OF THE SKIN

DESCRIPTION	DISORDER
Acanthosis nigricans	An excessive pigmentation and hypertrophy of the skin following internal cancer or an endocrine disorder; groin, axillae, genitalia, and neck seem to be the most commonly affected parts of the body
Epidermolysis bullosa	A condition of the skin characterized by formation of deep-seated bullae appearing after rubbing, irritating, or applying pressure on the skin
Erysipelas	A skin infection caused by·group A stretococci; usually affects the head and face but can affect other areas; affected area becomes red, hot, edematous, and glistening
Erythema multiforme	An acute inflammatory condition in which the patient has redness of the skin in connection with an involvement of one or more systems; fever, aching, respiratory symptoms, and vomiting frequently are present; symptomatic measures may be combined with steroid therapy, depending upon the severity
Erythema nodosum	Nodules that are red and tender appear on such parts of the body as the thighs, forearms, upper arms, head, face, and eyes; this condition is thought to be a hypersensitivity reaction
Seborrheic dermatitis	Dandruff is the common term for this condition; person has an oily scalp that itches and forms greasy scales
Toxic erythema	A redness of the skin resulting from capillary congestion; patient experiences a toxic reaction to some substances, such as drugs, pathogens, or foods; the involvement varies widely; treatment is directed toward removing the underlying cause

cises involving the graft site are avoided. The graft area is not washed or cleansed unless there are specific orders to do so. The dressing over the graft may remain undisturbed for 24 to 48 hours. Any fluid, pus, or blood that has collected under the mesh gauze should be evacuated gently by rolling the graft with a sterile cotton-tipped applicator before the site is redressed. The donor site should be kept as clean and dry as possible. Heat lamp applications several times a day may be prescribed. All suction drains should be kept patent.

Prosthetic devices such as silicon implants may be used in both cosmetic and reconstructive surgery.

Patients with massive injuries or deformities may require several operations over an extended period. For example, breast reconstruction is an option for many women following a mastectomy for breast cancer. The patient with radical neck surgery for cancer also may require multiple-stage surgery for reconstruction. Such patients can be expected to experience a number of behavioral changes related to the original illness and surgery as well as the new appearance created by reconstructive surgery. The nurse's warmth, understanding, and compassion can be helpful in assisting the patient to recover. A description of other skin disorders can be located in Table 24.7.

Case Study Involving an Ulcer of the Skin

Mrs. Alice Elms, a 76-year-old woman, was admitted to the hospital with chief complaints of shortness of breath and chest pain. She has a history of diabetes mellitus extending back for 15 years and has taken an oral hypoglycemic agent at home. Upon helping Mrs. Elms to bed, the nurse noticed a 3-cm open lesion on Mrs. Elms' right ankle. The admitting diagnosis for Mrs. Elms was congestive heart failure and diabetes mellitus.

QUESTIONS
1. What underlying condition could have predisposed to the development of an open lesion on Mrs. Elms' leg?
2. The physician ordered a proteolytic enzyme, TRAVASE ointment, to be applied to the ulcer following irrigation with normal saline. Describe the method to be used in applying TRAVASE ointment to Mrs. Elms' open lesion (decubitus ulcer).
3. What supplies are needed to apply a dry dressing to an open ulcer?

4. Describe the steps to be taken in changing the dressing on an open decubitus ulcer.
5. What is the relation of diet to the treatment of an individual with a decubitus ulcer?

Case Study Involving a Burn

John Jones, a 25-year-old electrical worker, was admitted to the hospital with partial- and full-thickness burns involving the face and neck, chest, arms and hands, and legs.

The physician's orders are:

- Intake and output q1h
- Foley catheter
- 1000 ml of 5 percent dextrose and lactated Ringer's solution intravenously
- CBC, BUN, SMA-12
- DEMEROL, 100 mg q3h prn, for pain IM
- Penicillin, 1 gm IV q6h
- Observe for symptoms of respiratory difficulty

QUESTIONS

1. List at least four symptoms that might indicate respiratory difficulty.
2. Realizing that the front of both arms and legs are burned, describe several ways the nurse can position Mr. Jones to promote comfort and prevent contractures.
3. What possible psychosocial problems could be experienced by Mr. Jones?

Suggestions for Further Study

1. Discuss the possible impact of a disfiguring skin disorder on an adult.
2. What methods of treating persons with burns are currently being used in your vicinity?
3. Mason, Mildred A.; Bates, Grace F.; and Smola, Bonnie K,: *Workbook in Basic Medical-Surgical Nursing,* 3rd ed. Macmillan Publishing Company, New York, 1984, Exercise 24.

Additional Readings

Acris, Cathleen, and Kraft, Edward R.: "Skin Transplantation." *American Journal of Nursing,* 81:1466–67 (Aug.), 1981.

Ahmed, Mary Cooke: "Op-Site for Decubitus Care." *American Journal of Nursing,* 82:61–64 (Jan.), 1982.

Conlee, Darien: "Put a New Face on Your Care of Cosmetic Surgery Patients." *Nursing 81,* 11:90–95 (Nov.), 1981.

Gaston, Susan F., and Schumann, Lorna Lou: "Inhalation Injury: Smoke Inhalation." *American Journal of Nursing,* 80:94–97 (Jan.), 1980.

Heckel, Patricia: "Teaching Patients to Cope with Psoriasis: The Unshared Disease." *Nursing 81,* 11:49–51 (June), 1981.

Kadlowec, Noreen; Price, James; and Forouzesh, Hohammed: "Systemic Lupus Erythematosus." *Journal of Nursing Care,* 14:6–9 (Aug.), 1981.

Koch, Sharon Johnson: "Augmentation Mammoplasty." *American Journal of Nursing,* 80:1480–84 (Aug.), 1980.

Larrow, Lonnie, and Noe, Joel M.: "Port Wine Stain Hemangiomas." *American Journal of Nursing,* 82:786–90 (May), 1982.

Levy, Donald M.: "Cosmetic Surgery Patients." *Journal of Practical Nursing,* 30:13–17 (Oct.), 1980.

Lyons, Michele: "Skin Cancer and the Sun." *Journal of Practical Nursing,* 32:16–20 and 40 (June), 1982.

McHugh, Mary L.; Dimitroff, Karen; and Davis, Nancy Dismore: "Family Support Group in a Burn Unit." *American Journal of Nursing,* 79:2148–50 (Dec.), 1979.

Rambo, Beverly J., and Wood, Lucile A. (eds.): *Nursing Skills for Clinical Practice,* 3rd ed. W. B. Saunders Co., Philadelphia, 1982, pp. 210–30.

Romm, Sharon; Smith, Charlotte; and Ritchie, Jean: "Nursing and Plastic Surgery." *Journal of Nursing Care,* 14:10–12 (Aug.), 1981.

Schulmeister, Lisa: "Screening for Skin Cancer." *Nursing 81,* 11:42–45 (Oct.), 1981.

"Test Yourself: Systemic Lupus Erythematosus." *American Journal of Nursing,* 82:783, 874 (May), 1982.

Woolridge, Maribeth, and Surveyer, Judith A.: "Skin Grafting for Full-Thickness Burn Injury." *American Journal of Nursing,* 80:2000–2004 (Nov.), 1980.

Glossary

ABDOMINAL PARACENTESIS. Withdrawal of fluid from the peritoneal cavity by the use of a hollow needle or a trocar.

ABDOMINOPERINEAL OPERATION. Surgical removal of the rectum, anus, and part of the colon through abdominal and perineal incisions.

ABORTION. Interruption of pregnancy before the fetus is viable.

ABSCESS. A collection of pus.

  STITCH ABSCESS. That which occurs around a skin suture.

ACCOMMODATION. The adjustment of an organ, an organism, or a part of the body; especially the ability of the eye to focus on objects at varying distances.

ACNE VULGARIS. An inflammatory condition often affecting the face and characterized by the formation of blackheads, papules, and pustules; also known as pimples.

ADHESION. An abnormal union of surfaces that are normally separate.

ADJUVANT. Assisting.

ALBUMINURIA. The presence of albumin in the urine.

ALKYLATING AGENT. Drug used to slow down the activity, growth, and multiplication of cells, especially in neoplasms.

ALLERGEN. A substance that causes an allergic reaction.

ALLERGY. An overly sensitive reaction to a substance normally considered harmless.

ALPHA-FETOPROTEIN. AFP; an experimental laboratory test that produces a specific antigen performed to aid in discovering a malignancy.

AMENORRHEA. A condition in which a woman has an absence of menstruation.

AMINO ACIDS. Chemical compounds obtained from proteins.

AMPERES. Number of electrons passing a specific point per second.

AMPULLA OF VATER. A short, dilated tube formed by the common bile duct and pancreatic duct as they enter the duodenum.

AMPUTATION. Removal of an appendage, limb, or outgrowth of the body.

ANAL FISSURE. An ulcerating crack or crevice in the mucous membrane of the anus.

ANALGESIC. An agent used to relieve pain.

ANAPHYLACTIC SHOCK. A state of shock that follows the injection of a substance to which the person is allergic; anaphylaxis.

ANEMIA. A decrease in the number of red blood cells, or in the amount of hemoglobin; both may be reduced.

ANESTHETIC. A drug that causes a loss of feeling.

ANEURYSM. A dilation of the wall of an artery, such as a dilation of the aorta caused by syphilis.

ANGINA PECTORIS. A condition in which a person has attacks of chest pain caused by an insufficient blood supply to the heart muscle.

ANGIOCARDIOGRAPHY. An x-ray study of the heart and great blood vessels following the injection of an appropriate medium.

ANGIOGRAPHY. An x-ray study of some part of the vascular tree following the injection of a radiopaque substance.

ANGIONEUROTIC EDEMA. Localized, swollen areas of the skin or the mucous membrane sometimes caused by a food allergy; giant urticaria.

ANKYLOSIS. Stiffness of a joint; union of the bones in a joint.

ANOREXIA. Loss of appetite.

ANTACID. A drug that neutralizes acids.

ANTIBIOTIC. A substance made from certain microorganisms that either checks the growth or kills other microorganisms.

ANTIBODY. Immunoglobulin; protein that reacts with an antigen to destroy it. The five major classes of antibodies are IgG, IgA, IgM, IgD, and IgE.

ANTICOAGULANT. A drug used to prevent the clotting of blood.

ANTIGEN. A foreign substance that causes the body to form antibodies.

ANTIMETABOLITE. An agent that slows down the growth of malignant cells by interfering with the cells' metabolism and growth.

ANTISPASMODIC. A substance that relieves convulsions or spasmodic pains.

ANTITUSSIVE. Drug used to relieve or suppress coughing.

ANURIA. Lack of urinary output caused by failure of the kidneys to excrete urine or by an obstruction in the urinary tract.

ANUS. External opening of the colon.

ANXIETY. A feeling of discomfort in response to some anticipated threat or danger.

AORTOGRAPHY. An x-ray study of the aorta following the injection of an appropriate medium.

APHASIA. Either the loss of speech or an impairment of speech.

APHONIA. Inability to speak; loss of the voice.

APICAL. Referring to the apex, which is the top of an organ or the pointed portion.

APNEA. A temporary absence of breathing.

APPENDECTOMY. Surgical removal of the vermiform appendix.

APPENDICITIS. An inflammation involving the vermiform appendix.

ARRHYTHMIA. A disturbance of either the rate or the rhythm of the heartbeat.

ARTERIOGRAM. X-ray examination of an artery after the injection of a suitable dye. For example, the arteries in the brain may be examined in this manner.

ARTERIOGRAPHY. An x-ray study of specific arteries following the injection of an appropriate medium.

ARTERIOSCLEROSIS. A condition of the arteries in which soft, fatty substances are deposited on the inside of the vessels causing the walls to become thicker. As calcium is deposited in these areas, it causes the artery to become rigid, hard, brittle, and less elastic. Hardening of the arteries.

ARTERIOSCLEROTIC HEART DISEASE. An abnormal heart condition caused by hardening of the coronary arteries.

ARTHRITIS. An inflammatory condition of one or more joints.

DEGENERATIVE JOINT DISEASE. A chronic condition of the joints that is less likely to cause deformity than is rheumatoid arthritis. Generally progresses slowly. The patient may have an increase in the size of the bones of the affected joints and spur formation. The inflamed joints are usually painfull, stiff, and enlarged. The joint changes are not as marked as those associated with rheumatoid arthritis. It is more common in late middle life. Also known as hypertrophic arthritis and osteoarthritis.

RHEUMATOID ARTHRITIS. A chronic condition that can affect many joints. The patient usually has general symptoms of inflammation such as fever and malaise. The inflamed joints generally are painful, swollen, and have a decreased ability to move. Ankylosis and deformity may occur. It is more common between 20 and 50 years of age.

ARTHRODESIS. Artificial fixation of a joint by fusing the surfaces.

ARTHROGRAPHY. X-ray examination following the injection of a radiopaque dye or air into a joint.

ARTHROPLASTY. Plastic surgery on one or more joints; forming joint capable of moving.

ARTIFICIAL PNEUMOTHORAX. The injection of air or gas into the pleural cavity to cause the lung to collapse. This technique was used in the treatment of pulmonary tuberculosis.

ASCITES. An abnormal collection of fluid in the peritoneal cavity.

ASTERIXIS. 1. A flapping tremor of the hands when the individual bends his hands back at the wrists while resting arms on a flat surface. 2. Liver flap.

ASTHMA. A condition in which the patient has attacks of dyspnea caused by spasm of air passages. Frequently refers to bronchial asthma.

BRONCHIAL ASTHMA. That caused by an allergy; allergic asthma.

CARDIAC ASTHMA. That caused by failure of the left ventricle, which results in congestion of the lungs.

ASTIGMATISM. Impaired vision resulting from an irregular curvature of either the cornea or the crystalline lens of the eye.

ATELECTASIS. Collapse of a portion of the lung.

ATHEROSCLEROSIS. A form of arteriosclerosis in which deposits of fat are made in the innermost wall of an artery.

ATHLETE'S FOOT. An inflammation of the feet and sometimes the hands caused by fungi. Tiny blisters filled with fluid form on the affected areas.

ATOPY. An allergic reaction strongly associated with heredity.

ATRIAL FIBRILLATION. Rapid uncoordinated quivering of atria resulting in rapid irregular pulse.

AUDIOMETER. An instrument used to measure a person's hearing ability.

AURA. A sensation that warns a person of an oncoming convulsion.

AUSCULTATION. The process of listening to sounds arising from within the body. Usually a stethoscope is used.

AUTOGENOUS. Originating within the individual's body.

BACTERIA. Microorganisms belonging to the plant kingdom. Some cause infectious disease such as tuberculosis and typhoid fever.

BEHAVIOR. The manner in which one acts.

BILE. A fluid secreted by the liver that aids in the digestion and absorption of fats.

BILIRUBIN. A red bile pigment normally found in bile and sometimes in the blood and urine. It is formed from the hemoglobin of red blood cells.

BIOPSY. Removal of tissue from the body for microscopic examination. This technique is often used to determine presence of cancer.

BLEPHARITIS. Inflammation of the edges of the eyelids.

BODY IMAGE. Picture of one's body.

BOTULISM. Acute poisoning caused by ingestion of toxins formed in foods by anaerobic bacteria called *Clostridium botulinum.*

BRADYCARDIA. Slow heart action. The pulse rate is usually below 60.

BRONCHOGRAM. X-ray examination of the bronchial tree after an iodized oil has been injected into the bronchi.

BRONCHOPNEUMONIA. An inflammation of the lungs distributed around the bronchi.

BRONCHOSCOPE. An instrument that can be inserted through the mouth, throat, and trachea into the bronchi. It enables the doctor to examine the bronchial walls; sometimes used in treatment.

BRONCHOSCOPY. An examination of the bronchial walls with a bronchoscope.

BURSA. A small sac containing fluid, which is located so as to prevent friction between surfaces that move upon one another.

BURSITIS. An inflammatory condition of a bursa.

CALCIFICATION. The deposit of lime salts in the body's tissues.

CALCULUS. A hard body formed in a cavity or elsewhere in the body; stone.
  RENAL CALCULUS. One located in the kidney; kidney stone; nephrolithiasis.

CALLUS. A gluey substance that forms around the fractured ends of a bone. Lime salts and bone cells are deposited in the callus and cause it to harden.

CANCER. A malignant tumor or one that threatens an individual's life.

CANNULA. A tube used for insertion into the body. The opening may have a trocar for insertion.

CARCINOEMBRYONIC ANTIGEN. CEA; an experimental laboratory test based on the production of antigens performed to discover the presence of certain tumors.

CARCINOMA. A malignant tumor of epithelial tissue.

CARDIAC CYCLE. The regular series of changes that occur in the heart with each heartbeat. Systole, diastole, and the rest period are the three phases that make up this series of changes.

CARDIAC ORIFICE. The opening between the esophagus and stomach.

CASEATION. Death of a group of cells that results in the formation of a cheeselike substance; occurs frequently in tuberculous infections.

CAST. 1. A substance that has assumed the shape of a cavity in which it was molded. A common example is seen in the casts found in urine. These casts are formed when a substance hardens in the tubule of the kidney and is later washed out by the flow of urine.
2. A mixture that becomes hardened as it dries, such as plaster-of-paris. This is used to immobilize parts of the body. Crinoline containing plaster-of-paris is moistened and molded over the affected area. As the plaster dries, it becomes hardened.

CATAMENIA. Menstruation.

CATARACT. Clouding of the crystalline lens of the eye.

CATHARTIC. An agent that increases motility of the intestines with a fluid evacuation.

CAUTERIZATION. The destruction of tissue by the use of a chemical or by using electricity that is passed through a thin blade or a wire loop.

CECOSTOMY. An operation in which an artificial opening is made into the cecum through the abdominal wall.

CECUM. The large pouch at the beginning of the large intestine.

CENTRAL VENOUS PRESSURE. CVP; pressure exerted by the blood in the venae cavae and right atrium.

CEREBRAL HEMMORRHAGE. Ruptured blood vessel in the brain; stroke.

CEREBROVASCULAR ACCIDENT. A disease of the arteries in the brain resulting in an inadequate blood supply; apoplexy; stroke; cerebral accident. It may be caused by hemorrhage, a thrombus, or an embolus.

CERUMEN. Earwax.

CERVICITIS. Inflammation of the cervix.

CHALAZION. Cyst of the meibomian gland located within the eyelid.

CHANCRE. A lesion that develops in an area through which invading microorganisms have entered the body. The term usually refers to the area through which spirochetes enter the body and cause syphilis.

CHEMOTHERAPY. The method of treating disease with either serum or drugs.

CHOKING. Obstruction within the throat or respiratory passage causing inability to breathe or swallow.

CHOLANGITIS. An inflammation of the bile ducts.

CHOLECYSTECTOMY. Surgical removal of the gallbladder.

CHOLECYSTITIS. An abnormal condition in which the gallbladder is inflamed.

CHOLECYSTOSTOMY. An operation in which an

opening is made into the gallbladder, usually to allow its contents to drain.

CHOLEDOCHOSTOMY. An operation in which an opening is made into the common bile duct.

CHOLELITHIASIS. The presence of gallstones in the gallbladder or in one of the bile ducts.

CHORDOTOMY. Surgery in which the pain-conducting pathways of the spine are severed.

CHROMOSOME. Rod-shaped body located in the nucleus of a cell. These bodies carry the basic units of heredity from parent to child.

CHRONIC OBSTRUCTIVE PULMONARY DISEASE. COPD; a group of conditions characterized by an obstruction in the normal exchange of gases within the lungs.

CILIA. Hairlike projections of mucous membrane in various parts of the body.

CIRCULATION. Movement from place to place in a set course, such as the flow of blood in the body's blood vessels.

PULMONARY CIRCULATION. The flow of blood from the right side of the heart through the lungs to the left side of the heart.

SYSTEMIC CIRCULATION. The flow of blood from the left ventricle through the blood vessels of the body and back to the heart again; general circulation.

CLIMACTERIC. Menopause.

COBRA. Type of poisonous snake.

COLECTOMY. Removal of the colon.

COLIC. Abdominal pain caused by muscle spasm.

COLITIS. An inflammation of the colon.

MUCOUS COLITIS. That characterized by the passage of mucus.

ULCERATIVE COLITIS. That characterized by ulceration of the mucous membrane.

COLLAGEN. A supportive protein found in skin, bones, tendons, cartilages, and connective tissues.

COLOSTOMY. An operation in which an opening is made through the abdominal wall into the colon and an artificial anus is formed.

COLPORRHAPHY. An operation in which the vagina is repaired by suture.

ANTERIOR COLPORRHAPHY. One is which a cystocele is repaired.

POSTERIOR COLPORRHAPHY. One in which a rectocele is repaired.

COLPOSCOPY. Examination of the cervix and vagina with a magnifying instrument.

COMA. A state of unconsciousness from which the person cannot be aroused.

COMMISSUROTOMY. An operation in which a stenosed heart valve is made larger.

COMMON BILE DUCT. The tube formed by the hepatic and cystic ducts that leads to the duodenum.

COMMUNICATION. A process by which information is exchanged.

COMPENSATION. A defense mechanism in which anxiety is relieved by making up for a real or imagined personal lack or feeling of inadequacy by emphasizing some personal, social, or physical attribute.

COMPUTERIZED AXIAL TOMOGRAPHY. A type of x-ray during which a scanner moves systematically across the area being studied taking views with an x-ray beam while a computer collects, analyzes, and makes a picture of varying amounts of x-ray absorbed by the tissue. The result is detailed cross sectional views of the area being studied; also known by the initials CT scan or CAT scan.

CONCUSSION. Pertains to a severe shaking or jarring of a part of the body. The term is often used in referring to the condition that follows a fall or a blow on the head resulting in either partial or complete loss of consciousness.

CONDYLOMATA ACCUMINATA. Venereal warts; warts caused by a virus. The warts are usually found on the genitalia and around the anus.

CONGENITAL DEFECT. Abnormal developmental condition present at birth.

CONGESTION. An abnormal amount of blood in a part of the body.

CONGESTIVE HEART FAILURE. A condition in which the heart is unable to pump blood properly. This results in an abnormal collection of fluid in various parts of the body. Cardiac failure; cardiac decompensation.

CONIZATION. Removal of tissue by the use of electricity, especially of the cervix.

CONJUNCTIVA. The mucous membrane that lines the eyelids and covers the front part of the eyeball.

CONJUNCTIVITIS. An inflammatory condition of the conjunctiva.

CONSTIPATION. A condition in which the person has fewer stools than usual. There is a longer period of time between bowel movements.

ATONIC CONSTIPATION. Type associated with decreased muscle tone of the colon.

SPASTIC CONSTIPATION. Type associated with increased muscle tone of the colon.

CONVERSION. A defense mechanism in which the person expresses strong emotional conflicts through physical symptoms.

CONVULSION. Involuntary contractions of the muscles.

CORAL SNAKE. Type of poisonous snake.

CORONARY ARTERIES. The blood vessels that supply the heart with blood.

CORONARY OCCLUSION. A heart attack caused by closure of a coronary artery that nourishes the heart; coronary thrombosis; myocardial infarction; "a coronary."

CORTEX. The external or outer layer of an organ or some other part of the body.

COUGH. A violent, involuntary exhalation of air following a deep inspiration.

CRANIUM. The bony case that protects the brain and its meninges; skull.

CRETINISM. Hypothyroidism that started during fetal life or early infancy.

CRISIS. A turning point.

CRYOSURGERY. Use of extreme cold to destroy tissue.

CULDOSCOPY. Examination of the uterus, oviducts, and some of the surrounding tissue following incision into the upper portion of the vagina. The examination is performed with an instrument having a light on the end.

CULTURE. 1. Pertaining to the growth of microorganisms on an artificial nutrient substance, such as bouillon, agar, gelatin, or blood serum. Microorganisms from the throat, blood, urine, and other parts or secretions of the body are grown frequently in the laboratory to determine the cause of illness. 2. Patterns of group behavior, values, language, art, and rituals that are transmitted from one generation to the next.

CYANOSIS. A bluish color of the skin and mucous membranes caused by an inadequate amount of oxygen in the hemoglobin of the blood.

CYST. An abnormal sac that contains liquid or semifluid material.

CYSTECTOMY. 1. The surgical removal of the urinary bladder or the gallbladder.
2. The surgical removal of a cyst.

CYSTIC DUCT. The tube leading from the gallbladder.

CYSTITIS. An inflammation of the urinary bladder.

CYSTOCELE. A condition in which the urinary bladder has prolapsed into the vagina.

CYSTOSCOPE. An instrument used by the doctor to examine and to treat conditions of the urinary bladder, ureters, and kidneys.

CYSTOTOMY. An operation in which an incision is made into the bladder.

CYTOLOGY. Study of cells, especially their structure, function, and origin.

DEAFNESS. A loss of hearing that may be either partial or complete.
  CONDUCTIVE DEAFNESS. That which occurs when the sound waves do not reach the inner ear properly.
  PERCEPTIVE DEAFNESS. That which occurs when the sound waves go through the middle ear properly but are not received properly by the brain.

DÉBRIDMENT. Removal of eschar.

DECOMPRESSION. The removal of pressure; especially the surgical relief of intracranial pressure.

DEFECATION. Evacuation or emptying the contents of the rectum.

DEFIBRILLATION. Administration of an electrical shock to the chest wall to stop all electrical activity in the heart. The hope is that a less harmful rhythm will develop instead.

DEFORMITY. An abnormal size or shape of the body or a part of the body.

DEGENERATION. Progressive deterioration of the body's cells often associated with the aging process. It results in a loss of the cell's ability to function effectively.

DEHISCENCE. The act of splitting; separation of the edges of an incision.

DEHYDRATION. An abnormal loss of water from the body's tissues.

DELIRIUM TREMENS. An acute psychotic state following a prolonged drinking period.

DENIAL. A defense mechanism in which the person refuses to face some part of reality.

DEOXYRIBONUCLEIC ACID. Complex protein in chromosomes that is considered the chemical carrier of genetic information; DNA.

DEPRESSION. A state of feeling sad.

DERMABRASION. Surgical planing of the layers of the skin through the epidermis and dermis to level a scar.

DERMATITIS. A general term used to indicate an inflammation of the skin.

DERMATOLOGIST. A physician specializing in dermatology.

DERMATOLOGY. The branch of medicine dealing with the structure and function of the skin, its diseases, and the treatment of persons with these diseases.

DERMOID CYST. A sac containing different kinds of tissues, such as teeth and hair; teratoma.

DESENSITIZATION. Method of treating a patient with an allergy; hyposensitization. An extract of the allergen is given to the patient in an effort to help him to build up a tolerance to that substance or to become less sensitive to it.

DIABETES INSIPIDUS. A disorder associated with production of a decreased amount of antidiuretic hormone by the posterior lobe of the pituitary gland.

DIAGNOSIS. A statement or conclusion about the nature or cause of disease.

DIATHERMY. The use of a machine that sends an electric current into the tissues below the skin to produce local heat.

DILATATION AND CURETTAGE. An operation in which the cervix is dilated and the lining of the uterus is scraped with a curette; D and C.

DIPLOCOCCI. Oval-shaped bacteria that grow in pairs.

DISORIENTATION.   Loss of proper bearings or a mental state of confusion regarding identity of self and others, place, or time.

DIURETIC.   A substance that increases the output of urine.

DIVERTICULITIS.   An inflammation of a diverticulum.

DIVERTICULUM.   A pouch or sac branching off from a structure. For example, a diverticulum may be located in the esophagus, the stomach, or the intestine.

DUODENUM.   The upper part of the small intestine, beginning at the stomach.

DYSMENORRHEA.   Painful menstruation.

DYSPEPSIA.   Indigestion.

DYSPHAGIA.   Difficult swallowing, or an inability to swallow.

DYSPNEA.   Difficult breathing, or shortness of breath.

ECCHYMOSIS.   Small hemorrhagic, nonelevated spots in the skin or mucous membrane presenting a bluish or purplish appearance.

ECHOCARDIOGRAM.   A test to determine the size, shape, and position of cardiac structures utilizing ultrasound.

ECHOGRAM.   The use of ultrasound waves that are transmitted to certain parts of the body and reflected back to a special receiver that records the patterns of waves.

EDEMA.   Collection of fluid in the tissue; dropsy.

ELECTRICAL SHOCK.   Shock experienced by an individual when an electric current passes through the body.

ELECTRICITY.   Form of energy caused by electrons flowing through a conductor.

DYNAMIC ELECTRICITY.   Moving electrons along a conductor, as in motors, generators, and batteries.

STATIC ELECTRICITY.   Buildup of nonmoving electric charges on the surface of nonconductors.

ELECTROCARDIOGRAM.   ECG; EKG; graphic measurement of electric currents generated by the conduction system within the heart.

ELECTROENCEPHALOGRAM.   EEG; A tracing or graphic record of the electrical waves of the brain.

ELECTROLYTE.   Chemical found in body fluids that has the ability to carry an electric charge.

EMBOLISM.   The obstruction of a blood vessel by an abnormal particle that has been circulating in the bloodstream.

CEREBRAL EMBOLISM.   That which occurs in a blood vessel of the brain.

PULMONARY EMBOLISM.   That which occurs in a blood vessel in the lungs.

EMBOLUS.   An abnormal particle, such as a blood clot or clumps of bacteria, that circulates in the bloodstream until it lodges in a blood vessel and causes embolism.

EMERGENCY.   An unexpected, sudden occasion frequently associated with an accident. The person involved in an emergency has a pressing or urgent need for care.

EMOTIONS.   A person's feelings, such as love, hate, fear, anxiety, worry, anger, jealousy, disgust, depression, and joy.

EMPHYSEMA.   A chronic disease of the lungs characterized by an abnormal enlargement of the air spaces associated with destruction.

EMPYEMA.   A collection of pus in an organ, a cavity, or a hollow space. For example, pus may form in the pleural cavity or the gallbladder.

ENCEPHALOGRAPHY.   X-ray examination of the brain after some of the cerebrospinal fluid has been replaced by air or oxygen.

ENDOCARDITIS.   An inflammatory condition of the endocardium.

BACTERIAL ENDOCARDITIS.   That caused by bacteria.

ENDOCARDIUM.   The membrane lining the inside of the heart.

ENDOCERVICITIS.   An inflammation of the membrane lining the cervix; cervicitis.

ENDOMETRIUM.   The mucous membrane that lines the inside of the uterus.

ENDOSCOPY.   An examination of a part of the body through an instrument.

ENDOTOXIN.   A poisonous substance stored within a living microorganism and given off after this organism dies.

ENTEROSTOMAL THERAPIST.   Specialist in the care of ostomates.

ENTEROSTOMY.   An operation in which an artificial opening is made into the intestine through the abdominal wall.

EPICARDIUM.   Innermost layer of the pericardium.

EPIDIDYMITIS.   An inflammation of the epididymis usually caused by bacterial infection.

EPILEPSY.   An abnormal condition in which the person has an increased discharge of energy from the brain at various times. This abnormal discharge of energy may cause loss of consciousness, convulsions, or both.

EPISTAXIS.   Nosebleed.

ERUCTATION.   Burping or belching.

ERYTHROPOIESIS.   Formation of red blood cells.

ESCHAR.   Dead or sloughing tissue.

ESOPHAGEAL SPEECH.   A method of speaking by swallowing air and producing sound when the air is forced back from the stomach. It is used by a patient who has had a laryngectomy.

ESOPHAGOSCOPY.   A procedure done by the physician to enable him to visualize the mucous membrane of the esophagus with an endoscope.

ESTROGENIC HORMONE. A substance produced mainly by an ovarian follicle and causing changes in the uterine mucosa; follicular hormonel; estrone; THEELIN.

EVISCERATION. Removal of protrusion of abdominal organs through the incision; disembowelment.

EXOPHTHALMOS. An abnormal protrusion of the eyeballs.

EXOTOXIN. A poisonous substance excreted by a living microorganism.

EXPIRATION. Act of forcing air out of the lungs; exhalation.

EXTENSOR. A muscle used to straighten a part of the body.

EXTRACORPOREAL. Taking place outside of the body.

FARSIGHTEDNESS. *See* Hypermetropia.

FEAR. A feeling of being frightened. The reason for the feeling usually is known.

FENESTRATION. An operation in which an opening is made in the bone covering the inner ear. This opening is covered by tympanic membrane. Sound waves are then transmitted from the tympanic membrane to the inner ear.

FEVER. A rise in the body's temperature above normal.

FEVER BLISTERS. *See* Herpes simplex.

FIBRILLATION. An abnormal uncoordinated contraction of muscles.

FIBRINOGEN. A substance in the blood necessary for clotting.

FIBROMYOMA. A tumor of a muscle in which muscle tissue and white fibers are intermingled. It is frequently found in the uterus.

FIRST AID. The immediate care given to a person with a pressing or urgent need until more specific medical assistance can be obtained.

FLATULENCE. The presence of gas in the gastrointestinal tract.

FLEXOR. A muscle used to bend a part of the body.

FLUOROSCOPY. Special x-ray technique used to facilitate visualization of certain body parts during motion.

FOLLICLE-STIMULATING HORMONE. A substance secreted by the anterior part of the pituitary gland. This hormone stimulates follicles to grow in the female and aids in the development of mature germ cells in the male.

FOMITE. An object capable of harboring pathogenic microorganisms from one person and transmitting them to others.

FOOTDROP. A condition in which the foot falls. The foot is bent downward in an abnormal position.

FRACTURE. A broken bone.

FROSTBITE. An injury to tissue caused by exposure to low environmental temperature.

FULGURATION. The destruction of tissue by the use of electric sparks.

GALLBLADDER. A pear-shaped organ located under the liver for the storage of bile.

GANGRENE. Death of a portion of the body.

GASTRECTOMY. An operation in which part or all of the stomach is removed. The procedure is frequently called partial or subtotal gastrectomy when part of the stomach is removed.

GASTRIC GAVAGE. A method of giving liquid nourishment by means of a tube inserted through the throat and esophagus into the stomach. The tube may be passed through either the nose or the mouth to the throat.

GASTRIC LAVAGE. Washing out or irrigation of the stomach.

GASTROSCOPE. An instrument used to examine the inside of the stomach.

GASTROSCOPY. An endoscopic examination of the mucous membrane of the stomach, pylorus, and upper portion of the duodenum.

GASTROSTOMY. A permanent, artificial opening into the stomach.

GENE. Biologic unit of heredity located on definite places on the chromosome.

GENETICS. A branch of biology dealing with heredity and its relationship to variations in organisms.

GIGANTISM. Giantism; disorder of abnormal growth caused by hyperpituitarism.

GLAUCOMA. An eye disease in which the pressure within the eyeball is increased.

GLOMERULONEPHRITIS. An inflammation of the kidneys that involves the glomeruli.

GLYCOGEN. Form of sugar stored by the liver.

GLYCOSURIA. A condition in which sugar is present in the urine.

GOITER. An enlarged thyroid gland.

GOUT. A disease characterized by a disturbance of purine metabolism.

GRAAFIAN FOLLICLE. A small sac containing an ovum in the ovary; a mature ovarian follicle.

GRAND MAL SEIZURE. An attack of epilepsy characterized by loss of consciousness and a generalized convulsion.

GUMMA. A lesion that develops in a person with late syphilis.

GYNECOLOGIST. A physician specializing in gynecology.

GYNECOLOGY. A branch of medical science dealing with diseases of women, especially those of the reproductive organs.

HEAT CRAMPS. Painful muscle spasms following strenuous exercise during hot weather; heat exhaustion.

HEAT PROSTRATION. Vasomotor collapse caused by loss of fluid and sodium during vigorous exercise in hot weather.

HEMATEMESIS. Vomiting of blood.

HEMATOMA. A collection of clotted blood that readily becomes enclosed in a capsule.

HEMATURIA. The presence of blood in the urine.

HEMIPLEGIA. Paralysis affecting one side of the body.

HEMODIALYSIS. Removal of certain waste products from the blood with a semipermeable membrane.

HEMOGLOBIN. The coloring matter in red blood cells. It has the vital function of picking up oxygen and releasing it to the body's cells.

HEMOPHILIA. A disease characterized by a prolonged time for the blood to clot. This is a rare hereditary disease that occurs only in males but is transmitted only through females.

HEMOPTYSIS. The expectoration of blood from the respiratory tract.

HEMORRHOIDECTOMY. Surgical removal of hemorrhoids.

HEMORRHOIDS. Varicose veins of the anal canal and lower part of the rectum.
  EXTERNAL HEMORRHOIDS. Those located around the anal orifice.
  INTERNAL HEMORRHOIDS. Those located in the area of the junction of the anal canal and the rectum.

HEMOTHORAX. Collection of blood in the pleural space.

HEPATIC DUCT. The tube through which bile leaves the liver.

HEPATITIS. An abnormal condition in which the liver is inflamed.

HERNIA. An abnormal protrusion of part of the contents of a cavity through its wall; rupture.
  CONGENITAL HERNIA. One that is present at birth.
  INCISIONAL HERNIA. One that develops in an operative scar; ventral hernia.
  INGUINAL HERNIA. A protrusion of part of the abdominal contents through the inguinal canal in the groin.
  IRREDUCIBLE HERNIA. One that cannot be forced back into the cavity by gentle pressure.
  REDUCIBLE HERNIA. One that can be forced back into the cavity by gentle pressure.
  UMBILICAL HERNIA. An abnormal protrusion of part of the abdominal contents through the umbilicus.

HERNIORRHAPHY. An operation in which a hernia is repaired.

HERPES. A condition in which either the skin or mucous membrane is inflamed, and tiny blisters filled with fluid form.

HERPES SIMPLEX. That which is believed to be caused by a virus and occurs frequently about the lips; fever blisters.

HERPES ZOSTER. That which occurs along the course of a nerve and is associated with neuralgic pain; shingles.

HODGKIN'S DISEASE. An abnormal condition of the lymph nodes.

HOMEOSTASIS. Ability of the body to regulate and maintain a constant desirable internal environment.

HORDEOLUM. A stye.

HORMONE. A substance produced by an organ or a certain group of cells and carried by the blood to another part of the body where it has a specific effect on a target organ. For example, one hormone produced by the pituitary gland in the head is carried by the blood to the ovaries where it stimulates a follicle to develop. Another example is seen in the thyroid gland in the neck which secretes thyroxine. This hormone is carried by the blood to the body's cells to control their metabolism.

HYDROCELE. An abnormal accumulation of fluid in a sac within the scrotum.

HYDRONEPHROSIS. An abnormal collection of urine in the pelvis of the kidney because of an obstruction in the urinary tract.

HYDROTHERAPY. The use of water in the treatment of a patient.

HYPERCORTICISM. Overactive adrenal cortex.

HYPERGLYCEMIA. An increased amount of sugar in the blood.

HYPERIMMUNIZATION. Treatment of an individual with an allergy by building up tolerance to the involved allergen.

HYPERMETROPIA. A condition characterized by the ability to see objects better when they are at a distance; farsightedness.

HYPERTENSION. High blood pressure.
  ESSENTIAL HYPERTENSION. That occurring without a known cause; primary hypertension.
  MALIGNANT ESSENTIAL HYPERTENSION. A severe rapidly progressing case occurring without a known cause.

HYPERTENSIVE HEART DISEASE. Disease of the heart resulting from high blood pressure.

HYPERTHYROIDISM. An abnormal condition in which the thyroid gland is overactive; toxic goiter.

HYPERTROPHY. An abnormal increase in the size of an organ or a part.

HYPNOTIC. An agent that induces sleep.

HYPODERMOCLYSIS. The injection of a large amount of fluid into the tissue beneath the skin; subcutaneous infusion.

HYPOGLYCEMIA. A decreased amount of sugar in the blood.

HYPOKALEMIA. Low blood level of potassium.

HYPOPHYSIS. Pituitary gland; hypophyseal gland.

HYPOSENSITIZATION. Desensitization.

HYPOTHERMIA. Lowered body temperature. Hypothermia may be used as an anesthetic.

HYPOTHYROIDISM. An abnormal condition in which the thyroid gland is underactive.

HYPOVOLEMIA. Reduced blood volume.

HYPOXIA. Oxygen deficiency.

HYSTERECTOMY. Surgical removal of all or part of the uterus.

   ABDOMINAL HYSTERECTOMY. Removal is done through an incision in the abdomen.

   VAGINAL HYSTERECTOMY. Removal is done through the vagina.

IATROGENIC DISEASE. An abnormal condition caused by the physician in an effort to treat the patient.

ILEOCECAL VALVE. A muscular structure located between the small and large intestine which prevents material from returning to the small intestine.

ILEOSTOMY. An operation in which an artificial opening is made into the ileum through the abdominal wall.

ILEUM. The lower part of the small intestine leading from the jejunum to the large intestine.

ILIUM. The broad upper part of the hipbone.

IMMUNITY. The state of being resistant to disease.

IMPETIGO CONTAGIOSA. An infectious disease of the skin that may be caused by streptococci and staphylococci. Vesicles, pustules, and crusts form on the affected area.

INCENTIVE SPIROMETRY. Use of a machine with various-colored lights that become visible when the patient blows air into the mouthpiece. The patient is encouraged to increase respiratory strength by lighting increasingly higher lights with each breath.

INCONTINENCE. Loss of the control of natural evacuations, especially involuntary micturition and/or defecation.

INDWELLING CATHETER. A hollow tube left in the patient's bladder for drainage of urine; retention catheter.

INFECTION. Inflammatory process caused by a pathogen.

INFLAMMATION. A defensive reaction of the body to any injury.

INFUSION. The introduction of fluid into a vein by gravity.

INJURY. Damage or harm to the body produced by such factors as a blow, a foreign body, a chemical, electricity, heat, cold, or a pathogen.

INSPECTION. The process of looking for abnormalities that can be seen with the eyes. Certain instruments, such as an otoscope or ophthalmoscope, may be used to visualize smaller areas such as the eye and ear.

INSPIRATION. Act of taking air into the lungs; inhalation.

INTESTINAL OBSTRUCTION. An abnormal condition in which there is a hindrance to the normal flow of contents within the intestines.

INTESTINAL RESECTION. Surgical removal of part of the intestine.

INTRAVENOUS. Within the veins.

INTRAVENOUS HYPERALIMENTATION. Administration of a concentrated solution of dextrose containing amino acids, vitamins, and electrolytes into a large blood vessel having a high blood flow. The purpose of this administration is nutrition.

INTUSSUSCEPTION. The slipping of one part into another, especially the slipping of one portion of the intestine into another.

ISCHEMIC. Having an inadequate blood supply.

ISCHIORECTAL ABSCESS. An abscess in the soft tissue near the anus or the rectum.

ISOLATION. Separation of an individual from other persons because of an infectious disease or to protect an individual having a decrease in defense mechanisms.

JAUNDICE. Yellowness of the skin, eyes, mucous membranes, and body secretions caused by bile pigments in the blood.

   HEMOLYTIC JAUNDICE. That which occurs when the destruction of red blood cells is abnormally fast.

   NONOBSTRUCTIVE JAUNDICE. That which occurs when the liver cells are damaged and are unable to eliminate bile pigments properly.

   OBSTRUCTIVE JAUNDICE. That which occurs when the flow of bile through either the common bile duct or the hepatic duct is blocked.

JEJUNUM. The middle part of the small intestine, beginning at the duodenum and ending at the ileum.

KELOID. Overgrowth of connective tissue at site of a scar or injury.

KERATOPLASTY. Plastic surgery of the cornea, especially a corneal transplant.

LACRIMAL GLAND. A gland located above the eye that produces tears; tear gland.

LAMINECTOMY. An operation in which part of the vertebrae covering the spinal cord is removed.

LAPAROSCOPY. Passage of an instrument to permit visualization within the abdominal cavity.

The instrument is inserted through a small incision in the abdominal wall.

LAPAROTOMY. An operation in which an incision is made through the abdominal wall.

EXPLORATORY LAPAROTOMY. That which is done to allow the surgeon to search for the diseased area.

LARYNGOSCOPE. A hollow, lighted instrument used to permit visualization of the larynx. It also may be used for removal of a foreign body in the airway.

LARYNGOSCOPY. Examination of the larynx using a lighted mirror that is held in the pharynx.

LAXATIVE. An agent that causes excretion of a soft, formed stool.

LEUKEMIA. A group of diseases in which there is an abnormal increase of white blood cells.

LEUKOCYTOSIS. An abnormal increase in the number of white blood cells.

LEUKOPENIA. An abnormal decrease in the number of white blood cells.

LEUKOPLAKIA. White, thickened, plaquelike lesions of the vulva.

LEUKORRHEA. A vaginal discharge.

LIFE-STYLE. An individual's usual way of living.

LIGHTNING. Discharge of atmospheric electricity from one cloud to another or from a cloud to the ground.

LIPID. An organic substance that is not soluble in water, but is soluble in such substances as ether and alcohol, that serves as a source of fuel, and that feels greasy.

LOBECTOMY. Removal of a lobe of an organ. The term is often used in referring to removal of a lobe of the lung.

LOCOMOTOR SYSTEM. Parts of the body concerned with motion, especially bones, muscles, and joints; the muscular and skeletal systems.

LUMBAR PUNCTURE. A procedure in which the physician inserts a needle between two of the lumbar vertebrae into the spinal canal to remove cerebrospinal fluid, in order to determine the pressure of the fluid, or to inject medication; also called spinal tap or spinal puncture.

LUTEINIZING HORMONE. A substance produced by the anterior part of the pituitary gland. This hormone stimulates the corpus luteum to develop and to produce progesterone in the female. It also stimulates the testis in the male to produce testicular hormones.

LYMPHOGRAPHY. X-ray visualization of the lymphatic system from the level of the second lumbar vertebra to the toes following injection of a radiopaque dye.

LYMPHOMA. A tumor or neoplastic disorder of the lymphoid tissue. The term is frequently used to indicate a malignant tumor.

MACRO SHOCK. Flow of electric current through a large area of the body.

MACULE. A discolored, unelevated spot on the skin.

MALAISE. A general and indefinite feeling of discomfort or illness.

MALIGNANCY. Threatening to a person's life, such as cancer.

MAMMOGRAPHY. X-ray examination of the breast.

MASTECTOMY. Removal of the breast and nipple.

EXTENDED RADICAL MASTECTOMY. Radical mastectomy and removal of a portion of the sternum and ends of the ribs overlying internal mammary lymph nodes.

MODIFIED RADICAL MASTECTOMY. Removal of breast, pectoral fascia, and lymph nodes of the axilla.

RADICAL MASTECTOMY. Removal of the breast, pectoral muscles, and lymph nodes of the axilla.

MASTITIS. An inflammatory condition of the breast.

MASTOIDECTOMY. The surgical removal of part or all of the mastoid air cells.

MASTOIDITIS. An inflammation of the air cells in the portion of the temporal bone behind the ear that is known as the mastoid.

MEATUS URETHRAE. The opening of the urethra.

MEDULLA. The middle or inner portion of an organ or body structure.

MENINGES. The membranes covering the brain and spinal cord.

MENINGITIS. An inflammatory condition of the membranes covering the brain, the spinal cord, or both.

MENOPAUSE. The period in a woman's life when menstruation stops; climacteric.

MENORRHAGIA. Excessive menstruation.

MENSTRUATION. The normal, periodic discharge of bloody fluid from the uterus; catamenia.

MENTAL MECHANISMS. Common methods of adjusting to stress; defense mechanisms.

METABOLISM. Process by which foodstuffs are used to produce energy, changed into tissue elements, and stored in the body's cells; changes that occur to food from the time it is digested until it is eliminated.

METASTASIS. Transfer of disease from one area of the body to another.

METRORRHAGIA. Uterine bleeding between menstrual periods.

MICROORGANISM. A tiny body visible only through a microscope.

MICRO SHOCK. Passage of electrical current through a small area of the body.

MICTURITION. The act of discharging urine from the bladder; urination; voiding.

MILK LEG. Thrombophlebitis.

MULTIPLE SCLEROSIS. An abnormal condition in which the person has areas of degeneration in the brain and spinal cord. These areas are replaced by scar tissue. Parts of the body receiving their nerve supply from the diseased areas have disturbed function.

MURMUR. An abnormal heart sound heard by the doctor with a stethoscope.

MYASTHENIA GRAVIS. A syndrome characterized by muscle weakness.

MYCETISMUS. Mushroom poisoning.

MYELIN. The fatty substance that forms a sheath of covering around nerve fibers.

MYELOGRAM. X-ray study of vertebral column following injection of a gas, air, or a radiopaque dye into the spinal cord.

MYOCARDIUM. Muscle tissue of the heart.

MYOPIA. A condition characterized by the ability to see objects better at close range; nearsightedness.

MYRINGOTOMY. An operation in which an opening is made into the tympanic membrane.

MYXEDEMA. An advanced form of hypothyroidism in adults.

NARCOTIC. A substance that produces stupor or insensibility.

NAUSEA. A feeling of discomfort in the region of the stomach and a tendency to vomit.

NEARSIGHTEDNESS. *See* Myopia.

NEOPLASM. A new growth or an abnormal growth of cells; tumor.

NEPHRECTOMY. The surgical removal of a kidney.

NEPHRITIS. An inflammatory condition of the kidneys.

NEPHROLITHIASIS. Kidney stones.

NEPHROLITHOTOMY. The surgical removal of a stone from the kidney through an incision into that organ.

NEPHROTOMY. An operation in which an incision is made into the kidney.

NEURALGIA. Pain along the course of one or more nerves.

NEURITIS. An inflammatory condition of one or more nerves.

NEUROLOGIST. A physician specializing in neurology.

NEUROLOGY. The branch of medicine dealing with the structure and function of the nervous system, its diseases, and the treatment of persons with these diseases.

NOCTURIA. Increased voiding at night.

NURSING INTERVENTION. Taking deliberative action in response to nursing observation(s), the patient's request, and/or the physician's orders.

NURSING OBSERVATION. Comprehensive systematic noticing of the patient, family, and the related environment; leads to one or more nursing interventions.

OLIGURIA. Decrease in the amount of urine produced.

OOPHORECTOMY. Surgical removal of an ovary.

OOPHORITIS. An inflammation of either one or both ovaries.

OPHTHALMIA NEONATORUM. A gonorrheal infection of a newborn baby's eyes.

OPHTHALMOLOGIST. A physician specializing in ophthalmology; oculist.

OPHTHALMOLOGY. The branch of medicine dealing with the structure and function of the eyes, its diseases, and the treatment of persons with these diseases.

OPHTHALMOSCOPE. An instrument used to examine the inside of the eye.

OPTICIAN. An individual who makes lenses according to the doctor's recommendation.

OPTOMETRIST. An individual licensed to measure the visual powers of a person without the use of drugs.

ORCHIECTOMY. Removal of one or both testes.

ORTHOPEDICS. The branch of surgery concerned with the treatment of a patient with a deformity, a disease, or an ailment of the locomotor system.

ORTHOPEDIST. A physician specializing in orthopedics.

ORTHOPNEA. A condition in which the patient must sit up in order to breathe.

OSCILLOMETER. An instrument used to measure the amount of blood pumped to the extremity with each heartbeat.

OSTEOMYELITIS. An inflammation of the bone that frequently involves the marrow.

OSTEOPOROSIS. A condition in which the bones become more porous resulting in easy fractures.

OSTOMATE. An individual with an artificial opening, especially in the colon.

OTITIS MEDIA. An inflammatory process of the middle ear.

OTOLOGIST. A physician specializing in otology.

OTOLOGY. The branch of medicine dealing with the structure and function of the ear, its diseases, and the treatment of persons with these diseases.

OTOSCLEROSIS. An abnormal growth of new bone usually around the oval window between the middle ear and inner ear. This results in progressive loss of hearing.

OTOSCOPE. An instrument used to examine the

external auditory canal and the tympanic membrane.

PAIN. A complex personal experience of hurt involving physical sensations, feelings and thoughts, and behavioral response; affects the whole person.

PAIN, REFERRED. The presence of pain in an area of the body that is not the diseased place.

PALLIATIVE. Helping to relieve without curing.

PALPATION. The process of feeling with the fingers for abnormal growths and/or swelling.

PALPITATION. An awareness of heart action that may appear to be fast or fluttering.

PANCREATITIS. An inflammatory condition of the pancreas.

PANCREOZYMIN. A hormone secreted by the mucosa of the duodenum that stimulates the secretion of pancreatic juice.

PANHYSTERECTOMY. Removal of the entire uterus.

PAPANICOLAOU SMEAR. Microscopic examination of the body's secretions to determine presence of malignant cells; cytologic test for cancer.

PAPILLEDEMA. An abnormal condition in which the optic nerve becomes edematous; choked disk.

PAPULE. A small, rounded, raised area on the skin.

PARAFFIN-DIP TREATMENT. The use of melted paraffin for the application of heat.

PARALYSIS. Loss of muscle function often caused by injury to the nervous system.

PARALYSIS AGITANS. A chronic disease of the nervous system. Parkinson's disease; shaking palsy; parkinsonism.

PARALYTIC ILEUS. Loss of muscle function of the intestines; adynamic ileus.

PARAPLEGIA. Paralysis of the legs.

PARENTERAL. Outside of the gastrointestinal tract.

PARESIS. A slight loss of muscle function.

GENERAL PARESIS. A late form of syphilis in which the nervous system is affected. The patient has mental changes, tremors, and difficulty in talking.

PAROXYSMAL. A sudden return or recurrence of symptoms.

PAROXYSMAL ATRIAL TACHYCARDIA. Pulse rate of approximately 150 to 200 beats per minute. The impulse initiating the heartbeat starts in the area of the atrium other than the sinus node.

PATHOGEN. An agent that causes disease, usually a microorganism.

PEDICLE. A slender projection that acts as a stem.

PERCUSSION. The process of tapping body surfaces to produce sounds that are interpreted by the examiner.

PERENNIAL. Occuring throughout the year or for more than one year.

PERFUSION. Passing fluid through blood vessels of a specific organ or part of the body; pouring a liquid over or through some part of the body.

PERICARDIAL TAP. Withdrawal of fluid from the pericardium with a needle; paracentesis of the pericardium.

PERICARDIUM. Membranous sac covering the heart.

PERINEORRHAPHY. An operation in which the perineum is repaired by suture.

PERINEUM. 1. The part of the body between the pubic arch in the front and the coccyx in the back.
2. The portion of the body between the vulva and the anus in the female and between the scrotum and the anus in the male.

PERIOSTEUM. A membrane that covers most of the surface of a bone.

PERISTALSIS. Wormlike wave of contraction in hollow, muscular tubes, such as the intestine. This motion forces the contents of the tube toward its opening.

PERITONEAL CAVITY. The space between the two layers of the peritoneum that may become a cavity.

PERITONEUM. Serous membrane covering the abdominal organs.

PERITONITIS. An inflammation of the peritoneum.

PESSARY. An appliance that is fitted into the vagina.

PETIT MAL SEIZURE. An attack of epilepsy characterized mainly by a loss of consciousness for a short period of time.

PHLEBITIS. A condition in which a vein is inflamed.

PHONOCARDIOGRAM. Permanent written record of the heart sounds heard by the stethoscope.

PHYSICAL THERAPY. Treatment of a patient by use of physical agents and special procedures, such as message and exercise. Heat, cold, and electricity are examples of physical agents.

PIGMENTED NEVUS. Mole.

PIT VIPER. Type of poisonous snake with folding fangs and a pit or depression on each side of its head.

PLEURA. Serous membrane covering the lungs.

PLEURISY. An inflammation of the pleura. It is called "pleurisy with effusion" when fluid collects in the pleural cavity.

PNEUMOENCEPHALOGRAM. X-ray study of the ventricles of the brain following the injection of air into the spinal cord; air encephalogram.

PNEUMONECTOMY. Removal of an entire lung.

PNEUMONIA. An infection of the lungs causing the spongy lung tissue to become more solid.

BACTERIAL PNEUMONIA. That caused by bacteria.

BRONCHIAL PNEUMONIA. *See* Bronchopneumonia.

HYPOSTATIC PNEUMONIA. That caused by staying in one position too long.

LOBAR PNEUMONIA. An acute illness in which one or more lobes are involved.

PRIMARY ATYPICAL PNEUMONIA. Viral pneumonia.

PNEUMOPERITONEUM. 1. The injection of air into the peritoneal cavity for examination of the abdomen by x-ray or to push the diaphragm upward into the chest cavity causing the lung to collapse.
2. A collection of gas in the peritoneal cavity.

PNEUMOTHORAX. The presence of air in the pleural space.

POISON. Any substance that causes damage to the body or alters the function of a part of the body as a result of chemical action.

POLIOMYELITIS. An infectious disease caused by a filterable virus.

ACUTE ANTERIOR POLIOMYELITIS. A form in which the anterior portion of the gray matter in the spinal cord is affected. Muscles receiving their nerve supply from the diseased area may become weak and paralyzed.

BULBAR POLIOMYELITIS. A type in which the medulla of the brain is affected. The respiratory and circulatory centers may be involved.

POLLINOSIS. Hay fever, seasonal allergy induced by airborne pollens of trees, grasses, and weeds.

POLYCYTHEMIA VERA. Primary polycythemia; abnormal increase in the production of red blood cells, white blood cells, and platelets.

POLYDIPSIA. Extreme thirst.

POLYP. An abnormal growth of tissue that appears to be growing on a stalk.

POLYURIA. An excessive output of urine.

PREJUDICE. An opinion or belief about a person or subject based on incomplete knowledge.

PRESBYOPIA. Faulty vision in which the person can see distant objects better than close objects; occurs with the aging process.

PROCTOSCOPY. An examination of the rectum with a proctoscope.

PROGESTERONE. A substance produced by the corpus luteum. It causes changes in the uterine mucosa in preparation for the fertilized ovum.

PROGNOSIS. Prediction of the length, course, and outcome of a disease.

PROJECTION. A defense mechanism in which the individual unconsciously rejects an unacceptable idea or feeling and identifies it as coming from someone else.

PROSTATECTOMY. The surgical removal of part or all of the prostate gland.

PERINEAL PROSTATECTOMY. Removal through an incision in the perineum.

RETROPUBIC PROSTATECTOMY. Removal through an opening in the lower part of the abdomen. The surgeon reaches the gland by going behind the bladder.

SUPRAPUBIC PROSTATECTOMY. Removal through an incision in the bladder above the pubic region.

TRANSURETHRAL PROSTATECTOMY. Removal through a special cystoscope that has been inserted into the urethra.

PROSTHESIS. An artificial replacement for a missing part.

PROTOZOA. Microorganisms belonging to the animal kingdom.

PRURITUS. Itching.

PSITTACOSIS. An infection of the lungs caused by a microbial agent commonly found in birds.

PSYCHIATRIST. A physician specializing in psychiatry.

PSYCHIATRY. A branch of medicine dealing with the treatment of patients with mental disorders.

PSYCHOMOTOR SEIZURE. An attack of epilepsy characterized by temporary mental disturbances.

PSYCHOSOMATIC MEDICINE. A special branch of medicine that emphasizes the close relationship between the mind and the body of an individual.

PSYCHOTHERAPY. Treatment of an individual's mind.

PULMONARY ECHOGRAM. An examination in which ultrasound waves are transmitted to the lungs and reflected to a special receiver that records the echoes.

PULSE DEFICIT. A decreased pulse count of the radial artery when compared with the pulse counted at the apex of the heart.

RABIES. Hydrophobia. A acute viral infection of the central nervous system transmitted to man from the saliva of an infected animal.

RADIATION SICKNESS. Illness following radiotherapy. It also may follow exposure to radiant energy, such as that associated with explosion of an atomic bomb.

RADIOCARDIOGRAPHY. Tests involving use of radioactive isotopes following intravenous injection. Arrival and flow of blood containing the radioactive isotopes in the heart are measured with a special counter.

RADIOTHERAPY. Treatment of disease by the use of rays, such as x-ray and radium; radiation therapy.

RADIUM. Metallic element that gives off rays. For this reason, it is referred to as radioactive.

RADON. A gas given off by radium.

RADON SEED. Tiny tube filled with the gas given off by radium; radon implants. These tubes may be placed in the body tissue as a treatment for cancer and other diseases.

RALE. Abnormal sound in air passages in the thoracic cavity.

RAPE. Forced penetration against a victim's consent; in some states defined as entry of any portion of the penis into the female genitalia.

RATIONALIZATION. A defense mechanism in which the person unconsciously finds a good reason for his behavior.

RECTOCELE. A condition in which the rectum has prolapsed into the vagina.

RECTUM. Lower portion of the large intestine, leading from the sigmoid colon to the anal canal.

REDUCTION. The replacement of a broken bone or a dislocated joint to its normal position.

    CLOSED REDUCTION. That which is done by external manipulation.

    OPEN REDUCTION. That which is done through a surgical incision.

REFRACTION. 1. The bending of rays.
2. The bending of light rays as they pass through substances that have different densities. Light rays are bent as they pass through the eye so that they will be focused properly on the retina.

REGRESSION. A defense mechanism in which a person returns to previous, more satisfying methods of coping with stress.

REHABILITATION. Assistance given to help a person in regaining the greatest amount of usefulness and maximum degree of health possible with his handicap.

REPRESSION. A defense mechanism in which the person excludes from his consciousness unbearable ideas, thoughts, and feelings.

RESECTION. An operation in which a section or segment of an organ is removed.

RESIDUAL URINE. An abnormal amount of urine left in the bladder after urination.

RESPIRATION. Process by which the living exchange gases with their environment; breathing.

    CHEYNE-STOKES RESPIRATION. A type of breathing in which the respirations show a gradual increase in depth and rate, followed by a gradual decrease in depth and rate, and then apnea. The cycle starts again after the apnea. This type of respiration also may be described as periods of deep snoring respirations interrupted by periods of apnea.

RHINITIS. Inflammation of the mucous membrane of the nose.

RHINOPLASTY. Surgical procedure to correct a nasal deformity using tissue from another part of the body or synthetic material.

RHIZOTOMY. Surgical severance of a sensory root as it enters the spinal cord to relieve pain.

ROENTGENOGRAM. Still picture showing structures such as bones and other body organs; x-ray.

SALMONELLOSIS. Food poisoning caused by the ingestion of food contaminated with microorganisms of the genus *Salmonella*.

SALPINGECTOMY. Surgical removal of a fallopian tube.

SALPINGITIS. An inflammation of the fallopian tubes.

SALPINGO-OOPHORECTOMY. Surgical removal of either one or both fallopian tubes and ovaries.

SARCOMA. Malignant tumor of connective tissue, such as bone, cartilage, fat, and tendons.

SCABIES. Infection caused by a crab-shaped mite.

SCAN. A procedure in which a radioactive substance is introduced into the patient's body to facilitate location of a tumor. A machine is used to detect the location of the radioactive substance.

SCIATICA. A condition in which the patient has pain along the course of the sciatic nerve.

SCLEROSIS. A hardening of certain body tissues, such as the arteries and nervous system.

SEASONAL. Related to the seasons of the year.

SECRETIN. A hormone secreted by the mucosa of the small intestine, which, in turn, stimulates secretion of pancreatic juice.

SEDATIVE. An agent that relieves excitement and anxiety.

SENESCENCE. A period in one's life during which time the greatest amount of aging occurs.

SERUM SICKNESS. Hypersensitivity reaction following administration of a serum or drug for the first time.

SEQUESTRECTOMY. Surgical removal of dead bone tissue.

SHOCK. A condition in which the patient has an insufficient amount of blood circulating in the body, especially the vessels in the outer part of the body. It may be caused by a marked dilation of the blood vessels or by an actual loss of blood.

SICKLE CELL ANEMIA. An hereditary form of hemolytic anemia.

SICKLING TEST. Blood test done to determine the presence of sickle hemoglobin.

SIGMOIDOSCOPY. An examination of the sigmoid part of the colon with an instrument, a sigmoidoscope.

SINUS TACHYCARDIA. Pulse rate of 100 to 150 beats per minute.

SPORE. A microorganism covered with a tough membrane that causes it to be more difficult to kill.

SPUTUM. Material raised from the tracheobronchial tree.

SPUR. An outgrowth of tissue.

STAPEDECTOMY. Removal of the small bone in the middle ear called the stapes.

STAPHYLOCOCCAL ENTEROTOXIN POISONING. Food poisoning caused by the ingestion of food contaminated by toxin previously formed from staphylococci.

STAPHYLOCOCCI. Oval-shaped bacteria that grow in grapelike clusters.

STEATORRHEA. An excessive loss of fats in fecal material.

STENOSIS. A narrowing of a portion of the body such as a cavity or a tube.

STEROID. Hormone secreted by the pituitary gland and/or cortex of the adrenal glands.

STOMA. An opening formed in the abdominal wall.

STOMATITIS. An inflammation of the mouth.

STRABISMUS. An abnormal condition of the eyes in which the person is unable to direct both eyes toward the same object. It is caused by a lack of coordination between the muscles controlling eye movement; also called squint.

STRANGULATION. 1. Constriction of an area that checks the normal flow of blood, such as strangulation of an obstructed part of the intestine. 2. An obstruction of the air passages resulting in an oxygen deficiency, such as choking a person by pressing on the trachea.

STREPTOCOCCI. Oval-shaped bacteria that grow in chain formation.

STRESSOR. Any agent inside or outside the body that influences homeostasis.

STYE. An acute inflammation on the edge of the eyelid; also called hordeolum.

SUBCUTANEOUS. Under the skin; hypodermic.

SUPPURATION. Process of pus formation.

SYMPATHECTOMY. Surgical removal of a part of the sympathetic nervous system.

SYMPTOM. A change in the body or functioning of the body that indicates disease or a change in the disease.

OBJECTIVE SYMPTOM. That which is seen, felt, heard, smelled, or determined by others.

SUBJECTIVE SYMPTOM. That which is felt by the patient.

SYNCOPE. Transient loss of consciousness caused by a decreased supply of blood to the brain.

SYNOVIA. Clear fluid found in various joints and bursae; also known as synovial fluid.

SYNOVIAL MEMBRANE. Tissue lining the capsule that protects freely movable joints.

TACHYCARDIA. Rapid heart action.

PAROXYSMAL TACHYCARDIA. That which occurs periodically.

TARANTULA. Hairy spider whose bite causes the victim to have severe local damage and pain.

TELANGIECTASIA. A fine, often irregular red line caused by dilation of a normally invisible capillary.

TENESMUS. Painful straining without having a bowel movement.

TEST(S). A special procedure or method of examination.

CONCENTRATION TEST. A type of kidney function test used to determine whether the kidneys are concentrating the urine properly.

ELIMINATION DIET TEST. Diet used as an aid in determining specific food to which a person is allergic.

INTRADERMAL TEST. A type of skin test in which substances are injected between the skin layers to determine specific causes of allergy.

KIDNEY FUNCTION TEST. Various types of tests designed to determine whether the kidneys are removing the proper amount of waste materials from the blood in the proper length of time.

OPHTHALMIC TEST. Procedure to determine substances to which a person is allergic. An allergen is dropped into the conjunctival sac. Redness and swelling of the membrane indicate that the patient is allergic to that substance.

PHENOLSULFONPHTHALEIN TEST. PSP test; a type of kidney function test in which phenolsulfonphthalein, a harmless red dye, is injected intravenously or intramuscularly. This dye, which is removed mainly by the kidneys, colors the urine. Urine specimens are collected at specific times after the dye is injected. The amount of dye in the urine is determined in the laboratory.

SCRATCH TEST. A type of skin test to determine substances to which a person is allergic. Known allergens are dropped into scratches on either the back or arm.

SENSITIVITY TEST. A laboratory procedure used to determine which antibiotics will be effective against microorganisms growing in a certain part of the patient's body.

SEROLOGY TEST. Laboratory examination of blood serum to diagnose syphilis.

SKIN TEST. Procedure to determine the reaction of skin, especially to an allergen. It is useful in determining substances to which a person is allergic. The known allergens may be injected between the skin layers, dropped into scratched areas, or placed on the skin.

TUBERCULIN TEST. A test to determine whether a person has or has had a tuberculosis infection.

TEST DOSE. Administration of a small amount of a drug that is likely to cause an allergic reaction before giving the full dose.

TETANUS. 1. State of continuous muscular contractions.

2. Lockjaw; an infectious disease caused by the bacillus *Clostridium tetani,* which grows only in the absence of oxygen. Bacilli enter the body through a puncture or penetrating wound. This infection causes the patient to have almost continuous muscle spasms and is often fatal.

TETANY. A condition in which a decreased amount of calcium in the blood results in muscular spasms.

THORACENTESIS. The withdrawal of fluid from the chest cavity; chest aspiration.

THORACOPLASTY. An operation in which portions of the ribs are removed to reduce the size of the chest wall. The procedure may be used in the treatment of pulmonary tuberculosis.

THORACOTOMY. An operation in which an incision is made into the thoracic cavity.

THROMBOANGIITIS OBLITERANS. A chronic disease of the blood vessels, especially in the legs of young men; Buerger's disease.

THROMBOCYTOPENIA. Hemorrhagic disease characterized by areas of bleeding located in the skin and mucous membranes.

THROMBOPHLEBITIS. A condition in which a vein is inflamed and a thrombus is formed; milk leg.

THROMBOSIS. The formation of a blood clot in the heart or a blood vessel.

CEREBRAL THROMBOSIS. That which occurs in a blood vessel in the brain.

THROMBUS. A blood clot that has been formed within a blood vessel or the heart.

THYROID CRISIS. An acute condition that may follow removal of the thyroid gland. It is characterized by fever, restlessness, profuse perspiration, and a rapid pulse.

THYROIDITIS. Inflammation of thyroid gland.

TICK. Small brown, flat parasite with eight legs, which burrows its head under the skin and sucks blood from the host.

TINEA PEDIS. Athlete's foot; common superficial fungal infection.

TINNITUS. Unusual noise in the ears, such as ringing, roaring, buzzing, and clicking.

TOMOGRAM. An x-ray done on sections of a certain part of the body.

TONOMETER. An instrument used to measure tension or pressure, such as the tension within the eyeball.

TOTAL PARENTERAL NUTRITION. TPN; nutrition obtained totally by intravenous means.

TRACHEOSTOMY. Tracheotomy.

TRACHEOTOMY. An operation in which an opening is made into the trachea; tracheostomy.

TRACTION. Drawing or pulling, especially by the use of weights, cords, pulleys, and other special equipment.

TRANQUILIZER. A drug used to calm or quiet the patient without clouding his consciousness.

TRAUMA. Injury.

TROCAR. A surgical instrument used to puncture a cavity for the drainage of fluid.

TRUSS. An apparatus sometimes worn over a reduced hernia to keep it from slipping out again.

TUBERCLE. A small rounded growth. The term is frequently used in referring to the lesion caused by tubercle bacilli.

TUMOR. An abnormal growth of the body's cells; neoplasm.

BENIGN TUMOR. One that grows slowly, does not spread, and is surrounded by a capsule.

MALIGNANT TUMOR. One that grows rapidly, spreads, and is not surrounded by a capsule; cancer; malignancy.

WILMS' TUMOR. A tumor of the kidneys that occurs usually in infants and young children.

ULCER. An abnormal break in the continuity of a surface; an open lesion.

UMBILICUS. The navel.

UREMIA. Failure of the kidneys to remove urinary constituents from the blood; kidney failure.

UREMIC FROST. A white, powdery substance on the skin of a patient with uremia.

URETER. A long small tube that carries urine from the pelvis of the kidney to the urinary bladder.

URETEROLITHOTOMY. The surgical removal of a

stone from the ureter through an incision into this tube.

URETHRA. A small tube that carries urine from the urinary bladder to the external opening.

URINARY STASIS. A slackening or a stoppage of the normal flow of urine through the urinary tract.

URTICARIA. A skin condition in which the patient develops itching wheals; hives; nettle rash.

UVEITIS. An inflammation of the ciliary body, iris, and choroid of the eye. One or more of these structures may be affected.

VAGINITIS. An inflammatory condition of the vagina.

VARICOCELE. Varicose veins of the spermatic cord.

VARICOSE VEIN. A dilated and tortuous vein.

VASECTOMY. Ligation or transection of the vas deferens for the purpose of interrupting the transportation of sperm or preventing recurrent epididymitis.

VECTORCARDIOGRAM. Graphic measurement of the electric currents generated by the conduction system within the heart, utilizing three dimensions in the form of loops.

VEGETATION. An outgrowth of tissue that is similar to a plant in outline.

VEIN LIGATION. An operation in which the upper end of a vein is tied.

VEIN STRIPPING. An operation in which a portion of a vein is removed by pulling it from its bed beneath the skin.

VENTRICULOGRAPHY. X-ray examination of the brain after air or some other suitable substance has been injected into the small cavities in the brain.

VERMIFORM APPENDIX. Wormlike projection attached to the cecum.

VERTEBRAE. The bones that protect the spinal cord and its meninges; components of the vertebral column.

VESICLE. A small sac or blister containing fluid.

VIPER. Type of poisonous snake with long, hollow fangs.

VIRUS. A small microorganism seen by a highpower electron microscope and capable of reproduction only within another living cell.

VITILIGO. Loss of pigmented cells of the skin.

VOLTAGE. The driving force causing electrons to flow in one direction through a substance.

VOLVULUS. A twisting of the intestine.

VOMIT. Ejection of contents of the stomach through the mouth.

WART. Verruca; common skin tumor caused by a virus.

WET COLOSTOMY. An artificial opening through which both urine and feces drain.

WHEAL. A raised, swollen area of the skin that usually itches, tingles, or burns. This lesion often appears and disappears quickly in the patient with urticaria. It also may occur after an insect or an animal bite.

Index

Page numbers in boldface type indicate illustrations; *t* indicates a table.